Early's
Mental Health
Concepts and Techniques
for Occupational Therapy

SIXTH EDITION

Early's
Mental Health
Concepts and Techniques
for Occupational Therapy

SIXTH EDITION

Cynthia Meyer,
OTD, MED., MS, OTR/L, OTA
Dean of Health Science
South Arkansas College
El Dorado, Arkansas

Courtney S. Sasse,
PHD, MA EDL, MS OTR/L, MA DPS
Occupational Therapist, Psychologist
Maple Heights Behavioral Health Hospital
Fort Wayne, Indiana

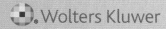 Wolters Kluwer

Philadelphia • Baltimore • New York • London
Buenos Aires • Hong Kong • Sydney • Tokyo

Acquisitions Editor: Lindsey Porambo
Development Editor: Amy Millholen, Tom Conville (freelance)
Editorial Coordinator: Remington Fernando
Editorial Assistant: Lauren Bala
Marketing Manager: Danielle Klahr
Production Project Manager: Kirstin Johnson
Manager, Graphic Arts & Design: Stephen Druding
Manufacturing Coordinator: Margie Orzech
Prepress Vendor: S4Carlisle Publishing Services

Sixth edition

Copyright © 2025 Wolters Kluwer.

9 8 7 6 5 4 3 2 1

Printed in Mexico

Library of Congress Cataloging-in-Publication Data

ISBN-13: 978-1-975189-89-1

ISBN-10: 1-975189-89-2

Cataloging in Publication data available on request from publisher.

shop.lww.com

QUADM0424

The sixth edition of *Early's Mental Health Concepts and Techniques for Occupational Therapy* is designed to provide the occupational therapy professional with information that frames knowledge across the spectrum of mental and behavioral health from an occupational therapy perspective. Perhaps most importantly, evidence-based approaches, models of practice, strategies, and skill sets are introduced that can be practically applied for use throughout the client-centered occupational therapy process. This text is unique in that it addresses the intraprofessional relationship between an occupational therapist and an occupational therapy assistant. While the previous five editions of this text have been primarily for the occupational therapy assistant, this edition is an intentional expansion that includes both types of occupational therapy professionals, highlighting the importance of this relationship to comprehensive occupational therapy services. Additionally, throughout the text, the role of the OT professional in the context of working with other health care professionals across disciplines is also addressed.

A note about terminology used in this edition: The person receiving occupational therapy services is mainly referred to as "client." The authors recognize that there are several terms for the people served by occupational therapy, and that different settings may encourage the use of different terms. The other term consistently used throughout the book is occupational therapy professional (OTP). This term includes both the occupational therapy assistant and the occupational therapist.

In 2022, the American Occupational Therapy Association (AOTA) addressed the question "What can Occupational Therapy do?" by releasing an infograph titled, *Occupational Therapy Addressing Mental and Behavioral Health in Non-Psychiatric Settings*. In this document, the AOTA underscored occupational therapy's core value, supporting clients' participation in meaningful occupation across settings, also emphasizing emergent roles in nontraditional psychiatric settings. They further acknowledged that the approach of an occupational therapy professional is to promote the clients' overall physical and mental health and wellness keeping occupation central as both the means of achieving optimal health and an outcome of optimal health. This textbook places occupational therapy practice in the midst of the current health care landscape and provides information that is critical in advocating for our expanding roles in areas such as population health and wellness, early intervention and long-term care, health promotion and suicide prevention, research, home health, and community practice, among others.

The writing style of the book follows the American Psychological Association's *APA Style Guide*, 7th edition. This includes an emphasis on equity and justice and the use of the third-person plural when referring to an individual, regardless of their biological sex identified at birth. The text has been updated to reflect the *American Occupational Therapy Association's Occupational Therapy Practice Framework: Domain and Process*, 4th edition (OTPF-4) and the *Diagnostic and Statistical Manual of Mental Disorders, Fifth Edition— Text Revised* (DSM-5-TR).

OVERALL CHANGES IN THE TEXT

This edition has several changes beyond expanding the audience to include all occupational therapy professionals. In the previous edition, the chapters about professional issues were removed, but one chapter on this topic has been reintroduced in this edition. This chapter focuses on the intraprofessional relationship between occupational therapy professionals, the varied roles of occupational therapy professionals, documentation, and managing a fast-paced, and often productivity-driven, career. The text has been divided into three sections. Section One focuses on fundamental information about mental health occupational therapy and information used across occupational therapy settings and service situations. In Section Two, the reader will be introduced to the occupational therapy domain and process using a "Domain" or "Home" metaphor and infograph to learn more about the nuts and bolts of an occupational therapy professional's role in psychosocial settings. The chapters in Section Three are organized around the *Pan Occupational Paradigm* and use *Doing, Being, Becoming, and Belonging* to articulate how OT professionals can move intervention plans into action.

Because research and the use of evidence has an overarching role in all aspects of health care provision, this edition features a full chapter (Chapter 10) on evidence-based practice within occupational therapy. The chapter covers the different uses of evidence, including research (with specific focus on occupational science), scholarship, evidence-based practice, and translation of knowledge.

Other changes include the following:

- Occupational therapy professionals are known for thinking outside of the box to creatively employ evidence-based strategies that support the occupations that people want and need to participate in. At the beginning and end of each chapter, the authors have created a section called *OT HACKS*. Through these sections, the content of the chapter is introduced and then later revisited or summarized. *OT HACKS* is designed to be a toolbox, so to speak, for planning and carrying out the OT process, highlighting important details, utilizing or engaging in related research, introducing population-specific topics, and studying case examples.

- Chapters 2, 3, and 6 provide goal writing templates and examples for the various theories, frames of reference, and practice models often applied in occupational therapy.
- Reflection Questions presented at the end of the chapters require more specific responses that review chapter content while also assisting the student with both course-related and National Board for Certification in Occupational Therapy (NBCOT) test preparation.

ORGANIZATION OF CONTENT

Unit One (Chapters 1–3) focuses on occupational therapy history and concepts, current professional considerations, and theories, frames of reference, and practice models used in occupational therapy.

Unit Two (Chapter 4) is dedicated to mental disorders and the information and revision of the *DSM-5-TR*.

Unit Three (Chapters 5–7) discusses the aspects of service provision. It begins by looking at our clients according to their development over time and then progresses to how aspects of occupational therapy may apply to clients across the life span, specifically with regard to the relationship between occupational engagement and optimal health. The methods and occupational therapy models that are considered in our work with clients are also considered. Finally, the environments, areas, and focuses of our practice are discussed.

Unit Four (Chapters 8–11) covers professional practice considerations. Safety issues are addressed, as are medical treatment, medication use, and complementary health approaches. The application and use of evidence are discussed and presented as a systematic process spanning from determining what to investigate, to how research is conducted, and finally moving to how evidence is located and used in everyday job tasks. The scholarship of translation describes how evidence is translated to, and for, various audiences.

Unit Five (Chapters 12–16) incorporates the *Home Metaphor* to examine the OT process more closely and learn more about *what we do* as occupational therapy professionals when we collaborate with our clients to help them optimize their occupational participation. Readers will be introduced to specific occupational therapy evaluation strategies and assessment tools that are useful in psychosocial settings and learn more about recommended types and approaches to intervention. Chapters 14 and 15 prepare the learner to transition from evaluation to intervention planning, implementation, and to considerations of the outcomes of occupational therapy, emphasizing distinctive aspects of OT such as occupational performance analysis and therapeutic use-of-self. Unit Five concludes with a chapter dedicated to one of the most frequently utilized intervention types used in psychiatric or behavioral health settings by occupational therapy professionals: group interventions.

Unit Six (Chapters 17–23) focuses on the "how-to" of psychosocial occupational therapy intervention. The chapters synthesize what the reader has learned about the occupational therapy domain and process in mental health arenas and shifts into occupational therapy intervention implementation. Since the central focus of occupational therapy intervention and outcomes is occupation, and ***not*** diagnosis, the chapters in Unit Six provide practical evidence-informed intervention strategies, activities, and approaches that target the common symptoms of prevalent mental health conditions that most often disrupt occupational participation.

Many of the text's past features have been revised to reflect current occupational therapy best practices, and these features have been retained. *What's the Evidence* sections have been updated with current evidence and research. *The Point-of-View* boxes remain in different chapters. Suggested resources are located at the end of each chapter and include, as appropriate, articles, books, videos, and websites.

OT HACKS

O   Occupation as a means and an end
T   Theoretical concepts, values, and principles, or historical foundations
H   How can we Help? OT's role in serving clients with mental illness or mental health needs
A   Adaptations
C   Case study includes
K   Knowledge: Keeping mental health OT practice grounded in evidence, in occupational science, and in research
S   Some terms that may be new to you

Acknowledgments

Because this is the sixth edition of this book, and this edition is completed by two new authors, we wish to acknowledge and thank, first and foremost, the previous author, Mary Beth Early. The first edition of this book came out in 1987, over 35 years ago. Due to her work, this book has become a staple item in occupational therapy assistant mental health education. Mary Beth Early has provided thousands of occupational therapy professionals not only information about mental health and mental disorders but also practical information that is "clinic ready." By providing intervention-centered planning concepts and implementation techniques, this book eases the transition of student to working professional.

Next, we encourage you to review the Acknowledgments in the previous editions. We would like to thank all of the professionals that assisted Mary Beth Early with content and writing suggestions.

We would also like to extend much appreciation to those who reviewed the textbook prior to commencing on this edition. Their willingness to reflect and share their insight was a valuable component of bringing this work to fruition.

The creation of this edition would not have the quality and strength if not for those who provided input and support throughout the writing process. In this list we include: Samuel Allen, Patricia Henton, Shirley O'Brien, Camille Skubik-Peplaski, and Gina Schwarz.

A special word of thanks goes to all from Wolters Kluwer who worked on this project.

Finally, we would like to thank our spouses and children. No work that we, as professionals, complete is done so without the support of our families. Occupational therapy professionals pour out all of who we are to our work and clients. We regroup and replenish ourselves through our loved ones.

Contents

List of Figures

List of Tables

List of Boxes

Principles of Occupational Therapy in Mental Health

Section One emphasizes the foundations of mental health occupational therapy, the connection occupational therapy has to other professions, what occupational therapy service delivery encompasses, and how we can spread the work of occupational therapy in the future.

Seen throughout this section is the historical and current conceptual and practical information about occupational therapy and health care. Consideration is given to the use of terminology for those with mental disorders and terminology associated with mental health concerns. Time is taken to address statutes and public policymaking that influence how occupational therapy is provided to those with mental disorders and mental health problems.

There are theories and approaches that come from other psychiatric-based or psychiatric-affiliated professions. These ideas and concepts help the profession of occupational therapy build its own frames of reference and approaches—ones with a focus on occupational performance and occupational participation. Some are specific, such as the sensory integrative frame of reference, some have a stronger focus in a particular area (such as the person environment occupation model and the ecology of human performance model), and some, like the model of human occupation, strive to align all our thinking and doing to be centered on our primary domain of occupation.

Understanding the psychiatric diagnoses our clients have is another piece to understanding how best to provide occupational therapy to those the profession serves. Thus, emphasis is placed on knowing the criteria used to diagnose mental disorders and how to best use occupational therapy to address the deficits associated with mental disorders.

As with all service areas (eg, physical dysfunction or pediatrics) within occupational therapy, the development of humans throughout the life span is a key factor. This section identifies connections between the personal factors associated with the stages of life and occupational therapy service delivery. Specific attention is paid to the use of co-occupation at various times of life.

How occupational therapy is practiced includes the methods employed by occupational therapy professionals and the approaches used for intervention, which are cast in the light of models both within and outside of occupational therapy. As the profession of occupational therapy moves forward, the models of public health, population health, and community health will impact the way occupational therapy is presented to others and how others view the work of occupational therapy professionals.

Procedural and pragmatic topics covered in this section are medical concerns covering medication, medical treatments, complementary medicine practices, detoxification, safety, and professional issues. All these topics include practical knowledge needed by the occupational therapy professional for effective and efficient service delivery.

Section One lays the foundation for our service delivery, offering the reader a view into the breadth of what is included in the practice of mental health occupational therapy.

CHAPTER

1

History and Foundational Concepts

OT HACKS OVERVIEW

O: Occupation as a means and an end

Occupation is the foundation for the Philosophical Base of Occupational Therapy.

T: Theoretical concepts, values, and principles, or historical foundations

The history of occupational therapy includes a foundation in moral treatment and the mental hygiene movement. Theoretical concepts of mental health occupational therapy include consideration toward people's innate drive to produce meaningful occupation.

H: How can we Help? OT's role in serving clients with mental illness or mental health needs

How does OT look in mental health practice?

A: Adaptations

Not applicable for this chapter

C: Case study includes

Case studies about the role of the occupational therapist and the occupational therapy assistant (OTA)

K: Knowledge: keeping mental health OT practice grounded in evidence, in occupational science, and in research

Knowledge of how to provide occupational therapy comes from occupational science and occupational therapists such as Mary Reilly, A. Jean Ayres, Lorna Jean King, Claudia Allen, and Gary Kielhofner.

S: Some terms that may be new to you

Epigenetics
Mental disorder
Mental health
Narrative reasoning
Parity
Psychiatric rehabilitation
Public health
Recovery movement
Redistributive policies
Reductionistic
Transinstitutionalize

INTRODUCTION

A common view is that people with mental health problems have trouble controlling their feelings, thoughts, and behavior. What is less obvious is that many people with mental disorders also have trouble doing everyday activities that the rest of us take for granted. Occupational therapy professionals address this part of human life—how people carry out the occupations that are important to them, how well they do their occupations, and how satisfied they feel about their occupational performance. Occupation is individualized and people perform occupations both individually and with others. Occupations occupy people's time, are purposeful, and are meaningful (27). Occupational therapy views meaningful engagement and participation in occupation as essential to physical, mental, and social health and to well-being. Occupational therapy professionals evaluate occupational functioning; work with clients and their families and caregivers

to identify goals; and intervene to help troubled individuals, families, and communities learn new skills, engage in occupation, maintain successful and adaptive habits and routines, explore their feelings and interests, and control their lives and destinies.

MENTAL HEALTH AND MENTAL ILLNESS

Before we look at the occupational therapy process for persons with mental health problems, it is useful to examine what we mean by the terms **mental health** and **mental illness**. The World Health Organization (WHO) has defined **mental health** as "a state of well-being in which every individual realizes his or her own abilities, can cope with the normal stresses of life, can work productively, and is able to make a contribution to her or his community" (138, para. 3). The mentally healthy person can manage daily affairs despite the stresses of internal difficulties and of the external world and is able to respond constructively and creatively to the changing demands and opportunities of life.

If mental health is relative, defined in relation to changing life conditions, at what point can we say that someone has mental health problems? Throughout recorded history, **mental illness** has been defined and redefined, reflecting increases in knowledge and understanding and changes in cultural beliefs and values. The American Psychiatric Association has defined mental disorder as follows:

> a syndrome characterized by clinically significant disturbance in an individual's cognition, emotion regulation, or behavior that reflects a dysfunction in the psychological biological, or developmental processes underlying mental functioning. Mental disorders are usually associated with significant distress or disability in social, occupational, or other important activities. (31, p. 14)

A mental disorder (mental illness) typically causes problems in thinking, as well as significant emotional discomfort (extreme anxiety, sadness, or rage) and/or impairment in the ability to function, such as to hold a job. We learn that the causes of the disorder may be psychological, biologic, or developmental. There is sometimes a risk to oneself, such as the risk of being imprisoned, or of dying by suicide, or as a result of carelessness and failure to use "common sense."

Important for occupational therapy is the recognition of disability or impairment in important areas of life activities: caring for oneself, working or being productive, engaging in effective and satisfying relationships with others, and pursuing valued leisure activities. Occupational therapy is an appropriate intervention for such problems because performance in human occupation and daily life activities is its main concern. Also, because occupational therapy uses occupation as a means of intervention as well as an outcome, clients must act and perform and thus prove to themselves and to others that indeed they *can* function (18).

RELATION OF OCCUPATION TO MENTAL HEALTH

The notion that involvement in occupation can improve mental health is not new; it appears in records of ancient civilizations from China to Rome. It is such an excellent idea that it is continually rediscovered and acclaimed. At the 1961 annual conference of the American Occupational Therapy Association (AOTA), Mary Reilly expressed it this way: "That man, through the use of his hands as they are energized by mind and will, can influence the state of his own health" (117, p. 1).

Every person is born with a drive to act on the environment, to effect change, to produce things, to work, to engage and participate with life, and to use hands and mind. The satisfaction of having an effect and the challenge and pleasure of solving problems give life meaning and purpose. We know that both the unemployed and those employed in routine jobs experience stress and may develop mental disorders because they lack the stimulation of challenging activity. Their drive to act is denied, frustrated, and weakened. We know too that those diagnosed with mental disorders grieve because they cannot do what they once did; disease and social stigma have obstructed their capacity to engage in valued occupations as they would like. Unhappiness and inactivity reinforce each other; those who are not afforded the opportunity to act become increasingly less able to do so.

Occupational therapy uses occupation to reverse the negative cycle of inactivity and disease. Occupation requires attention and energy; it has a unique meaning to the person performing it (7). Activity that engages the entire human being—heart, mind, and body—is powerful therapy. Not every activity is therapeutic, only those that ignite the person's interest and empower the will, strengthen skills, and improve the ability to act. Helping the client explore, discover, master, and manage the occupations that give that individual's life purpose and direction is the essence of psychiatric occupational therapy.

A FEW WORDS ABOUT LANGUAGE

In this book, we use the phrase "persons with mental disorders" to refer to clients and consumers we encounter in mental health practice. This "person-first" phrase limits the stigma associated with having a psychiatric diagnosis. It puts the person first and the disorder second. Historically, however, different words were used that would be highly stigmatizing today.

- moron, imbecile, idiot—these were historical descriptors through the 1970s with specific meanings for persons who today would be diagnosed with intellectual disabilities
- mad, lunatic, crazy—now used casually, but once had specific meanings
- of unsound mind, mentally ill—terms that were historically accurate in their eras

This is not an exhaustive list. To avoid confusing the reader and generating more stigma, the authors have not used these terms in the history that follows.

THOUGHTS ABOUT TERMINOLOGY

Several terms have already been introduced in this text. **Mental health**, **mental illness**, and **mental disorders** are terms that have been used and defined. The word *problems* has been added to the mix and presented as the term **mental health problems**. The use of terminology to describe the practice of occupational therapy within mental health and with those who have mental disorders deserves some reflection and consideration. There is more terminology associated with this type of occupational therapy practice delivery. Presented here will be current terminology used within the occupational therapy profession and associated psychological, psychiatric, and mental health organizations. Unfortunately, there is not a consensus on terminology use, and that can lead to confusion for both new and seasoned practitioners.

It is understandable that terminology changes over time. New governmental legislation and new policy changes from entities outside of the profession of occupational therapy impact our professional language. These changes have a ripple effect in how we refer to our practice activities. Table 1.1 presents terminology from entities outside of the profession of occupational therapy. This encompasses organizations such as the Substance Abuse and Mental Health Services Administration (SAMHSA), the American Psychiatric Association, the American Psychological Association, the Centers for Disease Control and Prevention (CDC), Mental Health America (MHA), and the National Alliance on Mental Illness (NAMI).

Language within our profession also changes over time. Terminology changes in relationship to current events, and documents are modified to address these changes. The AOTA uses various terms throughout its website and documents, as does the National Board for Certification in Occupational Therapy (NBCOT). Each organization uses its own terminology for mental health practice in its publications. Table 1.2 presents terminology used from the occupational therapy profession.

These differences, and similarities, are important to consider because education standards, certification examinations, licensing laws, advanced certifications, and reimbursement legislation also use their own terminology. If the terminology used does not match, or is not consistent, the effect is, at best, confusion and, at worst, a failure to learn, which can lead to not providing clients the best possible occupational therapy services.

Table 1.1. Terminology From Entities Outside the Profession of Occupational Therapy

Entity	Terminology
Substance Abuse and Mental Health Services Administration	**Mental Health** services for adults are defined "as receiving treatment or counseling for any problem with emotions, nerves, or mental health … or the use of prescription medication for treatment of any mental or emotional condition that was not caused by the use of alcohol or drugs" (123, p. 138). **Behavioral Health** refers to mental disorders and substance use disorders (37).
American Psychiatric Association	**"Behavioral health** refers to the array of professional services delivered to populations suffering with mental illnesses, substance use disorders and maladaptive health behaviors, such as lack of exercise, poor dietary habits and lackluster engagement in care" (61, para. 5).
American Psychological Association	**Psychological health** is connected to the Department of Defense and is associated with positive psychology. It addresses posttraumatic stress disorder and psychological wounds of combat. The four key focus areas are: • clinical care and prevention; • resiliency, strength building, and coping strategies for deployed service members and families; • scientific and clinical application research; and • service redundancy and overlap (106). **Behavioral health** is addressed with mental health and aligned with behavioral health disorders, behavioral health problems, behavioral health difficulties, behavioral health disparities, behavioral health challenges, behavioral health diagnoses, behavioral health prevention, and behavioral health needs. It encompasses behavioral health care, behavioral health programs, behavioral health interventions, behavioral health treatment, and behavioral health promotion. It includes psychology, health, and well-being. There are behavioral health providers and behavioral health workers. It has an importance in children's healthy development and in their social emotional health. It has a connection to substance use and social services (49). **Psychosocial** factors connected to the homeless include poverty and substance abuse (114). **Psychosocial** programs for the military are identified for obesity and eating disorders (54).

(continued)

Table 1.1. Terminology From Entities Outside the Profession of Occupational Therapy (*continued*)

Entity	Terminology
Centers for Disease Control and Prevention	**Mental health** includes emotional, psychological, and social well-being. It impacts our thoughts, feelings, and actions. It influences how we cope with stress, how we relate to other people, and how we choose to live our lives. Mental health and mental illness and not the same. One can have poor mental health and not have a mental illness. In the same manner, a person with a mental illness diagnosis can have periods of physical, social, and mental well-being (90). **Psychological health** is addressed through the COVID-19 pandemic. It is identified as a population health approach for public behavioral health and addressed psychological well-being. Psychological health is provided through psychological health care and is done so to provide early psychological skill development and prevent psychological disorders (60). **Psychological health** can be affected by the practice of female genital mutilation or cutting (62). **Psychological health** is considered for first responders in natural disaster response work and is assessed to determine their ability to continue relief work for the weeks following an initial event (74). **Social and emotional health** is associated with population health. It involves "experiencing stress, isolation, loss, or systemic social inequities" (58, para. 1). The goal to increasing social and emotional health is "improving emotional well-being, social connectedness, and resiliency" (58, para. 1). **Emotional health** is identified as a component of coping needed during a stressful time, such as during the COVID-19 pandemic. Stress, anxiety, grief, and worry can be associated with emotional health. Distress can be a component and includes problems with • fear, worry, sadness, numbness, anger, or frustration; • appetite, energy, or activity; • concentration and decision-making; • sleep; • physical symptoms or chronic health conditions; or • substance use (125). **Behavioral health** can be seen as a population health concern. It encompasses traditional mental health, substance use, psychological well-being, as well as behaviors that impact physical health and mental health. Other components of behavioral health include emotional well-being, behavioral adjustments, anxiety-free living and relationships, and the ability to cope with everyday stressors. "Obtaining and maintaining behavioral health requires flexibility, the ability to understand and manage emotions, engaging in behaviors that are healthy for the body and the mind, awareness of one's relationship to others and recognition of one's responses, and effectively employing strategies to deal with the demands of living" (90, para. 4). Because behavioral health is integrated into a population's needs, it is important to also address social determinants of health (90). **Psychosocial** interventions for children with attention-deficit/hyperactivity disorder include parent-driven behavior therapy, social skills training, peer support intervention, and cognitive behavioral therapy (110). **Psychosocial** population-based situations can include the everyday stressors associated with ensuring physiologic needs, social interaction, health, and well-being (96). **Psychosocial** considerations for those who are victims of traumatic population-based events refer to the emotional motivations and behaviors of people. Actions taken within the psychosocial realm are done to protect oneself and to protect those with whom they are in relationships. These actions are meant to diminish stress and anxiety, while improving overall well-being (43).

Table 1.1. Terminology From Entities Outside the Profession of Occupational Therapy (*continued*)

Entity	Terminology
Mental Health America	**Mental health** is a part of overall health and well-being. Mental health is part of the holistic approach of biology, psychology, and social environment considerations toward health. Major mental health conditions include depression and schizophrenia. Profoundly stressful events and situations such as abuse, traffic accidents, crime, disasters, war, and terroristic incidents are also part of mental health. Mental wellness includes items such as resiliency and coping (100). **Behavioral health** can include those with substance use and abuse problems, mental health problems, and mental illnesses (102). **Psychosocial** activities with elders are done to promote positive development, cope with mental health conditions, and stimulate wellness. Examples of psychosocial activities include caregiver education, support groups, leisure pursuits, community programs, quality-of-life interests, exercise, and educational pursuits (101).
National Alliance on Mental Illness	**Psychosocial** considerations include psychotherapy and social and vocational training. The goal is to support, educate, and guide those with mental illness and their families. Psychosocial interventions are designed to improve quality of life; decrease hospitalizations; and improve interactions at school, work, and home (115).

Table 1.2. Terminology From Occupational Therapy Professional Entities and Documents

Entity	Terminology
National Board for Certification in Occupational Therapy	**Mental health** should be addressed through interventions completed to support engagement in occupations that are meaningful to the person (108, 109). The person's mental health status should be considered as meaningful occupations are selected (109) and integrated (108) during occupational therapy service delivery for assistive technology and adaptive devices. **Mental health** status should be considered by the occupational therapy assistant candidate when implementing environmental modifications (108). Also, a person's **emotional regulation** should be considered by the occupational therapist candidate when recommending environmental modifications (109). **Psychosocial** skills and abilities should be addressed through interventions completed to support engagement in occupations that are meaningful to the person (108, 109). **Emotional regulation** and **behavioral reactions** should be considered during clinical decision-making when intervention plan modifications occur and when prioritizing client goals (108, 109).
Accreditation Council for Occupational Therapy Education (ACOTE)	**Mental health:** "A state of well-being in which every individual realizes his or her own potential, can cope with the normal stresses of life, can work productively and fruitfully, and is able to make a contribution to her or his community (WHO, 2014)" (as cited by ACOTE [25], p. 51). Mental health is identified as a population for the generalist occupational therapist and occupational therapy assistant (25). **Behavioral health:** "Refers to mental/emotional well-being and/or actions that affect wellness. Behavioral health problems include substance use disorders; alcohol and drug addiction; and serious psychological distress, suicide, and mental disorders (Substance Abuse and Mental Health Administration, 2014)" (as cited by ACOTE [25], p. 47).

(*continued*)

Table 1.2. Terminology From Occupational Therapy Professional Entities and Documents (*continued*)

Entity	Terminology
	Behavioral health and psychosocial: The entry-level occupational therapist must be able to "Design and implement intervention strategies to remediate and/or compensate for … psychosocial and behavioral health deficits that affect occupational performance" (25, pp. 29–30). The entry-level occupational therapy assistant must be able to "Demonstrate an understanding of the intervention strategies that remediate and/or compensate for … psychosocial and behavioral health deficits that affect occupational performance" (25, pp. 29–30). In addition, both the occupational therapist and occupational therapy assistant student must have a fieldwork experience that "addresses practice in behavioral health, or psychological and social factors influencing engagement in occupation" (25, p. 40). **Psychosocial factors:** "Psychosocial as pertaining to the influence of social factors on an individual's mind or behaviour, and to the interrelation of behavioural and social factors" (Martikainen et al., 2002, p. 1091)" (as cited by ACOTE [25], p. 52). All occupational therapy student fieldwork experiences must have a learning objective regarding psychosocial (25). Occupational therapy professionals are concerned with evidence-based practice involving occupational therapy interventions for psychosocial performance associated with people's engagement in everyday activities (25).
American Occupational Therapy Association (AOTA). Occupational Therapy Practice Framework: Domain and Process	**Social and emotional health:** "Identifying personal strengths and assets, managing emotions, expressing needs effectively, seeking occupations and social engagement to support health and wellness, developing self-identity, making choices to improve quality of life in participation" (27, p. 3). Emotions are regulated as a part of managing the symptoms and conditions associated with mental health needs (27). Emotional stability is tied to one's temperament, one's personality (9, 27), and one's ability to self-regulate (27). In the AOTA's current terminology structure, social and emotional health is considered a part of the occupation of health management (27). **Regulation of emotions:** This is specifically defined in the following ways: • Specific mental function (Mental Functions of Sequencing Complex Movement). "Mental functions that regulate the speed, response, quality, and time of motor production, such as restlessness, toe tapping, or hand wringing, in response to inner tension" (27, p. 52). • Specific mental function (Emotional). "Regulation and range of emotions; appropriateness of emotions, including anger, love, tension, and anxiety; lability of emotions" (9, p. 22; 27, p. 52). • Social interaction skill (Regulate). "Does not demonstrate irrelevant, repetitive, or impulsive behaviors during social interaction" (27, p. 48). • Performance skill (Emotional Regulation Skill). "Actions or behaviors a client uses to identify, manage, and express feelings while engaging in activities or interacting with others" (8, p. 640). **Psychosocial:** Using and developing the "General mental functions … over the lifespan, required to understand and constructively integrate the mental functions that lead to formation of the person and interpersonal skills needed to establish reciprocal social interactions, in terms of both meaning and purpose" (27, p. 52).
AOTA	**Mental health:** The AOTA webpage for mental health practice highlights mental illness, mental health treatment, and mental health prevention (4). Mental health when working with children and youth includes areas such as • social competence, • social-emotional learning skills, and • identifying early signs of mental illness (14).

Table 1.2. Terminology From Occupational Therapy Professional Entities and Documents *(continued)*

Entity	Terminology
	Mental health can be focused on evidence-based practice such as social skills, parenting programs, and structured recreation and activity programs with children who are timid (3). Mental health can also be connected to multiple areas of occupational therapy of practice, including but not limited to polytrauma, community mental health, sleep, mental health recovery, restraint reduction or elimination, sensory integration with adults, oncology, disaster relief, depression, and recovery for those with drug and alcohol abuse (5). **Social and emotional health:** Social and emotional learning can be identified as part of mental health (67). Social and emotional learning includes children becoming self-aware and socially aware so they can recognize and manage emotions and challenges. They want to be able to think about their feelings and how they should act toward others by regulating their behavior, make thoughtful and responsible decisions, and thus build their relationship skills (67). **Behavioral health:** Occupational therapy professionals have been identified as key members of community behavioral health teams. Because of occupational therapy professionals' client-centered holistic background knowledge and work with those with mental illness, cognitive impairments, and environmental context needs, they are well positioned to participate in the delivery of practice under community models of service delivery (6). Barriers associated with behavioral health that occupational therapy professionals can provide intervention to help remediate or compensate for include: • functional cognitive impairments, • medication management, • self-management of wellness concerns, • health promotion, • chronic disease management, • social interactions and community participation, • vocational pursuits, and • educational activities (11). **Psychosocial:** Guilt and perceiving self as a burden are identified as components of the psychosocial adjustment to a disability (93).

HISTORICAL UNDERSTANDING

The history of the occupational therapy profession is intertwined with that of psychiatry. It is useful to look back and consider the important threads that tie the two professions together. Furthermore, reviewing the history of occupational therapy in mental health can reveal the core values and interests of the profession—values and interests that are still strong today. The moral treatment movement, discussed in the next section, fueled the growth of both professions.

The Moral Treatment Era

Moral treatment was a pivotal stage in the development of psychiatry as a separate medical discipline. It was based on ideas developed in France by Pinel and in England by Tuke (116) and was first practiced in the United States at McLean Hospital in Massachusetts and at Frankford Asylum in Pennsylvania in the early 19th century (39). Tuke (116) wrote that insanity could originate in the body as well as in the mind and further believed that persons with mental disorders, despite some impairment of "intellectual powers," were nonetheless capable of autonomy and the exercise of choice. The philosophy of moral treatment included respect for the individual and a belief that clients would benefit most from a regular daily routine and the opportunity to contribute productively to their own care and to the welfare of society in general through involvement in occupation. Before the advent of moral treatment, such individuals were housed in large asylums where they were neglected; observers noted that they were ill-fed, unclothed, and often found lying in their own body wastes. It was not unusual for persons with mental disorders to be subjected to restraint and torture.

In contrast, early moral treatment hospitals provided a prescribed routine of daily hygiene, craft work, recreation, and regular meals, sometimes prepared by those who lived there, with crops grown on the hospital grounds. Efforts were made to engage as many clients as possible in regular employment or occupation, such as kitchen upkeep, laundry, general cleaning, grounds maintenance, or building repair within the hospital. The effect of such employment was described by Adolph Meyer, a physician and one of the founders of occupational therapy:

> It had long been interesting to see how groups of a few excited patients can be seated in a corner in a small circle of two or three settees and kept wonderfully contented picking the hair of mattresses, or doing simple tasks not too readily arousing the desire for big movements and uncontrollable excitement and yet not too taxing to their patience. Groups of patients with raffia and basket work, or with various kinds of handwork and weaving and bookbinding and metal and leather work, took the place of the bored wall flowers and of mischief makers. A pleasure in achievement, a real pleasure in the use and activity of one's hands and muscles and a happy appreciation of time began to be used as incentives in the management of our patients, instead of abstract exhortations to cheer up and to behave according to abstract or repressive rules. (105, p. 81)

Moral treatment, as described by Tuke (116), was founded on three principles.

1. Development of "self-restraint" using rewards, which aimed to increase clients' self-esteem and confidence. By complying with the rules and contributing through productive occupations, clients earned the right to privileges and more comfortable conditions.
2. Elimination of the use of force
3. Provision of a comfortable and humane environment to all

Occupational therapy arose out of the moral treatment movement. Early occupational therapy professionals based their work on moral treatment principles and used a variety of occupations, such as arts and crafts, classroom instruction, manual labor, games, sports, social activities, and self-care activities. These were designed to provide a balanced daily program that incorporated work, rest, and leisure. Occupations were planned and graded for the needs and abilities of individuals. Formation of habits and the development of skills and attention were emphasized.

The personality of the occupational therapist was important; kindliness, modeling of correct habits, and the ability to analyze and adjust occupations to suit the interests and capacities of clients were valued professional characteristics (92).

Ever since the beginning of occupational therapy in mental health, the profession has been greatly influenced and restrained by physician referral and the practice of psychiatry. For this reason, we will look at the history of American psychiatry before returning to the development of occupational therapy later in the chapter.

Psychiatry in the 20th and 21st Centuries

The medical specialty of psychiatry has shifted its techniques and interests several times since the moral treatment era. Early in the 20th century, the theories of Sigmund Freud (see Chapter 2) and other psychoanalytic theoreticians dominated the field. But psychoanalysis, which relies on talking, was not practical for those with severe disorders. Clients were simply too ill and symptomatic. Several pseudoscientific methods were used to try to limit the severity and effects of psychotic symptoms. Some of these methods, such as ice water baths and confinement in wooden restraints, were efforts to compel clients to submit to the rules of the institutions in which they lived.

Through the 1950s, physicians' treatments of major mental disorders aimed at changing the brain by changing the biology of the body. Some examples included the following treatments:

- prefrontal lobotomy (a kind of brain surgery, often crudely executed)
- insulin shock treatment (inducement of coma by lowering blood sugar with injections of insulin)
- electroconvulsive therapy (ECT)

A critical development during the 1950s was the discovery and introduction of the major tranquilizers. It seemed that finally a way had been found to control and diminish psychotic symptoms and extreme behaviors. The discovery and use of the tranquilizing drugs led indirectly to the passage in 1963 of the *Community Mental Health Act* (also known as the *Community Mental Health Centers Construction Act*) (Public Law 88–164). This law was designed to establish community-based treatment facilities and to move the clients from institutional settings to community living, now that their more extreme symptoms were controlled by medications. Unfortunately, inadequate planning and funding resulted in large numbers of deinstitutionalized clients with mental disorders being released into communities that lacked resources to meet their needs.

Historians later suggested that persons with chronic psychiatric disorders were not really *de*institutionalized by the 1963 legislation but rather were **transinstitutionalized**. In other words, they were moved from one kind of institution (psychiatric hospitals) into other kinds of institutions (jails, prisons, and nursing homes) and not into the community at all (127, 128). To complicate matters, the enactment of Medicaid and Medicare legislation in 1965 changed the incentives for the states. Mental health care had been, up to 1965, a state responsibility, but the new legislation made it possible to shift responsibility to the federal government once clients were discharged from the state hospitals (127). Thus, many were transferred to nursing homes (128).

The social and political climate of the 1960s and 1970s generated increased interest in and funding for mental health research, but much of this was directed toward those with mild conditions (thus, away from those with the most severe disorders). With increased attention on those with less serious problems, mental health professionals, including occupational therapy professionals, used newer theories (gestalt therapy, milieu therapy, behavioral therapy, and family therapy) during those years.

The 1960s and 1970s saw an explosion of interest in and studies of the biologic foundations of mental disorders. There had long been an interest in the genetics of the major brain disorders (schizophrenia, depression, manic depression). Research with diagnosed individuals and their families and the study of the human genome have enabled a better understanding of the link between genetics and the development of mental disorders. Since the beginning of the 21st century, there has been additional recognition of the role of **epigenetics**. Although a gene for a given condition (eg, schizophrenia) may be present in the genotype of an individual, this does not invariably lead to the development of schizophrenia. **Epigenetics** is the study of the events and circumstances that mediate gene expression. Events and circumstances may be prenatal or may occur after birth through disease, stress, or trauma, and possibly also exposure to chemicals in the environment. The consensus at present is that a genetic predisposition often results in disease in vulnerable individuals, but that environmental factors, including viruses and stressors, are also involved (57).

The medical specialty of psychiatry remains oriented strongly toward biologic and biochemical research and pharmacologic (drug) interventions. Imaging studies, conducted since the 1990s using positron emission tomography (PET), computed tomography (CT), and magnetic resonance imaging (MRI), have shown changes in the cerebral cortex, ventricles, and other brain structures (and brain activity) of persons with major mental disorders. Both functional MRI and magnetoencephalography (MEG) can detect brain activation patterns in various brain lobes for those with schizophrenia (45). Pharmaceutical companies fund major research to demonstrate the effectiveness of competing drugs aimed at the considerable market represented by people with psychiatric disorders. Furthermore, drug companies advertise and market directly to consumers. The volume of studies published requires physicians to review results constantly and to adjust their interventions according to published evidence. Many studies suggest that the medications used in psychiatry may themselves be responsible for altering the brain, causing an increase in receptors for specific neurotransmitters. Over time, the brain adapts to medication, which then is needed on a long-term basis (128). Concern has been raised that the rise in the percentage of persons with mental disorders in the population receiving Supplemental Security Income (SSI) and Social Security Disability Insurance (SSDI) may be attributed, at least in part, to the long-term use of these drugs (128).

A prevalent form of intervention for persons with serious mental disorders is associated with the **psychiatric rehabilitation** movement (33). Psychiatric rehabilitation uses evidence-based interventions such as cognitive behavioral rehabilitation and wellness recovery. Psychiatric rehabilitation has introduced mental health counselors, psychiatric rehabilitation practitioners, and other health professionals to methods of intervention that are very similar to the traditional methods of occupational therapy and that in many ways echo the principles of moral treatment. Psychiatric rehabilitation has been adopted by some states, including New York, under the name *intensive psychiatric rehabilitation treatment* (IPRT) (111). Psychiatric rehabilitation, discussed further in Chapter 2, is defined as helping persons with mental disorders improve their role functioning and their ability to function in the environments of their choice. Methods include skill development, provision of supports and resources, and the use of external structures to enable more community engagement (130).

Clients, Families, and Mental Health Parity

One of the most important forces at work on behalf of persons with mental disorders is the combined effort of clients, their families, and concerned professionals. Represented most prominently by the NAMI, this movement has helped reduce stigma associated with mental disorders and improve the quality of life for persons with mental disorders (107). Since 1979, the NAMI has advocated for policy changes to better the lives of those with mental disorders. There are NAMI affiliate organizations across the country working to better people's lives impacted by mental disorders. The millions of Americans with mental disorders see themselves not as outcasts but rather as members of the community with a voice and with a vision for their future.

The NAMI and similar organizations, clients, families, and professionals together advocate for appropriate housing, community care, supported employment, and culturally competent health care. In addition, families and consumers provide peer and family support and education (107).

Another organization, MHA, is dedicated to addressing the needs of those with mental disorders and promoting better mental health for all people. In the early 1900s, Clifford Whittingham Beers, who was affected by a mental disorder and was hospitalized (36), led the work of the mental hygiene movement within the original MHA organization, the National Committee for Mental Hygiene (99). The mental hygiene movement began with the Quakers' concern for persons with mental disorders to receive humane treatment. MHA works to promote the mental hygiene components of wellness and mental health, integration of mental health care and community supports, prevention and early identification for at-risk populations, and recovery (98, 99).

The **recovery movement** promotes the idea that people can recover from mental disorders, given sufficient time and support. Within the recovery movement those with mental disorders recognize the importance of person-centered care; the need for self-determination; and the idea that people can have restored function, moving beyond simply focusing on symptom management (53). Recovery is a personalized process and gives hope and power to individuals that they hold the control of their psychiatric care and solutions to problems and barriers in their daily life. Furthermore, within the recovery philosophy, those with mental disorders can decide when to accept psychiatric services and when not to do so. Mental health professionals are seen as professional services that can be accessed when needed and should play a role in building social and community systems to foster engagement and support (113).

Mental health parity has been an important aspect of consumer-focused activities. In 1996, the *Mental Health Parity Act* (MHPA) was signed into law in the United States, requiring insurance companies to reimburse mental health care to the same extent as physical health care. In 2008, the *Mental Health Parity and Addiction Equity Act* (MHPAEA) was enacted to curb abuses associated with loopholes in the 1996 MHPA. Although there are exceptions for some entities, generally, the coverage rules of the MHPAEA include equal coverage in group health insurance plans for physical and mental disorder needs. Parity between physical and mental health care includes inpatient services, outpatient services, emergency services, and prescription drug coverage (44). In addition, in 2010, the *Affordable Care Act* (ACA) included coverage for substance abuse treatment for those receiving services under that law.

Occupational Therapy in Mental Health: History and Trends

In the early history of occupational therapy, the profession was very dependent on physicians. From 1917 to the 1950s, psychiatric occupational therapists provided comprehensive programs of occupation based loosely on principles of moral treatment within institutional settings. The physician prescribed occupational therapy, often ordering specific activities for clients, and the occupational therapist carried out the treatment. After World War II, interest in rehabilitating veterans led to an emphasis on workmanship and vocational readiness (69).

During the 1940s and 1950s, occupational therapy was attacked by the medical profession for failing to have a "scientific basis" (84, 119). In response to that criticism, occupational therapy adopted the vocabulary, concepts, and some techniques of psychoanalysis, the prevailing psychiatric theory. Although occupational therapists continued to work under the prescription of physicians, Gail Fidler, Jay Fidler, and others began to use activities to evaluate their clients' psychodynamics (emotions and psychological defenses) (65). They analyzed activities for their capacity to meet clients' unconscious needs. Activities were matched symbolically to psychic content—for example, clay resembles feces and may symbolize anal stage concerns (see "Psychoanalytic Theory: Model of Object Relations" section in Chapter 2). This psychoanalytic application of occupational therapy in mental health followed the trend of using occupation to enhance medical outcomes (69) after World War II.

With the introduction of the major tranquilizers in the 1950s, occupational therapists were able to work with hospitalized clients whose behavior without medication made treatment difficult or impossible. At first, the main emphasis continued to be psychoanalytic. The theories developed by other disciplines, primarily psychology, during the 1960s and 1970s did not always include a focus on occupation. Of these new therapies, the behavioral approach was the one favored by occupational therapy professionals. The applied techniques of **behavioral therapy** became a part of the occupational therapy performed with persons diagnosed with mental disorders and intellectual disabilities to diminish acting out and to promote healthy behaviors. By reinforcing desired behavior through carefully selected rewards and by enforcing limits on undesirable behavior, occupational therapy professionals thought they could improve their clients' functioning. Behavioral approaches are discussed in detail in Chapter 2.

During the 1970s, sensory integration (SI), developed by occupational therapist A. Jean Ayres, was applied by occupational therapist Lorna Jean King in the treatment of clients with chronic psychiatric disorders. King proposed that poor functioning and grossly abnormal posture in those with chronic schizophrenia could be attributed to errors in sensory processing, which might be corrected or at least ameliorated by carefully designed sensorimotor programs. SI is rarely used today for this population. Instead, the focus in the 21st century is on **sensory processing** or **sensory modulation**, the ways individuals perceive and respond to sensation. Occupational therapists such as Dunn, Champagne, and Brown have contributed to the development of this area of intervention (40, 41, 46, 47) (see Chapters 3 and 21).

Sensory modulation provides low-cost options for occupational therapy intervention. Everyday activities, equipment, and supplies can be used to arouse or calm, allowing for emotional regulation. In addition, therapeutic use of self can be incorporated into intervention sessions, thus enhancing the service delivery of sensory modulation activities. Sensory modulation also incorporates a highly client-driven intervention situation, because of the specific sensory strategies and environmental modifications being integrally connected to specific self-regulation needs identified for each individual (77).

During the 1980s, occupational therapist Claudia Allen outlined and developed her practice model for **cognitive disabilities**. Allen proposed that a person's performance in a task indicates the quality of their thought processes. She identified six levels of cognitive functioning, which can be evaluated through performance of unfamiliar small crafts, such as leather lacing or mosaics. The six levels were later elaborated and expanded. Diagnosis of cognitive level can contribute to the psychiatric diagnosis and can be used to predict future functioning and to identify interventions and supports that may be effective (2). Allen's cognitive disabilities model is described further in Chapter 3.

Sensory modulation and **cognitive disabilities** attribute the occupational functioning problems, for persons with severe and persistent mental disorders, to defects in nervous system structures or functions. The questions for occupational therapy professionals are to what extent can these defects be corrected or remediated and to what extent can the person work around the defects. Correction is termed **remediation** and working around the deficit is termed **compensation** (alternately, **adaptation**). Defects that cannot be remediated must be compensated for, if the person is to function. The **sensory modulation** approach can be either remedial or compensatory; Allen's cognitive disabilities model is almost entirely compensatory; activities are modified and/or social support from others is provided to allow for occupational performance.

Both sensory modulation and cognitive disabilities emphasize activity or occupation as a focus for evaluation and intervention. The theories applied in the 1950s and 1960s were criticized for the absence of this focus. In addition, they were considered **reductionistic** (reducing the client's problems to isolated elements such as insight or behavior). During the 1960s and 1970s, Mary Reilly (117) and others attacked these approaches, arguing for a more comprehensive theory of occupational therapy practice that would focus primarily on the occupational nature of human beings. Since the 1980s, Kielhofner (84–86), Kielhofner and Burke (87), and others built on Reilly's work with the **model of human occupation (MOHO)**. This frame of reference organized research findings and traditional occupational therapy beliefs to create a comprehensive frame of reference for use in all practice areas, including physical medicine, developmental disabilities, and psychiatry. The frame of reference proposes that human response to the environment occurs because of an interaction among three systems: (a) volition (motivation), (b) habituation (roles and habits), and (c) performance (skills of the mind, brain, and body). The interactions among the three systems are dynamic, with each system affecting the other two systems. The MOHO is discussed in Chapter 3.

Some occupational therapy professionals during the 1980s began to apply cognitive behavioral principles (81). This approach, discussed in Chapter 2, investigates the events and associated feelings and thoughts that drive behavior. The client is taught to recall the chain of events and feelings and ideas and to challenge erroneous ideas. Once the ideas are proven false, there is an opportunity to change the behavior. Cognitive behavioral therapy and dialectical behavioral therapy, which is derived from it, show strong research evidence of effectiveness.

Also, beginning in the 1980s, occupational therapist Florence Clark (50) and others (80) developed a new scientific discipline, *occupational science*, for the systematic study of the occupational nature of humans. Research in occupational science is beginning to generate data that help occupational therapy professionals understand the nature of occupation and that validate the effectiveness of occupational therapy.

In 1996, a group of Canadian occupational therapists published the foundation article about the Person-Environment-Occupation (PEO) model, which considers transactions between the person, the environment, and the occupation. This model relates to occupational science research and is similar to the MOHO in many respects. The PEO model is discussed further in Chapter 3 (89).

Around the turn of the 21st century, as discussed previously, **sensory processing** regarding mental health began to be identified in the occupational therapy literature (40, 41, 46, 47). The *Adult Sensory Profile* was developed as an evaluation instrument to help identify sensory sensitivities and differences in adults and adolescents and includes documented strategies to compensate for these. This is important for persons with serious mental disorders, some of whom are acutely sensitive to environmental factors such as noise or odors. Others may have an insensitivity to surrounding stimulations and are unaware of sensations coming in from the environment, which causes them to miss cues from other people. People seek ways to self-regulate themselves and increase their level of comfortableness within their environment. Some people will need more stimulation to feel better and some will need to decrease their sensory stimulation to feel more comfortable with and around others (59, 104, 129).

The client-driven approach to mental health care and intervention for those with mental disorders has fueled an interest in exploring the phenomenology of illness or how the person views what is happening. The telling of a personal story and the appreciation of this story by the occupational therapy professional are the foci of **narrative reasoning**. Narrative reasoning is a way to study how people understand and tell the stories of their lives; it has enriched our appreciation and analysis of occupation and its relation to individuals (95). Occupational therapy professionals also use narrative reasoning to "make sense" of the client's story. As occupational therapy professionals trying to understand all the pieces of a client's life and daily situations, we can use narrative reasoning to organize our own thoughts about the client. This helps put intervention planning into an order meaningful to the client and prioritize how we will plan our therapeutic interventions with our clients. This type of narrative reasoning can be done as a professional discussion with a professional peer, and we can then glean new perspectives or identify aspects we may not have previously homed-in on with our clients (78).

Although occupational therapy professionals have been striving to clarify the theoretical understanding of occupation and refine their assessment and intervention techniques, they have also been aware about the proliferation and growth of other activity-oriented mental health therapies, all of which, to some extent, share occupational therapy techniques and theoretical concepts. Vocational rehabilitation counseling and dance, art, music, and poetry therapies focus on activities that once primarily concerned only occupational therapy professionals. Increasingly, nursing, social work, psychology, psychiatry, and even physical therapy are addressing the daily life activities and occupational functioning of persons with mental disorders. This sounds so much like occupational therapy that it can be hard for the layperson to see the difference. Occupational therapy professionals employed in psychiatric or psychosocial rehabilitation programs have a unique scope of practice and a skill set in activity analysis of occupation that is not part of the preparation of members of other professions.

The passage of the Americans with Disabilities Act of 1990 (ADA) (Public Law 101–468) allowed for new opportunities in mental health occupational therapy, working with clients trying to gain access to employment, supported housing, community mobility, and other everyday life opportunities.

The ADA mandates that qualified persons are not excluded from employment and work activities because of disability owing to physical or mental impairments. Occupational therapy professionals can help prepare persons with mental impairments for the world of work through training in work, self-advocacy, and attitudinal and behavioral skills and by collaborating with employers to analyze job functions and to determine reasonable accommodations (51, 68, 112). Occupational therapy intervention can focus on increasing self-confidence and self-identity for those with mental disorders regarding transitioning into community living (32). Stigma is still present, and discrimination (subtle or not) occurs. Advocacy from clients and from professions such as occupational therapy can increase social and political awareness. Occupational therapy professionals have the education, training, and background to assist employers and persons with disabilities to interpret and apply the law in a cost-effective and reasonable fashion.

The SAMHSA has begun to focus on behavioral health. They are working to integrate behavioral health services into primary care, community health, and **public health** (121). Behavioral health conditions include typical mental disorders such as anxiety, attention-deficit/hyperactivity disorder, bipolar disorder, depression, eating disorders, and psychosis (72). Other behavioral health situations include suicide prevention and substance abuse intervention (72). Behavioral health in these arenas includes promoting good mental health, resiliency, and well-being; providing intervention for those with mental disorders and substance use disorders; advocating for clients with mental disorders; supporting recovery work for those with mental disorders; and working with families of those with mental disorders and within communities where these individuals live. As the SAMHSA works to help integrate therapeutic services for those with behavioral health needs, there can be a greater emphasis placed on improving these clients' physical health as well (121). Occupational therapy can coordinate with other members of the behavioral health team while focusing on meaningful and productive life occupations for those experiencing recovery, enhancing community living independence through work on performance skills, and consulting with other professionals regarding performance patterns (63).

Public health is a newer practice area for occupational therapy professionals. The WHO has identified public health as a method to encompass promoting greater and sustainable health and well-being, strengthening services offered through public health systems, and decreasing inequities (136). A particular initiative of the WHO's public health work includes mental health strategies such as policy work toward developing and improving mental health initiatives and increasing quality of mental health services (137). The AOTA has also identified public health initiatives when working with those with mental disorders. Public health for occupational therapy professionals can include use of recovery model activities in the community, targeting intervention for those in the community experiencing trauma and violence, and providing wide-reaching programming including education about the role of occupational therapy and mental health, coping with everyday stress, environmental modifications to enhance social situation participation, and mental health literacy (13).

With a focus on public health, occupational therapy professionals have begun to have a more societal and global perspective. On a societal level, we have begun to focus more on areas such as disaster readiness and response (15). When considering mental health needs of a population and disaster preparedness, we can be advocates for policies and legislation that include the needs of those with mental disorders. We can also address the needs of populations experiencing occupational disruption, such as during times of sheltering in place and the barriers this causes to people being able to interact socially with others and remain connected to their daily occupational routines (132). Beyond considering victims of public disasters, we also think of how we can assist first responders. The World Federation of Occupational Therapists (WFOT) has identified occupational therapy professionals' work toward identifying first responder worker burnout and promoting therapeutic activities such as meditation, mindfulness techniques, and diaphragmatic breathing (134). As a part of disaster work, occupational therapy professionals can work with the mental health considerations of displaced persons through interventions for anxiety and depression, suicide awareness, and regaining a "normalcy" connected to occupational performance patterns (135).

Recent political gains for the profession of occupational therapy enhances our efforts and contributions for those with mental disorders. Some of this positive legislation includes the following:

- Centers for Medicare & Medicaid, in 2013, required occupational therapy be offered in all community mental health centers that bill for partial hospitalization services under Medicare guidelines (97).
- SAMHSA, beginning with fiscal year (FY) 2015, included occupational therapists as suggested staff for *Primary Behavioral Health Care* integration grants (55).
- SAMHSA, in 2015, included occupational therapists as suggested staff for *Certified Community Behavioral Health Centers* (122).
- The congressional reauthorization of the *Behavioral Health Workforce Education Training* grant initiative in 2016 allowed occupational therapy educational programs to become eligible for mental health–specific fieldwork

funding (1). In addition, in 2018, the *Health Resources Services Administration* (HRSA) included the profession of occupational therapy as a part of the behavioral health workforce (54).

The future of occupational therapy in psychiatry cannot be foretold. The limited number of occupational therapy professionals in mental health can lead to a smaller number of available fieldwork placements in mental health (82). Practice acts in some states, such as New York, have restricted the practice of occupational therapy to physician referrals, obstructing the occupational therapy profession from moving independently into community positions outside the medical model (23).

Leaders in occupational therapy mental health practice remind us, however, that the coming years provide many opportunities for occupational therapy in mental health under the ACA (76, 120). More occupational therapy education needs to be focused on the assessment and intervention skills needed for providing prevention in the community and within the wellness and recovery models.

The AOTA has identified our profession's distinct value within the arena of mental health as:

- developing and maintaining people's positive mental health,
- preventing individual's mental ill health, and
- assisting those with mental disorders in their recovery from mental health challenges so they may experience full lives and enjoy a productive life (13).

Fine (66) in 1999 wrote that the 21st century will test the profession with bottom-line economics and frequent re-engineering of staff configurations in mental health practice. Hospital-based practice has declined because of decreased client populations and decreased lengths of stay, staff shortages, and reduced reimbursement. Managed care has limited hospital stays and benefits for mental health care. Occupational therapy professionals are advised to develop and maintain awareness of political change regarding mental health parity and to help advocate on behalf of consumers (70).

Despite reduced reimbursement and the movement away from hospital practice, persons with mental disorders will continue to need and benefit from occupational therapy. We increasingly see these clients in their homes, workplaces, and communities. The occupational therapy professional frequently serves as consultant or manager rather than as provider of direct service. Occupational therapy professionals teach clients and families to manage symptoms and maximize occupational functioning. Opportunities in mental health for occupational therapy professionals are likely to expand. These opportunities have been and will continue to be found primarily in the community as well as in long-term care facilities. The reader is encouraged to consider ideas such as:

- wellness and health promotion for persons with mental disorders and for the general population (12, 16, 71, 91, 124);

- direct interventions and prevention programs to address the occupational problems of victims of domestic violence and youth violence (17, 18, 20, 75, 79, 83);
- interventions in schools and in community after-school programs for school-aged children with mental health problems (34, 35);
- forensic services for people with mental disorders who have become inmates and parolees of the prison system (56, 118, 131);
- life coaching and motivational services on a fee-for-service basis (88);
- outreach and community integration for those who are homeless (10, 48, 73);
- telehealth services to promote healthy living habits and routines, as well as quality-of-life experiences (22, 94);
- education within social systems to increase awareness of the occupational injustice associated with human trafficking and individual interventions to reestablish meaningful occupations and participation with others (42, 126); and
- occupational profile to build trust, empower clients, and collaborate using a trauma-informed approach with clients (19, 64).

Opportunities for occupational therapy provision expand as we become more familiar and comfortable with public policy and policymaking. Public policy is made because there is a recognition of a public problem (38). The policies a government creates are meant to be solutions and are done so on the public's behalf. Policies can lead to laws (statutes and regulations). Those outside the government can influence policymaking and thus can advance a particular direction of the final draft of a policy. **Redistributive policies** can allocate monies to be used for those with a limited voice and with limited resources, such as those with mental disorders and their families. It can also target areas such as public health, societal mental health initiatives, and livable communities. As occupational therapy professionals, we can utilize organized efforts such as the AOTA's advocacy and policy tools to contact our legislators, urging them to support policy initiatives that concern providing better mental health services for our clients (28). One such activity was the political efforts on the AOTA's part to have occupational therapy practitioners recognized as mental health professionals. A federal legal change identifying us as mental health professionals would help local and state policy efforts and thus expand our opportunities to be reimbursed for providing mental health services (29).

Policies are developed based on several societal needs. Contextual factors such as the culture of a group of people living in a particular geographic region can influence policymaking. Socioeconomic status is another contextual factor influencing policy activities. For instance, legislative work can be enhanced through the work of a lobbyist associated with a particular organization or agency. Funds to secure and maintain a lobbyist are required to utilize this resource.

A leading mental health policy topic is equitable consideration and treatment for those with mental disorders (103). Societal policy should be inclusive of all people's occupational needs. Equitable policymaking ensures initiatives are created by people coming from structurally disadvantaged backgrounds and that policy includes language that is reflective of the populations in need of service and support (103). Current mental health policy recommendations from the MHA include:

- prevention programming for all people,
- identification of those who are "at risk" and intervention for these population needs,
- integration of mental health care services for those in need of such services, and
- utilization of recovery programming (103).

Occupational therapy's greatest challenges are to maintain its professional visibility, claim its unique expertise in occupation (52, 133), and communicate effectively to make clients, insurance companies, and federal agencies aware of its special skills in evaluating and intervening effectively to address mental health problems. Figure 1.1 gives an overview of the parallel histories of psychiatry and occupational therapy.

THE ROLE OF THE OCCUPATIONAL THERAPY ASSISTANT AND THE OCCUPATIONAL THERAPIST

Students sometimes question how the OT differs from the OTA. Some job tasks are similar, or even the same, which can make the distinction between the roles cloudy. It can seem as if the OT completes all the paperwork and the OTA provides more of the intervention with clients. There can be confusion about the difference between the professional and the technical levels of occupational therapy education. If they are to work together effectively, both levels of occupational therapy professionals must understand the role differences.

Among the many factors affecting the entry-level roles of the OTA and the OT in the 21st century are the official educational standards and role expectations, descriptions, and responsibilities (25, 26, 30); the licensing and certification guidelines of the various states for occupational therapy professionals; and the local market availability for not only occupational therapy professionals but also other baccalaureate-level activities for therapists (such as recreation therapists and music therapists), as well as other mental health practitioners. In addition, the regulations and needs within mental health treatment facilities and community agencies and the experience and skills of individual occupational therapy professionals influence their roles. To clarify the roles of the OTA and the OT, the AOTA has in the past conducted several projects on *role delineation*. The purpose

of these projects was to outline precisely, or to delineate, the roles of entry-level OTAs and OTs. *Entry level* refers to new graduates of training programs as differentiated from experienced practitioners. The AOTA has consequently published *role guidelines* to help practitioners structure job tasks in a way that reflects the preparation of the OT or OTA to perform these tasks. These documents include, for instance, the *Value of Occupational Therapy Assistant Education to the Profession* (2019) (24) and the *Guidelines for Supervision, Roles, and Responsibilities During the Delivery of Occupational Therapy Services* (2020) (26). The *Standards for Occupational Therapy Education* are periodically reviewed and revised, the most recent version having been adopted in 2018 (25). In 2021, the AOTA's representative assembly redefined the *Standards of Practice for Occupational Therapy* (30). These documents provide a framework for discussing the role of the OTA and the OT in a mental health setting.

As a starting point, the entry-level OTA learns to have a collaborative partnership with the supervising OT. This ensures a provision of occupational therapy services that are recognized as skilled and a value to the client (24). The OT and the OTA are prepared to perform complementary job functions. Both are involved in all stages of the occupational therapy service delivery process from screening and assessment to discharge planning, but their roles and the areas for which each is responsible are distinct, with the OT taking the leadership role. Differing educational experiences prepare the OTA and the OT. The partnership between the two professionals must include teamwork and respect for one another's knowledge (21). The OTA commits to this partnership by demonstrating service competency with the job duties the OT indicates for the OTA to perform. This most often happens with administering assessment tools; however, service competency is a needed component for all aspects of client care.

The OT initiates the evaluation process and determines the appropriate assessments. The OTA can assist in assessment administration as well as gathering client data and reporting that data to the OT. The OT analyzes the occupational performance data and synthesizes the information to formulate the intervention plan. The intervention plan of care is determined by the OT and is developed in collaboration with the client and the OTA. Intervention is performed through a collaborative process with the OTA selecting, implementing, and modifying intervention interactions throughout the intervention implementation process. The OTA contributes information and documentation to the OT, assisting with the process of the OT determining the need to continue, change, or cease current occupational therapy services. Targeted occupational-based outcomes are collaboratively identified by the OT, OTA, and client. OTAs provide information regarding progress toward these outcomes and may assist with completing identified outcome measures (21).

The education and fieldwork training of the OTA and the OT prepare them to work in a complementary fashion, as the following situation illustrates.

Case Study – Supported Employment

The setting is a community day treatment center. The clients range in age from 25 to 65 years. Many are inactive and, if left to their own devices, would spend their days sitting unoccupied in the lounge. Two OTAs work at the center, leading a variety of groups such as lunch preparation, horticulture, physical fitness, nutrition management, and crafts. The supervising OT, who works 8 hours per week at this facility, has a strong interest in supported employment and has persuaded the director of the agency to fund the development of a program to help clients prepare for some level of work in the community. One of the OTAs has an interest in this area and has recruited two community businesses, a fast-food restaurant and a chain drug store, to hire clients part-time.

An occupational profile is initiated by the OT, and the OTA collects chart information to assist with completing the occupational profile process. The OT completes social skills and vocational skills assessments with the clients. The OTA also completes a vocational interest inventory with the clients. The OT and OTA identify six clients who may be ready for this program. The OTA now runs a job performance and work skills group 5 days a week for 1 hour a day, geared to prepare clients to begin the specific available jobs. The group employs a psychoeducational approach, focusing on social interaction skills and process skills in situations members may encounter while on the job (eg, acknowledging and responding to a request for assistance from a customer). Other topics include proper dress and hygiene, expectations, and job performance responsibilities (managing time use, maintaining required work patterns, initiating inquiries about work procedures) needed for employment. The OTA meets with the OT once a week to review clients' progress. The OTA is concerned that clients may need a staff member with them on the job, at least for the first few days. The OT agrees and helps the OTA lay out a schedule to place the clients into the jobs one at a time, with the OTA initially attending work with the clients as a job coach. The long-term plan is to train peer counselors (clients who know the jobs well and are reliable) to take over as job coaches.

The clients' response to the employment intervention is monitored every 3 months. Those clients who have not transitioned into a community vocational setting are reassessed to determine their skill progression and interest in the facility's vocation program. The client, OT, OTA, and facility social worker meet as an interdisciplinary team to discuss transition out of the supportive employment program either to a community vocational setting or to a different type of programming at the facility. The OT shares with the social worker the intraprofessional discussions the OT and OTA have while reviewing the clients' needs. This information, along with other possible community resources and information about the environment of other programs, helps the team determine the best place for the client to complete their transition.

The collaboration between OT and OTA in this situation makes use of their different skills. The OT and the OTA have completed the evaluation process with the clients, the OTA performing parts of assessments as directed by the OT supervisor. After analyzing and synthesizing the evaluation process results, the OT has matched clients' individual psychological assets and interests with the requirements of the job program. The OTA is carrying out a psychoeducational training regimen designed by both the OT and the OTA. The OTA makes good use of supervision to explore questions related to client progress. The specifics reported by the OTA are useful to the OT when conferring with the restaurant and drug store manager about the need for more physical space to perform occupational therapy services (eg, workspace to provide side-by-side coaching between the OTA and the client and also to train peer counselors). This sort of complementary relationship is only one example of the ways in which the OTA and OT work together.

By education, the OTA's area of greatest expertise is performance in areas of occupation. These include work, play, leisure, rest and sleep, activities of daily living, health management, instrumental activities of daily living, education, and social participation. The OTA is also trained extensively for intervention implementation for performance skills and performance pattern needs. The OT is also educated in these areas, with this level of education having a greater academic focus toward assessment, evaluation, and interventions in client factors and specific performance skills, understanding theoretical constructs, and applying theoretical concepts. The OTA is trained in structured techniques used with assessments. The OTA is thus able to carry out large segments of the occupational therapy program with supervision from the OT, who is better prepared to design the overall program and to evaluate and plan interventions for complex problems involving a combination of performance skill deficits and problems in client factors.

What the occupational therapy professional working in a mental health setting actually does on a day-to-day basis varies widely, depending on the experience of the occupational therapy professional, state law, the setting or facility, and reimbursement structure of the practice setting. Hypothetically, the occupational therapy professional could plan and carry out programs of independent self-care activities, selecting clothing and accessories, shopping and meal preparation, financial management, community mobility, communication management, safety and emergency maintenance, home establishment and management, care of others, job performance and maintenance skills, and play and leisure participation. The occupational therapy professional may teach coping skills and self-identity skills or provide interventions for performance skills such as social interaction skills or cognitive process skills. Consider another example of an OTA in mental health practice.

Occupational Therapy Events That Shaped Mental Health Practice

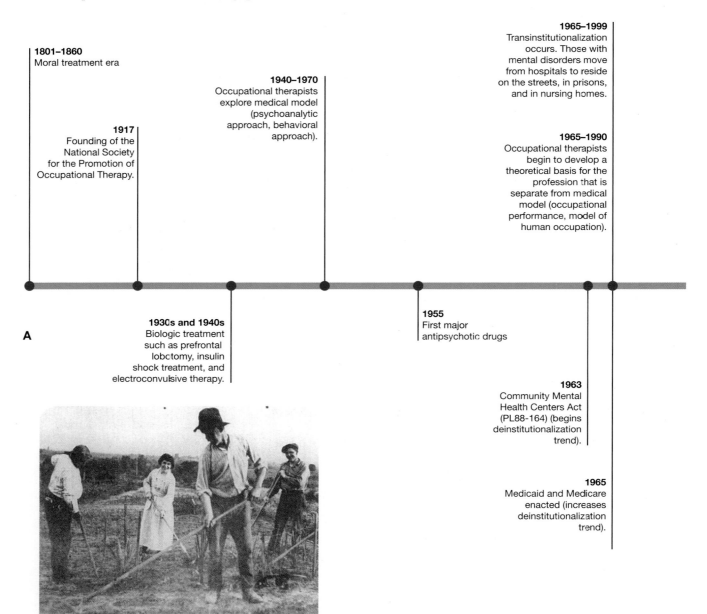

1801–1860
Moral treatment era

1917
Founding of the
National Society
for the Promotion of
Occupational Therapy.

1940–1970
Occupational therapists
explore medical model
(psychoanalytic
approach, behavioral
approach).

1965–1999
Transinstitutionalization
occurs. Those with
mental disorders move
from hospitals to reside
on the streets, in prisons,
and in nursing homes.

1965–1990
Occupational therapists
begin to develop a
theoretical basis for the
profession that is
separate from medical
model (occupational
performance, model of
human occupation).

A

1930s and 1940s
Biologic treatment
such as prefrontal
lobotomy, insulin
shock treatment, and
electroconvulsive therapy.

1955
First major
antipsychotic drugs

1963
Community Mental
Health Centers Act
(PL88-164) (begins
deinstitutionalization
trend).

1965
Medicaid and Medicare
enacted (increases
deinstitutionalization
trend).

B

Figure 1.1. A, Timeline. Selected Key Events in the History of Psychiatry, Medicine, Law, and Occupational Therapy in Mental Health. (Photo credit and info: U.S. Public Health Service Hospital, St. Louis, MO—1921.) B, A Garden (Practical OT). (Photo courtesy of Archives of the American Occupational Therapy Association, Inc. Bethesda, MD.)

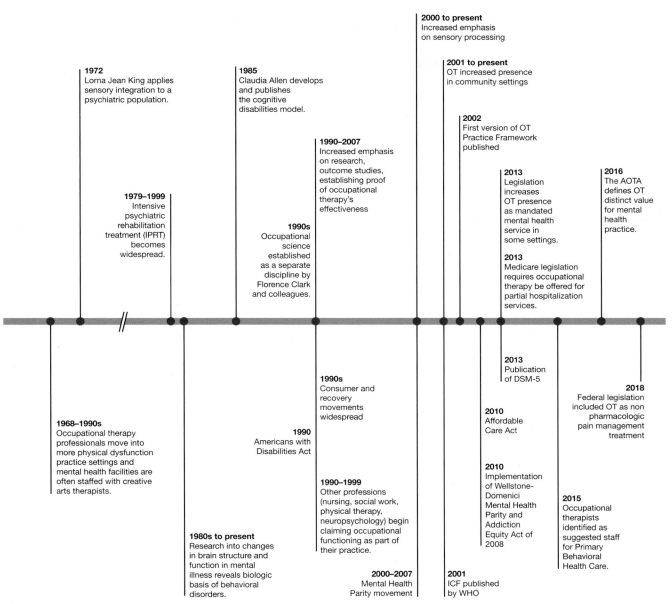

2000 to present
Increased emphasis
on sensory processing

2001 to present
OT increased presence
in community settings

1972
Lorna Jean King applies
sensory integration to a
psychiatric population.

1985
Claudia Allen develops
and publishes
the cognitive
disabilities model.

2002
First version of OT
Practice Framework
published

1990–2007
Increased emphasis
on research,
outcome studies,
establishing proof
of occupational
therapy's
effectiveness

2013
Legislation
increases
OT presence
as mandated
mental health
service in
some settings.

2016
The AOTA
defines OT
distinct value
for mental
health
practice.

1979–1999
Intensive
psychiatric
rehabilitation
treatment (IPRT)
becomes
widespread.

1990s
Occupational
science
established
as a separate
discipline by
Florence Clark
and colleagues.

2013
Medicare legislation
requires occupational
therapy be offered for
partial hospitalization
services.

2013
Publication
of DSM-5

1990s
Consumer and
recovery
movements
widespread

2010
Affordable
Care Act

2018
Federal legislation
included OT as non
pharmacologic
pain management
treatment

1968–1990s
Occupational therapy
professionals move into
more physical dysfunction
practice settings and
mental health facilities are
often staffed with creative
arts therapists.

1990
Americans with
Disabilities Act

2010
Implementation
of Wellstone-
Domenici
Mental Health
Parity and
Addiction
Equity Act of
2008

1990–1999
Other professions
(nursing, social work,
physical therapy,
neuropsychology) begin
claiming occupational
functioning as part of
their practice.

2015
Occupational
therapists
identified as
suggested staff
for Primary
Behavioral
Health Care.

1980s to present
Research into changes
in brain structure and
function in mental
illness reveals biologic
basis of behavioral
disorders.

2000–2007
Mental Health
Parity movement

2001
ICF published
by WHO

Figure 1.1. (continued)

Case Study – Service Agency

The setting is a large community service agency. The clients who attend its programs have serious and persistent mental disorders such as schizophrenia and bipolar disorder. Many have a dual diagnosis with a substance abuse history as well. Among the many programs provided here are a psychosocial clubhouse, a supported employment program, and a transitional employment program. One OT serves as consultant to the agency 6 hours per week.

An experienced OTA has recently been hired for the psychosocial clubhouse program. This is a new position; the four OTAs working in the employment programs have not had the time to provide any services in the clubhouse. The new OTA began by sitting down with client members of the club and formulating a plan for services; the OT sat in on the first meeting as an observer. In accordance with suggestions from the members, the OTA helps the member leader with the lunch program 5 days a week, providing information and guidance on nutrition and smart shopping. Another major responsibility is facilitating a photography workshop and gallery; members expressed a strong interest in taking digital photographs and editing them, with the possible goal of having a gallery with rotating public display shows. The OTA also meets with individual members to address specific needs such as selecting appropriate clothing for work, maintaining and repairing work clothing, identifying leisure opportunities for interests such as strength training, interpreting medication instructions, and locating 12-step groups near members' residences. One day a week, the OTA accompanies members on a trip to a community resource, such as the YWCA, to learn what additional programs are available. The OTA meets with the OT once a week to review progress, discuss concerns, and prepare for the Level I OTA fieldwork student who will start the next month. Just the past week, the OT commented that the OTA had such a full program that it was hard to believe that the position did not even exist 6 months ago.

OT HACKS SUMMARY

O: Occupation as a means and an end

Occupations are used as meaningful engagement and participation and are essential to overall well-being.

T: Theoretical concepts, values, and principles, or historical foundations

Moral treatment was based on the belief that people with mental disorders could benefit from daily regular routine activities and they could participate productively in their daily life.

Mental hygiene movement included working toward humane treatment for those with mental disorders.

Psychiatric treatments started with psychoanalysis and moved to medical treatments such as insulin shock treatment and ECT.

Community practice began in the 1960s and over the next 20 years the focus was on moving people out of large institutions and into small community home–like settings. Psychiatric-based health care centered around such theories and practice models as gestalt therapy, milieu therapy, behavioral therapy, and family therapy.

Occupational therapy began to focus on cognitive deficits, sensory processing issues, and aligning intervention with people's internal drive to participate and master occupations within their environment.

H: How can we Help? OT's role in serving clients with mental illness or mental health needs

Occupational therapy is provided in all settings, such as inpatient, outpatient, and community-based centers. Clients receive services to allow them to lead more productive lives, cope with the problems associated with the mental disorder, and regain connections to others. Mental health is a concern for all people and the ability to remain motivated to produce valued occupations. Services can focus on cognitive or sensory processing skills, environmental connections used by people to complete occupations, or work within social systems and the public health arena.

A: Adaptations

Not applicable for this chapter

C: Case study includes

Case studies were about the practice setting of supported employment and the practice setting of a community service agency. They highlighted the differences between the role of the occupational therapist and the OTA.

K: Knowledge: keeping mental health OT practice grounded in evidence, in occupational science, and in research

Knowledge of how to provide occupational therapy comes from occupational science (Florence Clark) and occupational therapists such as Mary Reilly, A. Jean Ayres, Lorna Jean King, Claudia Allen, and Gary Kielhofner.

S: Some terms that may be new to you

Epigenetics: the study of events and circumstance that mediate gene expression

Mental disorder: an impairment in which the person has significant distress with typical daily life activities and events and is unable to manage themselves regarding participation with others and regarding performing daily needed activities

Mental health: a person's well-being that allows someone to cope with everyday stresses so that the person remains a productive member of their community

Narrative reasoning: storytelling by the client about their life, done so occupational therapy professionals can better understand the client's view of their life; occupational therapy professionals telling the client's story in a "professional discussion" with peers so that they can better "make sense" of the client's life

Parity: the idea that there should be equal services provided for both physical health problems and mental health problems

Psychiatric rehabilitation: focuses on improving people's skills, which they use to function in their environment;

obtaining satisfaction with their occupational roles; and using external structures to enable community living

Public health: a system of health care and health initiatives for the whole community with a focus on providing needed services to all and on people's overall well-being

Recovery movement: a model of living centered around the concept of "recovery from a mental disorder"; it is person centered and focuses on self-determination and a person's restored function

Redistributive policies: policies made so that those with little voice in society can receive needed services and benefits

Reductionistic: viewing the client's problems in isolation and not approaching the client from a holistic occupational-based view

Transinstitutionalize: movement from one kind of institution to another

Reflection Questions

1. A new client has been diagnosed with a mental disorder. Relate three typical life conditions or situations that can become overwhelming to the point of the person being unable to manage daily life affairs, to specific occupational performance losses.

2. A client has worked in an entry-level clerical position for the past 5 years and is 30 years old. During high school the client's family did not have the financial means that would allow the client to attend college. The client has always wanted to be a paramedic. The client has become depressed and anxious. The question for the OTA student and OT student is different and will be provided by the instructor.

3. What aspects of moral treatment compare to occupational therapy service delivery?

4. To what does a lack of parity in mental health care lead?

5. Throughout the decades, occupational therapy services for those with mental health problems and mental disorders have changed. The question for the OTA student and OT student is different and will be provided by the instructor.

6. Describe the collaborative partnership between the OTA and the occupational therapist.

REFERENCES

1. 21st Century Cures Act of 2016. 42 U.S. C. § 9021. (2016). https://www.congress.gov/114/plaws/publ255/PLAW-114publ255.htm

2. Allen, C. (1985). *Occupational therapy for psychiatric diseases: Measurement and management of cognitive disabilities.* Brown and Company.

3. American Occupational Therapy Association. (n.d.). *Evidence-based practice.* Retrieved July 24, 2021, from https://www.aota.org/About-OccupationalTherapy/Professinals/EBP.aspx

4. American Occupational Therapy Association. (n.d.). *Mental health (practice).* Retrieved July 24, 2021, from https://www.aota.org/Practice/Mental-Health.aspx

5. American Occupational Therapy Association. (n.d.). *Mental health (professionals).* Retrieved July 24, 2021, from https://www.aota.org/practice/clinical-topics/mental-health

6. American Occupational Therapy Association. (n.d.). *Occupational therapy practitioners: A key member of the community behavioral health team.* https://www.aota.org//media/Corporate/Files/Advocacy/Federal/Overview-of-OT-in-Community-Behavioral-Health.pdf

7. American Occupational Therapy Association. (1993). Position paper: Purposeful activity. *American Journal of Occupational Therapy, 47*(12), 1081–1082.

8. American Occupational Therapy Association. (2008). Occupational therapy practice framework: Domain & process (2nd edition). *American Journal of Occupational Therapy, 62*(6), 625–683.

9. American Occupational Therapy Association. (2014). Occupational therapy practice framework: Domain & process (3rd edition). *American Journal of Occupational Therapy, 68*(Suppl. 1), S1–S48.

10. American Occupational Therapy Association. (2016). AOTA's societal statement on livable communities. *American Journal of Occupational Therapy, 70*(Suppl. 2), 1–2.

11. American Occupational Therapy Association. (2016). *Occupational therapy service outcome measures for Certified Community Behavioral Health Centers (CCBHCs): Framework for occupational therapy service with rationale for outcome measures selection and listing of occupational therapy outcome measure tools.* https://www.aota.org/-/media/Corporate/Files/Practice/MentalHealth/occupational-therapy-outcome-measures-community-mental-health-services.pdf

12. American Occupational Therapy Association. (2016). Occupational therapy services in the promotion of mental health and well-being. *American Journal of Occupational Therapy, 70*(Suppl. 2), 1–15.

13. American Occupational Therapy Association. (2016). *Occupational therapy's distinct value: Mental health promotion, prevention, and intervention across the lifespan.* https://www.aota.org/-/media/corporate/files/practice/mentalhealth/distinct-value-mental-health.pdf

14. American Occupational Therapy Association. (2016). *Occupational therapy's role with mental health in children and youth.* https://www.aota.org/About-Occupational-Therapy/Professionals/MH.aspx

15. American Occupational Therapy Association. (2017). AOTA's societal statement on disaster response and risk reduction. *American Journal of Occupational Therapy, 71*(Suppl. 2), 1–3.

16. American Occupational Therapy Association. (2017). Mental health promotion, prevention, and intervention in occupational therapy practice. *American Journal of Occupational Therapy, 71*(Suppl. 2), 1–19.

17. American Occupational Therapy Association. (2017). Occupational therapy services for individuals who have experienced domestic violence. *American Journal of Occupational Therapy, 71*(Suppl. 2), 1–13.

18. American Occupational Therapy Association. (2017). Philosophical base of occupational therapy. *American Journal of Occupational Therapy, 71*(Suppl. 2), 1.

19. American Occupational Therapy Association. (2018). AOTA's societal statement on stress, trauma, and posttraumatic stress disorder. *American Journal of Occupational Therapy, 72*(Suppl. 2), 1–3.

20. American Occupational Therapy Association. (2018). AOTA's societal statement on youth violence. *American Journal of Occupational Therapy, 72*(Suppl. 2), 1–2.

21. American Occupational Therapy Association. (2018). Importance of collaborative occupational therapist—Occupational therapy assistant intraprofessional education in occupational therapy curricula. *American Journal of Occupational Therapy, 72*(Suppl. 2), 1–18.

22. American Occupational Therapy Association. (2018). Telehealth in occupational therapy. *American Journal of Occupational Therapy, 72*(Suppl. 2), 1–18.

23. American Occupational Therapy Association. (2019, August). *Occupational therapy: Referral requirements.* https://www.aota.org/-/media/Corportate/Files/Secure/Advocacy/Licensure/StateRegs/referral-req.pdf

24. American Occupational Therapy Association. (2019). Value of occupational therapy assistant education to the profession. *American Journal of Occupational Therapy, 73*(Suppl. 2), 1–3.

25. American Occupational Therapy Association. (2020, December version). *2018 Accreditation Council for Occupational Therapy Education (ACOTE) standards and interpretive guide (effective July 31,*

2020). Accreditation Council for Occupational Therapy Education. Retrieved July 11, 2021, from https://acoteonline.org/accreditation-explained/

26. American Occupational Therapy Association. (2020). Guidelines for supervision, roles, and responsibilities during the delivery of occupational therapy services. *American Journal of Occupational Therapy, 74*(Suppl. 2), 1–62.

27. American Occupational Therapy Association. (2020). Occupational therapy practice framework: Domain and process—Fourth edition. *American Journal of Occupational Therapy, 74*(Suppl. 2), 1–87.

28. American Occupational Therapy Association. (n.d.). *Advocacy and policy.* https://www.aota.org/Advocacy-Policy.aspx

29. American Occupational Therapy Association. (2021, June 17). *Bill recognizing occupational therapy practitioners as mental health professionals reintroduced in congress.* https://www.aota.org/advocacy/advocacy-news/legislative-issues-update/legislation-re-introduced-recognizing-otp-as-mental-health-professionals

30. American Occupational Therapy Association. (2021). Standards of practice for occupational therapy. *American Journal of Occupational Therapy, 75*(Suppl. 3), 7513410030.

31. American Psychiatric Association. (2022). *Diagnostic and statistical manual of mental disorders* (5th ed., text rev.). https://doi.org/10.1176/appi.books.9780890425787

32. Angell, A. M., Goodman, L., Walker, H. R., McDonald, K. E., Kraus, L. E., Elms, E. H. J., Frieden, L., Jordan Sheth, A., & Hammel, J. (2020). "Starting to live life": Understanding full participation for people with disabilities after institutionalization. *American Journal of Occupational Therapy, 74*(4), 1–11.

33. Anthony, W. A., Cohen, M., & Farkas, M. (1990). *Psychiatric rehabilitation.* Boston University Center.

34. Arbesman, M., Bazyk, S., & Nochajski, S. (2013). Systematic review of occupational therapy and mental health promotion, prevention, and intervention for children and youth. *American Journal of Occupational Therapy, 67*(6), 120–130.

35. Barnes, K. J., Beck, A. J., Vogel, K. A., Oxford Grice, K., & Murphy, D. (2003). Perceptions regarding school-based occupational therapy for children with emotional disturbances. *American Journal of Occupational Therapy, 57*(3), 337–341.

36. Beers, C. W. (2004). *A mind that found itself* (eBook ed.). Project Gutenberg. https://www.gutenberg.org/files/11962/11962-h/11962-h.htm

37. *Behavioral health equity.* (n.d.). Substance Abuse and Mental Health Service Administration. Retrieved July 23, 2021, from https://www.samhsa.gov/behavioral-health-equity

38. Birkland, T. A. (2011). *An introduction to the policy process: Theories, concepts, and models of public policy making* (4th ed.). Routledge.

39. Bockoven, J. S. (1971). Legacy of moral treatment: 1880's to 1910. *American Journal of Occupational Therapy, 25*(5), 223–225.

40. Brown, C. (2001). What is the best environment for me? A sensory processing perspective. *Occupational Therapy in Mental Health, 17*(3–4), 115–125.

41. Brown, C., Tollefson, N., Dunn, W., Cromwell, R., & Filion, D. (2001). The adult sensory profile: Measuring patterns of sensory processing. *American Journal of Occupational Therapy, 55*(1), 75–82.

42. Bryant, C., Freeman, L., Granata, M., He, H., Hough, H., Patel, S., Stedman, A., Silvia, S., & Tran, M. (2015). Societal statement on the role of occupational therapy with survivors of human sex trafficking in the United States. *OCCUPATION: A Medium of Inquiry for Students, Faculty & Other Practitioners Advocating for Health through Occupational Studies, 1*(1), 1–4.

43. Centers for Disease Control and Prevention. (2005, December). *Roundtable on the psychosocial challenges posed by a radiological terrorism incident.* https://www.cdc.gov/nceh/radiation/emergencies/pdf/rt-psychosocial.pdf

44. Centers for Medicare & Medicaid Services. (n.d.). *The Mental Health Parity and Addiction Equity Act (MHPAEA).* Retrieved July 4, 2021, from https://www.cms.gov/CCIIO/Programs-and-Initiatives/Other-Insurance-Protections/mhpaea_factsheet

45. Cetin, M. S. (2015). *New approaches for data-mining and classification of mental disorders in brain imaging data* [Doctoral dissertation]. The University of New Mexico. Digital Repository.

46. Champagne, T. (2005). Expanding the role of sensory approaches in acute psychiatric settings. *Mental Health Special Interest Section Quarterly, 28*(1), 1–4.

47. Champagne, T., & Koomar, J. (2011). Expanding the focus: Addressing sensory discrimination concerns in mental health. *Mental Health Special Interest Section Quarterly, 34*(1), 1–4.

48. Chapleau, A., Seroczynski, A. D., Meyers, S., Lam, K., & Buchino, S. (2012). The effectiveness of a consultation model in community mental health. *Occupational Therapy in Mental Health, 28*(4), 379–395.

49. *Child and adolescent mental and behavioral health resolution.* (2019, June). American Psychological Association. https://www.apa.org/about/policy/child-adolescent-mental-behavioral-health

50. Clark, F. A., Parham, D., Carlson, M. E., Frank, G., Jackson, J., Pierce, D., Wolfe, R. J., & Zemke, R. (1991). Occupational science: Academic innovation in the service of occupational therapy's future. *American Journal of Occupational Therapy, 45*(4), 300–310.

51. Crist, P. A. H., & Stoffel, V. C. (1992). The Americans with Disabilities Act of 1990 and employees with mental impairments: Personal efficacy and the environment. *American Journal of Occupational Therapy, 46*(5), 434–443.

52. Darnell, J. L., & Heater, S. L. (1994). The issue is: Occupational therapist or activity therapist—Which do you choose to be? *American Journal of Occupational Therapy, 48*(5), 467–468.

53. Davidson, L. (2016). The recovery movement: Implications for mental health care and enabling people to participate fully in life. *Health Affairs, 25*(6), 1091–1097.

54. Department of Health and Human Services Health Resources and Services Administration (2019). *Justification of estimates for Appropriations Committees.* https://www.hrsa.gov/sites/default/files/hrsa/about/budget/budget-justification-fy2019.pdf

55. Department of Health and Human Services Substance Abuse and Mental Health Services. (2014). *Primary and behavioral health care integration.* Request for applications (RFA) No. SM-15-005. Catalog of Federal Domestic Assistance (CFDA) No.: 93.243. https://www.samhsa.gov/grants/grant-announcements/sm-15-005

56. Dittmann, M. (2003, March). *How to expand a psychosocial program.* American Psychological Association. https://www.apa.org/monitor/mar03/howtoexpand

57. Dupont, C., Armant, D. R., & Brenner, C. A. (2009). Epigenetics: Definition, mechanisms and clinical perspective. *Seminars in Reproductive Medicine, 27*(5), 351–357.

58. *Emotional well-being: Population health.* (2021, February 2). Centers for Disease Control and Prevention. Retrieved July 23, 2021, from https://www.cdc.gov/emotional-wellbeing/index.htm

59. Engel-Yeger, B., & Dunn, W. (2011). Exploring the relationship between affect and sensory processing patterns in adults. *British Journal of Occupational Therapy, 74*(10), 456–464.

60. Evans, A. C., & Bufka, L. F. (2020, August 6). *The critical need for a population health approach: Addressing the nation's behavioral health during the COVID-19 pandemic and beyond.* Preventing Chronic Disease: Public Health Research, Practice, and Policy. Centers for Disease Control and Prevention. https://www.cdc.gov/pcd/issues/2020/20_0261.htm

61. *FAQs for PCPs.* (n.d.). American Psychiatric Association. Retrieved July 23, 2021, from https://www.psychiatry.org/psychiatrists/practice/professional-interests/integrated-care/learn/faq

62. *Female genital mutilation/cutting (FGM/C).* (2020, May 11). Centers for Disease Control and Prevention. https://www.cdc.gov/reproductivehealth/womensrh/female-genital-mutilation.html

63. Ferlin, A., Fischer, H., Januszewski, C., & Hahn, B. (2018, December 24). *Occupational therapy integrated behavioral health care: A visual service framework.* American Occupational Therapy Association. https://www.aota.org/publications-news/opt/archive/2018/integrated-behavior.aspx

64. Fette, C., Lambdin-Pattavina, C., & Weaver, L. L. (2019). Understanding and applying trauma-informed approaches across occupational therapy settings. *OT Practice, 24*(5), CE1–CE9.

65. Fidler, G. S., & Fidler, J. W. (1963). *Occupational therapy—A communication process in psychiatry.* Macmillan.

66. Fine, S. B. (1999). Surviving the health care revolution: Rediscovering the meaning of "good work." In A. H. Scott (Ed.), *New frontiers in mental health*. Haworth Press.

67. Foster, L., & AOTA 2013 Mental Health Work Group. (n.d.). *Occupational therapy's role in mental health promotion, prevention, & intervention with children & youth: Social and emotional learning (SEL)*. https://www.aota.org/-/media/Corporate/Files/Practice/Children/SchoolMHToolkit/Social-and-Emotional-Learning-Info-Sheet.pdf

68. Frieden, L. (1992). The issue is: The Americans with Disabilities Act of 1990: Will it work? (Pro). *American Journal of Occupational Therapy, 46*(5), 468–469.

69. Friedland, J. (1998). Occupational therapy and rehabilitation: An awkward alliance. *American Journal of Occupational Therapy, 52*(5), 372–380.

70. Gallew, H. A., Haltiwanger, E., Sowers, J., & van den Heever, N. (2004). Political action and critical analysis: Mental health parity. *Occupational Therapy in Mental Health, 20*(1), 1–25.

71. Gitlin, L. (2017). Questions and answers. *OT Practice, 17*(12), 32.

72. Grant, K., Khan, S., Dutta-Gupta, I., Counts, N., Reinert, M., & Nguyen, T. (2019, August 1). *Reimagining behavioral health: A new vision for whole-family, whole-community behavioral health*. Mental Health America. https://www.mhanational.org/research-reports/reimagining-behavioral-health-new-vision-whole-family-whole-community-behavioral

73. Griner, K. R. (2006). Helping the homeless: An occupational therapy perspective. *Occupational Therapy in Mental Health, 22*(1), 49–61.

74. *Health hazard evaluation of police officers and firefighters after Hurricane Katrina*. (2006, April 28). Morbidity and Mortality Weekly Report. Centers for Disease Control and Prevention. https:cdc.gov/mmwr/preview/mmwrhtml/mm5516a4.htm

75. Helfrich, C. A., Lafata, M. J., MacDonald, S. L., Aviles, A., & Collins, L. (2001). Domestic abuse across the lifespan: Definitions, identification and risk factors for occupational therapists. *Occupational Therapy in Mental Health, 16*(3–4), 5–34.

76. Hildenbrand, W. C., & Lamb, A. J. (2013). Occupational therapy in prevention and wellness: Retaining relevance in a new health care world. *American Journal of Occupational Therapy, 67*(3), 266–271.

77. Hitch, D., Wilson, C., & Hillman, A. (2020). Sensory modulation in mental health practice. *Mental Health Practice, 23*(3), 10–16.

78. Humber, T. K. (2004). *The use of clinical reasoning skills by experienced occupational therapy assistants* [Doctoral dissertation]. The Pennsylvania State University. ProQuest Dissertations Publishing.

79. Humbert, T. K., Bess, J. L., & Mowery, A. M. (2013). Exploring women's perspectives of overcoming intimate partner violence: A phenomenological study. *Occupational Therapy in Mental Health, 29*(3), 246–265.

80. Jackson, J., Carlson, M., Mandel, D., Zemke, R., & Clark, F. (1998). Occupation in lifestyle redesign: The Well Elderly Study Occupational Therapy Program. *American Journal of Occupational Therapy, 52*(5), 326–336.

81. Johnson, M. T. (1987). Occupational therapists and the teaching of cognitive behavioral skills. *Occupational Therapy in Mental Health, 7*(3), 69–81.

82. Kautzmann, L. N. (1995). Alternatives to psychosocial fieldwork: Part of the solution or part of the problem? *American Journal of Occupational Therapy, 49*(3), 266–268.

83. Kessler, A. (2012). Addressing the consequences of domestic violence. *OT Practice, 17*(3), 6.

84. Kielhofner, G. (1985). *A model of human occupation: Theory and application*. Lippincott Williams & Wilkins.

85. Kielhofner, G. (1992). *Conceptual foundations of occupational therapy*. F.A. Davis.

86. Kielhofner, G. (2008). *A model of human occupation: Theory and application* (4th ed.). Lippincott Williams & Wilkins.

87. Kielhofner, G., & Burke, J. (1980). A model of human occupation. Part 1: Conceptual framework and content. *American Journal of Occupational Therapy, 34*(9), 572–581.

88. Klippel, L. (2006). A horse of a different color: Mental health occupational therapy and coaching. *Mental Health Special Section Quarterly, 29*(1), 1–4.

89. Law, M., Cooper, B., Strong, S., Stewart, D., Rigby, P., & Letts, L. (1996). The Person-Environment-Occupation Model: A transactive approach to occupational performance. *Canadian Journal of Occupational Therapy, 63*(1), 9–23.

90. *Learn about mental health*. (n.d.). Centers for Disease Control and Prevention. Retrieved July 23, 2021, from https://www.cdc.gov/mentalhealth/learn/index.htm

91. Letts, L., Edwards, M., Berenyi, J., Moros, K., O'Neill, C., O'Toole, C., & McGrath, C. (2011). Using occupations to improve quality of life, health and wellness, and client and caregiver satisfaction for people with Alzheimer's disease and related dementias. *American Journal of Occupational Therapy, 65*(5), 497–504.

92. Licht, S. (1983). The early history of occupational therapy: An outline. *Occupational Therapy in Mental Health, 3*(1), 67–88.

93. Lieb, L. C. (2019, February 19). *Occupational therapy and self-perceived burden: Facilitating psychosocial adjustment to disability*. American Occupational Therapy Association. https://www.aota.org/Publications-News/otp/Archive/2019/self-perceived-burden.aspx

94. Linder, S. M., Rosenfeldt, A. B., Curtis Bay, R., Sahu, K., Wolf, S., L., & Alberts, J. L. (2015). Improving quality of life and depression after stroke through telerehabilitation. *American Journal of Occupational Therapy, 50*(5), 338–346.

95. Mallinson, T., Kielhofner, G., & Mattingly, C. (1996). Metaphor and meaning in a clinical interview. *American Journal of Occupational Therapy, 50*(5), 338–346.

96. McKnight-Eily, L. R., Okora, C. A., Strine, T. W., Verlenden, J., Hollis, N. D., Njai, R., Mitchell, E. W., Board, W., Puddy, R., & Thomas, C. (2021, February 5). *Racial and ethnic disparities in the prevalence of stress and worry, mental health conditions, and increased substance use among adults during the COVID-19 pandemic—United States, April and May 2020*. Morbidity and Mortality Weekly Report. Centers for Disease Control and Prevention. https://www.cdc.gov/mmwr/volumes/70/wr/mm7005a3.htm

97. *Medicare program: Conditions of participation (CoPs) for community mental health centers*. 78 Fed. Reg. 64635 (October 29, 2013) (to be codified at 42 CFR pt. 485). https://www.federalregister.gov/documents/2013/10/29/2013-24056/medicare-program-conditions-of-participation-cops-for-community-mental-health-centers

98. Mental Health America. (n.d.). *About mental health America*. Retrieved July 4, 2021, from https://www.mhanational.org/about

99. Mental Health America. (n.d.). *Our history*. Retrieved July 4, 2021, from https://www.mhanational.org/our-history

100. Mental Health America. (2015, December 5). *Position Statement 17: Promotion of mental wellness*. Retrieved July 24, 2021, from https://mhanational.org/issues/position-statement-17-promotion-mental-wellness

101. Mental Health America. (2016, March 5). *Position Statement 35: Aging well: Wellness and psychosocial treatment for the emotional and cognitive challenges of aging*. Retrieved July 24, 2021, from https://mhanational.org/sites/default/files/Position-Statements/Position-Statement-35.pdf

102. Mental Health America. (2017, March 3). *Position Statement 59: Responding to behavioral health crises*. Retrieved July 24, 2021, from https://mhanational.org/issues/position-statement-59-responding-behavioral-health-crises#:~:text=All%20law%20enforcement%20personnel%20should,are%20available%20on%20every%20shift

103. Mental Health America. (n.d.). *Mental health policy*. https://www.mhanational.org/policy-issues

104. Meredith, P. J., Rappel, G., Strong, J., & Bailey, K. J. (2015). Sensory sensitivity and strategies for coping with pain. *American Journal of Occupational Therapy, 69*(4), 1–10.

105. Meyer, A. (1982). The philosophy of occupational therapy. *Occupational Therapy in Mental Health, 2*(3), 79–86.

106. Munsey, C. (2009, February). *Top psychologists will examine military's efforts to promote psychological health*. American Psychological Association. https://www.apa.org/monitor/2009/02/military

107. National Alliance on Mental Illness. (n.d.). *Home page*. Retrieved July 30, 2021, from https://www.nami.org/Home

108. National Board for Certification in Occupational Therapy. (2020). *2020 COTA matrix study*. https://www.nbcot.org/-/media/PDFs/Matrix_Report_COTA.pdf

109. National Board for Certification in Occupational Therapy. (2020). *2020 OTR matrix study*. https://www.nbcot.org/-/media/PDFs/Matrix_Report_OTR.pdf

110. *National treatment profile: What types of treatment do children with ADHD receive?* (n.d.). Centers for Disease Control and Prevention.

Retrieved July 24, 2021, from https://www.cdc.gov/ncbddd/adhd/features/kf-national-treatment-profile-adhd-nsdata.html

111. New York State Office of Mental Health. (n.d.). *Program type definitions*. Retrieved July 4, 2021, from https://omh.ny.gov/omhweb/par/program_type_definitions.html

112. Nosek, M. A. (1992). The issue is: The Americans with Disabilities Act of 1990: Will it work? (Con). *American Journal of Occupational Therapy, 46*(5), 466–467.

113. O'Hagan, M. (2009). *An update on recovery in Mental Health Today.* Mary's Writing and Free Downloads. http://www.maryohagan.com/publications.php

114. *Psychosocial factors and homelessness.* (2011). American Psychological Association. https://www.apa.org/pi/ses/resources/publications/homelessness-factors

115. *Psychosocial treatments.* (n.d.). National Alliance on Mental Illness. Retrieved July 24, 2021, from https://www.nami.org/About-Mental-Illness/Treatment/Psychosocial-Treatements

116. Raad, R., & Makari, G. (2010). Samuel Tuke's description of the retreat. *American Journal of Psychiatry, 167*(8), 898.

117. Reilly, M. (1962). The 1961 Eleanor Clarke Slagle lecture: Occupational therapy can be one of the great ideas of 20th century medicine. *American Journal of Occupational Therapy, 16*(1), 1–9.

118. Schindler, V. P. (2005). Occupational therapy in forensic psychiatry: Role development and schizophrenia. *Occupational Therapy in Mental Health, 20*(3–4), 1–171.

119. Serrett, K. D. (1985). Another look at occupational therapy's history. *Occupational Therapy in Mental Health, 5*(3), 1–31.

120. Stoffel, V. C. (2013). Opportunities for occupational therapy behavioral health: A call to action. *American Journal of Occupational Therapy, 67*(2), 140–145.

121. Substance Abuse and Mental Health Services Administration. (n.d.). *SAMHSA—Behavioral health integration.* https://www.samhsa.gov/sites/default/files/samhsa-behavioral-health-integration.pdf

122. Substance Abuse and Mental Health Services Administration. (2015). *Planning grants for certified community behavioral health clinics.* Retrieved July 4, 2021, from https://www.samhsa.gov/grants/grant-announcements/sm-16-001

123. Substance Abuse and Mental Health Services Administration. (2020). *Behavioral health barometer: United States: Volume 6.* https://www.samhsa.gov/data/report/behavioral-health-barometer-state-barometers-volume-6

124. Swarbrick, M. (2009). A wellness and recovery model for state psychiatric hospitals. *Occupational Therapy in Mental Health, 25*(3–4), 343–351.

125. *Taking care of your emotional health.* (2019, September 13). Centers for Disease Control and Prevention. Retrieved July 24, 2021, from https://emergency.cdc.gov/coping/selfcare.asp

126. Thompson, T., Flick, J., & Thinnes, A. (2020). Occupational injustice and human trafficking: Occupational therapy's role. *OT Practice, 25*(1), CE1–CE9.

127. Torrey, E. F. (1997). *Out of the shadows.* Wiley.

128. Whitaker, R. (2011). *Anatomy of an epidemic: Magic bullets, psychiatric drugs, and the astonishing rise of mental illness in America.* Broadway Books.

129. Whitcomb, D. A., Carrasco, R. C., Neuman, A., & Kloos, H. (2015). Correlational research to examine the relation between attachment and sensory modulation in young children. *American Journal of Occupational Therapy, 69*(4), 1–8.

130. White Swan Foundation. (2015, June 30). *What is psychiatric rehabilitation?* https://www.whiteswanfoundation.org/mental-health-matters/understanding-mental-health/what-is-psychiatric-rehabilitation

131. Whitford, G., Jones, K., Weekes, G., Ndlove, N., Long, C., Perkes, D., & Brindle, S. (2020). Combatting occupational deprivation and advancing occupational justice in institutional settings: Using a practice-based enquiry approach for service transformation. *British Journal of Occupational Therapy, 83*(1), 52–61.

132. Whitney, R. V., & Walsh, W. E. (2020). Occupational therapy's role in times of disaster: Addressing periods of occupational disruption. *OT Practice, 25*(5), CE1–CE8.

133. Wood, W. (1996). Legitimizing occupational therapy's knowledge. *American Journal of Occupational Therapy, 50*(8), 626–634.

134. World Federation of Occupational Therapists. (2019). *WFOT guide for occupational therapy first responders to disasters and trauma.* https://wfot.org/resources/wfot-guide-for-occupational-therapy-first-responders-to-disasters-and-trauma

135. World Federation of Occupational Therapists. (2019). *WFOT resource manual: Occupational therapy for displaced persons.* https://wfot.org/resources/wfot-resource-manual-occupational-therapy-for-displaced-persons

136. World Health Organization. (n.d.). *Public health services.* Retrieved July 4, 2021, from https://www.euro.who.int/en/health-topics/Health-systems/public-health-services/public-health-services

137. World Health Organization. (n.d.). *WHO special initiative for mental health.* Retrieved July 4, 2021, from https://www.who.int/initiatives/who-special-initiative-for-mental-health

138. World Health Organization. (2022, June 17). *Mental health.* https://www.who.int/news-room/fact-sheets/detail/mental-health-strengthening-our-response

SUGGESTED RESOURCES

Articles

American Occupational Therapy Association. (2013). AOTA's societal statement on health disparities. *American Journal of Occupational Therapy, 67*(Suppl. 6), S7–S8.

Peloquin, S. M. (1994). Moral treatment: How a caring practice lost its rationale. *American Journal of Occupational Therapy, 48*(2), 167–173.

Stoffel, V. C. (2013). Opportunities for occupational therapy behavioral health: A call to action. *American Journal of Occupational Therapy, 67*(2), 140–145.

Sujit Sarkeh, O. P., & Singh, M. A. (2021). Clinical practice guidelines for psychoeducation in psychiatric disorders: General principles of psychoeducation. *Indian Journal of Psychiatry, 62*(Suppl. 2), S319–S323.

Websites

American Occupational Therapy Association. *Occupational therapy service outcome measures for Certified Community Behavioral Health Centers (CCBHCs): Framework for occupational therapy service with rationale for outcome measures selection and listing of occupational therapy outcome measure tools.* https://www.aota.org/-/media/Corporate/Files/Practice/MentalHealth/occupational-therapy-outcome-measures-community-mental-health-services.pdf

American Occupational Therapy Association. *OT room at military hospital.* http://www.otcentennial.org/photo/workshops-for-veterans

American Psychiatric Association Foundation. *A website for the promotion of mental health in the workplace.* http://www.workplacementalhealth.org/?DID=70

Centers for Disease Control and Prevention. *Mental health.* https://www.cdc.gov/mentalhealth/

International Mental Health Collaborating Network. *History of recovery movement.* https://imhcn.org/bibliography/history-of-mental-health/history-of-recovery-movement/

Mental Health America. https://mhanational.org/

Mental Health Occupational Therapy Association. https://justinteerlinck.wixsite.com/mentalhealthot

National Alliance of Mental Illness. https://www.nami.org/Home

National Institute of Mental Health. https://www.nimh.nih.gov/

World Federation of Occupational Therapists. *Occupational therapy and mental health.* https://wfot.org/resources/occupational-therapy-and-mental-health

Medical and Psychological Theories, Frames of Reference, and Models of Mental Health and Mental Illness

OT HACKS OVERVIEW

O: **Occupation as a means and an end**

Occupational connection will be made through these theories and models: Object Relations, Development as identified by Erikson's, Behavioral, Cognitive Behavioral, Cognitive Enhancement, Client-Centered, Neuroscience Theories, and Psychological Rehabilitation.

T: **Theoretical concepts, values, and principles, or historical foundations**

Information will come from psychological-based theories, frames of reference, and models that align with mental health occupational therapy practice.

H: **How can we Help? OT's role in serving clients with mental illness or mental health needs**

How do we use theories, frames of reference, and models that are not born from occupational therapy?

A: **Adaptations**

Adapting to situations one cannot independently self-manage is a process built from the science of psychology.

C: **Case study includes**

Case studies and examples throughout the chapter present when and how psychology-based theories, frames of reference, and model information helps to guide our decision-making.

K: **Knowledge: keeping mental health OT practice grounded in evidence, in occupational science, and in research**

Knowledge presented will come from psychological theorists such as Freud, Erikson, Pavlov, Skinner, Beck, Ellis, Bandura, and Rogers.

S: **Some terms that may be new to you**

Key terms are summarized throughout the chapter.

INTRODUCTION

Medical and psychological theories attempt to explain how mental health problems develop and how occupational therapy professionals may help someone cope with them. These theories also help establish the basis for how we use ourselves with our clients, or how we use what is called therapeutic use of self (discussed more in Chapter 15). Historically, occupational therapists have used theories originally developed by psychologists or psychiatrists.[1] Although many of these theories are used less widely today, techniques based on them are still in use. Also, occupational therapy professionals often work in settings in which some of the staff employ one or more of the theories discussed in this chapter. Chapter 3 explores frames of reference and practice models developed specifically for use in occupational therapy practice.

First, however, why use a theory at all? One very good reason is that a theory provides ideas about what to do in a situation with a client. Imagine the following scenario.

Case Example

Your supervisor on level 1 fieldwork has asked you to cover her cooking group while she goes to a meeting. Because you are comfortable with cooking, you agree to do it. Everything seems to be going fine. All eight members are busy with their tasks. Suddenly one teenager starts drawing a knife across her wrist. She is not cutting open her skin, but just dragging the knife across her skin.

What would you do? Are you finding it hard to think of an answer? Maybe you would like to think about it for a while, but in a real situation, you would not have much time. You would have to respond quickly, and it might help if you had a theory to give you some ideas.

A theory is one way of looking at something, and because there are many ways of looking at how the mind works, we have many theories about it. A theory provides a set of principles and concepts that can be used to organize, explain, and predict observable phenomena—in this case, behavior and other aspects of mental health. A theory helps explain why

---

[1]Much of the material in this chapter derives from Early (30).

we work a particular way with a client. A theory is one explanation, but there is not yet any one "correct" theory that explains all we want to know about the human mind. Consequently, many theories try to explain the same thing. As an occupational therapy professional, you will use techniques based on these theories.

Major medical and psychological theories, frames of reference, and models used in mental health treatment are covered in this chapter. You will learn about the main ideas, special vocabulary, and some of the basic techniques of each theory.

Frames of reference refer to when a profession views a particular aspect or domain of its knowledge and teachings as a mechanism for client change. Change happens on a continuum and involves both functional change as well as lapses in function or an inability to function, known as dysfunction. It is important to note that function does not typically happen in a fast upward trajectory of skill and ability. It happens in a spiral fashion; in other words, when function improves, there can be setbacks or limitations because of decreased abilities or skills. Models take the philosophical base and theoretical concepts of a profession and synthesize them in accordance with the theoretical data of science(s) used by the profession. Models can be built around one theory's information or can be eclectic in nature, being built from various relevant theories. Models organize a way of thinking about a client's performance.

PSYCHOANALYTIC THEORY: MODEL OF OBJECT RELATIONS

The model of object relations is an approach based on the psychoanalytic theory work of Sigmund Freud and his followers, who believed that mental health and mental disorders are determined by our relations with objects in our environment. These objects may be physical (natural or human-made) or human (relationships with others). Our abilities to love and respond to other people and to take a working interest in the things in our environment are seen as expressions of object relations. The way a person relates to things and people gives clues about their lifelong pattern of object relations, which is believed to develop through relationships in very early childhood.

According to the model of object relations, the infant develops relationships with objects in the environment to satisfy needs, such as hunger and thirst. Humans have inborn tendencies, or *drives*, to try actively to satisfy needs. It is believed that humans are born with drives for self-preservation, pleasure, and exploration and that these inborn drives originate in the most primitive part of the self, the **id**. The id is not concerned about other people's feelings but only with satisfying its own needs. At birth, the personality is dominated by the id. It is only through experiences of and relationships with human or physical objects that other parts of the personality develop.

As an example, when infants are hungry, they cry. This is their way of expressing their drive for food and their terrible frustration at not being fed. As children develop, they are expected to express their needs in ways that are more socially acceptable. They are put under pressure to adapt to the rules of society. For instance, they must learn to talk about their feelings instead of just striking out. If they cry, they may be sent to their rooms. In the beginning, children's parents actively teach them to follow the rules of society, but gradually these rules become part of the children's personalities. Freud called this the **superego**. The superego acts as the conscience or moralizer and tells the person what is right and wrong.

As you might imagine, the id and the superego are often in conflict. For example, a person who is dieting may pass a bakery window and see a chocolate cake. Their id prompts them to eat that chocolate cake. The superego says, in effect, "You should not do that." The conflict between what the id wants and what the superego will allow can generate anxiety. The person may feel confused and tense, not knowing what to do. Fortunately, a third part of the personality, the **ego**, controls anxiety by compromising between the warring id and superego.

The word ego, as it is used in the model of object relations model, refers to something quite different from the everyday meaning. ("That person has a big ego.") The ego, the third main part of the personality, performs many mental functions that deal with reality and with the conflicting desires of id and superego. Memory and perception are two important functions of the ego. Another is reality testing, or the ability to tell the difference between reality and fantasy and to share the same general ideas about reality that most people do. For example, a student may say that a particular teacher does not like them, citing as evidence that the teacher frowns. Is it true that the teacher dislikes the student? Reality testing is needed; the student may gather evidence from other incidents or from feedback from peers. Willingness to consider other points of view (eg, that the teacher keeps saying they cannot hear the student when they speak so softly or that the teacher complained of having a headache) indicates good reality testing. Persistence in beliefs despite evidence to the contrary indicates denial of reality and suggests poor reality testing. Learning about reality and comparing or testing assumptions about reality consume much of the ego's time and attention.

The ego also helps control impulses and organize actions. In addition, the ego makes use of many **defense mechanisms**, which make a compromise among the id, the superego, and the demands of reality. Defense mechanisms ward off or defend against anxiety, frustration, guilt, and other uncomfortable or distressing feelings (19).

One defense mechanism is **displacement**, or the transfer of the id's drive to another object. In the case of the person looking in the bakery window, the ego might substitute another object, so that the person finds themselves thinking of a stylish outfit they saw the other day. All this happens without the person being aware of it because *all defense mechanisms operate unconsciously*. Some other defense mechanisms are listed in Table 2.1. Understanding the various defense mechanisms helps the occupational therapy professional speculate

Table 2.1. Selected Defense Mechanisms[a]

Defense Mechanism	Definition	Example
Denial	Refusing to believe something that causes anxiety	A mother plans for her child who has a severe intellectual disability to earn a doctoral degree.
Projection	Believing that an unacceptable feeling of one's own belongs to someone else	A self-isolating client in a work group says that others will not talk to him.
Rationalization	Making excuses for unacceptable behavior, actions, or feelings	A teenager says he did not do his homework because he did not have the right kind of paper.
Conversion	Conflicts turned into real physiologic symptoms	A girl with poor coordination gets a migraine headache when it is time for volleyball.
Regression	Functioning at a more primitive developmental level than previously; going back to an immature pattern of behavior	A 7-yr-old child who is hospitalized for major surgery begins to walk on tiptoes and suck his thumb.
Undoing	Trying to reverse the effects of what one has done by doing the opposite	A client accuses the professional of trying to run his life. Later he brings her flowers.
Idealization	Overestimating someone or valuing them more than the real personality and person seem to merit	A woman says that the group leader is the most handsome and kindest man in the world.
Identification	Adopting the habits or characteristics of another person	A teenage girl begins to wear her hair just like her therapist does.
Sublimation	Unacceptable wishes channeled into socially acceptable activities	A child who wants to cut things up to see how they work grows up to become a surgeon.
Substitution	A realistic goal or object substituted for one that cannot be achieved	A young man fails the examination for the police department and then takes a job as a security guard.
Compensation	Efforts to make up for personal deficits; this can also be a conscious effort	A woman, blind from birth, learns to travel without a cane or any other aid.

[a]All defense mechanisms operate unconsciously and should not be confused with other mental mechanisms, such as suppression, that are conscious.

on why someone is behaving in a certain way and then helps provide an effective response.

Most mental operations, like defense mechanisms, operate unconsciously. Even so, they may dominate behavior. The conflicting demands of the id and superego create anxiety, which the ego attempts to control, usually by unconscious defense mechanisms. Sometimes the ego consciously tries to control the anxiety through suppression (trying to keep the negative behavior, actions, or feelings from occurring), but whether conscious or unconscious defenses are used, occasionally the ego is overwhelmed and unable to resolve the conflict. According to the model of object relations, the extreme anxiety that results can cause a breakdown of ego functions—in other words, a mental disorder. *A mental disorder occurs when the ego is unable to achieve a successful compromise among the id, the superego, and the demands of reality.* In a mental disorder, a person's behavior is dominated by tremendous anxiety and by unconscious processes that are out of control.

The supposition that mental disorders are caused by unconscious processes creates problems for occupational therapy professionals. How do you help someone cope with something they are unaware of? The model of object relations proposes that to change a person's mental disorder, the unconscious conflicts must be brought to a conscious level and the person needs to become aware of them. Freud discovered that the analysis of symbols in clients' dreams provided clues to their unconscious feelings and that by talking with clients about their dreams he could sometimes make them conscious of these feelings. Freud believed that once this consciousness was achieved, the symptoms would be relieved.

Analysis of symbols relies on the fact that many symbols are universal, at least within a particular culture. A symbol is something that stands for something else. Some examples of symbols in American culture are the Statue of Liberty, which symbolizes freedom, and the color red, which symbolizes passion or anger. Red in Chinese culture, however, symbolizes weddings and celebrations, and white (which in Western culture symbolizes purity and is used for weddings) is associated with death. Some symbols seem universal across cultures; the circle, for example, symbolizes unity.

In the model of object relations, many symbols are used as keys to the meaning of unconscious conflicts. For example, food symbolizes the relationship with the mother, who is the first object to satisfy the hunger need. Thus, in our minds, food is often associated with love and trust. Most of us occasionally overeat, even when we are not hungry. Because food symbolizes comfort and motherly love, overeating may be a symbolic way to meet our unconscious needs for love and comfort. Tall, slender objects such as skyscrapers or spears may symbolize the phallus (penis) and may be associated with the phallic stage of development, in which the child explores his own genitalia and is curious about the genitalia of the opposite sex.

Occupational therapy professionals who apply the model of object relations use symbols expressed by clients in arts, crafts, and everyday activities (31, 36, 37). Using expressive mediums, clients can explore the use of mature defense mechanisms. Clients are motivated by their inner ideas and needs when choosing crafts and other expressive activities. These expressions help the occupational therapy professional better recognize and understand the internal reasons for clients' actions and behavior. The goal is to build mature and useful coping mechanisms to use in times of anxiety and stress (24).

As an example, ceramics can provide an opportunity to explore issues of self-control versus control by others. Because wet clay is so like feces in color and texture, it can symbolize the anal period, during which the child learns to control the bowels and to cooperate with their parents through self-control. People have widely varying reactions to ceramics. Some cannot wait to handle the clay; others shrink back and may try to avoid it altogether, as the following situation illustrates.

Case Example

The occupational therapy professional is working alone with a 35-year-old woman, Paula, in the ceramics shop. Paula is rolling out small beads, measuring each against the others. She avoids touching the clay with her hands, using tools and plastic gloves instead. When she finishes with each bead, she places it neatly in line with the others.

The occupational therapy professional comments, "The beads are very neat and precise."

Paula answers, "They have to match."

"Why is that?"

"It would look like a mess if they didn't."

The occupational therapy professional thinks for a few seconds and then responds, "I have seen some necklaces with beads of all different sizes."

"People who wear those are slobs."

"Oh?"

"They don't care about doing things right."

As this brief dialogue illustrates, there are many ways in which someone can relate to a symbol. A client's behavior toward an activity may reveal their attitudes and feelings about issues that activity symbolizes. Because people have their own personal occupational histories, they may also have individual or **idiosyncratic** symbols that are theirs alone. For example, beads may mean something to Paula because of some previous experience of hers, and although clay is a powerful symbol of anal issues, it may not mean this to everyone. Another person may use it to sculpt tall towers (possibly related to the phallic stage of development).

Occupational therapy professionals who employ the model of object relations successfully must understand the theories behind it. The model of object relations provides a structure for thinking about how the mind works. Table 2.2 provides examples of craft projects occupational therapy professionals can use therapeutically to assist clients to express emotions and begin to manage feelings that interfere with their participation with others. Though not the dominant theory it once was, the model of object relations continues to be studied and used today by professionals working with people who have psychiatric problems. A study by Warshawsky and Handelzalts (70) looked at the use of object relations to predict characteristics of teenage females with disordered eating and predicting motivation for recovery for the same population. Their research found the father was negatively related to a participant displaying eating characteristics if the father was thought of as "doing good as opposed to having or expressing intense ill will" and "as having good intent or effect on others" (70, p. 1737). Regarding the object relationship with the mother, "The more the mother was conceived as a source of conflicts, the more the participants exhibited eating disorder characteristics" (70, p. 1737). In addition, father support was positively correlated with the participants' motivation to recover (70). The occupational therapy professional can use this type of evidence from the model of object relations to help the client focus using the strength from one parental relationship to help cope with the losses associated with the other parental relationship. Table 2.3 provides examples of client goals based on the model of object relations.

Table 2.2. Model of Object Relations and Occupational Therapy			
Final Outcome Desired	**Occupation and Activity Demands**	**Relevance and Importance to the Therapeutic Process**	**Interventions (Projects to Make or Complete)**
Decrease hyperactivity	Objects used and their properties: • use items easy to control the outcome of their action(s) • limit use of sharps • at least semi-familiar items Social demands: • start with solo or partner activities to decrease demand on social interactions Sequence and timing demands: • use varied steps and steps with differing levels of simplicity and complexity	• release of energy into the function of the activity	• painting large space or area rocks for a garden • staining nonintricate furniture • tie fleece blankets

Table 2.2. Model of Object Relations and Occupational Therapy (*continued*)

Final Outcome Desired	Occupation and Activity Demands	Relevance and Importance to the Therapeutic Process	Interventions (Projects to Make or Complete)
	Required actions and performance skills: • repetitive actions and steps Required body functions: • use shoulder girdle joint area • use proximal joints of upper extremity		
Increase self-esteem	Objects used and their properties: • flexible inherent properties • distinct to the client Social demands: • partner or small group Sequence and timing demands: • complete in 1–2 sessions • construct or build product Required actions and performance skills: • match activity requirements to client's performance skill abilities	• quick success	• tote bag • stenciling • crayon art • sun-catcher • fuse bead project • scrapbooking (start with one page or small board projects)
Limit dependency on others	Objects used and their properties: • novel or new to the client • nonresistant materials Space demands: • small area to limit interaction and distraction Social demands: • solo work Sequence and timing demands: • orderly structure	• activities should require supervision and direction (which can be decreased over time) • initial portion of activity requires greater interaction with occupational therapy professional	• leather lacing • leather stamping • stenciling • paint by numbers • puzzle (start with 50 or under pieces)
Increase participation with others	Objects used and their properties: • multiple uses to allow for creativity by all participants • require use or participation by multiple people Space demands: • dependent on area needed to interact with others and complete task • consider if expanse of natural environment may be overwhelming Social demands: • start with smaller groups • move to medium and larger size groups Sequence and timing demands: • time inherent to activity to allow for multiple participants	• situations designed to involve others • ensure that others will accept client and their product	• physical activity • cooking • baking • decoration making • decorating for holidays and special events • paint/create murals
Decrease compulsivity	Objects used and their properties: • small-sized products to limit product size • inherent use parameters to dissuade client from enlarging product or altering end-product result of project • predictable in use and handling qualities • minimal flexibility and more controllable substances and materials	• ensure structure of project encourages constructive use of objects	• tile trivet top for jewelry box • sand art picture • soap carving • lacing projects • use of craft kits

(continued)

Table 2.2. Model of Object Relations and Occupational Therapy (*continued*)

Final Outcome Desired	Occupation and Activity Demands	Relevance and Importance to the Therapeutic Process	Interventions (Projects to Make or Complete)
	Space demands: • limited space to minimize changes or alterations with project structure Social demands: • solo • small group Sequence and timing demands: • repetitive with an easily visible product or purpose • organized steps		
Limit preoccupation with other thoughts	Objects used and their properties: • novel or new to the client • distinct to the client • complex • Sequence and timing demands: • changes in steps and actions • multiple steps	• grounded in reality • "real" not contrived or simulated	• leather lacing • leather stamping • stenciling • needlework • rugmaking
Express hostility	Objects used and their properties: • resistive properties Space demands: • area to move in gross motor patterns Social demands: • solo work Sequence and timing demands: • repetitive motions and movements Required actions and performance skills: • gross motor movements	• expresses hostility openly and knowingly, rather than on an unconscious level • constructive avenue for release of anger	• clay activity • stamping • kneading dough • lacing through thick cardboard or thick suede material
Decrease guilt	Objects used and their properties: • simplistic • mundane Space demands: • just enough room for project or task Social demands: • done alone Sequence and timing demands: • complete in one setting	• complete a task that requires minimal direction giving and does not require much supervision or interaction by occupational therapy professional • focus on prep time and cleanup time of project or task • altruistic nature attached to activity	• sanding wood • basket making • cooking or baking • making decorations for social gathering
Develop and strengthen self-concept	Objects used and their properties: • distinct to client • end-product that benefits self and/or others • multiple layers of project activity • creative in nature Space demands: • area to store project items Social demands: • start with solo or partner activities to decrease demand on social interactions Sequence and timing demands: • can evolve a few sessions to increase time for reflection	• establish personal identity and awareness • demonstrate one's individual value to self and others	• greeting cards • scrapbooking (start with one page or small board projects) • monogramming • fabric decorating craft (bag, purse, hat, t-shirt)

Concepts adapted from Milwaukee Area Technical College. (1990). *Guide for psychoanalytical and object relations theory in OT Asst 130 psychosocial dysfunction*. Author.

Table 2.3. Intervention Goals for Model of Object Relations

Aim of Intervention

Through the use of symbolic and expressive therapeutic modalities:
- Become aware of, and identify, mechanisms used to control unconscious conflicts, anxiety, frustration, guilt, and distress.
- Develop helpful mechanisms to cope with inner thoughts and emotions to complete daily occupations.

Goals

Client will complete expressive project with _____ (add needed amount or type of assistance)* and _____** within _____***.

Client will complete reflective activity with _____ (add needed amount or type of assistance)* and _____** within _____***.

Client will notice link between emotion and action during occupation of _____ with _____ (add needed amount or type of assistance)* and _____** within _____***.

Client will notice defensive action taken during occupation of _____ with _____ (add needed amount or type of assistance)* and _____** within _____***.

Client will identify positive coping strategy with _____ (add needed amount or type of assistance)* and _____** within _____***.

Client will demonstrate positive coping strategy, during time of stressful occupation of _____, with _____ (add needed amount or type of assistance)* and _____** within _____***.

* guidance, prompt, cue, direct supervision/contact, indirect supervision/contact
** structured environment, setup of activity, participation of a peer, no peer involvement, no direct involvement from practitioner for ____ (amount of time), ____ amount of redirection
*** number of minutes, number of attempts, number of sessions, number of weeks

Concepts Summary

1. Humans are born with drives for self-preservation and pleasure. These drives reside in the id, the most primitive and childish part of the personality.
2. Children develop control over the id drives by learning the moral standards of society from their parents. These standards form the superego, a second part of the personality.
3. The id and the superego often conflict because they desire different things: the id wants to satisfy its own needs, and the superego wants to follow the rules. Beyond this, reality may not permit either desire to be satisfied, adding to the conflict.
4. The ego, a third part of the personality, attempts to resolve the conflicting demands of the id, the superego, and reality. It does this through ego functions such as memory, perception, reality testing, and defense mechanisms.
5. The id, ego, and superego operate unconsciously. We are not normally aware of their functioning.
6. When the ego cannot resolve unconscious conflict, anxiety becomes overwhelming, and the ego cannot operate normally. This breakdown of ego functions is recognized as a mental disorder.
7. Ego functions can be strengthened or restored if the person can become conscious of the unconscious conflict that is causing the anxiety.
8. One method of identifying unconscious processes is by the analysis of symbols.

VOCABULARY REVIEW

analysis of symbols
One of the methods used in object relations therapy. The therapist analyzes symbols in the client's dreams or artwork to discover their unconscious meanings.

anxiety
An uncomfortable feeling of tension that may arise from unconscious conflict

conflict
Opposition between simultaneous demands, such as those of the id and the superego or the self and reality

conscious
Mental functions of which we are aware. Suppression is one example.

defense mechanism
Any of several methods used by the ego to control anxiety and conflict. All defense mechanisms operate unconsciously (Table 2.1).

ego
The part of the personality that regulates behavior by compromising among the demands of the id, the superego, and reality. The ego contains many functions, such as memory, perception, reality testing, and defense mechanisms. These work together in a continuous process of adapting to reality. Many ego functions operate unconsciously.

id
The part of the personality that contains the drives to self-preservation and pleasure. The id is present from birth or before and operates unconsciously.

object
> Anything toward which the id directs its energies to satisfy a drive. Objects may be human (people) or nonhuman (animals and things).

reality testing
> The ability to tell the difference between reality and fantasy and to share the same general ideas about reality as everyone else. Reality testing is an ego function.

superego
> The part of the personality that contains standards for behavior. The superego is thought to be a representation of rules learned from parents and other authorities. It operates unconsciously.

suppression
> An attempt to control anxiety and conflict by *consciously* controlling or denying it. Suppression is conscious, unlike the defense mechanisms, but it may serve the same purpose regarding anxiety.

symbol
> Something that represents something else. Symbols may be universal, cultural, or idiosyncratic.

unconscious
> Mental functions of which we normally are not aware. These include the id, the superego, and the defense mechanisms.

DEVELOPMENTAL THEORY

There are several versions of developmental theory. The best known are those of Erikson, Piaget, and Gesell. This section outlines the main concepts common to all developmental theories and then explores Erikson's theory of psychosocial development.

The first developmental concept is that *a person matures through a series of stages that occur in a fixed sequence*. At each stage, the person encounters specific **developmental tasks** that, when mastered, provide a foundation for later development. For example, a child learns to stand before learning to walk. The standing stage must come before the walking stage. Physical, social, emotional, and intellectual growth happen simultaneously, but each in a fixed sequence. In other words, children can develop social skills as they are learning to walk, but they cannot walk before they stand. In the normal growth process, development is gradual and spontaneous and eventually results in a mature and functional adult.

However, many factors can interrupt the growth process. Physical disease, poverty, malnutrition, trauma, or emotional or social deprivation can keep a person from mastering the developmental tasks of a particular stage. When this happens, a **developmental lag** may result. A developmental lag is a discrepancy (difference) between a person's behavior and the behavior one would expect of a person of that age. In other words, a person who has a developmental lag has fallen behind in development and is not as mature as their peers. In this respect, development level or ability is considered from the perspective of "stage," not of "age." Take, for example, the case of David.

> ### Case Example
>
> David is a 29-year-old man who has attended several colleges, majoring in a variety of subjects but never graduating. He has had a succession of jobs that seem unrelated: dishwasher, produce clerk, busboy, crewman on a sailboat, handyman, horse groom, waiter, messenger, and house painter. David has acquired a lot of skills over the years but does not stick to anything, and he does not know what to do about it. He sees friends his own age are establishing themselves in careers and settling down in marriage and family life. David feels increasingly distant from his friends. He is extremely depressed and has twice attempted suicide.

As part of the evaluation process, an occupational therapist using Erikson's theory of psychosocial development would first analyze where David was lagging in development. According to Erikson, at around 3 years of age the child enters a developmental stage termed **initiative versus guilt**. In this stage, the developmental task is for the child to establish a sense of purpose and direction (initiative) in activities. The child feels pleasure and power at the ability to affect the world around them. This stage lays a foundation for setting goals and working to accomplish them in later life, but this can happen only if the child is permitted to follow their own direction.

However, the child's direction may be unacceptable to the parents, who may have their own ideas about what the child should be doing. For example, David's history revealed that his parents pushed him to read at an early age and constantly compared him with his older brother, who could read before he was age 3. David was an active child and good at sports and games, but his parents discouraged these interests and stressed reading as the preferred activity.

Because David was not permitted to pursue his own interests as a child, his sense of purpose (initiative) remained confused and vague. During adolescence, this confusion was reactivated when he attempted to choose a career. Because he had little previous experience in setting his own direction and following it through to success, he was unsure of himself and uncertain of his direction and how to proceed. This pattern repeated itself over the years. For example, David felt guilty when he enjoyed crewing on the sailboat; he thought he should be doing something "more important" with his life and went back to college but dropped out after one semester.

According to Erikson's theory, mental health problems occur when developmental tasks are not successfully mastered. Failure at one stage of development does not prevent the person from continuing to develop, but problems may result because the foundation is weak. To help a person who has problems because of a developmental lag, the occupational therapy professional designs situations that will facilitate growth in the deficient area. In other words, if a person has failed to develop adequately in a given area, the occupational therapy professional can make it easier for the development to occur by creating conditions that encourage growth. For example, in David's case, an occupational therapy professional might expose him to a variety of activities that fit his skills and interests, helping him choose and get involved in an activity that needs consistent effort over a long time (eg, woodworking). The occupational therapy professional would encourage David when he became disheartened and would try to sustain his interest in the activity by showing him new challenges or problems to solve. The occupational therapy professional might help him find new ways to use his skills by producing objects for sale or by having him instruct others. The occupational therapy professional would be careful not to push him too hard or instruct him in ways he "has to complete something"; this is a time for David to fulfill his sense of purpose in life. Long term, David would benefit from periodic reassessment to determine how he has incorporated his ability to control his initiation and maintenance of his sense of life direction and move toward healthy long-lasting intimate relationships.

This example focuses on one of the eight stages of psychosocial development proposed in Erikson's theory. The word **psychosocial** refers to the interaction between the self (**psyche** or **mind**) and society (or participation with others), an interaction that Erikson believed was the core of successful human functioning. As occupational therapy professionals we use this term, psychosocial, when discussing mental health and mental disorders. We provide therapeutic intervention toward a person's acceptance and maintenance of oneself, in turn providing a pathway toward participation with others. Table 2.4 lists and explains the eight stages. Erikson suggested that each stage is organized around a central crisis that has two possible but totally opposite resolutions. For example, the crisis of purpose and self-direction can be resolved as either **initiative or guilt**. In other words, a person can either "initiate," start planning to complete activities on their own and find success, or feel "guilt" as they continually fail at attempts to be independent with their own ideas of what they want to do and what they want to become throughout life. Erikson argued that there is a continuum of resolutions between these two extremes at any stage and

Table 2.4. Erikson's Eight Stages of Psychosocial Development

Approximate Age	Psychosocial Stage	Explanation
Birth–18 mo	Basic Trust vs Mistrust	Infants need nurturance from the mother. If they perceive her as reliable, they develop the capacity to trust others. If not, they tend to mistrust others, feel anxious about others' willingness to meet their needs, and so on. Mistrust involves not trusting that another person will complete the relationship actions we are seeking.
2–4 yr	Autonomy vs Shame and Doubt	During this period, children learn to control their bowel and bladder and become more independent in exploring the environment. Their sense of motivation and will is shaped by the parents' attitudes toward bodily functions and their willingness to allow their children to control themselves. Control comes by learning, which leads to becoming competent and then mastering a skill. The person needs to have the opportunity for success with trial-and-error learning.
3–5 yr	Initiative vs Guilt	Preschool and kindergarten children begin to combine skills and plan activities to accomplish goals. They begin to imitate adult roles, try out new ways of doing things, and develop a sense of self-direction. Self-acceptance and self-worth are established here, along with a sense of accomplishment. The child begins to learn they "can do."
6–12 yr	Industry vs Inferiority	During elementary school, children acquire skills and work habits. They compare themselves with their peers. Attitudes of parents, teachers, and other children contribute to their sense of competence. A lack of ability to be successful with attempted tasks can lead to decreased self-esteem.
Adolescence	Identity vs Role Confusion	Adolescents experiment with a variety of adult roles. Key issues include vocational choice and gender identification. Rebellion against parents is common, as teenagers try to assert a separate identity. This is a time for exploration of interests and for identification of future roles. Various opportunities need to be presented and attempted.
Young adulthood	Intimacy vs Isolation	The central concern of this period is to find a suitable partner with whom to share life. Emphasis is placed on how one presents oneself as trustworthy, self-controlled, and self-driven. One must know their own identity and feel comfortable in sharing it.
Middle adulthood	Generativity vs Stagnation	Adults look toward the future and try to contribute to it through work, community leadership, child rearing, and so on. Boredom or self-absorption can limit advancing through this stage.
Old age	Ego Integrity vs Despair	Faced with the prospect of death, older adults review and evaluate their life's choices to see whether they have done what they meant to do.

cautioned students not to think of the outcome in good–bad, either–or terms. He also noted that human development is continuous and that anyone facing a problem in the present must rely on the interconnected matrix or network of feelings about earlier developmental events. When a new crisis arises, a person may regress and reexperience the conflicts of earlier developmental stages.

Erikson's and other developmental theories are consistent with many of the basic ideas of occupational therapy. The concepts of gradation, of learning through successively more challenging and complex stages, and the focus on solving problems and acquiring skills make developmental theory an appealing choice for working with persons who have poor social relationships and weak skills (79). Similarly, occupational therapy professionals have long attempted to meet the client at their own level, matching tasks to abilities and interests. Table 2.5 presents goals for use within the developmental theory.

There are three major difficulties with this approach. The first is that some persons with major mental disorders (eg, those diagnosed in childhood or early adolescence) appear to lag in the earliest stage of psychosocial development; they have always had problems trusting others, as their histories show. To change fundamental and lifelong mistrust is a serious challenge. Second, like approaches based on object relations' theoretical concepts, which itself has a developmental orientation,[2] application of developmental theory to intervention is possible only over the long term because developmental change is a gradual process. Third, human development involves many complex and interrelated issues that can be understood only through rigorous study, and occupational therapy professionals must be exceptionally well trained in adept use of developmental theory. One model used in psychiatric occupational therapy that is related to developmental theory is **development of adaptive skills**. This practice model is described in Chapter 3.

Concepts Summary

1. Human beings mature through a series of stages that occur in a fixed sequence. Specific developmental tasks arise at each stage; the person's experience with these tasks provides a foundation for later development.
2. Problems occur when developmental tasks are not mastered sufficiently well. This causes a lag in development that can interfere with a person's attempts to master other developmental tasks in future stages.
3. A developmental lag can be corrected by exposing the person to a situation that will encourage growth in the deficient area. If the proper conditions are created and the occupational therapy professional provides corrective guidance, the developmental task can be mastered.

VOCABULARY REVIEW

development
   A process of maturation occurring throughout life

developmental lag
   A delay in development demonstrated by failure to master a developmental task

developmental stage
   A specific level of development, generally believed to occur at a specific time in a human being's life. Various developmental psychologists postulate different theories, each containing several developmental stages. Erikson proposed eight stages of psychosocial development. Piaget proposed four stages of cognitive development. Regardless of the theory, the stages always occur in a fixed sequence.

developmental task
   A problem or crisis that arises during a developmental stage. Solving the problem shows mastery of the task. An example is choosing a career, traditionally a developmental task of adolescence.

psychosocial development
   The ongoing process in which the person resolves conflicts between personal needs and what society demands and permits

Table 2.5. Intervention Goals for Developmental Theories

Aim of Intervention

Rebuild foundation of missed developmental skills and abilities.
Psychosocial: Balance understanding of self (control and maintenance of self) with actions toward others (participation in occupations in society).

Goals

Client will attempt occupational activity of _____ at developmental stage of _____ with _____ (add needed amount or type of assistance)* and _____** within _____***.

Client will identify developmental stage need of _____ with _____ (add needed amount or type of assistance)* and _____** within _____***. (can use both for current stage in and next stage [when near time to transition to next stage])

Client will demonstrate developmental stage skill of _____ with _____ (add needed amount or type of assistance)* and _____** within _____***.

* guidance, prompt, cue, direct supervision/contact, indirect supervision/contact
** structured environment, setup of activity, participation of a peer, no peer involvement, no direct involvement from practitioner for ____ (amount of time), ____ amount of redirection
*** number of minutes, number of attempts, number of sessions, number of weeks

---

[2]The alert reader may have noticed that Erikson's developmental theory is in some respects similar to object relations theory. Erikson's training and background were psychoanalytic; therefore, much of his work is based on the writings of Freud. Freud's work focused on psychosexual rather than psychosocial development.

BEHAVIORAL THEORIES

The behavioral theoretical methods are derived from the work of Pavlov, a Russian physiologist who experimented with dogs, and Skinner, an American psychologist who studied how animals responded to stimulation. The central concept of these theories is that all behavior is learned. *Behaviors that have pleasurable results tend to be repeated.* Consider the following example.

Case Example

You are in a new class. The professor says something you do not understand, so you ask a question. The professor says they are glad you asked that question and gives you an answer that helps you understand. The next time you have a question, you raise your hand.

It seems almost common sense that people repeat actions that result in pleasure or rewards. Imagine what might happen if the professor gave a confusing answer or had in some way made you feel embarrassed for asking the question. You might feel that you should never ask another question. This illustrates a complementary concept: *Actions that have negative or unpleasant consequences tend not to be repeated.*

According to behavioral theories, each person develops through a process of learning from the results of their behavior. If adaptive behaviors are rewarded and maladaptive behaviors punished or ignored, the result should be a mature and responsible human being. Sometimes, however, ineffective behaviors are learned. Mental disorders, in these theories, are defined by abnormal behavior that results because normal or adaptive behavior was not rewarded or did not have pleasurable consequences. In some cases, abnormal behavior occurs because maladaptive behavior was reinforced. In occupational therapy, the outcomes of adaptive behaviors are seen as successful completions of everyday experiences, or as successful occupational performance.

As an example, take the case of a 2-year-old child who screams and cries when their mother goes out for an evening. Every time they cry, the babysitter gives them a piece of candy. The undesirable behavior (screaming) has had a pleasurable consequence (candy). Very quickly the child learns that screaming is an effective way of getting candy. In later life, they may carry on the pattern, screaming at other people to get what they want. More effective ways of managing this behavior might be to give a "time-out" until the behavior stops. Or the babysitter could just wait it out and "withhold reinforcement" by not providing a pleasurable reward.

Occupational therapy professionals use a variety of techniques based on behavioral theory. Sometimes this is called an **action–consequence** approach because the occupational therapy professional tries to change the person's behavior (action) by changing the consequences of the behavior. The occupational therapy professional may reward new adaptive behaviors or ignore or not reward (withhold reward) the maladaptive behavior. Some occupational therapy professionals use both methods. An example is the case of Chris, who repeatedly interrupts while the occupational therapy professional is working with other clients. Chris constantly asks for the occupational therapy professional's opinion of the craft project. Using the action–consequence approach, the occupational therapy professional directs Chris to work independently for 5 minutes, after which time the occupational therapy professional will provide feedback. During the 5-minute work period, the occupational therapy professional ignores any disruptive behavior by Chris, but after this there will be the "reward" of some individual time and attention provided to Chris.

A behavioral program allows the occupational therapy professional to use a structured format for helping the client change from using maladaptive behaviors to using adaptive behaviors. To begin, the occupational therapy professional completes **identification of the terminal behavior** (step one). Terminal behavior is the normal or adaptive behavior that the occupational therapy professional wants the person to perform. In the case of Chris, this might be working on his own for half an hour. Once the terminal behavior has been identified, the occupational therapy professional **determines a baseline via a method of recording** (step two). The baseline is a known standard or record of how the person behaved *before* the intervention was started. The baseline is a recording of the maladaptive behavior. For example, the occupational therapy professional might count how often Chris tries to interrupt during a half-hour period. Records of the client's behavior after intervention can be compared with this baseline to determine to what extent the intervention was effective.

Next the occupational therapy professional **selects a reinforcement**. Reinforcement is the name given to the occupational therapy professional's response (consequence) to the client's performance of the desired, or adaptive, behavior (action). In Chris's case, the occupational therapy professional already knows that attention from them will be an effective reinforcement. The occupational therapy professional then decides how often the reinforcement will be given (this is called the **schedule**). The occupational therapy professional may decide to reward Chris every time work is completed for 5 minutes without interruption. This would be a continuous schedule of reinforcement because a reward is given every time the action is performed. Usually, **continuous schedules** are used at the beginning of the intervention period when the occupational therapy professional is trying to get the person to do the desired action. Later, when the behavior is established, the reinforcement might be scheduled intermittently, not every time the action is performed but only now and then. **Intermittent schedules** are more effective than continuous schedules once the behavior has been learned. Table 2.6 shows the steps in designing a behavioral treatment program in occupational

Table 2.6. Steps in Developing a Behavioral Treatment Program

Step	Example 1	Example 2
1. Identify the terminal behavior jointly with the client. (adaptive behavior client will perform after intervention)	Complete an activity independently, without seeking reassurance.	Complete an activity independently, without seeking reassurance.
2. Determine the baseline of terminal behavior, prior to intervention, via a method of recording that behavior.	Count the number of times the client seeks reassurance during a 60-min occupational therapy session.	Record the amount of time between each occurrence of client seeking reassurance during a 60-min occupational therapy session.
3. Select a reinforcer that is meaningful to the client that will be provided when the client meets the goal.	The client receives 3 min of attention from the occupational therapy professional.	The client receives 1 min of attention from the occupational therapy professional.
4. Determine a schedule of reinforcement. (goal in bold)	Intermittent reinforcement. Attention from occupational therapy professional after **limiting reassurance-seeking to half the number of times reassurance-seeking was recorded in the baseline data, during 30 min of a 60-min session**.	Constant reinforcement. Attention from occupational therapy professional after **increasing the amount of time between reassurance-seeking occurrences, by 30 s, for a 5-min period**.

Adapted from Sieg, K. W. (1974). Applying the behavioral model. *American Journal of Occupational Therapy, 28*(7), 421–428.

therapy as identified by Sieg's behavioral treatment model (62) and gives examples.

It is important to consider the types of reinforcement. Reinforcement is done to increase the likelihood of the terminal behavior happening in the future. The reinforcement typically used, as in this example, is positive reinforcement. In positive reinforcement, something desired is added. The positive reinforcer is provided, or given, to the client or added to the situation. Negative reinforcement is about removing something already present, not adding something. It is the removal of something the person wants to avoid, or the removal of an adverse situation. As the person engages in the adaptive behavior, the adverse situation goes away. The person learns new adaptative behavior, which in turn leads to the adverse situation never even occurring. Here are some examples:

- One roommate continually asks another roommate to hang up their jacket (adverse situation). The roommate hangs up their jacket as soon as they walk in the apartment (adaptive behavior) and is not asked to hang it up (removal of negative reinforcement).
- A bill collector is calling you throughout the week (adverse situation). You pay the bill (adaptive behavior). The bill collector stops calling you (removal of negative reinforcement).
- As you travel to work in the morning, there is a great deal of traffic, which at times causes you to be late for work (adverse situation). One morning you leave 15 minutes earlier for work (adaptive behavior) and you arrive to work a few minutes early (removal of negative reinforcement) (47).

Often the terminal behavior seems very far from the way the person is acting now. For example, for Chris to sit still and work independently for half an hour appears to be a distant goal. To help Chris reach it, the occupational therapy professional might use **shaping**. Shaping is a method of working toward a terminal behavior through successive approximations, or small steps. In Chris's case, the occupational therapy professional might start with the expectation of 5 minutes of independent work, at the end of which time there is an interaction between the two. Once the 5-minute period of independent work has been established, it can be extended to 10 minutes. Then, Chris would have to work for 10 minutes to be rewarded. Gradually the half-hour goal would be reached through a series of steps or approximations, each one closer to the goal than the one before.

When the terminal behavior involves learning a complicated routine with several steps, the technique of **chaining** can be used. Chaining is teaching a multistep activity one step at a time. The person does the steps they know, and the occupational therapy professional does the rest. Gradually the person learns the whole activity. Chaining can begin with the first step (forward chaining) or the last step (backward chaining). Forward chaining has the client begin the task and the occupational therapy professional completes the later steps that the client is unable to complete. An example of backward chaining is having a person fold the laundry (last step) that someone else has washed. After learning to fold, the person learns how to use the dryer. Gradually, by working backward in this way, they learn the entire sequence of washing clothes. Adults with an intellectual disability appear to learn faster with backward chaining than with forward chaining (72), and this approach can also be effective with other learners who have cognitive disabilities or who lack experience or confidence in a task.

Other strategies that can be used include **systematic desensitization**. This is a technique for reducing fear (desensitizing) by guiding the person to relax, and then gradually increasing exposure to the fear-provoking stimulus. For example, if a child is afraid of dogs, the occupational therapy professional might first show pictures of dogs, or videos, and in another session have a dog brought to the door of the therapy room. It would take several more steps to reduce the child's fear sufficiently that the child could tolerate being close to the dog and perhaps playing with the dog.

Occupational therapy professionals have used behavioral techniques with hyperactive children (21), children with severe intellectual disability (73), and children with autism and related developmental disorders (71). Unlike therapies based on object relations or developmental concepts, behavioral therapies give quick results, as the following example of a child with hyperactivity described by Cermak et al. (21) illustrates.

Case Example

Tom spent a great deal of time lying on the floor kicking his legs and thrashing around. His behavior was disruptive to the group. In the classroom, this conduct disturbed the other children and made it difficult for Tom to sit long enough to finish his schoolwork. The occupational therapy professionals decided to give him the attention he wanted. When he was sitting on the bench, the leader or another member of the group sat next to him and put their arm around him. Surprisingly, after one play session of being on the floor 30 times, Tom was on the floor only twice the next session (21, p. 315).

Like many human efforts, a behavior modification program is only as effective as the thinking and planning behind it, and the consistency of its implementation (53). Occupational therapy intervention approaches based on modified behavioral concepts include Mosey's (52) **activities therapy** and the use of social skills training (16). Because these approaches are so widely used today, they will be discussed in more detail in "Role Acquisition and Social Skills Training" in Chapter 3.

Behavior therapies have been criticized for treating people like machines; for using unhealthful reinforcers, such as candy, coffee, and cigarettes; and for using aversive reinforcement (punishment). The idea that people will respond the way an occupational therapy professional "programs" them to is repugnant; it is also unrealistic. Occupational therapists who set goals with, rather than for, their clients and who explain the treatment program to them can hardly be accused of treating clients like machines. Although occupational therapy professionals at times have used unhealthy reinforcers to get clients to respond, other rewards, such as weekend passes and other privileges, are selected wherever possible. Finally, occupational therapy professionals do not use punishment unless there is no other way to stop clients from harming themselves. Table 2.7 provides examples of goals to use within the behavioral theories approach.

In summary, behavioral theories consist of a group of approaches that have in common the idea that people learn from the consequences of their behavior. Understanding how people learn is important to occupational therapy professionals who want to help people get rid of maladaptive behaviors and acquire new skills.

Concepts Summary

1. All behavior is learned.
2. Actions that have had pleasurable consequences tend to be repeated.
3. Normal behavior is learned if appropriate behaviors are rewarded and maladaptive behaviors are punished or ignored.
4. Abnormal behavior is learned if maladaptive behavior is reinforced or if adaptive behavior is punished or ignored.
5. Abnormal behavior can be changed if the occupational therapy professional changes the consequences of the behavior.

Table 2.7. Intervention Goals for Behavioral Theories

Aim of Intervention

Decrease unwanted maladaptive behaviors.
Increase wanted adaptive behaviors.

Goals

Client will complete occupational activity of _____ with _____ (add needed amount or type of assistance)* and adherence to behavioral treatment plan within _____***.

Client will complete occupational activity of _____ with _____ (add needed amount or type of assistance)* and _____** within _____***.

Client will complete occupational activity of _____ with _____ (add needed amount or type of assistance)* and no demonstration of maladaptive behavior of _____ (add client-specific maladaptive behavior) within _____***.

* guidance, prompt, cue, direct supervision/contact, indirect supervision/contact
** structured environment, setup of activity, participation of a peer, no peer involvement, no direct involvement from practitioner for ____ (amount of time), ____ amount of redirection
*** number of seconds, number of minutes, number of attempts, number of intervals, number of sessions, number of weeks

backward chaining

Chaining that starts with the final step(s) completed by the client. The occupational therapy professional completes the first step(s) of the task.

behavior

Any observable action

chaining

A method of teaching a complex activity one step at a time, starting with either the first or the last step. The occupational therapy professional performs the steps the client does not complete, until the client masters the entire sequence.

forward chaining

Chaining that starts with the first step(s) completed by the client. The occupational therapy professional completes the final step(s) of the task.

reinforcement

Positive (added) or negative (removed) to increase the likelihood the client will stop performing maladaptive behaviors and begin performing adaptive behaviors

schedule of reinforcement

The timing of the reinforcement. Schedules may be **continuous** (reinforcement follows every performance of the desired behavior) or **intermittent** (reinforcement is given only occasionally).

shaping

A method of approaching the terminal behavior gradually, using a series of steps (successive approximations) that lead to the goal

terminal behavior

The intervention goal, the adaptive behavior the person will show at the end of a successful treatment program

COGNITIVE BEHAVIORAL THEORETICAL CONTINUUM

Cognitive behavioral intervention is based on the work of the psychiatrist Aaron Beck (11–13) and others (9, 32, 76). The many variations on cognitive behavioral theories all share an underlying assumption: human behavior is based on what we think and believe. To put this another way, what we think (cognition) determines how we act (behavior). This theoretical continuum proposes that people with mental health problems and mental health disorders have maladaptive patterns of thinking (**cognitions**) that lead to unsuccessful behaviors. Cognitive behavioral interventions help the person understand and change negative cognitions, and this process brings about a change in behavior.

Negative cognitions include **automatic thoughts** that occur without the person recognizing them or challenging their logic. For example, someone who says hello to a neighbor and gets little or no response may think, "She doesn't like me. Nobody likes me. I'm just not someone that people like." The negative thought triggers negative feelings (anxiety or depression)

and maladaptive behaviors (avoidance of social situations, poor eye contact, and dysfunctional interactions with others).

Cognitive behavioral approaches link a precipitating event to a person's thoughts about the event and then to the feelings these thoughts evoke. Events are in themselves neutral; they receive their value from our thoughts about them. When an event occurs, a person has thoughts about it, although these thoughts may occur below the level of conscious awareness. These thoughts are evaluative, attaching an **attribution** or meaning to the event. For example, a raise in pay for most people is a positive event. When informed of a raise in pay, most people think, "That means they think I am doing a good job." However, some people attach a negative evaluation to a pay raise; a person might think "Uh oh, now they are going to expect me to work even harder. I will never be able to meet their expectations."

Thoughts lead to feelings. In the example of the pay raise, interpreting the raise to mean that others think one is doing a good job can lead to feelings of positive self-evaluation ("I feel really competent and successful"), contentment, excitement, and increased motivation. Ultimately, these feelings stimulate associated behaviors, such as confident posture, efforts to solve problems on the job, and pleasant and assertive interactions with coworkers.

Thinking that a pay raise indicates unreachable expectations can provoke feelings of anxiety, negative self-evaluation, and hopelessness. The person may elaborate and ruminate on the negative thoughts and associated negative feelings ("Once they find out I cannot really handle it, they will fire me for sure") and then act on these feelings—for example, by failing to concentrate because of ruminations, procrastinating or avoiding assigned tasks, or coming in late. Again, thoughts provoke feelings that affect the person's behavior, in this case adversely.

Cognitive behavioral intervention focuses on both cognition and behavior and on the relationship between them. Cognitive techniques involve challenging and modifying negative automatic thoughts and their underlying assumptions. Behavioral techniques focus on identifying behaviors, investigating their consequences, and evaluating their effectiveness. Traditional behavioral techniques such as systematic desensitization are also used.

Of all cognitive behavioral approaches, Beck's variation is the most widely recognized and practiced. The cognitive behaviorally trained occupational therapy professional can work one-on-one with the person to identify negative or distorted thoughts and examine their validity.

Occupational therapy professional and client also monitor the client's behavior and evaluate its effectiveness. Homework interventions are designed by the occupational therapy professional with input from the client, are carried out by the client, and the work toward completing the homework interventions is self-reported back to the occupational therapy professional. Beck discusses this approach as a sort of joint scientific effort of collecting data and testing hypotheses. Homework intervention in this approach includes bibliotherapy (assigned reading), graded tasks, and activity scheduling (11). These are familiar to occupational therapy professionals, as they have been traditional occupational therapy techniques since the beginnings of our profession.

Other techniques developed by Beck include cognitive rehearsal, self-monitoring, and reattribution. **Cognitive rehearsal** is employed with clients who have difficulty carrying out tasks, even when they know them well. The person is asked to imagine carrying out each successive step in the task. This helps the person attend to details that might otherwise escape attention and lead to task failure (eg, forgetting to bring exercise clothing to the gym). **Self-monitoring** requires that the client notice and record negative cognitions and their associated events with an aim to discovering the frequency of the problem and understanding the chain of events, thoughts, feelings, and behaviors. The person may utilize a diary, a structured record sheet, a smartphone or tablet, a laptop computer, or even a smart watch to collect data. **Reattribution** is used to challenge the client's belief that their personal shortcomings are responsible for negative external events. This is particularly helpful with individuals who are depressed, as they may think that they are responsible for things that are clearly outside their control.

The following is an example of Beck's treatment of a woman who was afraid of being in crowded places. This example shows the use of self-monitoring and desensitization.[3]

Case Example

Therapist: What are you afraid of when you're in a crowded place?

Client: I'm afraid I won't be able to catch my breath. . . .

Therapist: And?

Client: . . . I'll pass out.

Therapist: Just pass out?

Client: All right, I know it sounds silly but I'm afraid I will just stop breathing . . . and die.

Therapist: Right now, what do you think are the probabilities that you will suffocate and die?

Client: Right now, it seems like one chance in a thousand.

Beck asked this client to visit a crowded store and to write down her estimates of the probability of dying at various steps on the way to the store. The client's notations and consequent interactions with the therapist were as follows.[4]

---

[3]From Beck (11, p. 253). Used with permission of International Universities Press.
[4]From Beck (11, pp. 253–254). Used with permission of International Universities Press.

Case Example Continued

1. Leaving my house—chances of dying in store: 1 in 1,000
2. Driving into town—chances of dying in store: 1 in 100
3. Parking car in lot—chances of dying in store: 1 in 50
4. Walking to store—chances of dying in store: 1 in 10
5. Entering store—chances of dying in store: 2 to 1
6. In middle of crowd—chances of dying in store: 10 to 1

Therapist: So, when you were in the crowd you thought you had a 10 to 1 chance of dying.

Client: It was crowded and stuffy and I couldn't catch my breath. I felt I was passing out. I really panicked and got out of there.

Therapist: What do you think—right now—were the actual probabilities that you would have died if you stayed in the store?

Client: Probably one in a million.

With continued treatment the client learned to remind herself that she had already thought about this rationally and that she was as safe in the store as she was elsewhere. Eventually, she was able to visit stores and crowded places with only minimal discomfort.

In addition to Beck, other leaders in the development of cognitive behavioral treatment include Albert Ellis and Albert Bandura. Ellis (32) is the founder of rational–emotive therapy (RET), which works with the ABCDEs of human experience. An activating event (A) has cognitive, emotional, and behavioral consequences (C). People view or experience A in terms of their beliefs (B). The focus of therapy is on the beliefs (B), which Ellis divides into rational and irrational beliefs. Rational beliefs express personal desires or preferences ("I would like people to like me.") in contrast with irrational beliefs ("People *must* like me or I will not be able to go on."). Irrational beliefs typically begin with words such as *should*, *ought*, and *must*. Ellis linked these irrational beliefs to cognitive distortions such as all-or-none thinking, personalizing, fortune telling, and overgeneralization.

The aim of RET is for the client to realize that we create our world through the way we interpret experience. Thus, one's own psychological experience is self-created and can be changed. The RET therapist helps the client to dispute (D) the irrational beliefs to bring about a corrective emotional (E) experience (Table 2.8). The therapist using this approach directly challenges the person's spoken or even unspoken irrational beliefs. The aim is to dispute this thinking and replace it with more rational ideas. Ellis encouraged therapists following his technique to use an active, highly directive, and confrontational approach. Indeed, transcripts of Ellis's therapy sessions reveal techniques that may seem brutal, such as poking fun at the client and using profanity and insults. According to Ellis, such methods are necessary to challenge and disrupt irrational thinking.

Table 2.8. Cognitive Behavioral Model Based on Rational–Emotive Therapy of Ellis

A	Activating event	Student is assigned to present a speech to a class of 50.
B	Belief	"I can't do this. I'll make a fool of myself."
C	Consequence	Frightened student stammers, forgets speech, and performs poorly.
D	Disputation	"What do you mean by 'I can't'?" "You are always well prepared." "You can rehearse this in front of friends." "Have you considered learning some relaxation techniques?" "Have you thought about using cue cards or other memory aids?"
E	Corrective emotional experience	Student brings cue cards, uses deep breathing and visualization to relax. Performance is excellent. Everyone applauds loudly.

WHAT'S THE EVIDENCE?

Efficacy of simplified-cognitive behavioral therapy for insomnia (S-CBTI) among female COVID-19 patients with insomnia symptom in Wuhan mobile cabin hospital.

The article referenced below is a study of 66 women with mild or common type COVID-19 experiencing insomnia while in a mobile cabin hospital. Approximately half the participants had chronic insomnia and approximately half the participants had acute insomnia. The S-CBTI treatment included education on COVID-19, education on sleep hygiene; behavioral therapy for stimulus control, sleep restriction, and self-suggestion relaxation training (imagining a relaxing scene or recalling a familiar bedroom and applying multiple senses to the scene); and psychological therapeutic sessions regarding group separation, future supports, and management of the disease process. Significant results were found for those with acute insomnia to have decreased symptoms of insomnia as measured by *The Insomnia Severity Index* and decreased sleep latency (the time from going to bed to falling asleep) as measured by the use of a sleep diary. How does this information help occupational therapy professionals address the occupation of sleep? What cognitive behavioral principle can we add into our sleep intervention, and how can we use it?

From He, J., Yang, L., Pang, J., Dai, L., Zhu, J., Deng, Y., He, Y., & Li, H. (March 23, 2021). Efficacy of simplified-cognitive behavioral therapy for insomnia (S-CBTI) among female COVID-19 patients with insomnia symptom in Wuhan mobile cabin hospital. *Sleep and Breathing,* 25(4), 2213–2219.

Bandura (10) investigated the effects of social modeling, which uses a skilled model to teach behavior. The model, which may be a person, a video, or a cartoon, demonstrates the behavior, which is then copied by the client. Learning occurs through imitation. This training method is more effective for humans than trial-and-error learning with external reinforcement (rewards and punishments). Originally, Bandura was trying to show that modeling is a more powerful training method than trial and error or operant conditioning (behavioral techniques). Bandura's work explained why children imitate adults even when the behavior they are copying is not appropriate for their age. He also argued convincingly that television violence, even with symbolic models such as cartoon characters, is a potent teacher of violent behavior.

He attacked the cathartic (release of emotion) methods used in psychoanalytic approaches, stating that it made no sense to encourage angry people to act out their anger because this increases rather than decreases their anger. Bandura's work is especially relevant to occupational therapy because modeling techniques are used extensively in teaching skills to clients (see "Role Acquisition and Social Skills Training" section in Chapter 3 and "Psychoeducation" section in Chapter 6).

The cognitive behavioral approaches can be applied throughout occupational therapy practice.

One example is the use of negative reinforcement and learning how to facilitate change in daily life. This process can be used with clients to help them identify an adverse situation impacting occupational behavior and then identify adaptive behaviors that can allow them to be successful with the desired occupation. They can practice the adaptive behaviors to better cope with the adverse situation in the future.

1. Identify the adverse situation you want to change (or remove).
2. Identify the adaptive behavior you want to engage in.
3. Identify the unwanted maladaptive behaviors you are performing that keep the adverse situation (the negative reinforcement) occurring.
4. Plan how you will learn to manage the adverse situation differently, so the adaptive behavior becomes a habit.
5. Arrange for times when you can practice the adaptive behavior.
6. Complete the practice and reflect on how well using the adaptive behavior worked toward the removal of the negative reinforcer.
7. Revamp your practice work as needed until the adverse situation is gone and all that remains is the adaptive behavior (43).

Cognitive behavioral theoretical principles have been applied in occupational therapy by Johnston (42) and Taylor (67) and others (56, 66, 68, 77). Johnston described the teaching of communication skills, assertive training, problem-solving, and feeling management in a day treatment setting. These skills were taught in groups and individually. Interventions included role-playing; teaching of behaviors; and monitoring of beliefs, assumptions, and self-talk (automatic thoughts).

Taylor's work (67) focused on anger intervention. From a cognitive behavioral perspective, the link between anger and aggression is learned. One can be angry and act aggressively—or not. Anger intervention teaches nonaggressive management of anger. The major techniques used are (a) monitoring physiologic arousal, (b) practice in arousal control methods, (c) monitoring escalating self-talk (angry automatic thoughts), (d) promotion of neutral or calming self-talk via humor and diversional activities, (e) identification of anger-arousing stimuli, and (f) learning strategies to avoid these conditions.

In Taylor's approach, the client first learns to identify and contain arousal. Only after arousal has been controlled to some extent are the cognitions behind the arousal addressed. Clients are exposed to activities that induce high and low states of arousal (eg, physical exercise is generally energizing while listening to soothing music is generally calming). Clients are taught to use both high- and low-arousal activities for reducing anger. Although Taylor employed crafts and other traditional activities in her approach, she molded them to the goals of cognitive behavioral therapy. For example, if physical exercise or wedging clay is used, the client is cautioned not to dwell on angry thoughts because these will perpetuate and accelerate angry arousal. The occupational therapy professional teaches more appropriate self-talk so that the client can learn to use the activity to promote a calm state.

Once arousal has been controlled, the client explores the cognitive components of anger and learns to change anger-producing cognitions. The emphasis is on problem-solving, stress management, and positive and neutral self-talk.

Babiss (8) reported her work using cognitive behavioral methods and dialectical behavior therapy (DBT). The DBT approach, developed by Marsha Linehan for borderline personality disorder clients (46), helps the client acknowledge and tolerate unpleasant thoughts and self-destructive impulses and not act on the impulse, even though it may be strong. Controlled studies demonstrate that DBT may be more effective than other approaches (27). In the group described by Babiss, an emotion is the focus of a particular session. Participants identify precipitating events that may bring on that emotion; they then list the behaviors that they use to respond to that emotion. The group helps participants identify constructive or neutral ways of behaving (taking a walk, texting a friend), to substitute for negative and self-destructive ways (drinking, shouting, cutting self).

Table 2.9 provides examples of occupational therapy goals to use with clients that follow the principles of the cognitive behavioral theoretical continuum.

Table 2.9. Intervention Goals for Cognitive Behavioral Theoretical Continuum

Aim of Intervention

Human behavior can be changed based on what we think and believe.
Cognitive processes can determine behavior (actions).
People can understand and change negative thinking, thus bringing about a behavior change.

Goals

Client will identify negative thoughts limiting occupational activity of _____ with _____ (add needed amount or type of assistance)* and completion of homework activity within _____***.

Client will complete behavior change of _____ during occupational activity of _____ with _____ (add needed amount or type of assistance)* and _____** within _____***.

Client will complete cognitive rehearsal for occupational activity of _____ with _____ (add needed amount or type of assistance)* and _____** within _____***.

Client will complete self-monitoring for occupational activity of _____ with _____ (add needed amount or type of assistance)* and _____** within _____***.

Client will identify the source for negative events with _____ (add needed amount or type of assistance)* and _____** within _____***.

Client will complete occupational activity of _____ with _____ (add needed amount or type of assistance)* and use of RET principles within _____***.

Client will complete occupational activity of _____ with _____ (add needed amount or type of assistance)* and use of negative reinforcement principles within _____***.

Client will communicate assertively during occupational activity of _____ with _____ (add needed amount or type of assistance)* and _____** within _____***.

Client will communicate/socially interact appropriately during occupational activity of _____ with _____ (add needed amount or type of assistance)* and _____^ within _____***.

Client will problem-solve completion for occupational activity of _____ with _____ (add needed amount or type of assistance)* and cognitive skill of_____^^ within _____***.

(continued)

Table 2.9. Intervention Goals for Cognitive Behavioral Theoretical Continuum (*continued*)

Client will demonstrate emotional regulation during occupational activity of _____ with _____ (add needed amount or type of assistance)* and with_____^^^ within _____***.

Client will demonstrate anger management during occupational activity of _____ with _____ (add needed amount or type of assistance)* and with_____** within _____***.

* guidance, written prompt, cue, direct supervision/contact, indirect supervision/contact
** structured environment, setup of activity, participation of a peer, no peer involvement, no direct involvement from practitioner, assistive technology device, identification of negative impacting environment/situation, self-monitoring, self-talk
^ complete X number of turn-taking interactions, approach/start X number of comments/questions, remain and participate for X number of minutes, conclude/disengage, turn toward, question, reply, disclose appropriate amount of self-information, by placing self at appropriate distance to others, by speaking for a reasonable length of time, acknowledge and encourage others
^^ judgment, concept formation, cognitive flexibility, insight
^^^ decreased impulsivity, decreased repetitive behaviors, decreased irrelevant behaviors, appropriate displays of affection, polite expression of differing opinions, without disruptive behavior
*** number of attempts, number of sessions, number of weeks

Concepts **Summary**

1. Thinking and behavior are linked.
2. Automatic thoughts and their associated feelings generate behavior.
3. Identifying automatic thoughts and challenging their validity allow us to consider and learn alternative patterns of thinking and behavior.
4. We create our own experience of the world and can change it by becoming aware of how we think and feel.
5. Social models (parents, peers, the media) are powerful teachers of what we think, believe, and feel.

VOCABULARY REVIEW

activity schedule
Used to describe a written self-report of how the person is spending time. Alternatively, it is a planned or projected schedule the person is assigned to follow as **homework**.

assumptions
The unarticulated rules by which a person orders and organizes experience. These assumptions are arbitrary and are learned or acquired during development. Assumptions may be, for instance, adaptive, maladaptive, or **depressogenic** (leading to depression).

attribution
The meaning attached by the person to an event. Attributions may be either positive or negative.

automatic thoughts
Thinking that occurs involuntarily and that is provoked by specific events and situations. For persons with psychiatric disorders, these thoughts are often negative and based on faulty assumptions or errors in reasoning.

bibliotherapy
A homework intervention of reading books and articles that reinforces material covered in therapy sessions

cognitions
Thoughts, both rational and irrational

cognitive distortions or cognitive errors
Mistakes in reasoning such as overgeneralization, all-or-nothing thinking, and personalization

cognitive rehearsal
The technique of carrying out a task in one's imagination

graded tasks
A stepwise series of tasks graded from simple to complex, the purpose of which is to promote engagement in activities, realistic self-assessment, and positive self-evaluation of ability to reach a goal

homework
Intervention for the person to work on between therapy contacts. Ideally, homework is designed collaboratively by the client and occupational therapy professional. Homework is most effective when the occupational therapy professional shows a genuine interest and reviews it regularly.`

reattribution
A technique used by Beck to challenge the self-blaming thoughts of those who are depressed. The purpose is to show that events perceived as negative may not be the person's fault.

self-monitoring
Noting and recording negative cognitions and the events that precede them.

self-talk
One's personal cognitions or internal thoughts. See also **automatic thoughts**. One of the goals of cognitive behavioral therapy is to identify negative, maladaptive self-talk and replace it with positive, adaptive self-talk.

COGNITIVE ENHANCEMENT THERAPY: A NEURODEVELOPMENTAL APPROACH

Cognitive enhancement therapy (CET) is a neurodevelopmental-based approach for improving cognitive abilities, processing speed, and social cognition. It is appropriate to use with those with schizophrenia, schizoaffective disorder, and similar cognitive disorders. The focus of intervention is on maximizing success with cognitive social recovery activities, thus increasing the potential to engage in meaningful social roles and live more independent and satisfying lives in the community (20). CET is recognized as an evidence-based intervention technique by the Substance Abuse and Mental Health Services Administration (SAMHSA) (60).

Research foundations for CET come from the disciplines of psychology, neurophysiology, sociology, neuropsychology, and psychiatry. Practice areas associated with CET include social work, vocational rehabilitation, and cognitive remediation. In addition, CET is based on traumatic brain injury rehabilitation and the principles of neuroplasticity (the ability of the brain to repair itself after trauma or repair itself from developmental delays) (20).

Evidence has shown that 12 months after a CET training program participants showed significant improvements in cognitive social abilities, and after 36 months, participants were able to retain those cognitive abilities. Beneficial outcomes for participants included:

- processing speed needed for learning;
- cognitive skills such as attention and concentration, memory (working and verbal), cognitive flexibility, mental stamina, motivation, initiation, energy, and problem-solving;
- social cognitive skills such as perspective taking of self and of others, understanding verbal and nonverbal themes and meanings, not digressing with unimportant details, "thinking on your feet," abstract and active thinking, role flexibility, humor, recognition and appreciation of spontaneity, and understanding and mastering social norms;
- meaningful adult role socialization;
- self-management of mental and physical health; and
- adjustment and acceptance of disability (40, 41).

The CET activity included software training exercises in attention, memory, and problem-solving. The participants worked in small groups and in pairs. They also had social cognitive group exercises and online Socratic coaching (a method of asking questions to encourage critical thinking) (40).

CET is built around holistic tenets and brings together cognitive thinking skills and social interaction skills. "Cognition and social cognition are so closely related that they influence and support each other. For example, CET challenges participants to pay attention (a cognitive capacity) so they can understand people better (a social-cognitive capacity)... when participants understand other people better, it is easier for them to pay attention" (20, p. 4). The occupational therapy professional who uses CET is considered a coach, helping clients set goals and successfully meet occupational challenges (20).

Socialization is a key component of CET. It utilizes the concept that social cognition is used to interact wisely with other people. When we socialize with others, we learn the informal rules of how to wisely and effectively socially participate with others. As adults, if people do not quickly "get the gist" of how to appropriately socially interact with others, they are excluded from social activities. Thus, learning how to detect, evaluate, and use the unwritten and unspoken social rules is important to success with social participation and to role success. CET training challenges clients to guided, but not rehearsed, social situations where they can experience and practice social interactions to increase their social cognitive ability (20). The occupational therapy professional as CET coach is not directive and does not continually "instruct" the client about what to do or not do. Rather, the occupational therapy professional interacts with the client as an "adult," allowing the client to "read" social cues and learning (and becoming successful) through trial-and-error experiences (20). Table 2.10 provides examples of CET occupational therapy goals to use with clients.

Concepts **Summary**

1. The brain has neuroplasticity properties and has the capacity to learn cognitive and social skills.
2. CET approach uses group interventions, computerized training, and coaching by the practitioner.
3. Learning in guided, but not rehearsed, trial-and-error experiences allows for "reading" of social cues.

Table 2.10. Intervention Goals for Cognitive Enhancement Therapy

Aim of Intervention

Improve cognitive skills.
Improve social cognitive.
Engagement is appropriate social roles and satisfying community life activities.

Goals

Client will complete cognitive skill of _____* for occupational activity of _____ with _____** and _____*** within _____.^^

Client will complete social skill of _____^^^ for occupational activity of _____ with _____** and _____*** within _____.^^

* attention, initiation, memory, mental stamina, cognitive flexibility, processing speed, disability adjustment, disability acceptance
^^^ understanding themes, understanding meanings, understanding messages, "thinking on your feet," abstract thinking, role flexibility, humor, demonstration of spontaneity, demonstration of social norms, role adjustment, role acceptance, role socialization
** Socratic questioning, peer interaction, small group interaction, computerized training
*** coaching, adult interaction, trail-and-error learning, modeling, guided experiences
^^ number of sessions

CLIENT-CENTERED HUMANISTIC THERAPY

One of several humanistic therapies, client-centered therapy was developed by psychologist Carl Rogers. Humanistic therapies are concerned with the person's view of life and with helping people find satisfaction in whatever way makes most sense for them. Rogers used the word *client* to convey a greater sense of self-determination. The word *patient* suggests a dependent role in a medical relationship. He believed that the client's personal development is best fostered by a relationship with a warm, nondirective therapy professional who accepts the client as the client wishes to be accepted.

A central tenet of client-centered therapy is that human beings possess the potential for directing their own growth and development. No matter how psychotic or disorganized the behavior may appear, the client is capable of self-understanding and ultimately of changing behavior.

Another concept is that people direct their own lives. The occupational therapy professional does not tell the client what to do; the client must determine what action to take. By being *nondirective*, the occupational therapy professional allows the client to take an individual direction. The occupational therapy professional does help the client, however, by making the client more aware of feelings and by helping the client explore the possible consequences of contemplated action. Rogers believed that only when clients are aware of how they feel and what is likely to happen are they truly free to choose what to do (58).

For example, a high school student, Karen, may plan to go to college because that is what her family expects her to do, even though she is confused and not particularly interested in college. She has suppressed these feelings and is not aware of them. A client-centered occupational therapy professional would listen to her and reflect the hidden feelings that they hear. The student, now aware of the feelings, might feel freer to choose not to go to college, or at least to explore other possibilities.

A third and related concept is that mental health problems occur when a person is not aware of feelings and of the available choices. In other words, people who do not know how they feel about the people and events in their lives are likely to act in disorganized, confused, or maladaptive ways.

A fourth concept is that a person can become more aware of feelings and choices by experiencing them in a relationship with an occupational therapy professional who genuinely accepts themselves and the client. Professionals must be aware of their own feelings and attitudes and be comfortable expressing them. They must be able to provide **unconditional positive regard**—that is, they must continue to like the client no matter what the client does. By accepting the client as is, no matter how bizarre the attitudes or behaviors of the client, the occupational therapy professional helps the client accept themselves. Gradually, the client's self-perception changes, and their behavior becomes more organized and more consistent with their feelings. The client adapts better to new situations; in short, their mental health improves.

The client's relationship with a warm, empathic occupational therapy professional is the key to client-centered approach. **Accurate empathy** involves constantly being in the moment with the client so that one can "feel with" the client, sensitively tuning in to the client's feelings and thoughts (22). Client-centered occupational therapy professionals use several techniques that facilitate clients' awareness and expression of feelings. These techniques can be used when interviewing and conversing with clients; five are discussed here (38).

One technique is the open invitation to talk. This invitation to talk is conveyed through **open questions**, questions that are designed to require more than a one-word answer. They encourage the client to talk freely and at length. Two examples are "What were your feelings when that happened?" and "Tell me about your family."

The opposite is **closed questions**, such as "Are you married?" and "Were you angry when that happened?" Sometimes closed questions are the quickest way to get specific details from a client. However, closed questions require only one- or two-word answers and limit self-expression because the person is likely to stop after that; using closed questioning is not a client-centered technique.

A second technique used by client-centered occupational therapy professionals is the **minimal response**, which shows that the occupational therapy professional is listening to the client and that the client should go on talking. Some examples are nodding the head, or saying "Uh-huh" or "Go on." These responses let the client know that the occupational therapy professional is tuned in to what the client is saying. Using minimal response is like displaying active listening skills with the client.

A third technique is **reflection of feeling**. Through this technique, the occupational therapy professional puts the client's feelings into words and helps them experience the emotional content. An example is given here:

Case Example

Client: My husband doesn't mean anything by it, by the things he does that, well, you know. [Client looks down at her hands and sighs deeply.] It's just that I feel a certain way that he just can't see. Maybe he doesn't want to. But he's too busy with his work and everything. He works so hard.

  Occupational therapy professional: You're sad that your husband is too busy to see how you feel. You feel that maybe he works so hard so that he doesn't have to see.

Just as reflection of feeling focuses on the emotional aspect of the client's words, a fourth technique focuses on the narrative content or story. Using **paraphrasing**, the occupational therapy professional restates in different words what the client has said. This lets the client know that the occupational therapy professional has been listening and helps the them check out whether they understood what the client meant. An example is given here:

> **Case Example**
>
> Client: So, then Jack said he would take care of it, but he never did. You'd think he would do what he said, but no. So, I had to take time off from work to go to the state energy department and pay the bill.
>
> Occupational therapy professional: Because Jack let you down, you had to lose time from work.

Paraphrasing can help the occupational therapy professional sort out what the client has been saying, which is particularly valuable when the client speaks for a long time or in a disorganized fashion.

A fifth technique is **withholding judgment**. The occupational therapy professional refrains from giving an opinion about the client's remarks or behaviors. Clients often look to the occupational therapy professional for advice, praise, approval, or rejection. The following is an example:

> **Case Example**
>
> Client: My mother says I dress too sexy; that's why I have so much trouble. It's none of her business. My clothes are okay, don't you think?
>
> Occupational therapy professional: What do you think?

Here, the occupational therapy professional is not only withholding judgment but also encouraging the client to evaluate the situation themselves. If the occupational therapy professional had said, "Your clothes are okay," or "You dress nicely," or "Maybe your mother has a point there," the client might react to the comment instead of thinking out the problem on their own. The occupational therapy professional is letting the client know that they must decide for themselves.

All five of these techniques are derived from similar techniques used in object relations therapy. Like object relations therapy, client-centered therapy requires many sessions and is most practical in long-term treatment situations. Client-centered therapy, because it relies on the clients' ability to direct themselves, seems inappropriate for persons with, for instance, severe intellectual disabilities, who may not use words and may appear unable to make some decisions. This issue is at the heart of the persistent debate over the use of the word *client* in occupational therapy practice and literature. Sharrott and Yerxa (61) argue that a client would be capable of choosing and securing occupational therapy services; in contrast, some of the persons served by occupational therapy are so disabled that they are incapable of acting in their own best interests and for that reason should be called patients. On the other hand, since the 1990s, persons with mental health problems have organized politically and often prefer (when living in the community) to be called consumers.

Despite these concerns, although it is unusual for an occupational therapy professional to solely embrace humanistic-based therapy, psychiatric occupational therapy professionals continue to use client-centered techniques, which are effective for getting people with mental health problems to express themselves and for establishing a solid therapeutic relationship. This approach is often combined with other approaches, such as behavioral techniques, which may give faster results in changing a person's behavior (29).

Chapter 15, "Therapeutic Use of Self," describes and illustrates further how Rogers's techniques can be applied by the occupational therapy professional. Table 2.11 provides examples of client-centered humanistic occupational therapy goals to use with clients.

Table 2.11. Intervention Goals for Client-Centered Humanistic Therapy

Aim of Intervention

Helping the client find satisfaction in occupation performance in whatever way makes the most sense to the client.
Helping the client become more aware of their feelings by helping the client explore possible consequences of contemplated actions.
Helping the client genuinely accept themselves and providing unconditional positive regard toward the client.

Goals

Client will express self-awareness of feelings regarding occupational activity of _____ with _____ (add needed amount or type of assistance)* and _____** within _____***.

Client will identify possible barriers for success with occupational activity of _____ with _____ (add needed amount or type of assistance)* and _____** within _____***.

Client will identify possible solutions to obtain occupation of _____ with _____ (add needed amount or type of assistance)* and _____** within _____***.

* guidance, prompt, cue, direct supervision/contact, indirect supervision/contact
** use of open questions, use of reflection of feeling, use of paraphrasing, structured environment, group environment, no direct involvement from practitioner
*** number of attempts, number of sessions, number of weeks

1. Each human being has the potential to direct their own growth and development.
2. Each person is free to choose their own course of action.
3. Mental health problems can occur when a person is not aware of their own feelings and of their available choices.
4. A person can become more aware of feelings and choices by exploring them in a relationship with a warm, empathic occupational therapy professional who genuinely accepts themselves and the client.

VOCABULARY REVIEW

accurate empathy

Understanding the feelings and actions of another person, staying attuned to the person's thoughts and feelings. This is contrasted with sympathy, which includes a sense of *feeling* what the other feels.

genuineness

A sense conveyed by the occupational therapy professional that the occupational therapy professional is really the way they appear and is not just putting on an act for the client's benefit

minimal response

A brief verbal or nonverbal action of the occupational therapy professional that gives the message that they are actively listening and want the client to keep talking. Examples are nodding, saying "Go on," and leaning forward in the chair.

nondirective behavior

A behavior of the occupational therapy professional in which they refrain from giving an opinion on anything the client says or does

open invitation to talk

An interviewing technique in which questions are worded to require a response longer than one or two words. This encourages the client to talk.

paraphrasing

The occupational therapy professional's restatement of the *story* or narrative content conveyed by the client's words

reflection of feeling

The occupational therapy professional's restatement of the *feeling* conveyed by the client's words or nonverbal expression

unconditional positive regard

A sense conveyed by the occupational therapy professional that they accept, like, and respect the client regardless of the client's feelings or actions

warmth

A sense conveyed by the occupational therapy professional that they feel concerned about the client's well-being

withholding judgment

The occupational therapy professional's deliberate abstinence from giving opinions on the client's behavior, feelings, or intention

NEUROSCIENCE THEORIES

Neuroscience refers to the entire body of information about the nervous system—how it is organized, what it looks like, and how it operates. Use of neuroscience theories to plan and perform intervention requires knowledge of the anatomy and physiology of the nervous system. Much of current medical practice in psychiatry is based on neuroscience; the physician may determine the diagnosis and choose medications based on brain imaging studies of the client or on blood tests. And some occupational therapy practice models in mental health reflect a neuroscience foundation.

How much of our mental and emotional experience results from physical, biologic, and chemical events in the brain? Freud himself explored this possibility during his earliest years in medicine, when he worked on the neuroanatomy of the medulla (75). Research since that time has demonstrated many associations between behavior and brain activity. The central concept of neuroscience theories is that the phenomena we think of as mind and emotion are explained by biochemical and electrical activity in the brain.

Neuroscience theories assume that normal human functioning requires a brain that is anatomically normal, with normal neurophysiology and brain chemicals in the proper proportions. Neuroscientists are finding that some mental disorders are associated with variations from these normal conditions. This is particularly obvious in the case of schizophrenia and other severe and persistent mental disorders. Ventricular enlargement has been found in the brains of persons with schizophrenia, and abnormalities of brain anatomy and neurotransmitter mechanisms are suspected of contributing to the symptoms of the disease (4, 14, 25, 45). Brain imaging techniques provide views of deep brain structures in sufficient detail to show atrophy and reduced blood flow in the brains of persons with Alzheimer disease (50, 80). Other techniques measure the magnetic fields produced by electrical activity in the brain. Still another measures blood oxygenation by shining near-infrared light (not visible to humans) through the skull (26). The research evidence has been so plentiful and convincing that some leading research psychiatrists have proposed regrouping the major mental disorders with other disorders of the central nervous system (ie, multiple sclerosis, Parkinson disease)—in other words, reclassifying these conditions as medical problems rather than problems of mental health (69). The National Alliance on Mental Illness (NAMI) had designated the 1990s as the decade of the brain, but research since then has been so active, productive, and promising that perhaps the 21st century will be the century of the brain (78).

If mental disorders are caused by brain defects, then intervention must be directed at the brain itself. Treatment of mental disorders, according to the neuroscience model, involves changing the abnormal *somatic* (bodily) conditions through somatic intervention. These interventions include pharmacotherapy (drugs), psychosurgery, and electroconvulsive therapy (ECT). Despite their negative side effects, drugs have been useful in controlling psychotic and affective (mood) symptoms that might otherwise prevent people from participating in rehabilitation. However, there is evidence that use of antipsychotic medications may be associated with brain atrophy and other changes (48, 74).

Psychosurgery (stereotactic and laser surgery on the brain) has been used successfully to stop abnormal rage in persons with temporal lobe epilepsy. In addition, ECT (sometimes incorrectly called "shock treatment") is effective in reversing extreme suicidal depressions that fail to respond to drugs (51). All these treatments were discovered serendipitously (by fortunate accident) and were used for years with little understanding of how they worked; one of the major contributions of recent neuroscience is to demonstrate some of the mechanisms behind them (39). In clients with treatment-resistant depression, psychiatrists have found success in stimulating brain centers using technology such as transcranial magnetic stimulation (TMS), vagus nerve stimulation (VNS), and deep brain stimulation (DBS) (26, 49, 55, 64).

Only physicians can prescribe or provide drugs, surgery, and brain stimulation. The traditional role of occupational therapy in the neuroscience approach has been to monitor the effects on functional performance of the somatic treatments prescribed by the physician. By observing how the person performs in activities, the occupational therapy professional can collect information to help the doctor determine or verify the diagnosis and later decide whether the medical treatment is working and whether it should be increased, decreased, or modified. Occupational therapy professionals also help clients adjust their approach to activities to cope with the side effects of drugs and ECT (63). This topic is discussed in Chapter 8.

Among the exciting new hypotheses in neuroscience are those relating to *neuroimmunomodulation* (33) and *psychoneuroimmunology* (PNI) (15, 65). Research indicates an interaction between the central nervous system and the immune system; it is this interaction that regulates the immune response of the body. Depression as a diagnosis often occurs with diagnosed medical illnesses such as cardiovascular disease (65). Farber (33) suggested that occupational therapy may strengthen the immune response by reducing helplessness and hopelessness and helping the person establish positive attitudes. Techniques may include stress management education and mindfulness meditation.

Several occupational therapy intervention approaches have ties to neuroscience theory. One was Lorna Jean King's sensory integration approach to intervention with those with schizophrenia. King (44) proposed that games and postural exercises can bring about changes in the sensorimotor functioning of persons with certain types of chronic schizophrenia. She argued that these activities stimulate the part of the central nervous system that processes and organizes sensory information.

A second occupational therapy approach related to neuroscience was developed by Allen (1), who proposed that the problems psychiatric clients have functioning in daily life originate in physical and chemical abnormalities of the brain. She argued that the role of occupational therapy should be to define the person's functional level very precisely and to modify the environment to help the person function as well as possible. She believed that occupational therapy cannot change the client's level of function and should instead work on adapting the environment to the disability.

More recently, Brown and coworkers (17, 18), building on the work of Dunn and Westman (28), developed an evaluation of sensory processing for adults and adolescents. These writers offer strategies for modifying the environment and one's behavior to compensate for sensory differences. Two key notions for this approach are neurologic threshold and behavioral response. The neurologic threshold may be high or low and is a measure of how easily a person registers sensation from the environment. The person with a low threshold notices sensations very easily, and someone with a high threshold does not notice sensations that are obvious to most everyone else.

The behavioral response is the kind of action taken regarding the sensory information. For example, one person may be very sensitive to odors (low threshold) and another quite insensitive (high threshold). The behavioral response for the person with low threshold may take the form of avoiding department store perfume and cosmetic counters. The person with high threshold may not be aware of their own bodily odors or of the need to bathe regularly, with a behavioral response of low registration, or not noticing unpleasant odors. Although olfactory sensation (smell) is the example here, Brown also addresses other sensory systems (vision, taste, hearing, touch). The sensory processing and modulation approaches now in use also may promote helpful changes in behaviors associated with the autonomic nervous system (excitation vs relaxation).

American Psychiatric Association (2022) provides information derived from neuroscience research (3).

Concepts Summary

1. All mental processes, including behavior and emotion, originate in biochemical and electrical activity in the brain.
2. Abnormal behavior and abnormal emotional states (mental disorders) are caused by defects either in the anatomy or in the level of chemicals in the brain.
3. Abnormal mental conditions can be controlled by changing either the anatomy or the chemical and electrical activity of the brain. Treatments include surgery, drugs, and ECT.

behavioral response
Action taken by a person in reaction to sensory information

chemotherapy
A treatment in which chemical substances (drugs) are introduced into the body to cure a disease or control its symptoms

electroconvulsive therapy (ECT)
A treatment in which an electrical current applied to the brain causes a brief seizure. ECT is used most often to treat severe depression that does not respond to medication.

neuroimmunomodulation
The proposed interactive regulation of immune responses through the combined actions of the neurologic, endocrine, and immune systems

neurologic threshold
The degree to which the person's nervous system registers sensation from the environment

neurotransmitter
A chemical that transmits nerve impulses from one neuron to another within the central nervous system. Examples are serotonin, dopamine, norepinephrine, and acetylcholine.

organic
Referring to the brain, the organ of mind and emotion

psychoneuroimmunology
The study of the interaction of the immune system and the central nervous system

psychosurgery
Surgery on the brain in which nerve fibers are cut or destroyed to control abnormal behavior or mood disturbances

PSYCHIATRIC REHABILITATION AND PSYCHOSOCIAL REHABILITATION

Psychiatric rehabilitation and psychosocial rehabilitation are competing names for what is essentially the same approach. Psychiatric rehabilitation (PsyR) is an approach documented by William Anthony and others (5–7) and Farkas and others (34, 35) at the Sargent College of Allied Health Professions, Boston University. It combines principles and concepts from the fields of physical rehabilitation, client-centered therapy, behavioral psychology, and psychosocial rehabilitation (7, 57). Unlike the other models described in this chapter, PsyR is *eclectic* (drawing on many sources for techniques). As such, it is **atheoretical** (without theory), although it uses techniques associated with several theories. It is not a **treatment theory** and does not attempt to explain why or how mental disorders occur. Rather, it is a **rehabilitation approach** that focuses on how best to help the person with a mental disorder function optimally in their life situation (Table 2.12).

"Psychosocial rehabilitation" is a term preferred by many health professionals who are not psychiatrists (psychologists, nurses, occupational therapy professionals). Because many of the methods and principles have a social emphasis, this term does seem more descriptive. However, the literature for PsyR is much more extensive than for psychosocial rehabilitation. A search in August 2014 across multiple medical and psychological databases yielded 1,962 articles that contained one term or the other or both. Of these, 1,233 (63%)

concerned "psychiatric rehabilitation," 686 (35%) concerned "psychosocial rehabilitation," and 42 (2%) included both terms. The literature for psychosocial rehabilitation appears to contain many articles about adjustments to physical disorders or disabilities (cancer, burns, traumatic brain injury), whereas the literature for PsyR seems exclusively concerned with mental disorders. For the purposes of this chapter, we will continue to use the term PsyR. In later chapters concerning rehabilitation, we will use either or both terms, depending on the contextual situation.

PsyR is uncannily like occupational therapy in that it is oriented to the present and future, focuses on the development of skills and resources, and uses activities and environmental adaptations as a base for intervention.

PsyR is included in this text because it has become a popular model for design of mental health programs and occupational therapy programs, because it has a developing research base, and because the occupational therapy professional is likely to encounter the model in settings that serve persons with mental health problems. Some states in the United States have adopted PsyR as the model for mental health service delivery statewide (5, 54).

Because PsyR is not allied with or based on any theory, we cannot examine its theoretical underpinnings so we will instead look at goals, values, and guiding principles (34, 57). Instead of addressing how clients came to be ill, PsyR focuses on aiding them in achieving a better quality of life, in recovering and integrating themselves in their communities. The *goals* are recovery, community integration, and quality of life (57). The *values* of PsyR are strongly oriented toward client self-direction (self-determination, dignity, and hope). The *guiding principles* include the following:

- client-centered, individual approach
- services that emphasize normal functioning in the community
- focus on the strengths of the client
- assessment based on the clients' situations
- coordination of services accessible to clients
- focus on work
- focus on skills development
- environmental modifications and supports
- family involvement
- research and outcome orientation

Competencies are achieved by two methods: developing the client's skills and improving environmental supports and resources. Many intervention techniques, including psychotropic medication, are considered compatible with this approach, but interventions must be individualized. The client is expected to participate actively in their own rehabilitation, with appropriate support from the mental health system and the environment. Because work is a significant organizing theme of adult life, the client's participation and satisfaction in a vocational role are targeted for major intervention.

PsyR is conducted in a three-stage process of *rehabilitation diagnosis, rehabilitation planning*, and *rehabilitation intervention*. The rehabilitation diagnosis is a statement of the

Table 2.12. Intervention Goals for Psychiatric Rehabilitation

Aim of Intervention

Helping the client achieve a better quality of life, in recovering and integrating themselves in their communities.

Goals
Recovery
Community integration
Quality of life

Values
Client self-direction (self-determination, dignity, hope)
Focus on: community living, vocation, skill development, environmental modifications and supports, family support

Goals

Client will identify community living skill of _____ to complete occupational activity of _____ with ____ (add needed amount or type of assistance)* and _____** within _____***.

Client will complete community living skill of _____ to complete occupational activity of _____ with ____ (add needed amount or type of assistance)* and _____** within _____***.

Client will identify vocational skill of _____ to complete occupational vocation of _____ with ____ (add needed amount or type of assistance)* and _____** within _____***.

Client will complete vocational skill of _____ to complete occupational vocation of _____ with ____ (add needed amount or type of assistance)* and _____** within _____***.

Client will identify community environment support of _____ to complete occupational activity of _____ with ____ (add needed amount or type of assistance)* and _____** within _____***.

Client will secure community environment support of _____ to complete occupational activity of _____ with ____ (add needed amount or type of assistance)* and _____** within _____***.

* guidance, prompt, cue, direct supervision/contact, indirect supervision/contact
** perceiving a need for change, a desirable view of change, being open to establish new relationships/strengthen relationships, having sufficient self-understanding to reflect on new learning; family support, case management
*** number of attempts, number of sessions, number of weeks

environment in which the client—say, Kenji—would like to function and the resources and skills he will need for this environment. The rehabilitation diagnosis disregards the symptoms and pathology of disease and thus differs from a medical or psychiatric diagnosis. It is situation specific and individualized.

In the rehabilitation diagnosis stage, on first meeting the client, the PsyR practitioner sets the stage for collaboration by explaining to the client how they can participate in evaluation and planning. The first step in a PsyR diagnosis is setting the *overall rehabilitation goal* (ORG), a statement of the environment and role in which the client would like to live, work, study, and so on. An example is, "Kenji would like to live at Livingston Arms, a supported residence." The occupational therapist and the client jointly determine the ORG.

Once the ORG is chosen, the focus shifts to evaluating the client's functional skills. The question to be answered in this phase is, "Which of the skills needed in this environment can the client perform and which can he not perform?" Occupational therapy professional and client work together to list specific skills that correspond to the behavioral requirements of the chosen role and environment. One example might be speaking in turn at community meetings. Client and occupational therapy professional can then assess Kenji's skill level and evaluate the level needed in the supportive living environment. If Kenji has the needed level of skill, this is listed as a strength. If he lacks it or does not perform it with sufficient frequency or accuracy, it is listed as a deficit.

Because community supports are needed for successful functioning in any environment, a resource assessment is also performed. Again, client and practitioner together list the elements needed for the client to function successfully in the chosen environment. These might include things (spending money, clothing, medication), people (sponsor, buddy, home group), and activities (day treatment, evening leisure program). Again, resources that are available at the required level are listed as strengths and those that are less than adequate are listed as deficits. Thus, the rehabilitation diagnosis yields a list of skill strengths and deficits and resource strengths and deficits in relation to an ORG.

The next stage is the formulation of the rehabilitation plan. The typical diagnosis yields many deficit areas; here, the occupational therapy professional and client must determine which ones are to be the priorities for intervention. They might select, for example, "Kenji will say what he thinks in community meeting" and "Kenji will wait until his turn to speak at community meetings." Occupational therapy professional and client then discuss and select appropriate interventions, such as direct skills teaching.

The third stage, rehabilitation intervention, is the enactment of the plan. Here the client may, for example, attend a class or individual session to learn a new skill and do homework or other assignments to practice or reinforce the skill. The client may enter a new environment and practice using a skill that they understand but do not consistently use. The occupational therapy professional works on resource development with the client in this stage, which may mean helping the client find an exercise class in the community, secure spending money from parents, or obtain food stamps.

One of the most important concepts of PsyR is that evaluation and intervention make sense only in relation to the environment in which the client is functioning or intends to be functioning. A client may be "lacking in social skills," but the only social skills that matter are those that are relevant to the environment in which they interact. Defining the environment establishes a context in which further evaluation of the client's skills and resources makes sense.

The two main areas of intervention in PsyR are (a) developing the client's functional skills and (b) modifying the environment to maximize functional use of skills (5). These interventions occur after assessment and are targeted at moving the client toward the established ORG. PsyR practitioners also assess the client's **rehabilitation readiness**, defined as "a reflection of consumers' interest in rehabilitation and their self-confidence, not of their capacity to complete a rehabilitation program" (23, p. 644). The six dimensions of rehabilitation readiness are shown in Box 2.1.

Although PsyR is atheoretical, it does make certain identifiable assumptions. The first is *functioning adequately in the environment of one's choice is possible for everyone.* By analogy with physical rehabilitation, the person with a bilateral upper extremity (BUE) amputee can live in the community, can hold a job, and can enjoy leisure activities.

The second is *to function successfully, one must possess the needed skills and resources.* Again, by analogy with physical rehabilitation, to dress oneself, the person with the BUE amputee must learn a new motor pattern (skill) and may need certain adaptive equipment and the assistance of another person (resources) to don the prostheses and the harness that supports them. To live in a supported living situation, the person with a psychiatric disability may have to learn when and how to care for their clothing (skill); will need money to purchase laundry products, services, and dry-cleaning; and may need support and reminders from a case manager (resources).

The third is *skills that are lacking can be developed through training, and skills that are present but that are weak can be strengthened through practice.* For skills to make sense, they should be learned and practiced in the environment in which they will be used or one as similar to it as possible. For example, to learn to speak in turn in a group meeting, the client should attend such meetings and practice the skill while there.

The fourth is *environmental supports and resources enable and facilitate successful functioning.* Just as grab bars and a tub-transfer seat make bathing easier for a person with physical weakness and limited standing tolerance, so too can environmental supports make things easier for the person with a psychiatric disability. For example, the support of a case manager can make it easier for the client to avoid relapse and rehospitalization by enabling the client to obtain a prescription for medication or by assisting the client to join a self-help group. In addition to providing supports, the case manager can help the client learn to use them. The client who can recognize that they are at risk for a relapse and who knows how to obtain medication or to reach out to a support network is better able to remain in the community.

The fifth assumption is *belief in and hope for the future facilitated rehabilitation outcomes.* In other words, a sense of motivation and personal investment is necessary; the client must have a positive expectation that they can indeed function.

PsyR is compatible with the **recovery movement**, a model of behavioral health promoted by SAMHSA (59). SAMHSA promotes prevention and rehabilitation programs and is a clearinghouse resource for government programs related to behavioral health.

As stated previously, occupational therapy has a natural fit with PsyR, which is a multidisciplinary approach. Regardless of professional credentials or certification, all practitioners provide similar services. Anthony (5) indicates that an activities-oriented background is desirable. As a PsyR practitioner, the occupational therapy professional would work with the client to develop the rehabilitation diagnosis and rehabilitation plan. Occupational therapy professionals may provide many different rehabilitation interventions, including skills instruction and training, general programming, and development and adaptation of environment supports.

BOX 2.1 Six Dimensions of Rehabilitation Readiness

The consumer will:

1. perceive a need for rehabilitation
2. view change as desirable
3. be open to establishing relationships
4. have sufficient self-understanding
5. be aware of and able to interact meaningfully with the environment
6. have significant others who support their participation in rehabilitation

Adapted from Cohen, M. R., Anthony, W. A., & Farkas, M. D. (1997). Assessing and developing readiness for psychiatric rehabilitation. *Psychiatric Services, 48*(5), 644–646.

Case Study – College Student

You are working with a client using the PsyR approach. The client lives at home, is 25 years, has a part-time job at a local grocery store, and attends the local university. She wishes to complete her degree in engineering. She would like to live in the dorm next year. In the past, the client has become withdrawn from friends, overspent and has credit card debt, has not maintained healthy eating or sleeping habits, and failed several college courses because of not attending and not completing coursework. It is currently 2 months before the next college semester begins and you see the client weekly.

Concepts Summary

1. Functioning adequately in the environment of one's choice is possible for everyone.
2. To function successfully, one must possess both the skills and the resources needed to do so. The selection of skills and resources is highly individual, depending on the person and the immediate context. Persons with chronic psychiatric disorders often lack the necessary skills and resources for functioning in their chosen environments.
3. Skills that are lacking can be developed through training. Skills that are present but weak can be strengthened through practice. Both practice and training make sense only in the environment of choice.
4. Environmental supports and resources enable and facilitate successful functioning. Persons with psychiatric illness can function better when such supports are available, and they know how to use them.
5. Belief in and hope for the future facilitate rehabilitation outcomes.

VOCABULARY REVIEW

overall rehabilitation goal (ORG)
An agreement between the client and practitioner about the environment and roles the client would like to occupy (where the client intends to live, learn, or work)

rehabilitation diagnosis
A process to identify the client's ORG. The ORG becomes the basis for evaluating the client's skills (functional assessment), resource strengths, and deficits (resource assessment), in relation to this goal.

rehabilitation intervention
Processes for developing client skills and environmental resources specified in the client's rehabilitation plan. This may include direct skills teaching, skill refinement and practice, coordination and linking of existing resources, and development of new resources.

rehabilitation planning
A process that identifies and prescribes high-priority skill and resource goals, the interventions for achieving them, and the personnel responsible

rehabilitation readiness
"a reflection of consumers' interest in rehabilitation and their self-confidence, not of their capacity to complete a rehabilitation program" (23, p. 644)

EXPLANATORY MODELS FROM OTHER CULTURES

The information presented thus far originated within the context of Western (European and American) culture. But only about 15% of the planet's population lives in these areas. Approximately 85% of humans live elsewhere. In addition, within these countries there exist ethnic and cultural groups that do not share in the ideas and beliefs of Western culture. The United States is a nation of immigrants, and the occupational therapy professional may encounter individuals from other cultures in a variety of settings, including mental health. Recognizing that the client may not agree with the views of mental health professionals is a critical element in learning how the client views their symptoms or behaviors.

It is important for the health professional to accept that the person truly believe in their cultural explanation, just as someone from the West with a neuroscience orientation may believe that brain chemistry is a reasonable explanation.

According to the American Psychiatric Association, **culture** "refers to systems of knowledge, concepts, values, norms, and practices that are learned and transmitted across generations" (3, p. 860). The American Occupational Therapy Association (AOTA) identifies the **cultural context** to include "customs, beliefs, activity patterns, behavioral standards, and expectations accepted by the society of which a client is a member" (2, p. S9). How are mental disorders explained in other cultures and in other parts of the world?

Some of the reasons given for emotional distress and abnormal behavior in different countries and cultures are (3, 10) as follows:

- possession by spiritual forces, ghosts, animals, evil spirits;
- sorcery and witchcraft;
- loss of semen (real or imagined);
- belief that one's genitals are shrinking or withdrawing into the body;
- wind in the body or the head;
- thinking too much;
- sickness sent by others;
- constitutional vulnerability to stress;
- departure of the soul from the body; and
- fear that one is offensive to others, particularly in body odors.

Three examples of cultural syndromes of distress are shown in Box 2.2. Many of the specific syndromes share aspects with diagnoses used in the *DSM-5-TR*. But some do not. Because culture is a shared experience, the client experiencing mental or emotional distress would expect to be understood by others within a given cultural community and likely not so much by a psychiatrist or mental health professional from outside that culture. The *DSM-5-TR* includes a framework for assessing cultural aspects of a person from the view of their culture, as well as some specific culture-bound concepts of distress (3). The occupational therapy professional may not be directly involved in assessing cultural beliefs of an individual but may learn of the person's beliefs while conducting routine assessments and interventions.

BOX 2.2 Three Examples of Cultural Concepts of Distress

- **Dhat syndrome**—anxiety or upset because of loss of semen, one of the seven essential bodily fluids in Ayurvedic (Hindu) medical system—South Asia, India, Pakistan (syndrome also recognized historically in other cultures)
- **Kufungisisa**—anxiety and depression caused by thinking too much, which damages the mind—Zimbabwe, Nigeria
- **Susto**—a fright or trauma causes the soul to leave the body, causing multiple forms of mental, emotional, and physical distress—Mexico, Central America, South America

From American Psychiatric Association. (2022). *Diagnostic and statistical manual of mental disorders* (5th ed., text rev., pp. 873–879). https://doi.org/10.1176/appi.books.9780890425787

OT HACKS SUMMARY

O: **Occupation as a means and an end**

Behavioral theories focus on how we can present learning occupational task behavior that can be repeated and learned over time.

Client-Centered therapy embraces client-driven choices for occupational choices.

Cognitive behavioral theoretical continuum emphasizes that new occupational behavior can be learned and used in various situations.

Cognitive enhancement therapy uses social role learning, and cognitive skills learning, to improve the social cognition used during social participation and with a person's roles.

Erikson's developmental theory presents the concept of psychosocial and the idea of an interplay between oneself and their participation with others around them.

Model of object relations presents the idea that the client's occupational need is centered around the loss of or damage to a relationship with someone (or something) in their lives and the client is using defense mechanisms to shift their focus onto another object (human or nonhuman) to cope with the client's anxiety. We want to use meaningful and expressive activities as a means toward the client reaching an occupational end that will allow the client to fully manage life's stressors and participate with others.

Neuroscience theories focus on the neuroanatomy of the brain and nervous system processes that impact mental health.

PsyR approach is centered on occupational tasks of daily life and community living.

T: **Theoretical concepts, values, and principles, or historical foundations**

Nonoccupational therapy theoretical methods and approaches' alignment with occupational therapy practice includes the object relation focus on relationships and participation with others, the developmental focus on sequential skill obtainment, behavioral tenets that actions can be learned, cognitive behavioral principles that maladaptive patterns of thinking can be changed, CET work on linking social and cognitive skills together for community living, client-centered principles that people self-determine their own actions, neuroscience theories and occupational supports that can enhance daily living for those with mental disorders, and the PsyR focus on daily life activities and community living.

H: **How can we Help? OT's role in serving clients with mental illness or mental health needs**

Behavioral approaches used by occupational therapy professionals provide practice to the client to learn how to change their behavior during occupational activities.

Client-centered therapy methods utilize our therapeutic use of self and our ability to help facilitate client's self-discovery of their feelings and how best to make behavior changes.

Cognitive behavioral methods used in occupational therapy allow learning and reflection on the part of the client to find new ways to manage oneself and cope with internal and external stressors and problems.

Cognitive enhanced therapy gives us the opportunity to use cognitive and social intervention learning strategies (small group work, use of paired peer interactions, computerized learning modules) to focus on appropriate role performance with occupations involving others and to gain the problem-solving needed to complete the cognitive aspects of occupations.

Developmental theories indicate a person has a "lag" in development and once that "lag" is realized and developmental skills are rebuilt, the person can complete desired and necessary occupations.

Model of object relations uses expressive modalities to explore reasons for defense mechanisms and to begin to find new alternatives to coping.

Neuroscience theories help us use information about the nervous system to understand how to affect behavioral changes with our clients.

PsyR approach is a natural fit for occupational therapy professionals. We help clients identify how best to live quality lives within their communities (identifying client's strengths and deficits) and how they can use resources to support themselves.

A: **Adaptations**

By using psychological theoretical knowledge, we analyze and determine what is missing or what foundational functional capability is not operating in a manner to allows the person to complete desired occupations.

We use psychological concepts to build occupational therapy frames and models for our practice to guide our clients complete their desired occupations.

C: **Case study includes**

Cases presented:
   Model of object relations: use of clay beads
   Developmental: Erikson's stage of initiative vs guilt
   Behavioral: group member seeking reassurance from professional
   Cognitive behavioral: client with fear of crowded places
   Client-centered: various relationship difficulties
   PsyR: supported residence living; college student living on campus

K: **Knowledge: keeping mental health OT practice grounded in evidence, in occupational science, and in research**

Behavioral theory is from scientific research completed from Pavlov and Skinner.

Client-centered therapies come from Carl Rogers's principle that people find satisfaction in whatever way of doing that makes the most sense for them.

Cognitive behavioral theoretical continuum is based on the work of Aaron Beck, Albert Ellis, and Albert Bandura.

Cognitive enhancement therapy comes from the disciplines of psychology, neurophysiology, neurophysiology, sociology, and psychiatry.

Erikson's developmental stages theory is based on concepts of developmental sequence.

Model of object relations grew from Freud's psychoanalytical theory.

Neuroscience theories come from the disciplines of anatomy and physiology.

S: Some terms that may be new to you

Key terms are summarized throughout the chapter.

Reflection Questions

1. A new family moves in next door. The preteen daughter begins to act and dress like the teenager of the family living next door. The preteen daughter is displaying what defense mechanism?

2. Explain a compromise the ego would need to make between the id and superego when the person is displaced after a natural disaster. What is the role of the id? What is the role of the superego?

3. What is an appropriate intervention modality to use with a person in the Autonomy vs Shame and Doubt stage?

4. Your client enjoys nature, music, and tennis. They wish to talk more with others when they are in the community. The question for the OTA student and the OT student is different and will be provided by the instructor.

5. Complete the questions in the *What's the Evidence?* box. How does this information help occupational therapy professionals address the occupation of sleep? What cognitive behavioral principles can we add into our sleep intervention?

6. During a group session a client is reserved and turns their body away from others. The topic is: making good use of free time. What are good, open questions the occupational therapy professional can use with this client?

References

1. Allen, C. K. (1985). *Therapy for psychiatric disorders: Measurement and management of cognitive disabilities.* Little, Brown and Company.
2. American Occupational Therapy Association. (2014). Occupational therapy practice framework: Domain & process (3rd edition). *American Journal of Occupational Therapy, 68*(Suppl. 1), S1–S48.
3. American Psychiatric Association. (2022). *Diagnostic and statistical manual of mental disorders* (5th ed., text rev.). https://doi.org/10.1176/appi.books.9780890425787
4. Andreasen, N. C., Paradiso, S., & O'Leary, D. S. (1998). Cognitive dysmetria as an integrative theory of schizophrenia: A dysfunction in cortical-subcortical-cerebellar circuitry? *Schizophrenia Bulletin, 24*(2), 203–218.
5. Anthony, W. A. (1982). Explaining "psychiatric rehabilitation" by an analogy to "physical rehabilitation". *Psychosocial Rehabilitation Journal, 5*(1), 61–65.
6. Anthony, W. A., Cohen, M., & Farkas, M. (1982). A psychiatric rehabilitation treatment program: Can I recognize one if I see one? *Community Mental Health Journal, 18*(2), 83–96.
7. Anthony, W., Cohen, M., & Farkas, M. (1990). *Psychiatric rehabilitation.* Center for Psychiatric Rehabilitation, Boston University.
8. Babiss, F. (2002). An ethnographic study of mental health treatment and outcomes: Doing what works. *Occupational Therapy in Mental Health, 18*(3–4), 1–146.
9. Balhara, Y. P. S. (2011). Culture-bound syndrome: Has it found its right niche? *Indian Journal of Psychological Medicine, 33*(2), 210–215.
10. Bandura, A. (1965). Behavioral modifications through modeling procedures. In L. Krasner & L. P. Ullmann (Eds.), *Research in behavior modification: New developments and implications* (pp. 310–340). Holt, Rinehart & Winston.
11. Beck, A. T. (1976). *Cognitive therapy and the emotional disorders.* Meridian.
12. Beck, A. T. (1988). *Love is never enough.* Harper & Row.
13. Beck, A. T., Rush, J. A., Shaw, B. F., & Emery, G. (1979). *Cognitive therapy of depression.* Guilford.
14. Benes, F. M. (1998). Model generation and testing to probe neural circuitry in the cingulate cortex of postmortem schizophrenic brain. *Schizophrenia Bulletin, 24*(2), 219–230.
15. Black, P. H. (1995). Psychoneuroimmunology: Brain and immunity. *Scientific American, 272*, 16–25.
16. Brady, J. P. (1984). Social skills training for psychiatric patients. I: Concepts, methods, and clinical results. *Occupational Therapy in Mental Health, 4*(4), 51–68.
17. Brown, C. (2001). What is the best environment for me? A sensory processing perspective. *Occupational Therapy in Mental Health, 17*(3–4), 115–125.
18. Brown, C., Tollefson, N., Dunn, W., Cromwell, R., & Filion, D. (2001). The adult sensory profile: Measuring patterns of sensory processing. *American Journal of Occupational Therapy, 55*(1), 75–82.
19. Carson, N. (2020). *Psychosocial occupational therapy.* Elsevier.
20. Center for Cognition & Recovery. (2017). *Cognitive enhancement therapy: An overview of evidence-based practice.* Retrieved August 16, 2021, from http://cetcleveland.org/marketing/
21. Cermak, S. A., Stein, F., & Abelson, C. (1973). Hyperactive children and an activity group therapy model. *American Journal of Occupational Therapy, 27*(6), 311–315.
22. Client-centered therapy. *Harvard Mental Health Letter, 22*(7), 1–3.
23. Cohen, M. R., Anthony, W. A., & Farkas, M. D. (1997). Assessing and developing readiness for psychiatric rehabilitation. *Psychiatric Services, 48*(5), 644–646.
24. Cole, M. B., & Tufano, R. (2020). *Applied theories in occupational therapy: A practical approach* (2nd ed.). SLACK.
25. Csernansky, J. G., & Grace, A. A. (1998). New models of the pathophysiology of schizophrenia. *Schizophrenia Bulletin, 24*(2), 185–187.
26. Demitri, M. (2016, May 17) *Types of brain imaging techniques.* PsychCentral. Retrieved August 15, 2021, from https://psychcentral.com/lib/types-of-brain-imaging-techniques#1
27. Dialectical behavior therapy. (2002, August). *Harvard Mental Health Letter, 19*(2), 1–3.
28. Dunn, W., & Westman, K. (1997). The sensory profile: The performance of a national sample of children without disabilities. *American Journal of Occupational Therapy, 51*(1), 25–34.
29. Dunning, R. E. (1973). The occupational therapist as counselor. *American Journal of Occupational Therapy, 27*(8), 473–476.
30. Early M. B. (1981). *T.A.R. Introductory course workbook. Occupational therapy: Psychosocial dysfunction.* LaGuardia Community College.
31. Eklund, M. (2000). Applying object relations theory to psychosocial occupational therapy: Empirical and theoretical considerations. *Occupational Therapy in Mental Health, 15*(1), 1–26.
32. Ellis, A. (1994). *Reason and emotion in psychotherapy.* Birch Lane.
33. Farber, S. D. (1989). Neuroscience and occupational therapy: Vital connections. 1989 Eleanor Clarke Slagle lecture. *American Journal of Occupational Therapy, 43*(10), 637–646.
34. Farkas, M., & Anthony, W. A. (2010). Psychiatric rehabilitation interventions: A review. *International Review of Psychiatry, 22*(2), 114–129.

35. Farkas, M. D., Cohen, M. R., & Nemec, P. B. (1988). Psychiatric rehabilitation programs: Putting concepts into practice? *Community Mental Health Journal, 24*(1), 7–21.

36. Fidler, G. S., & Fidler, J. W. (1963). *Occupational therapy: A communication process in psychiatry.* Macmillan.

37. Fidler, G. S., & Velde, B. P. (1999). *Activities: Reality and symbol.* SLACK.

38. Hays, J. S., & Larson, K. (1963). *Interacting with patients.* Macmillan.

39. Hedaya, R. J. (1995). *Understanding biological psychiatry.* Norton.

40. Hogarty, G. E., Flesher, S., Ulrich, R., Carter, M., Greenwald, D., Pogue-Geile, M., Kechavan, M., Cooley, S., DiBarry, A. L., Garrett, A., Parepally, H., & Zoretich, R. (2004). Cognitive enhancement therapy for schizophrenia: Effects of a 2-year randomized trial on cognition and behavior. *Archives of General Psychiatry, 61*(9), 866–876.

41. Hogarty, G. E., Greenwald, D. P., & Eack, S. M. (2006). Durability and mechanism of effects of cognitive enhancement therapy. *Psychiatric Services, 57*(12), 1751–1757.

42. Johnston, M. T. (1987). Occupational therapists and the teaching of cognitive behavioral skills. *Occupational Therapy in Mental Health, 7*(3), 69–81.

43. King, J. (2019, May 15). *Let's talk about reinforcement.* CMC: Center for Motivation & Change. https://motivationandchange.com/lets-talk-about-reinforcement/

44. King, L. J. (1974). A sensory-integrative approach to schizophrenia. *American Journal of Occupational Therapy, 28*(9), 529–536.

45. Kyriakopoulos, M., & Frangou, S. (2007). Pathophysiology of early onset schizophrenia. *International Review of Psychiatry, 19*(4), 315–324.

46. Linehan, M. (1993). *The cognitive behavioral treatment of borderline personality disorder.* Guilford Press.

47. Lumen. (n.d.). *Reinforcement and punishment.* Introduction to Psychology. Retrieved August 2, 2021, from https://courses.lumenlearning.com/waymaker-psychology/chapter/operant-conditioning/

48. Madsen, A. L., Keidling, N., Karle, A., Esbjerg, S., & Hemmingsen, R. (1998). Neuroleptics in progressive structural brain abnormalities in psychiatric illness. *Lancet, 352*(9130), 784–785.

49. Mayberg, H. S., Lozano, A. M., Voon, V., McNeely, H. E., Seminowicz, D., Hamani, C., Schwalb, J. M., & Kennedy, S. H. (2005). Deep brain stimulation for treatment-resistant depression. *Neuron, 45*(5), 651–660.

50. McNeil, C. (1995). *Alzheimer's disease: Unraveling the mystery.* National Institutes of Health.

51. Meissner, M. (2021, April 1). *What to do when your antidepressant isn't helping enough.* PsychCentral. Retrieved August 15, 2021, from https://psychcentral.com/depression/treatment-resistant-depression

52. Mosey, A. C. (1973). *Activities therapy.* Raven.

53. Norman, C. W. (1976). Behavior modification: A perspective. *American Journal of Occupational Therapy, 30*(8), 491–497.

54. Office of Mental Health, New York State. (2014). *Data book for behavioral health carve-in and health and recovery plans (HARP), draft, January 21, 2014.* Retrieved May 16, 2022, from https://www.health.ny.gov/health_care/medicaid/redesign/behavioral_health/plan_process/docs/data_book_behav_hlth_carve-in_harps.pdf

55. O'Reardon, J. P., Cristancho, P., & Peshek, A. D. (2006). Vagus nerve stimulation (VNS) and treatment of depression: To the brainstem and beyond. *Psychiatry, 3*(5), 54–63.

56. Phillips, M. E., Bruehl, S., & Harden, R. N. (1997). Work-related post-traumatic stress disorder: Use of exposure therapy in work-simulation activities. *American Journal of Occupational Therapy, 51*(8), 696–700.

57. Pratt, C. W., Gill, K. J., Barrett, N. M., & Roberts, M. M. (2007). *Psychiatric rehabilitation* (2nd ed.). Elsevier.

58. Rogers, C. (1961). *On becoming a person: A therapist's view of psychotherapy.* Houghton Mifflin.

59. SAMHSA. (2020, April 16). *Community mental health services block grant.* Retrieved August 15, 2021, from https://www.samhsa.gov/grants/block-grants/mhbg

60. SAMHSA's National Registry of Evidence-Based Programs and Practices. (n.d.). *CET training, LLC.* Retrieved August 16, 2021, from https://www.cognitiveenhancementtherapy.com/samhsa/

61. Sharrott, G. W., & Yerxa, E. J. (1985). Promises to keep: Implications of the referent "patient" versus "client" for those served by occupational therapy. *American Journal of Occupational Therapy, 39*(6), 401–405.

62. Sieg, K. W. (1974). Applying the behavioral model. *American Journal of Occupational Therapy, 28*(7), 421–428.

63. Smith, D. A. (1981). Effects of psychotropic drugs on the occupational therapy process. *Mental Health Special Interest Section Quarterly, 4*(1), 1–3.

64. Somani, A., & Kumar Kar, S. (2019). Efficacy of repetitive transcranial magnetic stimulation in treatment-resistant depression: The evidence thus far. *General Psychiatry, 32*(4), e100074.

65. Spollen, J. J., & Gutman, D. A. (2006). *The interaction of depression and medical illness.* Medscape. Retrieved August 15, 2021, from https://www.medscape.org/viewarticle/457165

66. Sullivan, A., Dowdy, T., Haddad, J., Hussain, S., Patel, A., & Smyth, K. (2013, March). Occupational therapy interventions in adult mental health across settings: A literature review. *Mental Health Special Interest Section Quarterly, 36*(1), 1–3.

67. Taylor, E. (1988). Anger intervention. *American Journal of Occupational Therapy, 42*(3), 147–155.

68. Toal-Sullivan, D., & Henderson, P. R. (2004). Client-oriented role evaluation (CORE): The development of a clinical rehabilitation instrument to assess role change associated with disability. *American Journal of Occupational Therapy, 58*(2), 211–220.

69. Torrey, E. F. (1997). *Out of the shadows.* Wiley.

70. Warshawsky, D., & Handelzalts, J. E. (2014). Object relations and relationships with parents as predictors of motivation to recover from eating disorders. *Psychology, 5*(15), 1730–1742.

71. Watling, R., & Schwartz, I. S. (2004). Understanding and implementing positive reinforcement as an intervention strategy for children with disabilities. *American Journal of Occupational Therapy, 58*(1), 113–116.

72. Weber, N. J. (1978). Chaining strategies for teaching sequenced motor tasks to mentally retarded adults. *American Journal of Occupational Therapy, 32*(6), 385–389.

73. Wehman, P., & Marchant, J. A. (1978). Improving free play skills of severely retarded children. *American Journal of Occupational Therapy, 32*(2), 100–104.

74. Whitaker, R. (2011). *Anatomy of an epidemic: Magic bullets, psychiatric drugs, and the astonishing rise of mental illness in America.* Broadway Books.

75. Winson, J. (1985). *Brain and psyche.* Anchor Doubleday.

76. Wright, J. H., & Beck, A. T. (1995). Cognitive therapy. In R. E. Hales, S. E. Yudofsky, & J. A. Talbott (Eds.), *American psychiatric press textbook of psychiatry* (2nd ed., pp. 1083–1114). American Psychiatric Association.

77. Yakobina, S., Yakobina, S., & Tallant, B. K. (1997). I came, I thought, I conquered: Cognitive behaviour approach applied in occupational therapy for the treatment of depressed (dysthymic) females. *Occupational Therapy in Mental Health, 13*(4), 59–73.

78. Yuste, R., & Church, G. M. (2014). The new century of the brain. *Scientific American, 310*(3), 38–45.

79. Zemke, R., & Gratz, R. R. (1982). The role of theory: Erikson and occupational therapy. *Occupational Therapy in Mental Health, 2*(3), 45–63.

80. Zubenko, G. S. (1997). Molecular neurobiology of Alzheimer's disease (syndrome?). *Harvard Review of Psychiatry, 5*(4), 177–213.

SUGGESTED RESOURCES

Articles

Watling, R., & Schwartz, I. S. (2004). Understanding and implementing positive reinforcement as an intervention strategy for children with disabilities. *American Journal of Occupational Therapy, 58*(1), 113–116.

Yuste, R., & Church, G. M. (2014). The new century of the brain. *Scientific American, 310*(3), 38–45.

Books

Pratt, C. W., Gill, K. J., Barrett, N. M., & Roberts, M. M. (2014). *Psychiatric rehabilitation* (3rd ed.). Academic Press.

Videos

Cognitive Behavioural Therapy (CBT) *techniques.* https://www.youtube.com/watch?v=HoFNs-3-0Go

UNC *occupational science—Client centered therapy.* https://www.youtube.com/watch?v=AR9EDA0fO68

Yellow *duck books—Wipe away therapeutic stores.* https://www.youtube.com/watch?v=a5k4NKSH30I

Websites

Association for Behavioral and Cognitive Therapies. https://www.abct.org/

Beck Institute. *The home of cognitive behavior therapy and recovery-oriented cognitive therapy.* https://beckinstitute.org/

Center for Object Relations. https://www.nwfdc.org/?v=e2ae933451f4

Changing Minds. *Coping mechanisms.* http://changingminds.org/explanations/behaviors/coping/coping.htm

Get Self Help. *Cognitive behavior therapy resources.* https://www.getself-help.co.uk/?fbclid=IwAR19yaR7nCW_BmdG5fR9o-xRAOI9eq-te-KW7QwTvfT-JwAk-yDKWkx87fXA

Psychology Tools. *CBT worksheets, handouts, and skills-development audio: Therapy resources for mental health professionals.* https://www.psychologytools.com/downloads/cbt-worksheets-and-therapy-resources/

SimplyPsychology. *Jean Piaget and his theory & stages of cognitive development.* https://www.simplypsychology.org/piaget.html

Society of Clinical Psychology. *Cognitive behavioral therapy for schizophrenia.* https://www.div12.org/treatment/cognitive-behavioral-therapy-cbt-for-schizophrenia/

Therapist Aid. *Essential tools for mental health professionals.* https://www.therapistaid.com/

CHAPTER

3

Occupational Therapy Frames of Reference and Practice Models

Patricia Henton and Cindy Meyer[1]

OT HACKS OVERVIEW

| **O:** | **Occupation as a means and an end** |

Through occupational therapy–based frames of reference and practice models, occupation is an end goal and is also used as an intervention focus to improve the overall functional performance.

| **T:** | **Theoretical concepts, values, and principles, or historical foundations** |

Theoretical concepts are the foundation of occupational therapy frames of reference and practice models.

| **H:** | **How can we Help? OT's role in serving clients with mental illness or mental health needs** |

Occupational therapy frames of reference and practice models guide how we help clients use their internal abilities and the influence of external factors to support occupational performance.

| **A:** | **Adaptations** |

Adaptations to people's disability status and situation can be achieved via the basic principles and assumptions of various frames of reference and practice models.

| **C:** | **Case study includes** |

Case studies and examples presenting how occupational therapy–based frames of reference and practice model information help guide our decision-making.

| **K:** | **Knowledge: keeping mental health OT practice grounded in evidence, in occupational science, and in research** |

Knowledge connected to occupational therapy frames of reference and practice models grows out of the medical and psychological theories, frames of reference, and models.

| **S:** | **Some terms that may be new to you** |

Key terms are summarized throughout the chapter.

INTRODUCTION

Chapter 2 presented some of the many medical and psychological theories, frames of reference, and models of how the mind works. Each one gives us a way of looking at mental health and mental disorders—a way to organize, explain, predict, and intervene with behavior. We can think of theories as being similar to eyeglasses with a variety of colored lenses. The world looks different through each color, and we respond differently to what we see when we wear them. Theories are like this; when we look at a client through the lens of a particular theory, we pay attention to the things that theory says are important and we ignore everything else, just as red lenses make green things prominent and make red things fade away. It can be fascinating to try on these different points of view, but we must ultimately decide which one gives us the most useful view of the person and their problems and how to address

them through occupational therapy. As occupational therapy professionals, we must consider which one is most consistent with what we know of the individual and their goals and problems and which one is best supported by research. At the same time, we must appreciate that no one theory, frame of reference, or model is sufficient and that each forces us to ignore some aspects that might be important.

Because participation in occupation is the chief concern of occupational therapy, any theory, frame of reference, or practice model useful to occupational therapy professionals must explain how people's performance of occupations affects their mental health and how their mental health affects their performance of occupations. None of the theories, frames of references, or models discussed in Chapter 2 addresses occupation specifically, although their ideas can be applied in occupation-centered intervention. For instance, the object relations model focuses on the symbolic content of activities as a mirror of unconscious processes. This approach works best with those who have good insight and good verbal skills.

---

[1]We thank Katherine McGinley for helpful suggestions pertaining to the content of this chapter.

As an occupational therapy approach, client-centered therapy has been criticized for being a talking therapy, not a doing therapy, and for lacking the activity core on which occupational therapy is based. Similar to and derived from psychoanalytic therapy, client-centered therapy also works best with those who are articulate and whose cognitive functions are not greatly disturbed. Thus, it cannot be applied effectively with many of the clients seen in occupational therapy mental health practice (21, 55). However, occupational therapy is a client-centered profession, and for this reason, many of the techniques of client-centered therapy are reflected in the occupational therapy professional's therapeutic use of self (102).

Like client-centered therapy, developmental theories, such as Erikson's, used in mental health are derived from psychoanalytic foundations. They emphasize social and sexual development. Because some of these theories address the development of the motivation, skills, habits, and attitudes that enable full participation in occupation and activity, occupational therapy professionals have used developmental concepts in their practice. Later in this chapter, we look at this more closely, with Mosey's model for development of adaptive skills.

Although the behavioral approach has been used in occupational therapy with persons with intellectual disabilities, conduct disorders, and cognitive disabilities, it focuses on learning as a consequence of external rewards. In this, behaviorism conflicts with one of the central assumptions of occupational therapy—the internal reward implicit in the intrinsic motivation for activity. Nonetheless, many of the techniques used in behavioral approaches (role modeling, shaping, chaining) have been applied successfully by occupational therapy professionals. We consider these later in the chapter, when we look at social skills training and Mosey's role acquisition model, which include concepts and techniques aligned with behavioral and cognitive behavioral theory.

Neuroscience theories focus on brain anatomy and chemistry. There is much to be learned about the effects of the brain's structure and metabolism on participation and performance of human activity. Because occupational therapy professionals are not trained to perform surgery or prescribe drugs, our contribution to this theory is our skill in observing and describing the client's functional behavior as it may be affected by neurosurgical or neurochemical interventions. Another aspect of neuroscience theory proposed by occupational therapy leaders since the time of Adolph Meyer is that participation in activity may affect brain metabolism, changing the client's behavior and emotion. We look at both aspects later in this chapter, with Allen's model of cognitive disabilities and sensory integration (SI) developed by A. Jean Ayres.

This chapter describes seven occupational therapy frames of reference and practice models that have been used successfully with persons with psychiatric disorders. They are as follows:

- **Development of adaptive skills** (also called recapitulation of ontogenesis) is based on developmental concepts.
- **Role acquisition** is based on developmental and behavioral concepts used together with *social skills training*, which is based primarily on behavioral concepts.

- **Cognitive disabilities model (CDM)** is based on neuroscience foundations.
- **Model of human occupation (MOHO)** is based on occupational behavior theory.
- **Person–Environment–Occupation (PEO) Model** is based on occupational behavior theory.
- **Ecology of Human Performance (EHP)** has a focus on the environment's role, mixed with the client-context relationship, toward task performance.
- **Sensory integration (SI)** is based on neuroscience foundations.

Each of these frames of reference and practice models uses occupation or activity in interventions, and each considers functional performance in occupation and daily life activities to be important to mental health. However, most of these models have features that limit their application to only some of the clients seen in mental health settings. The exceptions are MOHO, PEO, and EHP.

All these frames of reference and practice models embody the philosophical base and theoretical concepts of the occupational therapy profession. The philosophical base of our profession begins with the idea that all people want to participate in their desired occupations and in turn engagement in these occupations is connected to people's health and well-being. Occupations happen over the life span and are considered within various factors of environmental contexts and personal contexts. As occupational therapy professionals, we target people's therapeutic engagement, through various approaches, so that people can achieve meaningful occupational performance unique to their individual needs and concerns (11). Concepts at the center of our profession include the following (105):

- People should be considered from a holistic view and not in a reductionist manner.
- People are active beings.
- Occupation is essential and critical for people's well-being, health, and quality of life.
- Learning includes doing, thinking, feeling, and the experience itself.
- The occupational process includes the participation in occupation, which includes occupation used therapeutically as a means and an end within the occupational therapy process.
- People have the potential for change. Habits can be formed and adaptation, through a balance of work–rest–play, is possible.
- The client-centered approach allows for active participation from the client, family, and significant others.
- Humanistic values lay the foundation for occupational therapy and include: altruism, equality, freedom, justice, dignity, truth, and prudence (12).

These frames of reference and practice models also demonstrate the theoretical foundations of the occupational therapy profession (137). The therapeutic process is the planned purposeful activity of the client, which is connected to their occupational roles. Doing is purposeful, involves a relationship, and creates an end product. Analysis of activity allows for selection of intervention for the specific needs, interests, and abilities of the client. Therapeutic intervention addresses the client's need for a balance of life's occupational desires and responsibilities—leading to quality interactions with self, others, and the environment. These theoretical concepts include the following ideas:

- There is an innate and spontaneous urge, or drive, to explore one's world. People want to identify the roles they wish to have and to experience those roles within everyday activities and within the environment. This leads to achieving competence with these roles and satisfaction with their occupational behavior associated with these roles (73).
- The client interacts and engages with the environment—which includes relationships with people and objects, as well as patterns of interaction connected to time use and the impact of time connected to the activity itself. The environment includes family and others we socially interact with and to whom we have a civic responsibility.
- Occupation is based on functional skills and abilities gained in a developmentally sequential manner. Development occurs over time and simultaneously across multiple aspects of life (such as social, cultural, physical, psychological, and cognitive). Foundation skills allow for occupational performance and occupational performance allows for role fulfillment.
- Body systems and body functions must be intact or integrated for movement and learning and change to occur. When body systems and functions are not intact or integrated, an inability to perform desired occupations can occur. Trauma, injury, disease, and insufficiencies in opportunities and resources can cause disruption in development and satisfaction with occupational performance and occupational role fulfillment.
- Function is a by-product of organized occupation and dysfunction is a by-product of disorganized occupation. Occupation includes physical, social, cognitive, psychosocial, context, and environmental concerns. Occupational therapy can fill the gaps in development, assist with occupational adaptation to a client's disrupted or dissatisfied occupational performance situation, and help to increase a person's occupational function (73).

We call these frames of reference and practice models rather than theories because they are ways to organize our thinking about problems in clinical practice, just as a cardboard or plastic frame or model helps architects organize thoughts about the design of a physical space. As occupational therapy professionals, you will need to know the evaluation (the occupational therapist being responsible for administering the evaluation process and the occupational therapy assistant often being asked to assist with the administration of assessments) and intervention techniques, or what to do with the client under each frame of reference or practice model (13).

The focus of this text is on the intervention principles used with the frames of reference and practice models. Each frame of reference and practice model provides a powerful lens, offering a unique view of the client. Included with each frame of reference and practice model discussed here are intervention goals, based on the information presented about that frame of reference or practice model. This chapter attempts to use identity-first language regarding autism as preferred by the autistic community (130). Person-first language is used with other mental conditions in this chapter (1, 114).

DEVELOPMENT OF ADAPTIVE SKILLS

The **development of adaptive skills** model, which was conceived by Anne Cronin Mosey (101, 102) and is also called recapitulation of ontogenesis, means the stage-by-stage progression of development. Mosey (101) identifies six areas of adaptive skills and lists stages of development within each skill. The skills are as follows[2]:

- **Sensory integration skill.** The ability to receive, select, combine, and use information from the balance (vestibular), touch (tactile), and position (proprioceptive) senses to perform functional activities
- **Cognitive skill.** The ability to perceive, represent, and organize sensory information for thinking and problem-solving
- **Dyadic interaction skill.** The ability to participate in a variety of relationships involving one other person
- **Group interaction skill.** The ability to participate successfully in a variety of groups; generally, this means being able to act as a productive member of the group.
- **Self-identity skill.** The ability to recognize one's own assets and limitations and to perceive the self as worthwhile, self-directed, consistent, and reliable.
- **Sexual identity skill.** The ability to accept one's sexual nature as natural and pleasurable and to participate in a relatively long-term sexual relationship that considers the needs of both partners.

Each of these skills, acquired in a series of stages, follows a developmental sequence. In typical development and in occupational therapy, stages are encountered and mastered in order, and no stage can be skipped.

Table 3.1 gives the breakdown of stages for Mosey's developmental skills. Mosey gives much detail on cognitive skills. However, the reader should be aware that her terms and descriptions differ from those in the American Occupational Therapy Association's (AOTA) *Occupational Therapy Practice Framework: Domain and Process—Fourth Edition* (OTPF-4E) (14).

According to Mosey, the development of adaptive skills is a suitable practice model for clients who have not mastered all the stages of development appropriate for their chronologic

---

[2]These skills are paraphrased from Mosey (102). Mosey's earlier work included a seventh skill, drive-object skill. For a discussion of this skill, see Mosey, A. C. (1970*). Three frames of reference for mental health.* SLACK.

Table 3.1. Stages in the Development of Selected Adaptive Skills

Adaptive Skill	Age of Mastery
Sensory integration	
1. Ability to integrate tactile subsystems	0–3 mo
2. Ability to integrate primitive postural reflexes	3–9 mo
3. Maturation of righting and equilibrium reactions	9–12 mo
4. Ability to integrate two sides of the body, be aware of body parts and their relationship, and plan gross motor movements	1–2 yr
5. Ability to plan fine motor movements	2–3 yr
Cognition	
1. Ability to use inherent behavioral patterns for environmental interaction	0–1 mo
2. Ability to interrelate visual, manual, auditory, and oral responses	1–4 mo
3. Ability to attend to the environmental consequence of actions with interest, to represent objects in an exoceptual manner, to experience objects, to act on the basis of egocentric causality, and to seriate events in which self is involved	4–9 mo
4. Ability to establish a goal and carry out means, to recognize independent existence of objects, to interpret signs, to imitate new behavior, to apprehend influence of space, and to perceive other objects as partially causal	9–12 mo
5. Ability to use trial-and-error problem-solving, to use tools, to perceive variation in spatial positions, to seriate events in which self is not involved, and to perceive causality of other objects	12–18 mo
6. Ability to represent objects in an image manner, to make believe, to infer a cause given its effect, to act on the basis of combined spatial relations, to attribute omnipotence to others, and to perceive objects as permanent in time and space	18 mo–2 yr
7. Ability to represent objects in an endoceptual manner, to differentiate between thought and action, and to recognize the need for causal sources	2–5 yr
8. Ability to represent objects in a denotative manner, to perceive viewpoint of others, and to decenter	6–7 yr
9. Ability to represent objects in a connotative manner, to use formal logic, and to work in realm of hypothetical	11–13 yr
Dyadic interaction	
1. Ability to enter into trusting familial relationships	8–10 mo
2. Ability to enter into association relationships	3–5 yr
3. Ability to interact in an authority relationship	5–7 yr
4. Ability to interact in a chum relationship	10–14 yr
5. Ability to enter into a peer, authority relationship	15–17 yr
6. Ability to enter into an intimate relationship	18–25 yr
7. Ability to engage in a nurturing relationship	20–30 yr
Group interaction	
1. Ability to participate in a parallel group	18–24 mo
2. Ability to participate in a project group	2–4 yr
3. Ability to participate in an egocentric-cooperative group	5–7 yr
4. Ability to participate in a cooperative group	9–12 yr
5. Ability to participate in a mature group	15–18 yr
Self-identity	
1. Ability to perceive self as worthy	9–12 mo
2. Ability to perceive assets and limitations of self	11–15 yr
3. Ability to perceive self as self-directed	20–25 yr
4. Ability to perceive self as a productive, contributing member of a social system	30–35 yr
5. Ability to perceive self as having an autonomous identity	35–50 yr
6. Ability to perceive one's own aging process and ultimate death as part of life cycle	45–60 yr

(continued)

Table 3.1. Stages in the Development of Selected Adaptive Skills (*continued*)

Adaptive Skill	Age of Mastery
Sexual identity	
1. Ability to accept and act according to one's pregenital sexual nature	4–5 yr
2. Ability to accept sexual maturation as positive growth	12–16 yr
3. Ability to give and receive sexual gratification	18–25 yr
4. Ability to enter into a sustained sexual relationship characterized by the mutual satisfaction of sexual needs	20–30 yr
5. Ability to accept the sex-related physiologic changes that occur as a natural part of the aging process	35–50 yr

Exoceptual representation, memory of stimuli as an action or motor response; *egocentric causality*, belief that one's own actions are completely responsible for object response; *endoceptual representation*, memory of stimuli in terms of felt experience; *denotative representation*, memory of stimuli in terms of words that stand for or name objects; *connotative representation*, memory of stimuli in terms of a more complex set of associations that are associated with an object; *decenter*, distinguish several features or characteristics of an object (be flexible enough to see it from several perspectives).
Adapted with permission from Mosey, A. C. (1987). *Psychosocial components of occupational therapy*. Raven.

age. Mosey specifically states, however, that this model does not directly address performance in occupation. The focus is instead on the general skills and behaviors needed to negotiate one's environment successfully (101); these skills in turn support performance in occupation. The aim of this model is to help the person master, step-by-step, occupation-supporting skills not yet acquired. Four basic concepts guide the use of this model[3]:

1. *The occupational therapy professional must provide an environment that facilitates growth.* The details and features of the environment depend on the particular subskill. For example, if the subskill of perceiving the self as self-directed is the focus, the clients must be given freedom to make their own decisions and to explore a variety of options. This is best practiced outside the clinic-based intervention setting, where the options of everyday life can be found in ample supply. A simulated experience, such as an arts and crafts group, is less likely to develop this skill, regardless of the variety of crafts available.

2. *The subskills are mastered in order.* This follows from item number 1; unless clients have already come to recognize and appreciate their assets and limitations, they have great difficulty making choices in an unstructured environment. One cannot develop a sense of self-direction until one understands one's own capacities and limitations.

3. *Subskills from different areas may be addressed at the same time, provided they are normally acquired at the same chronologic age.* Thus, the person needing to develop a sense of their assets and limitations might also work on cooperative group skills but not as easily on mature group skills, which depend on learning both self-assessment and cooperative skills.

4. *The client's intrinsic motivation or desire for mastery of the subskills must be engaged.* Caution must be taken by the occupational therapy professional to be exquisitely

sensitive to evidence of the client's motivation or lack thereof. For example, anxiety and frustration may suggest that the environment and activities are not motivating or suitable for the person at this time. When the proper environment, activities, and subskill behaviors are present, the person appears engaged, involved, and interested.

Case Example

Judi has been a client at a suburban community day treatment center for 2 months. She is a 27-year-old unemployed high school graduate who has taken some courses at a local community college but has not declared a major. She has worked in the past, but never for more than a few weeks at a time and has held many kinds of jobs—warehouse package handler, grocery store clerk, lifeguard, assembly line worker, and administrative professional. She has been hospitalized twice for suicide attempts and has attended several different outpatient programs. She lives at home with her widowed mother; they are financially comfortable with the pension and life insurance income from Judi's father, who was a business executive.

Judi's physical appearance is clean and her hair is well brushed. Her clothing is new and fashionable, but not well coordinated with color selection. Judi appears to relate well to other clients in social situations but often says that she feels left out and that others dislike her. Alternately, she reports that she feels superior to everyone else and totally inadequate. She has also had problems relating to staff members. Often, she seems to agree with a staff suggestion but fails to follow through. At other times, she argues with staff over every detail and has several times left the center very abruptly and angrily.

After interviewing Judi and her mother, reviewing her record, and administering a task skills assessment (done by the occupational therapy assistant), the occupational therapist summarizes the findings on the *Adaptive Skills Developmental Chart* (101). The following subskills are targeted for development in occupational therapy:

- **Dyadic interaction skill**: subskill 3, the ability to interact in an authority relationship

---

[3]Mosey lists these as three concepts, combining the second and third into one.

- **Group interaction skill**: subskill 3, the ability to participate in an egocentric-cooperative group
- **Self-identity skill**: subskill 2, the ability to perceive the assets and limitations of the self

Because the first two of these are normally learned at the same chronologic age, 5 to 7 years old, they were the first to be addressed. Judi agreed to participate in the jewelry production group, an egocentric-cooperative group that meets three afternoons a week for 2.5 hours each time. She was also to meet weekly with Paulette, the occupational therapy assistant, to review progress in the group and to discuss expectations and goals. She was expected to sign in each day in Paulette's office on her arrival at the treatment center.

The activity purpose of the jewelry group was to produce items for sale in the center's gift shop. The goal was to help the members develop egocentric-cooperative skills. Design and production decisions were delegated to the group members, who needed some assistance to get started.

Evelyn, an occupational therapy assistant assigned to lead this group, provided suggestions and guided the group in making their decisions and generating new ideas. Because group members lacked experience in estimating needs, ordering supplies, and pricing items for sale, Evelyn shared resources and experiences with them and encouraged them to look online at prices for similar items. As the group became more confident and as members learned more skills, Evelyn began to step back from the group and let them work things out by themselves. As needed, she intervened in a nonauthoritarian manner to help group members recognize each other's needs for approval and for respect from other group members. For example, when Judi complained that she never got a chance to participate in design work, Evelyn helped her problem-solve and practice how to ask for it from the group. Judi was surprised and pleased when they agreed to give her a turn.

In her weekly sessions with Judi, Paulette developed initial rapport and encouraged Judi to identify areas she would like to improve in the jewelry group. As trust was developed within their relationship, Paulette would provide feedback on Judi's skills to encourage further development. Paulette noticed that Judi was frequently late, both for individual sessions and for attendance at the center, but Paulette made little mention of this at first. As a trusting relationship developed, Paulette provided feedback on Judi's lateness and how it impacted herself and others in the group. Paulette used this opportunity to allow Judi to express her feelings about the constructive feedback. Initially resentful, Judi gradually accepted this, and was able to collaborate with Paulette to come up with solutions. She asked to be placed in a second group, the clerical production group, so that she could work on computer and office skills. Paulette considered it reasonable for Judi at the time and thought it would give her the experience of working with another authority figure. She recommended it to the occupational therapist.

The case example of Judi shows how the development of adaptive skills model can be applied by the occupational therapy professional in both individual sessions and with

group activities. The example takes place in a long-term community setting, where a client could comfortably attend for many months. This lengthy period is necessary for the development of these adaptive skills, which are ideally learned over quite a long period in the child's life. Therefore, this developmental approach may not be as effective in short-term settings.

The development of adaptive skills model targets client functions and performance skills as described in the OTPF-4E (14).

In settings using the development of adaptive skills model, the occupational therapy professional can be highly instrumental in providing interventions that help clients progress with performance skills solidly connected to occupational participation. Occupational therapy professionals wishing to apply this practice model should obtain regular mentorship in its use and would benefit from further study of Mosey's work (100-102). Box 3.1 provides examples of development of adaptive skills occupational therapy goals to use with clients.

BOX 3.1 Adaptive Skills Intervention Goals

Aim of Intervention

Adaptive skills are acquired in a development sequence. Can address different area subskills at the same time. Adaptive skills are mastered step-by-step.

Does not directly address occupational performance.

These are the general occupation-supporting skills and behaviors needed to successfully negotiate one's environment.

The occupational therapy professional must provide an environment that facilitates growth.

The client's intrinsic motivation or desire for mastery of the subskills must be engaged.

Goals

Client will explore motivating activities to increase success with adaptive developmental skill of _____ for success with completing occupational activity of _____ with _____* (add needed amount or type of assistance) and _____^ within _____***.

Client will identify adaptive developmental skill abilities and limitations for success with completing occupational activity of _____ with _____* (add needed amount or type of assistance) and _____^ within _____**.

Client will complete adaptive developmental skill of _____ for success with completing occupational activity of _____ with _____* (add needed amount or type of assistance) and _____** within _____***.

* guidance, written prompt, written directions, cue, direct supervision/contact, indirect supervision/contact
** structured environment, everyday environment of _____, setup of activity, participation of a peer, no peer involvement, no direct involvement from practitioner, assistive technology device, self-monitoring, self-talk
^ use of inventory checklist tool, self-reporting assessment tool, self-reflection
*** number of attempts, number of sessions, number of weeks

Concepts Summary

1. The occupational therapy professional must provide an environment that facilitates growth as defined by the subskill or subskills to be developed.
2. Subskills are mastered in order.
3. Subskills from different areas may be addressed at the same time, provided they are normally acquired at the same chronologic age.
4. The client's intrinsic motivation, or desire for mastery of the subskills, must be engaged.

VOCABULARY REVIEW

Cognitive skill
The ability to perceive, represent, and organize sensory information for thinking and solving problems

Dyadic interaction skill
The ability to participate in a variety of relationships involving one other person

Group interaction skill
The ability to participate successfully in a variety of groups; generally, this means being able to act as a productive member of the group.[4]

Recapitulation of ontogenesis
Mosey's title for this practice model; refers to the return to or review of early stages of development

Self-identity skill
The ability to recognize one's own assets and limitations and to perceive the self as worthwhile, self-directed, consistent, and reliable

Sensory integration skill
The ability to receive, select, combine, and use information from the balance (vestibular), touch (tactile), and position (proprioceptive) senses to perform functional activities

Sexual identity skill
The ability to accept one's sexual nature as natural and pleasurable and to participate in a relatively long-term sexual relationship that considers the needs of both partners

ROLE ACQUISITION AND SOCIAL SKILLS TRAINING

Role acquisition, a term coined by Mosey (100-102), is the learning of the daily life, work, and leisure skills that enable one to participate in roles that are social and/or productive. Examples are student, worker, volunteer, family member, leisure participant, retiree, and many others.

Success in roles depends to some extent on social skills. Social skills training refers to the teaching of interpersonal skills needed to relate to other people effectively in situations as varied as dating and applying for a job (27). Role acquisition and social skills training focus on here-and-now behaviors—how the person is functioning in the present. For example, Mark, a 52-year-old man, has been in institutions for much

of his life. In institutions, his needs for food, clothing, and shelter are taken care of by the staff. To live in the community successfully, Mark must acquire daily living skills, such as doing the laundry and shopping for food, and social skills, such as how to talk to cashiers and neighbors.

Because both role acquisition and social skills training use techniques derived from behavioral and especially from cognitive behavioral theory, the reader may find it helpful to review those sections of Chapter 2 before proceeding further. Role acquisition and social skills training view behavior as motivated from within. The client's needs, wants, and goals are seen as a starting point for clinical intervention. Role acquisition is based on developmental concepts to explain the sequence and methods by which skills are acquired (100).

Role Acquisition

The aim of intervention under the role acquisition model is to help the person gain the specific skills needed to function in the occupational and social roles they have chosen. Clients also need to develop an awareness of what they are doing and why. This awareness must extend to the environmental context, with an understanding of what is expected and appropriate for that context. To continue with the example of Mark, although he needs to learn ways to care for his clothing, he also must develop a sense that caring for his clothing will affect how other people see him as a neighbor and member of the community. What Mark believes and understands about what he is doing is just as important as his physical actions. (The reader may note here a similarity to cognitive behavioral theory.)

Role acquisition is based at least in part on the idea that all behavior is learned. By extension, what has been learned can be unlearned, and new behaviors can be learned to take their place. What has not been learned previously can be learned for the first time. Occupational therapy professionals have long been concerned with how best to help people learn and with discovering under what circumstances learning is most likely to occur. Their collected experience and wisdom can be translated into the following set of 10 principles for planning and providing intervention (22, 102, 111).

Principle 1: Client Participation

The person should participate in identifying problems and goals for intervention and in addressing their own progress (22, 102). This conveys the idea that clients are ultimately responsible for themselves and that their ideas about what they need are important. Not all clients can participate equally in this. Some can tell the occupational therapy professional exactly what their problems and goals are and spontaneously assess their own progress during intervention, but this is rare. Others have such limited awareness of their own deficiencies and needs that developing this awareness itself is a goal of intervention. An example is an individual with schizophrenia who is experiencing active hallucination episodes and is currently unhoused. They have adopted a costume of twisted and knotted rags held together with duct tape. Persuading this

---

[4]Mosey's levels of group interaction are further explained in Chapter 16.

person to give up the outfit can be quite difficult. Improving basic hygiene and grooming is a goal the occupational therapist chooses because it is necessary for community living and the person appears unable to meet this need. Obviously, the occupational therapy professional should try to explain it and to engage the person's interest and motivation.

Involving clients in identifying problems and setting goals can be structured into the first meetings with them. From the start, the occupational therapy professional should try to learn the client's view of the situation and what they want out of the intervention. Checklists and questionnaires that the client can complete and score independently are useful. Also, the occupational therapist can present the results of the evaluation process to the client and incorporate the client's responses into the intervention plan. An example is sharing the results of a vocational interest assessment with a client who is unemployed and discussing the need for further assessment of skills and aptitudes before a training program is selected. If the client wants to try a training program before the full evaluation process is finished, a compromise plan can be arranged.

Some clients have a general view of what they want to achieve but little sense of the steps they must take to get there. An example is a person in their early 20s with an intellectual disability who wants to have an intimate partner relationship. Although they can identify their goal, they can partner with the occupational therapy professional to create goals with intermediate steps. These may include learning to share interests with others and the social expectations of a date. Once they appreciate how these skills are connected to their goal of having an intimate partner, they may be more interested in learning them.

Some clients are preoccupied with an idealized role. An example is the harried parent of three preschool children who wants to have a perfect home, picture-perfect children, an athletic figure, and dinner on the table at exactly 6:30 PM every evening. Nothing less will satisfy their image of what a parent should be; consequently, they are frequently tense and depressed. In this situation, the occupational therapy professional helps the client examine their goals and reason through their implications, perhaps in a discussion group with others.

Occasionally, a person appears apathetic and unmotivated to identify any goals at all or chooses ones that present no challenge. An example is a 34-year-old client who wants to live with their parents and collect public assistance rather than return to their own apartment and their job as a content analyst in a law office. If the person cannot imagine suitable goals, the occupational therapist must. Furthermore, the occupational therapist may have to cajole and persuade the person to become involved in activities at all. Helping clients take the first steps toward involvement in occupation when they feel hopeless and incompetent can dramatically improve the quality of the person's life and their motivation for rehabilitation. It is important that occupational therapy professionals recognize this responsibility and be willing to be assertive with the client in such a situation.

Getting clients to assess their own progress, or lack thereof, is equally important. For decades, the treating professional was seen as all-powerful and the client as a passive receiver of treatment. This view has gradually shifted and given way to a more consumer-driven health care model. Older clients and those with cognitive disabilities may still depend on the psychiatric system to make their decisions for them. In occupational therapy, the client, by engaging in occupation, is carrying out their own plan. The occupational therapy professional is responsible for making sure clients know what they are supposed to be doing and why. But clients benefit from developing attention to their performance and their feelings about the activities in which they participate. Being able to assess one's own reaction and to reflect on how an activity feels, how competent one feels doing it, and whether it achieves what one set out to do are skills that help one maintain a balanced, flexible, and satisfying life.

Principle 2: Personalized Goals

Choose goals and activities that reflect the client's interests, personal and cultural values, and present and future life roles (22, 102). No two people are alike, and the occupational therapy professional must not assume that they can predict what is best for the client. Information about the client's interests and values can be obtained through interview or assessment (such as the *Modified Interest Checklist*) and sometimes from the medical record or from family members.

Clients' values may be shaped in part by their ethnicity, social class, and culture. Ethnicity refers to person's heritage and national origin, for example, Native American, Uzbek, Polish, Jamaican, Korean, Mexican, and Brazilian. Social class refers to the person's rank or status within the larger society. This rank is based in part on educational level and family background and in part on vocation and personal wealth. For example, those whose earnings fall below the poverty level are generally considered to be in the lowest social class, but a Harvard-educated farm worker from a wealthy family would be considered upper class even though their earnings fall in the poverty range.

Culture is a complex and constantly changing concept that includes the customs, beliefs, and objects associated with specific groups of people (91). As in all health professions, occupational therapy professionals need to recognize their limitations regarding cultural knowledge. Each ethnic group has many cultural variations, because family traditions and new customs acquired from association with members of other cultural groups are often quite individual. Consider, for example, the situation of American Jews, who may be Orthodox, Conservative, or Reform in their religious practices; some are so distant from Jewish tradition that they have a Christmas tree in their homes, exchange Christmas gifts, and go to work on Jewish holidays such as Yom Kippur. Likewise, Black men from the West Indies can have expectations of their wives that are different from those of Black men born in the United States.

In addition to the specific cultural group to which the client belongs, the values and trends of the larger culture must be considered. The best contemporary occupational therapy practice reflects this by involving clients in occupations that are meaningful today and that are meaningful to that person. Weaving, basketry, and copper enameling were adopted by occupational therapy professionals when the practice of these crafts by artisans was diminishing and when home use of crafts was advocated to preserve them. Arts and crafts have risen and fallen in popularity over the years. Scrapbooking, quilting, friendship bracelets, and cooking were popular in the second decade of the 21st century—aided by videos and other resources available through the Internet.

Nonetheless, crafts will not be the primary modality for many clients. Instead, the occupational therapy professional must identify and help the client engage in occupations that are personally meaningful, whether these be gardening; using a computer, smart phone, or video game system; performing yoga or tai chi; caring for pets; or managing time and a schedule.

The person's present and future life roles also influence the choice of activity. Activities used in occupational therapy should be geared to helping clients acquire needed skills and making them competent at something they need to do in everyday life. The best activities are those that will enable the person to handle the everyday demands of life. For example, a high school student hospitalized for a brief period will probably benefit most from keeping up with schoolwork and learning better notetaking and study skills.

Principle 3: Ability-Based Goals

Choose goals and activities that provide a realistic challenge but are consistent with the client's present level of ability (22, 102). Some people who have psychiatric disorders are unable to perform their usual occupations as effectively as they once did. Their thinking may be slow or confused; they may hallucinate (see or hear things that are not there); they may have to make a conscious effort to perform simple motions; and they may have incorrect ideas (delusions) and be so preoccupied with their own concerns that they have trouble attending to what is going on around them. Nonetheless, they may expect themselves to accomplish tasks that are beyond their current capability; they may see less-demanding tasks presented by the occupational therapy professional as a sign that others think very little of them. The occupational therapy professional should express hope and optimism that the person will recover and will be able to accomplish more in the future. At the same time, the occupational therapy professional should explain the purpose of the activity and its relation to the client's condition and goals.

Activities should require some effort from clients; otherwise, they may just go through the motions without becoming intrinsically involved. The activities should not be so simple and routine that clients do not have to pay attention to what they are doing. On the other hand, they should not require such intense effort that the person quickly becomes tired or frustrated.

Principle 4: Increasing Challenges

Increase challenges and demands as the person's capacity increases. At the beginning, many clients can work for only short periods or on only simple activities. Positive support from the occupational therapy professional may be needed to encourage the client's first efforts. After a person feels comfortable and reasonably successful, they generally are willing and ready to try more difficult tasks. Some improve only slowly, whereas others improve so rapidly that they get bored or tune out unless quickly given new challenges.

Principle 5: Natural Progression

Present skills in their natural developmental sequence (22). All skills are developed in a predictable direction from simple to complex. This is true of motor skills, which begin as gross, generalized motions and progress gradually to finely coordinated movements. Similarly, the ability to interact in a group starts with being able to tolerate other people and only gradually develops into a varied repertoire of ways of relating to those people. In both cases, there are many steps along the way to full mastery of the skill. It is important to keep this principle in mind when teaching skills to clients. Moving from simple to complex and following a natural, step-by-step sequence strengthens learning because the skills are built on a solidly developed foundation.

Principle 6: Client Knowledge

Clients should always know what they are supposed to be learning and why. The occupational therapy professional should orient the person to each new activity, never assuming the person sees the connection between the immediate activity and the intervention goal. Orientation should include an explanation of why the activity is being done, what steps are involved, how long the activity will take, and what is required for successful performance. Someone who has never had a job and who is placed in a prevocational setting may have little idea of what behaviors are expected on the job. Unless the importance of being on time for work is explained, the person may resist or ignore the occupational therapy professional's emphasis on punctuality. In addition, if asked to perform unfamiliar tasks, such as entering data into a spreadsheet, the process must be explained to the person.

Principle 7: Client Awareness

Clients should be made aware of the effects of their actions (22). Many clients lack the skill or perspective necessary to assess their own performance; if so, the occupational therapy professional must do so for them. All people need to recognize their actions have consequences and those consequences hold meaning and importance (102). You can appreciate this yourself just by thinking of how eagerly you await the results of tests, especially those in which you are uncertain of your performance. Similarly, clients need to know whether they have achieved, to what extent, and how they can improve. If the person seems unsure about what to do next and does not comment on their own success or failure, the occupational therapy professional has ample evidence that the client needs feedback and guidance from someone else.

Some individuals with disabilities may make slow progress, and improvements may be so slight as to be barely perceptible. Here the occupational therapy professional must be especially alert to small changes in behavior so that they can be rewarded immediately. Consider, for example, the person whose social anxiety is such that they keep eyes downcast and fail to make eye contact with others. To increase this person's confidence during interactions, the occupational therapy professional should respond positively to even the smallest gains made in social interactions.

There are many ways of responding to a client's efforts and giving feedback. One is through the systematic use of reinforcement, as discussed in Chapter 2. Occupational therapy professionals need to be aware of their emotional reactions to the client and of the verbal and nonverbal responses they communicate. Tolerance, acceptance, positive support, and a sense of humor are extremely important in motivating people. At the same time, the occupational therapy professional must remain in a professional role and maintain boundaries with the client during the therapeutic relationship. Because of the powerful effects of the occupational therapy professional's reaction on the client's motivation and future behavior, it will be discussed separately in Chapter 15.

Principle 8: Practice Makes Perfect

Skills must be practiced repeatedly and then applied to new situations (22, 102). There is truth to the old saying, "Practice makes perfect"; and although we do not expect our clients to achieve perfection in everything they attempt, we do want to make sure they know a skill well enough to use it in the future. To ensure this, the occupational therapy professional must provide opportunities for clients to practice until they are comfortable. A single correct performance cannot be taken as evidence that someone has learned a skill; for instance, if Mark does the laundry correctly today, this does not guarantee that he can do so next week. Performing a skill repeatedly strengthens learning and helps transform skills into habits.

Once a skill or habit is well established through practice, variations and shortcuts can be attempted. It is crucial that the client be encouraged to practice new skills and habits in their own environment and that someone monitor the efforts there. When, for example, Mark attempts to do the laundry at home, he may discover that the machines in his local laundromat operate differently from the one on which he learned. If Mark has trouble asking others for help and is unable to solve problems on his own, he may give up on doing his laundry altogether.

Practicing a skill in a variety of situations helps the client see that what works in one situation can work in others. This is called generalization. For example, assembling the necessary supplies before beginning an activity is a skill that works just as well in studying for a test as in doing the laundry. People can be helped to apply learning from one situation to another similar situation by being involved in varied activities and environments. In addition, this variety can help the person learn that a given behavior or skill does not work in all situations. This ability to recognize what behavior is appropriate or effective for a given situation is called *discrimination*. For example, according to societal standards, athletic shoes and sweats should be worn for athletic activities and not for a job interview.

Principle 9: Parts of the Whole

If a task is too complex or time consuming to learn all at one time, teach one part at a time, but always do or show the whole activity. Many tasks that clients need to learn are long, complicated multistep operations. Doing the laundry is an example. The major steps are sorting the clothes by color and type of fabric, assembling laundry supplies (including knowing which laundry products to use and in which order) and money, getting to the laundry area, loading the clothes in the washer, inserting the coins or card, adding the detergent and perhaps bleach, running the machine, unloading the washer, loading the dryer, inserting the payment and turning on the dryer after selecting the appropriate settings, removing the dry clothes, and folding or hanging and/or ironing them. Further refinements include using spot removers and fabric softeners, using net bags for lingerie, clipping sock pairs together, adjusting water and dryer temperature, and using special cycles on the washer. The client must also learn which clothes can be washed in a machine and which must be dry-cleaned or washed by hand.

The most effective way to help someone learn a complex task like this is to go through the entire process with the person many times. However, because of other demands on an occupational therapy professional's time, this is often not possible, and a complex task can seem overwhelming if presented all at once. The recommended approach is to teach only what can be learned in a single session—for example, folding clothes immediately after removing them from the dryer. Taught in isolation, this step may not make much sense to the client but connecting this step to the rest of the activity will demonstrate why it is important. This may be done in a variety of ways.

One method for showing how a step or subskill relates to the larger complex activity of which it is a part is to talk it through. In this example, it would necessitate a brief verbal overview of the whole process of doing the laundry, emphasizing why, when, and how the clothes should be folded. To maintain the person's interest and attention is important to keep the overview brief and to the point. Because some people have trouble following spoken descriptions and directions, other learning aids such as posters, printed handouts, samples of how a project looks at various stages, photos, or video recordings can also be used. Chaining, as described in Chapter 2, can be incorporated with these techniques.

Another technique is to simplify the activity by removing all but the most basic steps. For example, starting with a load of mixed-color wash-and-wear items in a washer with only one temperature setting, using only detergent (omitting all other laundry products), and using a dryer with a single temperature setting focus attention on the essential key steps of the activity and reduces confusion.

Activities make most sense when they are presented in context. For example, a makeup class for an adolescent becomes more motivating if it is followed by a dance or other activity for which makeup is appropriate. Similarly, a trip to an actual destination enhances learning how to use the bus or subway and doing the laundry when the client's clothes are dirty makes more sense than just washing things to show how it is done (22).

Principle 10: Imitation

People learn how to do things by imitating others. It is easy to see this in small children, who mimic their parents' actions, words, and even intonations. The tendency to learn through imitation continues throughout life; watching how someone does something and then trying to do the same thing is familiar to all of us. This is no less true for people with mental disorders, but with an important difference: in some cases, their experience may have included few good role models. Consider the person who was abused by their parents when they were a child; this is the only behavior they are familiar with, and one that they are likely to repeat when they have children of their own. To learn other ways of parenting, they must be exposed to better role models. In a child-care skills group, they can learn how to manage their own feelings, reduce stress, and communicate effectively by watching other parents and imitating what they do.

Clients often look to staff for role models. Being a good role model is demanding. It requires that the occupational therapy professional embody the qualities they are trying to get the client to develop. A tense occupational therapy professional cannot help someone relax, and a nonassertive occupational therapy professional is likely to have trouble developing assertiveness in their clients because they lack it themselves. This is discussed further in Chapter 15.

Fellow clients can also serve as models for imitation. Encouraging a person to observe and copy the behavior of another client reaps a double reward because it increases the confidence of the one being imitated. Clients can also be taught to imitate positive role models from their past. For example, a childhood teacher or a favorite uncle may possess characteristics useful in the present; in that case, the occupational therapy professional helps the person remember and focus on the model while attempting the activity. Box 3.2 provides examples of role acquisition occupational therapy goals to use with clients.

BOX 3.2 Role Acquisition Intervention Goals

Aim of Intervention

The learning of daily life, work, and leisure skills

Enables client's need to fulfill social roles and productive roles.

Focus on here-and-now behaviors.

Use behavioral and cognitive behavioral principles.

Start with the client's needs, wants, and goals.

Develop awareness of what it is the client is doing and why.

Develop awareness of what is expected and appropriate to do in the environmental context.

Goals

Client will identify role acquisition goals for success with completing occupational activity of _____with _____* (add needed amount or type of assistance) and _____^ within _____***.

Client will complete role acquisition activity of _____ for success with completing occupational activity of _____ with _____* (add needed amount or type of assistance) and _____** within _____***.

* guidance, written prompt, written directions, verbal directions, cue, direct supervision/contact, indirect supervision/contact
** structured environment, everyday environment of _____, setup of activity, participation of a peer, no peer involvement, no direct involvement from practitioner, observation of staff, observation of peers, imitation of past mentor, assistive technology device, self-monitoring, self-talk, _____ amount of effort, step-by-step progression/complexity of task, developmental progression of ability, increased/decreased complexity of task, remedial practice sessions, adapted practice, rehearsal, practice in varying environments, sample, whole to part teaching-learning process, reinforcement of _____, use of homework activity
^ use of inventory checklist tool, self-reporting assessment tool, self-reflection, realistic discussion of performance patterns, connection to personal/cultural values, connection to present/future roles
*** number of attempts, number of sessions, number of weeks

Social Skills Training

As mentioned previously, social skills training refers to the teaching of interpersonal skills needed to relate effectively to other people. Some persons with mental disorders have problems in this area. They may fail to look at others or fail to reply to questions asked of them, or they may produce speech that is too loud or may place themselves too close to others or may not regulate what they say to others. Such behavior is a serious disadvantage when applying for (and keeping) a job, asking someone for a date, meeting new people, or just shopping for food or clothing. Figure 3.1 illustrates someone who strongly desires relationships with others but does not understand the rules of social conduct that lead to mutually positive interactions.

Social skills are the readily known and clearly identifiable actions and behaviors that people use when interacting and communicating with others. Social participation is completed to stay interactive and connected with one's

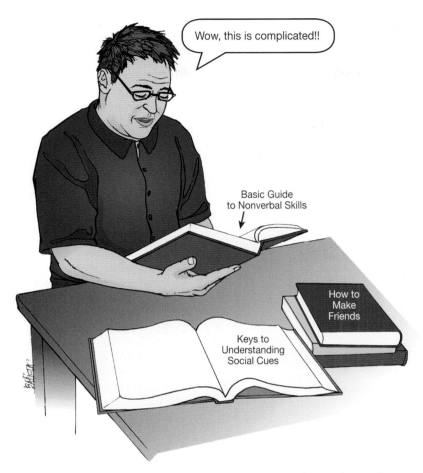

Figure 3.1. Some People Find Social Behavior Very Hard to Understand.

environment. By performing and interacting skillfully with others, a person can have their interpersonal needs met (68). Others respond to the way a person acts, and the more awareness and regulation a person has over their social behavior, the more success they are likely to have in conversing and working with other people.

Kelly (68, p. 3) defines social skills as "those identifiable, learned behaviors that individuals use in interpersonal situations to obtain or to maintain reinforcement from their environment." In other words, social skills help us get what we want from others. Others respond to the way we act, and the more awareness and regulation a person has over their social behavior, the more success they are likely to have in conversing and working with other people.

Social skills have been classified in many ways. One way is to group the behaviors that are needed in different situations. For example, in a job interview, the necessary skills include looking (eye contact), expressing emotion appropriate to the situation, producing speech that is clear and audible, matching the language of others, listening, replying to questions, heeding the topic under discussion, disclosing one's qualifications positively, acknowledging the other person in the conversation, and requesting relevant information from others.

Another way of grouping skills is by content or purpose. This approach recognizes that the same social skills may apply in a variety of interactions; for instance, showing interest is important in friendship and dating as well as on the job. Generically, social skills can be classified into four groups (127):

- self-expressive skills,
- other-enhancing skills,
- assertive skills, and
- communication skills.

Table 3.2 states the specific examples of skills associated with each of these four groups.

Assessment of social skills is performed by an occupational therapist. However, the occupational therapy assistant has many opportunities to observe the client and can contribute to a discussion of the person's social skills. The occupational therapy assistant may also be asked to participate in or even take a lead role in social skills training (intervention to remedy social skills deficits).

A social skills training session usually consists of four distinct phases: motivation, demonstration, practice, and feedback. These phases are probably already quite familiar to occupational therapy professional students, as they are

Table 3.2. Social Skills for Each Type of Group Purpose	
Social Skills Groups	
Self-expressive skills: disclosing feelings and opinions disclosing positive things about oneself disclosing one's values and beliefs	*Other-enhancing skills:* giving compliments smiling and expressing interest empathizing with others by giving support and encouragement
Assertive skills: questioning and making requests disagreeing with another's opinion or statement of fact refusing requests questioning another's behavior setting limits on another's aggressiveness	*Communication skills:* matching language of others by controlling the tone and quality of one's voice producing speech by clearly articulating words choosing the proper words for a situation

Adapted from social skills group purpose concepts from Stein, F. (1982). A current review of the behavioral frame of reference and its application to occupational therapy. *Occupational Therapy in Mental Health, Occupational Therapy in Mental Health, 2*(4), 35–62. OTPF-4E language from American Occupational Therapy Association. (2020). Occupational therapy practice framework: Domain and process—Fourth edition. *American Journal of Occupational Therapy, 74*(Suppl. 2), 1–87.

not unlike those used in the traditional occupational therapy method of instructing someone in an activity (126).

- **Motivation** consists of identifying the behavior to be learned and explaining why it is important. The occupational therapy professional should give examples of the desired behavior and discuss why it is relevant to the person's goals. If the client can state reasons it is important, so much the better.
- In the **demonstration phase**, the occupational therapy professional shows the person how the behavior is performed. Methods include modeling by the occupational therapy professional, role-playing by the occupational therapy professional and another person (client or staff person), and recorded models. Regardless of the method, during this phase the person watches and observes but does not attempt the behavior until the practice phase.
- **Practice** can be structured to improve learning. One way is to ask the person to rehearse the desired behavior by talking it through. This can reduce anxiety before the actual performance. For example, if the target behavior is asking relevant questions on a job interview, the person would be asked to identify some questions first. Then they might try the questions out in role-playing with another client.
- Additionally, the client can write down what they intend to say or ask. These items can be ordered, or prioritized, based on the practice situation. An innovative way for the person to remember identified questions or statements is to use cue words or phrases that could be placed on a physical or an electronic tablet they will use to take notes during the job interview.

- **Feedback** is given at the end of the intervention session and summarizes what the person has learned. Feedback also may focus attention on what is to be learned next. Throughout the session, the occupational therapy professional should also provide immediate feedback on the client's performance. It is important that the feedback be immediate and specific, emphasizing positive aspects of the person's performance and providing concrete details about how to improve it. To illustrate, following the client's role-playing of interviewing for a job, the occupational therapy professional might say, "You appeared confident and your answers to the questions were brief and to the point. Some interviewers would like people to show enthusiasm. Would you like to work on this skill?"

Training in social skills should involve not only learning the appropriate behaviors but also learning to perceive when and where they are appropriate (80). Social perception requires reading subtle variations in others' behavior and in the immediate environment. For example, if two people are seated in a room conversing with each other and a third person comes in, several things can happen, depending on the situation and who is involved. One of the seated people might look at the entering person, stand up, and greet them. This would be good manners in many situations, especially if the entering person has authority (eg, is the boss or an older person). However, if the scene is a student lounge and all three people are students who know each other well and have spent all day together, it may appear rude or strange for one person to stand up, in effect concluding the conversation.

WHAT'S THE EVIDENCE?

Development and Validation of Vellore Assessment of Social Performance Among Clients With Chronic Mental Illness

This study reviewed the use of an assessment for verbal and nonverbal social skills and for receptive, processing, and expressive social competence. The assessment tool was tested for psychometric measures of reliability and validity. It was also tested for its correlation with psychopathology. The *Vellore Assessment of Social Performance* was developed to provide a client's baseline performance, as well as to assess progression with social skills and social competence. The benefits and limitations of its use can be found in the study: Thamaraiselvi, S., Priyadarshini, A., Arisalya, N., Samuel, R., & Jacob, K. S. (2020). Development and validation of Vellore Assessment of Social Performance among clients with chronic mental illness. *Indian Journal of Psychiatry, 62*(2), 121–130.

To summarize, social skills training is a structured approach for teaching interpersonal behaviors. It fits within the general framework of role acquisition and uses behavioral concepts and techniques. Both role acquisition and social skills training can be used as intervention approaches within occupation-based practice models; both approaches recognize that the occupational therapy professional must first motivate the client and that skills and habits are acquired through learning within a social environment. Both approaches assume that if the input from the environment is changed, the client's behavior will change. The case example of Howard illustrates the application of both role acquisition and social skills training.

Case Example

Howard is a 45-year-old single man who lives with his widowed mother in a two-bedroom apartment in a low-income neighborhood of a large city. Howard was first hospitalized at age 14 and has been in and out of the hospital many times in the intervening years. He has received a dual diagnosis of schizophrenia and intellectual disability.

Until 3 weeks ago, Howard was employed for 25 years by a messenger service. His job was to pick up and deliver packages via the subway and bus system. He got this job following successful vocational rehabilitation during one of his hospitalizations. Recently, however, the old manager, who was fond of Howard, retired, and his replacement found Howard's hygiene "unbearable." This was given as the reason for dismissal. After being terminated, Howard began to hallucinate and became afraid to leave his apartment. His mother took him to the emergency room, and after an overnight stay, he was referred to the outpatient day hospital program.

On meeting Howard, the occupational therapy assistant, Gloria, immediately observed that his hygiene was quite poor. His clothes fit badly, his pants were buttoned but unzipped, he had several days' growth of beard, and his hair was uncombed. He wore a dirty yarmulke, which was lopsided despite three bobby pins. He had noticeable body odor and visible food particles stuck in his teeth. He walked with a shuffling gait and kept his eyes downcast. He did answer Gloria's questions, although his answers were often long, rambling, and difficult to follow. At the end of the interview, Howard followed Gloria to the door and continued talking and asking her questions even though she had 3 times told him that she had to leave to run a group.

During the assessment of daily living skills, it became evident that Howard knew how to perform basic hygiene and grooming routines but did not always remember to do them and had trouble keeping his attention on what he was doing. He was easily distracted by the presence of other people and would interrupt whatever he was doing to talk to them. An evaluation of task skills revealed similar patterns. Once instructed, Howard was able to perform simple tasks, such as stuffing envelopes, but often stopped in the middle to talk to others and had to be reminded to return to his task. The content of his speech was egocentric and tangential; he talked mostly about himself, TV shows he had seen, and things he had done. He frequently sought approval of his task performance from staff members.

After receiving written permission from Howard to do so, Ben, Gloria's supervising occupational therapist, interviewed by telephone both Howard's mother and his former employer. The employer said that he felt bad about firing Howard but did not know how to deal with his poor hygiene and incessant talking. He agreed to take Howard back on a trial basis if these problems were resolved. He also stated that the company's insurance policy, under which Howard was still covered, provided for 14 days annually of inpatient psychiatric hospitalization and up to 6 months of outpatient treatment. No new information was obtained from Howard's mother.

Ben assessed Howard's social skills during a social skills group, using structured role-playing in which other clients played the parts of Howard's employer and various customers. The following problem behaviors were noted: interrupting others who are speaking, introducing inappropriate topics, and failing to perceive and act on the other's desire to end the interaction.

Ben and Gloria discussed the evaluation results with Howard. Howard was most interested in returning to work and agreed to the following goals:

- To perform daily hygiene and grooming routines
- To learn conversational skills appropriate for a job situation

Because social contact was so important to Howard, one-on-one meetings with Gloria were selected as the main reinforcer. Gloria also thought this would provide opportunities for her to explore other aspects of Howard's social behavior in various environments, such as the hospital coffee shop and local stores and parks.

Specific training included a day-long job skills group run by Andre, another occupational therapy assistant, and a daily morning hygiene group run by Gloria and Paul, a nurse's aide. Howard was also scheduled for evening recreation groups. All staff were asked to give Howard feedback on incorrect behaviors and to praise and support any improvements.

The first target behavior in the job skills group was learning not to interrupt others. Andre explained this to Howard, giving several examples and indicating other clients who had mastered this skill and whom Howard could watch as role models. During discussion periods at the end of each day's work, Howard reviewed and assessed his behavior that day and listened to feedback from Andre and the group members. Other behaviors were taught in the same fashion.

In the daily hygiene skills group, Howard practiced his hygiene and grooming under supervision. He gradually relearned the entire sequence of brushing his teeth, showering, shaving, using deodorant, and combing his hair. After Howard had practiced the routine daily for several weeks, he no longer needed reminders.

Howard achieved his work skill goal and was able to transition back to his job after a month, first 2 d/wk, gradually increasing to 5 d/wk. Gloria visited him twice at work to observe and give him feedback on his behavior at the job. She also coached Howard's employer on how to give constructive feedback. On discharge from day hospital, Howard was enrolled in the evening aftercare program, which he continued to attend for 3 months, at which point he made a successful transition to an evening psychosocial club program near his home.

Throughout his intervention, Howard participated in selecting his own goals and evaluating his own progress. Because his role as a worker was so important to him, this became the focus of the intervention plan. New skills and behaviors were taught sequentially, allowing Howard to succeed first at easy tasks before attempting more difficult ones. Each task was explained to Howard, and role models were provided. Finally, the newly acquired skills were carried over to the job, with staff support and supervision.

This example also shows how various levels of occupational therapy staff can work together and with nursing staff to carry out an intervention plan. Both role acquisition and social skills training are approaches well suited to an interprofessional team effort because the goals and methods are easily understood and carried out by all levels of staff.

Both social skills training and role acquisition are consistent with the OTPF-4E (14). They address the development and maintenance of occupational roles, social participation, performance skills, and performance patterns.

It appears that behavioral change transfers best to environments similar to those used for training (57, 58). Therefore, skills should be taught either in the environment in which they will be used or in an environment carefully designed to mimic the final environment of action. Social skills training may be more motivating in the context of job placement and training. Arbesman and Logsdon (15), in a systematic review of the literature, reported that social skills training strengthens the effectiveness of individualized job placement.

Box 3.3 provides examples of social skills training occupational therapy goals to use with clients.

BOX 3.3 Social Skills Intervention Goals

Aim of Intervention

Teach interpersonal skills needed to effectively relate to others.

Clients are able to get what they need in a given situation and for specific purposes.

Improve social skills of: self-expression, enhancing relationships with others, assertiveness, and overall communication.

Motivate client, demonstrate the behavior, client to practice behavior, occupational therapy professional to provide feedback.

Goals

Client will identify social skill need/behavior, and state its importance, for success with completing occupational activity of _____^^ with _____* (add needed amount or type of assistance) and _____^^^ within _____***.

Client will increase social skill of _____^ for success with completing occupational activity of _____^^ with _____* (add needed amount or type of assistance) and _____** within _____***

^ self-expression, relationship enhancement, assertiveness, communication (can use specific subskill such as identified in Table 3.4)
^^ include connection of occupational activity to client's chosen role(s)
* guidance, written prompt, written directions, verbal directions, cue, direct supervision/contact, indirect supervision/contact
** demonstration/modeling by occupational therapy professional, observation of role-playing by others, viewing recording; practice by stating components of skill/communication situation; practice by role-playing skill/communication situation; immediate feedback throughout the session
^^^ staff-provided examples, social skills instructional material, self-assessment tool
*** number of attempts, number of sessions, number of weeks

Schindler (120, 121) has provided extensive guidelines for *role development*, a model based on role acquisition. Schindler applied the role development model for clients with schizophrenia in forensics (prison settings). Schindler's specific examples and explanations of methods may be helpful to occupational therapy professionals using the models discussed in this section.

Concepts Summary

1. The person should be involved in selecting problems and goals for therapy and in assessing their own progress.
2. Choose goals and activities that reflect the client's interests, personal and cultural values, and present and future life roles.
3. Choose goals and activities that provide a realistic challenge but are consistent with the client's present level of ability.
4. Increase challenges and demands as the person's capacity increases.
5. Present skills in their natural developmental sequence.
6. Clients should always know what they are supposed to be learning and why.
7. Clients should be made aware of the effects of their actions.
8. Skills should be practiced repeatedly and then applied to new situations and environments.
9. If a task is too complex or time consuming to learn all at one time, one part should be taught at a time. Always, initially, have the occupational therapy professional do or show the whole activity to the client.
10. People learn to do things by imitating other people.
11. Skills should be taught in a four-stage process consisting of motivation, demonstration, practice, and feedback.
12. Feedback should be given throughout the learning process and should be immediate, specific, positive, concrete, and directive.

VOCABULARY REVIEW

behavior
Any observable action

chaining
A method of teaching a complex activity one step at a time, starting with either the first or the last step. The occupational therapy professional performs the remaining or initial steps, respectively, until the person masters the entire sequence.

demonstration
The second stage in the cycle of skills training, in which the target behavior is demonstrated to the person via role-play, recording, or another example

discrimination
The ability to recognize differences in situations that call for a change in behavior

extinction
Discouraging an undesired behavior by removing any reinforcement. An example might be the occupational therapy professional ignoring a child's temper tantrum instead of responding to it. This technique is called planned ignoring.

feedback
> This word has several meanings. In the cycle of skills training, it is the fourth stage, in which the person's performance of the target behavior is reviewed and summarized. More generally, however, feedback means information from the environment about the effects of one's action. When given by a person, feedback is most effective when it occurs immediately after the behavior is performed, includes positive aspects of the performance, and gives specific information on what can be done to improve it.

generalization
> The ability to apply a skill or behavior to new situations that are similar to the one in which it was learned

imitation
> A method of learning by copying or mimicking the behavior of another person

motivation
> The first stage in the cycle of skills training, in which the target behavior is identified and its importance explained

practice
> The third stage in the cycle of skills training, in which the person attempts the target behavior and repeats it until they become comfortable.

reinforcement
> Consequences of behavior that either encourage or discourage the repetition of the behavior

shaping
> A method of approaching the terminal behavior gradually, using a series of steps (successive approximations) that lead to the goal

skills
> Basic action patterns that can be combined into a variety of more complex actions

social skills
> Those skills that are used to relate to other people in a variety of situations

target behavior
> The new behavior to be learned in the immediate treatment situation. The target behavior is a short-term goal, which is distinguished from the long-term goal known as the terminal behavior, a desired behavior that will be mastered by the completion of the treatment program.

COGNITIVE DISABILITIES MODEL

The CDM, developed by occupational therapist Claudia Kay Allen, focuses on the functional effect of impaired cognition—a frequent symptom of mental disorders—on task performance (2–4, 6, 9). The central concept is that some people with psychiatric and neurologic disorders suffer from a disturbance in the mental functions that guide motor actions. Allen states: "just as physical disabilities restrict the physical ability to do a voluntary motion action, a cognitive disability restricts the cognitive ability to do a voluntary motor action" (3, p. 31). In other words, a person's mental disorganization can impair performance of tasks such as leather lacing and getting dressed.

Allen believed that the reason some persons with psychiatric diagnoses cannot perform these activities correctly is that they have a cognitive disability. She further stated that cognitive disabilities may prevent some people from successfully adapting to life outside a hospital or supervised living situation. She argued that task performance, even of seemingly unrelated tasks such as crafts, reflects ability to function and to take ordinary care in the community. Persons who demonstrate impaired task performance may be at risk of injury to self or others because they do not understand cause and effect and do not anticipate ordinary dangers, such as fire danger from storing too many flammable objects in the home (9). One might question whether crafts provide the best tasks to test performance; why not use ordinary familiar activities, such as dressing or cooking? Allen used crafts precisely because they are unfamiliar to many people. Familiar tasks may have been overlearned—that is, practiced so frequently that they have become habits. An unfamiliar task, such as a craft, gives a better measure of how well the person can solve problems and process new information.

People with cognitive disabilities may experience difficulties understanding, learning, and remembering information. Some individuals may have a hard time understanding what people are saying when following dialogue on a television show or during a class lecture. Some people with cognitive disability may find it extremely challenging to concentrate or remember information, such as when studying for a test or solving a problem. These kinds of challenges happen throughout the day and may interfere with completing a variety of daily activities and occupations. Cognitive disability can occur to various degrees with diagnoses such as schizophrenia, affective disorders, dementia, substance abuse, traumatic brain injury, and cerebral vascular accidents.

Allen (3) originally defined six **cognitive levels** (of ability and disability) related to task performance. These range from level 1 (severe impairment) to level 6 (no impairment). These have been further expanded into 26 modes, permitting greater sensitivity in rating task performance. A decimal system organizes the modes within the original six levels (eg, level 4.4, level 5.0) (8). For simplicity's sake, the following discussion is limited to the original six levels. Readers who wish more information may consult Allen's publications on the cognitive performance modes (4, 8).

Persons functioning at levels 1 through 4 have difficulty living unassisted in the community because they cannot perform the necessary routine tasks, such as paying bills, obtaining adequate nourishment, and finding their way to an unfamiliar place. The lower the cognitive level, the more difficulty the person has and the more assistance they require.

Cognitive level is assessed by observing the motor actions the person performs during a task and by inferring the sensory cue that the person was paying attention to at the time. In other words, the occupational therapy professional observes what the person does (motor action) and tries to identify what sensory information provoked or started that action. The sensory cues progress from internal at the lowest cognitive levels to external and more complex and abstract at the higher levels. Motor actions are automatic at the lowest level and become more refined at higher levels. Table 3.3 outlines the motor actions and associated sensory cues for the six levels.

Identification of a person's cognitive level requires careful assessment, which must be directed and interpreted by an occupational therapist, although the occupational therapy assistant may assist by performing some parts of the evaluation process. Instruments used in this model include the *Routine Task Inventory-Expanded* (RTI-E) (67), the *Cognitive Performance Test* (CPT) (32), the *Allen Cognitive Level Screen-5* (ACLS-5) (7), the *Large Allen Cognitive Level Screen-5* (LACLS-5) (7), and the *Allen Diagnostic Module*, 2nd Edition (ADM-2) (50). The RTI-E is a screening instrument that includes tasks in four areas (physical activities of daily living [ADLs], community instrumental ADLs [IADLs], communication, and work readiness). The person's performance is observed or reported. The RTI-E may be completed by any of three methods: client's self-report, caregiver's report, or observation of client's performance. Alternately, the RTI-E may be completed by a team. The RTI-E may not provide an accurate assessment of cognitive level because daily practice and habitual performance make many tasks routine and habitual. For each of the tasks, the behaviors typical of the cognitive levels are described. For example, using a map is typical of level 6 and not knowing one's destination is characteristic of level 3. The RTI-E may yield a falsely high score because performance of ADLs does not involve new learning. The RTI-E is discussed further in Chapter 12.

Individuals scoring at or estimated to be capable of scoring at levels 3 through 5 on the RTI-E may be assessed with the ACLS-5. The person is asked to imitate the occupational therapy professional's demonstration of leather lacing stitches, graded in complexity from the running stitch (level 3) to the single cordovan stitch (level 5). A person's performance on this assessment must be interpreted cautiously because visual deficits and drug side effects can impair performance (3). An enlarged version, the LACLS-5, with larger, more widely spaced holes and larger lacing material that is more easily grasped is also available to be used with persons who are older or with persons with low vision deficits.

The CPT (21) evaluates cognitive level by observing the client's performance in seven structured tasks (dressing, shopping, medication management, using the phone, travel, washing, and making toast). The CPT has been shown to be a good predictor for those who had cognitive deficits and needed to retire from driving or drive with restrictions (34). It should be noted the CPT score scale is to 5.6, thus those scoring in the level 5 and high level 4 range on the CPT cannot be directly correlated with the scoring descriptors for those level with the original CDM ACL-5 assessment scoring information (33).

The ADM was developed to provide alternative tasks to assess and reassess cognitive levels and to avoid the practice effect (tendency to perform better as the task is practiced) of repeated use of the ACLS-5 and LACLS-5 (7). The ADM-2 includes 35 craft projects that have been analyzed and clinic tested against the 26 modes (50). An ADM-2 task such as

Table 3.3. Cognitive Levels: Motor Actions and Associated Sensory Cues

Action	Level 1: Automatic Actions	Level 2: Postural Actions	Level 3: Manual Actions	Level 4: Goal-Directed Actions	Level 5: Exploratory Actions	Level 6: Planned Actions
Spontaneous motor actions	Automatic	Postural	Manual but not goal directed	Goal directed	Exploratory (experimentation, trial and error)	Planned
Imitated motor actions	None	Approximate imitations	Manual or manipulative	Copy or reproduction of an example, rote learning	New steps are imitated	Often unnecessary; actions can be initiated without demonstration
Examples of motor action	Sniffing, withdrawal from noxious stimuli, swallowing	Walking, gesturing, calisthenics	Picking up or touching objects, stringing beads	Chopping carrots, sanding wood	Spacing of tiles, blending of makeup colors	Budgeting, building a project from a diagram
Attention to sensory cues (inferred from observation)	Subliminal recognition of familiar objects (arousal must be stimulated)	Proprioceptive (movements and position of the body), effects of gravity	Tactile (touchable cues), objects that can be touched and moved	Visible (what is not in plain sight is ignored)	Related (relations between two visible cues)	Symbolic (abstract or intangible)
Examples of sensory cues	Hunger, thirst, or discomfort	Posture, gesture, motion	Texture, shape	Color, size, discomfort	Overlapping, color mixing, spatial relations	Evaporation, electrical current, heat, time, gravity

Adapted from Allen, C. K. (1985). *Occupational therapy for psychiatric diseases: Measurement and management of cognitive disabilities* (p. 34). Little, Brown and Company.

placing mosaic tiles can be used to verify an ACL score obtained by one of the other instruments, and the variety of ADM-2 tasks allows for introducing different tasks to track changes in cognitive level (eg, when medications take effect). The ADM-2 is discussed in more detail in Chapter 12.

Allen describes each of the levels in detail. Only an occupational therapist can use this model to assess the client and plan interventions. The occupational therapy assistant who has service competency may conduct parts of the assessment under the direction of a supervising occupational therapist (50) and may carry out the interventions. The following descriptions, which are brief, summarize and illustrate only the six original levels (3, 7):

- *Level 1.* The person seems mostly unaware of what is going on and may be in bed with the side rails up. The person pays attention for only a few seconds but carries out automatic habitual motor routines, such as self-feeding when food is presented. The person is very slow to respond to the occupational therapy professional's request or cue but may respond by rolling over or holding up a hand, for example.

- *Level 2.* The person seems to be aware of movement and position and of the effects of gravity. The person sits and initiates some gross motor actions. Someone at this level is not aware of environmental factors and thus may wander off. The person may assume off-balance or unstable physical positions or perform untypical-looking movements.

- *Level 3.* At this level, the person is interested in what is going on. Easily distracted by objects in the environment, the person enjoys touching them and manipulating them. The person engages in a simple repetitive craft or other activity but is likely to be surprised to see that something has been produced. The person has difficulty understanding cause and effect except in their own simple actions. The person may be easily disoriented and may get lost. Figure 3.2 illustrates the repetitive actions

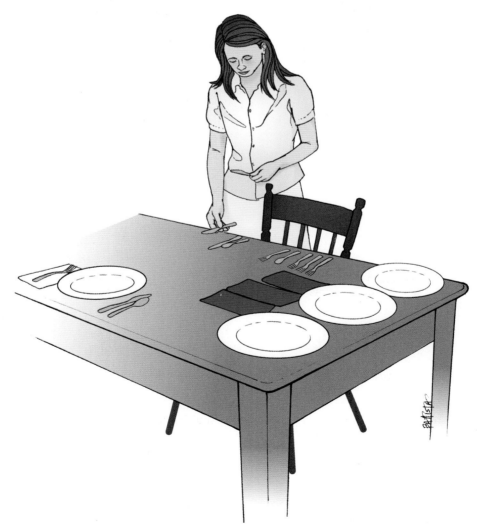

Figure 3.2. Allen's Level 3. A Repetitive Action With Disregard for a Goal. (Adapted from Allen, C. K. (1985). *Occupational therapy for psychiatric diseases: Measurement and management of cognitive disabilities* (p. 88). Little, Brown and Company.)

of a person at level 3, who would not stay focused on the task of setting the table and would instead enjoy repeating the placing of utensils in a line.

- *Level 4.* The person can copy demonstrated directions presented one step at a time; can visualize the goal of making something; and is interested in doing simple two-dimensional projects, such as mosaic tile trays with a checkerboard pattern. However, the person does not plan for such details as spacing between the tiles. The person tends to rely on prior learning and finds it easier to imitate a sample than to follow a diagram or picture. The person cannot recognize errors and may not be able to correct them when they are pointed out. The person does not understand that objects can be hidden from view (eg, may not look under the bed for shoes). See Figure 3.3 for an example of level 4. Similarly, the person does not notice glue sticking to the bottom of a tile tray.

- *Level 5.* The person shows interest in the relationships between objects. However, the relationships must be concrete and obvious. Some examples are overlapping edges in paper folding or woodwork, space between tiles, and matching colors in makeup or clothing. The person is interested in the effects that can be produced using the hands and may vary the pressure or the speed of hand motions. The person can generally perform a task involving three familiar steps and one new one. New steps must be demonstrated by the occupational therapy professional. The person at level 5 may appear careless because of inability to anticipate the possible consequences of actions. For example, the person may damage a garment when removing the price tag or label by pulling too hard or cutting through the fabric. The person who functions at level 5 may benefit from social skills training to improve attention to the nuances of expected social

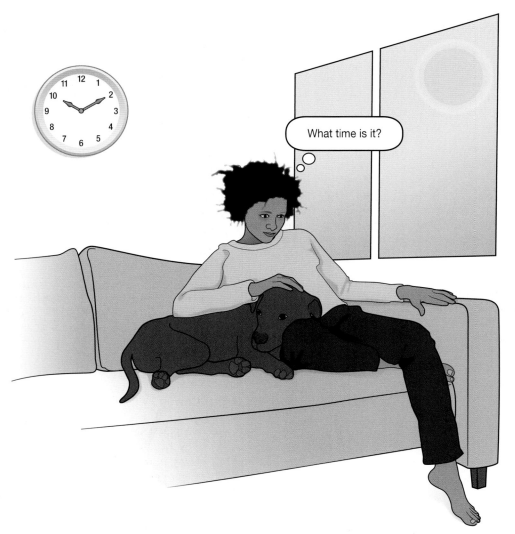

Figure 3.3. Allen's Level 4. The Person Does Not Notice What Time It Is Because the Clock Is Behind the Person's Line-of-Sight. (Adapted from Allen, C. K. (1985). *Occupational therapy for psychiatric diseases: Measurement and management of cognitive disabilities.* Little, Brown and Company.)

behavior. Allen believed that level 5 is sufficient for a person with limited occupational performance expectations to function in the community, although she warned that the person at a level 5 may not take ordinary and reasonable care regarding the rights of others.

- *Level 6.* The person appreciates the relationships between objects even when they are not obvious. Some examples are anticipating that a dark-colored, hand-dyed garment may bleed when washed and planning to have enough money for infrequent expenses, such as car repairs or doctor bills. At level 6, the person can anticipate errors, reason why they may occur, and plan ways to avoid them. Level 6 is associated with those who have had a greater depth and breadth of educational, vocational, and social experiences.

Goals for intervention based on the CDM are in Box 3.4.

BOX 3.4 CDM Intervention Goals

Aim of Intervention

Identify cognitive leve through assessment (via task or observation of occupational performance).

Monitor changes in cognitive level that may result from medical treatments.

Adapt the environment to compensate for cognitive loss (such as for safety, attention, direction following, and sensorimotor actions). This includes caregiver education and training.

Goals

Level I:

Client will respond to presented stimulus of _____ to participate in occupational activity of _____ with maximum of _____ physical/verbal/demonstration cue and additional time of _____ seconds within _____ attempts/days.

Level II:

Client will imitate motor action of _____ to participate in occupational activity of _____ with maximum of _____ physical/verbal/demonstration cue and _____* within _____ attempts/days.

Client will complete motor action of _____ to participate in occupational activity of _____ with maximum of _____ physical/verbal/demonstration cue and _____* within _____ attempts/days.

* additional time of _____ seconds within, peer modeling, handling techniques, key points of control, placement of extremity, postural support

Level III:

Client will complete manual activity of _____ to participate in occupational activity of _____ with _____* cue (add needed amount) and _____** within _____ attempts/days.

* verbal, demonstration, written, physical
** setup of items within client's reach, use of a timer, quiet environment, use of a sample

---

Level IV:

Client will copy/complete activity of _____ to complete/participate in occupational activity of _____ with _____* cue (add needed amount) and _____** within _____ attempts/days.

* verbal, demonstration, written

** setup of items within client's visual field, use of a timer, quiet environment, small group, use of a sample, discussion of directions prior to completing activity, provision of error identification

Level V:

Client will complete activity of _____ to complete occupational activity of _____ with _____* cue (add needed amount) and _____** within _____ attempts/days.

* verbal, demonstration, written

** written instructions, small group, use of a sample, discussion of possible effects prior to completing activity, provision/demonstration of _____ new task steps

---

Since first publishing in 1985, Allen and colleagues have elaborated on the six levels, creating sublevels within them. These sublevels are termed *modes*. Modes are defined in the following format: " . . . pays attention to [_____], motor control of [_____], and verbal communication by [_____]" (6). An example of a mode is given in Box 3.5. The mode shown, 4.2, is the level at which Allen judges a person sufficiently competent for discharge for community living, because the person can ask for help.

BOX 3.5 Mode 4.2: Engaging Abilities and Following Safety Precautions When the Person Can Differentiate the Parts of the Activity

Abilities

The person's best ability to function at this time has been observed in the following behaviors:

Pays attention to part of a single activity: For example, aware of objects in plain sight and within 24 inches
Motor control of matching one striking cue: For example, matches the sample one feature at a time
Verbal communication by following social rituals inflexibly: For example, recognizes the rules of give and take

Adapted and condensed from Allen, C. K., Blue, T., & Earhart, C. A., (1995). *Understanding cognitive performance modes*. In Allen Conferences (p. 77).

Allen suggested that cognitive levels cannot easily be changed by occupational therapy intervention. However, over the long term (years), environmental change and time may enable a person to function at a higher level; this may result in a measurable change in cognitive level. Allen maintained that the proper roles of occupational therapy are to (a) identify the cognitive level through assessment, (b) monitor changes in cognitive level that may result from other treatments such as medications, and (c) adapt the environment to help the person compensate for or accommodate to their disability. This may include caregiver education and training.

To illustrate the effect of medication on cognitive level, consider a person who on admission to an inpatient hospital unit is overactive, has trouble concentrating even for brief periods, is distracted by objects in the environment, and has little awareness of their own effect on others but can do repetitive manual tasks like stringing beads. Such behavior, which is characteristic of level 3, is typical of a person with mania. Someone with this diagnosis may be given lithium carbonate; when this drug reaches therapeutic levels, the person's cognitive level returns to the premorbid level (whatever it was before the manic episode, perhaps level 5 or 6). Occupational therapy staff can observe improvements in task performance, which should be reported to the physician as evidence that the drug is taking effect (3).

The environment must be modified to allow a person functioning at a lower cognitive level to succeed. Many people diagnosed with schizophrenia need supervised living situations because, at their best, they function only at level 4. They may dress oddly because they do not coordinate clothing colors and styles, and they do not always recognize what clothing is appropriate for a given situation. Similarly, although they can wash and groom themselves, they may neglect hidden parts such as the underarms, neck, and back of the head. They may burn themselves on hot cooking equipment and lack financial literacy skills such as budgeting money and paying bills. They may not be able to manage their own medication, forgetting to take pills or forgetting to get prescriptions refilled. For all these and many other reasons, they need assistance and supervision.

Depending on what is available, the person may live with family, in a group home or supervised residence, or in an apartment with other clients. In the latter case, daily visits from a care partner are advisable.

Another example of environmental modification or compensation is setting up supplies and tools for activities in a manner that allows for a person's disability. At levels 3 and 4, clients are easily distracted by anything visible. Consequently, supplies that are not needed for the current stage of an activity should be placed out of sight on a separate table. Because clients at these levels focus on what is visible, these clients should have individual sets of their own tools and supplies (within their reach for level 3 and within their line-of-sight for level 4). By contrast, at level 5, a person can be expected to share tools and to focus only on the supplies needed for the current step, allowing for supplies of other steps to remain visible to the client. How the occupational therapy professional sets up the client's occupational working area is called the **usable task environment** (3). The usable task environment enlarges as the cognitive levels increase. For each cognitive level, the usable task environment is identified here.

- Level 1: within or on the person's body (sensations)
- Level 2: amount of functional range of motion the person has
- Level 3: area within arm's reach
- Level 4: area within the person's visual field (line-of-sight)

- Level 5: the area in which the activity is occurring (includes physical area not immediately seen by the person, but used during the activity)
- Level 6: the possible, or potential, area needed or used to complete an occupation

Allen's model of cognitive disabilities is summarized in nine propositions [(3), quotes and adaptations of the propositions come from p. 368]:

1. The observed routine task behavior of clients with cognitive disabilities will differ from the observed behavior of those without cognitive disabilities. Persons with cognitive disabilities do not perform as well as those without cognitive disabilities in occupations needed for independent community living.
2. "Limitations in task behavior can be hierarchically described by the cognitive levels." In other words, the degree of disability is more severe at level 4 than at level 5 and is more severe at level 3 than at level 4, and so on.
3. "The choice of task content is influenced by the diagnosis and the disability." Although people functioning at level 6 typically prefer some balance of work (vocation), self-care, and leisure activities, those functioning at lower levels may find work too difficult. They may, instead, prefer crafts or hobby activities. Crafts allow persons with lower cognitive functioning to produce something tangible because of their efforts; these tangible products may compensate in some way for the loss of self-esteem from not being able to work in competitive employment.
4. The task environment may have a positive or a negative effect on a client's ability to regulate their own behavior. In general, tasks that are unstructured and creative tend to make those with limited cognitive functioning worse. Because the directions are not clear, those who lack good internal organization have no way to organize their efforts and may become confused and distressed. An example is asking someone with psychotic symptoms to draw a picture of themselves. They are likely to reject the task totally, to perform it in a perfunctory fashion (eg, by drawing a stick figure), or to produce something that reflects their hallucinations and other symptoms (eg, drawing a huge mouth with jagged teeth). When someone appears uncomfortable with a task because it is beyond their capabilities, the occupational therapy professional should adjust the directions or the steps involved and sometimes should substitute a different task altogether.
5. "People with cognitive disabilities attend to those elements of the task environment that are within their range of ability." This is another way of saying that people ignore whatever they do not understand or cannot make sense of. For example, those functioning at level 4 or 5 cannot be expected to construct a project from a three-dimensional plan, such as a working drawing or mechanical diagram; they cannot conceptualize how to proceed from such directions, although this would be a reasonable task for someone at level 6. Similarly, persons at level 4 may not recognize that they can get up and look

in a closet or ask the occupational therapy professional for a tool; because they cannot see the tool, they assume it does not exist or is unavailable.

6. Occupational therapy professionals can select and modify a task so that it is within the person's range of ability through the application of task analysis. In other words, the occupational therapy professional can re-structure the directions, materials, or nature of the ac-tivity so that the person can perform it. As an example, when teaching the sanding of wooden kits, the occupa-tional therapy professional can expect persons at level 6 to sand with the grain once the concept of grain is ex-plained. Persons at level 5 can be told to sand up and down, the long way or other similar wording; after a few experiences of sanding and more verbal instruction, they should be able to understand and apply the concept of grain. For persons at level 4, on the other hand, because they can follow only demonstrated directions presented one at a time, the sandpaper must be part of the demon-stration. They must be instructed to turn the project over and sand the other side. Persons functioning at level 3 can sand once the motion is demonstrated but may sand back and forth as well as up and down and have difficulty learning to sand in just one direction. Similarly, unless the occupational therapy professional intervenes, clients may continue sanding until they have reduced the project to toothpicks, because they do not recognize the purpose of the sanding or that they should stop at a given point.

7. "An effective outcome of occupational therapy services occurs when successful task performance is accompa-nied by a pleasant task experience." In other words, the occupational therapy professional should help clients feel good about what they have done, both during the pro-cess and afterward. In part, this is achieved by present-ing only achievable tasks. A person faced with a task that is too difficult is likely to feel overwhelmed, ashamed, frustrated, or angry. Sometimes, it is helpful to select an activity that the person has performed well in the past and feels good about performing. When a new task is introduced, it should be analyzed and presented at the person's level of comprehension (see proposition 5).

8. "Steps in task procedures that require abilities above a person's level of ability will be refused or ignored." Someone who can-not do something will find a way to avoid it. For example, a person at level 4, when shown how to braid the upper edge of a basket, instead substitutes a less involved finishing method, such as making simple loops. They cannot follow the over/under multistrand demonstration of braiding.

9. "The assessment of the cognitive level can contribute to the legal determination of competency." Because people functioning at level 4 or below have identifiable problems that prevent them making sound judgments about their own welfare, assessment of a person's cognitive level may be useful in a court of law. Persons at levels 1 and 2 typi-cally behave in ways that make their disabilities obvious, but the person functioning at level 3 or 4 may appear

reasonably intact, especially if they have good verbal skills. At these levels of disability, there is serious ques-tion about a person's competence to manage financial affairs or to stand trial for a crime.

In summary, the CDM provides a system for classify-ing a person's ability to carry out routine occupational tasks needed for successful community adjustment. The model provides instruments for assessment of cognitive level and prescriptions for how to modify tasks, environment, levels of assistance, and therapeutic approach for those with levels of disability that are incompatible with independent function-ing. The following case example illustrates the CDM.

Case Example

Marvin[4] has been hospitalized twice in the past month. On the last admission, his diagnosis was adjustment disorder, based on his report of a recent separation from his wife. During the current admission, it was learned that Marvin and his wife have been separated for 5 years, that his wife lives out of state, and that Marvin is concerned about his two children. He has threatened to harm his wife. The social worker has been unable to locate Marvin's wife or anyone else who can verify his story.

Marvin is 45 years old, tall, overweight, and sloppily dressed. He needs a shave. He says that he knows eight foreign languages, which he learned in his 20 years as a business consultant. He can speak some of them, according to staff fluent in foreign languages. His diagnosis is major depressive episode with suicidal ideation. On the unit, he has shown a good appetite at meals, has slept soundly, and does not appear depressed. Marvin scored at level 3 on the ACLS-5. He was placed in a basic skills group. During his first week in this group, the following behaviors were observed:

- When asked to cut apart strips of mailing labels, he held the scissors upside down but was able to perform the task.
- When asked to cut rags into 7-inch squares, after being given a sample, he cut pieces of varying sizes ranging from 10 to 18 inches. None of the pieces were square. When this error was pointed out to him, Marvin apolo-gized, and his eyes appeared wet. He then tried to cor-rect his error by trimming the edges but did not attempt to trace the sample size on to the squares or otherwise measure them.
- After satisfactorily completing a decoupage project, Mar-vin attempted to attach the hanger to the front of the plaque but had the attachment prongs facing up and was using the round end of a ball-peen hammer.

Having observed the misuse of scissors and hammer and the failure to recognize the proper positioning of the hanger, the occupational therapist recommended that the client be evaluated for a neurocognitive disorder. Misuse of common tools is not usually seen in depression but is often a feature of neurocognitive disorders. Marvin's teary-eyed apology for cutting the rags incorrectly was seen as evidence to support the diagnosis of depression. The occupational therapist also recommended that Marvin be placed in supervised living be-cause he was indeed functioning at mode 3.4.

As this case example illustrates, assessment of cognitive level is very useful for diagnostic, transition, and discharge planning purposes.

In relation to the OTPF-4E, the model of cognitive disabilities addresses occupations, performance skills, client factors, and the environment. Occupations mainly include ADLs, IADLs, work, and social participation. Mental functions such as attention and perception are important in the explanation for how this model may be applied toward safety with occupations and caregiver education and training.

In the almost four decades since the CDM was first published, research and development have supported and expanded some aspects of this practice model (33, 35, 40, 43, 65, 95, 108, 109, 124, 129). In addition, Allen and colleagues have provided detailed and specific intervention guidelines for persons at each level (4, 8, 9, 51, 52, 87-89, 113).

More recently, the CDM has been identified to consider the capacity of the person who is cognitively impaired to be able to improve in function over time (49). The brain is remarkably plastic (able to reshape itself and to recover functions after injury) even in adult life. It appears that functional abilities and cognitive levels do increase for many persons in the months and years following injury and that these increases are not owing to medication or other somatic intervention. This is true of persons with traumatic brain injury as well as for some of those with severe and persistent mental disorders (59).

Before concluding a discussion about Allen and cognitive disabilities, it is important to mention the Allen Cognitive Disability Model, or the ACDM. The ACDM is the latest conceptual framework Allen used to describe cognition. It is different from the CDM information presented thus far. The ACDM includes the following ideas (5):

- The person with a cognitive disability participates in activity that makes the person occupied and happy.
- Once the person's cognitive functional ability is assessed, adjustments to how they participate can be made, allowing them reengagement with activity.
- If a cognitive disability is present, but not identified, the person can experience low motivation or apathy and, in turn, stops completing activities they are accustomed to doing.
- Consideration must be made toward individual differences and caregivers must be educated and trained about how to make activities achievable, or completed, as needed, through support from the caregiver.
- For the person with a cognitive disability, we want to center on activities that engage the brain and arouse attention. We want to provide the correct quality of sensorimotor information, so the person's aroused attention is engaged and maintained.
- The six cognitive levels are a categorization of the quality of sensorimotor information that arouses attention. It is a hierarchy of ability. Sensorimotor information must be presented at the level of the person. If too much is asked of the person, the action takes too much energy and is ignored. If too little is asked of the person, the action takes too little energy and can be relaxing or boring.

- Who the "person is now" comes from a reduced amount of information that arouses their attention. This information is their sense of identity and their memories. What they do and how they perceive others is connected to their sense of identity and their memories. Their senses of space, direction, and time are an integral part of how to decide what they will do and how they will do it. They also do not realize all that they can no longer do. All this put together is an **obsolete identity**, or not realizing the reduction in their abilities. Their self-report of activity and ability can be misleading, because the person believes they can do more, and are capable of doing more, than they actually do.
- The obsolete identity is based on how they performed occupations prior to their cognitive disability. Lacking the ability to internalize new and abstract information into their sense of self causes their current identification of themselves to be who they were before the cognitive disability. Activities presented to the person must be appealing to them, as viewed from their obsolete identity. In addition, activities must be graded to meet the abilities demonstrated by the person's cognitive level.
- There are six cognitive ability levels, which are similar to the CDM, and focus on how sensorimotor information is perceived by the person and connected to the person's motor actions.
- The Allen Cognitive Level Screen, 6th Edition (ACLS-6) uses observation of numerous standardized activities. There is also a leather lacing component. The assessment is scored via an electronic application. There are differences, including that the lacing tool is hard plastic, and the scoring includes recording the total amount of time it takes the person to complete the lacing stitches.
- Assessment information includes 10 profiles. Each cognitive level (levels 1–5) has a high and a low profile. The profiles offer practical information for discharge recommendations.

Information regarding how to access the ACDM app, which is needed to learn more about the ACDM and for using the ACLS-6 assessment and scoring, is available at the end of the chapter in the *Suggested Resources*.

Concepts Summary

1. The observed routine task behavior of persons with cognitive disabilities differs from the observed behavior of those without cognitive disabilities.
2. Limitations in task behavior can be hierarchically described by the cognitive levels.
3. The choice of task content is influenced by the diagnosis and the disability.
4. The task environment may have a positive or a negative effect on a person's ability to regulate their own behavior.
5. Persons with cognitive disabilities attend to the elements of the task environment that are within their range of ability.
6. Occupational therapy professionals can select and modify a task so that it is within the person's range of ability through the application of analyzing the task and the environment.

7. An effective outcome of occupational therapy services occurs when successful task performance is accompanied by a pleasant task experience.
8. Steps in task procedures that are above a person's level of ability will be refused or ignored.
9. The assessment of the cognitive level can contribute to the legal determination of competency.

VOCABULARY REVIEW

Allen Cognitive Level (ACL) test
An assessment in which the person is asked to imitate the occupational therapy professional's demonstration of leather-lacing stitches graded in complexity from the running stitch to the single cordovan stitch

cognitive disability
Lack or impairment of ability to carry out motor actions, caused by a disturbance in the thinking processes that direct motor acts. Cognitive disability can be observed in the way a person performs routine tasks.

cognitive level
The degree to which the mind is capable of responding to task demands. Allen identifies six cognitive levels, ranging from level 1 (severe impairment) to level 6 (no impairment).

competence
A legal term meaning having sufficient mental ability to manage one's own financial affairs, safeguard one's own interests, and understand right and wrong

environmental compensation
Modification of the environment to permit successful completion of a task. An example is seating a distractible person away from other people.

practice effect
The tendency to perform better as a task is practiced

Routine Task Inventory-Expanded (RTI-E)
A checklist of task behaviors in 32 specified and 8 unspecified categories, used as a guide for observing and classifying a person's task abilities and cognitive level

routine tasks
ADLs, such as grooming, dressing, bathing, walking, feeding, toileting, housekeeping, preparing food, spending money, taking medication, doing laundry, traveling, shopping, and telephoning

task abilities
What the person can do successfully; the tasks or parts of tasks that the person can complete adequately in the present state

task demands
The degree of complexity present in the materials, tools, and skills needed to perform a task. Task demands vary from simple (eating a sandwich) to complex (providing for adequate income at retirement).

task directions
Oral, written, or demonstrated instruction about how to perform a task

task environment
The people, objects, and spaces in which the person performs a task. Psychological and emotional aspects of the environment must be considered along with physical aspects.

THE MODEL OF HUMAN OCCUPATION

The *MOHO*, developed by Gary Kielhofner and his colleagues beginning in 1976 (21, 71-73), provides a broad view of human occupation in relation to health. Based on concepts introduced by Mary Reilly and others in the 1960s and 1970s, this model analyzes and describes the development of occupational behavior. It considers the roles of culture and of environment in shaping occupation and addresses specifically the health-maintaining and health-restoring aspects of activity. It emphasizes the effects of choice, interest, motivation, and habits on human activity. The model is particularly useful because it can be applied in all areas of occupational therapy practice and used with other models (73). In addition, because it is an occupational performance model, it overlaps with all the domains in the OTPF-4E (14).

Human Occupation[5]

Human occupation comes from our internally driven need to act. We have a desire for **action** and that desire is seen outwardly through the occupations we perform, or what is called our occupational participation. Our **volition** system houses our motivation toward our occupations. Occupations are organized into patterns and routines via our **habituation** system. And our **performance capacity** system includes the mental and physical abilities we possess to complete skilled occupational performance. The **environment** influences each of these three components, in turn, the environment is continually influencing occupational participation.

Volition

Volition includes our unique thoughts, feelings, and personal history. It is a mix of the following three parts.

Personal causation is *one's sense of personal capacity* of *self-efficacy*. This involves knowing and understanding what we can do (sense of capacity), the power to effectively make change and achieve desired outcomes (efficacy), and the belief in oneself or sense of oneself in having this power to effect change (self).

Values are grounded in the cultural messages we receive. They are the *personal convictions* that come from our worldview and how we view life. Values stir our emotions and encourage us to take action. This strong emotional disposition to act on what we perceive as correct, and right, is called a *sense of obligation*.

Interests are what we find enjoyable or satisfying to do. We see it as what we find preferable. We find *enjoyment* in performing simple daily rituals such as taking care of a treasured pet to intense, emotion-filled sky-diving adventures. Through our experiences we accumulate a unique configuration of things we prefer to do; this is called an *interest pattern*. Interest patterns for a person can hold a theme, such as

---

[5]Unless otherwise noted, information presented from this subsection through the subsection "Doing" is from Taylor, R. R. (Ed.) (2017). *Kielhofner's model of human occupation* (5th ed.). Wolters Kluwer.

a musical interest that is woven throughout the majority of what we do, or it can be diverse, and we can have wide variety of interests.

This process of volition is ongoing and occurs over time. Through the volitional process (during and as a reflection of the process) we **experience** feelings (such as happiness while attending a wedding or sadness while attending a funeral) and thoughts (such as self-awareness of what steps to take during a task or self-control when managing anger). Interpreting occupational performance occurs as we recall what occurred and what we did, reflecting on the experience and its impact on us and others. There are hundreds of possibilities and expectations for actions we can take both now and in the future. The ones we notice and react to are the ones we have **anticipation** for performing and completing.

Activity choices are what we decide to do now and in the near future. These are activities such as washing the dishes from dinner, exercising later with a friend, and attending this weekend's sporting event or neighborhood party. It does not take long for us to decide to do an activity, but much of our time is taken up completing them. **Occupational choices** are for longer commitments of time and become extended or permanent parts of our lives. These include establishing new roles, making a new activity part of our permanent routine, or deciding to participate in a long-term project. "Occupational choices are thus defined as deliberate commitments to enter an occupational role, acquire a new habit, or undertake a personal project" (131, p. 14). Activity choices and occupational choices largely influence the type of occupational performance we have throughout our daily lives.

As occupational therapy professionals, we utilize the parts of a client's volitional system to keep our therapy client-centered. We want to present an atmosphere aligned with a client's interests and values so they feel a desire to make activity choices and occupational choices that they will have an anticipation for doing. Our client's sense of, or belief in, their own ability or power to impact, or affect, or change their situation or circumstance, in other words, their personal causation, is always an underlying consideration of our time with them. So often our client feels powerless, is afraid, is uncertain what to do or even think (or decide). By helping them "find their way" and by setting up our therapy session with them to give them success and time to reflect on what they have accomplished, we give them the chance to increase or mature their belief in themselves.

Habituation

Habituation is our internalized readiness, our way of behaving that is connected to what we find familiar—what we "do" daily without thinking about doing, what we assume will happen (because it always does), and how we "normally" interact with others. This is associated with, and we take notice to, the factor of time (such as when and how often something occurs), our physical environment (such as the layout of our home or workspace), and our social movements and interactions intertwined with social expectations that make up

our culture. All this interaction is done within a stable world around us, which in turn allows us to function in a stable manner within our habits and roles.

Habits are the acquired tendencies in which we respond to and perform in a particular and consistent way within the environments and the situations we find familiar. We internalize the way we do things through repeated performance and consistently doing the same thing within the same environment and regarding the same personal factors. When this activity starts, it requires attention and concentration, but in time it becomes automatic. Thus, our actions must be repeated enough so that they become a pattern and this activity must be done within an environment that is consistently the same. There are three types of habits.

- *habits of occupational performance*: how we choose to perform routine daily activities
- *habits of routine*: consideration of when and where (space and time) we perform activities
- *habits of style*: the individualized and unique manner in which we complete activities

We behave and act in certain ways, with certain people, at certain times, in certain situations, because of **internalized roles**. We perform particular actions because of how we learned to do so, because of a particular social status or particular identity we have. Over time, through socialization, we begin to recognize roles for ourselves. These are roles that others have put on us and include specific expectations. Other roles are self-identified and are in response to what we individually and personally see as our responsibilities. These roles arise out of a particular circumstance or out of necessity. Thus, we have internalized roles that can be either socially or personally defined and each role we have has its associated behaviors and attitudes. Our roles are connected to others, to places, to time, and to tasks.

Within occupational therapy, we can take advantage of a client's healthy and *supportive habits*. These types of habits can help a client rebuild or regain capacities, activities, or occupations. In contrast, *unhealthy and harmful habits* can cause difficulty for a client. Examples of unhealthy habits are a non-nutritious diet or a cluttered and unsanitary home. Harmful habits are taking unnecessary risks such as not keeping a home emergency kit or having unprotected sexual intercourse with numerous partners. As occupational therapy professionals, we may also work with a client who has not had the opportunity to establish habits. Consider a person who is without permanent housing and has had to move from one physical environment to another on a regular basis. Without a consistent and familiar living environment, the person has not had the chance to build habits. Likewise, we may work with a client who has not had the opportunity to form internalized roles. The person may have lacked a consistent environment with social expectations from which to learn and practice actions and responses. We may provide that stable environment, first as a model and then as a place to practice those interactions. It may also be that a client has self-identified a necessity-based role as a protector of an abused sibling or parent, or as a family provider even though the client is still well under the age of 18 years. We know these roles have now become tightly knit with their volitional system, but we also know these roles can include habits that are unhealthy or harmful. In these cases, we most likely will find ourselves working within an interprofessional team to help these clients find a balance and determine a course of action that will benefit them and those connected to their roles.

Performance Capacity

Performance capacity is being able "to do" things, combined with identifying the objective physical and mental components of the performance, and personal and individualized subjective experience. Being able to do something, anything, and everything depends on the objectively measured physical and mental capacities that we have and the abilities we use during the performance. This comes from our client factor body functions such as mental functions (specific and global), sensory functions, neuromusculoskeletal and movement-related functions, and cardiovascular and respiratory functions. Being able "to do" also involves how that action is experienced solely by the person doing it, or the subjective experience.

Considering what we do, objectively and subjectively together, is to look at our actions through the concept of the **lived body**. The MOHO posits that the lived body includes these two ideas:

- The mind and body are a unit. We know things (mind) about our actions and our world by doing things with our body (body). They work together and cannot be separated. This is *mind–body unity*.
- The subjective experience of doing something is not an "extra" or a result of the objective components performing the act. How it feels to do something, how it is experienced by us, forms our capacity for doing it.

Take, for example, when you see freshly cut grass on a cool autumn evening. You remove your shoes and socks and walk barefoot. You wiggle your toes. You may close your eyes. You may stop and smell the grass. Your thoughts may travel to another time when you enjoyed the pleasure of walking or sitting in a similar place with loved ones and friends. You did this because you saw and smelled the fresh cut grass. You felt the cool breeze. You registered the early evening time approaching. You slowed your pace and rubbed your feet on the ground. You experienced it. What did not happen was you just identifying the range of motion or strength needed to perform the action. Or the amount of energy it would take to complete the act.

Although we may focus on the objective pieces of our actions while we learn something new, once we know the component parts we start to move faster, practice it over, and start to "feel" it. We practice it with different movements and timing. Again, we feel the experience of it. In occupational therapy, our clients have had a disruption in the objective physical and mental components of the actions they wish to do. Thus, their focus or concentration is on the specific component

parts, and we are helping them rebuild or build a new way to feel the experience once again. It could also be that they are so focused on the components of parts of an activity, they are disrupted from feeling it or experiencing it. For instance, they are so absorbed with the details of a trip and counting down the miles, they do not enjoy the experience of traveling.

Environment

The **environment** (OTPF-4: Context: Environment Factors and Personal Factors) in which actions and occupations occur is many layered, complex, involves interactions with others, includes space and objects, offers possibilities, and holds meanings. Our unique volitional system, habituation system, and performance capacity system determine how the environment will influence us. All the parts of the environment influence each other and act together to influence us. The **environmental impact** includes the opportunities, supports, demands, and constraints the environment provides and places on each of us. Again, the environment has many layers and is complex. It includes the following.

- dimensions: physical, social, occupational
- factors: economic, political, cultural
- attitude: social
- aspects: geographical, ecologic
- contexts: where people operate, and the following are experienced:
  - physical space
  - objects involved
  - relationships
  - interactions
  - occupations
  - activities
  - expectations
  - opportunities
- cultural context unique to each person involving all aspects of context

There are three levels of interaction among the environmental dimensions, you, and across all three levels.

- *immediate context*: places where you are and go most of the time
- *local context*: the geographic area closest to you
- *global context*: involves the factors of economic, political social, legal, climate, and geography

As occupational therapy professionals we consider environment from concepts such as accessibility, respect for an individual's cultural context, and inclusivity.

Interaction of Person and Environment: A Dynamic System

Current MOHO concepts stem from dynamic systems theory in that people move, or have action, so they can self-organize, because of their interactions with multiple systems that cause fluctuations of continuity. We seek stable patterns of behavior, but when there is a **perturbation**, a shift or disturbance, we feel a sense of discomfort and that gives us a signal to change. Our clients often have experienced a perturbation in their patterns of behavior; thus, we are working to help them develop a new pattern to change with the new set of circumstance. We are all influenced by the multiple variables within our internal environment and external environments, and we want to respond. We perform physical and cognitive operations from which we then receive feedback from other people and from various variables within our environment. This continual process over time becomes more complex and involves more aspects of our environment. Figure 3.4 depicts this dynamic system.

This dynamic interaction that occurs among our internal systems and the environment, and the deep desire we have to change are of tremendous importance to the MOHO. In consideration of this dynamic interaction and the process of change, there are five guiding principles for the MOHO:

- Occupational actions, thoughts, and emotions arise out of the dynamic interaction of volition, habituation, performance capacity, and environmental context.
- Change in any aspect of volition, habituation, performance, capacity, and/or the environment can result in change in the thoughts, feelings, and doing that make up one's occupations.
- Volition, habituation, and performance capacity are maintained and changed through what one does and what one thinks and feels about doing.
- A particular pattern of volition, habituation, and performance capacity will be maintained so long as the underlying thoughts, feelings, and actions are consistently repeated in a supporting environment.

- Change requires that novel thoughts, feelings, and actions are sufficiently repeated in a consistent environment to coalesce into a new organized pattern. (131, p. 26)

There are several key points to consider as part of these guiding principles. Each system within us and all the aspects of our environment working together and being linked together to form a dynamic whole is called a **heterarchy**. Each aspect is contributing to the process and the environment is central to this interplay. This dynamic interplay comes about because we think and feel about what is occurring to us, what we are doing, who we are doing it with, and where it is happening. Our reactions and reflections, as well as others' reactions and opinions shape what we do in the future. This **emergence** of actions, thoughts, and feelings is spontaneous and happens because everything is interacting together. Over time what we wish to do and what we must do change. What we think and feel over time influences our patterns of behavior, as well as what we do and accomplish, and what is expected of us. As we take on new roles and projects, our patterns (habits and routines) change, as do our performance capacities. Our sense of being an *occupational being*, or the sense of who we are and who we wish to become, that develops and accumulates over time, based on our repeated patterns of engagement, and reflects our life experiences is called **occupational identity**.

When we provide occupational therapy services, we are providing the support and opportunities to adjust for the demands and constraints the client is experiencing. As clients reflect on what they are doing and how it makes them feel, new actions emerge from the volition, habituation, and performance capacity systems. This leads to new occupational

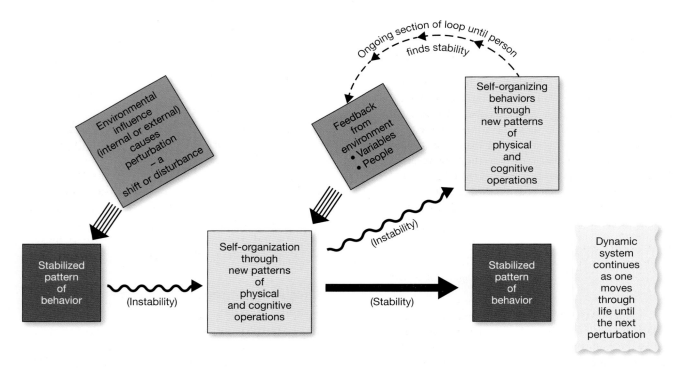

Figure 3.4. The Dynamic System Process of Interaction. (Adapted from Taylor, R. R. (2017). *Kielhofner's model of human occupation* (5th ed.). Wolters Kluwer.)

choices, or what is called **occupational shift**. You may recall how we can provide the path to help our clients increase their self-efficacy, or to practice their skills to increase their belief in their power to change themselves. As people practice their chosen occupations over time, while participating in their various social roles, their chosen occupations become something they can skillfully and easily perform. This is called **occupational competence**.

We can stop for a moment and consider that the changes our clients are incurring can be led by a *control parameter*, or a factor that creates a dynamic interaction or shift in thoughts, feelings, and actions. We can utilize this control parameter to further encourage change, assuming the control parameter is positive for the client. However, if the control parameter is harmful or damaging to the client, we can work to help the client maneuver around or away from that control parameter. Next, we consider someone's **resiliency**, or their responding ability toward changing and adapting, or recovering, from a specific situation or event. Again, we may work to help a client increase their resiliency. This can include providing interventions designed to support occupations. This includes interventions such as mindfulness, stress management techniques, or self-awareness skills. This is done so the client can withstand environmental barriers during chosen occupations. The change process a client does so that they can engage in their chosen activities or so they can develop new activities is called occupational adaptation. **Occupational adaptation** is the dynamic combination of environmental impact, a positive occupational identity, and the occupational competence developed over time that corresponds with one's occupational identity.

Doing

The MOHO concepts go beyond our thoughts, feelings, and actions. It also includes the concept of "doing." We will introduce "doing" here and continue this discussion in Chapter 6, as a model of our service provision. **Doing** involves three levels, including occupational participation, occupational performance, and occupational skills.

Occupational participation involves our everyday engagement in *productivity* (working, volunteering, studying, providing knowledge or services), *play* (done for its own sake; done freely; done to explore, pretend, celebrate, and engage), *ADLs* (life tasks of self-care and self-maintenance). The OTPF-4E (14) would define occupational participation through these occupations:

- *productivity* as work and education;
- *play* as play, leisure, and social participation; and
- *ADLs* as ADLs, IADLs, health management, and rest and sleep.

Occupational participation is influenced by the personal factors of volition, habituation, and performance capacity, and by the contextual factors found within the environment.

Occupational performance is the discrete acts of doing, or the discrete units of doing that we perform. Think about that act or unit as engaging in an *occupational form*.

To engage in an occupational form, you must complete all the discrete acts, all the steps that make up the whole activity. When you make the bed, you must pull and place both the fitted sheet and flat sheet around and across the entire bed. You also must place the blanket on top and maybe a bedspread on top of the blanket. In addition, you must tuck pillows into pillowcases and place those at the head of the bed. In fact, before you started those acts, you had to ensure you had the items needed to make the bed, they were clean, and that you could move around the area near your bed so that you could make it. Over time, the acts we choose to do become habits and they are done within our environment.

Occupational skills are the observable, goal-directed actions that we complete during occupational performance. There are three types and include the following:

- *Motor*: moving parts of the body or the moving of objects within an environment
- *Process*: logical sequence of actions over time, appropriately selecting and using items
- *Communication and interaction*: conveying intentions and needs, expressing self for involvement in coordinated social interactions

We need now to step back to occupational participation and bring within the dynamic system of occupational participation the pieces of occupational performance and occupational skills. To do this, we will view occupational participation as having six dimensions:

- **participation** in roles
- **occupational form**, or choosing an activity within a role
- **occupational performance**, or participating in a chosen activity
- participation in all the **steps of that activity**
- **occupational skills**, or the specific actions that make up a step of the activity
- **subjective experience** (feeling of doing the activity) and **objective assessment** of components involved from the performance capacity

If occupational participation is dynamic, and includes where our occupations are and how we "do" and how we "think" and "feel" about our participation, then it influences and helps build our occupational identity and our occupational competence. You may recall how occupational identity and occupational competence lead to, and are a part of, occupational adaptation and also the occupational shifts that occur and resiliency needed to continually adapt to our occupational situation. All these concepts and ideas are intertwined, are a part of each other, and impact one another. When you hear that occupation is complex, these past few pages are a good example of that complexity. This is what we must remember as we work with our clients. A disease process that robs them of being able to partake in any aspect along the way is where we come in to provide the missing pieces so they can continue their journey through and to occupation. Figure 3.5 illustrates the occupational adaptation process and how all the pieces are linked and fit together.

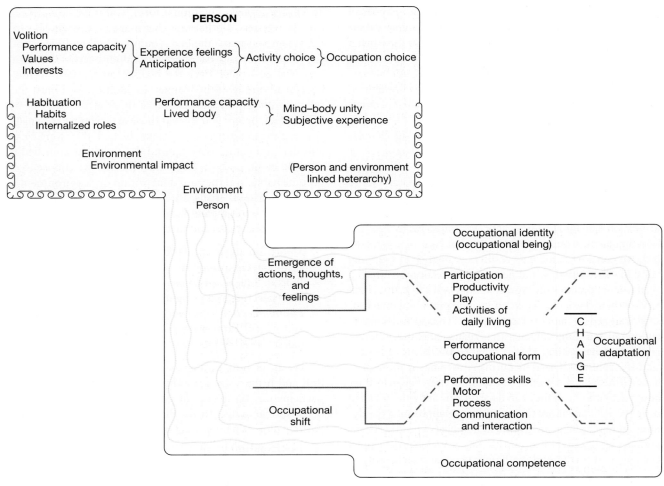

Figure 3.5. The Process of Occupational Adaptation. (Adapted from Taylor, R. R. (2017). *Kielhofner's model of human occupation* (5th ed.). Wolters Kluwer.)

Case Example

Rose, a 20-year-old mother of two, was admitted to the in-patient psychiatric unit with a diagnosis of depression following a suicide attempt. Over the past 3 weeks, she had begun to neglect the housework and the children. She spent long periods sitting around "thinking." She was able to feed and clothe her two children, a boy aged 4 and a girl aged 2, but she paid little attention to her own grooming. Her husband, Larry, took her to the emergency room. Staff documented that her hair was oily and dirty, and her clothes were food stained. She admitted to feeling depressed.

Larry and Rose married almost 5 years ago, when she was pregnant with their first child. Because both were still in high school, they lived with Larry's parents until Larry got his high school diploma; they then moved to a one-bedroom apartment nearby. Since then, Larry has been working for his uncle, who installs aluminum siding, and since the birth of the second child, he has had a second job at a gas station at night. Rose, who is a year younger than Larry, did not complete high school.

Rose's parents, who are extremely religious, disapproved of Rose and Larry's and the out-of-wedlock pregnancy. They

have not seen Rose since she married Larry and she left their home; they have never seen their grandchildren.

During the first day of her hospitalization, Rose was quiet and subdued. She isolated herself from other clients but responded when spoken to by others. After several reminders from nursing staff, she carried out her morning grooming in a superficial and inattentive manner. She ate little, pushing the food listlessly around on the plate.

The supervising occupational therapist, Raquel, assigned James (an occupational therapy assistant) to collect background information. James reviewed Rose's medical chart, looking through the admitting information, the history, and the nursing notes for any information about Rose's feelings about herself, her interests, past and present roles, habits, and skills. He then introduced himself to Rose, briefly explained what occupational therapy is and how it might help her, and then asked her a series of questions from the *Occupational Performance History Interview-II* (75) about her childhood, past productive activities, and present home life. Rose spoke softly, sometimes hesitating, but answered all the questions. She said she was willing to fill out some questionnaires. James left her with the *Role Checklist-Version 3* (123) to complete on her own. He also gave her a schedule of general activity groups and scheduled a meeting for the following day to collect and review the questionnaires.

Later that same day, after reviewing James's interview notes, Raquel met with Rose and explained that she would be working with James to schedule the occupational therapy interventions. She followed up on some points from James's notes and discussed the *Role Checklist-Version 3*. She encouraged Rose to talk about her child-care and homemaking responsibilities and asked her about her goals for the hospitalization. The next day, Raquel and James went over the results of all the assessments and arrived at the following conclusions.

- **Volition**. Rose feels that she has no control over her life. She is overwhelmed by the responsibilities of caring for her home and family; she loves her children but feels she cannot handle them. She checked several group sports activities and computer programming on the interest checklist but says she has no time for these things. On the *Role Checklist-Version 3*, she listed religious participant, friend, and hobbyist as past and future but not present roles.

- **Habituation**. Rose is having difficulty with her homemaker and child-care roles. She wanted to study computer science in college and to become a computer programmer but now sees this as impossible. She performed well in the student role, completing her junior year in high school despite her advanced pregnancy. She has difficulty completing household chores before beginning others, does not have a routine schedule for housework, and has trouble managing money (pays bills late, buys unnecessary items).

- **Performance capacity**. Rose seems to have adequate motor skills but has trouble sequencing and continuing with tasks. She complains that she cannot concentrate. She seems not to plan things before she does them. She is personable and pleasant to others but waits for them to approach her rather than taking the first step (does not initiate or assert herself). She evaluates her own performance negatively.

- **Environment**. According to Rose and Larry, home life is very disorganized. Although Rose rarely leaves home, the small apartment is crowded with furniture, dirty clothes and dishes, unanswered mail, and children's toys. The disorder increased when Rose started to become ill 3 weeks ago. Larry's parents visit about twice a week, and Larry's mother tries to help but has recently been frustrated with Rose, who does not follow her advice to keep things organized. Rose and Larry both had friends during high school but have not seen any of them in the past 6 months.

Because Rose's hospitalization insurance allows for only a 1-week stay, Raquel and James arranged for continued care with a community mental health agency that provides occupational therapy services. They contacted the local agency and scheduled an appointment for Rose to visit the center and meet the occupational therapist. James and Rose together outlined a series of goals on which Rose could begin to work while still in the hospital and that she would continue and complete at home.

1. Work with Rose to develop self-care routines adequately and on time each day. Increase Rose's sense of self-control by allowing her to choose, with guidance, the occupational therapy groups she will attend during the next few days. Encourage her to try out games and word processing on the occupational therapy department's computer. Encourage her to discuss her situation in social groups with other clients, especially with those who are parents.
2. Establish a daily routine for self-care, housekeeping, and childcare at home, scheduling only necessary tasks and leaving time for leisure.
3. Review Rose's plans for the future. Explore options for her to resume friendships, to return to church activities, and to complete school and help her consider how she might approach these goals.
4. Recommend that the community occupational therapist visit Rose and Larry at home after discharge to evaluate the home environment and discuss ways it could be reorganized. Recommend community follow-up, a parent support group, and a play group for the children. Recommend that Rose be taught streamlined routines for housework and self-care and that she be helped to establish a weekly and seasonal housekeeping schedule and a child-care schedule.
5. Support Rose's interest in group sports by helping her explore opportunities for volleyball and softball at the local community fitness center.

On the day of discharge, Rose smiled as she said to James, "It seemed so hopeless to me before. Nothing is really different yet, but now I feel like I can make it different. Maybe that's what matters."

This case example illustrates some principles for using the MOHO. First, in a dynamic system, all parts affect the others. Requiring Rose to demonstrate adequate self-care routines activates habituation and performance capacity. Engaging in these customary occupational routines can support more normal functioning and engagement in other tasks. Second, change in the relevant environment can support or precipitate a change in the various human systems. Rose's home environment is critical to her ability to get and stay organized; the home visit will provide information so that the occupational therapist can suggest ways to make it more manageable and supportive for Rose. Furthermore, learning simplified housework routines will help her establish efficient habits and will free her time for other pursuits, such as sports or finishing school.

The example also shows the role of the occupational therapy assistant in this model. The occupational therapy assistant carries out the structured parts of the assessment, gathers data from the medical record, and collaborates with the occupational therapist to develop the intervention plan. The occupational therapy assistant works closely with the client to schedule intervention activities. Either in the hospital or in the community, the occupational therapy assistant could provide training in household management or leisure planning, could teach child-care and self-care skills, and could help Rose reorganize her home environment.

Intervention goals for the MOHO are in Boxes 3.6 and 3.7.

BOX 3.6 MOHO Intervention Goals (Non–System Based)

Aim of Intervention for: self-organization, resiliency, occupational identity, occupational competence, occupational adaptation, occupational participation, occupational performance, and occupational skills

Self-organization for stable patterns of behavior

Resiliency toward changing and adapting for recovery

Complete occupational identity, occupational competence, and occupational adaptation

Occupational participation through occupational performance and occupational skills

Goals

Client will improve self-organizing behavior to complete occupational participation of _____ with _____* (add needed amount or type of assistance) and _____** within _____***.

** structured environment, everyday environment of _____, setup of activity, participation of a peer, no peer involvement, no direct involvement from practitioner, assistive technology device, self-monitoring and reflection; mindfulness, stress management techniques, self-awareness

Client will improve resiliency to complete occupational participation of _____ with _____* (add needed amount or type of assistance) and _____^ within _____***.

^ structured environment, everyday environment of _____, setup of activity, participation of a peer, no peer involvement, no direct involvement from practitioner, assistive technology device, self-monitoring and reflection; mindfulness, stress management techniques, self-awareness

Client will improve occupational identity to complete occupational participation of _____ with _____* (add needed amount or type of assistance) and _____^^ within _____***.

^^ structured environment, everyday environment of _____, setup of activity, participation of a peer, no peer involvement, no direct involvement from practitioner, assistive technology device, self-monitoring and reflection, use of inventory checklist tool, self-reporting assessment tool, self-reflection, identifying new/needed roles, completing new project of _____, establishing new habit of _____, establish new routine for _____

Client will improve occupational competence to complete occupational participation of _____ with _____* (add needed amount or type of assistance) and _____^^^ within _____***.

^^^ structured environment, everyday environment of _____, setup of activity, participation of a peer, no peer involvement, no direct involvement from practitioner, assistive technology device, self-monitoring and reflection, performing occupations in various environments, performing occupations for various roles

Client will improve occupational adaptation to complete occupational participation of _____ with _____* (add needed amount or type of assistance) and _____^^^^ within _____***.

^^^^ completion of occupational identity, completion of occupational competence, increased resiliency, identification of control parameter, adaptation to harmful control parameter

Client will improve occupational performance to complete occupational participation of _____ with _____* (add needed amount or type of assistance) and _____+ within _____***.

+structured environment, everyday environment of _____, setup of activity, completion of _____ steps, backward chaining, forward chaining, work simplification/energy conservation/joint protection techniques

Client will improve occupational skill of _____ to complete occupational participation of _____ with _____* (add needed amount or type of assistance) and _____++ within _____***.

++structured environment, everyday environment of _____, setup of activity, participation of a peer, no peer involvement, no direct involvement from practitioner, assistive technology device, backward chaining, forward chaining, grading _____/adapting_____ intervention for client factor need (physical, cognitive, sensory, perceptual, emotional, communication interaction, social [specify areas of need])

* guidance, written prompt, written directions, cue, direct supervision/contact, indirect supervision/contact, physical assistance
*** number of attempts, number of sessions, number of weeks

BOX 3.7 MOHO Intervention Goals (System Based)

Aim of Intervention for: personal volition, habituation, performance capacity

Doing, or occupational participation through recognition and use of volitional, habitual, and performance capacity system

Goals

Client will improve sense of personal capacity to complete occupational participation of _____ with _____* (add needed amount or type of assistance) and _____** within _____***.

** structured environment, everyday environment of _____, self-monitoring and reflection; mindfulness, self-awareness

Client will improve self-efficacy to complete occupational participation of _____ with _____* (add needed amount or type of assistance) and _____^ within _____***.

^ structured environment, everyday environment of _____, setup of activity, participation of a peer, no peer involvement, no direct involvement from practitioner, assistive technology device, self-monitoring and reflection; mindfulness, self-awareness, self-needs awareness, self-worth/esteem

Client will identify values/interests of occupational identity to complete occupational participation of _____ with _____* (add needed amount or type of assistance) and _____^^ within _____***.

^^ use of inventory checklist tool, self-reporting assessment tool, self-reflection, identifying of beliefs, identify of interest pattern

Client will identify habits of style to complete occupational participation of _____ with _____* (add needed amount or type of assistance) and _____^^^ within _____***.

^^^ identification of roles, identification of role expectations, awareness of temporal factors, awareness of self and environmental supports/barriers (limitation), acceptance of limitations, adapted technique

Client will improve routines to complete occupational participation of _____ with _____* (add needed amount or type of assistance) and _____^^^ within _____***.

^^^ identification of roles, identification of role expectations, awareness of temporal factors, awareness of self and environmental supports/barriers (limitation), acceptance of limitations, adapted technique

Client will improve supportive habits to complete occupational participation of _____ with _____* (add needed amount or type of assistance) and _____*^ within _____***.

*^structured environment, everyday environment of _____, setup of activity, health management techniques, work simplification/energy conservation/joint protection techniques

Client will limit/decrease unhealthy habit/harmful habit to complete occupational participation of _____ with _____* (add needed amount or type of assistance) and _____**^ within _____***.

**^ structured environment, everyday environment of _____, setup of activity, participation of a peer, no peer involvement, no direct involvement from practitioner, assistive technology device, grading _____/adapting_____ (of client function or performance skill), self-awareness of negative consequences of actions

Client will identify roles to complete occupational participation of _____ with _____* (add needed amount or type of assistance) and _____**^^ within _____***.

**^^ use of role checklist tool, self-reporting assessment tool, self-reflection, identify routines, identify social expectations

Client will improve role performance to complete occupational participation of _____ with _____* (add needed amount or type of assistance) and _____*^^^ within _____***.

*^^^structured environment, everyday environment of _____, setup of activity, participation of a peer, no peer involvement, no direct involvement from practitioner, assistive technology device, backward chaining, forward chaining, grading _____/adapting_____ intervention for client factor need (emotional, communication interaction, social [specify specific areas of need])

Client will identify physical/mental functional needs performance to complete occupational participation of _____ with _____+ (add needed amount or type of assistance) and _____++ within _____***.

+use of inventory tool, self-reflection, observation, self-reporting

++ structured environment, everyday environment of _____, setup of activity, participation of a peer, no peer involvement, no direct involvement from practitioner, assistive technology device, backward chaining, forward chaining, grading _____/adapting_____ intervention for client factor need (physical, cognitive, sensory, perceptual, emotional, communication interaction, social [specify areas of need])

Client will improve physical/mental functional needs performance to complete occupational participation of _____ with _____++ (add needed amount or type of assistance) and _____++ within _____***.

++ structured environment, everyday environment of _____, setup of activity, participation of a peer, no peer involvement, no direct involvement from practitioner, assistive technology device, backward chaining, forward chaining, grading _____/adapting_____ intervention for client factor need (physical, cognitive, sensory, perceptual, emotional, communication interaction, social [specify areas of need])

Client will identify subjective expression feelings to complete occupational participation of _____ with _____* (add needed amount or type of assistance) and _____+++ within _____***.

+++self-monitoring and reflection, mindfulness, interoception, self-awareness skills

Client will improve awareness/use of subjective expression feelings to complete occupational participation of _____ with _____* (add needed amount or type of assistance) and _____+++ within _____***.

+++self-monitoring and reflection, mindfulness, interoception, self-awareness skills

* guidance, written prompt, written directions, cue, direct supervision/contact, indirect supervision/contact
*** number of attempts, number of sessions, number of weeks

The MOHO gives us a good basic design for understanding the occupational nature of human beings. The description of the model as presented here has been brief and is intended to help the occupational therapy professional student obtain a general sense of the clinical reasoning an occupational therapy professional might apply to a person's problems. The model itself is much more complex; an entire text has been written to explain it (70-73, 131). In addition, much research has explored the effectiveness of the model and has attempted to develop it further (60, 61, 74, 79, 104, 135) and analyze its value (56, 79, 85, 86). We expect continued changes and growth in this model.

Concepts **Summary**

1. Human beings are internally driven to act.
2. Humans act within a dynamic system to self-organize because of multiple system interactions that cause fluctuations in the continuity we experience throughout our daily life.
3. Human action is called human occupation. Human occupation is organized into three systems, each of which affects and is affected by the others. All three systems interact with the environment.
4. Volition, or motivation, initiates action.
5. Habituation organizes actions into predictable routines and patterns.
6. Performance capacity is the ability to act, consisting of objective physical and mental capacities for action and the subjective experience of this capacity.
7. Doing involves occupational participation, occupational performance, and occupational skills.
8. Through occupational identity and occupational competence, which occurs through participation, performance, and skills, people move to occupational adaptation.

VOCABULARY REVIEW

dynamic system of interaction
Humans engage in self-organization because of interactions with multiple systems that cause fluctuations in continuity.

environment
The physical, social, and occupational dimensions; and the economic, political, and cultural factors of the immediate, local, and global societal contexts that impact occupational motivation, organization, and performance

habits
Particular and consistent performances and responses we have acquired, completed within environments and situations we find familiar

habituation
Internalized readiness to perform patterns of behavior that are guided by our habits and roles and connected to the environment

human occupation
An internally driven act toward doing, or participation in, productivity, play, or ADLs

interests
Personal preferences in activity or people. Interests are pleasurable and motivate actions accordingly.

internalized role
How we have learned to act at certain times with certain people, in certain situations

lived body
Considering what we do, objectively and subjectively together

occupational adaptation
Dynamic combination of environmental impact, a positive occupational identity, and occupational competence that corresponds with one's occupational identity

occupational competence
Skillful and easily performed chosen occupations because of being practiced over time within various social roles

occupational identity
Our sense of being that develops over time, based on repeated patterns of engagement and reflect our life experiences

occupational participation
Everyday engagement in productivity, play, and ADLs

occupational performance
Discrete acts of doing, or the discrete units of doing that we perform

occupational skills
Observable, goal-directed actions that we complete during occupational performance

performance capacity
Abilities to do things, to perform actions, combined with identifying the objective physical and mental components and the subjective experience of the action

personal causation
The individual's sense of their own competence and ability to be effective

values
Internalized images of what is correct and right

volition
Motivation; the thoughts and feelings that are involved with selecting, enacting, and continuing an occupation or activity

PERSON–ENVIRONMENT–OCCUPATION MODEL

The **PEO** model is, like the MOHO, an occupational performance model. It was developed during the 1980s in Canada by occupational therapists Mary Law, Barbara Cooper, Susan Strong, Debra Stewart, Patricia Rigby, and Lori Letts (84). It is a person-centered model that focuses on the occupational performance that results from **transactions** among the person, the different contexts of the environment, and the occupations in which the person engages (18). We will define these terms.

The PEO views the **person** in a holistic way and the person is considered through the various roles they complete. More than one role can be completed at a time, and different roles take precedence at different times, depending on the occupational demands of the person. The person includes the body (physical self), the mind (the cognitive self and the affective self), and the spiritual self. Performance skill competencies (motor, cognitive, and sensory) are considered part of the person, as are acquired life experiences and personal factors. The person is viewed as dynamic and changing through time and experience. A person makes choices as to what occupations they want to do and when to do those occupations, based on the limiting factor of what opportunities are available (18).

Within the PEO, the **environment** includes physical, social, cultural, institutional, and virtual components (18). Environment is fundamental to occupational performance. As in the MOHO, the "same" occupation performed in a different environment results in a different occupational performance. The environment suggests how one may behave, what one may do, and in this way cues behavior (84).

Within the PEO, **occupation** represents "groups of self-directed functional tasks and activities in which a person engages over the lifespan" (84, p. 16). Occupations are composed of tasks. *Tasks* are sets of activities. *Activities* are the basic unit. Occupation includes the temporal aspects of habits and time use patterns (routines), both of which are connected to the usage of space. Time is considered on the macrolevel of "periods of time" and on the microlevel of time needed to complete tasks, actions, and occupations and create our use of time (18). An example of these concepts is located in Table 3.4.

Occupational load "is applied to the number of roles, tasks, and occupations that an individual undertakes in the course of a specific time span, such as a day or a week" (18, p. 145). Consideration must be given to the number of roles one has and the amount of work, expectations, and responsibilities associated with each role. The occupational load can become overwhelming, and it can become difficult to cope (or manage) one's emotions and emotional response to this load. Our clients experience losses such as chronic conditions, acute injuries, and mental disorders. This can make their occupational load unmanageable. As occupational therapy professionals, rethinking about a client's life situation through the PEO lens can help readjustment occur and help us collaborate with the client to help them find a new balance and organization. The options possible within the environment can be considered along with their role needs and occupational desires (18).

Occupational performance is the point at which the person, the environment, and the occupation intersect (23) (see Figure 3.6). Occupational performance may be limited or expansive. The extent of occupational performance reflects the compatibility between the person, the environment, and the occupation. For example, a person who is depressed, like Rose in the previous example, may have little motivation to engage in self-care. And, a disorganized environment presents many obstacles to performing self-care and homemaker tasks. At one point in her life, perhaps when she was living at home before she met Larry, Rose may have engaged easily and competently in self-care. Figure 3.6 shows the variability of occupational performance throughout the life span. At one point it may be full and at another time restricted. Later (or earlier) in life (eg, as the figure shows), occupational

Table 3.4. Occupational Pieces, Space Considerations, and Temporal Aspects

Occupation and Its Parts	Space Considerations	Temporal Aspects	Time Level
Activity: Searching for evidence in databases	Computer station or desk Home study area or college library or public library	Habit: Always starting with a particular database or only looking for full-text articles	Microlevel: Amount of time needed to - set up material to use databases - log-in and databases to "open" - search any given database
Task: Producing a research paper	Computer station or desk Home study area or college library or public library Kitchen table or private home office space Quiet space or noisy space Area to store office supplies needed to produce the research paper	Habit: Using certain phrases or vocabulary within the text Routine: Completing it in steps: (1) General research in books. (2) Narrowed down topic research in databases. (3) Use of index bibliography cards. (4) Start with conclusion. (5) Make an outline. (6) Complete the body. (7) Write the introduction. (8) Proofread. (9) Make sure it is electronically submitted.	Microlevel: Amount of time needed to: - write bibliography cards - write sections of research paper - proofread paper - log-in, open learning management system and ensure electronic submission of research paper
Occupation: Being a student who produces research papers and completes other tasks such as passing a test	Living: - on campus - close to campus - an hour from campus Living: - alone - with peers - with parents - with small children	Routine: Doing small amounts of research papers each day vs waiting until 48 hours before it is due and then starting. Studying in chunks, starting with prereading for class	Microlevel: Amount of time to: - study for a test - read and prepare for a class discussion - complete a research paper - finish an assignment or project Macrolevel: Period of time one is a college student

Adapted from concepts from Baptiste, S. (2017). The person-environment-occupation model. In J. Hinojosa, P. Kramer, & C. Brasic Royeen (Eds.), *Perspectives on human occupation: Theories underlying practice* (2nd ed., pp. 137–159). F.A. Davis.

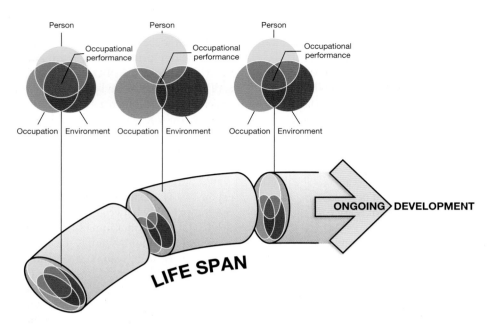

Figure 3.6. Person–Environment–Occupation Model. (Reprinted with permission from Law, M., Cooper, B., Strong, S., Steward, D., Rigby, P., & Letts, L. (1996). The person-environment-occupation model: A transactive approach to occupational performance. *Canadian Journal of Occupational Therapy, 63*(1), 9–23 (Figure 1b, p. 15).)

performance may become easier and fuller. Occupations and roles also shift throughout the life span and priorities change during different stages of life.

Within occupational therapy, the occupational therapy professional collaborates with the client so they can engage in the occupations they choose. An optimal occupational plan includes objectives identifying (a) how the person wants to perform their occupations (rated a particular level of performance ability between "not being able to complete the occupation at all" to the level of "completing the occupation just the way the person wants to do so") and (b) how satisfied the person is with how well the person completes the occupation (18). Because our client's occupations and role expectations shift, their occupational priorities shift, and this change can cause them conflict with their occupational performance. That conflict can be in how they view themselves, occupation considerations, and environment aspects and how that view may no longer be balanced, or how it has become disorganized.

Transactions, as described earlier, are the ongoing adjustments and changes that occur during occupational performance, as the person and the environment act and react to each other. A transaction is more than an interaction. It includes changes that continually occur as the person and the environment adjust to each other during occupational performance. In contrast, an interaction is time-limited, not considered to be ongoing and dynamic. As these transactions occur, the effect is to modify the occupational performance.

The **PEO** model is concerned with person–environment fit, or the extent to which the environment is a good match

for the person's interests and abilities. The better the fit, the better the occupational performance. The poorer the match, the less satisfactory the occupational performance.

Basic Assumptions of the Person–Environment–Occupation Model (84)

The person is dynamic, complex, continually developing, and always interacting within and with the environment. The unique characteristics of the person influence the ways in which that person performs occupations and the way that person interacts with the environment. For instance, the cultural background of the person is one of the unique characteristics and will always be present in that person, although the person may modify their behavior in a new cultural environment. To illustrate, Leila is a college student from the United States who studied abroad in Egypt. She learned that modesty was viewed differently and may require wardrobe adjustments to be respectful. Leila learned from her peers at the university what was expected, and she made appropriate adjustments to participate in activities with her class and within the community.

The person's occupational performance takes place within the context of the environment, which can facilitate or restrict performance. For example, consider that getting around in one's community in a wheelchair is easier where sidewalks exist, are level, and have curb cuts at street crossings. Another environment, with unpaved gravel roads and no sidewalk, restricts community mobility for someone in a wheelchair. Similarly, as we discussed about Rose, a complex environment may be overwhelming to someone who is depressed and has low energy. Simplifying the environment may facilitate transactions that improve performance.

The environment is more easily changed than is the person (84). This may mean a change to a completely different environment. In the example of the person in a wheelchair, a move into town may be necessary so that stores and services can be accessed and so that the wheelchair can be operated easily on smoother surfaces. It is easier to move to a new environment than to get the person who needs a wheelchair to somehow not need it anymore, or a person with depression to have more energy and ability to concentrate and plan.

Occupations meet the human need for self-maintenance and the expression of achieving the occupations that occur within the context of one's roles and within the environment. Occupations include self-care, productivity or work, leisure, and rest or sleep (18). Many occupations exist, with tasks and activities within them. A person may engage in multiple occupations over a day or over a lifetime.

Occupational performance occurs in time and space and is continually changing. Changes occur because of transactions among the person, environment, and the occupation in which the person has engaged.

A person's occupational performance must balance the ever-changing needs and priorities of the self and the needs and priorities that are presented in the environment. Throughout one's life, the meanings one attaches to occupation and the environment must be renegotiated with the view of the self and the view of role expectations and role responsibilities. Aspects of occupational performance can be objectively measured through observation of performance components. Self-report is required for the subjective components of performance satisfaction (18).

For example, consider a client who has had multiple orthopedic injuries and surgeries involving both upper extremities. They enjoyed many manual activities prior to their injuries. They had the idea to resume playing piano, something they had once done daily. But now they are frustrated by pain and incoordination and have begun to blame themselves for not being able to get past these challenges and make it work. They become depressed each time they attempted playing the piano, because their fingers and wrists no longer respond as they once did. At a previous time in their life, their available range of occupational performance was broad and diverse. Now, though they have lots of time, they find little to do that they want to do and have a very restricted range of occupational performance.

The better the fit between person and environment, the better the occupational performance. Fitting the environment to the person may involve minor adjustments or major ones. For example, a person who is older and whose vision is more limited than when they were younger may find it very challenging and frustrating to read or use a computer in a home office that was perfectly fine at an earlier point in their life. Purchasing a floor lamp with a higher light output might be all that is needed to enable performance.

The PEO is a person-centered model. A large variety of assessment instruments are used within the PEO, examining various aspects of the person, the environment, and the occupation. Many assessments were not designed by occupational therapists. One of the appeals of the model is that occupational therapists can use existing assessment tools with documented reliability and validity (see Chapter 12 for explanation of these terms).

The Canadian Occupational Performance Measure (COPM) (83) is a PEO-associated assessment tool, designed by Canadian occupational therapists for use with the PEO model. It is a client-centered subjective assessment that documents the client's own perception of their occupational performance, over time. In the initial meeting, the occupational therapist engages the client in a discussion of self-care, leisure, and productivity. The client names and describes tasks or activities they normally do. The occupational therapist engages the client to select five problems identified as most important to them. The client is then asked to assign a rating from 1 to 10, indicating *how well* they do the activity and *how satisfied* they are with the performance. It is possible to see yourself as doing an activity in an average way (rating of 5) and at the same time feel that the performance is adequate (rating of 10). Alternatively, one can see performance as being performed close to excellent (rating of 9) while also feeling highly dissatisfied with the performance (rating of 2).

The results of the COPM are used to determine goals for intervention. The client chooses which goals have highest priority. Interventions may address person factors, environmental factors, or occupation factors, and sometimes more than one of these. A variety of intervention methods may be used.

Goals for intervention to use with the PEO are listed in Box 3.8.

BOX 3.8 PEO Intervention Goals

Aim of Intervention

Seek balance and organization with simultaneous role expectations and responsibilities.

Develop habits and routines for prioritized occupational performance.

Seek environments, and adjust as needed, for optimal occupational performance.

Identify performance level for desired occupations.

Complete occupations at self-chosen satisfaction level.

Goals

Client will identify:

occupational performance level

occupational performance satisfaction level

role expectations and responsibilities

habits

routines

person factor of physical self/performance skill of _____

person factor of cognitive self of _____

person factor of affective self of _____

person factor of spiritual self of _____

task

activity

to complete occupational performance transaction of _____

with _____ (add needed amount or type of assistance)

  guidance

  written prompt

  written directions

  cue

  direct supervision/contact

  indirect supervision/contact

  physical assistance

and _____

  use of self-inventory tool

  use of client-centered occupational performance rating scale

  use of life experiences

  physical environmental component of _____

  social environmental component of _____

  cultural environmental component of _____

  institutional environmental component of _____

  virtual environmental component of _____

  environmental options of _____

  space considerations of _____

  coping skills of _____ for management of occupational load

  readjustment/reprioritization for management of occupational load

within _____.

  number of attempts

  number of sessions

  number of weeks

Client will develop/complete:

  role expectations and responsibilities

  habits

  routines

  person factor of physical self/performance skill of _____

  person factor of cognitive self of _____

  person factor of affective self of _____

  person factor of spiritual self of _____

  task

  activity

to complete occupational performance transaction of _____

with _____ (add needed amount or type of assistance)

  guidance

  written prompt

  written directions

  cue

  direct supervision/contact

  indirect supervision/contact

  physical assistance

and _____

  self-reflection

  use of life experiences

  physical environmental component of _____

  social environmental component of _____

  cultural environmental component of _____

  institutional environmental component of _____

  virtual environmental component of _____

  environmental options of _____

  space considerations of _____

  coping skills of _____ for management of occupational load

  readjustment/reprioritization for management of occupational load

within _____.

  number of attempts

  number of sessions

  number of weeks

Case Example

Evangeline lives in supported housing in a metropolitan area. She is single, never married, is 47 years old, and has a history of mental disorders since age 30. She is unable to work because of multiple disabling conditions, including asthma and arthritis. Currently diagnosed with bipolar disorder and borderline personality disorder, she has had difficulty sustaining stable relationships with friends and family. She has a history of polysubstance abuse (alcohol and cocaine) and is presently taking several prescription medications. These include a narcotic painkiller and many psychotropic drugs (an antidepressant, an antiseizure drug, an antipsychotic, and a stimulant). She has been enrolled in a grant-funded program that provides occupational therapy services to unemployed persons living in supported housing.

Evangeline met three times with the occupational therapist, Shawn, to complete the COPM. The goals she identified were to develop social relationships with other people, maintain her sobriety, decrease her use of medication, and secure a job.

Evangeline's education and work history up to the first psychotic episode showed a bachelor's degree in psychology, and steady employment in a variety of social service and human resources positions. She has not worked in a full-time paid position in the past 17 years but has attempted a variety of part-time office and retail jobs. She was terminated for cause from every one of these jobs, most typically because of disagreements with management and failure to adhere to workplace rules and schedule. She states that she is generally the smartest person around and that it is tiresome to deal with people who "will not get out of their own way."

Given Evangeline's stated interest in sobriety, and her polydrug use, Shawn explored with her how she might achieve and maintain sobriety. Because she has done this in the past, she agreed to resume attending Alcoholics Anonymous (AA) and/or Narcotics Anonymous (NA) meetings daily, to have a full medical workup, and to cooperate with medical doctors and the psychiatrist regarding medication reduction. She was motivated by her desire to maintain her position in the supported housing program. She risked losing her housing if she continued to use drugs the way she had been.

Shawn recommended that Evangeline enroll in a living skills program (LSP) for sobriety management and stress management. The program was coordinated by the occupational therapy assistant, Crystal, who conducted sessions jointly with a peer counselor (person who has a mental health diagnosis who is now helping others). Before beginning the program, Evangeline expressed impatience about getting a job and said she did not see how this was going to help her. She said she wanted to work as a volunteer peer counselor herself.

After 6 weeks, Evangeline had made progress in reducing her use of prescription pain medications to one pill per day at bedtime and was using over-the-counter anti-inflammatories instead. Crystal observed that Evangeline had several outbursts during the LSP classes, often criticized the peer counselor within the group, and was making it difficult for other students to progress. She seemed uncomfortable with the group and with the content of the program. Shawn thought that a dialectical behavior therapy (DBT) group to work on coping skills might be a better fit, given the diagnosis of borderline personality disorder. With Evangeline's consent, he contacted a clinic nearby that offered DBT groups, and she enrolled there. The DBT groups there were limited to 4 people, whereas the life skills classes accommodated up to 12. She continued to meet with Shawn, to attend AA/NA, and to work on reducing further her medication use.

A year later, Evangeline has remained sober and has been able to develop and continue a few friendly relationships with other women she has met. She got involved in a sexual relationship with a man she met at an NA meeting and went through a difficult time as he began to abuse her. It almost cost her sobriety and her place in supported housing. After discussing the situation with Shawn, Crystal, who had herself been a victim of domestic abuse, reached out to Evangeline, who decided to break off the abusive relationship. Evangeline says she is not presently interested in beginning another romantic relationship.

She has begun to attend the life skills classes on a limited basis, as she still finds the group size too large to tolerate anything more frequent. She has been volunteering at an animal rescue shelter three mornings a week and would like to get a job working with animals, perhaps as a veterinary technician. She says the animals make her feel peaceful. She says she loves stroking their fur, grooming them, taking them for walks, and playing with them. She is particularly fond of several pit bull mix dogs that were rescued from a dog-fighting arena. Her current goals are to continue to maintain sobriety, to continue her social life, to continue her volunteer animal rescue work, and to apply to school. She is still attending the DBT group and says it is hard work to manage her feelings, and even to feel her feelings. She recognizes the importance of learning to do this if she is to succeed in school and in her volunteer work, and eventually to get a job.

This case example demonstrates how the PEO model starts intervention from the client's stated goals. If Evangeline had not identified sobriety as a goal, the medication problem would not have been addressed as it was. The model is compatible with other occupational therapy and mental health models and techniques. The LSP group aims to help the client learn or acquire basic life skills (103). Such a group might be based on role acquisition or psychoeducation (see Chapter 6). The DBT group is a cognitive behavioral method, and occupational therapy professionals can seek advanced training to do this work (90).

The case shows how powerful the motivation for a productive life can be in prompting a person to change self-destructive behaviors. Movement toward this goal may be impaired by client factors that need to be addressed first. In this case, Evangeline's substance use and her volatile emotionality, were impediments to successful engagement in school or volunteer work.

Another aspect of the case is the importance of Crystal's therapeutic use of self. It is not always appropriate to share one's personal challenges with clients (called self-disclosure). But, in this case, Crystal's own history of domestic abuse caused her to feel protective of Evangeline and to reach out and help her get assistance to end the relationship with her abuser. Involving Shawn in the decision as to whether to share her own experience with Evangeline shows Crystal's professional maturity and her understanding of teamwork and the supervisory relationship.

Evangeline was uncomfortable in the LSP group (a poor fit of environment to person). She was unable to learn there, so Shawn identified another environment that would be a better fit. Despite this environmental change, much of the intervention addressed aspects of the person. Client factors impeded Evangeline's pursuit of sobriety, social interaction, and productive activity. Thus, changing these client factors was a primary focus of occupational therapy.

The setting here is long term and in the community. The PEO model can be used within the hospital and in the community, both long term and short term, depending on the person's goals and available resources. The PEO model has been applied in occupational therapy mental health practice primarily in Canada, but it is used internationally, and has been the subject of many research studies (24, 96, 110). An occupational therapy program in the United States using the

PEO model, with those without permanent housing, was found to promote involvement in productive roles such as student, volunteer, or worker (103).

Concepts Summary

1. The person is complex and continually developing.
2. Occupations meet basic human needs and are basic to being human.
3. The person's occupational performance takes place within the context of the environment, which can facilitate or restrict performance. It occurs in time and space and is continually changing.
4. Occupational load includes role expectations and occupations undertaken. Occupational load can become overwhelming.
5. The purpose of any intervention is to improve occupational performance, based on the occupational choices of the client, within the opportunities presented in the environment.
6. Interventions may be targeted at the level of the person, the environment, and/or the occupation.
7. The better the fit of the environment to the person, the better the occupational performance.
8. The environment is more easily changed than is the person.

VOCABULARY REVIEW

environment
    Includes physical, social, cultural, institutional, and virtual components. Environment is fundamental to occupational performance.

occupation
    "Groups of self-directed functional tasks and activities in which a person engages over the lifespan" (84, p. 16). Occupations are composed of tasks. Tasks are sets of activities. Activities are the basic unit.

occupational load
    The roles, tasks, and occupations that we complete within a particular time span

occupational performance
    "The outcome of the transactions of the person, environment and occupation" (84, p. 17).

person
    "A unique being who assumes a number of roles simultaneously" (83, p. 15). The person includes the body, mind, and spiritual self. Performance skills are considered part of the person, as are acquired life experiences and person factors. The person is viewed as dynamic and changing through time and experience.

person–environment fit
    The degree to which the environment is compatible with the person and supportive of the best level of occupational performance for that person.

transaction
    The ongoing and dynamic relationship that occurs during multiple interactions that have mutual effects on the person and the environment as occupational performance occurs

ECOLOGY OF HUMAN PERFORMANCE

EHP is considered an ecologic model, recognizing influences of the person, environment, and task on functional performance. It was initially developed by occupational therapists Dunn, Brown, and McGuigan (47) as a framework that emphasized the critical nature of a person's contexts in performing functional tasks. The EHP utilizes terminology of "task" instead of occupation as it was intentionally created for interdisciplinary collaboration and access by professionals of other disciplines. In the EHP model, the person is portrayed within the context, and tasks that surround them. Tasks within a specified performance range are highlighted, as they represent specific tasks that are available to the person because of their own abilities, skills, and experiences within a supporting environmental context. Tasks outside of the performance range are considered outside of the person's reach. As the person's occupational performance increases because of the development of new skills, the performance range to accomplish tasks also increases. Likewise, when the person's occupational performance decreases because of injury or a loss of skills, the performance range decreases (46).

Contextual changes may also increase or decrease the performance range, depending on whether they support or hinder occupational performance. Because of the dynamic nature of variables related to person factors and context, changes in occupational performance (and the client's performance range) may occur with new or restored skills, altered tasks, or modified environments. Additionally, strategies may be applied to create or promote occupational performance, establish or restore skills, maintain performance capacity, modify context or activity demands, or prevent barriers to performance. These strategies of the EHP have informed the OTPF-4E and are viewed as five separate approaches to intervention (Dunn, McClain, Brown, & Youngstrom, 1998, as cited in OTPF-4E [14]).

The EHP provides an occupational therapy perspective when used in collaboration with other disciplines (48) and demonstrates the value of occupational therapy. It considers the uniqueness of the individual performing a task within specific sociocultural and temporal contexts (such as chronologic age and developmental level). It also provides a framework for occupational therapy evaluation and intervention.

For evaluation, the EHP emphasizes information about the client's contexts, as well as their skills. It also guides occupational therapy professionals to identify the client's functional performance needs to determine what the client desires or needs to do. The occupational therapy professional completes a task analysis and observes the client in a variety of settings. Dunn's Sensory Profile assessments (Adolescent/Adult Sensory Profile [A/ASP], Sensory Profile, Infant-Toddler Sensory Profile, School Companion, Sensory Profile-2 [SP-2]) are based on SI theory and the

EHP (30, 45). The relationship between the client's sensory processing patterns, tasks, and contexts determines whether or not the client is able to function optimally. For example, if a client is demonstrating difficulties in dressing tasks because of sensory sensitivity and sensory avoiding patterns, the occupational therapist must evaluate specific contexts where the client performs the dressing tasks to determine whether it is supporting or hindering occupational performance.

For intervention, the EHP identifies intervention strategies to improve the client's performance range. Based on the evaluation findings and interpretation, the occupational therapist collaborates with the client to set goals. Depending on the client's identified outcomes and needs, the occupational therapist will provide a variety of intervention options. Five specific intervention strategies may address the person/context/task relationship to: (i) restore skills, (ii) alter the environment, (iii) adapt the task, (iv) prevent problems, and (v) create opportunities to support optimal performance (48). "According to the framework, understanding the person-environment transaction is the basis for designing interventions that support engagement in chosen tasks" (48, p. 260). Using the example of a client with sensory processing and dressing difficulties, the interaction of the client's sensory processing patterns and contextual factors of the dressing environment must be assessed to determine their occupational performance. Intervention may be applied to restore the client's function by increasing their (or the caregiver's) awareness of sensory processing patterns affected by the environmental context. Other types of strategies may involve altering, adapting, or creating an optimal fit between the client's sensory processing patterns and the environmental context (48). In this example, intervention may also include adapting the task by offering choices of different types of clothing styles or fabrics. Intervention may involve modifying the environment to provide additional physical or social support, or to provide a calm and relaxing room to promote the "just-right" level of arousal for dressing. Altering the type of detergent or fabric softener may also assist the client. Thus, the EHP provides a variety of intervention strategies to promote the client's occupational performance and quality of life.

According to Dunn et al (48), each person's context is unique and complex, and the occupational therapy professional must understand it to understand the person. Therefore, understanding the personal factors, including their culture, age, development, and experiences, as well as the physical, social, and attitudinal environmental factors is key to learning about the person and their occupational performance. In the EHP, the person functions in different ways depending on their context; however, actions of the person also change the context. In this dynamic system, intervention that is applied to any component (person, task, or context) has the potential to change their performance outcome. The EHP acknowledges performance differences in natural and contrived contexts. Because of the variability of performance in contrived contexts, natural environments provide optimal locations for both evaluation and intervention. The EHP also promotes self-determination and inclusion in all aspects of life. An example of an EHP intervention goal is shown in Box 3.9.

BOX 3.9 Ecology of Human Performance Intervention Goal

Aim of Intervention

Complete occupational tasks within client's performance range.

Restore skills.

Alter the environment.

Adapt the task.

Prevent problems.

Create opportunities to support optimal performance.

Goal

Client will complete occupational task of _____ with _____* (add needed amount or type of assistance) and _____** within _____***.

* guidance, written prompt, written directions, verbal directions, cue, physical assistance, direct supervision/contact, indirect supervision/contact, setup
** new learned skill of _____, restored skill of _____, grading (explain type), adaptation (explain what), modified environment of _____, health promotion strategy of _____, prevention of _____
*** number of attempts, number of sessions, number of weeks

Concepts Summary

1. Ecology model recognizes the influence of person, environment, and task on functional performance.
2. EHP is an interdisciplinary-based model designed for collaboration among disciplines.
3. The person is portrayed within the context and tasks that surround them.
4. A person's context is unique and complex. It must be understood by the occupational therapy professional and the person.
5. Tasks are considered within a specified performance range, and tasks the person is unable to perform are considered outside the person's reach.
6. Occupational performance increases or decreases, based on skills gained or lost.
7. Context influences performance range and can also enhance or hinder performance range.
8. Five main intervention strategies are a part of EHP: restore (skill), alter (environment), adapt (task), prevent (problem), or create (opportunity).
9. A person's function changes based on their context and a person's actions can change the context.

natural environments
  Optimal location for both evaluation and intervention

performance range
  Specific tasks that are available to the person because of their own abilities, skills, and experiences within a supporting environmental context

personal factors
  Includes items such as culture, age, development, and experiences

task
  How occupational performance is defined

SENSORY INTEGRATION FRAME OF REFERENCE

Sensory Integration Background and General Information

Sensory integration (**SI**) is a frame of reference initially developed in the early second half of the 20th century by the occupational therapist A. Jean Ayres (16, 17) as an intervention to use with children with learning disorders. SI is the smooth working together of all the senses to provide information needed for accurate perception and motor action. A. Jean Ayres addressed not only the five senses that are commonly recognized (sight, hearing, taste, smell, and touch) but also proprioception and vestibular awareness. Identified here are two other internal senses that occupational therapy addresses—kinesthesia and interoception.

Proprioception is the sense that helps us identify where parts of our bodies are positioned in space, even if we cannot see them. For example, you do not have to look under your desk to know where your feet are; you have a built-in sense, proprioception, which keeps you informed of their location and position.

Kinesthesia is the sense of knowing where and how a body part is moving. For instance, when you move your arms to clap at a concert or to brush your hair, kinesthetic awareness helps you know where your arms are moving (in front of your body or around your head) and how well that movement is being performed (for instance, with a full amount or a lack of range of motion) (36, 54).

Vestibular awareness is the sense that detects motion and the pull of gravity during movement. For instance, when you fall while learning to roller skate or ride a bicycle, you sense that you have gotten off-balance and you have a feeling for what speed you are going and in what direction you are likely to fall. You get this information from your vestibular system, which coordinates sensations of balance, velocity, and acceleration.

Interoception is an internal sense that has recently begun to be addressed by occupational therapy. As defined by the OTPF-4E, it is "internal detection of changes in one's internal organs through specific sensory receptors" (14, p. 53). Interoception allows us to feel the sensations occurring inside of our bodies (93). Being aware of how our internal body feels helps us to be more self-aware of our emotions, mood, motivation, and conscious behavior (39). Afferent (sensory) neurons carry sensory information from the internal organs to the central nervous system, which then provides information for the autonomic nervous system (39). The sense of interoception, and using internal body awareness and internal body sense as a predictive mechanism, may be helpful toward achieving allostasis and making adaptive changes to maintain body homeostasis (20, 38). Further discussion of how this sense adds to processing of sensory information will be addressed in the next section.

SI is a neurologic process that allows us to take in all the information from the five basic senses and the proprioceptive and vestibular systems so that you can accurately interpret what is going on around you and act on it. Ayres's initial concepts were based on the neurologic ideas that sensory systems build upon one another hierarchically, requiring organization of the foundational layers (such as the tactile, proprioceptive, and vestibular) before there could be organization in higher order functional systems. In this theory, the lower brainstem level functions needed to be integrated first, so that higher level functional skills could then be integrated in a hierarchical fashion (Ayres, 1979, as cited in Cole [37]), at a largely unconscious level. With advancing knowledge of neuroscience, the original hierarchical theory is no longer held. Further discussion of current SI theory will be addressed in the next section ("A Shift in the Framework").

It should be noted that SI intervention has not generally been found effective in mental health research studies. However, occupational therapy professionals continue to apply it and study its effects. Research around SI and those with mental illness began with research by occupational therapist Lorna Jean King (76); however, at present, there is little research evidence to support the use of this model with the psychiatric population (57). Reisman and Blakeney (112), in a study of five clients with schizophrenia, demonstrated significant improvement in measures of ward behavior (social interest and reduction of psychopathology) following SI intervention of just a few weeks' duration. SI has been attempted with clients who have dementia without evidence of significant therapeutic benefit (115). SI techniques applied as part of a sensory-based hatha yoga program for military veterans with posttraumatic stress disorder (PTSD) were found to be helpful in reducing anxiety. The techniques used in the study that were found to be helpful included:

- deep touch pressure through the palms and feet and
- enhanced proprioceptive input throughout the torso and throughout all four limbs by using:
  - slow and rhythmic dynamic flow during specific asanas (body postures used were downward dog and upward dog) and coordinated breathing and
  - props use of strapping and wood blocks (128).

Intervention grounded in SI has shown positive effects with children with sensory processing difficulties and with learning disabilities (136). In a review of the literature, regarding autism spectrum disorder (ASD), there was strong evidence to support the efficacy of using Ayres Sensory

Integration (ASI) (discussed later in this section) intervention to improve individual goals of functioning and of participation, as measured by the *Goal Attainment Scale* (GAS), and moderate evidence for using ASI interventions to decrease a child's caregiver assistance needs for social skills and self-care (118). There was insufficient evidence to support ASI intervention as a mechanism for client outcome changes in the skills of play, sensorimotor, perceptual, cognitive, and language (118). The study also reported moderate evidence of ASI for decreasing autistic mannerisms (118). It is important to note that the autistic community currently opposes the viewpoint of decreasing autistic mannerisms (66).

Because of the powerful and occasionally unpredictable effects on the central nervous system, SI intervention programs must be designed and monitored by an occupational therapist. SI assessments and interventions must be identified by the occupational therapist. Occupational therapy assistants, under the occupational therapist's supervision, can help by carrying out the intervention once the plan has been designed.

Occupational therapy for SI dysfunction requires extensive training for assessment and intervention. The AOTA has taken the position that occupational therapists desiring to use SI techniques should receive advanced training, because SI is based on more advanced knowledge than is provided in entry-level professional education programs (10).

A Shift in the Framework

As stated earlier, the SI frame of reference, originally developed by A. Jean Ayres, was based on the neurologic knowledge of the time and looked at foundational layers of the sensory system developing and organizing first, with higher order sensory functions integrating later. Over the decades, and with advances in neuroscience, there has been a paradigm shift. When conceptualizing how the brain perceives, interprets, and organizes sensory information, the principles of neuroplasticity and a systems view of brain function are currently the underpinnings for SI. Neuroplasticity is considered in current SI theory in that our nervous system can adapt and change in response to sensory input or challenges, such as through child-directed, sensorimotor play opportunities (82). The concept of a systems approach focuses on numerous factors (such as sensorimotor activity, cognition, and task demands) that intertwine to cause an outcome or behavior (31). In this line of thinking, consideration is given to the context of chosen activities and developing methods to manage one's behaviors within those contexts (31). Another consideration of SI is the interaction between the person and the contexts of temporal, cultural, and physical (natural and fabricated environment). Variables that impact a person's performance within a physical environment can be regarded within their personal factors and the contextual barriers and supports (31).

Distinct Approaches Using a Sensory Integration Frame of Reference

Theoretical foundations of ASI frame of reference are seen in new sensory frames of reference and approaches in occupational therapy. Three main lines of thinking about sensory processing that apply SI theory include the SI approach, sensory-based/self-regulation approaches, and the sensory processing approach. Each of these will be considered individually. Figure 3.7 is a delineation of the different sensory approaches that apply SI theory and the terminology used in each.

1. Sensory Integration Approach

The SI approach primarily utilizes SI as its foundational theory. The **ASI** frame of reference continues with the same guiding principles of A. Jean Ayres's early work in SI and integrates data-driven decision-making to guide the ASI intervention. The SI approach remains as a clinical intervention targeting sensorimotor actions through child-directed activities of play (119), with the goal of establishing functional abilities and participation in meaningful activities. ASI separates SI dysfunction into common patterns of *poor sensory perception* (difficulty discriminating and interpreting sensory information), *somatodyspraxia, vestibular and bilateral integration deficits, visuodyspraxia,* and *difficulties with sensory reactivity (hyperreactivity, hyporeactivity, tactile defensiveness,* and *gravitational insecurity)* (119). Additional categories of common SI problems identified by the ASI frame of reference include dyspraxia, language-based dyspraxia, and ideational dyspraxia (125).

The following principles of ASI have been identified by occupational therapists Schaff and Mailloux (119):

- Use of individually tailored, sensory-rich experiences and environment to foster active participation in physical, social, and functional activities
- Development is supported and facilitated by developmentally appropriate activities.
- Sensory information is integrated for development and for using skills in all aspects of participation.
- Sensation can be constructive and beneficial, or sensation can be disorganizing and insufficient. Sensation is considered regarding its nature, quality, and amount. How sensation is received is dependent on age, need, and neurologic characteristics.
- Sensory information is integrated through the organization of the sensation, the response to the sensation, and the interaction with the sensory information.
- Adaptation and neuroplasticity are promoted through brain-behaviors.
- Interaction occurs in a playful and motivating context between the child and the occupational therapy professional.
- Focus is on improvements in sensorimotor skills, functional skills, and daily activity participation.
- Sensorimotor factors impact participation in daily activities.

When using ASI, there is a systematic step-by-step sequence by which the occupational therapist uses clinical and professional reasoning to determine the best intervention

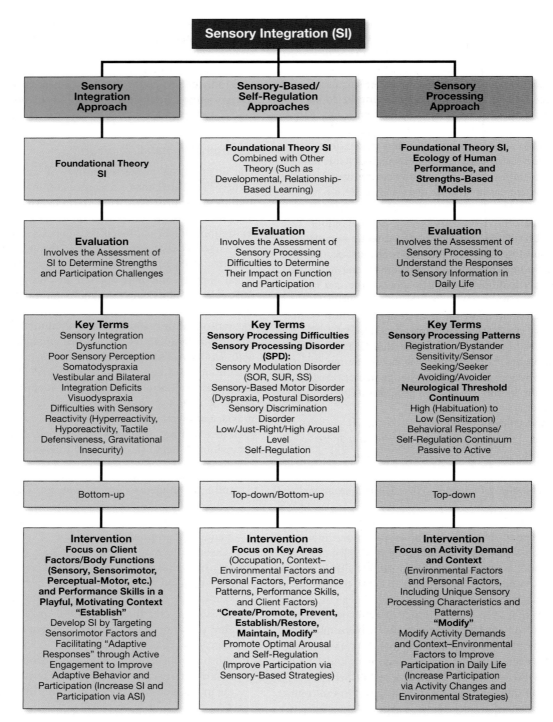

Figure 3.7. Delineation of Sensory Integration, Approaches, and Terminology Used in Occupational Therapy Practice. (Based on terminology of American Occupational Therapy Association. (2020). AOTA 2020 occupational therapy code of ethics. *American Journal of Occupational Therapy*, 74(Suppl. 3), 1–13; Ayres, A. J. (1979). *Sensory integration and the child*. Western Psychological Services; Bodison, S. C., Stein Duker, L. I., Cermak, S. A., & Balance, E. I. (2019). An examination of sensory-related terminology across disciplines: Part one. *SIS Quarterly Practice Connections*, 3(2), 14–16; Dunn, W. (2014). *Sensory profile*-2. Pearson; Miller, L. J., Anzalone, M. E., Lane, S. J., Cermak, S. A., & Osten, E. T. (2007). Concept evolution in sensory integration: A proposed nosology for diagnosis. *American Journal of Occupational Therapy*, 61(2), 135–140; Parham, L. D., Cohn, E. S., Spitzer, S., Koomar, J. A., Miller, L. J., Burke, J. P., Brett-Green, B., Mailloux, Z., May-Benson, T. A., Smith Roley, S., Schaaf, R. C., Schoen, S. A., & Summers, C. A. (2011). Fidelity in sensory integration intervention research. *American Journal of Occupational Therapy*, 61(2), 216–227; Schaaf, R. C., & Mailloux, Z. (2015). Clinician's guide for implementing *Ayres Sensory Integration®: Promoting participation for children with autism*. AOTA Press; Tomcheck, S. D., & Koenig, K. P. (2016). *Occupational therapy practice guidelines for individuals with autism spectrum disorder*. AOTA Press; Wilbarger, 1991; Williams, M. S., & Shellenberger, S. (1996). *How does your engine run?* Therapy Works.)

for the child (119). To begin, the child's strengths and participation challenges are identified. Participation challenges are those activities the child and the adults in the child's life would like to have happen, but are currently difficult. Next, a comprehensive assessment, based on ASI, is completed. Then, based on the assessment data, a hypothesis is developed, based on the sensorimotor factors that contribute to the other information already gathered. The hypothesis links assessment data with the strengths and participation challenges data. Fourth, goals are developed and scaled using a quantitative system. Next, outcome measures are identified. This includes sensorimotor factors that can be assessed via ASI-based testing (proximal outcome) and other outcome measures that can be used to assess changes with participation activities (distal outcome). After the goals and outcome measures are determined, the stage is set for intervention. This includes several of the indicators from the *Fidelity Measure* (which will be discussed next). Once the intervention stage is set, the intervention can be conducted by individually "tailoring" and adjusting sensorimotor activities (with emphasis on tactile, proprioceptive, and vestibular sensory systems) at the "just-right challenge" to actively engage the individual in play. Finally, proximal outcomes are assessed by monitoring progress of sensorimotor factors, and distal outcomes are assessed by using the previously determined outcome measure.

Extensive training is required to effectively provide ASI intervention, and the therapy process should adhere to ASI *Fidelity Measure* specifications (106). The following items are requirements of ASI (119):

- **Therapist qualifications**, including specific training and supervision
- **Safe environment**, including particular equipment maintained to a certain level of integrity
- **Records review**, of particular documents including historical and current information about the client
- **Physical space**, requirements for a certain amount of available area
- **Available equipment**, of specific amount and types
- **Communication with parents and teachers**, about what is occurring during intervention and connections between sensorimotor factors and participation activities
- **Process elements,** including the occupational therapist's integration of the following SI principles: presenting sensory opportunities (with a focus on tactile, vestibular, and proprioceptive); supporting a sensory modulation/regulated state; challenging ocular, postural, oral, and/or bilateral motor control; praxis and behavioral organization; collaborating on activity choice; presenting/tailoring activities at the just-right challenge; ensuring physical safety and success in achieving an adaptive response; supporting intrinsic motivation; and establishing a therapeutic alliance (106, 119).

It should be noted that provision of ASI requires extensive evaluation, which must be selected by the occupational therapist and carried out by an occupational therapist or by an occupational therapy assistant under an occupational therapist's supervision. The *Evaluation in Ayres Sensory Integration* (EASI) is an assessment of the underlying sensory functions that can impact participation and occupational performance. The battery of tests included in the EASI address sensory perception; praxis; ocular, postural, and bilateral motor integration; and sensory reactivity (94). The occupational therapist is the qualified occupational therapy professional to initiate an ASI intervention program.

2. Sensory-Based/Self-Regulation Approaches

Sensory-based/self-regulation approaches also apply SI foundational theory. There are protocol-based or intervention regimens, which are applied by the occupational therapy professional and tend to follow a specific procedure in the application of the sensory input. Sensory strategies can focus on self-regulation activities that are completed by the person to regulate themselves during a sensory-challenging time, or can focus on specifically targeted sensory inputs to promote optimal arousal for participation in daily life. These persons or their caregivers (including persons such as teachers) are taught how to perform these sensory strategies in the environment and in relationship to the time of when the person is involved in occupations that present with sensory challenges. One final consideration toward these approaches includes changes in surroundings. This can include modifications to the general environment, adaptations to an individual's personal space and activities, or the provision of multisensory options for the person to access within their physical space. Examples of sensory changes within the environment can include adjusting lighting or sound levels near the person, as well as providing adapted seating such a therapy ball chair (26).

Foundational theory of sensory-based/self-regulation approaches include the SI frame of reference (from A. Jean Ayres), in combination with other theories, such as developmental, cognitive, relationship-based, and ecologic. Evaluation is holistic and focuses on all OTPF-4E domains relevant to the individual's occupations, context, performance patterns, performance skills, and client factors. Generally, occupational therapy professionals utilize the terminology of "sensory processing difficulties" when describing specific challenges related to the processing of sensory information, including tactile, proprioceptive, vestibular, visual, auditory, olfactory, gustatory, and interoceptive. These approaches also use terminology of "sensory processing disorder" and further differentiate the types of sensory processing problems as *sensory modulation disorders, sensory-based motor disorders*, and *sensory discrimination disorders* (97). Additionally, these approaches consider the individual's arousal level (such as low, just right, high) in response to sensory information and their ability to self-regulate within specific contexts. The occupational therapist develops an individualized and client-centered intervention plan using a problem-solving approach. Sensory-based strategies may involve changing the activity, environment, and/or contexts to achieve an optimal arousal level for participation in daily life activities. Strategies are best applied in a proactive manner. This means that the occupational therapist considers the timing and application of sensory strategies prior to or during specific sensory challenges. Sensory strategies can include using sensory equipment and materials that provide immediate sensory input to help regulate the sensory system. Individual interventions can include the use of weighted vests or blankets, oral motor chewing devices, fidget toys, and stretching bands (25). There are numerous programs that also provide a more structured sensory experience. These programs are designed to help the person, and caregiver, learn how to identify sensory abilities and needs, and then identify sensory-oriented activities to support self-regulation and participation in daily activities. Four examples of sensory-based/self-regulation approaches include Lucy Jane Miller's *Sensory Therapies and Research* (STAR) *approach*, Patricia and Julia Wilbarger's *Sensory Diet*, Diana Henry's *Tool Chest* and *Sensory Buffet*, and Williams and Shellenberger's *Alert Program*. Additionally, multisensory interventions, including sensory enrichment and a Snoezelen multisensory environment, are also considered sensory-based interventions. Research evidence compiled from studies on individualized sensory strategies and multisensory activities supports the use of sensory-based interventions for improving occupational performance and regulation of behavior with autistic individuals (134). Research on noncustomized sensory strategies, multisensory environments, and single-sensory interventions is insufficient.

"Sensory Therapies and Research"

The *STAR* approach by Lucy Jane Miller is a frame of reference used in pediatric occupational therapy for children with sensory processing difficulties (98). It uses principles of SI along with developmental, dynamic systems, relationship-based (Developmental, Individual differences, Relationship based [DIRFloortime]), and other theories to guide parents in applying individualized sensory strategies for children experiencing sensory difficulties (98, 122). This frame of reference uniquely focuses on the parent–child relationship when applying sensory-based intervention to enable participation in daily occupations and "joie de vivre, (joy in life)" (98, p. 163). The occupational therapist works with the parent to create an individualized sensory plan (or sensory lifestyle) and provides education to equip parents to perform the sensory plan with their child. The STAR frame of reference can be beneficial for children with relational and sensory processing difficulties that are often experienced with developmental conditions of ASD and attention-deficit/hyperactivity disorder (ADHD) (98).

To apply the STAR frame of reference, the OT completes an evaluation that includes a detailed history, interview of parents and caregivers in natural settings (home, school), observations, and specific assessments of sensory processing, motor skills, social–emotional development, and the parent–child relationship. The occupational therapist involves parents in the evaluation, goal-setting, and intervention. The intervention process (known as Play, Relationships, Organize, Communicate, Enjoy, Sensation, Success [PROCESS]) engages parents in the therapy with the child in a supportive environment. A multisensory therapeutic environment and environmental supports (such as visual and routine-based transitions) are set up to promote an optimal arousal level of the child and to encourage active engagement in child-directed play activities. Parents learn to follow the lead of the child in play to develop the child's sensory processing abilities, self-regulation, and the parent–child relationship. During each session, the occupational therapist provides parent education to apply specific sensory strategies during daily life activities in a manner that supports the child's social–emotional development and promotes coregulation and self-regulation of the child. Sensory-based strategies are applied at the "just-right level" (optimal level of arousal) using a problem-solving process of "ASECRET," which stands for *Attention, Sensation, Emotion Regulation, Culture, Relationship, Environment, and Task* (98). Additional therapies can include sound-based therapy, mental health, and family treatment, provided through an interdisciplinary team. Occupational therapists that use the STAR approach must be trained in SI and DIRFloortime therapy. They may also benefit from a mentorship program at the STAR Institute. A fidelity measure is also available for this approach (98).

"Sensory Diet"

The *Sensory Diet* was developed by occupational therapist Patricia Wilbarger in 1984 (138). The aim of the "sensory diet" strategy is to improve participation in daily life activities for individuals with sensory processing difficulties, and more specifically sensory defensiveness. The "sensory diet" strategy involves creating an individualized plan of therapeutic sensory-based activities in collaboration with the person or caregiver. The strategy is designed to decrease the person's sensory defensiveness and increase self-regulation (139). The goal of this strategy is to attain an optimal level of arousal for participation in daily activities at home, school, or work. The occupational therapist employs a comprehensive evaluation using an interview process and analyzes sensory processing difficulties within the context of physical and social environments.

The interview is considered a first level of treatment as it promotes the person's (or caregiver's) awareness of sensory defensiveness. The "sensory diet" is a second level of treatment consisting of carefully selected sensory-based activities that promote optimal arousal level throughout the day. "Sensory diet" activities provide a specific type of sensory input, based on the person's identified sensory needs. "Sensory-based activities provided at regular intervals are the cornerstone of the sensory diet" (139, p. 336). The "sensory diet" requires the occupational therapist to closely monitor the effect of certain sensory-based activities, in collaboration with the person (or caregiver). General principles of safety, precautions, and recommendations for developing consistent routines, predictable schedules, and preparing for transitions are also provided by the occupational therapy professional. Training to provide the "sensory diet" strategy involves in-depth information relative to theoretical foundations of SI and neuroscience. Thus, as with all sensory-based/self-regulation approaches, the occupational therapy professional needs training specific to understanding SI theory, and the application of specific sensory strategies that may be individualized and applied by the person or caregiver throughout the day (139).

A third level of treatment, developed by the Wilbargers, includes a protocol-based intervention that applies deep pressure and proprioceptive input every 1.5 to 2 hours during the daily routine. This intervention uses a prescriptive protocol with a specific pattern, duration, and frequency of deep pressure stimulation via a soft surgical brush and light joint compressions, and requires specialized training and supervision (139). However, this prescriptive protocol has insufficient research support.

"Tool Chest" and "Sensory Buffet"

The *Tool Chest* program by occupational therapist Diana Henry includes use of the assessment tools, *Sensory Processing Measure* (SPM) and *Sensory Processing Measures-Preschool* (SPM-P). There are numerous educational products within the program to teach parents and teachers how to help identify sensory processing problems and then identify specific sensory strategies to help with improved attention, coordination, social participation, and behavior and mental health. The strategies target the different sensory systems and include activities for areas such as calming touch pressure activities with use of heavy pillows, functional positioning with a ball chair, use of playground equipment for vestibular input, and particularly designed playlists to listen to through headphones to increase learning preparedness (62, 64).

Diana Henry also developed the strategy of the *Sensory Buffet*, which provides a variety of sensory-based activities to meet the unique sensory needs of children with sensory processing difficulties (63). This strategy emphasizes the use of a variety of sensory-based activities tailored to address sensory challenges and to promote self-regulation. Environmental and task modifications are used to increase participation in daily life activities at home, school, and the community. Specific training for occupational therapy professionals includes knowledge on SI and the application of sensory-based strategies for children, parents, and caregivers. A comprehensive evaluation is completed by the occupational therapist and includes SPM or SPM-P. An individualized intervention plan may be designed specifically by the occupational therapist; however, general sensory strategies are provided for parents and teachers to facilitate self-regulation in children and youth with sensory processing difficulties (62, 64).

The "Alert Program"

The *Alert Program* developed by occupational therapists Mary Sue Williams and Sherry Shellenberger teaches children to identify their level of alertness, and then the child and the adults in the child's life can identify activities to support a level of alertness needed for the skill of attending to information and to learning (132, 140). It is based on the analogy of a car engine (but wording can be changed based on the child's preferences), allowing the child to identify, for instance, if their engine runs high (having problems with self-regulation or with sensory overload) or if their engine runs low, or if their engine is running "just right." The program helps the adults identify signs of how the child's "engine" is running, through signs such as pupil dilation, sweating, or finger-flaring. Often heavy-work pattern activities are encouraged, because they help "engines running on high to cool down," as well as "engines running on low" to rev-up, helping the child return to a "just-right" state of alertness. A heavy-work pattern activity is one such as stacking and carrying textbooks across the classroom over a period of time (133). The *Alert Program*, in a study with a small sample size of children with emotional disturbances, was shown to positively impact adapting to sensory environmental contexts in the classroom (19).

Another program that is similar to the *Alert Program* is the *Brain Works* program. This program, created by occupational therapist Gwen Wild, also is designed to help children self-regulate through identifying if they are under-responding or over-responding to their environment. Through the use of a tachometer, the child can identify if their sensory "engine" is going too fast (green), just right (yellow), or too sluggish (red). Based on a comprehensive OT evaluation that includes assessment of the child's sensory processing difficulties, the OT develops an individualized treatment plan that includes specific sensory activities to promote the optimal arousal of the child. The occupational therapist develops an individualized visual folder with premade activity cards and then provides education and training to the child, parents, and caregivers for its use at home or school. During training, the child learns to identify their sensory "engine" on the tachometer, and then the child selects appropriate activities to perform (based on premade activity cards), to adjust, or maintain, their engine for optimal arousal. For instance, if their engine is too fast, the child learns to pick activities to help them slow down or to calm themselves. The occupational therapy professional carefully monitors the child's responses to the sensory activities during intervention and provides additional education and training as needed. There is both a hard copy and an electronic application of the program. The occupational therapy professional needs to have specific training in sensory processing to effectively use the Brain Works program (28).

Multisensory Interventions and Environments

Education and exploration about the effect of the environment on one's personal level of arousal is another very important aspect of a sensory processing intervention. Sensory rooms (see Chapter 14) can provide a safe place in which the individual can select from multiple sensory options to create an environment that is comforting and secure (92). The client can partake in a therapeutic environment designed to help them modulate for their sensory needs. The client can request, actively choose, and arrange preferred colors, textures, aromas, music, weighted blankets, and activities that provide the desired modulation of sensation. Exploring options within a sensory room will increase self-awareness of preferences. The occupational therapy professional and client can discuss the experience and consider how preferences might be met in the home environment or out in the community. For example, the client might paint their bedroom a different color, purchase bed linens of a specific weight or texture, use a white noise or sound machine, reduce or increase the level of lighting, etc.

Sensory strategies and interventions that have been found to be beneficial for those with dementia and apathy include aromatherapy (lemon balm), multisensory stimulation, and music (81). Additionally, for those with dementia and agitation, aberrant motor behavior, and irritability, beneficial strategies include aroma therapy (lavender) and live music (81). Also, in a study with inpatient clients on a general psychiatric unit and inpatient clients on a geriatric neuropsychiatry unit, the following client self-chosen sensory activities were found to make a significant change in blunted affect, emotional withdrawal, and somatic concerns (78):

- aromas
- music recordings
- rocking chairs
- tactile stimulation (such as squeeze ball, sand table, and tactile surfaces)
- visual stimulation (such as watching a fish tank or watching a calming video)

Now let us shift our attention back to the sensory function of interoception, which was introduced in the previous section. People with lower interception awareness can miss their body's cues regarding emotions they are feeling, and invertedly, those with a higher interoceptive awareness (or sensitivity) can "feel" their body's emotions too intensely, causing the person to feel overwhelmed (93). As occupational therapy professionals we, for instance, provide coping skill interventions to persons who need to regulate their response to internal feelings too great for them to process and adjust their outward response (self-regulation). Better interoception awareness can enhance a person's ability to identify their needs during an overwhelming situation and then be able to focus on using learned coping skills during the situation. The use of mindfulness (being more present and attentive to body signals) is an example of a strategy that can help to increase interoception awareness (93).

There is a beginning body of knowledge to support the use of interoception intervention use toward the improvement of occupational performance. A study of physicians making therapeutic decisions early on during the COVID-19 pandemic, without the benefit of proven evidence-based treatments, was found to rely on "listening to" and trusting their internal signals to make treatment decisions for their clients (117).

In a review of randomized controlled studies, interoception interventions for a variety of mental disorders were found to decrease negative behaviors associated with the disease process and to increase interpersonal skills (69).

- Interoceptive exposure (being exposed to feared body sensations) significantly decreased panic attack frequency and panic severity in those with panic disorder, and demonstrated good results to decrease symptoms for those with irritable bowel syndrome.
- The use of self-help strategies such as self-monitoring of binge-eating triggers and finding pleasure from eating was found to significantly decrease binge-eating behaviors in those with eating disorders.
- For those with substance use disorders, at 3 months postintervention of mindful awareness in body-oriented therapy (versus those without the intervention) had fewer days using the substance.
- Mindfulness-based cognitive therapy used by those with chronic pain with a comorbid diagnosis of depression demonstrated increased self-regulation, emotional awareness, and nondistracting thoughts (thus allowing greater interoceptive skills); the increase in nondistracting thought ability was correlated to improvement in the depression diagnosis.

3. Sensory Processing Approach

The sensory processing approach is based on research by Winnie Dunn and the development of the *Sensory Profile* assessments (30, 44, 45). This approach utilizes a SI perspective along with the theoretical framework of the EHP and strengths-based models (45). According to Dunn's Sensory Processing Framework (SPF), sensory processing can be measured in two areas: **threshold of sensory experiences** and **behaviors responding to sensation**. There is a continuum associated with the extent to which a person registers sensory information. This continuum is a neurologic threshold and its two extremes are a high threshold and a low threshold. A **high threshold** indicates the person has a slow recognition of a sensation, thus needing more sensory input to detect it. A **low threshold** indicates the person more quickly recognizes a sensation, thus needing less sensory input to detect it.

One student, for example, may find it difficult to concentrate when television or other noise is present (low threshold [needing less sensory input to register it]), whereas a classmate says they can study only when the television is on (high threshold of sound [needing more sensory input to register it]). You may recall an incident in which you or someone else asked "what is that smell?" (low threshold of odors), but others present did not smell anything unusual (high threshold for odors). Compare the person who sleeps through an earthquake (high threshold of vibration) to someone else who startles when a heavy truck goes by (low threshold of vibration).

As the previous examples suggest, the SPF includes all senses (the five basic ones and proprioception and vestibular awareness). A given individual may be highly sensitive in one area and not in others. For example, the student who can only study when the television is on may be very irritated by tags, zippers, and seams in clothing (high threshold for sound, low threshold for tactile sensation).

The second area of the SPF concerns behavior in response to sensation. There is a continuum for behavior responses, with two end extremes. At the ends of the continuum for active responses there are: **sensation seeking, or seeker,** versus **sensation avoiding, or avoider.** Active behavior responses are differentiated into actively looking for more stimulation (**sensation seeking**) versus those who actively try to get away from it (**sensation avoiding**). Consider the person who enjoys spending time in a perfume shop experiencing the different intense scents (sensation seeking for odors), versus the person who will cross the street to get away from the aromas that waft through the door of the perfume store (sensation avoiding for odors). Another example is the person whose idea of fun is riding a huge roller coaster (vestibular sensation seeking), and his friend who avoids anything that moves too much (vestibular sensation avoiding). Sensation seeking and avoiding are active measures of behavior, or how a person responds to sensation. At the end of the continuum for passive responses there are: **registration** versus **sensory sensitivity.** If a person has a low threshold for detecting sensory input, a passive response would be sensory sensitivity. **Sensory sensitivity, or sensor,** is when the person does not provide an immediate response to the sensory experience. For example, when a person is given their lunch tray in a cafeteria, they may not make much, or really any, acknowledgment of some of the food, but later on they display irritation or make an inappropriate outburst. If a person has a high threshold for detecting sensory input, a passive response would be registration. **Registration, or bystander,** is when the person does not detect or notice the sensory stimulus, thus missing needed information, and needs to have their attention drawn to the stimulus. For instance, a person who is talking to another person in a library may miss a subtle or small cue from the librarian indicating the need to lower their voice. The person in this example may need the librarian to come over to the person and specifically ask the person to be quiet. Table 3.5 organizes sensory registration and behaviors by threshold type.

How is sensory processing measured? Brown and Dunn (30) developed an evaluation instrument, the A/ASP, a paper-and-pencil test that can be administered and scored in less than 1 hour. The A/ASP uses the individual's or the caregiver's responses concerning the individual's sensory processing characteristics and behaviors in response to sensation. Information is gathered about each of the senses, and the results are organized into four quadrants of sensory processing patterns (sensory sensitivity, registration, sensation seeking, sensation avoiding) that reflect the two different continua of sensory processing. For children 14 years and younger, the SP-2 (45) is available. It is designed in the same manner as the A/ASP; however, it has scoring suited for various age brackets, such as infant, toddler, and child. These are completed with the assistance of the parent. It also has a scoring model designed for school use, which is completed with assistance from the teacher (45). More detail on such assessments can be found in Chapter 12.

In a study using the *SP-2*, with children 6 to 11 years old in the general population, it was found that higher results for sensation avoiding were positively correlated as a predictor for depression, negatively correlated as a predictor for adaptability (being able to adjust oneself to routine changes and with shifting from one task to another task), and negatively correlated as a predictor for resiliency (ability to overcome obstacles through the use of supports). It was also found that higher results for sensation seeking were negatively correlated as a predictor for depression and positively correlated as a predictor for resiliency (41).

Individuals in the population will vary tremendously in neurologic threshold for sensation and in behavioral response to stimulation. You need only consider your classmates, family, and friends to recognize a range of normal differences. However, the A/ASP yields information about the extent to which someone differs from the general population. Threshold levels, active behaviors, and passive behaviors are all on a continuum, and as such, behavior responses will vary in type and intensity, based on the threshold level for any given sensory experience.

Table 3.5. Sensory Registration and Behaviors Based on Threshold Type

	Low Threshold for Detecting Sensory Stimulus	High Threshold for Detecting Sensory Stimulus
Recognition of sensory input	More quickly recognizes a sensation	Slower to recognize a sensation
Amount of sensory input needed for a person to recognize the sensory input	Less	More
Active behavior response	- Sensory avoiding - Avoider	- Sensory seeking - Seeker
Passive behavior response	- Sensory sensitivity - Sensor	- Registration - Bystander

Adapted from Thompson, S. D., & Ralsor, J. M. (2013). Preschool and primary grades: Meeting the sensory needs of young children. *Young Children, 68*(2), 34–43; Dunn, W. (2014). *Sensory profile-2.* Pearson.

Many people with psychiatric disabilities fall outside the normal range in one or more of the four quadrants of high or low registration, sensation seeking, and sensation avoiding. Brown (29) gives several very interesting examples of personal narratives of people with schizophrenia or other disorders describing their distractibility and increased time needed for comprehension. Another study suggests that people with PTSD symptoms may experience problems with both sensation seeking and sensation avoiding (53).

A sensory processing intervention is designed to improve awareness and develop effective and appropriate behavioral responses to sensation. The results of the A/ASP are shared with clients, and the occupational therapist can help the client to develop an individualized plan. The plan may aim to compensate for sensory registration problems and attempt to promote the level of registration. Or occupational therapy may be targeted at changing the behaviors associated with seeking or avoiding. If a client has a high threshold for detecting, for example, odors, then the occupational therapy professional will suggest ways to increase or enhance these sensations and to improve **discrimination** of a variety of odors. The ability to notice and identify different smells is critical for safety in the community; one must be able to identify the smells of smoke, natural gas, and spoiled food.

On the other hand, if a client has a low threshold for detecting visual and auditory sensory inputs, the occupational therapy professional would guide the client in selecting environments and situations that are not so overwhelming in sensation. The goal is to help the client **modulate** (moderate or control) the sensation that is being received and the behavioral response. **Sensory modulation** is the regulation (control or moderation) of sensation itself or of behavioral responses to sensory stimulation (77).

It is often the case that people who have low thresholds of sensation detection become over-aroused by too much stimulation and may react emotionally. Existing in a constant state of feeling overwhelmed by sensation can be exhausting. The effort to avoid encountering excessive stimulation may cause the person to remain isolated, which leads to problems in community living and social participation. Or the person may become angry when overstimulated. Too much stimulation feels threatening when no escape seems possible.

Many people express interest in finding nonmedical and nonpharmacologic (no drugs) strategies for relieving their symptoms and helping them pursue the things they enjoy doing. It helps to develop self-awareness about one's own sensory threshold and learn how to control behavioral responses. Working within the SPF, the occupational therapist would assess the client, and the two would plan a program together. The occupational therapy assistant might be asked to administer and score the A/ASP; the occupational therapist would then interpret it and share the results with the client. The occupational therapy assistant might be involved in a meeting in which the results are discussed. This is especially helpful when the occupational therapy assistant is charged with carrying out any part of the plan.

What kinds of interventions are used in the SPF? Several options exist. One is an educational and training process, in which the occupational therapy professional helps the client learn about their sensory registration and sensation-related behavior. Along with education and sensory processing, the occupational therapy professional would provide training by teaching the client strategies for modifying the environment, seeking support from others, and controlling sensory input. Here are some examples:

- For a high threshold of odors, the occupational therapy professional may introduce an array of scented items and engage the client in identifying differences and naming the scents. The aim here is to increase awareness, registration, and discrimination of odor.
- For a client with a high threshold for tactile and proprioceptive input, the occupational therapy professional may teach self-massage techniques, application of lotion, and playing with different textures and objects that vary in weight (99).
- For a client with a low threshold of sound, the occupational therapy professional may discuss options for limiting sound in the environment and for communicating one's own needs to others in a respectful but assertive way (29).

Education and training can also be done for caregivers through a coaching model including individual and group sessions. Coaching with caregivers can include strategies for improving the client's participation toward achieving intervention goals, providing knowledge about sensory processing, collaborating with ongoing intervention goal planning, and guiding the caregiver on how to problem-solve in new sensory-challenging situations for the client (107). Educating and training other professionals within psychiatric facilities on the use of sensory modulation approaches can also be beneficial for clients. Areas specifically identified to address with other professionals include the following (113):

- education and training (initial and periodic refresher sessions) for using sensory rooms and sensory equipment to ensure skills and confidence in using the strategies
- keeping enough sensory equipment readily available on the client's inpatient unit

The occupational therapy professional could also provide staff on client inpatient units a "cheat sheet" of sensory strategies and sensory equipment beneficial for specific client behaviors.

The SPF is a strengths-based approach. The SPF's assessments and interventions are built on the idea that we all have strengths that can assist us during challenging situations and in challenging environments. "From a strengths-based perspective, knowing a person's patterns creates a tool for gaining insights about what settings and activities are likely to be easier or more challenging, and reveals possibilities for navigating successfully in everyday life" (45, p. 14). In accordance with the EHP model, we consider the personal factors (past experiences, values, interests, and skills for sensorimotor, cognitive, and psychosocial) interconnected to the context (temporal, cultural, and physical environment [natural and fabricated]) (46). As noted earlier, we would look to modify the activity demands of environmental context; prevent potential barriers in the environment; and modify, or adjust, the features of the task to match the sensory preferences identified for that individual person (42). We can even take this concept a step further and look to create environments that provide benefits to a population as a whole, such as stores or restaurants within a community that match sensory preferences (42). For instance, a restaurant could have a multisensory rich environment for bystanders. A grocery store that did not routinely change aisle traffic patterns or placement of products, and has large aisles to decrease overcrowding and unnecessary socialization would benefit avoiders.

Box 3.10 provides an example of how to use a sensory processing goal with clients.

BOX 3.10 Sensory Processing Framework Intervention Goal

Aim of Intervention

Registration of sensory experiences through the neurologic threshold. (high and low)

Behaviors responding to sensations. (active and passive)

Goal

Client will successfully complete the occupation of _____ with _____ (add needed amount of type of assistance)* and _____** strategies within _____***.

* independently, no cuing, supervision, assistance
** multisensory, auditory, visual, taste, smell, touch, activity level
*** number of attempts, number of sessions, number of weeks

Case Example

Amanda is 32 years old, the youngest of five siblings. Her family has a military background, and all her siblings have served in the armed forces. She has a history of learning disabilities since middle school, with difficulty reading and concentrating. After graduating from high school, she enlisted in the Army, completed basic training, and served 3 years, mostly stateside. She was briefly deployed in Iraq but was returned to stateside duty after manifesting extreme symptoms of PTSD after witnessing a suicide bombing attack. She was not injured physically, but several members of her unit were killed, and others seriously injured. She helped evacuate the dead and wounded. At present, she is in a day program at a veteran's hospital, for treatment of her PTSD.

Occupational therapy is part of the day program. Janice, the occupational therapist, met with Amanda to discuss her concerns and goals. She noted that Amanda's eyes and body alerted to the smallest sound in the environment and that it was difficult to keep her focused. She appeared highly distractible. Ashanti, the occupational therapy assistant, administered the A/ASP to Amanda individually, rather than in

a group as is customary in this outpatient setting. Amanda took more time than is usual to finish the A/ASP, as she got up several times to get a drink of water and look out of the window.

After Ashanti scored the A/ASP, Janice studied the results and shared them with Amanda in a meeting also attended by Ashanti. They discussed the general purpose of the assessment and laid out the results. Amanda's A/ASP showed the following:

- Higher sensory sensitivity to all stimuli compared to most people, with greatest registration of tactile sensation, sounds, and smells.
- Greater than average sensation seeking and sensation avoiding than most people, but these scored just outside the normal range.

Janice shared with Amanda that these same patterns were noted in a research study of veterans with PTSD (53). She then explained each pattern in more detail. Amanda agreed that she has "always been super-sensitive" and that this seems involved with the ADHD that she has had since childhood. She admitted that she does at times "shut down" when there is too much going on (sensation avoiding). She said that she does not seek sensation so that she can explore it; she does not really enjoy too much stimulation. Rather, she is always on the alert for signs of trouble; the world feels dangerous to her. In this sense, her hypervigilance leads her to seek out sensations that worry her.

Her goals, she said, are to gain admission to a training program for emergency medical technicians (EMTs), to complete the program, and to get a job with an ambulance service. She is concerned about not being able to concentrate and about how this will affect her class work and job prospects.

Janice explained the purpose of sensory processing interventions and gave some examples. Amanda said she was interested, especially if the occupational therapy professional could help diminish her anxiety and help her concentrate. Together with Amanda, the occupational therapy professionals laid out a plan of activities. Ashanti was responsible for carrying out these interventions with Amanda. Some of the goals and activities included the following:

- To address sensory sensitivity—explore options for environmental control, using items in the sensory room; explore the use of weighted blankets and self-massage to dampen tactile oversensitivity; possibly use noise-dampening drapes, sound-cancelling headphones, and a white noise machine to filter out extraneous sound; consider gradual safe immersion in normal stimulating environments, to desensitize to these environments, thus permitting more access to life in the community.
- To address sensation seeking—learn and use mindfulness meditation techniques, and controlled breathing for self-calming.
- To address sensation avoiding—keep a personal journal of sensory experiences and behavioral responses to identify events that lead to avoidance. Learn ways to reduce the amount of sensory input from the environment or locate a quite area when you feel overwhelmed by the sensory input from the environment (take a break).

After Ashanti introduced Amanda to the sensory room and its contents, she was able to self-schedule personal use of the room three times a week for 30 minutes. Amanda met twice weekly in a discussion group with other veterans with PTSD, focusing on strategies for managing stress and dealing with overstimulation. She attended a mindfulness meditation class twice a week. She met once a week for an individual session with either Ashanti or Janice, to review her sensory experiences of the previous week and to learn new techniques to better self-manage sensory-based situations.

Six weeks later, Amanda had established regular habits of daily meditation and personal journaling. She found that she enjoyed certain scents, such as lavender, and that white noise was essential for her to sleep soundly. Consequently, she purchased a sleep machine (to generate white noise) and lavender-scented toiletries.

In her meetings with Janice and Ashanti, she began to examine whether EMT was the right career choice for her. She expressed that she was worried that the sirens and noise, and the experience of being at scenes of trauma, were perhaps too much and that she would not be able to cope. She was worried about flashbacks. At this point, she is considering a career in massage therapy, because she is finding self-massage to be calming and would like a career where she serves other people.

This brief example illustrates the roles of the occupational therapist and the occupational therapy assistant in the sensory processing approach. As in other frames of reference, the occupational therapist has overall responsibility for designing and directing the interventions. The occupational therapy assistant plays a partnership role and can contribute by administering assessment tools, by carrying out the intervention plan, and by collaborating with the client and the occupational therapist.

Concepts Summary

1. SI is the smooth working together of all the senses to provide information needed for accurate perception and motor action.
2. Successful motor output depends on accurate reception and interpretation of sensory input.
3. According to SI theory, activities that provide increased vestibular, tactile, and proprioceptive input can help reorganize the way the central nervous system organizes and interprets sensory input.
4. Activities selected for SI intervention programs should be pleasurable and should be presented in a noncompetitive, unpressured, and cheerful manner.
5. Sensory-rich environments can be designed to complement a person's sensory preferences.
6. SI intervention can have a powerful and unpredictable effect on the central nervous system.
7. Current neuroscience concepts include the consideration of neuroplasticity and a systems approach.
8. ASI uses a systematic step-by-step sequence toward intervention identification for the child.

9. Intervention applied in a sensory-based/self-regulation approach can be performed through sensory strategies, cognitive or learning strategies, and environmental changes.
10. Individuals differ in neurologic threshold for sensation and in behavioral response.
11. Neurologic thresholds are experienced on a continuum from low to high.
12. Behavioral responses are experienced on a continuum from active responses of sensation avoiding to sensation seeking to passive responses of sensory sensitivity and registration.
13. Extremes of neurologic threshold may cause the person to feel out of control and lead to behavior that appears to others to be antisocial, disorganized, overly emotional, or isolating.
14. Extremes of behavioral response may cause problems living in the community and participating in occupations.
15. Meeting sensory needs can help a person who feels out of control regain a sense of control.
16. Developing awareness of one's own sensitivities and behavioral responses enables a person to better meet sensory processing needs and preferences.

VOCABULARY REVIEW

bilateral motor coordination
The ability to perform activities that involve the use of both sides of the body, particularly when the two sides perform different motions, as in swimming or tying one's shoes

interoception
The sensory mechanism that allows one to feel the sensations occurring inside the body

kinesthesia
The sensory mechanism for knowing where and how a body part is moving

neurologic threshold
The point at which the nervous system registers a sensation; can be low or can be high

post-rotatory nystagmus
Rapid eye movements normally occurring immediately after vestibular stimulation that includes rotation

proprioception
The sensory mechanism for locating body parts in space without visual clues and for integrating our relationships to gravity

protocol-based interventions
Interventions that follow a set regimen

registration
Not detecting or noticing a sensory stimulus

self-regulation
Client factor relating to the control of emotional responses, including intensity experienced and appropriate match of behavior and expression to the situation

sensation avoiding
Taking action to prevent experiencing sensation

sensation seeking
Taking action to experience sensation

sensation seeking versus sensation avoiding
A continuum of active behavioral responses to sensation

sensory discrimination
The ability to recognize and identify different sensations; the ability to notice a difference between different sensations

sensory integration (SI)
The process of receiving and organizing sensory information within the central nervous system

sensory modulation
Taking action to control and moderate the amount and kind of sensation experienced, as well as one's behavioral response

sensory processing
The process of receiving and organizing sensory information within the central nervous system and responding to this information through behavior.

sensory sensitivity
Not providing an immediate response to experiencing sensation

sensory sensitivity versus registration
A continuum of passive behavioral responses to sensation

tactile defensiveness
A variety of aversive responses displayed by a person because of an over-reaction or defensive response to non-noxious tactile stimulation (36). Touch is perceived as unpleasant (116).

vestibular awareness
The sensory mechanism for receiving information about balance, velocity, and acceleration of the body

vestibular stimulation
Sensory input to the balance system. Such input may include rocking, spinning, and other movement.

SUMMARY

This chapter introduces seven frames of reference and practice models used by occupational therapy professionals for interventions with persons who have mental health problems:

- Development of adaptive skills
- Role acquisition and social skills training
- Cognitive disabilities
- Model of human occupation
- Person–environment–occupation
- Ecology of human performance
- Sensory integration

MOHO, PEO, and EHP are occupational performance models compatible with the use of other models. It is important to employ a frame of reference or practice model that complements the client's situation. Selection of an appropriate frame of reference or practice model is the responsibility of the occupational therapist; the occupational therapy assistant gains service competency and depth of understanding by observation and discussion with the occupational therapist and by continued professional development and study.

As a final note, two additional models will be introduced in Chapter 6. The Kawa model is centered in Japanese culture and has a view of life experiences different from Western society and culture. These ideas will be addressed and developed as we consider culture and how it influences our way of practicing occupational therapy. The Occupational Adaptation model focuses on how we, as people, adapt to our life situations, considering who we are, who we need to be, and the environment in which we must participate.

Case Study – Mr Velasquez

A 22-Year-Old Man with Schizophrenia and Intellectual Disability

J. Velasquez
Case #085562

This 22-year-old Hispanic man with a diagnosis of schizophrenia and mild intellectual disability was referred to a community day treatment center in a large East Coast city. The referral originated at another mental health clinic in a different part of the city. He had been attending that clinic for medication management, and the staff there believed he could benefit from a structured day program and family therapy.

DSM-5-TR Diagnosis at Admission
F20.9 Schizophrenia

F17 Intellectual disability, mild

Z code
V60.3 Acculturation difficulty (does not speak English after 6 years in the United States)

Mr Velasquez was born in Colombia, South America. His parents were teenagers when he was born and have subsequently divorced (the father is reported to have an addiction to both illicit drugs and alcohol). The client, who has four younger sisters and a younger brother, lived with his maternal grandparents in Colombia while his mother emigrated to the United States when he was 10 years old. The rest of the family emigrated 6 years ago. Immediately after the move, the client became ill but was never hospitalized. He was followed at an outpatient clinic and stabilized on haloperidol (Haldol) and benztropine (Cogentin). Mr Velasquez dropped out of school at age 16, without completing his high school education.

On admission, the social worker obtained the following information from the family. The mother is employed in a factory job. Mr Velasquez, who speaks no English, stays home and masturbates throughout the day. He sees only family members and has not been able to care for his own hygiene. His 14-year-old sister has been washing and dressing him. He appears to be hallucinating, says he is in the space shuttle, and has frequent loud outbursts of inappropriate laughter. Mr Velasquez was also seen by the psychiatrist, who changed his medication to Risperdal.

The occupational therapy evaluation was performed 3 days later by an occupational therapy student under the supervision of the therapist. Assessment instruments used were the Occupational Role History Interview-II and the ACL screening test. Results were as follows.

Interview

Mr Velasquez appeared for the interview neatly dressed but with the back of his hair uncombed and his pants unzipped. He closed the zipper at the student's reminder to do so.

Occupational Role History Interview-II

In the Occupational Role History Interview-II, Mr Velasquez often gave tangential and irrelevant replies to questions asked by the student. He spoke of violent events, such as being beaten by a man with a club in school and having been accused by a classmate of killing her grandmother. When asked about school, he stated that he was good at drawing but bad at biology and physics. Mr Velasquez said emphatically that he had no friends and could think of no one whom he had looked up to in the past as a role model.

Mr Velasquez attended school in Colombia but had no further schooling since his family moved to this country when he was 16. He has never had a job. He has extremely limited understanding of English; the interview was conducted in Spanish.

Allen Cognitive Level Screening Test

In the ACL screening test, the client was able to complete three whip stitches. When asked, he found a twisted lace on the back of leather and corrected it by removing the leather lacing. He was unable to complete the single cordovan stitch. This performance was scored at cognitive level 4.2.

For an abbreviated version of the Occupational History Interview-II, see Chapter 12.

Additional resources needed to understand case study: from the website *OT-Innovations.com*, from *The ACL Battery* page, download the *Allen Cognitive Level Caregiver Guides* for *Levels 4.0–4.4* and *Levels 4.6–4.8* at https://www.ot-innovations.com/clinical-practice/cognition-2/the-allen-cognitive-level-battery/. This case example/case study is loosely based on an actual case. The names and certain other facts have been changed to protect the client's identity. Minor adaptations were made to the case by Meyer, C. (2021).

OT HACKS SUMMARY

O: Occupation as a means and an end

ASI focuses on sensory integrative skills needed for occupational performance, most noticeably in academic occupational performance in children with learning disorders.

CDM considers the environment, including educating and training caregivers, and how it is set up to allow clients with cognitive limitations to complete occupations safely and with as much independence as possible.

Dunn's SPF connects the person's threshold to sensory information to how the sensory information received during the sensory experience influences the person's active and passive responsive behaviors during occupational performance.

EHP highlights the occupational task performed by the person and the context factors that influence the person's performance range.

MOHO's central tenet is occupation. It is a part of the occupational skills needed to build the occupational performance that in turn supports overall occupational participation.

Mosey's Development of Adaptive Skills focuses on the skills needed throughout life to complete one's chosen occupations (SI, cognition, dyadic interaction, group interaction, self-identity, and sexual identity).

PEO is an occupational performance model. It considers the transactions among the person, the environment, and the occupations the person chooses to perform.

Role Acquisition model emphasizes client-chosen goals and reflection on progress. Tasks are presented in a natural developmental sequence, full examples of tasks are shown to the client, and the client is given numerous opportunities to practice. Social skills are integral to accomplishing one's roles and skills are taught in a four-stage process of motivation, demonstration, practice, and feedback.

Sensory-Based/Self-Regulation Approach includes protocol-based procedures applied to the person and sensory strategy interventions completed by the person to promote self-regulation to improve occupational performance.

SI frame of reference

Social Skills Training is a part of role acquisition. Social skills include self-expression, other social communication enhancements, assertiveness, and communication with others. Social skills training involves the four steps of motivation, demonstration, practice, and feedback.

T: Theoretical concepts, values, and principles, or historical foundations

Doing is purposeful and is integral to people's roles and tied to time, the environment, and relationships with others.

There is an internal desire to explore one's world and become competent in performing one's life activities.

People's abilities and functions are developed in a systematic and organized order and when there is a disruption in this development, therapeutic intervention can help restore or adapt for limitations.

H: How can we Help? OT's role in serving clients with mental illness or mental health needs'

All occupational therapy–based frames of reference and practice models center around the outcome of occupational performance. Frames of reference and practice models organize our professional (clinical) reasoning, helping to keep our focus on how occupational needs and demands influence our clients and how our clients' occupational performance influences our clients' roles and lived experiences. The frames of reference and practice models help to explain to other professions the role of occupation in the therapeutic process.

A: Adaptations

Although a model such as Mosey's Development of Adaptive Skills obviously is centered on adaptation (per the wording in the title), most occupational therapy frames of reference and practice models have a connection to "adaptation" (be it small or short term, or be it the main enhancement or focus).

ASI: promotes adaptation and neuroplasticity through brain-behaviors

CDM: occupational performance is adapted by analyzing the mechanics of the occupation for safety concerns, attention considerations, and sensorimotor actions. Caregivers are educated and trained on how best to set up the occupational environment so that the client can safely complete as many steps or aspects of the client's chosen occupations as the client is able to do so.

Dunn's SPF considers a multisensory approach including environmental changes to better match a person's sensory threshold.

EHP: includes intervention approaches to alter the environment and adapt the task

MOHO: occupational adaptation is the product of an interconnected positive occupational identity and occupational competence.

Mosey's Development of Adaptive Skills: as people develop they "adapt" to life roles and situations; people approach completing life occupational expectations by adapting themselves, their responses, and their abilities to the requirement of the situation.

PEO: Adjustments may be made by the person to complete occupation with the limits of the environment. The environment available to the person, based on the person's needs, may need to be adjusted.

Role Acquisition: how we present occupational activities to clients is based on their current level of ability; we "adapt" our presentation to present the pieces, in the mode that best allows the client to learn the steps and sequence of the entire occupation.

Sensory-Based/Self-Regulation Approaches include modifications to the general environment and adaptations to personal space and activities.

Social Skills: people's initiations to others and responses are an adaptation to how others present themselves and to how different situations are framed

C: Case study includes

Cases presented:

CDM: Marvin—ACL level 3.4; limited problem-solving ability; difficulty with tool use and completing simple projects; needs 24-hour supervised living arrangements

CDM: Mr Velasquez—ACL level 4.2: difficulty with socially appropriate behavior and ability to retain employment

Development of adaptive skills: Judi—building a relationship with a new client in a suburban community day treatment center

MOHO: Rose—mother and wife with feelings of loss of control over life activities, disorganization with routines and home environment, difficulty with cognitive-based tasks

PEO: Evangeline—substance misuse and bipolar disorder and borderline personality disorder; difficulty retaining employment and maintaining relationships with others; participating with LSP, AA/NA, and DBT

Role Acquisition and Social Skills Training: Howard—self-care and vocational skills completed with transition to previous work environment; client self-assessment of skill

progress; interdisciplinary teamwork with nursing assistant to ensure hygiene self-care tasks were completed

SI Frame of Reference: Amanda—veteran hospital day program for PTSD where an A/ASP was completed with results of higher sensory sensitivity to all stimuli and greater than average sensation seeking and sensation avoiding; intervention plan to reduce sensory sensitivity, reduce fear-linked sensation seeking, reduce sensation seeking and sensation avoiding, and reduce "shutting down" when wanting to avoid sensations

K: Knowledge: keeping mental health OT practice grounded in evidence, in occupational science, and in research

CDM and **SI** are based on neuroscience concepts.

MOHO, PEO, and **EHP** are based on client-centered therapeutic concepts.

Mosey's Adaptive Skills and Role Acquisition models are grounded in developmental theory.

S: Some terms that may be new to you

Key terms are summarized throughout the chapter.

Reflection Questions

1. If your client is exhibiting Mosey's adaptive skill of perceiving themselves as self-directed, how would you address becoming competent in the next self-identity adaptive skill?
2. Using the role acquisition model, if your client wants to set unrealistic, inappropriate, too simplistic goals for themselves, what can you do?
3. Complete the question provided by your instructor about the article discussed in the *What's the Evidence* box.
4. For a client with a low threshold for gustatory sensations, the occupational therapy professional could suggest what type of intervention?
5. Clients with the following CDM levels are on the occupational therapy professional's caseload. What is an activity that is appropriate for a client at each level and why?
   Level 2
   Level 5
6. If the client was demonstrating difficulty with completing all the individual steps or acts that make up a whole activity, you would determine the client is having difficulty with what aspect of occupational performance?
7. As you are working with a client on determining what tasks or activities are a priority for the client, what considerations and actions should you take with the client, according to the PEO model?
8. During sessions with the occupational therapy assistant, it has been difficult for the client to gain acceptance of their mental disorder and the changes the client will need to make. According to the EHP model, the occupational therapist would encourage the occupational therapy assistant to focus on what?

REFERENCES

1. ADA National Network. (2017). *Guidelines for writing about people with disabilities.* http://adainfo.us/ADANNwriting

2. Allen, C. K. (1982). Independence through activity: The practice of occupational therapy (psychiatry). *American Journal of Occupational,* 36(11), 731–739.

3. Allen, C. K. (1985). *Occupational therapy for psychiatric diseases: Measurement and management of cognitive disabilities.* Little, Brown and Company.

4. Allen, C. K. (2017). *Structures of cognitive performance modes.* S&S Worldwide.

5. Allen, C. K. (2018). *Allen App* (Version 1.16). [Mobile application software]. Retrieved September 23, 2021, from https://acdmweb.com

6. Allen, C. K., & Allen, R. E. (1987). Cognitive disabilities: Measuring the consequences of mental disorders. *Journal of Clinical Psychiatry,* 48(5), 185–191.

7. Allen, C. K., Austin, S. L., David, S. K., Earhart, C. A., McCraith, D. B., & Riska-Williams, L. (2007). *Manual for the Allen Cognitive Level Screen-5 (ACLS-5) and Large Allen Cognitive Level Screen-5 (LACLS-5).* ACLS and LACLS Committee.

8. Allen, C. K., Blue, T., & Earhart, C. A. (1995). *Understanding cognitive performance modes [Presentation].* In Allen Conferences.

9. Allen, C. K., Earhart, C. A., & Blue, T. (1992). *Occupational therapy treatment goals for the physically and cognitively disabled.* AOTA Press.

10. American Occupational Therapy Association. (2015). Occupational therapy for children and youth using sensory integration and methods in school-based practice. *American Journal of Occupational Therapy,* 69(Suppl. 3), 1–20.

11. American Occupational Therapy Association. (2017). Philosophical base of occupational therapy. *American Journal of Occupational Therapy,* 71(Suppl. 2), 7112410045P1.

12. American Occupational Therapy Association. (2020). AOTA 2020 occupational therapy code of ethics. *American Journal of Occupational Therapy,* 74(Suppl. 3), 1–13.

13. American Occupational Therapy Association. (2020). Guidelines for supervision, roles, and responsibilities during the delivery of occupational therapy services. *American Journal of Occupational Therapy,* 74(Suppl. 2), 1–62.

14. American Occupational Therapy Association. (2020). Occupational therapy practice framework: Domain and process—Fourth edition. *American Journal of Occupational Therapy,* 74(Suppl. 2), 1–87.

15. Arbesman, M., & Logsdon, D. W. (2011). Occupational therapy interventions for employment and education for adults with serious mental illness: A systematic review. *American Journal of Occupational Therapy,* 65(3), 238–246.

16. Ayres, A. J. (1972). *Sensory integration and learning disorders.* Western Psychological Services.

17. Ayres, A. J. (1979). *Sensory integration and the child.* Western Psychological Services.

18. Baptiste, S. (2017). The person-environment-occupation model. In J. Hinojosa, P. Kramer, & C. Brasic Royeen (Eds.), *Perspectives on human occupation: Theories underlying practice* (2nd ed., pp. 137–159). F.A. Davis.

19. Barnes, K. J., Vogel, K. A., Beck, A. J., Schoenfeld, H. B., & Owen, S. V. (2008). Self-regulation strategies of children with emotional disturbance. *Physical & Occupational Therapy in Pediatrics,* 28(4), 369–387.

20. Barrett, L. F., Quigley, K. S., & Hamilton, P. (2016). An active inference theory of allostasis and interoception in depression. *Philosophical Transactions of the Royal Society,* 371(1708), 20160011.

21. Barris, R., Kielhofner, G., & Watts, J. H. (1983). *Psychosocial occupational therapy: Practice in a pluralistic arena.* Ramsco.

22. Barris, R., Kielhofner, G., & Watts, J. H. (1988). *Bodies of knowledge in psychosocial practice.* SLACK.

23. Baum, C., & Law, M. (1997). Occupational therapy practice: Focusing on occupational performance. *American Journal of Occupational Therapy,* 51(4), 277–287.

24. Bejerholm, J., & Ekland, M. (2006). Engagement in occupations among men and women with schizophrenia. *Occupational Therapy International,* 13(2),100–121.

25. Bodison, S. C. (2018). A comprehensive framework to embed sensory interventions within occupational therapy practice. *SIS Quarterly Practice Connections,* 3(2), 14–16.

26. Bodison, S. C., & Parham, L. D. (2018). Specific sensory techniques and sensory environmental modifications for children and youth with sensory integration difficulties: A systematic review. *American Journal of Occupational Therapy,* 72(1), 1–11.

27. Brady, J. P. (1984). Social skills training for psychiatric patients. I: Concepts, methods and clinical results. *Occupational Therapy in Mental Health,* 4(4), 51–68.

28. BrainWorks. (n.d.). *Brain works sensory diet kit.* Sensational Brain.

29. Brown, C. (2001). What is the best environment for me? A sensory processing perspective. *Occupational Therapy in Mental Health,* 17(3–4), 115–125.

30. Brown, C., & Dunn, W. (2002). *Adolescent/Adult sensory profile.* Psychological Corp.

31. Bundy, A. C., & Murray, E. A. (2002). Sensory integration: A. Jean Ayres' theory revisited. In A. C. Bundy, S. J. Lane, & E. A. Murray (Eds.), *Sensory integration: Theory and practice* (2nd ed., pp. 3–33). F.A. Davis.

32. Burns, T. (2013). *Cognitive performance test.* Maddak Inc.

33. Burns, T., & Haertl, K. (2018). Cognitive performance test: Practical applications and evidence-based use. *SIS Quarterly Practice Connections,* 3(4), 17–19.

34. Burns, T., Lawler, K., Lawler, D., McCarten, J. R., & Kuskowski, M. (2018). Predictive value of the Cognitive Performance Test (CPT) for staging function and fitness to drive in people with neurocognitive disorders. *American Journal of Occupational Therapy,* 72(4), 1–9.

35. Cairns, A., Hill, C., Dark, F., McPhail, S., & Gray, M. (2013). The large Allen Cognitive Level screen as an indicator for medication adherence among adults accessing community mental health services. *British Journal of Occupational Therapy,* 76(3), 137–143.

36. Case-Smith, J., & O'Brien, J. C. (2015). *Occupational therapy for children and adolescents* (7th ed.). Elsevier.

37. Cole, M. B. (2018). *Group dynamics in occupational therapy: The theoretical basis and practice application of group intervention* (5th ed.). SLACK.

38. Corcoran, A. W., & Hohwy, J. (2019). Allostasis, interoception, and the free energy principle: Feeling our way forward. In M. Tsakiris & H. De Preester (Eds.), *The interoceptive mind: From homeostasis to awareness* (pp. 272–292). Oxford University Press.

39. Craig, A. D. (2002). How do you feel? Interoception: The sense of the physiological condition of the body. *Nature Reviews Neuroscience,* 3(8), 655–666.

40. David, S. K., & Riley, W. T. (1990). The relationship of the Allen Cognitive Level test to cognitive abilities and psychopathology. *American Journal of Occupational Therapy,* 44(6), 493–497.

41. Dean, E. E., Little, L., Tomcheck, S., & Dunn, W. (2018). Sensory processing in the general population: Adaptability, resiliency, and challenging behavior. *American Journal of Occupational Therapy,* 72(1), 1–8.

42. Dean, E. E., Little, L. M., Wallisch, A., & Dunn, W. (2019). Sensory processing in everyday life. In B. A. Boyt Schell & G. Gillen (Eds.), *Willard and Spackman's occupational therapy* (13th ed., pp. 942–964). Wolters Kluwer.

43. Decker, M. D. (1996). Evaluating the client with dementia. *Mental Health Special Interest Section Quarterly,* 18(4), 1–2.

44. Dunn, W. (1997). The impact of sensory processing abilities on the daily lives of young children and their families: A conceptual model. *Infants & Young Children,* 9(4), 23–25.

45. Dunn, W. (2014). *Sensory profile-2.* Pearson.

46. Dunn, W. (2017). The ecological model of occupation. In J. Hinojosa, P. Kramer, & C. Brasic Royeen (Eds.), *Perspectives on human occupation: Theories underlying practice* (2nd ed., pp. 207–235). F.A. Davis.

47. Dunn, W., Brown, C., & McGuigan, A. (1994). The ecology of human performance: A framework for considering the effect of context. *American Journal of Occupational Therapy,* 48(7), 595–607.

48. Dunn, W., Brown, C., & Youngstrom, M. J. (2003). Ecological model of occupation. In P. Kramer, J. Hinojosa, & C. Brasic Royeen (Eds.), *Perspectives in human occupation: Participation in life.* Lippincott Williams & Wilkins.

49. Earhart, C. A. (2013, June 04). *A brief history of the cognitive disabilities model and assessments.* Allen Cognitive Group. https://allencognitive.com/history/

50. Earhart, C. A. (2015). *Using Allen diagnostic modules—2nd edition assessments.* S&S Worldwide. Retrieved August 22, 2021, from https://cdn.ssww.com/share/S52_How_to_use_the_Allen_Diagnostic_Module.pdf

51. Earhart, C. A. (2016). *Summary of the modes of performance in the Allen scale.* Allen Cognitive Group. http://allencognitive.com/wp-content/uploads/Summary-of-Modes-of-Performance-101216-1.pdf

52. Earhart, C. A. (2017). *Analysis of modes of performance for the Allen cognitive scale's hierarchies of functional cognition and activity demands.* Allen Cognitive Group. http://allencognitive.com/wp-content/uploads/Analysis-of-Modes-of-Performance-for-the-Allen-Cognitive-Scales-Hierarchies-of-Functional-Cognition-and-Activity-Demands.pdf

53. Engel-Yeger, B., Palgy-Levin, D., & Lev-Wiesel, R. (2013). The sensory profile of people with post-traumatic stress symptoms. *Occupational Therapy in Mental Health, 29*(3), 266–278.

54. Fitts, D. (n.d.). *Kinesthesia vs. proprioception: What's the difference?* The Sensory Toolbox. Retrieved September 12, 2021, from https://thesensorytoolbox.com/kinesthesia-proprioception/

55. Hagedorn, R. (1992). *Occupational therapy: Foundations for practice—Models, frames of reference and core skills.* Churchill Livingstone.

56. Hagulund, L., & Kjelberg, A. (1996). A critical analysis of the model of human occupation. *Canadian Journal of Occupational Therapy, 66*(2), 102–108.

57. Hayes, R. (1989). Occupational therapy in the treatment of schizophrenia. *Occupational Therapy in Mental Health, 9*(3), 51–68.

58. Hayes, R., Halford, W. K., & Varghese, F. N. (1991). Generalization of the effects of activity therapy and social skills training on the social behavior of low functioning schizophrenic patients. *Occupational Therapy in Mental Health, 11*(4), 3–20.

59. Helfrich, C. A., Chan, D. V., & Sabol, P. (2011). Cognitive predictors of life skill intervention outcomes for adults with mental illness at risk for homelessness. *American Journal of Occupational Therapy, 65*(3), 277–286.

60. Helfrich, C., Kielhofner, G., & Mattingly, C. (1994). Volition as narrative: Understanding motivation in chronic illness. *American Journal of Occupational Therapy, 48*(4), 311–317.

61. Henry, A. D., & Coster, W. J. (1997). Competency beliefs and occupational role behavior among adolescents: Explication of the personal causation construct. *American Journal of Occupational Therapy, 51*(4), 267–276.

62. Henry, D. (2001). *Tool chest: For teachers, parents, & students.* Henry Occupational Therapy Services.

63. Henry, D. A., Wineland, M. K., & Swindeman, S. (2007). *Tools for tots: Sensory strategies for toddlers and preschoolers.* Henry Occupational Therapy Services.

64. Henry Occupational Therapy Services, Inc. (2016). *Welcome.* Retrieved October 9, 2021, from http://www.henryot.com/

65. Josman, N., & Bar-Tal, Y. (1997). The introduction of a temporal variable to the Allen Cognitive Level (ACL) test in adult psychosocial patients. *Occupational Therapy in Mental Health, 13*(2), 25–34.

66. Kapp, S. K., Steward, R., Crane, L., Elliott, D., Elphick, C., Pellicano, E., & Russell, G. (2019). 'People should be allowed to do what they like': Autistic adults' views and experiences of stimming. *Autism, 23*(7), 1782–1792.

67. Katz, N. (2006). *Routine task inventory—Expanded.* Manual 2006. Allen Cognitive Network. Retrieved August 22, 2021, from http://www.allen-cognitive-network.org/pdf_files/RTIManual2006.pdf

68. Kelly, J. A. (1982). *Social-skills training: A practical guide for interventions.* Springer.

69. Khoury, N. M., Lutz, J., & Schuman-Olivier, Z. (2018). Interoception in psychiatric disorders: A review of randomized controlled trials with interoception-based interventions. *Harvard Review of Psychiatry, 26*(5), 250–263.

70. Kielhofner, G. (Ed.). (1985). *A model of human occupation: Theory and application.* Lippincott Williams & Wilkins.

71. Kielhofner, G. (Ed.). (1995). *A model of human occupation: Theory and application* (2nd ed.). Lippincott Williams & Wilkins.

72. Kielhofner, G. (Ed.). (2002). *A model of human occupation: Theory and application* (3rd ed.). Lippincott Williams & Wilkins.

73. Kielhofner, G. (Ed.). (2008). *A model of human occupation: Theory and application* (4th ed.). Lippincott Williams & Wilkins.

74. Kielhofner, G., & Forsyth, K. (1997). The model of human occupation: An overview of current concepts. *British Journal of Occupational Therapy, 63*(3), 103–110.

75. Kielhofner, G., Mallinson, T., Crawford, C., Nowak, M., Rigby, M., Henry, A., & Walens, D. (1998). *Occupational Performance History Interview (OPHI-II).* MOHO Web. Retrieved October 31, 2021, from https://www.moho.uic.edu/productDetails.aspx?aid=31

76. King L. J. (1974). A sensory-integrative approach to schizophrenia. *American Journal of Occupational Therapy, 28*(9), 529–536.

77. Kinnealey, M., Koenig, K. P., & Smith, S. (2011). Relationships between sensory modulation and social supports and health-related quality of life. *American Journal of Occupational Therapy, 65*(3), 320–327.

78. Knight, M., Adkison, L., & Stack Kovach, J. (2010). A comparison of multisensory and traditional interventions on inpatient psychiatry and geriatric neuropsychiatry units. *Journal of Psychosocial Nursing and Mental Health Services, 48*(1), 24–31.

79. Kramer, J., Kielhofner, G., Lee, S. W., Ashpole, E., & Castle, L. (2009). Utility of the model of human screening tool for detecting client change. *American Journal of Occupational Therapy, 25*(2), 181–191.

80. Krupa, T., Kirsh, B., Pitts, D., & Fossey, E. (2016) *Bruce & Borg's psychosocial frames of reference: Theories, models, and approaches for occupation-based approaches* (4th ed.). SLACK.

81. Kverno, K. S., Black, B. S., Nolan, M. T., & Rabins, P. V. (2009). Research on treating neuropsychiatric symptoms of advanced dementia with non-pharmacological strategies, 1998–2008: A systematic literature review. *International Psychogeriatrics, 21*(5), 825–843.

82. Lane, S. J., Mailloux, Z., Schoen, S., Bundy, A., May-Benson, T. A., Parham, L. D., Smith Roley, S., & Schaaf, R. C. (2019). Neural foundations of Ayres Sensory Integration®. *Brain Sciences, 9*(7), 1–14.

83. Law, M., Baptiste, S., Carswell, A., McColl, M. A., Polatajko, H. J., & Pollock, N. (2014). *Canadian occupational performance measure* (5th ed.). CAOT Publications ACE.

84. Law, M., Cooper, B., Strong, S., Steward, D., Rigby, P., & Letts, L. (1996). The person-environment-occupation model: A transactive approach to occupational performance. *Canadian Journal of Occupational Therapy, 63*(1), 9–23.

85. Lee, J. (2010). Achieving best practice: A review of evidence linked to occupation-focused practice models. *Occupational Therapy in Health Care, 24*(3), 206–222.

86. Lee, S. W., Taylor, R., Kielhofner, G., & Fisher, G. (2008). Theory use in practice: A national survey of therapists who use the model of human occupation. *American Journal of Occupational Therapy, 62*(1), 106–117.

87. Levy, L. L. (1987). Psychosocial intervention and dementia, Part II: The cognitive disability perspective. *Occupational Therapy in Mental Health, 7*(4), 13–36.

88. Levy, L. L. (1990). Activity, social role retention, and the multiply disabled aged: Strategies for intervention. *Occupational Therapy in Mental Health, 10*(3), 2–30.

89. Levy, L. L., & Burns, T. (2011). The cognitive disabilities reconsidered model: Rehabilitation of adults with dementia. In N. Katz (Ed.), *Cognition, occupation, and participation across the life span: Neuroscience, neurorehabilitation, and models of intervention in occupational therapy* (3rd ed., pp. 407–441). AOTA Press.

90. Linehan, M. M. (1993). *Skills training manual for treating borderline personality disorder.* Guilford Press.

91. Litterst, T. A. E. (1982). A reappraisal of anthropological fieldwork methods and the concept of culture in occupational therapy research. *American Journal of Occupational Therapy, 39*(9), 602–604.

92. Loukas, K. M. (2011). Occupational placemaking: Facilitating self-organization through use of a sensory room. *Mental Health Special Interest Section Quarterly, 34*(2), 1–4.

93. Mahler, K. (2019, March 10). *What exactly is interoception? What is interoception?* Retrieved September 18, 2021, from https://www.kelly-mahler.com/resources/blog/what-exactly-is-interoception/

94. Mailloux, L., Parham, D., Smith Roley, S., Ruzzano, L., & Schaaf, R. C. (2018). Introduction to the Evaluation in Ayres Sensory Integration (EASI). *American Journal of Occupational Therapy, 72*(1), 1–7.

95. Mayer, M. A. (1988). Analysis of information processing and cognitive disability theory. *American Journal of Occupational Therapy, 42*(3), 176–183.

96. McWha, J. L., Pachana, N. A., & Alpass, F. (2003). Exploring the therapeutic environment for older women with late-life depression: An examination of the benefits of an activity group for older people suffering from depression. *Australian Journal of Occupational Therapy, 50*(3), 158–169.

97. Miller, L. J., Anzalone, M. E., Lane, S. J., Cermak, S. A., & Osten, E. T. (2007). Concept evolution in sensory integration: A proposed nosology for diagnosis. *American Journal of Occupational Therapy, 61*(2), 135–140.

98. Miller, L. J., Schoen, S. A., & Spielmann, V. (2020). A frame of reference for sensory processing difficulties: Sensory therapies and research (STAR). In P. Kramer, J. Hinojosa, & T.-H. Howe (Eds.), *Frames of reference for pediatric occupational therapy* (4th ed., pp. 159–204). Wolters Kluwer.

99. Moro, C. A. (2007). A comprehensive literature review defining self-mutilation and occupational therapy intervention approaches: Dialectical behavior therapy and sensory integration. *Occupational Therapy in Mental Health, 23*(1), 55–67.

100. Mosey, A. C. (1970). *Three frames of reference for mental health.* SLACK.

101. Mosey, A. C. (1973) *Activities therapy.* Raven.

102. Mosey, A. C. (1987). *Psychosocial components of occupational therapy.* Raven.

103. Muñoz, J. P., Dix, S., & Reichenbach, D. (2006). Building productive roles: Occupational therapy in a homeless shelter. *Occupational Therapy in Health Care, 20*(3–4), 167–187.

104. Neville-Jan, A. (1994). The relationship of volition to adaptive occupational behavior among individuals with varying degrees of depression. *Occupational Therapy in Mental Health, 12*(4), 1–18.

105. O'Brien, J. C. (2018). *Introduction to occupational therapy* (5th ed.). Elsevier.

106. Parham, L. D., Cohn, E. S., Spitzer, S., Koomar, J. A., Miller, L. J., Burke, J. P., Brett-Green, B., Mailloux, Z., May-Benson, T. A., Smith Roley, S., Schaaf, R. C., Schoen, S. A., & Summers, C. A. (2011). Fidelity in sensory integration intervention research. *American Journal of Occupational Therapy, 61*(2), 216–227.

107. Pashazadeh Azari, Z., Hosseini, S. A., Rassafiami, M., Samadi, S. A., Hoseinzadeh, S., & Dunn, W. (2019). Contextual intervention adapted for autism spectrum disorder: A RCT of a parenting program with parents of children diagnosed with autism spectrum disorder (ASD). *Iranian Journal of Child Neurology, 12*(4), 19–35.

108. Penny, N. H., Mueser, K. T., & North, C. T. (1995). The Allen Cognitive Level test and social competence in adult psychiatric patients. *American Journal of Occupational Therapy, 49*(5), 420–427.

109. Raweh, D, V., & Katz, N. (1999). Treatment effectiveness of Allen's cognitive disabilities model with adult schizophrenic outpatients: A pilot study. *Occupational Therapy in Mental Health, 14*(4), 65–77.

110. Rebeiro, K. L. (2001). Enabling occupation: The importance of an affirming environment. *Canadian Journal of Occupational Therapy, 68*(2), 80–89.

111. Reed, K. (1984). *Models of practice in occupational therapy.* Lippincott Williams & Wilkins.

112. Reisman, J. E., & Blakeney, A. B. (1991). Exploring sensory integrative treatment in chronic schizophrenia. *Occupational Therapy in Mental Health, 11*(1):25–43.

113. *Representative observable attributes of functional cognitive abilities and intervention guidelines for cognitive levels.* (n.d.). Allen Cognitive Group. Retrieved September 22, 2021, from http://allencognitive.com/wp-content/uploads/Representative-Observable-Attributes-of-Functional-Cognitive-Abilities-and-Intervention-Guidelines-for-Cognitive-Levels.pdf

114. Research and Training Center on Independent Living. (2020). *Guidelines: How to write about people with disabilities (9th edition).* The University of Kansas. https://rtcil.org/guidelines

115. Robichaud, L., Hébert, R., & Desrosiers, J. (1994). Efficacy of a sensory integration program on behaviors of inpatients with dementia. *American Journal of Occupational Therapy, 48*(4), 355–360.

116. Royeen, C. B. (1985). Domain specifications of the construct tactile defensiveness. *American Journal of Occupational Therapy, 39*(9), 596–599.

117. Salvato, G., Ovadioa, D., Messina, A., & Bottini, G. (2021). Health emergencies and interoceptive sensibility modulate the perception of non-evidence-based drug use: Findings from the COVID-19 outbreak. *PLoS One, 16*(8), e0256806.

118. Schaaf, R. C., Dumont, R. L., Arbesman, M., & May-Benson, T. A. (2018). Efficacy of occupational therapy using Ayres Sensory Integration: A systematic review. *American Journal of Occupational Therapy, 72*(1), 1–10.

119. Schaaf, R. C., & Mailloux, Z. (2015). *Clinician's guide for implementing Ayres Sensory Integration®: Promoting participation for children with autism.* AOTA Press.

120. Schindler, V. P. (2004). Occupational therapy in forensic psychiatry: Role development and schizophrenia. *Occupational Therapy in Mental Health, 20*(3–4), 1–175.

121. Schindler, V. P. (2008). Developing roles and skills in community-living adults with severe and persistent mental illness. *Occupational Therapy in Mental Health, 24*(2), 135–153.

122. Schoen, S. A., Miller, L. J., Camarata, S., & Valdez, A. (2019). Use of the STAR PROCESS for children with sensory processing challenges. *The Open Journal of Occupational Therapy, 7*(4), 1–17.

123. Scott, P. J. (2019). *Role checklist version 3: Participation and Satisfaction (RCv3).* MOHO Web. Retrieved October 31, 2021, from https://www.moho.uic.edu/productDetails.aspx?iid=6

124. Secrest, L., Wood, A. E., & Tapp, A. (1995). A comparison of the Allen cognitive level test and the Wisconsin card sorting test in adults with schizophrenia. *American Journal of Occupational Therapy, 54*(2), 129–136.

125. Smith Roley, S., Schaaf, R. C., & Baltazar-Mori, A. (2020). Ayres Sensory Integration® frame of reference. In P. Kramer, J. Hinojosa, & T-H. Howe (Eds.), *Frames of reference for pediatric occupational therapy* (4th ed., pp. 87–158). Wolters Kluwer.

126. Spackman, C. S. (1981). Methods of instruction. In H. S. Willard & C. S. Spackman (Eds.), *Occupational therapy* (4th ed.). Lippincott.

127. Stein, F. (1982). A current review of the behavioral frame of reference and its application to occupational therapy. *Occupational Therapy in Mental Health, 2*(4), 35–62.

128. Stoller, C. C., Greul, J. H., Cimini, L. S., Fowler, M. S., & Koomar, J. A. (2012). Effects of sensory-enhanced yoga on symptoms of combat stress in deployed military personnel. *American Journal of Occupational Therapy, 66*(1), 59–68.

129. Su, C.-Y., Tsai, P.-C., Su, W.-L., Tang, T.-C., & Tsai, A. Y.-J. (2011). Cognitive profile difference between Allen cognitive levels 4 and 5 in schizophrenia. *American Journal of Occupational Therapy, 65*(1), 453–461.

130. Taboas, A., Doepke, K., & Zimmerman, C. (2023). Preferences for identity-first versus person-first language in a US sample of autism stakeholders. *Autism, 27*(2), 565–570.

131. Taylor, R. R. (Ed.). (2017). *Kielhofner's model of human occupation* (5th ed.). Wolters Kluwer.

132. The Alert Program. (2016, May 15). *Brief overview of the Alert Program® for parents.* https://www.alertprogram.com/brief-overview-of-the-alert-program-for-parents/?doing_wp_cron=1633804346.4707748889923095703125

133. The Alert Program. (2016, July 26). *Alert Program® overview: Supporting children with autism.* https://www.alertprogram.com/alert-program-overview-supporting-children-with-autism/?doing_wp_cron=1633804159.5869460105895996093750

134. Tomcheck, S. D., & Koenig, K. P. (2016). *Occupational therapy practice guidelines for individuals with autism spectrum disorder.* AOTA Press.

135. Turner, N., & Lydon, C. (2008). Psychosocial programming in Ireland based on the model of human occupation: A program evaluation study. *Occupational Therapy in Health Care, 22*(2/3), 105–114.

136. Vargas, S., & Camilli, G. (1999). A meta-analysis of research on sensory integration treatment. *American Journal of Occupational Therapy, 53*(2), 189–198.

137. Walker, K. F., & Ludwig, F. M. (2004). *Perspectives on theory for the practice of occupational therapy* (3rd ed.). Pro-Ed.
138. Wilbarger, P., & Wilbarger, J. (2002). Clinical application of the sensory diet. In A. C. Bundy, S. J. Lane, & E. A. Murray (Eds.), *Sensory integration: Theory and practice* (2nd ed., pp. 339–341). F.A. Davis.
139. Wilbarger, P., & Wilbarger, J. (2002). The Wilbarger approach to treating sensory defensiveness. In A. C. Bundy, S. J. Lane, & E. A. Murray (Eds.), *Sensory integration: Theory and practice* (2nd ed., pp. 335–338). F.A. Davis.
140. Williams, M. S., & Shellenberger, S. (1996). *How does your engine run?* Therapy Works.

SUGGESTED RESOURCES

General

Krupa, T., Birsh, B., Pitts, D., & Fossey, E. (2016). *Bruce & Borg's: Psychosocial frames of reference: Theories, models, and approaches for occupational-based practice* (4th ed.). SLACK.
Occupation focus conceptual frameworks. https://vula.uct.ac.za/access/content/group/9c29ba04-b1ee-49b9-8c85-9a468b556ce2/Framework/intro.htm
OT Theory. *Theories and models.* https://ottheory.com/theories-and-models

Development of Adaptive Skills

Mosey, A. C. (1970). *Three frames of reference for mental health.* SLACK.
Mosey, A. C. (1987). *Psychosocial components of occupational therapy.* Raven.

Role Acquisition and Social Skills Training

Brady, J. P. (1984). Social skills training for psychiatric patients: I. Concepts, methods, and clinical results. *Occupational Therapy in Mental Health, 4*(4), 51–68.
Mosey, A. C. (1973). *Activities therapy.* Raven.
Schindler, V. P. (2004). *Occupational therapy in forensic psychiatry: Role development and schizophrenia.* Routledge.
Schindler, V. P. (2008). Developing roles and skills in community-living adults with severe and persistent mental illness. *Occupational Therapy in Mental Health, 24*(2), 135–153.

Sensory Integration Frame of Reference

Brown, C. (2001). What is the best environment for me? A sensory processing perspective. *Occupational Therapy in Mental Health, 17*(3–4), 115–125.
Champagne, T. (2005). Expanding the role of sensory approaches in acute psychiatric settings. *Mental Health Special Interest Section Quarterly, 28*(1), 1–4.
Henry Occupational Therapy Services Inc. http://www.henryot.com/
OT-Innovations: Sensory modulation. https://www.ot-innovations.com/clinical-practice/sensory-modulation/
Sensational Brain. www.sensationalbrain.com
Sensory Integration Global Network. https://www.siglobalnetwork.org/
Sensory Processing Foundation. http://www.spdfoundation.net/
The Alert Program. https://www.alertprogram.com/
The Collaborative for Leadership in Ayres Sensory Integration®. https://www.cl-asi.org/

The Sensory Connection Program. http://www.sensoryconnectionprogram.com/index.php
Therapeutic brushing techniques. https://www.ot-innovations.com/clinical-practice/sensory-modulation/therapeutic-brushing-techniques/

Cognitive Disabilities

ACDMweb. https://acdmweb.com/uk
Allen, C. K. (1985). *Occupational therapy for psychiatric diseases: Measurement and management of cognitive disabilities.* Little, Brown and Company.
Allen, C. K., Earhart, C, A., & Blue, T. (1992). *Occupational therapy treatment goals for the physically and cognitively disabled.* AOTA Press.
Allen Cognitive Group. http://allencognitive.org/
Allen Cognitive Mentors. *Mary Platt: ACL at a glance beginner's tips.* https://www.allencognitivementors.com/shared-resources
Allen Cognitive Network. *Ability to function* http://www.allen-cognitive-network.org/
Crisis Prevention Institute. *Stage-specific therapeutic gardening activities.* https://www.crisisprevention.com/Platform/Dashboard/Products/Stage-Specific-Therapeutic-Gardening-Activities
Interview with Catherine Earhart about the Claudia Allen scale. https://www.youtube.com/watch?v=qz2tNF3X-4g
Katz, N. (2018). *Cognition and occupation across the life span.* AOTA Press.
S & S Worldwide. *Using Allen diagnostic modules—2nd edition assessments.* https://cdn.ssww.com/share/S52_How_to_use_the_Allen_Diagnostic_Module.pdf
Welcome to OT-Innovations. https://www.ot-innovations.com/clinical-practice/cognition-2/the-allen-cognitive-level-batte

The Model of Human Occupation

Helfrich, C., Kielhofner, G., & Mattingly, C. (1994). Volition as narrative: Understanding motivation in chronic illness. *American Journal of Occupational Therapy, 48*(4), 311–317.
Johnson, H., Kielhofner, G., & Borell, L. (1997). Anticipating retirement: The formation of narratives concerning an occupational transition. *American Journal of Occupational Therapy, 51*(1):49–56.
Model of Human Occupation. *MOHO in Motion—Story of Ramona—Model of Human Occupation.* https://www.youtube.com/watch?v=-Qo2jHJSQow
MOHO Web. https://www.moho.uic.edu/
Taylor, R. (2017). *Kielhofner's model of human occupation* (5th ed.). Wolters Kluwer.

Person–Environment–Occupation

Law, M., Cooper, B., Strong, S., Steward, D., Rigby, P., & Letts, L. (1996). The person-environment-occupation model: A transactive approach to occupational performance. *Canadian Journal of Occupational Therapy, 63*(1), 9–23.
Letts, L., & Rigby, P. (2003). *Using environments to enable occupational performance.* SLACK.
Rebeiro, K. L. (2001). Enabling occupation: The importance of an affirming environment. *Canadian Journal of Occupational Therapy, 68*(2), 80–89.

Understanding Psychiatric Diagnoses

OT HACKS OVERVIEW

O: Occupation as a means and an end

Occupational deprivation (not experiencing adequate meaningful occupational participation) is perhaps the most primary consequence for people who are diagnosed with mental illnesses classified in the *Diagnostic and Statistical Manual of Mental Disorders Fifth Edition Text Revision* (*DSM-5-TR*). Dr Adolf Meyer, a well-known psychiatrist and an advocate for occupational therapy (OT), embraced a theory of psychobiology. Dr Meyer's psychobiologic view proposed that "mental disorders represented reactions of the personality to psychological, social, and biological factors" (11, p. 5). Meyer's belief in the psychobiologic theory influenced the original *Diagnostic and Statistical Manual of Disorders* published in 1952, and his belief in a holistic practical approach to classifying, diagnosing, and treating mental illness is still evident in the latest publication of the *DSM-5-TR*.

Occupational deprivation is a serious problem that has the potential to exacerbate the symptoms of mental illness and hinder recovery. The person may be unable to participate in work or school, or may do so only sporadically. Leisure and social, or community, engagement may be entirely lacking. OT interventions, where participation in occupation is central, provide structure and realistic opportunities to participate in valued roles and occupations. Peer mentoring, individualized instruction, and modeling can clarify and encourage new and more healthy behaviors while effectively helping the client develop coping and resiliency skills (5).

T: Theoretical concepts, values, and principles, or historical foundations

In psychiatric and behavioral health settings, the recovery movement has sparked an evolving paradigm shift in our understanding about how to best support the health and well-being of clients with mental illness. Recovery-related concepts and terminology that help define aspects of recovery for people with mental health diagnoses should always be a highly individualized process. Applying an occupational model of practice to collaborations with clients, while also having a general understanding of common characteristics of particular illnesses, grounds our work in the value of occupation, rather than on the person's diagnosis.

H: How can we Help? OT's role in serving clients with mental illness or mental health needs

There are so many roles that the OT professional can fulfill as a member of a mental or behavioral health team. This is due to our focus on occupational participation and occupational outcomes. So much of what OT can offer through provision of services is inherent to the skill sets that are a natural part of our professional standards of practice (7, 8).

The following quote is an excerpt from a research study by Faulkner and colleagues (2022) titled, *A Mixed Methods Expert Opinion Study on the Optimal Content and Format for an Occupational Therapy Intervention to Improve Sleep in Schizophrenia Spectrum Disorders*. It captures the dynamic ways that OT can support the recovery needs of people with mental health diagnoses by applying our unique occupational perspective. A link to the full article can be found in the *Suggested Resources* at the end of the chapter.

"Occupational therapists focus already on activities, routines, and meaningful occupation, environmental adaptation, holistic assessments and consideration of complex systems, and work around personal motivations (volition)" (31, p. 2).

A: Adaptations

Each client must have clearly written goals that can be met through occupational engagement, and an intervention program must be designed to meet these goals. The goals and the program must be reevaluated at intervals. It is not at all uncommon to encounter a client record that lists three, four, or even more psychiatric diagnoses simultaneously. A primary objective of OT is to determine what the client's priorities are for their recovery.

C: Case study includes

The case example of Matthew, given in Box 4.2, shows how a diagnosis might be made according to the parameters of the *DSM-5-TR*. It also illustrates how psychiatric disorders may be impacted by client factors, occupational history, substance use, and social structures and contexts.

K: **Knowledge: Keeping mental health OT practice grounded in evidence, in occupational science, and in research**

A scoping review of OT intervention studies analyzed OT interventions for adults with severe mental illness (SMI). Thirty-five studies met the inclusion criteria. The findings indicated that psychosocial intervention was the most investigated type of OT intervention applied with adults with SMI, closely followed by psychoeducational approaches to intervention, and by interventions focused on specific client factors such as cognition. Group interventions with clients with schizophrenia were a common format for intervention implementation, and cooperation from a multidisciplinary team in which an OT professional collaborates was found to be typical. Average timeline and service provision for the OT interventions with this population were 2- to 3-weekly 60-minute sessions and a duration of 3 to 6 months (60).

One of the strengths of this study, articulated by the authors and researchers, is that they provided a detailed description of four types of OT intervention that have been studied, and that are a part of current OT practice with this population. However, although scoping reviews such as this are becoming more abundant, there remains a need to continue to build evidence regarding OT intervention with clients who experience SMI, to highlight both our unique contribution and to grow our resources for provision of evidence-based care.

S: **Some terms that may be new to you**

Active phase
Alogia
Anhedonia
Apnea
Biomarkers
Bipolar
Cataplexy
Catatonia
Communication
Compulsion
Cultural concepts of distress
Delusions
Depression
Duration
Frequency
Hallucinations
Hyperactivity
Hypervigilance
Hypomania
Hypopnea
Impulsivity
Language
Mania
Negative symptoms
Obsession
Occupational deprivation
Positive symptoms
Prodromal phase
Provisional diagnosis
Rapid-cycling
Residual phase
Self-direction
Specific learning disabilities
Specifiers
Speech
Subtypes
Torpor

INTRODUCTION

The occupational therapy professional who works in a mental health setting might naturally expect to encounter clients who have received a psychiatric diagnosis; however, the increasing number of clients who have one or more mental health diagnoses means that all occupational therapy professionals, regardless of the setting, are more likely to encounter this group. Understanding how such diagnoses are reached can help the OT team appreciate our own role(s) in collaborating with and serving this population, and it can improve our understanding about how other disciplines approach these clients (7, 8). Although occupational therapy (OT) professionals are concerned with clients' ability to engage in occupation in everyday life and major occupational roles, other professionals may be more focused on clients' symptoms and expressed feelings, or other exacerbations of illness. To understand how OT fits within the treatment team in a mental, behavioral, or psychosocial health care setting, one must first appreciate the larger framework of psychiatric diagnosis.

The American Psychiatric Association's (APA) *Diagnostic and Statistical Manual of Mental Disorders* (*DSM*) formulates a structure and system to classify and categorize mental health diagnoses and is used in the United States. The international standard for classifying diseases is the World Health Organization's (WHO) *International Classification of Diseases, Tenth Edition, Clinical Modification* (*ICD-10-CM*). Because mental illness occurs around the world, the *DSM-5 and the DSM-5-TR* provide appendices with keyed codes to align with the diagnostic codes of the *ICD-10-CM*, which went into effect in the United States in October 2015 (10, 24). Also of note, the Centers for Disease Control and Prevention's National Center for Health Statistics (NCHS) implemented new diagnosis codes related to the COVID-19 pandemic into the *ICD-10-CM* in April of 2022. The new codes Z28.310, Z28.311, and Z28.39, allow health care practitioners the codes for reporting COVID-19 vaccination status (25).

In February of 2022 the WHO released the *ICD-11*. This is the 11th revision of the ICD coding set. The *ICD-11* is entirely digital, with integrated application programming interface (API) tools to facilitate its implementation. Members of the WHO report extraordinary involvement of health care providers from almost 100 countries in developing and modifying the *ICD-11*, making it scientifically vetted and designed for use in an increasingly globally connected digital world. The timeline for a U.S. transition to using the *ICD-11* for reporting health care claims is unclear, but in September 2021, the National Committee on Vital and Health Statistics (NCVHS) issued recommendations to the secretary of the U.S. Department of Health and Human Services (USDHHS) proposing an agenda to evaluate the implementation and transition of *ICD-11* in the United States. International agreement on diagnostic criteria is essential for shared research, to track health care data and statistics, and for accurate billing of medical services.

In 2022, the APA released the *DSM-5-TR*, which is the first published revision of the *DSM-5* (published in 2013). The APA states that, "The clinical and research understanding of mental disorders continues to advance. As a result, most of the *DSM-5-TR* disorder texts have had at least some revision since the 9 years from original publication in *DSM-5*, with the overwhelming majority having had significant revisions" (11, preface, p. xxi). One can infer from this statement that mental health diagnosis is an ongoing and ever-changing process that evolves as we gain a better understanding of mental illness through innovations in research, technology, and practice, and that the *DSM* follows suit, developing in tandem with our understanding.

This edition of the *DSM-5-TR* integrates all prior online updates made to the *DSM-5* since 2013, including updates to incorporate and align with the WHO and the *ICD-10-CM* codes. Other changes include the addition of a new diagnosis, prolonged grief disorder, which is not without controversy (20), as well as the addition of symptom codes for reporting self-injurious nonsuicidal behavior, or suicidal behavior. Importantly, the revision of the updated *DSM-5-TR* is the first *DSM* to be reviewed (and revised) to evaluate its ethnoracial equity and inclusion qualities, and to ensure that adequate attention to client risk factors related to experiences of racism and discrimination are properly addressed. Additionally, multiple work task groups were assigned to assess the text for consistent use of nonstigmatizing language (11).

Nevertheless, because a complete description of the underlying pathology of many psychiatric conditions remains unclear, the *DSM* is an evolving document that practitioners can use as a standard reference and reliable guide to clinical diagnostics and practice in psychiatry. Although occupational therapy professionals do not diagnose psychiatric conditions, a general understanding of the structure and function of the *DSM* allows us access to a resource that presents a concise and explicit set of criteria for psychiatric illnesses and their typical presentations. OT professionals can synthesize these considerations with the data collected while completing an occupational profile to get a more accurate and holistic evaluative picture of the occupational needs of clients in this population.

Clients entering the mental health system in the United States are usually assigned a diagnosis from the *DSM* by a treating medical doctor, such as a psychiatrist. However, as will be discussed throughout the text, because of health disparities and other confounding factors, the literature indicates that more than half of adults with a mental disorder do not receive the treatment that they need. This is the case for over 27 million adults in the United States alone (59). This chapter introduces the major concepts and overall structure of the *DSM-5-TR* presented with pertinent information about the structure and function of the *ICD-10-CM*. The reader will learn some of the underlying assumptions of psychiatric diagnosis while simultaneously becoming more familiar with the diagnostic coding process used in the United States. We will explore the structure and organization of the *DSM-5-TR* emphasizing some of the major diagnostic categories that are commonly encountered in modern OT practice, regardless of the setting. For each diagnostic category, we will briefly outline some of the problems that result in occupational disruption and some of the ways that the OT professional typically addresses the barriers to occupational engagement. More specific occupation-based interventions that target common symptoms of psychiatric illnesses, and that therefore impede occupational engagement, will be presented in Chapters 17 to 23. Throughout this chapter, we will use the term **diagnostician** to refer to the individual who is responsible for the psychiatric diagnosis. Depending on the practice setting, this may be a psychiatrist, a physician with another practice specialty, a psychologist, a psychiatric nurse practitioner, or a psychiatric social worker.

PSYCHIATRIC DIAGNOSIS: AN EVOLVING SCIENCE

From the 1800s, when all mental disease was categorized as idiocy, to the mid-20th century, when a few diagnostic categories were listed in the *ICD*, very little information was available to guide the diagnostician in determining the cause and nature of a person's mental distress or abnormal behavior. The *DSM*, first published in 1952, was an attempt to offer more guidance. Since that time, the *DSM* has undergone many revisions in an effort to improve the accuracy and usefulness of each diagnosis. The *DSM-5* was published in 2013 and the current manual, the *DSM-5-TR*, in 2022; both employ the categorical approach of previous *DSMs*. The *DSM-5* series (2013 and 2022) removed the multiaxial system that was present in the *DSM-IV* series and instead utilized two new terms, *Subtypes* and *Specifiers*, to further cultivate diagnostic impressions and descriptions; both subtypes and specifiers work toward specificity in describing a condition (19). Subtypes in the *DSM-5* are used to describe a subordinate category of a disorder, and subtypes of particular conditions are considered distinct disorders (12). Specifiers, as used in the *DSM-5* series, are used to extend a diagnosis to further describe or clarify the condition. Specifiers are typically used to make clear the course, severity, or special features of an illness (12, 32). Although the *DSM-5* is considered a categorical classification system, most psychiatric illnesses, like other illnesses, are as unique as we are as human beings. The psychiatric illness may not fit neatly inside the boundaries of a single condition; in fact, that is rarely ever the case. Some *DSM-5* authors argued that similar signs and symptoms of individual mental disorders are found in different diagnoses, and for that reason the categorical approach is too restrictive. To allow for research of these similar signs and symptoms, the *DSM-5* series included a separate section (Section III) for measurement and further study of these "cross-cutting" symptoms. Depression, anger, sleep disturbance, and substance use are examples of cross-cutting symptoms. (Cross-cutting refers to cutting across diagnostic lines.)

In cases where symptom clusters span across diagnostic categories, these often indicate vulnerabilities that fall under the umbrella of a larger category of disorders, such as the symptoms of anxiety and depression, which can be characteristic of multiple diagnoses stemming from a variety of *DSM* conditions. Because of this, the disorders in the *DSM-5* were arranged into a new organizational system with other enhancements in the text that encourage a broadened use of the text by various disciplines across psychiatric settings. Following a brief overview in the next section about how clinicians in the United States use *ICD-10* codes to bill for services related to specific *DSM-5-TR* diagnoses, the reader will be provided with a summary of the latest updates included in the *DSM-5-TR*. These updates were developed and peer-reviewed by experts in the mental health field over the past decade.

DSM-5-TR and *ICD-10-CM*: Applying Diagnostic Codes in Psychiatric Practice

Prior to the publication of the *ICD-10-CM* by the WHO in 2015, the *ICD-9-CM* had been utilized for over 30 years, and so the new version of the ICD markedly changed how health care practitioners across disciplines documented for reimbursement of their services. The *ICD-10-CM* has up to seven digits per code. In some settings, and for some practitioners, including rehabilitation professionals using the *ICD-10* codes for billing, each condition is coded to a specific diagnosis, but must also be coded with a particular etiology, severity, body location, or intervention (contact/treatment) code. This results in great variation in both the length of the code and to how the category/type of diagnoses are documented. *The ICD-10-CM* is divided into 26 sections, one for each letter of the alphabet. Thus, the 26 sections are considered alphabetic, and begin with A, B, C, D, etc. Each lettered section also corresponds with different medical specialty areas. For example, sections A and B cover infectious diseases, whereas section C is oncology. The mental health codes appear in section F (and for practitioners in the United States are more fully described and aligned with the *DSM*). Therefore, most mental health diagnostic codes begin with the letter F. The *ICD-10-CM* "F Section" for mental illness is further divided into subsections. See Box 4.1 for a summary and description of the *ICD-10-CM* mental health F subcategories.

DSM-5-TR: Developmental Issues and Diagnosis

The chapters and the order in which the diagnoses or conditions appear in the *DSM-5-TR* text have been rearranged chronologically to reflect a life span approach. Childhood disorders, or disorders that are more frequently diagnosed in pediatrics, such as neurodevelopmental disorders, are placed near the beginning of the text. Disorders more commonly diagnosed in older adulthood, like neurocognitive disorders, are placed closer to the end of the text. Subheadings labeled "development and course" are listed for each condition with descriptions of how the disease presentation may change over time. Other potential age-related changes that may occur, such as the prevalence of a condition among a particular

BOX 4.1 *ICD-10-CM* Mental Health F Code Subcategories and Description of Subcategory Condition(s)

ICD-10-CM Mental Health F Code Subcategory	Description of Subcategory Condition(s)
F01–F09	Mental disorders because of clear physiologic conditions
F10–F19	Mental disorders because of substance abuse
F20–F29	Schizophrenia, schizotypal, delusional, and other psychotic processes
F30–F39	Mood disorders
F40–F48	Anxiety, dissociative, stressor-related, and somatoform disorders
F50–F59	Behavioral syndromes with physical factors
F60–F69	Personality disorder
F70–F79	Intellectual disabilities
F80–F89	Pervasive developmental disorders
F90–F98	Disorders of childhood and adolescence
F99–F99	Unspecified mental disorders

ICD-10-CM, International Classification of Diseases, Tenth Edition, Clinical Modification.
Adapted from Buser, S. (2022). *DSM-5-TR insanely simplified: Unlocking the spectrums within DSM-5-TR and ICD-10* (pp. 161–162). Chiron Publications.

age group, have also been added and updated. In some conditions, like posttraumatic stress disorder (PTSD) or insomnia disorders, the age-related factors have been added to the specifiers and criteria sets, so that professionals have a more accurate idea of how a diagnosis may show up in a particular age group. In other words, the symptoms of PTSD may be different in young children, adolescents, young adults, and older adults.

DSM-5-TR: Integration of Current Evidence and Research

The integration of scientific findings from the latest research in genetics, epigenetics, neuroscience, and neuroimaging significantly informed the revision of the chapters in the *DSM-5-TR*. The consistently emerging new research supports the notion that there may be genetic links between diagnostic groups. Furthermore, the evidence is mounting that there are physiologic and genetic indicators and risk factors for certain diagnoses. Placing this information with each diagnosis will assist health care professionals to identify and perhaps clarify, especially conditions that exist on a spectrum (ie, autism or schizophrenia) by assessing common neurocircuitry, genetic factors, or environmental exposure (10, 11).

DSM-5-TR: Classification of Bipolar and Depressive Disorders

Considering that bipolar disorders and depressive disorders are among the most diagnosed disorders in the United States and around the world, the presentation of these disorders has been reconfigured in the *DSM-5* series to help both diagnosticians and practitioners to improve client treatment plans. The streamlining of the information about these conditions aims to enrich client and practitioner education. In the *DSM-IV*, the definitions of manic, hypomanic, and major depressive *episodes* were separate from the definitions of the *disorders*, that is, bipolar I disorder (BPD-I), bipolar II disorder (BPD-II), and major depressive disorder (9). This created confusion and often prolonged the diagnostic process. In the *DSM-5-TR*, the major components are listed with the criteria for each one of the disorders (instead of separating out information about episodes). Similar changes were made to streamline information for distinguishing between bereavement and major depressive disorder; and more comprehensive explanations or narratives were added for the new specifiers anxious distress and mixed features, both of which are listed in the text under criteria for these individual diagnoses.

DSM-5-TR: Substance Use Disorders

Substance use disorders have been restructured and redefined in the *DSM-5* series to establish improved consistency and a better understanding of these conditions. When the *DSM-5* replaced the *DSM-IV-TR* in 2013, the terms "substance abuse" and "substance dependence" were eliminated and replaced with the broad category called "substance use disorders." Also, in the *DSM-5* series, the specific substance that the person ingests defines the specific disorder and so can be referred to as a specifier. However, the lack of understanding and frequent confusion in differentiating between **substance dependence** and **addiction**, as well as the frequency with which the terms were used interchangeably, adds another layer of misunderstanding about this group of conditions. When a client demonstrates dependence on a substance, according to the definition of dependence, it is typical for the client to build a tolerance and to show signs of withdrawal from the substance that they are dependent upon (especially with pain medicine and other prescription drugs that impact the central nervous system), but that does not automatically signify that an addiction is present. The latest version of the text aims to continue to clarify the criteria for substance use disorders to improve the overall understanding of the diagnoses in this category (11).

DSM-5-TR: Major and Mild Neurocognitive Disorders

Tremendous expansion and explosive growth in the branches of neuropsychology, the development and use of advanced brain imaging techniques, and increased understanding of the neurobiologic systems led to the need for the *DSM-5* and the *DSM-5-TR* chapters to have enhanced specificity in describing major and mild neurocognitive disorders to support practitioners in understanding, diagnosing, and treating these conditions (10, 11). In former versions of the *DSM* texts, many types of organic brain disorders were grouped under the broad category referred to as "the dementias," with very little distinction between the subtypes. Advanced clinical diagnosis, enhanced understanding, and therefore more specific treatment plans for variants of the types of dementia and other diseases that impact the brain were often not possible.

Advances in the identification of biologic markers and in findings of links to specific genetic markers have advanced our diagnostic capacity, which has a direct carry over into our capacity to deliver evidence-based interventions in practice. One example of this advanced ability to link research to practice is found in a research study that focused on the self-monitoring ability of adults who had been diagnosed with dementia. The authors of this study took into consideration that prior research had indicated that there was a possible neuronal substrate associated with a person's ability to self-monitor, and that this was related to the human capacity of demonstrating empathy, which is also a central aspect of forming and maintaining social relationships. With this information in mind, the research team designed a study with 77 clients who had been diagnosed with various types of dementia. The participants were screened using voxel-based morphometry (a type of advanced imaging) to assess for any possible volume reduction in the brain structures of clients who had self-monitoring problems, the decrease of social or emotional expressiveness, and any degree of change in their self-presentation habits. These characteristics (self-monitoring, self-presentation, social and emotional expressiveness) were assessed using the *Revised Self-Monitoring Scale*. Using regression analysis, the correlation between gray matter loss in these individuals and deficient performance of self-monitoring was determined. The results of this study suggested that clients with dementia have a decreased ability to initiate or maintain self-monitoring. Based on the imaging and correlations drawn from this study, these findings implicate an impaired insula and orbitofrontal cortex, as well as a disconnection from structures of the salience network of the brain, to the deficiencies in self-monitoring (56). It is this type of research that has fed the advancement in our understanding of the central nervous system and created the need to enhance the specificity of description in the *DSM-5* to support the evolution of our diagnostic capacity.

DSM-5-TR: Section III Emerging Measures and Models

Section III of the *DSM-5-TR* consists of assessment methods and tools, such as the *DSM-5 Self-Rated Level 1 Cross-Cutting Symptom Measure for Adults*, and a similar cross-cutting symptom measure for parents or guardians of children ages 6 to 17 to utilize. Other techniques and tools included in this section are shared to encourage improved understanding among practitioners of the multidimensional context of mental illness, including the impact of culture, environment, and the sociopolitical conditions that these clients face. Another helpful tool included in this section of the *DSM-5-TR* is the *Clinician-Rated Dimensions of Psychosis Symptom Severity* (11). The severity of symptoms in schizophrenia and other psychotic disorders often gives the behavioral and mental health care team, and the client and their loved ones, important predictive information about what to expect regarding aspects of the illness like cognitive deficits. This instrument provides a practical way to capture a client's patterns and track the severity of symptoms over time. The tool provides scales that assess the primary symptoms of psychosis, including hallucinations, delusions, disorganized speech, abnormal psychomotor behavior, and negative symptoms. Ongoing research indicates that people who experience psychotic disorders also tend to experience cognitive limitations or impairments in a range of cognitive domains. Capturing dysfunction in the cognitive domains can support prediction about future prognosis and functional abilities, thus this scale can be used to help practitioners with treatment planning and setting realistic functional goals.

The *DSM-5-TR* also includes in Section III the *World Health Organization Disability Assessment Schedule* (WHODAS 2.0) (75), which is compatible with the *International Classification of Functioning, Disability and Health* (ICF), also developed by the WHO (10, 11). The purpose of the WHODAS 2.0 is to provide a measure of disability that can be implemented even when a mental disorder is mild or not able to be diagnosed (10, 11). A given diagnosis (in most cases) does not by itself indicate the extent of disability, and a separate measure of disability and functioning helps to document

need for services and to describe barriers to occupational engagement. The WHODAS 2.0 is available in seven versions, which differ in length and intended mode of administration. The assessment contains many items about occupational performance (self-care, mobility, social interaction, functioning in school and work, and household tasks) and may alert diagnosticians that OT services are warranted. A link to the WHODAS 2.0 is available in the additional resources at the end of this chapter (75).

DSM-5-TR: Section III Culture and Psychiatric Diagnosis

As occupational therapy professionals, our domain of concern includes understanding a client's occupational history, or life experiences. Evaluation of the client's successful engagement in desired occupations, and determining what factors may be limiting or inhibiting occupational performance, requires that we understand their contexts, including environmental contexts and personal factors. As defined by the fourth edition of the Occupational Therapy Practice Framework: Domain and Process (*OTPF-4*), some of the personal factors that are an inherent part of context include chronologic age, sexual orientation, gender identity, race and ethnicity, cultural identification and attitudes, social background, social and socioeconomic status, upbringing and life experiences, education, profession, and professional identity, among other factors (6).

The updated chapter, *Culture and Psychiatric Diagnosis*, in Section III of the *DSM-5-TR* provides information and suggestions for developing knowledge about the client's cultural and social context that is helpful to include in the evaluation and diagnosis of mental health conditions. The chapter introduces and defines relevant key terms to help practitioners understand the cultural context of the illness experience and includes an expanded version of *The Outline for Cultural Formulation* that was initiated in the *DSM-IV* (9). *The Outline for Cultural Formulation* provided an initial structure for assessing information about the cultural features of a client's mental health problem(s) and how that relates to the client's social and cultural context and history. Included in this chapter of the *DSM-5-TR* is the *Cultural Formulation Interview*, which is an interview protocol designed and field-tested to operationalize the integration of culture and social context into clinical diagnosis of mental health conditions (10, 11). Readers may see some parallels between the domain of concern and process of occupational therapy, and the need to evaluate and carefully consider how culture and social context are in relationship with a client's mental health condition during the psychiatric diagnostic process. The case example of Matthew, given in Box 4.2, shows how diagnosis might be made according to the parameters of the *DSM-5-TR*. It illustrates how psychiatric disorders may be compounded by substance use and by social context.

Another section in the *Culture and Psychiatric Diagnosis* chapter of the *DSM-5-TR* that is particularly helpful for

BOX 4.2 *DSM-5-TR* Case Example: Matthew

A 27-year-old Caucasian Jewish male named Matthew was admitted through a city hospital emergency room to Garden of Eden State Psychiatric Center in New York City 2 days after the police found him wandering on the street in a neighborhood known for its illegal drug trade. When the police apprehended him, he was naked, shouting, "The ozone layer is gone! Global warming is heating up the Earth. God is burning us up for our sins!" and "I am the son of God. I can heal the ozone layer. Only by my touch can global warming be stopped."

Matthew was restless and required restraint during the initial examination to prevent injury to self and others. He was 40 pounds underweight, poorly nourished, and unkempt. Matthew had open wounds on his upper and lower extremities.

A family history revealed that a paternal uncle had been hospitalized for an unspecified mental illness in late adolescence and who never subsequently lived outside of a psychiatric hospital. A cousin on his maternal side has experienced several acute schizophrenic episodes, and is stabilized with medication, living semi-independently with supports in her community. Matthew's parents and older sister are all professionals. He has had 17 admissions to both public and private psychiatric and drug rehabilitation facilities; follow-through with treatment recommendations has been inconsistent.

Previous records indicate that Matthew was a difficult child who argued and fought with playmates from an early age. By the time Matthew entered kindergarten, his pediatrician had recommended a psychiatric consultation because of concerns about destructive behaviors, although no definitive diagnosis was established. Matthew reported to his parents that he sometimes heard voices that told him what to do. His parents observed him "talking to himself" at times. The psychiatrist told the parents that their son had an above-average IQ (IQ of 133), but was developing a severe and chronic behavioral disorder. Various therapies during childhood had poor results; Matthew was first hospitalized at age 13 when he tore the house apart after a teacher asked him to rewrite a composition. At that time, his parents agreed to inpatient treatment. On discharge after 90 days (the extent of insurance coverage), the hospital recommended that treatment be continued at a public psychiatric hospital. The family rejected this recommendation because they found the public facility frightening.

This was the first instance in a repeating pattern of treatment that was followed by inconsistent adherence to treatment recommendations. Matthew began to experiment with alcohol and marijuana at age 15, which served as a gateway to using more illicit drugs. Matthew dropped out of school in 10th grade and ran away from home many times. He would, each time, come home and ask for food, a hot shower, and money. When refused money, he would often attempt to steal from his parents and sister. When Matthew was 19 years old, the family told him that he could not come home again. Matthew has been living on the street for much of the 8 years since. He tried five community residential rehabilitation programs for people who are mentally ill chemical abusers (MICAs), but because he was unwilling or unable to comply with the rules, the programs were unsuccessful each time. He has since been rejected for treatment by five other residential programs. At times, Matthew has been through detox and with appropriate medication management, a decrease in symptoms was documented. He states that his problems are really simple: "People should just be allowed to do whatever they want as long as they do not hurt others. I could do just fine if the police would mind their own business."

Matthew's Social Security benefits have been discontinued because he failed to report for an annual evaluation. His parents refuse to allow him to return to their home.

DSM-5-TR Diagnosis
F20.9	Schizophrenia, continuous
F10.20	Alcohol use disorder, moderate
F12.20	Cannabis use disorder, moderate

Z Codes
Z91.19	Nonadherence to medical treatment
Z91.83	Wandering associated with mental disorder
Z59.02	Unsheltered Homelessness

DSM-5-TR, Diagnostic and Statistical Manual of Mental Disorders Fifth Edition Text Revision.
Adapted from a case example contributed by Hermine D. Plotnick and Margaret D. Rerek.

occupational therapy professionals and others who collaborate with and care for individuals with psychiatric or behavioral health problems is the section that explains **cultural concepts of distress**. Cultural concepts of distress are ways that individuals experience, understand, and communicate about their suffering, behavioral problems, or difficult thoughts and emotions. According to the *DSM-5-TR*, it is essential that practitioners and diagnosticians understand cultural concepts of distress. The concepts are critical to psychiatric diagnosis for the following reasons:

- To enhance identification of individual's concerns and detection of psychopathology
- To avoid misdiagnosis
- To obtain useful clinical information
- To improve clinical rapport and engagement
- To improve therapeutic efficacy
- To guide clinical research
- To clarify cultural epidemiology (11, pp. 872–873)

For examples of common cultural concepts of distress, see Table 4.1.

Table 4.1. Common Cultural Concepts of Distress

Cultural Concept of Distress	Description and Related Conditions in *DSM-5-TR*
Ataque de nervios "attack of nerves"	**Description:** Syndrome found in Latinx characterized by symptoms of intense emotional upset. A general feature of an ataque de nervios is a sense of being out of control. **Related Conditions in *DSM-5-TR:*** Panic attack, panic disorder, other specified or unspecified dissociative disorder, functional neurologic symptom disorder, intermittent explosive disorder, other specified or unspecified anxiety disorder, other specified or unspecified trauma- and stressor-related disorder
Dhat syndrome	**Description:** Dhat syndrome is a term that was coined in South Asia more than 50 years ago to account for common clinical presentations of young men who attributed their various symptoms to semen loss. Although the name indicates a distinct syndrome, this is instead a cultural explanation of distress with symptoms like anxiety, fatigue, weakness, weight loss, erectile dysfunction, depressed mood, and other somatic symptoms. The distinguishing feature is anxiety and distress about the loss of "*dhat*" (related to the concept of *dhatu*, or semen). Dhatu is described in the Hindu system of medicine, Ayurveda, as one of seven essential bodily fluids whose balance is necessary to maintain health. **Related Conditions in *DSM-5-TR:*** Major depressive disorder, persistent depressive disorder, generalized anxiety disorder, somatic symptom disorder, illness anxiety disorder, erectile disorder, early (premature) ejaculation disorder, other specified or unspecified sexual dysfunction, educational problems
Hikikomori (a Japanese term composed of *hiku* [to pull back] and *moru* [to seclude oneself])	**Description:** Hikikomori is a Japanese term derived from *hiku* [to pull back] and *moru* [to seclude oneself]. Hikikomori is a syndrome of lingering and severe social withdrawal observed in Japan that may result in a person completely withdrawing from face-to-face interactions with others. Hikikomori typically presents with a narrative that describes an adolescent or young male who does not leave his room in his parent's home and has no face-to-face social interactions. The condition leads to distress over time, and is often associated with high intensity of Internet usage, decreased interest or willingness to occupational engagement in school or work. **Related Conditions in *DSM-5-TR:*** Social anxiety disorder, major depressive disorder, generalized anxiety disorder, posttraumatic stress disorder, autism spectrum disorder, schizoid personality disorder, avoidant personality disorder, schizophrenia, or other psychotic disorder. The condition may also be associated with Internet gaming disorder and, in adolescents, school refusal.
Khyâl cap "wind attacks"	**Description:** Khyâl attacks is a syndrome found in Cambodian contexts. Common symptoms include panic attacks, such as dizziness, palpitations, shortness of breath, cold extremities, and other symptoms of autonomic arousal. A person experiencing these khyâl attacks (wind attacks) may have catastrophic thoughts that khyâl will rise up in the body along with the blood and cause serious effects like asphyxiation, or dizziness, blurry vision, or even death. **Related Conditions in *DSM-5-TR:*** Panic attack, panic disorder, generalized anxiety disorder, agoraphobia, posttraumatic stress disorder, and illness anxiety disorder
Kufungisisa (thinking too much in Shona)	**Description:** This is an idiom of distress and a cultural explanation among the Shona of Zimbabwe of causes of anxiety, depression, and somatic problems, but also can be used to explain psychosocial distress like interpersonal and social difficulties. A primary symptom of Kufungisisa is that the client ruminates on troubling thoughts, especially worries about chronic illness and disease such as HIV-related disorders. **Related Conditions in *DSM-5-TR:*** Major depressive disorder, persistent depressive disorder, generalized anxiety disorder, posttraumatic stress disorder, obsessive–compulsive disorder, and prolonged grief disorder
Maladi dyab (literally "devil/Satan illness," also referred to as "sent sickness")	**Description:** A cultural explanation in Haitian communities for diverse medical and psychiatric disorders and problems with occupational function. "In this explanatory model, interpersonal envy and malice cause people to harm their enemies by having sorcerers send illnesses such as psychosis, depression, social or academic failure, and inability to perform activities of daily living" (11, p. 876). **Related Conditions in *DSM-5-TR:*** Problems related to the social environment or educational problems with the presence of other psychiatric disorders, and the cultural explanation of supernatural forces, may lead to misdiagnosis of delusional disorder, persecutory type, or schizophrenia.

(continued)

Table 4.1. Common Cultural Concepts of Distress (*continued*)	
Cultural Concept of Distress	**Description and Related Conditions in *DSM-5-TR***
Shenjing shuairuo ("weakness of the nervous system" in Mandarin Chinese)	**Description:** A cultural syndrome that integrates conceptual categories of Traditional Chinese Medicine with the Western construct of neurasthenia. Fewer diagnoses of Shenjing shuairuo and increased reference to the *ICD-10* and *ICD-11* have created more instances of replacing the use of Shenjing shuairuo as an illness category with the use of various forms of anxiety or depression. **Related Conditions in *DSM-5-TR*:** Major depressive disorder, persistent depressive disorder, generalized anxiety disorder, somatic symptom disorder, social anxiety disorder, specific phobia, and posttraumatic stress disorder
Susto ("fright")	**Description:** A cultural explanation for distress and misfortune prevalent in some Latinx cultural contexts in North, Central, and South America. *Susto* is an illness attributed to a frightening event that causes the soul to leave the body and results in unhappiness and sickness, and difficulty performing tasks associated with one's occupational roles. **Related Conditions in *DSM-5-TR*:** Major depressive disorder, posttraumatic stress disorder, other specified or unspecified trauma and stressor-related disorder, or somatic symptom disorder

DSM-5-TR, *Diagnostic and Statistical Manual of Mental Disorders Fifth Edition Text Revision*; HIV, human immunodeficiency virus; ICD, *International Classification of Diseases*.

Adapted from American Psychiatric Association. (2022). *Diagnostic and statistical manual of mental disorders* (5th ed., text rev., pp. 873–879). https://doi.org/10.1176/appi.books.9780890425787

THE DIAGNOSTIC CATEGORIES OF THE *DSM-5-TR*

Information in this section follows the organization of the *DSM-5-TR*. Selected disorders or categories are summarized. Inclusion of selected diagnostic categories in this textbook is based on the prevalence of the disorder and the likelihood that it will be encountered by the entry-level occupational therapy professional working in a clinical or community setting. Not every *DSM-5-TR* diagnosis is included here; this is not intended as an exhaustive list of diagnoses. Details and descriptive illustrations are incorporated to provide a holistic introduction of the illnesses. Common problems and characteristics of the illnesses, and concerns addressed by OT are also briefly discussed, whereas interventions related to specific symptoms that present barriers to occupation for clients with mental illness are further expanded in *Section Three* of the text. The reader should note that duration and frequency of symptoms are considered by the diagnostician and are part of the operational criteria for each diagnostic entity. **Duration** refers to "how long" the symptoms have been present. **Frequency** refers to "how often" the symptoms are felt. Also, although some of the diagnostic criteria are described for each diagnosis, it is beyond the scope of this text to list the complete diagnostic and health-related information. The reader is encouraged to consult the most updated *DSM* for more information related to conditions when needed (11).

Neurodevelopmental Disorders

Neurodevelopmental disorders occur when the development of the central nervous system (CNS) is disrupted. These disorders occur in infancy and early in life, and they can have profound effects often revealing neuropsychiatric, motor, learning, language, or nonverbal communication problems throughout the person's life (11, 41). Conditions such as the autism spectrum disorder (ASD) and attention-deficit/hyperactivity disorder (ADHD) are examples of neurodevelopmental disorders that can impair the growing child's ability to perceive, interact with, and respond effectively to the environment. Thus, these conditions significantly affect learning and skill development. Although these disorders were once thought of as being categorically defined, modern techniques used to measure the symptoms demonstrate apparent levels of severity and sometimes lack of distinction from typical development. For this reason, these diagnoses require both the presence of symptoms and occupational dysfunction (11). There are six categories of neurodevelopmental disorders that occur in this group (frequently occurring together):

- Intellectual Developmental Disorders (Intellectual Disability)
- Communication Disorders
- Autism Spectrum Disorder
- Attention-Deficit/Hyperactivity Disorder
- Specific Learning Disorder
- Motor Disorders

Intellectual Development Disability

Intellectual developmental disability (intellectual disability, or ID) is a disorder with onset during the developmental period that includes both intellectual and adaptive functioning deficits in the conceptual, social, and practical domains. ID is characterized by (a) deficits in intellectual functioning as confirmed by both clinical assessment and individualized, standardized intelligence testing, (b) deficits in adaptive functioning (in daily life activities and roles) that result in failure to meet developmental and sociocultural standards for personal independence and social responsibility, and (c) onset of intellectual and adaptive deficits during the developmental period (typically before age 18). The more severe the disability, the greater the impairment in adaptive function. The various levels of severity are essentially defined based on adaptive functioning, and not by the parameters of IQ. It is adaptive functioning that determines the amount of support that a client needs, and OT professionals are well suited to assess function in everyday occupational engagement. Those with severe and profound ID are likely to have significant impairment in motor functions, skills, and physical development, and may have increased challenge with mobility and self-care. Typical problems addressed by the OT for a person with this condition may include the following:

- Deficits in self-care
- Impaired social functioning
- Impaired or absent vocational functioning
- Perceptual–motor deficits

Disorders of Communication

Disorders of communication include deficits in language, speech, or communication and are diagnosed when impairment of speech or language is significant enough to interfere with academic or daily life functioning. According to the *DSM-5-TR*, **speech** is the expressive production of sounds including the characteristics of the sound such as articulation, fluency, voice, and resonance. **Language** focuses on a conventional use of symbols embedded with rules of form and function and synthesized to produce communication. **Communication** is the transfer of ideas and information using verbal and nonverbal behaviors to influence another individual (11). Children with communication disorders may or may not be seen by OT, particularly in the absence of other concurrent diagnoses; pediatric clients with communication disorders or with swallowing disorders are among those who are most frequently cotreated by a speech language pathology professional and an OT professional.

Autism Spectrum Disorder

In the *DSM-5-TR*, autistic disorder, Asperger disorder, and pervasive developmental disorder, once considered as separate conditions, have now been consolidated into one condition as **autism spectrum disorder** (ASD) (11, 44). "Symptoms of these disorders represent a single continuum of mild to severe impairments in the two domains of social communication and restrictive repetitive behaviors/ interests" (11, p. xxiv, Preface to *DSM-5*). The diagnosis of ASD (using the *DSM-5-TR* criteria) requires the documentation of at least two of the following characteristics:

- Repetitive actions or speech
- Insistence on sameness
- Restricted fixated interests
- Increased or decreased sensitivity to sensory stimulation

Additionally, the client may require support in either or both of the two domains of social communication and restrictive repetitive behaviors/interests, at the following three levels:

- Level 1—requires support
- Level 2—requires substantial support
- Level 3—requires very substantial support

By increasing the sensitivity and specificity of the criteria for diagnostic purposes in ASD, intervention plans can be designed to target and focus on more specific aspects of the impairment (11). Severity of ASD ranges from high to low functioning, in both cognitive domains and in social skills, interaction, and communication (48).

The spectrum of disorders in this category may be characterized by (a) impairment in social communication and relationships, generally including a decreased level of awareness of others, of contexts, and of social cues; (b) restricted and repetitive interests and activities, such as rituals and distinct motor mannerisms; (c) evidence of these problems early in life, even if not diagnosed until later; (d) significant impairment in social and occupational functioning; and (e) problems distinct from ID (which may be diagnosed as a co-occurring disorder). Areas addressed by OT include the following:

- Dysregulated sensory processing, registration, modulation, or regulation that interferes with occupational participation
- Perceptual–motor deficits such as postural control, gravitational insecurity, or gross or fine motor coordination that interferes with occupational participation
- Deficits in social interaction that interferes with occupational participation
- Self-care deficits that interfere with occupational participation
- Independent living skills deficits or needs that interfere with occupational participation
- Behavioral and social interaction skills necessary for success in school such as attention and following rules and routines
- Emotion regulation when it interferes with optimal occupational participation

Sensory-integrative, developmental, or behavioral frames of reference are often useful to consider in occupational therapy intervention planning with clients who have an ASD diagnosis. Nevertheless, the *DSM-5-TR* reminds professionals that "descriptive severity categories should not be used to determine eligibility for and provision of services . . . individuals with relatively better skills overall may experience different or even greater psychosocial challenges. Thus, service needs can only be developed at an individual level and through discussion of [the client's] personal priorities and targets" (11, p. 59).

A mild ASD may be diagnosed in someone who functions fairly well in their overall occupational roles and engagement. Some clients with ASD may only experience mild language delay; misinterpretation of what is being said to the client (or their receptive language skills) may be the only deficiency. Social deficits are more often a primary feature. Individuals with an ASD diagnosis who are functioning at the high end of the autism spectrum possess good to excellent verbal abilities, yet they have difficulty interacting with others. Typically, they have specific interests that they pursue, and often to the exclusion of all others. These interests become preoccupations that can dominate behavior, or at a minimum limit their experience of occupational balance (48, 49). The disorder may not be as apparent in early childhood, but sometimes becomes a problem when the child enters school and they are unable to relate effectively to peers and teachers, or experience problems with appropriately transitioning to new tasks and environments. Typically, the older child or adolescent with ASD will desire friendships, but they may have difficulty communicating or with developing social interactions, making it hard to make new friends. Sometimes the social isolation or the difficulty of adjusting in school or in their job leads to depression and/or anxiety (49).

ASD is a lifelong condition that may cause significant impairment in performance of work occupations and in social interactions and the person's relationships. An overwhelmed sensory system may significantly impact occupational engagement. The *Adolescent/Adult Sensory Profile* (17, 29) supports evaluation that explores how a client's sensory modulation and dysregulation may be impacting occupational participation. Interventions can be planned so that strategies for managing sensory needs and responses, particularly by modifying the environment, can be implemented. Wallace et al (73) suggest that sensory-based treatment may have the additional benefit of helping to alleviate anxiety and depression. Certainly, social skills training seems appropriate; however, the sensory deficits and lack of awareness of social cues and nonverbal communication are barriers to understanding and applying appropriate social skills and responses. Featured in the *Point-of-View* box, writer and autism advocate Christine Condo shares what it feels like from her perspective to move through life as a person with ASD (28). She was diagnosed in 2015. A link to the full article by Condo is available in the *Suggested Resources* at the end of the chapter.

POINT-OF-VIEW

I have high-functioning autism, and this means that I usually look normal on the outside. But I'm here to tell you that I am fundamentally different on the inside. ...

If there's a loud TV, my brain cannot tune it out. Actually, I cannot tune out anything. Ever. That smell of popcorn from a co-worker's desk? It hijacks my brain to the point that I have to take my work to another room if I am to have any hope of concentrating.

Imagine having the acuity of your senses turned up to 11. Imagine being keenly aware of every single element of your environment, all the time, especially those you normally, reflexively ignore. Imagine that every time you walk out your front door, it is like being forced to walk too close to a wall of spikes that constantly threaten to impale you.

Then imagine that, under this assault, you concentrate on maintaining an elaborate performance to relate to those around you while suppressing your natural mode of speaking and acting.

—Christine M. Condo, writer and autism spokesperson, diagnosed with ASD in 2015

Although the etiologic factors that cause or contribute to ASD remain elusive, research in the last decade found hundreds of genes associated with the condition(s). Genetic studies involving twins have also demonstrated a strong genetic correlation among ASD disorders (27, 74), which informs us that these disorders are highly heritable. **Biomarkers** are categorized into several major types, including genetic, immune, behavioral, metabolic, neuroimaging, neurophysiology, nutritional, or medical history. Research by Frye and colleagues (2019) suggests that the discovery of some promising biomarkers of ASD potentially offer something more, beyond observation of behaviors, which may lead to improving treatments and developing better interventions (35).

Attention-Deficit/Hyperactivity Disorder

Attention-deficit/hyperactivity disorder may be diagnosed in clients with a persistent pattern of **inattention** or **hyperactivity** that interferes with function or development for at least 6 months, typically with an onset of symptoms beginning before age 12. Diagnostic criteria for children require client demonstration/presentation of six or more symptoms of inattention or hyperactivity/impulsivity. For older adolescents and adults (ie, those who are age 17 and above) at least five of the symptoms must be present (11). The prevalence rate for ADHD is in the 3% to 7% range for school-aged children (44). Twins' studies have demonstrated a 70% to 90% heritability rate with ADHD, and researchers believe that a person is 2 to 8 times more likely to be diagnosed with ADHD if a first-degree relative has the condition (69). Three forms of ADHD are recognized in the *DSM-5-TR*:

F90.0 ADHD, Inattentive Type
F90.1 ADHD, Hyperactive/Impulsive
F90.2 ADHD, Combined

Children who have the **inattentive** form may seem not to listen, not to be attending. They may lose things or become distracted easily. They have trouble staying organized and may forget about responsibilities or appointments. They fail to persist in tasks and have trouble staying focused.

Hyperactivity means being more active than is normal, particularly when it is not appropriate to the situation. Fidgeting, talking, and being restless are examples. **Impulsivity** refers to acting quickly without regard for consequences, taking actions that may be harmful to self and others without thinking about the results. Behaviors may include interrupting others frequently and intrusively, making unnecessary purchases, and jumping to decisions without investigating the situation carefully.

Some typical problems addressed in OT include the following:

- Limited or unreliable attention span and problems with organization
- Poor impulse control
- Deficient age-appropriate skills for academic, social, and occupational roles
- Social skills deficits

ADHD for many continues into adult life, causing difficulties not just in school but also in the workplace. Occupational therapy should focus on occupational performance, appropriate for the age/stage and goals of the individual. Sample interventions include the following:

- Use of scaffolding techniques and implementing a consistent structured schedule
- Use of visual reminders, lists, and cues
- Use of smartphone devices and apps to cue behaviors
- Parent and teacher education about the need for scheduled breaks and gross motor activities
- Sensory-integrative activities and sensory processing education
- Modifications to home, classroom, or workplace context

In 1997, the National Institute of Mental Health (NIMH) launched what has become a pioneering research study involving 579 pediatric participants from all across the United States who were diagnosed with ADHD and were between the ages of 7 and 10 years. The purpose of the study was to evaluate the impact of multiple differing treatment modalities, including the following:

- **Medication management**—Medication only, using different doses of methylphenidate, commonly known as Ritalin
- **Behavioral treatment**—Behavioral interventions delivered by parents, counselors, and schools in a coordinated process
- **Combined treatment**—Children received both the medication and behavioral treatment.
- **Community care**—This was the control (or nontreatment) group.

Children who participated in the study were assigned to one of four different treatment groups for 14 months, followed by an evaluation of the impacts of the treatments. The research findings indicated that ADHD symptoms of hyperactivity and inattention are more responsive to pharmacologic intervention (alone) than behavioral intervention (alone), and as the researchers had hypothesized, the combined treatment that included both pharmacologic and behavioral intervention was "statistically superior in terms of core symptoms and oppositional/defiant behaviors" (41, p. 221).

The *DSM-5-TR* notes multiple functional consequences for people who are diagnosed with ADHD. ADHD is a risk factor for suicidal ideation and behavior in children. Adults with ADHD are at increased risk for suicide attempt when comorbid conditions such as mood or substance use disorders are present. Children with ADHD have an increased risk of developing conduct disorders in adolescence, often leading to poor job stability, elevated risk of unemployment, instability in relationships, and higher rates of incarceration as adults (11). The functional consequences and associated risks that come with a diagnosis of ADHD open many opportunities for occupational therapy professionals to collaborate with these individuals to positively impact their participation in life's occupations.

Specific Learning Disabilities

Specific learning disabilities are disorders that negatively affect the learning process. The disorder may be related to impairment in reading, impairment in written expression, or impairment in mathematics. Some children have specific learning disabilities in a combination of these areas. Children with these problems are educated with their nondisabled peers in the **least restrictive environment** (LRE) that can adequately meet their needs. Occupational therapy interventions for these children should address the major occupational roles of the child, particularly functional student performance throughout the school day. Occupational therapy may also provide services related to family and home life and peer relationships.

Gutman et al (37) provide occupational therapy guidelines for interventions in children with *regulatory disorders*, which include conduct disorders, ASD, and ADHD. **Regulatory disorders** share the common quality of difficulty in modulating or controlling one's response or reaction to sensation to interact effectively with the environment. The child may overreact to stimulation or fail to notice things that are important. Moods may fluctuate wildly. The guidelines given include the following:

- *Building a trusting and accepting relationship with the child.* The child may be slow to trust because of previous experiences. Accepting the child as a unique being and showing an interest in the child's perspective is a good start.
- *Helping the child recognize which behaviors are a problem.* It is essential for the child to hear that the *behavior* is not working, rather than that they are "bad."
- *Giving the child a vocabulary with which to describe what they are feeling.* Typically, the child feels uncomfortable in some way and immediately reacts with a behavior that gets them in trouble. If the child can learn to say, for example, "I feel mad—Jason is standing too close," then it becomes possible to ask Jason to move or have the child move to a less crowded space. Similarly, if the child can recognize that their heart is racing, they can learn breathing techniques to help it to slow down, indicating they are calmer.
- *Helping the child identify situations that will cause problems.* For example, the child can learn they do not like the feeling of zippers in pants or of labels in the necks of shirts and sweaters. The parent can be advised to purchase pants with elastic waists and to remove the offending labels.
- *Building impulse control and frustration tolerance.* When the child feels pushed and does not see any alternative, they will act out. Teaching the child what is required in different situations (school, church) and helping with gradual building of self-control are important. The OT professional might coach the child to "say it another way" or "use other words."
- *Building the ability to tolerate change.* Change is part of life, but transitioning from one activity to another is very

difficult for these children. Similarly, a change in the environment (a new piece of furniture) may be greeted with a tantrum. Telling the child in advance can be helpful so that the change is anticipated. Also, the child can be rewarded for any successful attempt to control negative behavioral expressions regarding change.

- *Helping the child acquire social interaction skills.* Taking turns, asking rather than grabbing, and making eye contact are just some of the skills that can be taught and practiced. Children need to learn the skills to be able to "use your [their] words," instead of acting out.

The neurodevelopmental disorders discussed here are commonly first seen in childhood and adolescence, and they shape how the individual grows and develops. Some disorders such as simple phobias (fears of, eg, spiders) or night terrors (nightmares that wake the child from sleep and are persistent) may diminish as the child develops. With other disorders, the effects can be profound and lifelong. For example, learning disorders that create stress in school may result in poor self-esteem and feelings of inadequacy and depression, and interfere with acquiring life skills. In other words, in many cases, a psychiatric disorder in childhood may place the person at risk throughout life. The case example of Matthew illustrates the relationship between childhood psychiatric history and functioning in later life.

SCHIZOPHRENIA SPECTRUM AND OTHER PSYCHOTIC DISORDERS

Although the word "schizophrenic" is sometimes incorrectly applied as a catch-all for bizarre behaviors, a diagnosis of schizophrenia or other psychotic disorders requires a person to meet specific criteria, and this spectrum of disorders is notoriously complex to diagnose. Not every person with psychotic symptoms receives a diagnosis of schizophrenia. In fact, in many cases an initial diagnosis, also called a **provisional diagnosis**, of schizophrenia is later revised to a different diagnosis, sometimes with less serious implications for prolonged dysfunction. It is essential for occupational therapy professionals to be able to clearly articulate information to the client, and about the client's conditions to other members of the interdisciplinary health care team. Therefore, it is equally as important to understand the sometimes subtle differences in the use of terminology. Whereas "psychotic disorder" is a psychological condition that is diagnosable, the word "psychosis" is used to describe a symptom, something that can be described behaviorally. Furthermore, psychosis is a symptom that occurs in the schizophrenia spectrum, and in other conditions outside of the schizophrenia spectrum, in other disorders and diagnoses (41). In the *DSM-5-TR*, the schizophrenia spectrum and other psychotic disorders includes schizophrenia, other psychotic disorders (delusional disorder, brief psychotic disorder, schizophreniform disorder, schizoaffective disorder, substance-induced psychotic disorder, postpartum psychosis, psychotic depression, age-related psychosis), and schizotypal personality disorder

(11, 41). These disorders are defined by dysfunction in one or more of five domains:

1. **Delusions**—Fixed beliefs that are not open to change even in light of conflicting evidence. The type of delusion can often be categorized by the content, and the delusion can be identified as *atypical* if they are not understandable to similarly aged, same-culture peers, if they do not arise from ordinary life experiences, or if they are clearly unbelievable (11). The following examples are common types of delusions that are recognizable.
   a. **Persecutory**—the belief that one is going to be harmed, harassed, and so forth by an individual, an organization, or other group
   b. **Referential**—belief that certain gestures, comments, environmental cues are directed at oneself
   c. **Somatic**—focus on preoccupations about one's health or organs
   d. **Grandiose**—when an individual believes that they have exceptional abilities, wealth, or fame
   e. **Erotomanic Delusions**—when an individual believes falsely that another person is in love with them
   f. **Nihilistic Delusions**—involve the conviction that a major catastrophe will occur

   It is important to recognize that people who have experienced extreme violence, abuse, torture, war, or discrimination can report fears that can be misunderstood as persecutory delusions, but these may represent posttraumatic stress symptoms, panic symptoms, or a response to intense fear (11).

2. **Hallucinations**—Hallucinations are experiences of perception, often extremely vivid that are not under an individual's voluntary control, and that occur with no external stimulus; auditory hallucinations, usually in the form of voices, are the most common type of hallucinations in the schizophrenia and related disorders, though hallucinations can originate from any sensory mode (11).

3. **Disorganized Thinking or Speech**—*Disorganized thinking* is also called formal thought disorder, and the diagnostician can typically document this characteristic during observation of the client's speech. However, because mildly disorganized speech can commonly occur with many conditions, and is somewhat nonspecific, the symptom must be severe enough to markedly disturb effective communication. Various forms of disorganized thinking that are notable in clients' speech include:
   a. **Derailment or Loose Association**—client switches from one topic to another, often abruptly.
   b. **Tangentiality**—answers to questions are only indirectly related, or completely unrelated.
   c. **Incoherence or "Word-Salad"**—terms used to describe speech that is so severely linguistically disorganized that it could be mistaken for receptive aphasia (11)

4. **Grossly Disorganized or Abnormal Motor Behavior (Including Catatonia)**—Grossly disorganized motor

behaviors can present problems in any of the client's goal-directed behaviors and can range from playful childishness to unpredictable agitation; these behavioral manifestations often lead to disruptions in occupational engagement (11). **Catatonic behavior** is when an individual demonstrates an obvious decrease in reacting to the environment or to contextual features of the environment. **Catatonia** is manifested in extreme psychomotor disturbance. This may be lack of movement, rigidity of movement, resistance to movement, an excited and apparently purposeless style of movement, or catatonic posturing in which abnormal postures are held. Repeated (perseverative) movement or speech may also be observed. This condition may be seen in combination with schizophrenia, or separately, or with other disorders (11).

5. **Negative symptoms**—Negative symptoms are most prominent in clients with schizophrenia, and less so in other psychotic disorders, particularly **diminished emotional expression** (reduced expression of emotions in facial expression, eye contact, or tone of voice) and **avolition** (a decrease in motivated, self-initiated purposeful activities). Negative symptoms can be thought of as the lessening or taking away of an aspect of an individual's personality, or way of being in the world. Other negative symptoms include **anhedonia** (a decreased ability to experience pleasure) or **alogia** (lessened speech output) (11). Positive and negative symptoms are further discussed in the following sections.

Prevalence and Burden of Schizophrenia and Psychotic Disorders

According to the NIMH and the WHO, more than 3.5 million adults, or 1.1% adult population in the United States, and more than 24 million people worldwide live with or are affected by schizophrenia (53, 77). Although schizophrenia and other psychotic conditions have a relatively lower prevalence rate, schizophrenia is one of the top 15 causes of disability worldwide, and people who experience schizophrenia often suffer extreme health inequities. Comorbid health problems, such as heart disease, liver disease, and diabetes, often go undetected or untreated in individuals with psychotic disorders, which leads to higher (and earlier) mortality rates. They are greater than twice as likely to die earlier than the general population, and internationally, two out of three people with psychosis do not receive adequate mental health care (53, 77).

The Progression of Schizophrenia Spectrum Disorders

The progression of schizophrenia falls into three phases: prodromal, active, and residual. In the **prodromal phase**, the level of functioning deteriorates. Usually, this can be observed by a decline in hygiene and grooming, interaction with others, and overall participation in life. In the **active phase**, the psychotic symptoms become increasingly apparent. Sometimes, a psychosocial stressor appears to precipitate, or bring on, the active phase. Following the active phase, the **residual phase** consists of the remission of the psychotic symptoms that are most disturbing to others (the person may still hear voices but may no longer be as reactive to the symptoms) and of a continuation and, in many cases, worsening of impaired functioning (11).

Positive and Negative Symptoms

Symptoms of schizophrenia have been divided into two classes: negative symptoms and positive symptoms. **Positive symptoms** include hallucinations, delusions, loosening of associations, and grossly disorganized speech and behavior. These symptoms are seen in the active phase of the illness. Though they may be present in the other two phases, they are not typically as severe or prominent. **Negative symptoms** include apathy and generally inexpressive mood (affective flattening), lack of goal-directed behavior (avolition), deterioration of hygiene, diminished functioning and participation in daily life, social isolation, and psychomotor slowing. These are seen in both the prodromal and the residual phases, and they appear to be related to physical changes in the brain (41).

Schizophreniform Disorder and Schizoaffective Disorder

Two of the conditions on the schizophrenia spectrum have similar features to schizophrenia: Schizophreniform Disorder (F20.81) and schizoaffective disorder, which in the *DSM-5-TR* can be classified as two types: **Schizoaffective Disorder, Depressive type** (F25.1); and **Schizoaffective Disorder, Bipolar type** (F25.0). **Schizophreniform disorder** is the classification of the diagnosis for an individual who experiences schizophrenic symptoms that last between 1 and 6 months (delusions, hallucinations, disorganized speech, grossly disorganized or catatonic behavior, or negative symptoms, and of which one of the symptoms must be delusions, hallucinations, or disorganized speech). **Schizoaffective disorders** are conditions that have characteristics of both schizophrenia and mood disorders. As with other psychotic disorders, a diagnosis of schizoaffective disorder carries a heavy burden; the individual is at high risk for self-harm and suicide (78). Schizoaffective disorder, depressive type is characterized by schizophrenic symptoms and depression symptoms that are present most of the time, having a minimum of 2 weeks of delusions or hallucinations *without* depression symptoms, yet experiencing depression symptoms for much of the duration of the illness. Schizoaffective disorder, bipolar type is characterized by schizophrenic symptoms and bipolar I symptoms that are present most of the time (ie, this subtype applies if a manic episode is part of the presentation, and a depressive episode may also be present), having a minimum of 2 weeks of delusions or hallucinations *without* bipolar symptoms, yet experiencing bipolar symptoms for much of the duration of the illness.

Another diagnosis, **schizotypal personality disorder**, is considered under the umbrella of the schizophrenia spectrum and is labeled as **schizotypal disorder** in the *ICD-10*, thus it is listed in this section of the *DSM-5-TR* text. Nevertheless, the full description and criteria for schizotypal personality disorder in the *DSM-5* series is listed in the chapter of the manual titled *Personality Disorders* (11).

Delusional Disorder

The most prominent feature of delusional disorder is the presence of one or more delusions that persist for at least 1 month. Delusional disorder diagnosis is not given if the person has *ever met Criterion A* for Schizophrenia, which is listed in the *DSM-5-TR* as follows:

a. Two (or more) of the following, each present for a significant portion of time during a 1-month period (or less if successfully treated). At least one of these must be (1), (2), or (3):
   1. Delusions
   2. Hallucinations
   3. Disorganized speech (e.g., frequent derailment or incoherence)
   4. Grossly disorganized or catatonic behavior
   5. Negative symptoms (i.e., diminished emotional expression or avolition) (11, p. 113–114)

Delusional disorder causes a person to be moderately unable to judge what is real and what is imaginary, which leads to delusions of various types (described previously), but the delusions are not at the schizophrenic level. Clients with delusional disorder tend to have otherwise good functional levels with fewer resultant bizarre behaviors (11, 19). People with **grandiose** and **persecutory** types of delusional disorder typically show organized delusional thinking around themes of persecution or specialness. Other aspects of thinking are usually unaffected. Affect and behavior are also more normal. Persons with these kinds of delusional disorders typically function better than those with other types of delusions, and many can live independently or semi-independently with supports in place. They may participate effectively in many aspects of community life, all the while needing to manage their systematized ideas often formulated around delusional thoughts.

Brief Psychotic Disorder

Essentially a brief psychotic disorder is diagnosed if the schizophrenic (or psychotic) symptoms continue for less than a month. Some of the characteristics of brief psychotic disorder are the involvement of at least one positive psychotic symptom: delusions, hallucinations, disorganized speech, or grossly abnormal psychomotor behavior, including catatonia. Brief psychotic disorder lasts a minimum of 1 day, but no more than a month. Additionally, the person diagnosed with brief psychotic disorder must meet an additional criterion of fully returning to their prior level of functioning, as it was prior to the onset of the psychotic symptoms (11). As mentioned in prior discussion, psychosis can be a symptom in several other conditions, and so the last criterion of brief psychotic disorder is an especially important one: "The disturbance is not better explained by major depressive disorder with psychotic features or another psychotic disorder such as schizophrenia or catatonia, and is not attributable to the physiological effects of a substance (e.g. a drug of abuse, a medication) or another medical condition" (11, p. 109).

The diagnostician must rule out other causes and make sure that the psychotic symptoms are not more reasonably explained by depressive or bipolar disorders with psychotic features, schizoaffective disorder, or schizophrenia. The diagnostician will also check to make sure that the psychosis is not attributable to the physiologic effects of a substance or other disease process. *The DSM-5-TR* underscores the significant importance of assessing cognition, levels of depression, and symptoms of mania (beyond the initial assessment of delusions, hallucinations, disorganized speech, and grossly disorganized or catatonic behavior) to make judicious distinctions between the various schizophrenia spectrum and other psychotic disorders. Table 4.2 summarizes the criteria, symptoms, and specifiers for the schizophrenia spectrum and other psychotic disorders.

Table 4.2. Diagnostic Indicators for Schizophrenia Spectrum and Other Psychotic Disorders

ICD-10 Code and Name of the Condition	Diagnostic Criteria and Indicators
F20.9 Schizophrenia	• Must have one positive symptom (hallucinations, delusions, or disorganized speech) for 1 mo • Two of the following: hallucinations, delusions, disorganized speech, disorganized behavior, or negative symptoms (ie, decreased emotion, decreased motivation) • Prior or residual poor functioning for at least 6 mo • Social or work impairment
F20.81 Schizophreniform Disorder	Schizophrenic symptoms with a duration between 1 and 6 mo
F25.1 Schizoaffective Disorder, Depressive type	• Schizophrenic symptoms and depression symptoms present most of the time • At least 2 wk of delusions or hallucinations without depression symptoms • Must have depression symptoms for the majority of the time

Table 4.2. Diagnostic Indicators for Schizophrenia Spectrum and Other Psychotic Disorders (*continued*)

ICD-10 Code and Name of the Condition	Diagnostic Criteria and Indicators
F25.0 Schizoaffective Disorder, Bipolar type	• Schizophrenic symptoms and bipolar I symptoms present most of the time • At least 2 wk of delusions or hallucinations without bipolar symptoms • Must have bipolar symptoms for the majority of the time

F23 Brief Psychotic Disorder	• Schizophrenic symptoms for <1 mo
	• Full return to premorbid level
	  • With marked stressors
	  • Without marked stressors
	  • With postpartum onset
	  • With catatonia

F22 Delusional Disorder	• Moderate delusions at least 1 mo, not schizophrenic level • Otherwise good functional level; no bizarre behavior • Erotomanic type • Grandiose type • Jealous type • Somatic type • Mixed type • Unspecified type • Persecutory type • Jealous type

ICD, *International Classification of Diseases.*
Adapted from American Psychiatric Association. (2022). *Diagnostic and statistical manual of mental disorders* (5th ed., text rev.). https://doi.org/10.1176/appi.books.9780890425787; Buser, S., & Cruz, L. (2022). *DSM-5-TR insanely simplified: Unlocking the spectrums within DSM-5-TR and ICD-10.* Chiron Publications.

Evidence-Based Occupational Therapy

The OT professional may encounter the client who is living with a schizophrenia spectrum disorder in inpatient or outpatient psychiatric care settings, and community mental and behavioral health settings; with the shift toward recovery-oriented approaches, now more commonly these clients are able to live in the community with supports. Because all occupational intervention planning is collaborative and client-centered, the intervention approach and type will be uniquely tailored to the person's level of occupational functioning in specific areas and based on recent events in the person's life. Regardless of the diagnosis, it is essential to focus on the person's strengths and priorities first, and to keep the occupational outcome in mind throughout the evaluation and intervention process (4). Every person has strengths that can provide support in recovery, and although much of the recent literature acknowledges that the symptoms of these disorders can be debilitating, some persons with schizophrenia already function quite well, particularly if they have had the necessary support in managing their illness. In such cases, intervention is directed at the problems that interfere with specific areas of occupational function, or with dyadic or group interaction skills. Researchers Hamm and colleagues "emphasize the importance of shifting away from an exclusively deficit-driven model of conceptualization and care, . . . and promoting increased attention to other aspects of the person, including strengths and resiliency" (38, p. 189).

Cognitive Function and Schizophrenia Spectrum Disorders

Client factors such as attention, concentration, problem-solving, working memory, and judgment are often impacted by schizophrenia (55). The OT professional may incorporate approaches to intervention that help **establish** or **restore** occupational function by targeting the client factors that are creating barriers to occupation. Or, in collaboration with the client, professionals may incorporate **compensatory approaches** to help improve the client's overall occupational performance as it affects daily life (6, 58, 63). Compensations may involve new technology such as smartphones, tablets, and electronic environmental systems or controls. The **remedial approach** involves direct teaching or improvement of specific occupational performance skills. The remedial approach may also employ techniques that can help the client to more effectively self-regulate if they experience hyposensitivity or hypersensitivity to sensory or environmental stimulation. Sensitivity to environmental input is a common barrier for clients who have been diagnosed with schizophrenia spectrum disorders, especially for clients who have a comorbid substance use disorder (80). The **compensatory approach** substitutes other abilities or provides external supports to compensate for diminished skills. The person might rely on a smartphone app, for example, to send alerts as reminders of daily tasks that may be forgotten.

Self-Direction, Communication and Interaction, and Daily Living Skills

Self-direction is a necessary component, and one of the core principles of the recovery process for people with mental illness. Essentially, self-direction means that the client has more autonomy in decision-making throughout the care process, including identifying priorities for the treatment plan and outcomes, and being considered as active agents in their own behavioral change process and life decisions. Occupational therapy professionals have the skills, knowledge, and training to support clients with mental illness in implementing self-direction into their recovery (31). In many ways, developing an occupational profile and a therapeutic alliance within an intentional relationship sets these core values of client-centeredness, collaboration, and autonomy in motion.

Evidence suggests that there are three critical tasks that individuals with schizophrenia spectrum disorders must accomplish for self-direction to become engaged (31, 38). Sometimes the first most critical task is also the most difficult; the individual must have enough self-awareness and esteem to believe that they deserve a qualitatively better life. They must have enough self-confidence and competence to express their preferences to make pragmatic and informed decisions toward reaching their goals. Next, the client must have the capacity to formulate ideas about their identity and their history, about their way of being in the world, who they are, where they have been, and what happened to them along the way. Lastly, the importance of the client with schizophrenia establishing a therapeutic relationship with a treatment team or care professional whom they trust cannot be overstated. To employ self-direction toward recovery, the client must possess the capability to come to an agreement with others on the defining problems. Furthermore, the problems must be realistic enough that treatment or intervention would support reasonable solution(s) (38).

Clients with more severe and long-term schizophrenia may perform poorly in basic and instrumental activities of daily living (IADLs). Research has consistently demonstrated the presence of metacognitive deficits in both early and late stages of schizophrenia spectrum disorders (38). Hygiene, dressing, and grooming can be coached, retaught, and practiced; behavioral and cognitive behavioral methods are among a few of the broadly incorporated approaches (31, 79). To make successful transitions into community life, adults with disabilities are likely to need specific instruction and practice in ecologically relevant contexts to develop necessary independent living skills in household management, housekeeping and cleaning, laundry, money management and budgeting, and community mobility. Because of the cognitive impairments that often accompany schizophrenia spectrum disorders, especially those that affect attention, occupational therapy professionals can play an important supportive role in assisting clients in developing independent living skills, safety behaviors, and emergency management skills.

Patterns and Routines, Development, and Maintenance of Habits

The structure provided by the patterns of habits, routines, and roles helps maintain a sense of continuity and occupational engagement. Schizophrenia can disrupt habits and role patterns in several ways: by distraction through hallucinations and delusions, or through apathy and other negative symptoms. Evidence indicates that the less routine, the less structure, and the fewer personally meaningful occupations, the less personal satisfaction the person is likely to experience (66). **Occupational deprivation** (not experiencing adequate meaningful occupational participation) is a serious problem that has the potential to exacerbate the symptoms of mental illness. The client may be unable to participate in work or school, or may do so only sporadically. Leisure and social or community engagement may be entirely lacking. Occupational therapy interventions should provide structure and realistic opportunities to participate in valued roles and occupations wherever possible. Peer mentoring, individualized instruction, and modeling can clarify and encourage desired behaviors while effectively helping the client develop coping and resiliency skills.

If time itself becomes disorganized, that is, if the person does not have places to go and things to do (work, school, or other organizing occupations and environments), strategies that help the client develop insight about their use of time can be applied. A time use diary, for example, can encourage the person to keep track of how time is spent, particularly if followed by an interview with the occupational therapy professional. Also, reshaping the environment to provide more cues that stimulate the person's familiar habits and patterns is an appropriate compensatory strategy to employ. Challenging and normal occupations should be available and encouraged; these reduce stigma and provide a source of positive self-evaluation. This means that rather than crafts or sheltered workshop situations, the client should be offered and expected to engage in activities of daily living (ADLs), work, leisure, and educational occupations typical of the client's same-aged peers and in ecologically relevant contexts (63, 66).

Chronicity of Illness

Schizophrenia follows a course of relapsing and remitting over time; periods of illness alternate with periods of better functioning and fewer symptoms. The person with a diagnosis of schizophrenia is likely to be a long-term recipient of mental health services, seen in both inpatient and outpatient settings for the remainder of their life. Enabling the person to remain in the community, functioning at the best possible, should be the goal. Persons with severe and persistent mental illness tend to require many social and environment supports; it is particularly important to identify potential crises and relapses before they occur and to reinforce and support self-management of medication and medical aspects of the disorder to prevent rehospitalization (63).

Assertive community treatment (ACT) is considered highly effective in preventing relapse and rehospitalization, and OT professionals have an evolving role in ACT teams (46). The deinstitutionalization movement of the 1950s and 1960s meant that individuals with chronic mental illness had the opportunity to live in their communities and outside of the walls of state and federal psychiatric hospitals and institutions. ACT was developed to support people's transitions between hospitalization and community life, with the goals being prevention of rehospitalization, maintenance of functional recovery, and occupational engagement that improves health and quality of life (14, 30). Individuals with serious mental illness who have consistently high or complex service needs can receive treatment and support from ACT services and teams (51). As mentioned previously, occupational therapy professionals have ever-evolving roles on ACT teams, and the increasing amount of research supporting the efficacy of the ACT service delivery model contributes to its continuing growth (65).

BIPOLAR AND RELATED DISORDERS

The *DSM-5-TR* begins the chapter on bipolar and related disorders with an explanation for the change in placement of this category of diagnoses in the *DSM-5* series. "Bipolar and related disorders are found between the chapters on schizophrenia spectrum disorders and depressive disorders in the *DSM-5-TR* in recognition of their place as a bridge between those two diagnostic classes in terms of symptomology, family history, and genetics" (11, p. 139). The word **bipolar** refers to the two poles or extremes of mania and depression. The person may be depressed (low mood), or manic (elevated mood), or alternate between the two cycles. **Mania** describes a mood that is elevated (high), expansive, and/or irritable. Although sleep patterns and routines are typically disturbed, the person's behaviors and reports may indicate that they feel rested despite the sleep deficit. The person may undertake many activities that are inconsistent with their prior behaviors (eg, compulsively spend money, travel, or seek attention). Cognitive functions are likely to be impaired, and the person shows poor judgment and insight during experiences of mania. Mania typically occurs in episodes, with periods of improved functioning alternating with episodic mania. There may also be depressive episodes and episodes of hypomania. **Hypomania** refers to a less severe or lasting episode of manic-like behaviors. Mania or hypomania may be present in conditions other than the bipolar disorders, and this symptom will be discussed in later sections. One example of this is the appearance of these symptoms with substance use, which can trigger symptoms of both mania and depressed mood (11).

Depression refers to a mood that is low and often disengaged, with loss of interest in activities that were previously pleasurable. As with mania, sleep is often disturbed. Appetite may be diminished or increased. Associated symptoms include low energy, suicidal thoughts, feelings of worthlessness, and restlessness or **torpor** (inactivity). Energy,

initiative, motivation (ie, volition) are low, cognitive functions can be slowed, and participation in ADLs and other occupations typically diminishes (11). Strategies and specific evidence-based interventions that the OT professionals can utilize for responding to the behaviors associated with mania and low or depressed mood will be addressed in Chapter 19.

Three main types of bipolar disorders and their diagnostic criteria (or symptomology) are important for OT professionals to recognize; each will be briefly introduced here and identified with its associated *ICD-10* code: BPD-I, BPD-II, and cyclothymic disorder. **F31.9, Bipolar I Disorder** is distinguished by episodes of mania, euphoric or irritable mood, and increased levels of energy that last at least a week. To meet the criteria for BPD-I during the episode of the inflated mood disturbance, three of the following seven symptoms must be present to a significant degree, and represent noticeable changes from the person's typical behavior (11). The symptoms are as follows:

1. Inflated self-esteem or grandiosity
2. Decreased need for sleep
3. More talkative than usual or pressure to keep talking
4. Flight of ideas or subjective experience that thoughts are racing
5. Distractibility (ie, attention too easily drawn to unimportant or irrelevant external stimuli), as reported or observed
6. Increase in goal-directed activity (socially, at work, or at school), or psychomotor agitation (purposeless non–goal-directed activity)
7. Excessive involvement in activities that have a high likelihood of having painful, illegal, or dangerous consequences

F31.81, Bipolar II Disorder is characterized by hypomania alternating with depression. **F34.0, Cyclothymic Disorder** is characterized by numerous hypomania and depression symptoms that are present most of the time, for a duration of 2 years; however, the client never reaches the full diagnostic criteria for hypomanic, manic, or depressive episodes. Clients with a diagnosis of cyclothymic disorder cannot be symptom free for greater than 2 months in the first 2 years of onset. Additionally, people with cyclothymic disorder experience and demonstrate "clinically significant" distress or impairment, as part of the criteria for the disorder (11).

BPD-I is considered more serious, and the functional deficits are typically worse than in BPD-II (11). Constant fluctuation of moods (in both bipolar disorders) often interferes with occupational functioning, and a **rapid-cycling** shift in the patterns of mood are associated with a poorer prognosis. Clients with BPD-I who experience four or more mood episodes (major depressive, manic, or hypomanic) within a year receive a specifier of BPD-I "with rapid cycling" (11, p. 146). The bipolar disorders are thought to exist on a spectrum, with a strong genetic component for predisposition to the disorders with heritability estimates around 90% in some twin studies. Members of a sibling group are at increased risk if one member has a diagnosis of bipolar disorder. At the less severe end of the spectrum are conditions with milder symptoms. The most recent data and genetic research support the notion that people inherit the traits of proneness to depression or mania separately, and that "bipolar disorder shares a genetic origin with schizophrenia" (11, p. 147).

Evidence-Based Occupational Therapy

During acute hospitalization, OT services are primarily directed at the following areas:

- Assessing cognitive levels
- Observing and reporting on present levels of function
- Managing behaviors and helping reduce expression of symptoms

In community settings, often a multidisciplinary behavioral health team will identify member roles. Occupational therapy will typically emphasize a return to function in desired occupational roles, with compensations and environmental modifications to reduce stress and improve attention and focus. Chapter 19 provides more detail about how the OT professionals might approach and manage the client who has active depressive or manic symptoms. Following a major episode of either mania or depression, once the symptoms have been reduced, the individual may benefit from OT directed at reestablishing life routines in self-care, work, and social and family life.

DEPRESSIVE DISORDERS

Depressive disorders, as suggested by their name, have low, sad, or irritable mood as a primary feature, often with related changes that significantly affect the individual's capacity to function. Changes in cognition or having somatic symptoms are common in several of the depressive disorders, but what distinguishes one disorder from another in these conditions is the duration, the timing, or the apparent cause(s) (11). Nevertheless, the disorders in this category of the *DSM-5-TR* are affective conditions that can seriously impact function and emotional regulation, motivation, and quality of life, and they are far more complex than historically understood. Disorders that affect mood (ie, depression and anxiety) account for nearly 65% of psychosocial disability worldwide (42). In fact, many medical experts encourage professionals to consider affective disorders more as a set of experiences, often exacerbated by environmental stressors or social conditions (41, 42, 62). "Depression is a reactive response to difficult situations like abuse, bullying, loneliness, or family breakdown. . . . Depression can be co-morbid with addiction, PTSD, trauma-related problems, insecure attachment, and, most commonly, anxiety" (36, 41, p. 187).

The conditions listed under the Depressive Disorders umbrella in the *DSM-5-TR* include: Disruptive Mood Dysregulation Disorder (F34.81); Major Depressive Disorder, single episode (F32.x); Major Depressive Disorder, recurrent (F33.x); Persistent Depressive Disorder (Dysthymia) (F34.1); Premenstrual Dysphoric Disorder (F32.81); Unspecified Mood Disorder (F32.A); Substance/Medication-Induced Depressive Disorder; and Depressive Disorder Due to Another Medical Condition (11). Although not an exhaustive list of symptoms of depression, the *DSM-5-TR* acknowledges the following as common to many of the depressive disorders.

- **S**adness—depressed mood, feelings of sadness (daily or most days)
- **I**nterest—anhedonia, loss of enjoyment or interest in occupations or activities that were once pleasurable
- **G**uilt—feelings of worthlessness
- **E**nergy loss—Lack of energy, feelings of fatigue (daily or most days)
- **C**oncentration loss—problems concentrating or difficulty making decisions
- **A**ppetite change—gain or loss of more than 5% of total body weight within a month, or significant change in appetite
- **P**sychomotor agitation or slowing—physical restlessness, agitation, or a change in energy levels that is noticeable to others
- **S**leep change—sleeping too much (hypersomnia) or not sleeping enough (insomnia)
- **S**uicidality—persistent thoughts of death, having a plan to commit suicide, or attempting to commit suicide

The common acronym SIG E CAPSS is often employed to help professionals remember the core symptoms of depressive disorders (19). A brief introduction and discussion of some of the most common depressive disorders follows.

Disruptive Mood Dysregulation Disorder

Disruptive mood dysregulation disorder was added to the *DSM-5* series, in part, to address trends over the last decade that leaned toward the overdiagnosis and intervention of the pediatric population with bipolar disorder. Disruptive mood dysregulation disorder was added to the depressive disorder spectrum for children up to 12 years old to indicate that children who demonstrate this pattern of symptoms typically develop unipolar depressive disorders, or anxiety disorders, more so than bipolar disorders in the teenage years and throughout adulthood. Disruptive mood dysregulation disorder is typified by recurring verbal or physical outbursts, rageful reactions (or temper tantrums) that seem out of proportion to the problem or situation, and are unusual of typical developmental expectations. For diagnostic purposes, the age range for this disorder is between 6 and 18 years, in other words the initial diagnosis for this disorder should *not* be made before 6 years or after 18 years. The outbursts usually occur at least 3 times per week for greater than a year, with the person demonstrating persistent irritability between outbursts that are not better explained by mania, depression, autism, or substance use (11).

Major Depressive Disorder: Single or Recurrent Episode

The coding for diagnosis of a major depressive disorder is based on whether the client has had a single episode or recurrent episodes, the current level of severity, presence of psychotic features, and the client's remission status. Although diagnosis can be made during a single episode, major depressive disorder is classically a multi-episodic disorder. According to the *DSM-5-TR*, "For an episode to be considered recurrent, there must be an interval of at least 2 consecutive months between separate episodes in which criteria are not met for a major depressive episode" (11, p. 184). Nevertheless, severity levels and psychotic features are only documented if the full criteria are already met for a major depressive episode, and remission specifiers are only indicated if the full criteria are not presently met for a major depressive episode. Although the occupational therapy professional will not be diagnosing a client with a depressive disorder, they may play a significant role on a behavioral health team in documenting and reporting how the SIG E CAPPS symptoms impact or are barriers to occupational function. A helpful summary of the specifiers, features, and severity levels for depressive episodes and conditions is presented in Table 4.3.

Table 4.3. Summary of Specifiers and Severity Levels of Depressive Disorders in the *DSM-5-TR*

Specifier and Definition: Depressive Disorder Specify If . . .	Symptoms/Criteria and Severity Specifier
With **anxious distress**: Presence of at least two symptoms during majority of the days of the current major depressive episode or current persistent depressive disorder **Special Note!** Occupational therapy professionals should be especially attuned to clients who experience anxious distress. This is a distinctive feature in bipolar disorders and major depressive disorders. Evidence suggests that clients with high levels of anxiety (anxious distress) are associated with increased risk of suicide, longer illness duration, and increased likelihood of nonresponse to treatment(s). It is very important to accurately document the presence and severity of anxious distress to improve and monitor occupational interventions and performance outcomes.	1. Feeling keyed up or tense 2. Feeling unusually restless 3. Difficulty concentrating because of worry 4. Fear that something awful may happen 5. Feeling that the individual might lose control of themselves Specify current severity: **Mild:** two symptoms **Moderate:** three symptoms **Moderate–severe:** four to five symptoms **Severe:** four to five symptoms and with motor agitation

With **mixed features**:
Special Note!
When mixed features are associated with a major depressive episode, there is a significant risk of the client developing bipolar I or bipolar II disorder. This is useful to know for the purposes of developing proactive and preventative occupational therapy treatment plans and occupational outcomes.
	a. At least three of the following manic/hypomanic symptoms present during majority of days of current major depressive episode (or most recent major depressive episode if major depressive disorder is currently in partial or full remission):
	  1. Elevated, expansive mood
	  2. Inflated self-esteem, grandiosity
	  3. Increased talking or pressure to keep talking
	  4. Flight of ideas or subjective experience of racing thoughts
	  5. Increase in energy or goal-directed activity (at work, school, or sexually)
	  6. Increase or excessive involvement in dangerous or risky activities
	  7. Decreased need for sleep
	b. Mixed symptoms are observable by others and are markedly different from a person's typical behavior.
	c. If a person's symptoms meet full criteria for mania or hypomania, the diagnosis should be bipolar I or bipolar II disorder.
	d. The mixed symptoms are not attributable to physiologic effects of substance use (ie, drug abuse or medication).

With **melancholic features**:
Special Note!
This specifier is applied if the features are present at the most severe stage of the episode. The client with melancholic features will experience almost a complete loss of capacity for pleasure; even highly motivating or desirable events do not bring about a higher or brighter mood. Melancholic features are qualitatively distinct. A description of a depressive episode that is more severe is not distinct enough to utilize the specifier. Psychomotor changes that may be observable to the OT professional and others are almost always present in depressive episodes with melancholic features.
	a. One of the following is present during the most severe period of the current major depressive episode (or the most recent major depressive episode if major depressive disorder is currently in partial or full remission):
	  1. Loss of pleasure in all, or almost all activities
	  2. Lack of reactivity to usually pleasurable stimuli (does not feel much better, even temporarily, when something good happens)
	b. Three or more of the following:
	  1. A distinct quality of depressed mood characterized by profound despondency, despair, and/or moroseness or by so-called empty mood
	  2. Depression that is regularly worse in the morning
	  3. Early morning awakening, at least 2 hr prior to normal time
	  4. Psychomotor agitation or slowing
	  5. Significant weight loss
	  6. Excessive or inappropriate guilt

(continued)

Table 4.3. Summary of Specifiers and Severity Levels of Depressive Disorders in the *DSM-5-TR* (*continued*)

Specifier and Definition: Depressive Disorder Specify If . . .	Symptoms/Criteria and Severity Specifier

With **atypical features**:
This specifier is applied when these features predominate during the majority of the days of the current major depressive episode (or the most recent major depressive episode if major depressive episode is currently in partial or full remission) or current persistent depressive disorder
	a. Mood reactivity (ie, mood brightens in response to actual or potential positive events)
	b. Two (or more) of the following:
	  1. Significant weight gain or increase in appetite
	  2. Hypersomnia
	  3. Leaden paralysis—heavy feeling in arms or legs
	  4. A long-standing pattern of interpersonal rejection sensitivity (not limited to episodes of mood disturbance) that results in significant social or occupational impairment
	c. Criteria are not met for "with melancholic features" or "with catatonia" during the same episode.

With **psychotic features**: Hallucinations and/or delusions are present at any time in the current major depressive episode (or the most recent major depressive episode if the major depressive disorder is in partial or full remission).	If psychotic features are present, specify if they are mood-congruent or mood-incongruent: **With mood-congruent psychotic features:** The content of all delusions and hallucinations is consistent with the typical depressive themes of personal inadequacy, guilt, disease, death, nihilism, or deserved punishment. **With mood-incongruent psychotic features:** The content of the delusions and hallucinations does not involve typical depressive themes of personal inadequacy, guilt, disease, death, nihilism, or deserved punishment, or the content is a mixture of mood-congruent and mood-incongruent themes.
With **catatonia**	This specifier is applied to the current major depressive episode (or the most recent major depressive episode if the major depressive disorder is in partial or full remission) if catatonic features are present during most of the episode.
With **peripartum onset**	This specifier is applied to the current major depressive episode (or the most recent major depressive episode if the major depressive disorder is in partial or full remission) if onset of mood symptoms occurs during pregnancy or in the 4 wk following delivery.
With **seasonal pattern**	This specifier applies to recurrent major depressive disorder. a. There has been a regular temporal relationship between the onset of major depressive episodes in major depressive disorders and a particular time of the year (like in the fall or winter). b. Full remissions also occur at a characteristic time of the year (eg, the depression seems to disappear in the spring or summer). c. In the last 2 yr, two major depressive episodes have occurred that demonstrate the temporal seasonal relationships defined earlier and no nonseasonal major depressive episodes have occurred during that same period. d. Seasonal major depressive episodes (as described earlier) substantially outnumber the nonseasonal major depressive episodes that may have occurred over the individual's lifetime.

DSM-5-TR, *Diagnostic and Statistical Manual of Mental Disorders Fifth Edition Text Revision*.
Adapted from American Psychiatric Association. (2022). *Diagnostic and statistical manual of mental disorders* (5th ed., text rev., pp. 210–214). https://doi .org/10.1176/appi.books.9780890425787

Persistent Depressive Disorder

When a mood disturbance caused by depressive episodes lasts for 2 years or more in adults, and 1 year or more in children, the depression can be considered chronic. Persistent depressive disorder is new in the *DSM-5* series (10, 11) and consolidates the *DSM-IV* diagnostic categories of chronic major depression and dysthymia (9). Clients with this diagnosis will have experienced at least two of the following symptoms: sleep changes, hopelessness, appetite change, low self-esteem, and concentration loss. Another important hallmark of this diagnosis is that the client will not have had months symptom free during the first 2 years. The OT professional will immediately recognize these clients by their significant distress and loss of meaningful roles, habits, and occupational patterns, which are likely to be observed as high rates of occupational deprivation or imbalance.

Premenstrual Dysphoric Disorder

Premenstrual dysphoric disorder (PMDD), after having been included in the *DSM-IV* series (9) as an Appendix under the category and title, "*Criteria Sets and Axes Provided for Further Study*," now after several decades of research has been added to the *DSM-5* series (11). The most recent evidence suggests that a specific and treatable form of depressive disorder with an onset prior to ovulation, cessation following menses, and a marked impact on function does exist. Criteria for the diagnosis include the client experiencing at least one of the following symptoms: mood swings, irritability/anger, sadness, or anxiety/tension; and a minimum of five of the following symptoms: mood swings, irritability/anger, sadness, anxiety/tension, loss of interest, poor concentration, fatigue, appetite change, sleep change, feelings of being overwhelmed, physical symptoms (breast tenderness, bloating, pain, and weight gain). PMDD creates distress and impairment for the client that interferes with most ADLs (57).

A rising interest in women's health issues and occupational therapy's role in supporting this population has led to an increase in the amount of research surrounding this topic. Estimates internationally using both prospective and retrospective reporting suggest a prevalence rate of PMDD somewhere between 1.2% and 7% (11, 57). A small cross-sectional study was undertaken at a public university to further explore the impacts of symptoms of PMDD on the occupational engagement, perceived competence, and value of occupations in university students. The researchers used a premenstrual symptom screening tool to detect premenstrual syndrome (PMS) and employed the *DSM-V* criteria to determine the presence of PMDD (57). Using the *Occupational Self-Assessment* (OSA) version 2.2 (13, 40), 35 students with PMDD were age-matched to 35 students without PMDD and evaluated to investigate their perceived occupational competence and value in daily occupations. The study found that university students with PMDD have lower occupational competence but similar occupational values compared to peers without PMDD. The findings support several potential roles for occupational therapy, particularly utilizing nonpharmacologic approaches, such as behavioral or cognitive interventions to support the goals of women with PMDD (57).

Unspecified Mood Disorder

Although this category is extremely broad, it serves an important role for clients who do not meet the full criteria for other mood disorders or depressive disorders. Unspecified Mood Disorders (F39) is often utilized when a client demonstrates symptoms indicative of a mood disorder and the symptoms are observed as the likely cause of significant distress resulting in disrupted social or occupational function and participation. The diagnosis appears in the *DSM-5-TR* in the chapter with depressive disorders (11), and immediately following the chapter on bipolar disorders, and is applied when the client does not meet the full criteria for any of the disorders in either the bipolar or the depressive disorders diagnostic classes at the time of evaluation. Occupational therapy professionals should develop an awareness of the general traits and characteristics of the depressive disorders to support the diagnostician who may be having difficulty choosing between unspecified bipolar and related disorder and unspecified depressive disorder (eg, acute agitation). Often diagnosticians rely on the reports of the members of the team (particularly the rehabilitation team) who have often spent more time with the client, and who may be able to comment on a person's level of independence or functional levels with critical tasks such as self-care and personal safety, or recovery-oriented tasks such as medication management.

Substance/Medication-Induced Depressive Disorder

According to the *DSM-5-TR*, the most critical feature of substance or medication-induced depressive disorder is a noticeable or ongoing disturbance in mood that predominates the client's overall presentation and participation in daily life activities. The client is likely to demonstrate a depressed mood and has obvious diminished interest in almost all of their daily occupations due to the direct physiologic effects of a substance (ie, a drug of abuse, a medication, or a toxin exposure). Lack of affect and significant lack of appreciation of pleasure or pleasurable activities is also a hallmark of this disorder, as is the case for many of the depressive disorders. Nevertheless, for a client to receive this diagnosis, the depressive symptoms must have onset during or immediately following substance intoxication or withdrawal, or have occurred after exposure to or withdrawal from a medication, and should be documented by a clinical history, physical examination, or laboratory results (*DSM-5-TR* criterion B1). Additionally, the involved substance/medication must be capable of producing the depressive symptoms (*DSM-5-TR* criterion B2). Lastly, if a client is living with this condition or has this diagnosis, according to the *DSM* criteria, the client's symptoms of depression cannot be better explained by a nonsubstance/medication-induced depressive disorder (11).

Because the neurochemical changes associated with intoxication and withdrawal states for some substances can be lengthy, and because powerful symptoms of depression or depressed mood can last well after a person stops using a substance, the diagnosis of a substance or medication-induced depressive disorder is still considered accurate throughout the detox or withdrawal period. However, this is an extremely complex illness to diagnose, and one of the most important roles for the occupational therapy professional is to accurately document and articulate to the multidisciplinary team any aspects of the client's occupational profile that may influence the diagnostician in obtaining the most clinically accurate diagnosis. In instances where this diagnosis is considered and the client presents with additional co-occurring physical or mental health problems, information from all members of the team is critical to provision of quality care.

Evidence-Based Occupational Therapy

For those with severe or persistent depression, ADLS and IADLS may be a focus of OT intervention. Bathing, dressing, eating, and personal hygiene and grooming often seem extremely difficult and unimportant to a person who experiences a deep depression, and these are often the tasks that the client will not be motivated to initiate. Reducing choices, simplifying routines, or beginning with easier or more motivating tasks is recommended. Gentle reminders about a single task sometimes motivates the person enough to perform more ADLs. Because these activities are likely linked to habits and routines, once the person has initiated the task, it is often much easier to continue.

Performance in school, work, and productive activities may be diminished or impaired. These occupations require energy and drive that may be lacking when a person is depressed. Interest in other people is diminished, which interferes with interpersonal relationships in the workplace and at home. Leisure and social participation may be especially problematic, with an inability to take pleasure in activities that once provided joy; this is a key feature of depression. Sleep and rest may be impaired, which impacts all other areas of occupational functioning.

Many adults with depressive disorders recover their ability to function once the depression is adequately treated. Habits, routines, roles, and occupational patterns may shift or change during depressive episodes, but with adequate treatment and support can generally be reassembled when the depressive mood lifts.

ANXIETY DISORDERS

Because many anxiety disorders start in childhood, in the *DSM-5-TR* the anxiety disorders are presented from a developmental perspective, with the disorders sequenced according to the typical age of onset. The features that are common symptoms of anxiety disorders are excessive fear, worry, or anxiousness, and the behavioral disturbances that occur secondary to the excessive anxiety or fears. A crucial part of understanding the anxiety disorders is understanding the difference between a normal feeling of being anxious, which happens when the sympathetic nervous system upregulates or fires up as a response to reasonable threats, concerns, or problems, and an anxiety disorder, when the escalation of the sympathetic nervous system fails to de-escalate once the threat is removed. For people with an anxiety disorder, the feelings of fear and worry do not calm down; in fact, in many cases the feelings of anxiousness intensify. Clients with these disorders often have sympathetic nervous systems that, over time, become consistently dysregulated and hyperresponsive to even perceived threats (41, 62, 71).

For the occupational therapy professional, our domain of concern focuses on what happens when the client's behavioral or physiologic disturbances disrupt occupational function. The Anxiety Disorders chapter in the *DSM-5-TR* includes the following diagnoses: Separation Anxiety

Disorder (F93.0); Selective Mutism (F94.0); Specific Phobias including:

- (F40.218) Animal fear (insects, snakes, dogs, etc.)
- (F40.228) Natural environment (heights, thunderstorms, etc.)
- (F40.230) Blood
- (F40.231) Needle injections
- (F40.232) Other medical fears
- (F40.233) Fear of injury
- (F40.248) Situational (elevators, planes, tight spaces)
- (F40.298) Other

Social Anxiety Disorder (F41.10); Agoraphobia (F40.0); Panic Disorder (F41.0); Generalized Anxiety Disorder (F41.1); Substance/Medication-Induced Anxiety Disorder; Anxiety Disorder Due to Another Medical Condition (F06.4); and Other Specified (F41.8) and Unspecified (F41.9) Anxiety Disorders. A brief introduction to anxiety disorders follows, with more specific interventions for clients who are experiencing anxiety discussed in Chapter 18.

Separation Anxiety Disorder and Selective Mutism

"The individual with separation anxiety disorder is fearful or anxious about separation from attachment figures to a degree that is developmentally inappropriate" (11, p. 215). To be considered developmentally inappropriate and receive the diagnosis of **separation anxiety disorder** a client (usually a child) demonstrates a minimum of three of the following characteristics: recurrent excessive distress when anticipating or experiencing separation from home or from parents or other attachment figures; persistent worry about losing attachment figures, or of harm coming to their loved one; persistent or excessive worry about events that may cause them to be separated from their loved one, such as being kidnapped or getting lost; reluctance or adamant refusal to go out (eg, to home, school, or work) because of fear of separation; excessive fear about being alone without attachment figures (at home or in other places); difficulty going to sleep when not in the presence of an attachment figure; nightmares involving a theme of separation; complaints of physical symptoms like headaches or nausea during separation from the attachment figures. To be clinically relevant for diagnostic purposes, the duration of the anxiety or fear response lasts at least 4 weeks in children and teens, and usually greater than 6 months in adults (11).

The onset of **selective mutism** normally occurs before the age of 5; however, it is often not recognized until the child reaches school age and enters a new social dynamic where there is an expectation of communication, an increase in social interactions, and tasks with novel occupational performance expectations. The main criterion for this disorder is that the person fails to speak in certain contexts or social situations, even though they speak in other situations. For example, a child may speak at home to parents and siblings, but consistently fails to speak to others at school or other similar venues. A diagnosis of selective mutism becomes increasingly obvious when the client's failure to speak in specific situations interferes with occupational engagement, whether in school or within the context of social participation, and when the mutism lasts at least 1 month (11). Readers are invited to learn more about the experience of selective mutism from the perspective of three families each raising a child with this diagnosis, in a documentary titled *Raising a Child With Selective Mutism: My Child Won't Talk.* A link to the video can be found in the *Suggested Resources.*

Panic Disorder and Agoraphobia

In **panic disorder**, a person may experience repeated, often abrupt, intense fear or discomfort that creates a feeling of panic, sometimes referred to as a **panic attack**. A panic attack reaches a peak within minutes, and during that time four (or more) of the common symptoms (listed later) occur. The anxiety and sense of fear or panic can be either expected (ie, anticipatory) or unexpected, and the persistent worry about having additional panic attacks, from a diagnostic standpoint, lasts for at least a month. Often the client will experience symptoms such as palpitations, sweating, trembling, shortness of breath, choking, chest pain, nausea, dizziness, derealization, fear of dying, numbness/tingling, and hot/cold flashes; and for clinical diagnosis of panic disorder, the client will have experienced at least four of these physiologic disruptions (11, 19). It is critical that the occupational therapy professional be aware of the fact that a "panic attack" can also be a specifier for other diagnoses, beyond just anxiety disorders. The *DSM-5-TR* presents common symptoms of a panic attack so that clinicians and diagnosticians recognize when a client may be experiencing a panic attack; however, a panic attack is not a mental disorder, and therefore does not have an associated *ICD-10-CM* code (11).

If a client experiences persistent panic attacks, they may become increasingly fearful of having further attacks, and are often especially fearful of being in an unfamiliar place when a panic attack occurs and being unable to recover. This fear can drive increasing levels of anxiety, with more serious physiologic reactions. In **agoraphobia**, which sometimes accompanies panic disorder, the client has an intense fear of being in strange places where a panic attack might occur. Specifically, the client is afraid of two or more of the following environments or structures: public transportation, open spaces, enclosed spaces (like theaters or coliseums), crowds, or simply being away from their own home. The real or imagined fear can become so pervasive that the person is unable to leave home, and consciously or unconsciously avoids these areas. To acquire a diagnosis of agoraphobia, the client will have these intensely fearful responses for more than 6 months, which impacts most occupations, but particularly work, school, and social participation (11).

Phobias are characterized by fears in response to a specific stimulus. Phobias, agoraphobia, and panic attacks all impair functioning by interfering with the performance of tasks related to occupational roles. The degree of impairment may be more or less severe, depending on the extent of the phobia. For example, a severe fear of school may prevent a child from attending, but if less severe, the child may only experience anxiety in specific situations at school, such as when called upon to read aloud or to perform a presentation in front of peers.

Social Anxiety Disorder

Over half a century ago, what was then called social phobia was differentiated from agoraphobia and other specific phobias. Today, the diagnosis of social anxiety disorder (SAD) has evolved from being a largely overlooked condition to being widely recognized and diagnosed (61). There is an approximate prevalence of SAD in the United States of 7%, and the prevalence rates seem to be increasing in the United States and in Eastern Asian countries, especially among adolescents ages 13 to 17 years. However, prevalence in the United States is lower in people of Asian, Latinx, African American, and Caribbean Black descent compared with non-Hispanic Whites (11). In the *DSM-5* series, the diagnostic criteria for SAD added (1) fear of acting in a way or showing anxiety symptoms that offend others or lead to rejection, and (2) fear of humiliation or embarrassment. The *DSM-5-TR* removed the "generalized subtype" and added the "performance only" specifier. Clients who experience performance only SAD typically experience the most detrimental effects of the disorder in school or work situations or in occupational roles where public speaking or presentations are frequently required tasks (10, 11).

SAD is perhaps one of the most significant precursory risk factors for developing bipolar disorder, substance use disorder, or other affective mood disorders (41). "Comorbid psychiatric disorders occur in up to 90% of patients with SAD. . . . Patients who have comorbid psychiatric disorders have an increased likelihood of greater severity of symptoms, treatment resistance, decreased functioning, and increased rates of suicide" (61, as cited in paragraph 11).

The most prominent feature of SAD, an obvious and persisting fear or sense of dread about social participation or performance, makes people with this disorder feel as though they are, or will be, under scrutiny and judged negatively in contexts that have a high degree of social elements. They often have intense fear of humiliation or embarrassment that causes them to avoid situations where the social demands are high, or they suffer high levels of distress during these situations. The OT professional must be keenly aware of the symptoms of this diagnosis and how it may lead to impairments of the client's developmentally and culturally appropriate and expected roles, habits, and routines (11, 41). Clients with SAD most often do not realize they have a defined mental health condition that is treatable, and so they do not seek treatment. Client education is a primary priority when treating and preventing this disorder (61).

Generalized Anxiety Disorder

Generalized anxiety disorder (GAD) is diagnosed when a person reports or is observed to be excessively worried or anxious on most days, for 6 months or longer. The person will also demonstrate at least three of the following common characteristics of anxiety: restlessness, decreased concentration, irritability, tenseness, insomnia, or fatigue. The *DSM-5-TR* reports that "Many individuals with generalized anxiety disorder report that they have felt anxious and nervous all their lives" (11, p. 252). An estimated 5.7% of adults in the United States experience GAD at some time in their lives (39, 54). Furthermore, GAD is responsible for 110 million disability days per year for the U.S. population because of its association with negative impacts on work performance, its link to higher use of medical resources, and the increased risk for coronary morbidity for people who have a diagnosis of GAD (11). Another way to think about a client with a diagnosis of GAD is that they are hypervigilant to a point that most of their occupations and occupational participation has self-imposed restriction creating interference in generally all aspects of their life (19).

Evidence-Based Occupational Therapy

Occupational therapy for anxiety disorders may focus on managing anxiety during life occupations, or it may focus on managing stressful situations to prevent anxiety. Regardless of the therapeutic approach, consideration of the physiologic system as a key client factor (ie, body structures and functions) should always be a central focus. One approach to the treatment of anxiety is to teach the person to recognize and engage in activities that are relaxing, not only at times of stress but perhaps, most importantly, on a regular basis to prevent the feelings of overwhelming anxiety or worry that evidence now tells us triggers more intense responses. This is known as a life balance or occupational balance approach (72). An effort can be made to teach the client the relaxation response and how to achieve it. When the anxiety is stimulus-specific and impairs function, as in agoraphobia, systematic desensitization and/or cognitive behavioral programs may be used to neutralize the anxiety response (54). Occupational therapy professionals are increasingly parts of teams that utilize these evidence-based approaches to support improved health for people who have anxiety disorders (33).

OBSESSIVE–COMPULSIVE AND RELATED DISORDERS

The *DSM-5* series removed obsessive–compulsive disorder (OCD) and PTSD from the Anxiety Disorders chapter, and created a new separate chapter for each: *Obsessive Compulsive and Related Disorders* and *Trauma and Stressor Related Disorders* (11). **Obsessive–compulsive disorder (OCD)** is characterized by obsessions and/or compulsions, which are time-consuming and distressing to the client and which interfere with functioning. An **obsession** is an unwanted intrusive thought or impulse that typically falls into categories (eg, the need to order things, worries about contamination or germs, worry about impending doom, or aggressive thoughts that threaten to disrupt the client's life). The person attempts to get rid of the obsession but often cannot do so. A **compulsion** is a repetitive behavior or ritualistic action performed in response to an obsession, often used by the person as an attempt to manage the obsessions (19). Hand washing and checking or touching things are examples. Related disorders that the OT professional may encounter in this class of disorders are:

- Body dysmorphic disorder
- Hoarding disorder
- Trichotillomania (hair pulling disorder)
- Excoriation (skin picking) disorder

In **Body Dysmorphic Disorder (F45.22),** the person focuses on imagined or minor bodily imperfections, to the point of obsession. Suicide is a risk. Eating disorders may be present as well. In **Hoarding Disorder (F42.3),** the person has difficulty discarding possessions (including those that are broken or useless) and may actively acquire more than can possibly be consumed. This leads to clutter and may pose a danger to self and others. **Trichotillomania (F63.3)** and **Skin Excoriation Disorder (F42.4)** may begin in adolescence or before. The person pulls out body hair (trichotillomania) or picks at or peels the skin (excoriation disorder) (11, 19).

Management of Obsessive–Compulsive and Related Disorders

Psychotherapeutic approaches, cognitive behavioral approaches, sensory approaches, and medication are used to treat obsessive–compulsive and related disorders. Behavioral and cognitive behavioral therapies (CBTs) are seen as more effective than other approaches, especially when combined with medication. For hoarding disorder, CBT may address the thoughts and fears that motivate the acts of acquiring and hoarding (50).

Evidence-Based Occupational Therapy

Occupational performance is the main agenda of any OT intervention (3). Compulsive behaviors may be minimal and not much of a problem. In other cases, these behaviors may be extremely time-consuming and disruptive to occupational routines. Systematic desensitization and a cognitive behavioral approach may be used. For hoarding disorder, the focus would be the home and the dangerous clutter, which puts the client in danger of increased fall risks along with other health risks related to unsafe or unsanitary conditions. It is difficult to engage the hoarder in disposing of accumulated items; the OT professional works as part of the team, and is often more available to visit the home than are other disciplines. Trichotillomania and excoriation disorder may be responsive to sensory-integrative or sensory processing interventions (11, 15).

TRAUMA AND STRESSOR-RELATED DISORDERS

As mentioned previously, *Trauma and Stressor-Related Disorders* were listed within the Anxiety Disorders chapter in the previous *DSM* (9, 10). What differentiates these disorders from the anxiety disorders is that they are caused or precipitated by a stressful event. Included in the Trauma and Stressor-Related Disorders chapter in the *DSM-5-TR* are the following disorders: Reactive Attachment Disorder (F94.1); Disinhibited Social Engagement Disorder (F94.2); Posttraumatic Stress Disorder (F43.10); Acute Stress Disorder (F43.0); Adjustment Disorders; and Prolonged Grief Disorder (F43.8). **Reactive Attachment Disorder (F94.1)** occurs in some children who have been neglected or separated from their caregiver. **Posttraumatic Stress Disorder (PTSD) (F43.10)** is a condition that follows the experience of severe trauma. Severe trauma, by *DSM-5-TR* standards, can be experienced trauma, witnessed trauma, learned about violent trauma to a loved one, or experiences of repeated or extreme exposure to aversive details of the traumatic event (eg, first responders repeatedly exposed to domestic violence, child abuse, or horrific automobile accidents) (11). Such traumatic events include war (especially combat), natural disasters, or personal or societal violence. Although returning veterans historically were among the first to be diagnosed with PTSD, in modern culture, violence is unfortunately happening more frequently, and severe trauma caused by environmental stressors in contexts removed from the battlefield are increasingly prevalent.

This condition affects family and loved ones as well as the person diagnosed with PTSD. The anxiety and other negative emotions provoked by the trauma are reexperienced in the form of intrusive memories, nightmares, and flashbacks. An avoidance response characterized by withdrawal, isolation, psychological numbing, constricted expression of feelings, and lack of interest in previously enjoyed activities reduces contact with the world and psychologically wards off the distressing feelings. Other associated symptoms may include **hypervigilance** (tense alertness), disturbed sleep, impaired concentration, feelings of guilt, emotional lability, or hyperarousal. Survivors of trauma are also more likely to self-medicate with alcohol and drugs, and have increased risk of suicide. Symptoms of PTSD are present for at least 1 month and create significant impairments across occupations (11).

Adjustment Disorders (F43.2x) is a category of disorders in which the client demonstrates the development of emotional or behavioral symptoms in response to an identifiable stressor that occurs within 3 months of the onset of the stressor. Once the stressor has been removed, or it stops, the symptoms of the disorder do not continue for longer than an additional 6 months. Specifiers in this category help describe the presentation and symptomology, as follows:

Adjustment Disorder

- **F43.21 With depressed mood:** Low mood, tearfulness, or feelings of hopelessness are predominant.

- **F43.22 With anxiety:** Nervousness, worry, jitteriness, or separation anxiety is predominant.
- **F43.23 With mixed anxiety and depressed mood:** A combination of depression and anxiety is predominant.
- **F43.24 With disturbance of conduct:** Disturbance of conduct is predominant.
- **F43.25 With mixed disturbance of emotions and conduct:** Both emotional symptoms (eg, depression, anxiety) and a disturbance of conduct are predominant.
- **F43.20 Unspecified:** For maladaptive reactions not classifiable as one of the specific subtypes of adjustment disorder (11, p. 319)

FEEDING AND EATING DISORDERS

Eating and feeding disorders categorized in the *DSM-5-TR* include: Anorexia Nervosa (F50.0x); Bulimia Nervosa (F50.2); Binge Eating Disorder (F50.81); Avoidant/Restrictive Food Intake Disorder (F50.82); Pica (children) (F98.3), Pica (adults) (F50.8). **Elimination disorders** include Enuresis (F98.0); Encopresis (F98.1). Diagnoses in this chapter are characterized by abnormal behavior in the consumption and retention of food (and in some cases nonfood items) (11). Infants and young children use their mouths as one way to explore the world and may put nonfood items in their mouths, which is developmentally appropriate. **Pica** is a diagnosis that would apply only after this developmental stage. In Pica, a person older than 2 years eats unusual and sometimes dangerous nonfood items like soil, soap, hair, paint, or other materials, for more than a month. **Anorexia nervosa** is characterized by abnormally low body weight, with refusal to take in food or to gain weight, a fear of gaining weight, and a disturbed body image (11). Two types of anorexia nervosa exist. In the **Restricting Type of Anorexia (F50.82)**, the person does not use binging and purging, instead uses purely fasting and exercising as a means to control their weight. In the **Binge/Purge Type of Anorexia (F50.02)**, the client is more likely to use binge eating or purging techniques to control their weight. **Bulimia nervosa** is characterized by binge eating, with the added criteria that there is very little sense of control during the binge. In bulimia nervosa the person will also use purging or overexercising as a way to control feelings of being out of control during the binge eating. With **binge eating disorder**, the differentiation is that although there is only a minimal sense of control during the binge, the person experiences loss of control that causes overeating on a weekly basis, but the person does not employ methods of purging or overexercising to try to compensate (11, 19).

Evidence-Based Occupational Therapy

In the United States, over 30 million people have an eating disorder, and that number is rising, particularly following the COVID-19 pandemic (25, 52). Occupational therapy focuses on the development of behaviors that support role performance and establishing or reestablishing healthy habits and routines. In addition, OT must address underlying problems related to distorted body image, low self-esteem, and limited assertiveness. Clients with disrupted eating also often have problems in performing ADLs and IADLs, in occupations such as grocery shopping, grooming and self-care, meal preparation, and eating (especially when eating involves social participation/social gatherings). Work or education tasks are ultimately impacted as well. When a person is consumed with thinking and behaviors, many of which are driven by cognitive distortions about food consumption and/or elimination, other occupations are likely to suffer. Ultimately, this can lead to both occupational imbalance and occupational deprivation (64). However, there is also recent evidence that suggests that occupations can be used in one of two ways by clients with eating disorders: (1) to continue to maintain disordered eating patterns; (2) with intervention and coaching, the same occupation may be used toward promotion of healthy habits and wellness.

The complexity of eating disorders demands careful treatment that considers a multifaceted approach by an interdisciplinary team. A small study was undertaken by Sørlie and colleagues (2020) with a 2-fold objective: to examine the roles of occupational therapy within a treatment team working with clients with eating disorders, and to report on the preliminary utility of an occupation-focused evaluation to highlight the relationship between occupations, self, and environment, using an assessment called the *Daily Experiences of Pleasure, Productivity, and Restoration (PPR) Profile* (64).

Having the client document their time use, such as when implementing tools like time use diaries, brings novel attention and awareness to the person regarding how their everyday lives are being impacted by their disordered habits of eating. The *PPR Profile* is an assessment that has roots in occupational science. Two formats of the PPR Profile are available, a self-report and a guided interview. Both formats ask the client to document or answer questions reporting the activities from the prior day. The PPR Profile captures objective and subjective dimensions of occupation in daily life, and therefore is useful in exploring how aspects of occupation and context are inexplicably linked and constantly influence one another. The *PPR Profile* was developed to investigate the dimensions of subjective experiences, including activities that the client enjoys (pleasurable experiences), activities that give agency to the client and make them feel accomplished (productivity), and occupations that refill the client's energy reserves (energy renewal). These dimensions are considered foundational to human flourishing (64). Sørlie et al explored the following research question: "What were the experiences and perspectives of individuals with eating disorders who used the PPR Profile with [follow-up by] an occupational therapist?" (64, p. 5).

The occupational therapy research team examined the reflections and data submitted by the participants using an inductive thematic analysis. Essential to their findings was that the participants acknowledged that the process of creating change was supported through focused attention and focused conversations with the occupational therapy professional about time use and daily habits, roles, and routines, which positively impacted self-awareness. In the follow-up conversations with the occupational therapist, often more detailed information was revealed as in this example: "One participant reported that after eating lunch she went to do an errand. As the senior therapist asked additional questions, the participant shared that she walked for several miles to get to the location, because she felt compelled to exercise since they had just eaten. This information would not have been discovered without the assistance of the occupational therapist" (64, p. 9). Among other contributions from this preliminary study, the critical importance of the therapeutic relationship between the OT professional and the client with an eating disorder was made clear (68).

SLEEP–WAKE DISORDERS

These disorders are related to the ability to obtain restful sleep in a regular pattern that is restorative and allows for participation in daily life. The *DSM-5* and the *DSM-5-TR* reorganized and recategorized *Sleep Disorders* to demonstrate and clarify the pathways between medical and psychological problems related to sleep (11). Ten disorders or disorder groups are recognized under three subcategory headings: *Sleep–Wake Disorders*, *Breathing-Related Sleep Disorders*, and *Parasomnias*. Categorizing the disorders this way helps clinicians in several ways: it helps both with knowing what certain observations may be indicative to support the diagnostician with differential diagnosis and with determining when a referral should be made to a sleep specialist (11).

Insomnia Disorder (F51.01) is diagnosed when people have difficulty initiating or maintaining sleep a minimum of 3 times per week, for at least a month. **Hypersomnolence Disorder (F51.11)** is a disorder where the individual may demonstrate excessive sleepiness, despite sleeping for 7 or more hours per night. For this diagnosis, the individual will also experience at least one of the following criteria: nonrestorative sleep lasting 9 hours or more, recurrent episodes of falling asleep through the day, or difficulty awakening. Furthermore, it is necessary to rule out other (or better) explanations such as sleep apnea, narcolepsy, or parasomnia (11).

Narcolepsy is coded by specific subtypes in the *DSM-5* series, and it occurs when sleep attacks that are not possible to resist happen at least 3 times a week for at least 3 months (10, 11). The other major criterion for narcolepsy to be diagnosed is that at least one of the following symptoms must be present:

- **Cataplexy**: sudden loss of muscle tone after laughing
- **Hypocretin deficiency** on spinal tap (Hypocretin is a brain hormone or neurochemical that is associated with the sleep–wake cycle.)
- Sleep study showing reduced rapid eye movement (REM) sleep latency

Circadian Rhythm Sleep–Wake Disorders (G47.2x) are disorders indicated by a disruption of the sleep pattern mostly because of an alteration of the circadian system or to a misalignment between the person's internal sleep–wake cycle and sleep disruption caused by an individual's physical environment or social or professional (work) schedule (11).

Breathing-Related Sleep Disorders

Breathing-related sleep disorders include the following diagnoses: **Obstructive Sleep Apnea-Hypopnea (G47.33); Central Sleep Apnea (G47.31);** and **Sleep-Related Hypoventilation (G47.31)**. All three of the disorders in this category can only be diagnosed through a sleep study (11). For this reason, it is important for the occupational therapy professional to recognize the symptoms of these disorders to detect when a referral may need to be made. Obstructive sleep apnea-hypopnea (OSAH or OSA) is one of the most common breathing-related disorders, yet it commonly goes untreated (47). OSAH is characterized by repeated episodes of upper pharyngeal airway obstruction during sleep. **Apnea** means temporary cessation of breathing, especially during sleep. **Hypopnea** means abnormally slow or shallow breathing. Each apnea or hypopnea represents a reduction in breathing of at least 10 seconds in adults or two missed breaths in children. Drops in oxygen saturation of greater than 3%, symptoms of snoring, and daytime sleepiness or headaches are likely (11). **Central sleep apnea** occurs because the CNS (brain) does not send proper signals to the muscles that control your breathing. This condition is different from OSAH in which you cannot breathe normally because of upper airway obstruction. Central sleep apnea is less common than OSA (47).

Parasomnias

Parasomnias are conditions marked by unusual behaviors, experiences, or physiologic changes that occur simultaneously with sleep, during specific sleep stages, or within the sleep–wake transitions. Common parasomnias include the **Non-Rapid Eye Movement (NREM) Sleep Arousal Disorders**: (F51.3) **Sleepwalking type**, characterized by a blank stare, where the person is relatively unresponsive, hard to awaken, and has no dream recall; and (F51.4) **Sleep Terror type** characterized by abrupt arousals, panic scream, intense fear, and autonomic arousal (19). (G47.52) **Rapid Eye Movement (REM) Sleep Behavior Disorder** is another common sleep problem that usually includes recurrent sleep arousals, often with sleep-talking or sleepwalking, but where the individual awakens alert, and not disoriented (11, 58). In **Nightmare Disorder** (F51.5), the person experiences terrifying awakenings with vivid recall and alertness, and has distress that results in disrupted occupations. Lastly, (G47.52) **Restless Legs Syndrome** is included in the *Sleep-Wake Disorders* chapter of the *DSM-5-TR*, because the symptoms of the disorder often are worse at night. Symptoms of restless legs syndrome may include urges to move the legs, experiencing unpleasant burning or tingling with a restless sensation in the legs, or muscle cramping or spasms in the legs.

A person's ability to get restful and healthy sleep has a profound impact on their engagement in all other aspects of occupation. Healthy sleep reduces the risk of physical and mental health problems, helps prevent accidents and injuries, and decreases disability and early mortality (2). With that in mind, the Office of Disease Prevention and Health Promotion (ODPHP), under the umbrella of the USDHHS, has composed several objectives related to improving sleep. The objectives are selected examples from the *Healthy People 2030* plan and can be found in Box 4.3 along with a selection of evidence-based practice resources from the American Academy of Sleep Medicine (AASM) and the USDHHS (2, 70).

BOX 4.3 *Healthy People 2030* **Examples of Sleep–Wake Related Objectives and Evidence-Based Practice Resources**

Healthy People 2030 Examples of Sleep–Wake Related Objectives	Evidence-Based Resources From the American Academy of Sleep Medicine (AASM)
1. Increase the proportion of adults with sleep apnea symptoms who get evaluated by a health care provider.	1. *Stroke & Obstructive Sleep Apnea,* Cathy Goldstein MD, MS. https://sleepeducation.org/wp-content/uploads/2021/04/nhsapstrokeosa.pdf AASM's *Patient Assessment. Self-assessment tool: Are you at-risk for obstructive sleep apnea?* https://sleepeducation.org/wp-content/uploads/2021/04/sleep-apnea-risk-assessment.pdf
2. Increase the proportion of adults who get enough sleep.	2. *For Clinicians: Practice Guidelines, Recommendations, and Policy Statements for Sleep and Sleep Disorders.* https://health.gov/healthypeople/tools-action/browse-evidence-based-resources/clinicians-practice-guidelines-recommendations-and-policy-statements-sleep-and-sleep-disorders
3. Increase the proportion of high school students who get enough sleep.	3. Printable Sleep Diary from the American Academy of Sleep Medicine (AASM). https://sleepeducation.org/resources/sleep-diary/
4. Increase the proportion of children who get sufficient sleep.	4. AASM's *Sleep Education: Bedtime Calculator.* A Resource for Parents. https://sleepeducation.org/healthy-sleep/bedtime-calculator/

Adapted from American Academy of Sleep Medicine. (2022). https://aasm.org/; United States Department of Health and Human Services, Office of Disease Prevention and Health Promotion. (2022). *Healthy People 2030: Building a healthier future for all.* https://health.gov/healthypeople

SUBSTANCE-RELATED AND ADDICTIVE DISORDERS

The *DSM-5-TR* removed the distinction between substance abuse and substance dependence, and the main diagnostic heading for this category of disorder became **substance use disorders**. Additionally, the number of criteria that a client with substance use disorder meets now determines the severity of the substance use disorder (19). Ten kinds of substances of abuse named in the *DSM-5-TR* and their corresponding *ICD-10-CM* codes are as follows:

- Alcohol (listed in the following section with its severity level criteria)
- Caffeine
- Cannabis; **Cannabis Use Disorder: Mild**—F12.10/**Moderate to Severe**—F12.20
- Hallucinogens; **Hallucinogen Use Disorder: Mild—F16.10/Moderate to Severe—F16.20**
- Inhalants; **Inhalant Use Disorder: Mild—F18.10/Moderate to Severe—F18.20**
- Opioids; **Opioid Use Disorder: Mild—F11.10/Moderate to Severe—F11.20**
- Sedatives, Hypnotics, Anxiolytics; **Sedative Use Disorder: Mild—F13.10/Moderate to Severe—F13.20**
- Stimulants; **Stimulant Use Disorder: Mild—F15.10/Moderate to Severe—F15.20**
- Tobacco; **Tobacco Use Disorder: Mild—Z72.0/Moderate to Severe—F17.200** *(Tobacco Use Disorder was added in the *DSM-5* series)
- Other (Unknown)

The diagnostician attempts to differentiate levels of use, from mild to severe, based on the number of symptoms or signs that are present (19). Each substance has a pattern of use and a particular group of associated behavioral features (ie, the criteria). The criteria are also arranged into the following subcategories:

Criteria 1–4: Related to cravings and overuse
Criteria 5–7: Impaired social functioning
Criteria 8–9: Failure to consider risks of use
Criterion 10: Tolerance
Criterion 11: Withdrawal

Alcohol use Disorder is diagnosed by severity as one of three levels: mild, moderate, or severe, as follows:

F10.10 Mild Alcohol Use Disorder = 2–3 symptoms
F10.20 Moderate Alcohol Use Disorder = 4–5 symptoms
F10.20 Severe Alcohol Use Disorder = 6 or more symptoms

Finally, **Gambling Disorder (F63.0)**, which shares many common features with the substance use disorders, was also added to this group in the *DSM-5* series (10, 11). Gambling disorder is characterized by continuous problematic gambling, despite having experienced significant impairment or distress because of the gambling. The person who is diagnosed with gambling disorder will, according to the *DSM-5-TR*, experience at least four of the following criteria: gamble with higher amounts of money over time, become irritated when they spend less time gambling, fail at efforts to stop gambling, are preoccupied With gambling, often gamble to feel better, "chase their losses," meaning they often continue to gamble at a later time to recuperate the money they lost, lie about their gambling, experience problems in relationships, work, or school, have to borrow money from others to compensate for their losses (11).

Many individuals who use a given substance are dependent on other substances as well (**polysubstance use**). Substance-related disorders are considered lifelong conditions as recurrence and relapse are unfortunately common. Substance-related disorders merit an extended discussion for several reasons. First, persons with such disorders typically demonstrate characteristic maladaptive occupational patterns, which are often reinforced or enabled by those with whom the substance user associates (ie, peers, family, employer). For this reason, a diagnosis of substance use disorder, and furthermore the evaluation and the intervention plan toward recovery, should be holistic enough to include more than just the individual who is using. Substance abusers have a higher than average incidence of other medical and psychiatric problems, impacting significantly the quality of their overall health care and increasing their mortality risk (21). **Comorbidity** (two or more disorders at the same time) is common; the *DSM-5-TR* includes a table that shows psychiatric diagnoses associated with specific substances (11, p. 545). In addition, substance users may have conditions that cause chronic pain, leaving them more vulnerable to self-medicate for pain and exacerbate their existing addiction problems.

The OT professional will certainly encounter persons with substance use disorders in settings as diverse as burn units, acute outpatient and acute inpatient settings, trauma units, physical rehabilitation centers, and mental or behavioral health settings. Occupational therapy has a specific focus with this group and can assume a significant role. In this section, we introduce a brief summary of the various abused substances, their effects, the mental and social characteristics of substance use, and common evidence-based OT approaches and interventions. More specific information about interventions can be found in Chapter 23.

The Effects of Abused Substances

Alcohol consumption is a socially sanctioned activity in America and in many cultures. Alcohol use is not considered an unhealthy occupation, and in the United States alcohol can be consumed legally by adults. Alcohol use, therefore, is not considered disordered until certain overuse conditions are met. Nonetheless, in the United States, alcohol causes approximately 140,000 deaths per year, according to the Centers for Disease Control and Prevention (22). In terms of comorbidity, alcohol is the substance most often involved, and 1 in 10 deaths among working-aged adults involves alcohol (22). "To reduce the risk of alcohol-related harms, the

2020-2025 Dietary Guidelines for Americans recommends that adults of legal drinking age can choose not to drink, or to drink in moderation by limiting intake to 2 drinks or less in a day for men or 1 drink or less for women, on days when alcohol is consumed" (22, p. 2).

There are varying degrees of *unhealthy* involvement with alcohol. Generally, alcoholics begin drinking in their teens or 20s, and the disease becomes progressive, leading to regular and excessive use. More males than females are heavy drinkers. There is a familial pattern of alcoholism, which may have a genetic component. However, one cannot discount the effect of observing, as a young child, the drinking behavior of family members. Three patterns of alcohol use are recognized: regular daily drinking, heavy weekend drinking, and periodic or episodic binge drinking. A person who uses alcohol excessively but who is not yet dependent on it can go for days, weeks, and even months of abstinence without suffering withdrawal symptoms. Once the disease has reached the dependence stage, however, the individual undergoes withdrawal when alcohol is withheld. Symptoms may include delirium tremens (the DT), characterized by fever, tremors, ataxia, and even hallucinations. Sweating and high blood pressure are other symptoms of withdrawal (11).

Chronic excessive alcohol use may lead to lasting neurologic damage and dementia. Medical disorders caused by alcohol include liver damage; gastric damage; premature aging; impotence and infertility; and increased risk of heart disease, respiratory disease, and neurologic disorders (22). Depression, which is associated with alcohol abuse, may be either a contributing factor or the result of alcoholism, which is a complex symptomology to unravel.

Marijuana is now legal in many states, and in addition is the most widely available illegal drug in the United States. It is often used in combination with alcohol or other drugs. Marijuana impairs a variety of cognitive and perceptual–motor functions, including concentration, judgment, short-term memory, perception, and motor skills. Marijuana may adversely affect reproduction and may exacerbate preexisting heart conditions. Because it is smoked and because it contains many known carcinogens, it may be more damaging to the lungs than tobacco. It has been linked to depression, and is suspected as the primary cause of amotivational syndrome in adolescents. This syndrome is characterized by loss of interest and initiative, difficulty concentrating, and diminished functional performance at school and work. It may also be associated with development of psychosis (11).

Among the stimulants that may be abused are cocaine and amphetamines and methamphetamine. Cocaine is derived from the leaves of the South American coca plant. As a white powder, it can be inhaled (snorted) through the nose or dissolved and injected. Crack, a smokable form of cocaine, produces a rapid high. Crack is more addictive than other forms of cocaine because the low that follows rapidly from the high intensely increases the desire for the drug. As with alcohol, cocaine use may follow either an episodic or a chronic daily pattern. Cocaine use may lead to serious medical problems, including frequent and tenacious upper respiratory infections, heart failure, reproductive problems (eg, miscarriage), stroke, seizures, personality changes, and violent psychosis. Newborns exposed to cocaine in utero may have the same physical problems as the mother, with serious birth defects and deformities. Furthermore, they may be irritable and have difficulty bonding with the mother or accepting nourishment (15).

Opioid narcotics, which may be either natural or synthetic, include heroin, morphine, and meperidine (Demerol). Illicit use of these drugs leads to addiction in about 50% of cases. Associated medical disorders include heart problems. Those who inject the drug run the risk of acquiring hepatitis C, human immunodeficiency virus (HIV), or other infections from contaminated needles. Children born to opioid-addicted mothers have withdrawal symptoms and may die of them (23). Synthetic opioids such as oxycodone (Percocet), hydrocodone (Vicodin), and oxycontin are prescribed for the treatment of severe pain, following surgery, for example. The number of prescriptions written for these medications has so significantly increased in the last decade that America is in the midst of an epidemic of opioid addiction (15). Drug seekers may visit many doctors to obtain more medication, users are more likely to engage in risky social behavior and may engage in criminal behavior, including prostitution, robberies, and violence, as a result of their addiction. When prescription opioids are in short supply or too expensive, users may turn to other drugs, such as heroin. Other commonly abused drugs include phencyclidine (PCP, also called angel dust), lysergic acid diethylamide (LSD), amyl nitrite (poppers) and other inhalants, and various prescription drugs (23).

Social Aspects of Substance Use Disorder

Social factors that impact alcohol or substance use disorders include codependency, enabling behaviors, and social and leisure deficits. **Codependency** refers to the unhealthy involvement of someone else in controlling or being controlled by a substance abuser. Codependent behavior is most common in spouses and immediate family members but may occur in others with whom the alcoholic associates. **Enabling** is a codependent behavior in another person characterized by making it easier for the substance user to continue to drink and/or take drugs. Examples of enabling include picking up the slack by taking care of the user's responsibilities (calling in sick for him or her) and providing money and other forms of material support.

After years of spending most leisure hours in drinking-related pursuits, the typical alcoholic has a network of drinking companions, a set of familiar drinking locations, and sometimes a repertoire of drinking-related activities (watching sporting events, gambling or playing cards, and so on). These habits related to the use of leisure time are a major problem for the recovering alcoholic, who must relearn how to enjoy leisure in a sober way (15).

Evidence-Based Occupational Therapy

In general, OT intervention aims to improve functioning and provide skill development in specific areas (7, 21, 33). Evaluation and intervention focus on these aspects:

- Performance patterns
- Use of time, especially leisure time
- Relapse prevention
- Cognitive and perceptual functions and skill development
- Social interaction, social skills, and self-expression
- Daily living skills
- Acquisition, development, and maintenance of valued occupational and social roles

Comorbidity of Substance Use and Other Psychiatric Disorders

Psychiatric comorbidity is the diagnosis of two or more psychiatric disorders in the same person. A high percentage of persons treated for a substance-related disorder are also diagnosed with another psychiatric disorder. This has been called **dual diagnosis**, but use of this term is discouraged because it implies only two diagnoses (and often there are more). The person may also be termed a mentally ill chemical abuser (MICA). People experiencing symptoms of mental disorder (eg, anxiety, depression, hallucinations) may use substances to "self-medicate."

Some persons with substance-related disorders also have been given diagnoses of schizophrenia or bipolar disorder. In general, substance users with comorbid conditions have fewer skills and correspondingly greater functional impairment than do those who have only the diagnosis of substance use disorder. Individuals diagnosed with a serious mental disorder and substance use disorder are more prone to relapse and require more structure than those with a single diagnosis (11, 21).

NEUROCOGNITIVE DISORDERS

In *DSM-IV*, these disorders were referred to as "dementia, delirium, amnestic, and other cognitive disorders." These terms may be more familiar to the reader than the term **neurocognitive disorder**. Neurocognitive disorders have as a primary feature a disturbance in cognition with a reduction from a previous level. These disorders are primarily acquired later life, after development to adulthood is completed. Another feature of these disorders is that the pathology is clearly related to the brain and the CNS (11).

A significant decline in cognition (specifically memory) is the main characteristic of disorders in this category. Other cognitive functions that may be affected, depending on the disorder and its severity, include attention, executive function, learning, language, and social cognition. All of these disorders involve temporary or permanent disruptions in the functioning of the brain. **Delirium (F05)**, the first disorder listed in this chapter of *DSM-5-TR*, is characterized by reduced alertness and awareness, disorganized thinking (impaired memory, incoherent speech), evidence of probable physiologic cause (eg, fever, head injury, or recent ingestion of toxic substance), and rapid onset of symptoms (11). Delirium is often associated with substance use. Delirium may last for only a few hours or for several weeks; clients are generally not seen in OT until the delirium has passed.

Major and mild neurocognitive disorders encompass a very large group of conditions that become increasingly common with advancing age. Among these are Alzheimer disease and similar disorders with different causes:

- Frontotemporal lobe atrophy
- Lewy bodies
- Vascular abnormalities
- Traumatic brain injury
- HIV infection
- Prion disease
- Parkinson disease
- Huntington disease
- Other medical conditions
- Multiple causes

These conditions are marked by the absence of delirium but a decline in cognitive function from a previous level, to the degree that independence in ADL or other occupations is impaired (11, 19). A **mild neurocognitive disorder** is diagnosed when evidence of cognitive decline exists but independence in daily life is still possible even for complex activities (although compensation or external support may be needed). For example, the person may be able to pay bills but might benefit from some oversight or assistance from another person. The person experiences these activities as more difficult or stressful than they were previously, but is still able to do them, for the most part.

Major neurocognitive disorder is the name now given to what in *DSM-IV* was termed **dementia**. Dementia (a term that is still in use) is marked by a severe impairment of short- and long-term memory as documented by the mental status examination. Additional criteria include evidence of impaired thinking or judgment, social or occupational impairment, absence of delirium, and probable organic cause (11, 19). Individuals with **major neurocognitive disorder** are seen in OT in mental health settings, physical medicine settings, skilled nursing facilities, assisted living, adult day care, and the home.

Major or mild neurocognitive disorder due to Alzheimer disease manifests in progressive and significant deterioration of intellectual, social, and occupational functioning. The person gradually is less and less able to function in daily life as the disease progresses. Alzheimer disease can be diagnosed using genetic testing or family history (11). On autopsy, the brains of clients with this type of dementia have shown clear and characteristic changes both on the gross level (eg, atrophy of the cerebral cortex) and the microscopic level (eg, neurofibrillary tangles). The typical age at first diagnosis is after age 70. The progression of the disease is gradual, with increasing loss of function. At the final stages, the person often loses the ability to speak or walk and can be bedridden. Death generally results from medical causes such as aspiration of food or liquid (11).

Major or mild frontotemporal neurocognitive disorder may be diagnosed on the basis of behavioral change, or decline in language ability, or both. The behavioral changes include **behavioral disinhibition** (lack of control over behavior) and personality change. The person declines in ability to empathize, loses interest in things, and may engage in compulsive behaviors. Also affected are social cognition and executive functions (11). If **language ability** is affected, the signs are a decline in the use of speech, in naming of objects, and in understanding words. The person may put inappropriate objects in the mouth (**hyperorality**). The average age at first diagnosis is 50 to 59 years, but may be as early as 20 years or as late as 80 years or more. Frontotemporal neurocognitive disorder progresses more quickly than does Alzheimer disease, with average survival of 6 to 11 years (10). Family history and genetic testing may aid in diagnosis (11). Work and family life are affected. The behavioral changes associated with this condition may make it impossible for the person to remain at home. For example, the person may wander, may masturbate or urinate in public, may shoplift, etc.

Major or mild neurocognitive disorder with Lewy bodies is characterized by impaired cognition that fluctuates, by visual hallucinations, as well as parkinsonism (motor problems such tremor, stiffness, and slow movement). Lewy bodies are clumps of protein in the brain and can be diagnosed only on autopsy. Various brain imaging techniques such as positron emission tomography (PET) and magnetic resonance imaging (MRI) may aid in diagnosis. Cognitive testing is needed in most cases. The cognitive impairment appears early in the disease, with the motor symptoms appearing later. This condition may also be called **dementia with Lewy bodies (DLB)** (10, 11). Persons with this disorder may faint frequently (syncope) and are at risk for falls. This is a progressive condition with both cognitive and motor symptoms.

Major or mild vascular neurocognitive disorder results from damage to the cerebrovascular system (blood vessels of the brain), usually caused by multiple small strokes or transient ischemic attacks (TIAs). The presence of cerebrovascular disease is established by history, examination, or neuroimaging (via MRI). Complex attention is the function most typically affected, but this depends on which brain areas have been injured. Executive functions and information processing may be impaired. In many but not all cases, the deterioration in function is stepwise or patchy rather than steadily progressive. Functioning varies from day to day, and although there may be significant problems in one area (eg, memory of names), other areas are relatively intact. The progression can sometimes be slowed by treating the underlying cause (eg, high blood pressure, high cholesterol).

As stated previously, major or mild neurocognitive disorder may also result from other conditions, such as infection with HIV, head trauma, Parkinson disease, and Huntington disease. Substance ingestion (usually alcohol, but also inhalants, sedatives, and others) may also cause the disorder. Some of these disorders result in permanent memory loss (23).

Evidence-Based Occupational Therapy

Neurocognitive disorders affect all areas of occupation. Occupational therapy interventions for persons with neurocognitive disorders generally address the following items:

- Prevention of further decline
- Roles, routines, and habits
- Decline in occupational performance in specific areas
- Memory deficits
- Limitations in judgment and other cognitive functions
- Deficits in social skills
- Emotional reaction to one's deteriorating mental state

A variety of occupations involving ADLs, IADLs, leisure, and social participation may be helpful, particularly when they are chosen by the client and embraced by the caregiver. Caregivers may appreciate recommendations about how to reimagine or reinvent a modified version of the client's previously enjoyed occupations (34). Attention should be given to fall prevention and environmental design to accommodate perceptual difficulties.

Depending on the severity of the neurocognitive disorder, certain approaches will be more appropriate than others. For example, individualized exercise is possible for persons with moderate dementia, whereas more staff involvement may be required for persons with more severe dementia. The *Cognitive Disabilities Reconsidered Model* is a modified version of *Allen's Cognitive Disabilities Model*, which while concentrating on the individual's remaining capabilities reverses the direction of a client's cognitive level of function to apply the constructs of the model to the declining levels of function and cognition experienced by individuals with dementia. The cognitive levels in the *Cognitive Disabilities Reconsidered Model* range from 1.0 to 5.6, with the lowest level being unresponsive and the highest level signifying normal function. *The Cognitive Performance Test* (CPT) (18) (introduced and briefly discussed further in Chapter 12) is the measure used to determine cognitive levels in the *Cognitive Disabilities Reconsidered Model*. Incorporating use of this model into OT practice is especially helpful for provision of caregiver education because it provides a way to gauge the client's ability to participate in various occupations and gives suggestions for the level and type of assistance that may be necessary for each cognitive level (16).

There is a temptation to imagine that forgotten skills can be drilled and practiced so that they can be retained. But research studies show that the effectiveness of such training is very weak. Ciro (26) argues convincingly, however, that training of specific tasks that are part of valued roles (cook, homemaker, etc.) can be effective because it draws on established **procedural memory**. Procedural memory (how to perform actions and routines) is generally better preserved in dementia than **declarative memory** (the names of things, facts to be recalled, for example). Tasks must be embedded in an occupation that is meaningful to and desired by the client. Each training session for a given task must be identical to the one before; variation in presentation will interfere with learning. This type of approach is recommended only at the mild stages of neurocognitive disorder.

Because improvement is not generally expected, occupational therapy interventions seek to maintain maximum functioning for as long as possible through the teaching of compensatory strategies and by careful environmental management. An example of a compensatory strategy is to perform a simpler version of the desired activity (eg, using a microwave to reheat prepared foods rather than cooking on a stovetop). Labeling drawers with pictures of their contents is a memory aid and an example of environmental management. When function declines so far that independence is no longer possible, the OT approach shifts to working with the family or other caregivers to assist them in encouraging as much independent function as possible (16).

PERSONALITY DISORDERS

The authors of *DSM-5* series (10, 11) distinguish between personality traits and personality disorders. The physician may list personality traits for someone who does not fully qualify for a diagnosis of personality disorder. **Personality traits** are enduring patterns of perceiving, relating to, and thinking about the environment and oneself that are exhibited in a wide range of social and personal contexts. Only when personality traits are inflexible and maladaptive and cause significant functional impairment or subjective distress do they merit a diagnosis of **personality disorder** (10). A continuum exists between personality traits as expressed in average individuals and the distressing conditions of personality disorder. In other words, a person may have a specific kind of personality that does not cause any dysfunction or distress or may have the same kind of personality in a more fixed and extreme way such that a diagnosis of personality disorder is made. A person may also experience an intensification of personality traits in the context of a specific event. This is referred to as **state** rather than **trait** disorder.

To merit a diagnosis of personality disorder, the traits must be stable and long-standing; in other words, a state disorder would not qualify because the symptoms or behaviors would not last beyond the experience of the causative event. For example, a child may be avoidant, fearful, and anxious around an event such as the death or illness of a parent. So long as the avoidant behaviors do not become a lifelong pattern, this would not be a disorder. The reader is cautioned that the personality, whether seen as "traits," a "state," or a "disorder," has traditionally been viewed as not easily changed. Because of great controversy and absence of agreement among experts, the *DSM-5* includes an alternative model for personality disorders (10, p. 761). In this model, the focus is on the maladaptive functioning and the more pathologic (more socially destructive) personality traits (such as antagonism).

The *DSM-5-TR* classifies the personality disorders into three clusters—A, B, and C (11). Cluster A disorders include paranoid, schizoid, and schizotypal types. Persons with these disorders may appear odd, eccentric, or different to others. Cluster B disorders include antisocial, borderline, histrionic, and narcissistic personality types. The common ground in these disorders is dramatic, erratic, emotional, self-centered behavior. Cluster C includes avoidant, dependent, and obsessive–compulsive personality disorders. The common feature is a fearful, anxious, or avoidant approach to life (11, 19).

The authors of *DSM-5-TR* recognize that many individuals diagnosed with personality disorders also display traits associated with other personality disorders. For example, someone who fits the criteria for borderline personality disorder may also report behaviors that are dependent or avoidant and are consistent with the Cluster C disorders. For this reason, the *DSM-5* allows for the listing of traits that cross the categories (45). In addition, significant comorbidity with other psychiatric or medical disorders may be present. The reader is encouraged to ask questions and listen to persons diagnosed with a given personality disorder, so that the most troubling symptoms and behaviors and the important goals that are unique to each person are understood.

Cluster A Disorders

Paranoid personality disorder is characterized by a tendency to interpret the actions of others as deliberately harmful to the self. Suspiciousness of others, including spouses and others who would normally be trusted, is common. Disturbances in routine may be seen as threatening. For example, the arbitrary rerouting of a bus or flight may be taken as intentionally directed at the person. Persons with this disorder may have problems functioning at work because of their suspicions of the intentions of managers and coworkers. Occupational therapy professionals may assist the person to learn and use new strategies to deal with problems at work. However, no overall change in attitude should be expected, as the paranoid stance is part of the person's adaptation to life.

A diagnosis of **schizoid personality disorder** is sometimes given to persons who have very limited social involvement with others. They live alone, avoid social contact, and seem uninterested in the social relations on which most people thrive. Occupational therapy intervention with persons with this diagnosis may be directed at assisting them to find and fit into a niche in life that is compatible with their personality structure. For example, a job with limited need for interpersonal relatedness and a high opportunity for independence may permit the schizoid individual to be socially productive and attain a sense of personal competence while avoiding the threatening experience of being with other people. Persons with this diagnosis may be slovenly in appearance and with housekeeping, and they may benefit from education and training in ADLs and IADLs.

Schizotypal personality disorder is characterized by the indifference to social involvement seen in schizoid personality disorder, coupled with peculiarities of behavior that are similar to those seen in schizophrenia. The OT approach is similar to that for the schizoid personality, with additional attention to improvement in self-care and the minimal social skills needed for community survival (11).

Cluster B Disorders

Antisocial personality disorder is diagnosed for those who have evidence of **conduct disorder** since before age 15 and who show a continuing pattern of antisocial acts after age 18 (11). Acts may include various crimes, deliberate cruelty to animals and people, failure to honor debts, lying, neglect of duties as a parent, and a pattern of impulsivity, among others. Persons with this diagnosis may be encountered in the criminal justice system or in the forensic units of hospitals, but also in other practice settings. Because of the developmental aspect of this disorder, they never really have the opportunity to acquire the behaviors, skills, and attitudes needed to succeed in life. Little has been written about OT treatment approaches to this population; however, trauma-informed care approaches are considered universally appropriate, especially in the juvenile justice system.

Borderline personality disorder is characterized by unstable and erratic relationships and a fluctuating sense of personal identity; the person has persistent fear of abandonment by others. Moodiness and chronic feelings of emptiness are common. The moodiness is often acted out in impulsive behavior such as overspending, substance use, sexual relations, and self-mutilation. Interpersonal relationships are highly intense and dramatic, with the partner in the relationship viewed as alternatively all good or all bad (11). Occupational therapy intervention is usually directed at reducing the symptoms with the aim of increasing the person's self-esteem and self-identity (15).

Skill groups that provide training in mindfulness, interpersonal effectiveness, and emotion regulation are considered particularly useful interventions for this population. Mindfulness is a technique for training the mind to observe and restrain or redirect its own activities. Interpersonal effectiveness techniques help the person communicate with other people to meet needs while maintaining a two-way positive relationship. Emotion regulation training educates the person about the nature of emotions and provides practical ways of recognizing and responding to emotions.

The central pattern of **histrionic personality disorder** is attention seeking and extreme emotionality. This diagnosis is more prevalent in women than in men. Typically, the individual with this diagnosis self-dramatizes, seeks center stage in all situations, and is uncomfortable when not the center of attention. The person may express very strong emotions that seem overexaggerated to others (11). Also, the histrionic person expresses global approval or disapproval without the usual details, for example, stating that a colleague is "a sadistic predator" but not providing any examples of incidents that led to this evaluation. This disorder may interfere with functioning in work, especially in positions of any responsibility, because impaired judgment is common. This disorder may be confused with borderline and narcissistic personality disorders (19).

Narcissistic personality disorder is characterized by extreme self-centeredness, shown in lack of understanding of other people's feelings, exploitation of others, grandiosity, and preoccupation with success. Fantasies of success may lead the person with this disorder to undertake unrealistic goals. Little has been written about occupational therapy intervention, but one focus might be to identify realistic goals by analyzing and modifying the unrealistic goals previously chosen. However, because a sense of special uniqueness is central to this condition, the person will resist relinquishing the fantasy, however far-fetched (11). Forcing a confrontation with reality before the person is ready is counterproductive. OT staff should use a gentle and consistent manner with firm limits and expectations.

Cluster C Disorders

The essential feature of **avoidant personality disorder** is fear and avoidance of social contact with others. This is an exaggerated form of the shyness or discomfort many people feel in unfamiliar social situations. Typically, the person has no close friends, is easily hurt by the mildest criticism, and avoids being evaluated (however briefly or fairly) by others (11). Understandably, this interferes with functioning in the work world and in social situations. Occupational therapy intervention for this and other Cluster C personality disorders may be directed at social skills training and realistic self-appraisal.

Dependent personality disorder is more commonly diagnosed in women than in men. It is characterized by a pattern of submission to the wishes of others and apparent inability to make decisions on one's own. Persons with this disorder seek guidance, reassurance, and support out of proportion to the situation (11). For example, an adult might let their spouse decide what they will eat when they are dining out and will permit or even seek recommendations as to what hobbies or social interests should be pursued. These individuals function well on the job, except when independent decision-making is needed. Persons with this diagnosis are not usually seen in OT in the absence of another psychiatric diagnosis.

Obsessive–compulsive personality disorder is characterized by perfectionism and is more often diagnosed in men than in women. Typical patterns of behavior include a preoccupation with details, inflexible insistence that others do things a certain way, overvaluing of productivity and undervaluing of social relations, miserliness, and overconscientiousness. These patterns can interfere with functioning at work because of the overall tendency to miss the main point, being sidetracked by the details.

Evidence-Based Occupational Therapy

Psychoeducational approaches to intervention are considered a gold standard especially when the intervention plan can be tailored to specific personality disorders (15). Social skills training and interventions such as role-play, journaling, and CBT aimed at increasing self-awareness, understanding, and skill in social participation may also be used.

APPLICATIONS OF DIAGNOSES TO OCCUPATIONAL THERAPY

The occupational therapy team practicing in mental health settings must appreciate the reality of psychiatric diagnosis and its relationship to reimbursement. Without a *DSM-5/ICD-10* diagnosis of sufficient severity, neither public nor private insurers will pay for OT intervention, which makes the psychiatric diagnosis an inescapable fact of practice today. The diagnosis provides useful information to OT staff that helps support a holistic and well-thought-out intervention plan. Each diagnosis has functional implications, and this helps professionals in targeting the occupations and client factors that might need attention (eg, work, social skills). Scores on the WHODAS 2.0 should provide clear information concerning the occupations affected and the degree of difficulty the client is experiencing (75, 76). These scores can justify the need for occupational therapy evaluation, intervention, and collaboration; they also further acknowledge the significant role that occupational therapy plays in holistic quality care.

OT HACKS SUMMARY

O: Occupation as a means and an end

Many psychiatric diagnoses share similar presenting symptoms, particularly in the acute phase of illness, before medication has taken effect. Reduction of symptoms and particularly diminishing problem behaviors that put the client or others at risk or in unsafe situations is a primary concern of the interprofessional behavioral health team in acute care settings. However, once the symptoms have remitted, the residual disability becomes the focus of treatment in a move toward the client's self-determinism and recovery. For most clients, occupational function is disrupted or unsatisfactory in some objective and describable way. To focus on the rehabilitation of these clients, we need clear problem and goal statements that are within our scope of OT practice, as well as the skills to perform an occupational performance analysis (4).

T: Theoretical concepts, values, and principles, or historical foundations

The Model of Human Occupation (MOHO) describes the process that leads to occupational adaptation. The core constructs of MOHO—volition, habituation, performance capacity, and environment—come together in nonlinear ways that allow clients to adapt to their life circumstances. **Volition** is considered a person's inherent motivation for occupational endeavors. **Habituation** refers to establishing occupational routines. **Performance capacity** suggests that the client possesses the necessary underlying physical, cognitive, and psychosocial skills to engage in occupations (43). For occupational adaptation to occur, occupational

competence and occupational identity must be established. Occupational therapy professionals can apply MOHO and other occupation-based theoretical concepts to the process of evaluation, intervention, and goal setting to highlight occupational therapy's unique approach to mental health recovery. Planning occupational outcomes for clients who have mental health conditions and who are in recovery leads to the development of both occupational competence and occupational identity. When the client engages in personally meaningful, relevant, and necessary occupations to achieve success in expected roles, and they are able to maintain patterns of occupation that are productive and satisfying, this inevitably leads to positive effects on overall health, well-being, and the development of the capacity for self-direction in the recovery process (38, 67, 68).

H: How can we Help? OT's role in serving clients with mental illness or mental health needs

Occupational therapy professionals' role in supporting the recovery process for clients is centered on enhancing occupational competence and occupational identity to promote occupational adaptation.

A: Adaptations

The focus of OT intervention for clients with psychiatric illness is **not** the client's diagnosis. Rather, the OT professional consistently focuses on what is creating a barrier to a person's optimal occupational engagement. This chapter provided guidance and direction for consideration of the psychiatric diagnosis in the development of OT problem and goal statements, as well as for forming occupation-based outcomes.

C: Case study includes

After reading Matthew's case example and his occupational history, and considering the information in this chapter, what role would an occupational therapy professional working with Matthew have throughout the various stages of his illness, and into his recovery? Using only the information given in the case study and within this chapter, which areas of occupation do you believe have been most impacted by Matthew's mental illness? Can you think of which occupational areas you might target for intervention planning?

K: Knowledge: Keeping mental health OT practice grounded in evidence, in occupational science, and in research

HOT Evidence Infographics, a resource from the American Occupational Therapy Association (AOTA), is an excellent way to make sure that OT practice stays grounded in the Evidence. Linked here, you will find one example, *Social Participation and Quality of Life of Adults with Serious Mental Illness*

https://www.aota.org/-/media/corporate/files/practice/hot-evidence/hot-evidence_social-participation-and-serious-mental-illness-final.pdf

S: Some terms that may be new to you

Active phase: second of three phases in the progression of schizophrenia, where psychotic symptomology becomes more pronounced

Alogia: lessened speech output

Anhedonia: loss of pleasure

Apnea: temporary cessation of breathing, especially while sleeping

Biomarkers: physiologic or behavioral characteristics that indicate genetic correlation or association with particular disorder(s)

Bipolar: the two poles or extremes of mania and depression

Cataplexy: sudden loss of muscle tone after laughing

Catatonia: extreme psychomotor disturbance

Communication: the transfer of ideas and information using verbal and nonverbal behaviors to influence another individual

Compulsion: a repetitive behavior or ritualistic action performed in response to an obsession; often employed to manage obsessions

Cultural concepts of distress: ways that individuals experience, understand, and communicate about their suffering, behavioral problems, or difficult thoughts and emotions

Delusions: fixed beliefs that are not open to change even in light of conflicting evidence

Depression: a mood that is low and often disengaged, with loss of interest in activities that were previously pleasurable

Diagnostician: individual responsible for the psychiatric (or other) medical diagnosis

Duration: how long the symptoms have been present

Frequency: how often the symptoms are felt

Hallucinations: experiences of perception, often vivid, that are not under an individual's voluntary control

Hyperactivity: being more active than normal, especially when the increased activity is not appropriate for the situation

Hypervigilance: tense alertness

Hypomania: a less severe or lasting episode of manic-like behaviors

Hypopnea: abnormally slow or shallow breathing

Impulsivity: acting quickly without regard for consequences

Language: conventional use of symbols embedded with rules of form and function and synthesized to produce communication

Mania: a mood that is elevated, expansive, and/or irritable

Negative symptoms: apathy and generally inexpressive mood (affective flattening), lack of goal-directed behavior (avolition), deterioration of hygiene, social isolation, diminished participation in daily life, and psychomotor slowing

Obsession: an unwanted intrusive thought or impulse

Occupational deprivation: not experiencing meaningful occupational participation

Positive symptoms: hallucinations, delusions, loosening of associations, and grossly disorganized speech and behavior

Prodromal phase: initial phase in the progression of schizophrenia where functional level begins to decline

Provisional diagnosis: initial diagnosis

Rapid-cycling: a quick shift in the pattern of moods

Residual phase: phase of progression of schizophrenia where the psychotic symptoms most disturbing to the client begin to remit; however, functional level may continue to decline, particularly if the individual does not have supports

Self-direction: client has more autonomy throughout the care process in directing their recovery, deciding priorities, and making decisions

Specific learning disabilities: disorders that directly affect the learning process

Specifiers: used to further extend, describe, or clarify a condition

Speech: expressive production of sounds including the characteristics of the sound such as articulation, fluency, voice, and resonance

Subtypes: used to describe a subordinate category of a disorder; subtypes of conditions are considered distinct disorders

Torpor: inactivity

Reflection Questions

1. Because occupational therapy professionals do not diagnose mental illnesses, explain the relevance of having a foundational understanding of the *DSM-5-TR*. What is the purpose of the *DSM-5-TR*?
2. What is the relationship between the *DSM* system and the *ICD* system?
3. Describe the categorical approach used in the *DSM-5-TR*.
4. Compare and contrast the *DSM-5-TR* and the *OTPF-4*.
5. Describe the *WHODAS 2.0*. Discuss the relevance of this assessment as it applies to occupational therapy daily psychosocial practice.
6. How might an understanding of *cultural concepts of distress* impact developing an occupational profile?
7. Choose and defend what you believe is the most relevant and important information that an occupational therapy professional can learn from a client's *DSM-5-TR* diagnosis.
8. Explain what is meant by *psychiatric comorbidity*. How do a client's psychiatric comorbidities affect occupational therapy evaluation and intervention?

REFERENCES

1. Aggarwal, N. K., Jarvis, G. E., Gómez-Carrillo, A., Kirmayer, L. J., & Lewis-Fernández, R. (2020). The Cultural Formulation Interview since DSM-5: Prospects for training, research, and clinical practice. *Transcultural Psychiatry, 57*(4), 496–514.
2. American Academy of Sleep Medicine. https://aasm.org/
3. American Occupational Therapy Association. (2020). AOTA 2020 Occupational Therapy Code of Ethics. *American Journal of Occupational Therapy, 74*(Suppl. 3), 7413410005.
4. American Occupational Therapy Association. (2020). Guidelines for supervision, roles, and responsibilities during the delivery of occupational therapy services. *American Journal of Occupational Therapy, 74*(Suppl. 3), 7413410020.
5. American Occupational Therapy Association. (2020). Occupational therapy in the promotion of health and well-being. *American Journal of Occupational Therapy, 74*, 7403420010.
6. American Occupational Therapy Association. (2020). Occupational therapy practice framework: Domain and process—Fourth edition. *American Journal of Occupational Therapy, 74*(Suppl. 2), 7412410010.

7. American Occupational Therapy Association. (2021). Occupational therapy scope of practice. *American Journal of Occupational Therapy, 75*(Suppl. 3), 7513410030.

8. American Occupational Therapy Association. (2021). Standards of practice for occupational therapy. *American Journal of Occupational Therapy, 75*(Suppl. 3), 7513410050.

9. American Psychiatric Association. (2000). *Diagnostic and statistical manual of mental disorders* (4th ed., text rev.). Author.

10. American Psychiatric Association. (2013). *Diagnostic and statistical manual of mental disorders* (5th ed., text rev.). Author.

11. American Psychiatric Association. (2022). *Diagnostic and statistical manual of mental disorders* (5th ed., text rev.). https://doi.org/10.1176/appi.books.9780890425787.

12. American Psychiatric Association. (2022). *APA Dictionary of Psychology.* https://dictionary.apa.org/subtype

13. Baron, K., Kielhofner, G., Iyenger, A., Goldhammer, V., Wolenski, J., Model of Human Occupation Clearinghouse. (2006). *A user's manual for the occupational self-assessment (OSA): Version 2.2.* University of Illinois.

14. Bond, G. R., & Drake, R. E. (2015). The critical ingredients of assertive community treatment. *World Psychiatry, 14*(2), 240–242.

15. Bonder, B. R. (2022). *Psychopathology and function* (6th ed.). SLACK.

16. Brown, C. (2019). Cognition. In C. Brown, V. C. Stoffel, & J. P. Munoz (Eds.). *Occupational therapy in mental health—A vision for participation* (2nd ed., pp. 385–402). F.A. Davis.

17. Brown, C., & Dunn, W. (2002). *Adolescent/Adult sensory profile.* Pearson.

18. Burns, T. (2006). *The cognitive performance test manual.* Maddak.

19. Buser, S., & Cruz, L. (2022). *DSM-5-TR insanely simplified: Unlocking the spectrums within DSM-5-TR and ICD-10.* Chiron Publications.

20. Cacciatore, J., & Francis, A. (2022). DSM-5-TR turns normal grief into a mental disorder. *The Lancet Psychiatry, 9*(7), e32.

21. Center for Behavioral Health Statistics and Quality. (2021). *Behavioral health equity report 2021: Substance use and mental health indicators measured from the National Survey on Drug Use and Health (NSDUH), 2015–2019* (Publication No. PEP21-07-01-004). Substance Abuse and Mental Health Services Administration. https://www.samhsa.gov/data/sites/default/files/reports/rpt35328/2021NSDUHBHEReport.pdf

22. Centers for Disease Control and Prevention, National Center for Chronic Disease Prevention and Health Promotion. *Excessive alcohol use.* https://www.cdc.gov/chronicdisease/resources/publications/factsheets/alcohol.htm

23. Centers for Disease Control and Prevention, National Center for Chronic Disease Prevention and Health Promotion. *Drug overdose: Other drugs.* https://www.cdc.gov/drugoverdose/deaths/other-drugs.html

24. Centers for Medicare and Medicaid Services. *ICD-10.* http://www.cms.gov/Medicare/Coding/ICD10/index.html?redirect=/icd10

25. Centers for Medicare and Medicaid Services. *COVID-19 update: April 1, 2022.* https://www.cms.gov/medicare/icd-10/2022-icd-10-cm

26. Ciro, C. (2013). Second nature—Improving occupational performance in people with dementia through role-based, task-specific learning. *OT Practice, 18*(3), 9–12.

27. Colvert, E., Tick, B., McEwen, F., Stewart, C., Curran, S. R., Woodhouse, E., Gillan, N., Hallet, V., Lietz, S., Garnett, T., Ronald, A., Plomin, R., Rijsdijk, F., Happe, F., & Bolton, P. (2015). Heritability of autism spectrum disorder in a UK population-based twin sample. *JAMA Psychiatry, 72*(5), 415–423.

28. Condo, C. M. (2020, March 3). "You don't look autistic": The reality of high functioning autism. *The Washington Post.* https://www.washingtonpost.com/lifestyle/2020/03/03/you-dont-look-autistic-reality-high-functioning-autism/

29. Dunn, W. (1999). *Sensory profile—User's manual.* Pearson.

30. Egan, M. Y., Kubina, L. A., Lidstone, R. I., Macdougall, G. H., & Raudoy, A. E. (2010). A critical reflection on occupational therapy within one assertive community treatment team. *Canadian Journal of Occupational Therapy, 77*(2), 70–79.

31. Faulkner, S. M., Drake, R. J., Ogden, M., Gardani, M., & Bee, P. E. (2022). A mixed methods expert opinion study on the optimal content and format for an occupational therapy intervention to improve sleep in schizophrenia spectrum disorders. *PLoS One, 17*(6), e0269453.

32. First, M. B., Yousif, L. H., Clarke, D. E., Wang, P. S., Gogtay, N., & Appelbaum, P. S. (2022). DSM-5-TR: Overview of what's new and what's changed. *World Psychiatry, 21*(2), 218–219.

33. Fox, J., Erlandsson, L. K., & Shiel, A. (2019). A systematic review and narrative synthesis of occupational therapy-led interventions for individuals with anxiety and stress-related disorders. *Occupational Therapy in Mental Health, 35*(2), 179–204.

34. Frankenstein, L. L., & Jahn, G. (2020). Behavioral and occupational therapy for dementia patients and caregivers. *GeroPsych: The Journal of Gerontopsychology and Geriatric Psychiatry, 33*(2), 85–100.

35. Frye, R. E., Vassall, S., Kaur, G., Lewis, C., Karim, M., & Rossignol, D. (2019). Emerging biomarkers in autism spectrum disorder: A systematic review. *Annals of Translational Medicine, 7*(23), 792.

36. Groen, R. N., Ryan, O., Wigman, J. T. W., Riese, H., Penninx, B. W. J. H., Giltay, E. J., Wichers, M., & Hartman, C. (2020). Comorbidity between depression and anxiety: Assessing the role of bridge mental states in dynamic psychological networks. *BMC Medicine, 18*, 308.

37. Gutman, S. A., McCreedy, P., & Heisler, P. (2004). The psychosocial deficits of children with regulatory disorders: Identification and treatment. *Occupational Therapy in Mental Health, 20*(2), 1–29.

38. Hamm, J. A., Buck, K. D., Leonhardt, B. L., Luther, L., & Lysaker, P. H. (2018). Self-directed recovery in schizophrenia: Attending to clients' agendas in psychotherapy. *Journal of Psychotherapy Integration, 28*(2), 188–201.

39. Harvard Medical School. (2007). *National Comorbidity Survey (NCS).* Retrieved August 21, 2017, from https://www.hcp.med.harvard.edu/ncs/index.php. Data Table 1: Lifetime prevalence DSM-IV/WMH-CIDI disorders by sex and cohort.

40. Hemphill, B. J., & Urish, C. K. (Eds.). (2020). *Assessments in occupational therapy mental health: An integrative approach* (4th ed.). SLACK.

41. Hill, R., & Dahlitz, M. (2022). *The practitioner's guide to the science of psychotherapy.* W. W. Norton.

42. Janiri, D., Moser, D. A., Doucet, G. E., Luber, M. J., Rasgon, A., Lee, W. H., Murrough, J. W., Sani, G., Eickhoff, S. B., & Frangou, S. (2019). Shared neural phenotypes for mood and anxiety disorders: A meta-analysis of 226 task-related functional imaging studies. *JAMA Psychiatry, 77*(2), 172–179.

43. Kielhofner, G. (2008). Dimensions of doing. In G. Kielhofner (Ed.), *Model of human occupation: Theory and application* (4th ed., pp. 101–109). Lippincott Williams & Wilkins.

44. Kilgus, M. D., Maxmen, J. S., & Ward, N. G. (2016). *Essential psychopathology & its treatment* (4th ed.). W. W. Norton.

45. Krueger, R. F. (2014). *The alternative DSM-5 model for personality disorders. Medscape Psychiatry and Mental Health, 2014.* https://www.medscape.com/viewarticle/826986

46. Lama, T. C., Fu, Y., & Davis, J. A. (2021). Exploring the ideal practice for occupational therapists on assertive community treatment teams. *British Journal of Occupational Therapy, 84*(9), 582–590.

47. Mayo Clinic. (n.d.). *Central sleep apnea—Symptoms and causes.* https://www.mayoclinic.org/diseases-conditions/central-sleep-apnea/symptoms-causes/syc-20352109

48. Mierau, S. B., & Neumeyer, A. M. (2019). Metabolic interventions in autism spectrum disorder. *Neurobiology of Disease, 132*, 104544.

49. Mughal, S., Faizy, R. M., & Saadabadi, A. (2020, November 18). Autism spectrum disorder. *StatPearls* [Internet]. https://www.ncbi.nlm.nih.gov/books/NBK525976

50. Muroff, J., Bratiotis, C., & Steketee, G. (2011). Treatment for hoarding behaviors: A review of the evidence. *Clinical Social Work Journal, 39*(4), 406–423.

51. Nakhost, A., Law, S. F., Francombe Pridham, K. M., & Stergiopoulos, V. (2017). Addressing complexity and improving access in community mental health services: An inner-city adaptation of flexible ACT. *Psychiatric Services, 68*(9), 867–869.

52. National Association of Anorexia Nervosa and Associated Disorders. (2019). *Eating disorder statistics.* https://anad.org/education-and-awareness/about-eating-disorders/eating-disorders-statistics/

53. National Institute of Mental Health. (n.d.). *Schizophrenia.* https://www.nimh.nih.gov/health/statistics/schizophrenia

54. National Institute of Mental Health. (2022). *Generalized anxiety disorder: When worry gets out of control.* https://www.nimh.nih.gov/sites/default/files/documents/health/publications/generalized-anxiety-disorder-gad/generalized_anxiety_disorder.pdf

55. Paquin, K., Wilson, A. L., Cellard, C., Lecomte, T., & Potvin, S. (2014). A systematic review on improving cognition in schizophrenia. *BMC Psychiatry, 14*: 139.

56. Parthimos, T. P., Karavasilis, E., Rankin, K. P., Seimenis, I., Leftherioti, K., Papanicolaou, A. C., Miller, B., Papageorgiou, S. G., & Papatriantafyllou, J. D. (2019). The neural correlates of impaired self-monitoring among individuals with neurodegenerative dementias. *The Journal of Neuropsychiatry and Clinical Neurosciences, 31*(3), 201–209.

57. Pekçetin, S., Özdinç, S., Ata, H., Can, H. B., Sermenli Aydın, N., Taş Dürmüş, P., & Çalıyurt, O. (2022). Perceived occupational competence and value among university students with premenstrual dysphoric disorder. *British Journal of Occupational Therapy, 85*(5), 327–331.

58. Perilli, V., Stasolla, F., Maselli, S., & Morelli, I. (2018). Occupational therapy and social skills training for enhancing constructive engagement of patients with schizophrenia: A review. *Clinical Research in Psychology, 1*(1), 1–7.

59. Reinert, M., Fritze, D., & Nguyen, T. (2021, October). *The state of mental health in America 2022.* Mental Health America.

60. Rocamora-Montenegro, M., Compañ-Gabucio, L. M., & Garcia de la Hera, M. (2021). Occupational therapy interventions for adults with severe mental illness: A scoping review. *BMJ Open, 11*(10), e047467.

61. Rose, G. M., & Tadi, P. (2022, July 4). Social anxiety disorder. *StatPearls* [Internet]. https://www.ncbi.nlm.nih.gov/books/NBK555890

62. Sapolosky, R. M. (2004). *Why zebras don't get ulcers.* Holt Paperbacks.

63. Shimada, T., Ohori, M., Inagaki, Y., Shimooka, Y., Ishihara, I., Sugimura, N., Tanaka, S., & Kobayashi, M. (2019). Effect of adding individualized occupational therapy to standard care on rehospitalization of patients with schizophrenia: A 2-year prospective cohort study. *Psychiatry and Clinical Neurosciences, 73*(8), 476–485.

64. Sørlie, C., Cowan, M., Chacksfield, J., Vaughan, E., & Atler, K. E. (2020). Occupation-focused assessment in eating disorders: Preliminary utility. *Occupational Therapy in Mental Health, 36*(2), 145–161.

65. Svensson, B., Hansson, L., & Lexén, A. (2018). Outcomes of clients in need of intensive team care in flexible assertive community treatment in Sweden. *Nordic Journal of Psychiatry, 72*(3), 226–231.

66. Swarbrick, M., & Noyes, S. (2018). Effectiveness of occupational therapy services in mental health practice. *American Journal of Occupational Therapy, 75*(5), 7205170010p1–7205170010p4.

67. Tan, B.-L., Zhen Lim, M. W., Xie, H., Li, Z., & Lee, J. (2020). Defining occupational competence and occupational identity in the context of recovery in schizophrenia. *American Journal of Occupational Therapy, 74*, 7404205120p1–7404205120p13.

68. Taylor, R. R. (2020). *The intentional relationship: Occupational therapy and use of self.* F.A. Davis.

69. Thapar, A., Cooper, M., Eyre, O., & Langley, K. (2013). What have we learnt about the causes of ADHD? *The Journal of Child Psychology and Psychiatry, 54*(1), 3–16.

70. United States Department of Health and Human Services, Office of Disease Prevention and Health Promotion. (2022). *Healthy People 2030: Building a healthier future for all.* https://health.gov/healthypeople

71. Van der Kolk, B. (2014). *The body keeps the score: Brain, mind, and body in the healing of trauma.* Viking Penguin Group.

72. Wagman, P., Hjärthag, F., Håkansson, C., Hedin, K., & Gunnarsson, A. B. (2021). Factors associated with higher occupational balance in people with anxiety and/or depression who require occupational therapy treatment. *Scandinavian Journal of Occupational Therapy, 28*(6), 426–432.

73. Wallace, S., Mactaggart, I., Banks, L. M., Polack, S., & Kuper, H. (2020). Association of anxiety and depression with physical and sensory functional difficulties in adults in five population-based surveys in low and middle-income countries. *PLoS One, 15*(6), e0231563.

74. Wicniowiecka-Kowalnik, B., & Nowakowska, B. A. (2019). Genetics and epigenetics of autism spectrum disorder: Current evidence in the field. *Journal of Applied Genetics, 60*, 37–47.

75. World Health Organization. (2012). *World Health Organization Disability Assessment Schedule 2.0. (WHODAS 2.0).* https://www.who.int/standards/classifications/international-classification-of-functioning-disability-and-health/who-disability-assessment-schedule

76. World Health Organization. (2021). *Comprehensive mental health action plan 2013–2030.* Author. License: CC BY-NC-SA 3.0 IGO.

77. World Health Organization. (2022, January 10). *Schizophrenia.* https://www.who.int/en/news-room/fact-sheets/detail/schizophrenia

78. Wy, T. J. P., & Saadabbadi, A. (2020, November 19). Schizoaffective disorder. *StatPearls* [Internet]. https://www.ncbi.nlm.nih.gov/books/NBK541012

79. Wykes, T. (2014). Cognitive-behavioral therapy and schizophrenia. *Evidence Based Mental Health, 17*(3), 67–77.

80. Zengin, G., & Huri, M. (2022). The sensory processing patterns of individuals with schizophrenia with comorbid substance use disorder. *Journal of Substance Use, 28*, 579–587.

SUGGESTED RESOURCES

Articles

Condo, C. M. (2020, March 3). "You don't look autistic": The reality of high functioning autism. *The Washington Post.* The article originally appeared in *The Washington Post* and lends itself well to a group discussion about perspective. Christine M. Condo is a writer and autism spokesperson who was diagnosed with autism spectrum disorder in 2015. She blogs about her autistic experience and is pursuing a master's degree in technical communication at George Mason University. This article is found at https://www.washingtonpost.com/lifestyle/2020/03/03/you-dont-look-autistic-reality-high-functioning-autism/

Faulkner, S. M., Drake, R. J., Ogden, M., Gardani, M., & Bee, P. E. (2022). A mixed methods expert opinion study on the optimal content and format for an occupational therapy intervention to improve sleep in schizophrenia spectrum disorders. *PLoS One, 17*(6), e0269453. This research study is mentioned in OT Hacks and provides a glimpse at the types of collaborative roles that OT professionals can have within mental health settings. Through participation in interdisciplinary research such as this, advocacy for OT's unique skill set will continue to grow. It is available at https://journals.plos.org/plosone/article?id=10.1371/journal.pone.0269453

First, M. B., Yousif, L. H., Clarke, D. E., Wang, S. P., Gogtay, N., & Appelbaum, P. S. (2022, June). DSM-5-TR: Overview of what's new and what's changed. *World Psychiatry, 21*(2), 218–219. This article presents a succinct overview and summary of the additions and changes to the *DSM-5-TR.* It is located at https://onlinelibrary.wiley.com/doi/pdf/10.1002/wps.20989

Oexle, N., Hum, B., & Corrigan, P. W. (2018). Understanding mental illness stigma toward persons with multiple stigmatized conditions: Implications of intersectionality theory. *Psychiatric Services, 69*, 587–589. In this article, the authors discuss the effects and consequences of disadvantage among people with mental illness who are members of multiple stigmatized social groups. Recommendations for more effective interventions for marginalized groups are discussed. The approaches to intervention suggested in this article, including both educational approaches and contact-based individualized interventions that consider the unique and diverse needs of the individual in community-based or natural environments, are roles where occupational therapy professionals' skill sets would be excellent matches for collaborating with this population. This article is found at https://ps.psychiatryonline.org/doi/epdf/10.1176/appi.ps.201700312

Books

Buser, S., & Cruz, L. (2022). *DSM-5-TR insanely simplified: Unlocking the Spectrums within DSM-5-TR and ICD-10*. Chiron Publications.

This book provides a summary of the key concepts of the new diagnostic schema introduced in the *DSM-5-TR*. The text is an excellent reference for mental health practitioners and students that is full of cartoons, mnemonic devices, and summary tables that will help occupational therapy professionals and those interested in working with clients with mental illness to understand the breadth and depth of concepts related to psychiatric diagnoses.

Videos

In May 2022, a press release announced that the American Psychiatric Association (APA) would collaborate with YouTube to develop mental health content based on facts and evidence. The APA received approval as an accredited health educator. The following link is the result of this ongoing collaborative project. https://www.youtube.com/c/AmericanPsychiatricAssociation

Learn more about the experience of selective mutism from the perspective of three families who are each raising a child with this diagnosis, in a documentary titled *"Raising A Child With Selective Mutism: My Child Won't Talk"* (Length of Video 48:40). https://www.youtube.com/watch?v=gONZsyo9Rdk.

Websites

The AOTA's evidence-based practice and knowledge translation link listed here has a wide variety of resources such as:
- The *American Journal of Occupational Therapy* (AJOT) Systematic Review Collection
- Critically Appraised Topics
- Occupational Therapy Practice Guidelines
- HOT Evidence Infographics
- Evidence Connection Collection

https://www.aota.org/practice/practice-essentials/evidencebased-practice knowledge-translation

The cross-cutting symptom measures, symptom severity rating scales, and other assessments such as the *Cultural Formation Interview* (CFI) that are covered in Section III of the *DSM-5-TR* are available online at: https://www.psychiatry.org/psychiatrists/practice/dsm/educational-resources/assessment-measures

Also available at the same address, practitioners can access the *DSM-5 Self-Rated Level 1 Cross-Cutting Symptom Measure–Adult*; the *Parent/Guardian-Rated DSM-5 Level 1 Cross-Cutting Symptom Measure–Child Age 6–17*; and the *Clinician-Rated Dimensions of psychosis Symptom Severity Scales.*

World Health Organization. (2012). *Measuring health and disability: Manual for WHO Disability Assessment Schedule (WHODAS 2.0)*. https://www.who.int/publications/i/item/measuring-health-and-disability-manual-for-who-disability-assessment-schedule-(-whodas-2.0)

CHAPTER

5

Human Occupation and Mental Health Throughout the Life Span With Those We Serve

OT HACKS OVERVIEW

O: Occupation as a means and an end

Occupational Performance and Occupational Participation over the life span

T: Theoretical concepts, values, and principles, or historical foundations

Skills and abilities associated with mental health and mental disorders

H: How can we Help? OT's role in serving clients with mental illness or mental health needs

How can Occupational Therapy help? Considerations across the life span when working with those with mental health difficulties and mental disorders

A: Adaptations

Adaptations and compensations can help those with mental health difficulties and mental disorders without the skills and abilities to complete desired occupational performance.

C: Case study includes

Case study of a child with Attention-Deficit/Hyperactivity Disorder and Oppositional Defiant Disorder

K: Knowledge: keeping mental health OT practice grounded in evidence, in occupational science, and in research

Knowledge gained with Evidence-Based Practice example

S: Some terms that may be new to you

Accumbens

Amygdala

Anterior cingulate cortex

Athleticism

Co-occupation

Environmental factors

Hippocampus

Parentified child

Prefrontal cortex

Realistic period

Splitting

Tentative period

Triangulation

INTRODUCTION

The desire to act upon the environment and to have an effect is a force that drives and shapes human behavior from birth to death. Occupation is essential for human growth and development. The focus and specifics of occupation change throughout life as the playing child matures into the working adult, who later retires and is occupied with nonwork activities. The foundation of occupation-related habits and skills formed in childhood profoundly influences all later development. Without participation in occupation, growth is frustrated and impaired. The ability to engage in occupation is one of the signs of mental health, and mental disorders can interfere with a person's ability to carry out daily occupations and to fulfill occupational roles. Because of factors such as mental health medical care and comorbidity of physical illness, those with serious mental disorders have a decreased life expectancy of 10 to 25 years (21).

This chapter considers how participation in occupation develops and changes as the person matures and ages. It looks at some of the common mental health problems and mental disorders[1] that arise in different life stages. It is an overview of the mental health needs of clients of various ages and the ways in which occupational therapy intervenes to help them. Take, for instance, the diagnosis of depression. During the early stage of life, children with depression experience difficulties such as problems at school, decreased social participation, losing interest in activities that were previously done for fun, changes with weight or in diet, anxiety, and having difficulty with family relationships. The adolescent can have the same

---

[1]All mental disorder diagnoses information is taken from the *DSM-5* (2), unless specified otherwise.

problems as a younger child and can incur lengthy mood changes, relationship problems with friends, lashing out at others and unusual levels of irritability, feeling worthless, having anger, sleeping or eating too much, and committing self-harm behaviors such as cutting or substance abuse. During adulthood, the person can have extended feelings of sadness and emptiness, experience irritability, and changes in cognition. In addition, adults may have violent behaviors toward others. The older adult can experience sleep difficulties, physical symptoms, social isolation, and suicide attempts (25).

This chapter particularly emphasizes the occupational aspects of these mental health problems and mental disorders and the role of occupational therapy in evaluation and intervention. Occupational therapy interventions for these groups focus on age-appropriate occupational roles and the skills that support them. The aim always is to promote participation in occupational performance to the extent possible. Consider again the diagnosis of depression. Apple has been noted to be working on depression symptom identification via recognition of changes in user facial features. Consider how people at different times in their lives interact with their cellular phone. As occupational therapy professions, we can utilize new technologies to assist our clients with sustaining mental well-being and helping them become more self-aware of their personal needs regarding a mental disorder (76).

This chapter also addresses the needs of family members (parents, siblings, partners, spouses, and children) of persons with severe and persistent mental illness. The chapter includes the needs of specialized populations within age categories, such as veterans with mental disorders.

While reading this chapter, the reader should examine Table 5.1, which summarizes aspects of human occupation for each age group and lists major mental disorders that typically make their first appearance in the respective age groups. A case study later in the chapter illustrates the interactions among developmental tasks (20), the development of human occupation, environmental risk factors, and age-specific vulnerabilities to mental illness.

Table 5.1. Some Aspects of Development of Human Occupation and Risks of Mental Disorders by Age Group

	Childhood	Adolescence	Adulthood	Later Adulthood
Percentage average of people experiencing mental health disorders during life stage[a]	35% between 11 and 15 yr of age	51% at age 21 48% at age 26	46% at age 32 44% at age 45	No data available
Onset of major mental disorders	Attention-deficit/hyperactivity disorder, autism spectrum disorder, obsessive–compulsive disorder, oppositional defiant disorder	Schizophrenia, substance-related disorders, bipolar and depressive disorders, personality disorders	Schizophrenia, bipolar and depressive disorders, substance abuse	Neurocognitive disorders such as Alzheimer, vascular, and other dementias; depression; polysubstance abuse (prescription medications, alcohol)
Volition	Personal causation developing through social interactions and play; values of culture taught; interests enacted through choice of activity	Increasing drive for autonomy; considering choice of occupation; weighing parental vs peer values; shifting interests affected by peer or environmental pressure	Maturation of personal causation, interests, values culminating in choice of occupation; values increasingly important in motivating behavior; interests possibly not addressed by work; avocational activities possibly especially fulfilling	Sense of efficacy possibly challenged by diminished physical capacity; importance (value) of work possibly declining as family and social values increase; opportunity in retirement to pursue interests more rigorously
Habituation	Self-maintenance habits; routines established by parental scheduling; gradual shift to more control by child; student, friend roles learned	Exploration of roles; role experimentation; expanded; more independent student role; first enactment of worker role; increasing self-regulation; acquisition of habits of time management	Multiple roles (spouse, parent, worker, friend, volunteer, church member); despite role conflict, multiple role involvement satisfying; habits and routines influenced by need to manage time for multiple involvements	Potential loss of major roles and role companions through retirement, physical disease, death (work role, spouse role, friend role); family roles and social roles increase in importance; habits of a lifetime well established; new habits hard to acquire

Table 5.1. Some Aspects of Development of Human Occupation and Risks of Mental Disorders by Age Group (*continued*)

	Childhood	Adolescence	Adulthood	Later Adulthood
Performance capacity	Tremendous development of skills transforming from helpless infant to active agent in worlds of family, play, school; age of exploration and increasing competence; co-occupations frequent	Continued development of skills in motor, process, communication, interaction; social relations with peers fostering expanded communication and interaction skills; co-occupations with peers	Peak abilities; mastery of many work-related skills; declining capacity may come from physical changes leading to reduced energy, need for eyeglasses, hearing aids; continued high level of involvement helping sustain greatest capacity and skill level; co-occupations within family, community, and workplace	Age-related changes in musculoskeletal, neurologic, cardiopulmonary systems varying in intensity; adjustments, adaptations to continue using skills (eg, energy conservation, pacing, rest periods); adaptive equipment, environmental aids helping sustain skills; may rely on others for personal care as capacities diminish
Occupational identity	Imagine their life story unfolding by narrating parts of their lives and sorting out meaning through stories; identity begins to emerge and by end of this stage the child has fairly well-developed sense of who they are	Greater ownership over forming own life story; early on focus is on enjoyment and then moves toward choosing roles and activities of adulthood; makes choices based on values	Regular reassessment of life story; move from an early focus on competence and achievement to a later focus of being concerned with value and personal satisfaction; seek control and direction over life with positive result of well-being or negative result of compromise, conflict, or catastrophe	Life story is organized and shared with others; a review of life needs to recognize its worth and importance; fulfilling cultural ideal of life instills comfort; transition to retirement and avocational activities
Occupational competence	Ability acquired to integrate past, present, and future; correlates to social norms and expectations; discover and pursue own interests and aptitudes	Connect present activities with the future outcomes and possibilities; make vocational and relationship choices; work on sense of capacity and feelings of efficacy	Change vocational roles, relationship type, or lifestyle based on change in occupational identity; explore worth of their lives' actions and life's meaning	Need for continued engagement in meaningful activities that being satisfaction with performance

Information from Taylor, R. R. (2017). *Model of human occupation* (5th ed.). Wolters Kluwer.
[a]Caspi, A., Houts, R. M., Ambler, A., Danese, A., Elliot, M. L., Hariri, A., Harrington, H., Hogan, S., Poulton, R., Ramrakha, S., Hartmann Rasmussen, L. J., Reuben, A., Richmond-Rakerd, L., Sugden, K., Wertz, J., Williams, B. S., & Moffitt, T. E. (2020). Longitudinal assessment of mental health disorders and comorbidities across 4 decades among participants in the Dunedin birth cohort study. *JAMA Network Open, 3*(4), 1–14.

CHANGES IN OCCUPATION OVER THE LIFE SPAN

Occupation develops and changes throughout life. This change occurs over a continuum from exploration to competence and finally to achievement (54).

- *Exploration* is the first stage of development and encompasses new roles, new environments, lifestyle changes, and reorganizing oneself after a major life event or circumstance. During this stage we try out new ways of learning and come to understand our capacities, preferences, and values. We make role changes, search for new meaning, discover new ways of doing, learn new ways to express our abilities, and come to understand our connection to life around us. This is a time period for trying new methods of performance and the requirements put on us by others are not overdemanding. We need to explore and

to discover in this safe environment because we are unsure of our capabilities and our desire to participate and perform in occupations. The environment should be one that offers resources and opportunities (67).

- *Competency* is the second stage of development, and it is a time to solidify new ways of doing that we discovered during the exploration stage. We want to improve our abilities and demonstrate that we can adequately meet the demands of various situations. We aim to adjust to the demands of the environment and the growing expectations of others. These newly gained abilities lead to developing new skills and to the refinement of skills that were learned during the previous stage. Our skills are organized into habits that support our occupational performance. We have a growing sense of personal control over our actions and our environment. We strive to organize our occupational performance into routines that demonstrate we are competent regarding how to perform within our chosen environments. We are moving toward a greater sense of self-efficacy, or the idea that we have control over our ability to produce the result we desire when working with others and within different environments (67).

- *Achievement* is the final stage of development, and when we are in this stage we have sufficient skills and habits for us to have full occupational participation in new situations, environments, and when asked to interact with new people and produce new meaningful outcomes. We are integrating new areas of occupational participation into our total life picture. Our occupational identity is reshaped to include new areas of occupational participation, alter current roles and current routines, and, thus, accommodate for a new overall pattern of occupational performance that will sustain our competence with our occupations (67).

Exploration, competency, and achievement form a continuum that gradually transform playful exploration into competent performance and ultimately into achievement and excellence. The skills that the child learns through play are gradually practiced and refined and finally polished and combined with other skills to enable more sophisticated and complex behavior to emerge.

Whenever the individual encounters novelty in the environment, these three levels of motivation are reexperienced in sequence. New situations and unfamiliar environments bring out the urge to explore, then to become competent, and then to achieve. This is as true of the working adult and the retiree as of the preschool child. For instance, when older persons move away from the vocational environment, they begin to explore the past and their own life's accomplishments; as they move forward, they begin to explore their present capabilities through avocational pursuits. This change encourages a desire for new competence and new achievement, beyond what was gained earlier in life (67).

At different times over the life span, there are different types of change. Change is ongoing and is both incremental and transformational. Different levels of development predominate at different stages in life. For instance, the child engages in occupation primarily because of a motive to explore, the adolescent does so to become competent, and the adult, to achieve. As a person develops and changes, and as various events and environments are a part of one's life span, change is transformational, or as sociocultural influences appear in one's life, one experiences different reasons for change. Exploration, competence, and achievement mix and overlap over the life span, making change a complex process that does not have clear start and stop points, but rather is an intertwined process that moves across the development continuum (67).

As one considers the life span and development, different occupational aspects take precedence and fill larger portions of our time. In childhood, more time is initially spent in play, activities of daily living (ADLs), and social participation. Time begins to shift toward education, some work occupations, and a beginning awareness of health management. In adulthood, work is the main consumer of time, along with instrumental ADLs and health management, with social participation remaining a constant consideration and a minimal amount of time spent toward leisure or play. During later adulthood, occupations such as ADLs, health management, and leisure are more heavily experienced, again, with social participation remaining a mainstay experience throughout this stage of life (67).

This picture of occupation over the life span in no way diminishes experiencing occupations such as education throughout adulthood, or work during later adulthood—each person's experience is individual to their personal factors and **environmental factors**. Every person is continually seeking to establish and enhance their occupational identity while gaining occupational competence with their desired participation in occupation (67).

THE ROLE OF CO-OCCUPATIONS THROUGHOUT THE LIFE SPAN

Before we can focus on the development of occupational performance and the influence of mental disorders on this process throughout the life span, we need to stop and consider co-occupation. For the most part, we are not lone islands existing in life with experiences circulating around us, rather than us participating with those experiences. We interact with others, depend on others, and seek others as a part of our occupational existence. Thus, we need to consider how co-occupations impact occupational development.

Co-occupations are those that involve two or more people and are by nature highly interactive and transactional (50). They are characterized by a back-and-forth involvement in which the actions of each participant shape the actions of another (50). A range of co-occupations exist, with varying degrees of sharing of physical space, emotions, intentions, time, and social influences and support (49, 50). Occupations done in a parallel fashion, such as reading near another person while the other person listens to music or plays a video game, are also considered co-occupations. In addition, co-occupations include shared occupations such as different people in the same kitchen preparing different dishes for an upcoming meal (79). Co-occupations provide opportunities for learning and change though the dynamic exchanges among the persons involved (51). Occupation throughout life comprises a mixture of co-occupation and solitary occupation.

At the beginning of life, the infant depends upon the parents for everything. Giving care to the child is a major occupation for parents. What has been the parents' solitary occupation or co-occupation with each other evolves into co-occupation with the child. As the baby develops, the parents engage them to participate as possible in feeding, communication, bathing, dressing, toileting, etc. These are occupations shared jointly by infant and caregiver, with the caregiver ideally serving in a teaching, assisting, and coaching role, allowing more participation as the child becomes capable. Studies show that co-occupation increases cognitive and emotional capacities, self-identity and awareness of self, and social interaction (51). Co-occupation is believed to foster brain growth and an increase in behavioral repertoire and expressed emotional range (51).

For the maturing child, co-occupations with peers and siblings include play and eventually chores, and as the child develops more ability and independence, it may expand to care of pets or the home, religious activities, shopping, etc.

The occupational life of the adolescent includes many co-occupations, generally with peers. School projects, clubs and sports, parties, and social life are some examples. Nonetheless, the adolescent also engages in some solitary occupations, such as study. The same is true of the adult, whose work may involve others or may be done alone, and who may become involved in a great variety of social and leisure and community activities.

As people age, and particularly as their performance skills diminish because of primary aging factors, co-occupations become more common. The older adult may require assistance with home management, meal preparation, functional mobility, ADLs, etc. Thus, often but not always, the older adult depends upon others to perform some part of occupations that were once done alone. If the person becomes more dependent because of deteriorating health and reduced capacities, the person may need others to perform some occupations on their behalf. Thus, an older adult may delegate to someone else the responsibility for paying bills (as an example).

INFANCY AND CHILDHOOD

Development

Babies start life with enormous needs and wants and absolutely no ability to satisfy them on their own. Parents must be able to figure out what babies want—whether the infant is hungry or thirsty or needs to be burped or cuddled or changed—and then provide it. To be able to relate to other people later and to engage in activities that involve others, infants and small children need to learn to trust their parents and then people in general. In addition, they need to learn to communicate their needs and feelings and to control their impulses. Thoughtful interaction and consistent discipline by the parents help the child acquire these skills. A stable, secure, and predictable environment is one of the most important factors in helping the child at any age to develop trust in self, other people, and the world in general.

While all this psychosocial development is going on, the child is developing in other ways too. Sensory abilities are becoming more refined, motor skills better coordinated, and perceptual and cognitive abilities more complex. The young child constantly uses and refines developing abilities to learn more about the world and how to interact with it.

All the experiences the developing infant and toddler are incurring create pathways within the brain toward continued occupational participation and performance. Motivation to experience events and situations, or to avoid them, starts early in a person's development and continues throughout life. The process of laying down neural pathways for the motivation system is as follows (39):

- **Prefrontal cortex, anterior cingulate cortex,** and **hippocampus** assess information coming in from the environment.
- When the child experiences a rewarding response to a situation, there is a surge of dopamine production. This is a signal to the child to expect being in a situation that is pleasing and valuable to seek out in the future.
- This dopamine surge also communicates to the substantia nigra and ventral tegmental area for dopamine to be released to structures such as the hippocampus, which assists with memory, and the **amygdala**, which is associated with emotions.
- Thus, the rewarding experience is connected to the memory of the pleasure received and strong positive emotions the child felt.
- The child can develop a "wanting" desire for the reward. This "wanting" desire is increased through the dopamine pathway. The dopamine pathway is robust and crosses various areas of the brain, such as the prefrontal cortex (which manages executive functions and self-regulating behavior), the anterior cingulate cortex (which tracks behavior and monitors the environment, alerting the child when behavior needs to be modified and stimulating the prefrontal cortex to manage behavior and decision-making), and the ventral tegmental area. Dopamine modulates the neural activity that occurs when the rewarding situation occurs. When behaviors or actions are done that elicit the rewarding situation, dopamine is increased, which in turn leads the child to seek out the rewarding experience again. The brain, over time, even when the stimulus is diminished or removed, still produces a "wanting" desire.
- The child can also develop a "liking" pleasure for the reward. This "liking" pleasure is a part of the serotonin pathway. Serotonin is produced by the raphe nuclei. Serotonin, in combination with other neurochemicals, must be received by specific areas of the brain to produce a "liking" feeling or emotion. This system is more fragile than the dopamine pathway and is less easily activated.
- Thus, it can be harder for a person to feel actual "liking" or pleasure versus feeling a "wanting" or desire. For instance, watching a show about being asked to a school dance or festival may trigger a "wanting" to attend such an event, based on memories of such activities. However, actually attending the dance or festival may not offer as much pleasure or "liking" as expected.
- A feeling of "liking" can trigger a "wanting." For instance, if the person finds attending the school dance or festival pleasurable, and is "liking" the experience, that can trigger a "wanting" desire to stay much longer than originally anticipated. The person may want to extend the whole social experience by continuing the social event—deciding

to "go out to eat" after the dance or festival or hang out for the rest of the evening at a friend's house.

- The repeated experiences a child has and the different associations the child has build different pathways, such as the dopamine pathway or the serotonin pathway.
- Pathways such as these link what the child does (actions and behaviors) and memories of the feelings and emotions associated with those actions and behaviors. Emotions, or "emotion triggers," are processed by the amygdala. This processed information then drives continued behavior, which is managed by the prefrontal cortex and the anterior cingulate cortex.
- A main task of the amygdala, when triggered by environmental information, is to alert the child of a situation to avoid. The amygdala quickly assesses the information and detects threats. If needed, stress hormones are released, leading the child to avoid continuing their current behavior or action.
- In the future, the child is motivated to repeat experiences that made them feel good and to avoid experiences that produced negative feelings or emotions. The evaluation of good feelings versus bad feelings, in response to a situation, is done by the nucleus **accumbens**, which acts as the "reward anticipator."

As the infant moves through the time of early development and into early childhood, play is the main occupation of the child. Research confirms that play is essential for later development (3). Studies of many species show that important neurologic connections are formed in their greatest numbers during the period when play is most vigorous in a young animal. These connections establish a foundation for skillful, responsive motor actions.

Play has been found to be a method for young animals to practice and rehearse the subtle social behaviors they will need as adults (3). Similarly, imitation and exploration of future occupational roles are enacted as child's play. Through fantasy and imitation, the child investigates and experiences various adult roles (parent, doctor, teacher, and so on). This experience is part of the fantasy period of occupational choice and is the first step toward choosing a career or adult vocation (23).

Gradually, as children are assigned chores and other responsibilities at home and in school, they spend some of their time in activities that must be classified as work. The purpose of play and work in childhood is distinctive. As children play, they explore their environments, learn about reality, and develop rules that are used to guide actions. For example, the child learns that objects fall to the floor when dropped, that a stove is sometimes hot, and that a favorite uncle or aunt will allow things that a parent will not. These rules about motions, objects, and people (55) are tools that the child uses to guide future action and to develop skills. This childhood learning about how the world functions is a foundation upon which later accomplishments are built. Thus, the playing child acquires knowledge and develops rules and skills that underlie and support the work of the student and the adult worker.

Although the child is not typically expected to do a great amount of work, the productive activities of the child are very important for later development. Studies have shown that industriousness in childhood is associated with job success and personal adjustment in adult life (72). Chores and schoolwork are the major productive activities of childhood. By engaging in these tasks over time, the child acquires habits of industry and responsibility and learns to schedule activities so that time also remains for play. Some tasks, such as handwriting, have clear associations with work. Even very young children can describe the difference between work and play and may describe their time in school as "work" (34). Although play remains the major occupation throughout childhood, the maturing child spends increasing amounts of time in activities that lay a foundation for the future role of adult worker. Habits and routines are developed and established.

During times of childhood play, joy can be experienced, because of the sense of having an effect on the world and on other people. These positive emotions associated with play help form an image of the self as personally effective and powerful, thus developing and enhancing a sense of personal causation. The pleasure that the child takes in one activity over another helps form interests that will motivate life choices.

As the child moves into the grade school years, the child refines growing abilities in many areas. The roles of student and contributing family member are gradually adopted. The child develops a more sophisticated awareness of social norms and expectations and of the needs of others, learning to delay gratification for increasingly longer and longer periods. In addition, the child becomes physically better coordinated and more intellectually sophisticated. Vast amounts of knowledge and increasingly complex skills are acquired through schoolwork and peer relationships. Habits and routines are improved and develop a greater complexity.

The child continues to need the love, support, and encouragement of parents and family to feel secure enough to attempt new challenges. Some mental health professionals have suggested that the family has such an effect on the mental health of the child that it may be the cause of emotional and behavioral problems. Others believe that the family is a factor but that biologic predisposition and experiences at school and elsewhere are also involved. Yet others suggest that the peer group is the most influential factor (26).

Mental Health Factors

Infancy and Early Childhood

It is unusual for mental health problems to be diagnosed in infancy. Often problems that are brought to the attention of psychiatric professionals are quite severe. Some of these problems are believed to have biologic causes, meaning that the behavioral or emotional disorder is caused at least in part by something physical within the body or the brain.

Intellectual disability, attention-deficit/hyperactivity disorder (ADHD), and autism spectrum disorder (ASD) are in this category.

Intellectual disability is characterized by general mental ability deficits and everyday activity functioning impairments. Forms vary from mild to profound. At the most disabled level, the child expresses desires and emotions nonverbally and may be totally dependent on others for physical care. Depending on the severity, the diagnosis may be made in infancy or during the school years.

ASD features include social–emotional reciprocity and social interaction with persistent impairment; behaviors, interests, or activities that are done in repetitive patterns and that are restricted; an onset from early childhood; and everyday functioning that is limited or impaired. Motor deficits may be noted, such as use of an odd gait or clumsiness. Intellectual impairment may also be seen. Children with ASD differ from children who do not have ASD, in the way they process and understand sensation (74). The child is usually slow to develop language skills, the learning of which seems to rely upon interactions with others.

Another serious mental health problem of early childhood is reactive attachment disorder, in which the child stops responding to other people because they have been neglected or ignored. If appropriate caregiving is not restored, social functioning problems can persist into the teenage years. It is easy to understand how the absence of normal co-occupation in early childhood would impair development and social attachment.

Middle Childhood

Centered in the middle childhood years are mental disorders of anxiety and impulse control. The median age of onset for these disorders is 11 years (29). Problems that are identified in children during these years are the disruptive, impulse control, and conduct disorders, in which the child behaves in an antisocial fashion (eg, stealing, skipping school). Other disorders may show up in physical behaviors (such as eating problems, stuttering, bedwetting).

Frequent and persistent patterns of angry and irritable moods, argumentative and defiant behaviors, or vindictiveness are features of oppositional defiant disorder (ODD). Children diagnosed with conduct disorder repetitively and persistently violate the basic rights of others, as well as violate other age-appropriate social norms or rules.

Social anxiety disorder includes an intense fear or anxiety of being scrutinized by others during social situations. Social situations are avoided, and their fear is out of proportion to an actual threat within the sociocultural context.

The child with obsessive–compulsive disorder (OCD) may be fearful and anxious and may use ritual behaviors (such as ordering, checking, or touching things) to cope with these feelings. The ritual behaviors interfere with success in school and may prevent the child from making friends. This disorder is generally treated with medication.

The child with ADHD has a shorter attention span than is normal for a child of similar age. Jumping from activity to activity, the child demonstrates a high level of energy (hyperactivity). It is difficult for the child to concentrate long enough to finish many of the tasks they have attempted. Impulsivity associated with ADHD manifests as hasty actions done without forethought that have a potential to be dangerous, social intrusions during others' conversations and activities, and important decisions made for future situations without consideration of possible long-term effects.

Regardless of diagnosis, it is common for children with mental health disorders to have deficits in **executive functions**, the skills used to plan, prioritize, make connections, and remember information (14). Children may be misperceived as lazy or unmotivated when the real problem is that they lack the thinking skills needed for a specific task, or for many tasks. The negative and lasting consequences may be poor performance in school and lifelong difficulties with work. Thus, when providing interventions, occupational therapy professionals should incorporate an awareness of how executive functions (or the lack thereof) may be affecting a child's occupational performance.

Occupational Therapy

Infancy and Early Childhood

Occupational therapy for children with these disorders presenting in early childhood often focuses on sensorimotor, sensory integrative, or sensory processing intervention approaches, which are believed to affect underlying physiologic systems. Occupational therapy assistants may carry out such interventions only under the direct supervision of occupational therapists with special training in these approaches. A behaviorally oriented treatment approach focuses on the development of self-care skills (eg, brushing teeth or shoe tying) through direct instruction and reinforcement.

Building a trusting relationship and modifying the environment to enable success are often the twin foundations of intervention with children. Baron (7) presented a case study of a 4-year-old boy who had ODD. A structured play experience with the occupational therapist over many weeks helped this child give up his resentful and argumentative behavior and develop a more spontaneous and genuine approach to play. Key elements of this intervention included a slow and careful building of trust through brief, frequent, one-on-one play with activities selected by the child from limited choices presented by the occupational therapy professional; modification of the social play environment so that competition was reduced; and teaching and reinforcement of social skills such as taking turns.

Very small children with mental health problems are seldom treated as inpatients. Because of the important role of parents and family life in a child's development, the philosophy is to keep the child with the family whenever possible. Therefore, children may attend day treatment centers, special preschools, or programs at community mental health centers or may be treated at home, often with the parents participating. Services provided in the community, where the young child lives and participates in various occupations, are considered early intervention (EI) programming. EI services are centered on the family, and goals, as well as intervention areas, are determined by the parents.

Occupational therapy for infants and small children with mental health problems is considered a very demanding and complex area of practice (15). In addition to emotional and social deficits, it seems that children with mental health problems are more likely than are other children to have developmental motor delays (33). The occupational therapist uses special developmental assessments and data collection instruments, such as the play history (9, 66), to assess the child's abilities, interests, and needs. Intervention is usually highly individualized, although some may take place in groups. Groups provide an experience of co-occupation, of working with others, sharing, waiting, and taking turns—skills that prepare the child to succeed during the school years to come.

Some of the goals of occupational therapy intervention with this very young population are developing trust and social interactions, increasing gross and fine motor coordination, improving sensory processing and perceptual skills, and facilitating spontaneous play. In addition to sensorimotor and sensory integrative methods, play therapy and expressive art activities are sometimes used to help children develop and express their fantasies.

Middle Childhood

Children whose mental disorders are so severe as to require hospitalization need a different approach. Children are hospitalized only when they are in danger of harming themselves or someone else. The occupational therapist would assess problems in occupational functioning and then discuss with the team the interaction of the disorder with the ability to function in self-care, work (school, chores), and play. Sensory processing assessment is often included. The occupational therapy assistant can assist with carrying out selected assessments, as directed by the occupational therapist, contribute to discussion of the child's occupational functioning, and help formulate transition and discharge recommendations. Children who have serious problems require intensive treatment and benefit from occupational therapy intervention to improve social engagement and emotional regulation (4). The goals of intervention may include increasing trust and social relatedness; developing cooperation; improving self-esteem and self-awareness; enhancing self-control; developing body awareness and sensorimotor skills; and improving coordination, perceptual skills, and cognitive abilities.

Children who have enough control over their behavior to live in the community may reside with their families or in special residences and participate in programs for children with special needs. Depending on the child's age and specific occupational deficits, occupational therapy programs may focus on life skills; social engagement, leisure, school-related skills; and/or sensory processing and modulation (4).

Occupational therapy professionals in the community can work with parents of children who have been discharged from the hospital after a stay for treatment of a psychiatric disorder. They may be seen in school settings, in the home, in day treatment settings, or in after-school programs. These facilities have particular staff, which may include one or more occupational therapy professionals as well as teachers, child psychologists, speech language pathologists, and the usual medical staff.

Development of age-appropriate skills may lag because of the mental disorder, and parents may not know what to expect from their child or how to help. Parent expectations may be too high or too low. Occupational therapy professionals can identify the child's skill level and suggest and model appropriate play, as well as help the parent engage in problem-solving around co-occupations. Another approach is the multifamily parent–child activity-based therapy group, which gives an opportunity for children with mental disorders and their parents to do activities with other children and parents in the same situation. Activities suggested by occupational therapy are simple but require some assistance from parents. Parents can get support from others, engage their children in a spontaneous and natural way, and learn techniques for responding positively and effectively to their children (43). Olson (44) stated that parents can learn positive and supportive parenting in occupation-based groups with their children but that this requires vigilance and persistence from the group leaders because families may have long-term negative expectations and behavior patterns.

Children with mild diagnoses may be enrolled in regular public or private schools and receive occupational interventions in the school and/or in after-school programs on an outpatient basis. Many children receiving occupational therapy services in the schools for other reasons (eg, learning disability, intellectual disability) can benefit from attention to their psychosocial and psychological needs (4, 8, 57). Occupational therapy services may address learning of social and emotional regulation skills, as well as stress management training, bullying prevention, and expressive arts (4).

When identified as needs in the Individualized Education Plan (IEP), coping, communication skills, sensory regulation, and social skills for group and interpersonal interaction should be addressed. Occupational therapy groups and individual sessions are usually worked around the school schedule; another model is for the professional to consult with the teacher or carry out the program in the classroom with the assistance of the teacher.

The *Occupational Therapy Psychosocial Assessment of Learning* (OT PAL) is an example of an assessment tool that may be used to observe and measure the child's ability to function appropriately for their age in the classroom (40, 69). Parents may be involved in the evaluation process and asked to complete a sensory profile, or the Canadian Occupational Performance Measure, or history assessments. Occupational therapy assessment and intervention for school-age children address the occupational roles of the child: family member, friend, player, student, and so on (13). Children and their families can learn how to better use the environment to make it easier for the student to do homework and chores successfully. Segal and Hinojosa (60) point out that families and situations require individual analysis and individualized support.

Emotional regulation interventions aim to improve the child's ability to recognize, control, and appropriately express feelings. Children with ASD typically have problems with emotional regulation, as do other children and adolescents with mental disorders. Traditional methods have focused on identification of emotions as shown in faces on a printed page and on coaching and behavioral methods. Olson (45) suggested that smartphones and tablets provide a great deal of versatility to customize for the problems of the individual. For example, apps that coach breathing or calming behaviors can be instantly available and used independently.

Executive functions may also be a focus. Children who have these deficits have difficulty deciding what to do, organizing their thoughts to decide what to do, or even to determine what to decide about. This impairs occupational functioning in school, in the home, and in social situations. Engaging the child in occupational performance, whether in school or in the home or the community, provides opportunities to observe difficulties with executive functions (14).

Children with ADHD or learning disabilities may be taught progressive relaxation and stress management techniques. Programs focusing on social emotional learning, activity-based social skills, bullying prevention, performing arts, and life skills may also be included (4).

Children who have few or no friends and limited social skills can benefit from the opportunity to interact with peers in groups, with leadership from a skilled occupational therapy professional. Activity-based group intervention closely simulates the normal play groups of childhood and can help these children learn and practice effective social skills (8).

Children with conduct disorder may benefit from activities that promote social participation, physical exertion, and rest (78). Activities that are structured and guided by adults (such as scouting, clubs, team sports, church groups, group lessons such as swimming or martial arts) may reduce behavioral problems (78).

Applied behavioral analysis (ABA) is an intervention that targets specific behaviors (eg, sitting down) with a highly structured training regimen. In an ABA program, several helpers, and the family, work with the child intensively, repeating the same instructions and giving the same reinforcements for at least 8 hours a day. Other methods include functional behavioral analysis (FBA) and positive behavioral support (PBS). FBA looks at the student's behavior, what purposes it may serve, and how best to intervene. PBS considers how the environment may be used to strengthen and support the student. The aim is to recognize a potential problem situation and prevent problem behavior by intervening early. Clearly communicating group rules, appropriately praising, and redirecting the student's focus are some examples of supports (11, 58).

Box 5.1 lists common focuses of occupational therapy intervention used with children who have psychosocial problems.

> **BOX 5.1 Children With Psychosocial Problems: Focus of Intervention**
>
> - Child-centered, occupation-based assessment and intervention, focusing on age-appropriate roles (player, friend, self-maintainer, family member, student)
> - Mutual collaborative goal setting, including child, family, and (when relevant) teacher
> - As needed, group programming for development of social skills and play behaviors
> - Child-centered positive supports: environmental strategies to promote success, sensory regulation, and intervention and redirection to prevent disruptions
> - As needed, special interventions (applied behavioral analysis, sensory integration)
> - Education of and consultation with parents regarding appropriate expectations, behavior management, and so on
> - Scheduling compatible with school schedule and needs of family

ADOLESCENCE

Development

Adolescents, like children, continue to spend more time playing than working. However, now motivated more by the desire to become competent than by the urge to explore, they choose activities in which practice and the habits of sportsmanship and craftsmanship make the difference between success and failure. Whether the activity is the track team, the chess club, social media, photography, or video gaming, the adolescent approaches it with determination to master and succeed. The biologic changes of puberty interact with the adolescent's use of occupation to motivate a growing interest in social activities that provide opportunities to explore and practice social and sexual behaviors.

The work of the adolescent continues to consist mainly of school and chores. School work becomes more rigorous and more time consuming, in keeping with the adolescent's growing cognitive capacity and discipline. Depending on the parents and the family situation, the chores may also be increasingly challenging. Many adolescents take on part-time jobs, which provide important experiences of what life is like in the adult working world and give feedback about the adolescent's readiness for work.

Adolescents are concerned about what they will do with their lives as adults, and vocational choice is generally viewed as one of the most important developmental tasks of adolescence. The process that began in the fantasy period of childhood now enters a new stage, known as the *tentative period*. During this time, the adolescent considers possible adult vocations in the light of their individual interests and the likelihood of their success. Finally, the adolescent weighs any choice in terms of personal values and achieved or expected place in the social system. From this overwhelming mass of factors, the adolescent must finally choose a job or career path but is likely to remake this decision several times throughout life.

Once the decision is made, the adolescent begins to work toward it, for example, by enrolling in a vocational training program, academic preparedness program, or looking for a job in their chosen field of work. This begins the *realistic period*, in which the choice of career is examined in light of personal needs for achievement, satisfaction, status, and economic security. For example, if the chosen career is one in which jobs are scarce (eg, acting) or the pay is low, the person may reconsider this decision and then must come up with alternatives and choose among them.

Thus, vocational choice is crystallized and acted upon during adolescence, although for adolescent children of affluent parents, the choice may be delayed into early adulthood. By contrast, adolescents from disadvantaged backgrounds may encounter overwhelming obstacles to realizing their vocational choice. In times of high unemployment, the adolescent with few skills may be denied employment or forced into a job that is experienced as demeaning and unsatisfying. The adult who decides or is forced to change careers later in life will need to repeat the process of vocational choice.

Mental Health Factors

The most important task of adolescence is to develop an identity separate from one's parents—a social and sexual identity that will support an independent life. Other important experiences center around the peer group of other adolescents. Through a variety of interactions and relationships with others of similar age, the adolescent explores values and interests and develops social skills. It is not unusual for an adolescent to experience insecurity, mood swings, loneliness, depression, and anxiety in response to hormonal and physical changes and the increasingly demanding expectations of others, or to experiment with smoking, alcohol, sex, and drugs. These are within the range of normal responses to a challenging life adjustment. Sometimes, however, the problems are severe.

Major psychiatric disorders such as schizophrenia and bipolar disorders often make their first appearance in adolescence. Schizophrenia (see Chapter 4) is a disorder that manifests itself in extreme personal disorganization. Its psychotic symptoms, hallucinations, and delusions can usually be controlled only with medications. But even with medication, many people who have schizophrenia have difficulty setting goals or structuring their time; their sense of self-identity is frequently compromised. When schizophrenia occurs as early as adolescence, it interferes with further psychosocial development. In other words, the developmental task of forming a separate identity is extraordinarily difficult for someone with schizophrenia, and, consequently, later development suffers.

Bipolar disorders (mania with or without episodes of depression) may also first appear in adolescence. There is a better prognosis, or predicted outcome, for bipolar disorders than for schizophrenia. Nonetheless, these are serious disorders, and suicide is a growing risk among adolescents, especially those with bipolar disorders or depression.

Substance-related and addictive disorders are mental health problems that are characterized by frequent use or excessive use of drugs, alcohol, inhalants, or other mind-altering substances. Adolescents may fall into substance abuse after experimenting with drugs or alcohol to be accepted by their peers. Some adolescents who have other mental health problems use these substances as self-medication to deaden their feelings of anxiety or depression.

Eating disorders affect some adolescents. Anorexia nervosa (abnormal restriction of energy-based items leading to extreme low body weight) and bulimia nervosa (inappropriate behaviors, such as vomiting, to relieve oneself of ingested food after binging) are more common in girls than boys. Real or perceived social pressure to look thin is a contributing factor. These conditions are discussed in Chapter 4.

Because forging a personal identity is the major task of the adolescent, gender identity may be a source of confusion. Experimentation with various sexual roles can be an expression of personal preference but may also be a way of acting out against one's parents. Adolescents who are gay or lesbian or who do not identify with their biologic sex face special challenges and may feel socially isolated. Suicide rates are higher in these groups.

WHAT'S THE EVIDENCE?

Association of outdoor artificial light at night with mental disorders and sleep patterns among U.S. adolescents.

The article referenced below is a study of 10,123 adolescents, between the ages of 13 and 18 years, and the association of outdoor artificial light at night (ALAN) to sleep patterns and past-year mental disorders. Those with the highest levels of outdoor ALAN were found to go to bed on weeknights 29 minutes later than those with the lowest amount of outdoor ALAN. Higher levels of ALAN were positively associated with an increased risk of experiencing mood disorders (major depressive disorder [MDD]/dysthymia and bipolar disorders) and anxiety disorders. Outdoor ALAN was also strongly associated with social determinants of health such as adolescents of racial/ethnic minorities, adolescents from immigrant families, and adolescents from families with lower family incomes (based on census data for median household income). Finally, there was a greater association between outside ALAN and delayed weekday bedtimes correlated in those assigned the sex of female at birth and increased years of age since menarche.

Based on this information, what would be an occupational therapy professional's initial professional reasoning about the personal and environmental factors associated with clients most impacted by outside ALAN regarding delayed bedtimes for weeknights? After reading the *Diagnostic and Statistical Manual of Mental Disorders Fifth Edition Text Revision* (*DSM-5-TR*) circadian rhythm sleep–wake disorder of delayed sleep phase type information, what aspects of this disorder would alert an occupational therapy professional of potential occupational deficits or difficulties?

Paksarian, D., Rudolph, K. E., Stapp, E. K., Dunster, G. P., He, J., Mennitt, D., Hattar, S., Casey, J. A., James, P., & Merikangas, K. R. (2020). Association of outdoor artificial light at night with mental disorders and sleep patterns among US adolescents. *JAMA Psychiatry, 77*(12), 1266–1275.

Occupational Therapy

Adolescents may be seen in outpatient or community settings, such as schools, but it is not unusual for them to be hospitalized, especially when they are psychotic and in need of medication. Separate units, facilities, or adolescent services are provided wherever there are sufficient numbers of adolescent clients to justify the expense.

Erickson stated that the developmental task of adolescence is establishing personal identity and avoiding role confusion. Adolescents are highly responsive to peer pressure and may be resistant to adult instruction. The adolescent who is trying to develop a separate identity will often act out or rebel against authorities (eg, treatment staff). Working with adolescents requires the ability to tolerate and set limits on provocative and rebellious behavior while supporting reasonable attempts at independence. If the staff is too permissive or inconsistent, the adolescent fails to grasp the boundaries of reasonable behavior; on the other hand, if the staff is too punitive and restrictive, the adolescent may become withdrawn and confused. Health professionals who work with adolescents receive additional and ongoing training to improve their ability to provide structure to support the adolescent's independence while setting firm limits on unacceptable behavior. Staff members may act as surrogates for parents or may be viewed by adolescents as parent-like authorities. Adolescents may have to work through many challenges as they attempt to exercise more freedom and take increasing responsibility for their own lives.

Adolescents can be quite skillful at manipulating adults and creating conflict through defense mechanisms known as *splitting* and *triangulation*. **Splitting** is a kind of thinking that is "all or nothing," or a way of thinking that is "all good or all bad." Instead of seeing people and situations as having good and bad parts, the person sees some people as all good and others as all bad. But these are not stable views: the person who is good one day may be viewed as bad on another day. Splitting is common in adolescence, but most people grow out of it as they come to understand the complexities of themselves and others.

Triangulation occurs when the person will not communicate directly with one person (the "bad one") but only with someone who is viewed as "good." Health care students and new staff may be flattered by the attention when seen as "the good one." But this is destructive to the team and to the client's welfare. It is important that staff communicate well with each other so that they can serve the needs of adolescents effectively. The key personal qualities needed to work well with adolescents are firmness, patience, flexibility, persistence, and a sense of humor.

Occupational therapy for adolescents is a specialized practice area. In addition to the occupational profile, the occupational therapist may use specialized assessment instruments such as the *Adolescent Role Assessment* (10) to learn how the adolescent is adjusting to school, family life, and friendships. Goals of intervention may include development of self-esteem and self-identity skills, development of occupational choices, training in daily living skills, development

of sensorimotor skills (especially in relation to body image), and acquisition of school and prevocational and leisure behaviors.

In selecting activities for adolescents, occupational therapy staff must keep up with current trends in activities and technology. Franklin (22), for example, in the 1980s reported that adolescents responded more favorably to a computer-based values clarification program than to a traditional paper-and-pencil version. This was the era in which computers were first becoming available to the public. Baron (6) (also in the 1980s) incorporated computers for word processing and graphics design into the tasks available to adolescent members of a newspaper intervention group. In this group, the variety of job tasks and the structure and rules helped members acquire and develop a sense of internal control and direction. Today, smartphones, tablets, and social media are popular and common. As technology continues to evolve, occupational therapy must keep pace. Social media and online behavior should not be neglected. Adolescents diagnosed with mental disorders may require education and practice in skills such as texting, use of Instagram and TikTok, awareness of sexual predation online, and identity theft. Teens have specific texting etiquette rules, for example, and these may not be obvious to someone who has difficulties with impulse control.

In working with adolescents who have mental health problems and mental disorders, the occupational therapy professional may lead self-care and other ADL groups, provide sessions on sex education and birth control, run vocational programs such as work groups and assembly lines, and provide training in social skills. Because adolescents are still in school most of the day, occupational therapy and other clinical services are scheduled to accommodate school hours. Students with mental health problems may present behavior problems in school; occupational therapy professionals can help identify the cognitive deficits and emotional regulation factors responsible and can work with the student to develop less disruptive and more appropriate ways of coping (17). Executive functions may be diminished, and activities such as calendar planning may be used to assess and address this (68).

Many adolescents benefit tremendously from role modeling and direct training in simple meal preparation and cleanup and also in simple home management tasks such as cleaning, home maintenance, and clothing care. Working in groups to plan and carry out meals, clean and decorate rooms, create seasonal decoration allows the clients to learn and practice skills and habits in a realistic situation with normal time pressures and performance expectations individually tailored to their capacities. Meeting social expectations on an individual level is also important. The adolescent should be expected to organize their own room and care for their own clothing and personal hygiene at a socially acceptable level. This is fundamental to establishing regular routines and habits.

Evidence exists that social skills programming is particularly effective for adolescents with severe disorders (7). Sensory regulation programs and cognitive interventions may be used with some groups. Leisure and physical education activities are essential. To promote free exchange of feelings and ideas about body image and self-esteem, it is recommended that males and females be seen, at least some of the time, in separate groups for physical activities such as weight training, aerobics, or yoga. Information about human sexuality and universal precautions can also be a part of the occupational therapy programming.

Adolescents experiencing the first onset of schizophrenia will generally have difficulty functioning in school and peer situations owing to sensory distractions from hallucinations and other perceptual distortions. When the teenager was previously functioning well, others may believe that they are simply not trying hard enough. Educating teachers, classmates, and family about the nature of the specific mental disorder can help adjust unrealistic expectations (18). These adolescents may benefit from accommodations such as a shorter school day with a later start, a distraction-free study area, a smaller classroom, and one-on-one tutoring. Stress management training, sensory regulation programs, and strategies from Allen's cognitive disabilities approach may be useful.

In general, the occupational therapy professional working with the adolescent who has a mental disorder will focus on the younger person's "occupations and interests of choice rather than the disorder" (24, p. 2). This is a client-centered practice in which the occupational therapy professional asks the person to identify goals that are personally important. Ideally, the activities should be identified by the adolescent as important, but often the person is unable to identify interests even with the aid of an interest checklist. The person may lack confidence and fear failure. With limited social skills and little history of success, this should not seem surprising. By attending to preferences of the adolescent, the occupational therapy professional may gradually introduce new activities and encourage development of communication and social skills. A study by Oxer and Miller (46) showed that providing choices of activities and objects facilitates participation. The occupational therapy professional then creates strategies and interventions to work toward those goals; the client is continually involved in evaluating whether the plan is working and in determining future goals of interest.

Box 5.2 lists common focuses of occupational therapy intervention used with adolescents who have psychosocial problems.

BOX 5.2 Adolescents With Psychosocial Problems: Focus of Intervention

- Occupation-based assessment and intervention, focusing on age-appropriate roles (player, friend, self-maintainer, family member, student, worker)
- Mutual collaborative goal setting, empowering adolescent to set goals for self, including family and (when relevant) teacher
- Attention to the development of occupational choice for education, training, and career

- As needed, group programming for development of communication and social skills
- Use of social media and technology as well as virtual communities, as appropriate
- Education in special needs of this age group (sexuality, gender identity, prevention of substance abuse)
- Education of and consultation with parents regarding appropriate expectations, coaching techniques, behavior management, and so on
- As appropriate, sensory regulation programming and cognitive retraining or compensation techniques
- Scheduling compatible with school schedule and needs of family

---

ADULTHOOD

Development

The adult spends many hours working, leaving little time for play or leisure. The work of the adult centers on the occupational role selected through the process of occupational choice. This work, which is not necessarily salaried (consider the homemaker), consumes much time and energy and allows for expression and gratification of the urge to achieve. For many adults, there is the additional work of parenthood.

Adults work to provide for their own needs and those of their families. Beyond this, they work to produce something of value to the rest of society. Having a productive work role is important for the self-esteem of the adult; it bestows a sense of identity, a place in the social hierarchy, and a reason for being. Adults who are unemployed or underemployed (working at jobs that are beneath their capacities) may hold negative views of their own abilities and worth. They may see themselves as incompetent and helpless rather than as competent and achieving members of society.

Despite working adults often having little time for play or leisure, the time they spend in leisure and recreation serves an important function: it restores and refreshes their energies to work again. Recreation is intended to restore a person's capacity to once again be able to labor. Different people feel different degrees of need for recreation; some people spend almost all their time working, leaving only negligible amounts for play, and appear to be quite satisfied and happy. Others limit their working hours precisely because they want to make time for leisure pursuits.

In middle and later adulthood, the individual looks toward the future and thus toward retirement. They begin to explore and plan for this next stage of their life. The major issue is the replacement of work with some other occupation that will fill the hours and compensate for the loss of the worker role and of the social relationships with coworkers. Statements of people anticipating retirement were analyzed and classified into three different types (30):

- regressive (anxious and uncertain, dreading the future)
- stable (expecting little change—may be either positive or negative)

BOX 5.3 Sample Statements of Persons Anticipating Retirement

Regressive: "I can't imagine not going to work. I don't have a plan for how to spend the time."

Stable (positive): "I do so many things now that I will be continuing [golf, volunteer at church], that I think very little will change except maybe I'll have more time."

Stable (negative): "Well, you know, I can't say that life will be different. Just more of the same. The same old, dreary routine."

Progressive (positive): "I have just been waiting so long for this. I'll have more time for the botanical garden and the arthritis group and travel and just everything that I want to do more of."

Progressive (negative): "Definitely retirement will be an improvement for me. My whole body aches after a long day at work, and frankly, I'm a little tired of the whole situation. It will be a relief."

Fictional composites, with acknowledgment to Jonsson, H., Kielhofner, G., & Borell, L. (1997). Anticipating retirement: The formation of narratives concerning an occupational transition. *American Journal of Occupational Therapy, 51*(1), 49–56.

- progressive (may be either positive, focusing on new activities, or negative, focusing on getting rid of unpleasant work situation)

Examples of statements reflecting these three styles of response to retirement are shown in Box 5.3. Successful adjustment to retirement may require a reassessment of interests and the development of new hobbies and goals. Without this preparation, the transition from full-time work to retirement can be stressful, even devastating.

Mental Health Factors: Early Adulthood

The ages from 18 years to approximately 40 years are filled with challenges and opportunities. Young adults, having engaged in the process of occupational choice, strive to obtain employment and succeed in their chosen careers. Having attained a sense of identity as a separate person, the young adult is able and eager to develop friendships and intimacies with others. The search for a marital or intimate partner is a primary task of this age group. Young adults with children are faced with the new role responsibilities of parenthood. Thus, early adulthood is a period characterized by a search for intimacy with others and a desire to achieve and contribute to the future in some way, whether through a career, raising children, or both.

Many of the clients seen in mental health settings are in this age range. Young adulthood is the period during which many of the major psychiatric disorders of adult life are first noted. It is a period in which alcohol or substance abuse may appear. Also, for those who are insecure in their jobs or in their personal and sexual or family lives, this can be a period of severe stress and difficult adjustment. Varying levels of employment/unemployment and uncertain job security can impede occupational success. The fact that there are more women than men in the population means that more women who desire male partners cannot find them. The process of choosing a partner is compounded by fears of infection by sexually transmitted infections (STIs). The rise in infertility problems, some a consequence of a prior STI, in this age group means that many couples cannot have their own biologic children. Persons who have hepatitis C or human immunodeficiency virus (HIV) may fear discrimination on the job and in society. All these factors are potentially stressful and may lead to mental health problems. Individuals with limited coping skills and limited exposure to effective role models may act out their stress and anxiety through domestic abuse and violence, substance abuse, or road rage (aggressive driving or cycling).

Among the mental health problems and psychiatric disorders often seen in young adults are adjustment reactions, alcohol and drug use, schizophrenia, mood disorders, eating disorders, anxiety disorders, and various personality disorders (see Chapter 4 for more information on diagnoses). Adjustment reactions or disorders are maladaptive or ineffective reactions to life stress; instead of dealing with the stress in a positive way (ie, by trying to solve problems and rise above the situation), the individual may feel overwhelmed by depression or anxiety, causing them to function poorly at work or in social situations. Along a continuum, some people may be reacting to stress; others may have mental disorders.

Substance use disorders are more prevalent among young adults than among adolescents (64). Alcoholism includes an excessive or uncontrolled use of alcohol, whether daily or episodically. Alcoholics may deny that they have a drinking problem; denial prevents them from seeking help or accepting it when it is offered, and this is considered part of the disease. Another problem alcoholics generally experience concerns their use of time; they spend their leisure hours drinking and often have no other consistent leisure pursuits. Alcoholics tend to become increasingly dependent on alcohol and are likely to have work-related problems and end up losing their jobs and relationships. Alcohol is not the only abused substance. Prescription drug dependence (opioids, sedatives or antianxiety drugs, sleep medications, and stimulants) and dependence on cannabis or street drugs are also epidemic.

Eating disorders include anorexia and bulimia. Anorexia is a disorder in which the person (usually female) restricts food intake to a dangerous degree, believing that they are fat even though they are emaciated. Bulimia, also mainly affecting women, is a disorder in which the person goes on eating binges and then makes themselves to vomit. It is believed that anxiety about self-control versus control by others is one of the factors in both conditions.

Many of the young adults seen in mental health settings have a diagnosis of either schizophrenia or mood disorder. For some, this is a continuation of a disease first diagnosed in adolescence, with multiple hospitalizations since then. Others have their first episode during their 20s or 30s. Some individuals are able to manage their condition with medication, so that the person leads a life free of severe episodes that require hospitalization. However, many cases of schizophrenia and mood disorders become classified as *chronic*, meaning that the disease continues throughout life. These conditions are commonly viewed as serious mental illness (SMI).

Clients with SMI have complicated and difficult lives and may be challenging to work with effectively. Some have a co-occurring diagnosis of a substance-related disorder or a comorbidity of another mental disorder such as borderline or another personality disorder, in addition to schizophrenia or an affective disorder. Although such individuals may have limited skills for independent living, they are usually street smart, being able to survive on their own in a marginal way. Some experience homelessness. Many of these individuals reject the label of mental illness, in part because of the stigma associated with it, and may move in and out of treatment. Involvement in criminal activities can occur; health care professionals must consider both possibilities of imprisonment and inpatient hospitalization (61).

The adult with a SMI may be single, living alone, and relying on social security income (SSI) and Medicaid, depending on the extent of the disability. Depending on the age at which the mental disorder first occurs, an adult may already be working. Many can continue working and may require accommodations, but are unable or unwilling to share their situations with their employers.

Mental Health Factors: Midlife

Ferol Menks (38, p. 31), an occupational therapist, identifies midlife as "a time of reassessment of former commitments and goals . . . as the person realizes . . . life does not lie limitlessly ahead. Physical and psychosocial changes, challenges, and options induce stress as the person feels the pressure of time, decisional conflict, and frustration." The goals that were selected and pursued during the early adult years may have been reached or may seem unattainable. Around age 40, the adult begins to reevaluate life's direction, feeling that this might be the last chance to make major changes. The midlife phase does not have a fixed end point, as many older adults continue to be active and employed after age 65.

Erikson (20) conceptualizes the major task of the middle adult years somewhat differently, terming it the crisis of *generativity versus stagnation. Generativity* is a "concern in establishing and guiding the next generation." Adults in the middle years who are unable to direct this energy successfully will feel stagnant or purposeless, cut off from the stream of human achievement that extends into the future.

One obvious avenue for achieving generativity is through one's children, but this path is not open to everyone. Mental disorders that impair social participation are a barrier to establishing intimate relationships. As a spouse and parent, the adult with a mental disorder may present problem behaviors that are disruptive and distressing to the rest of the family.

For those who are working, this need may be transformed into a concern with nurturing the careers of younger workers. Some adults seek out ways to contribute their expertise and energies through church or community organizations, tutoring, scouting leadership, and other activities.

The adult at midlife assesses whether work has been satisfying and worthwhile. If the work is found lacking either in opportunities for further achievement or in personal satisfaction, the individual may move into a second (or third or fourth) job path. This may necessitate a return to school, a transition that some find stressful.

Additional developmental stresses center around the process of primary aging. During this period, the adult undergoes a decline in physical capacities, a diminution in sexual energies, and cosmetic deterioration (wrinkles and so on). Women go through menopause, and men's sexual potency declines. All these changes signify that one is no longer young. Different people react differently to this. Some seek cosmetic surgery, subject themselves to intense exercise programs, look for younger sexual partners, and attempt to stay the forces of time. Others accept these changes gracefully as a condition of life and move on to other concerns.

Typically, the children of adults in this age group are teenagers or young adults. Dealing with the rebellion and turmoil of adolescent children can be a challenge and joy or a significant stress, depending upon the adult's coping skills. Eventually, these children mature, leave home, and create lives and families of their own; some adults find this prospect alarming because it means the end of their own roles as parents. Midlife adults also are frequently faced with the needs of their own aging parents, who may be dependent in some way on their care and whose deterioration is a reminder of the inescapability of death. Adults caught between the demands of their aging parents and demands of their own children have been named "the sandwich generation."

Thus, the stresses on the midlife adult are multiple. Successful negotiation of this stage entails understanding and accepting the aging process and identifying and pursuing goals in work or family or community life that enable one to contribute to the future in a way that feels significant to the individual.

Occupational Therapy

The goals of occupational therapy for alcohol and drug problems usually include development of self-awareness and self-responsibility, identification of personal goals, vocational assessment and work adjustment, and development of time management and leisure planning skills. Those recovering from alcohol disorders need to learn new activities and routines for their spare time to replace the empty hours once filled with drinking. Frequently, the occupational therapy professional works with a treatment team that may include medical staff, creative arts therapists, psychologists, and certified alcohol and substance abuse counselors. Programs and occupational therapy approaches to persons with alcoholism and other substance abuse disorders are discussed in more detail in Chapters 4 and 6.

Occupational therapy intervention for people who have adjustment disorders focuses on helping them identify and work toward specific goals, generally occupational goals. Interventions should be client centered and activity centered. A crisis intervention approach may be used.

When working with clients with eating disorders, occupational therapy usually includes assessment and modification of the person's habits and beliefs related to eating and food, education in nutrition and cooking, sensorimotor and expressive activities for development of a more positive body image, and training in daily living skills. Chapter 4 contains more information on these disorders and on occupational therapy approaches to intervention.

Occupational therapy goals for young adults focus on the development of adult life skills and the fulfillment of personal aspirations. Typical goals include completing one's education, identifying vocational interests and aptitudes, acquiring prevocational and vocational skills, obtaining and maintaining employment, developing daily living skills, improving social skills, developing coping skills, identifying and developing leisure interests, and structuring leisure time. The occupational therapist completes the assessments (which the occupational therapy assistant can perform with occupational therapist supervision and with service competency) and collaborates with the client to formulate the intervention goals and plan. Cognitive behavioral therapy and cognitive remediation may also be used (65).

The occupational therapy professional may aid with learning the student role while the person works toward a general equivalency diploma (GED) or other educational goal. The occupational therapy professional may lead classes or training programs for daily living skills, social skills, leisure skills, and job search skills and day-to-day supervision of work-oriented programs. Occupational therapy programming may include occupation-based interventions that use cognitive remediation or environmental cues (65).

When determining and selecting occupational therapy interventions, it is helpful to categorize the types of adults in midlife who have mental disorders into three groups:

- The first group consists of those who have had mental health problems for many years—problems that have continued and often worsened as they aged.
- The second group comprises persons with various adjustment disorders, those who have difficulty managing the crises and stresses of adult life and who resort to maladaptive behaviors such as drug and alcohol misuse, overeating, or withdrawal.
- The third group consists of individuals who are developing neurocognitive disorders such as Alzheimer disease (although these conditions more typically appear in late adulthood).

Each of these groups has different needs in terms of occupational therapy and mental health services.

Some of the middle-aged adults who have had mental health problems for many years are somewhat burned out. This means that they have little energy and seem passive and almost indifferent to what goes on around them. They will

go along with intervention programs but do not seem to have much invested in their own progress; getting through each day seems enough of a challenge. Not every person in this category is burned out, however. Some have come to identify themselves in the dependent "client" role; they use the mental health system to meet their needs for physical safety, food, shelter, and economic assistance. Others may view themselves as "consumers" of mental health services and feel that they have an important role in mentoring younger people with similar conditions. Occupational therapy intervention for adults with chronic disorders includes a focus on improving and maintaining daily living skills, providing opportunities for productive work in a supported environment, and facilitating as much independent function as the person can manage.

The second group, those who are experiencing difficulties with adjustments to the crises and stresses of adult life, need assistance in identifying and resolving the issues that confront them. As mentioned earlier, crisis intervention is a widely used approach. Menks (38) has described a *conflict resolution model* in which the occupational therapy professional guides the client through the following five-step process to resolve midlife conflicts and their associated pressures, and then builds adaptive responses to allow for continued competent occupational performance:

1. *Identifying the problem.* Information is gathered about the person's sociocultural factors, vocation and leisure history, life achievements, completed responsibilities, interests, and values. This information can be assembled from client and family interviews. The client may need assistance in realizing and accepting previous choices and the consequences of those choices. The occupational therapy professional takes a nondirective approach, providing the client with expressive methods to self-examine past decisions and reflect on emotions connected to current situations.
2. *Create alternative possibilities.* Through brainstorming, the client can determine alternative paths and options they can take with their lives. The occupational therapy professional is nonjudgmental during this process and assists the client to break down ideas that are too complex into manageable, understandable, and doable pieces.
3. *Considering the options.* Here the client evaluates the possibilities. The occupational therapy professional needs to monitor this process and ensure the person is not "jumping" too quickly toward an option that is too risky or unobtainable. The person may also not "see" all the possible solutions and thus may need gentle guidance in understanding the array of activities they could begin to undertake. The client may need time and small successful accomplishments to begin to realize what they can perform. Additional resource personnel may help the client learn details about various options and what is involved in making changes or undertaking certain activities. The client can use a "balance sheet" and list the positives and negatives of each solution and consider the impact of

each solution regarding cost, time, and other personal and sociocultural factors. The client is searching for an approach that will lead to a chosen solution, which likely is a compromise between what the person finds as an ideal life situation and what the person realistically can accomplish. This step is time consuming, and the person may vacillate between options prior to making a commitment to decide.

4. *The decision.* Decisions that involve losing something the person currently has, even if it negatively impacts the person, decisions with a certain amount of risk, or decisions that involve the unknown are difficult to make. Additionally, deciding between two options that bring different benefits can be difficult. At times, making a new decision can feel like a violation of a previous decision, the occupational therapy professional can help the client assess past choices and current implications of those choices. This ultimately can lead to seeing new decisions more clearly and reassure the person that a new course of action is not only healthy and positive, but also that it aligns with the life path the person had originally set out to take. The occupational therapy professional can also help the client identify negative consequences of rash decision-making or deciding too quickly and without all the relevant information.

5. *Implementing the decision.* Completion of the action is done in sequential steps. The occupational therapy professional can help the client prepare for feedback they will receive regarding their decision. Some feedback can be negative, and the person must be prepared to accept that feedback and still be secure in the decision they made. Self-efficacy is a key component to this process, and one which develops over time. As the person works within the various layers and aspects of their decision, the occupational therapy professional can provide reassurance that the client can learn to manage and benefit from their decision.

In the third category are people with neurocognitive disorders. Alzheimer disease, which is in this category, may show its first signs as early as age 40. Memory impairment or forgetfulness is usually the first symptom; the person first has trouble remembering details (dates, names, facts), and the memory loss becomes more profound as the disease progresses. Gradually, so much of the memory is lost that the person cannot complete simple activities, not remembering that the activities were even started. There are personality changes as well; though these are not always noticeable in the early stages, the behavior of persons with such disorders becomes less social and more inappropriate over time. Ultimately, they lose physical neuromotor control over their bodies, become incontinent and less mobile, and eventually die.

Because the symptoms of neurocognitive disorders may progress slowly at first, the person in the early stages of the illness can usually continue customary activities with a few minor adjustments. For example, at work, the person may have to be supervised more closely than before or switch to duties that require less attention to detail. Similarly, family members have to compensate for cognitive deficits in the home. The client who is the cook in the family, for instance, needs supervision to make sure they do not cause a fire. Occupational therapy professionals work with these early-stage individuals and their families in the home wherever possible. The goals of intervention are to assess what areas and activities are causing difficulty for the person, to identify current strengths and areas of need, and to help the family adapt the environment and provide the social support the person needs.

It is important that persons with neurocognitive disorders remain at home or in their accustomed environment for as long as possible because they are better able to function in familiar environments than in new ones (37). In the later stages of their illness, these individuals often do not remain in the community because they need either medical care or round-the-clock supervision. They may reside in nursing homes or some other long-term care facility. Occupational therapy professionals provide services that help these clients remain alert and function to the best of their present capacities. These might include sensory stimulation (eg, olfactory and tactile stimulation) and physical activities (exercise, gross motor movement, dancing).

Veterans

The occupational therapy professional will encounter military veterans across a variety of settings. The mental health problems of veterans, especially combat veterans, are of special interest. A traumatic reaction to battle is common. In World War I, this was known as "shell shock," which involved emotional numbing, fear, flight reaction, and problems sleeping. It is unclear whether shell shock was the result of brain injury or of psychological trauma. In World War II, a similar condition was termed "combat fatigue." Today, these conditions would likely be diagnosed as posttraumatic stress disorder (PTSD) or a traumatic brain injury (TBI), or both.

Veterans are, as a whole, intensely proud of their military service and identify strongly with the branch of the armed forces in which they served. They may look back on their years of service as an extremely important time of life. Those who experienced combat may be unable or unwilling to talk about what happened or to express their feelings.

In the third decade of the 21st century, the U.S. population includes veterans of several different foreign wars. As of September 2021, the oldest veteran of World War II was 112 years old (5). There are also veterans of wars in places such as Korea, Vietnam and Southeast Asia, Iraq, Afghanistan, Somalia, and Libya. The occupational therapy professional may come into contact with veterans diagnosed with mental disorders in hospitals (including military hospitals and Veterans Administration hospitals), in skilled nursing facilities, and in the community.

Typically, veterans of World War II and the war in Korea are in late old age, whereas those from the Vietnam War are in young or middle old age. Vietnam differed from other conflicts in several important ways. Over time, the Vietnam War became unpopular with much of the U.S. population. Demonstrations opposing U.S. involvement in Vietnam were frequent during the late 1960s and the 1970s. On returning from service in Vietnam, many veterans (including the two-thirds that enlisted) felt ostracized and scorned for having participated in an unpopular war. This contrasts with veterans of earlier wars, who were seen as having made a contribution to their country. The social stigma felt by Vietnam veterans is important to consider when meeting them.

Posttraumatic Stress Disorder and Suicide Risk

As a group, veterans who experienced combat in "the global war on terror" in Iraq and Afghanistan have high rates of PTSD, substance-related disorders, and MDDs. In addition, they may have sustained a TBI, as well as physical impairments such as amputations and spinal cord injury. In these wars, violence often occurs at a distance (drones, improvised explosive devices [IEDs]), and the person responsible for the violence may not observe the results of their actions.

Suicide is a serious risk for veterans. Approximately 6,500 veterans died in 2018 as a result of suicide (53). In 2018, the age-adjusted and sex-adjusted suicide rate for veterans was 28 per 100,000 (53). In contrast, for the general population, the rate was 18 per 100,000 (53). Preventing suicide and social isolation is a primary emphasis for occupational therapy intervention.

Occupational Engagement

According to Plach and Sells (52), veterans returning from Iraq and Afghanistan may face problems in occupational engagement. The top five challenges are in forming/maintaining leisure and social relationships, transitioning to the student or worker role, dealing with physical health issues, resolving problems with sleep and rest, and controlling risky or distracted behaviors while driving.

Reintegration into civilian life may be difficult. Because of the young age at which many service members enlist, development of personal identity may occur within the context of service. Thus, the young person may become identified with the military role, which is unlike most roles required in civilian life. The veteran may thus feel distanced from the skills needed to participate in community activities and family life. The veteran may feel pressure to enroll in an educational program and yet be unprepared to choose or participate in a program because of the gap since last being in the student role.

Employment opportunities may be limited if the veteran has no college degree. On the other hand, military service may provide veterans with special qualities and performance skills such as intense focus, loyalty, discipline, planning and organization, initiative, and ability to work with a team and within a structure or system. These are assets that may be attractive to employers. The occupational therapy professional can help the person explore skills that may be transferable to the civilian workplace.

The Military Culture

The culture of military service values **athleticism** and feats of physical and psychological courage. In contrast, civilian life affords little opportunity to experience the level of intense engagement required in a combat zone (56). High-intensity sports are an exception. "Ocean therapy" is a program (56) in which veterans learn surfing over 5 weeks, five times per week, and 4 hours per session. Surfing occurs in the natural environment (highly valued by veterans) and carries a sense of danger and significant risk. Education and practice of surfing techniques and skills are part of each session. In addition, the program includes group activities completed on land. Incorporated throughout the sessions are themes of role identity, leadership and trust, community building, problem-solving, and transition or generalization of learning into the context of daily life.

Another activity that incorporates the natural environment is horticulture or gardening. Involvement in a horticultural therapy group may benefit the veteran in several areas such as immersion in nature, community reintegration, development of new skills that may be transferred to employment, and practice in social interaction and group dynamics (73).

Some returning veterans have sustained a TBI as a result of blasts from IEDs or other combat-related causes. Significant comorbidity exists between TBI and PTSD and MDD. TBI may result in permanent deficits in memory or in behavioral problems. Veterans with a TBI may receive extended inpatient or residential care and yet continue to have problems in occupational performance (63).

Art and expressive activities permit nonverbal communication of feelings that might otherwise remain unexpressed. A program led by an art therapist at Walter Reed Army Medical Center involved veterans with TBI in making masks to illustrate hidden feelings. The masks created in the program are powerful icons of themes such as death and mutilation, blinding, emotional numbing, patriotism, physical pain, inability to speak or express oneself, etc. (1) (Figure 5.1).

Families of Veterans

Families of veterans have higher rates of diagnosed mental disorders and experience multiple difficulties (psychological, emotional, and financial) related to the deployment of their family member (12). Long and frequent separations disrupt family life and relationships. When the service member returns from deployment, the reintegration into civilian life may be highly stressful. Veterans with PTSD will be prone to reliving the trauma. They may feel emotionally numb and may be hyperalert and vigilant (12). Children may exhibit attention or behavior problems in school that are related to the parent's deployment or return.

Although the information presented here may suggest that all or most veterans experience difficulty on returning from service, this is incorrect. Many veterans never see combat and may welcome the release from service and the new freedom of living in the community. However, particularly for those who have seen combat, the "broken hero"

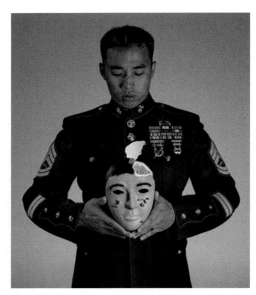

Figure 5.1. Marine Gunnery Sgt. Aaron Tam (Ret.), Holding the Mask He Made to Illustrate His Feelings About His Traumatic Brain Injury. (Reprinted with permission from Lynn Johnson.)

stereotype is an obstacle to community reintegration. Veterans may face discrimination from employers who fear workplace violence, as well as fear and stigma from the community at large (48). The portrayals of service members in movies and other media create an impression that these are violent, drug or alcohol-addicted, socially isolated individuals who might be dangerous. Chris Marvin, a retired veteran who was seriously wounded but who subsequently earned a business degree at a prestigious graduate program, advocates that veterans become involved in community service. He further recommends that communities see veterans as assets, with the capacity to make great contributions, even with diagnoses of (for example) PTSD (48).

See Box 5.4 for a summary of recommended interventions for veterans with psychosocial problems.

> **BOX 5.4 Veterans With Psychosocial Problems: Focus of Intervention**
>
> - Transition to community and family life
> - Reengagement, development, and maintenance of leisure skills and social relationships
> - Transitioning to worker or student role
> - Where relevant, identification of desired education or occupational training
> - Sleep hygiene
> - Analysis and management of risky driving behaviors
> - Where desired, engagement in activities that incorporate valued qualities, such as immersion in the natural environment, and high risk
> - Activities that permit or encourage appropriate verbal or nonverbal emotional expression, following recommendations of physician as well as preference of veteran

- Reduction of substance-related problems
- Suicide prevention
- Opportunities for altruism and community service

LATER ADULTHOOD

Development

During retirement and the latter part of life, the number of hours spent toward vocational work is typically much less than it had been between the ages of 18 and 65 years. More time suddenly becomes available, and decisions must be made about how to fill the hours. Leisure may replace work as the primary occupation, although many retirees who have the means to not work at all continue to serve productive social roles (eg, as volunteers) that can only be classified as work. After retirement, many adults also spend time in the co-occupation of child rearing, only now with grandchildren or great-grandchildren. Those in the later adulthood stage may also find they are providing self-care tasks for a spouse.

As of 2020, 10.6 million Americans age 65 years or older (19.4% of older Americans) were in the labor force, which is 6.6% of the overall U.S. labor force (71). Some continue in their life careers, full-time or with reduced hours. Others are employed in retail or other fields different from their experience. Reasons cited include the increase in life expectancy, the deferred age of eligibility to receive Social Security benefits, the economic recession that began in 2008, insufficient retirement savings, and anxiety about the stock market and about the security of savings.

Many continue to work because they have always done so, and they cannot imagine a different kind of life. During the later years of life, there can be various role losses. These include the role of worker, parent, and homemaker. These roles represent not just the loss of activities that once filled one's day but also of status, social identity, and customary avenues for social participation. To adjust, the older adult needs goals and occupations that provide satisfaction and opportunities for success and social contact and that support a sense of self-worth. Older adults find particular meaning in maintaining leisure activities that have been lifelong interests (28). Each older person lives in a particular environment, has a particular occupational history, and has specific interests. The ability to continue living with maximum independence in the community is highly individual and requires client-centered support (27).

In the words of the 18th-century poet William Cowper, "Absence of occupation is not rest; A mind quite vacant is a mind distressed." Thus, one of the important tasks of this stage of adult life is to identify and develop interests and challenges that will sustain one's sense of independence and self-worth after retirement.

Mental Health Factors

The most important psychosocial task of older adults is believed by many experts to be the development of an understanding and appreciation for what they have accomplished during their lives. Erikson (20) has called this the crisis of *ego integrity versus despair.* Erikson believed that to feel that life has been worthwhile, the older adult needs to see the self as only a small part of the human community, which will endure beyond one's own death.

In addition to this major developmental task, the older adult often must deal with significant life stress. One's aging body (primary aging), retirement and the loss of a career role, the deaths of spouses and cherished friends, economic worries, and the loss of one's home are just a few of the stresses that may press on the older adult's diminished energies. New hobbies, new friendships, and new roles as volunteer or grandparent may compensate for some of these losses, but many older adults find it difficult to make these adjustments.

Shimp (62) reminds us that many of our cherished "truths" about older people are in fact myths. Although many retirees are satisfied and relieved to give up their productive roles, many others happily undertake volunteer and paid jobs into their 90s. Also, the notion that those who are older cannot adapt to life stresses needs careful examination in each case. Even a severe stressor such as acute care hospitalization can be endured and managed successfully, given sufficient motivation and hope.

Depression is the most common psychiatric diagnosis in the elderly population (77). A person in a very deep or severe depression can become so withdrawn and self-involved as to appear to have dementia (cognitive impairment); for this reason, the condition is sometimes misdiagnosed as a neurocognitive disorder. In some cases, the depression is masked by multiple physical complaints—aches and pains, stomach problems, and so on—that can make it difficult to detect the underlying depression. When the depression is ultimately recognized and properly treated, usually with medication, the person's attention and cognitive functions return to normal. After depression, dementia is the psychiatric condition most diagnosed in older persons (77). Coincidentally and confusingly from a diagnostic point of view, depression is often a symptom of neurocognitive disorder. Even mild levels of depression and mild levels of cognitive impairment are associated with lower levels of occupational participation (47).

Substance misuse may also be present, which may involve the misuse of prescribed medications. This can be combined with alcohol or other drug use.

Occupational Therapy

The purpose of occupational therapy is to help the older adult maintain or achieve a feeling of competence or self-reliance and to prevent further deterioration in functioning. Older persons will experience age-related declines in memory functions and a general slowing of responsiveness, particularly in short-term memory. The occupational therapy professional should give the person time to respond and should anticipate that the person may have some difficulty recalling recent information (36). Reassurance that these are normal effects of aging and providing training in mnemonics (such as acronyms or other memory tricks) and the use of smartphones

and other technology can help these clients function more comfortably. Adaptations to the environment to organize tasks and make objects easier to find also help. However, any changes must be agreeable to the person and not insisted upon on them by the occupational therapy professional.

Another consideration toward acceptance of physical capabilities is the deficits associated with chronic medical and physical conditions. Decades of living with conditions such as arthritis, cardiac disease, and musculoskeletal disorders can require use of adaptive equipment and decrease physical endurance and activity. The older adult in this situation cannot "force" their body to perform at past levels of ability. It may be difficult for some to accept their current limitations and the assistance required to maintain living in their own home or accept when it becomes necessary to live in a long-term care facility. Remaining active in chosen occupations should be encouraged, at the physical level of ability.

Occupational therapy may be provided to the older adult in their home, an adult day center, a hospital, an assisted living facility, a community center, or a nursing home. Some larger medical center settings provide continuity of services from psychiatric inpatient to community aftercare. Such a comprehensive array of services, if well-coordinated, maximizes independent functioning and permits each person to be served in the least restrictive and most supportive environment (Box 5.5). The client may be admitted first for acute care and at this level be introduced to unit-level groups that address specific needs such as decreasing anxiety, promoting understanding of and adjustment to the hospital environment, and providing information and skills needed for successful community functioning (eg, obtaining benefits). At the next level, the person is encouraged to attend activities at a senior center on the hospital grounds. The third level is placement as an outpatient in the adult day center. Finally, at the fourth level, the consumer lives in the community and visits the center periodically and receives limited services at home.

> ### BOX 5.5 Elders With Psychosocial Problems: Focus of Intervention
>
> - Occupation-based assessment and intervention focusing on relevant age-appropriate roles (self-maintainer, leisure participant, friend, family member, homemaker, volunteer)
> - Mutual collaborative goal setting, encouraging the older person to identify valued goals, including family or another caregiver when relevant
> - Collaborative approach to intervention (eg, person asked to consider whether a suggested intervention is acceptable)
> - Education in special needs of this age group (eg, safety, fall prevention, nutrition)
> - Wellness and lifestyle redesign
> - Reconnection with previously enjoyed leisure activities
> - Education of and consultation with caregiver regarding appropriate expectations, behavior management

Community geriatric centers may provide activity programs, counseling, and meals; most participants do not have major mental disorders (eg, schizophrenia) but rather periodic or chronic depression or anxiety because of losses associated with aging. The centers may be housed in their own facilities or more typically within another community agency, such as a community-based fitness center or a church.

Some centers offer evening and night respite care, for example, from 7:00 PM to 7:00 AM, giving families a chance to get a good night's sleep while the family member stays overnight at a fully staffed program that can accommodate the nighttime restlessness common in persons with dementia. The person can sleep, of course, but if awake can participate in activities such as horticulture, card games, or listening to music.

Adult day care (16, 41) is a community-based, long-term service model for the elderly. Adult day care provides a group setting for leisure activities, avocational skills development, and social activities. Adaptive equipment and environmental modifications are provided to maximize functioning for clients who have physical and mental impairments. In adult day care, depending on state and local regulations, the occupational therapy professional may take on a managerial role; as director of programs and services, the occupational therapy professional may direct the activities of other activity therapy personnel and can create an occupation-oriented activity model. The preferences and interests of clients should lead the choice of activities, so that clients can participate to the greatest extent possible (19).

Environmental adaptations made by the occupational therapy professional can allow higher-functioning individuals to continue living in their own homes; this is very important for maintaining their sense of self-identity and a personal daily routine. In addition, the occupational therapy professional may provide leisure coaching, assist in the development of hobbies, and facilitate social involvement.

Older persons who have mental disorders with extensive functional losses (eg, schizophrenia or neurocognitive disorders) and who are unable to live in the community typically reside in nursing homes or in long-term geriatric units of large public institutions, where they can receive medical services.

Community-based residential facilities often involve occupational therapy provided by occupational therapy assistants, with the occupational therapist serving as part-time consultant; services may include orientation to the facility, reality orientation, memory training and assistance, sensory awareness, environmental modification, and training in daily living skills and use of assistive devices. An activity program, including social and recreational programming, music activities, and exercise and craft programs, may be provided by occupational therapy professionals or by recreational therapists or activity leaders.

One of the challenges of nursing home care is creating an atmosphere in which expectations and opportunities for independence are matched to the capabilities of the residents. The occupational therapy professional may use guidelines for environmental and social supports based on the Cognitive Disabilities Model (Chapter 3) and train nursing staff and volunteers to carry over such activities. Not all residents with psychiatric diagnoses in a nursing home have severe cognitive limitations. The occupational therapy professional must plan programs that allow people with different capacities to participate and plan for interventions that provide challenges to each person at their own cognitive ability level. The occupational therapist begins by assessing how well each person functions in terms of social, physical, and cognitive functioning and occupational skills, mainly focusing on self-care occupations. Intervention approaches and supports are often based on a cognitive-based intervention model. Activity groups may provide many different craft, leisure, and social activities that can be customized for individual members (32). As needed, occupational therapy professionals may provide or devise adaptive equipment to allow participation for those with physical impairments.

Sometimes, tasks that the resident can do (slowly perhaps, or only with supervision and cuing) are done for the resident because the staff is unaware of the additional time needed to allow participation by the resident. An occupational therapy professional can educate and train care personnel in the facility to help them meet a resident's needs and maximize the resident's participation and engagement. The occupational therapy professional can promote maximum independent performance in residents and can communicate to other staff the resident's real capabilities.

The occupational therapy professional who works with older adults must be receptive to the needs and concerns of the older individual. It is important to respect and accommodate the habits and beliefs that the person has built up over a lifetime. Because they have lost so many of the things that were once important to them, older people often fear the loss of their identity and self-direction and may feel threatened when a health care professional pushes them too far too fast. Also, because of a general slowing of physical capacities, older people may respond less quickly and often need more time to answer questions and learn new things. Finally, the older individual thinks often and deeply about the past and can enjoy telling stories about it; this recounting is an important psychological process for establishing a sense of ego integrity. It is important for the occupational therapy professional to recognize the value of this reminiscence and encourage it.

FAMILY MEMBERS

The medical model focuses on the client as the recipient of services and the center of intervention efforts. In a systems model, such as the model of human occupation, the perspective enlarges to include the person's environment, hence the family and the social support system. Occupational therapy professionals increase their effectiveness when they include the family in their clinical thinking and intervention efforts. As a member of the transdisciplinary health care team, the occupational therapy professional is sensitive to and ready to respond to family needs and issues. Working with families requires commitment and flexibility to schedule meetings when they are convenient for the family, sometimes in the evenings and on the weekends.

This can seem overwhelming to the entry-level professional, who may reason, "It is hard enough to concentrate on the client's problems; how can I include the family too?" Billing, documentation, and justifying communication with the family as real work are related concerns (12, 35). It takes time for new professionals to become skilled at communicating with families and to recognize that family members can yield useful information about the client, help support and maintain the person at optimum functioning, provide care in the home, and in other ways reinforce the interventions done in occupational therapy. An occupational therapy professional's involvement with the family may take many forms, ranging from no involvement to family as informant, to family as almost an "associate" therapy professional, to family as collaborator or team member or even as director of occupational therapy. Each of these forms of family participation requires specific skills and knowledge from the occupational therapy professional.

Families need help from mental health professionals because they must adjust to the situation of having a mentally ill family member, because they carry the greatest burden of care, and because they can be the most important and positive support in helping the person function. Families need to be partners in the planning and intervention process. Family involvement can be hampered by *Health Insurance Portability and Accountability Act* (HIPAA) regulations, in that the consent of the identified client is required, unless the person is a minor or is an adult with a legal guardian. Family members can serve as advocates and case managers and care providers; to perform these roles, they need education about the disease process and training about any compensations or modifications they can provide that will make things better. With sufficient information and guidance about possible options, family members will be better able to devote time and energy to securing reimbursement, housing, supported employment, and other supports for the ill family member. But this will happen only if they are involved in a systematic and collaborative manner (31).

Before we consider how occupational therapy professionals can work effectively with the family, or even the specifics of how family members can aid in interventions, we must first acknowledge that relatives of a person with a mental disorder face significant challenges and stresses. It is disturbing and difficult to accept that one's loved one has a lifelong mental disorder that may result in a chronic disability. Among the many issues faced are the following:

- guilt and fear,
- grief and feelings of loss over the relationship,
- uncertainty about setting limits,
- uncertainty about personal responsibilities and boundaries,

- fear of becoming sick oneself (if a genetic relative),
- fear of having children who may develop the illness (30), and
- fear that the family member will wander off or become homeless (70).

Parents

The parents of a person with a mental disorder, whether the identified client is a child, an adolescent, or an adult, may feel tremendous guilt and responsibility. Mothers especially may feel guilty, wondering if their own health habits during pregnancy contributed to the disorder in utero. Some parents may deny that there is any problem. It is important to understand and to reassure parents that the major mental disorders (schizophrenia, affective disorders, ADHD) are biologic, *not* caused by upbringing.

Parents may feel intense sadness when their child is compared with peers who do not have a mental disorder; the child's inability to proceed on a typical life course (relationships, career, children) is an ongoing loss. Parents may have difficulty setting realistic limits and expectations because it is hard to differentiate between disease-driven behaviors, for which the person is not responsible, and voluntary actions, which can be controlled.

Siblings

Siblings react differently, depending on their age at the time of the client's onset of illness and their own resources. Feelings may include confusion over the ill sibling's behavior, fear of possible violence, anger and resentment over the preferential treatment and parental attention given to the sibling with a mental disorder, sadness over the loss of the relationship, worries that one might become ill oneself, concerns about future liability and custodianship for the sibling, and worries about genetic risks to one's own offspring. One sibling may hide another's psychotic symptoms or strange behavior from the rest of the family, for fear of getting that sibling in trouble. As already mentioned, siblings may take on a life-long custodial responsibility, which in the co-occupation of caring for the sibling becomes a major occupational role. A disproportionate number of siblings of persons with mental disorders enter helping professions, working specifically in mental health; their childhood may have prepared them to tolerate behaviors associated with mental disorders and to read cues exceptionally well (59). On the other hand, siblings and children may have difficulty with assertiveness or with setting boundaries on inappropriate behavior, having experienced so much of it.

Spouses and Partners

Spouses and partners of persons who develop mental disorders may wonder whether they have made a bad choice and whether they should leave the relationship. Guilt, fears of personal responsibility in causing the breakdown, grief over the lost relationship, and concerns about any children are common. Spouses may have difficulty setting limits and expectations for the diagnosed spouse, not understanding which behaviors are the result of the disorder and which are not.

Children

Children react differently, depending on their age and level of cognitive development. Very young children may not recognize that the diagnosed parent's behavior is atypical, because it is the only thing they know. Older children recognize more clearly the absence of nurturing and the loss of a nurturing relationship. Some may wonder if they caused the parent's illness by their own misbehavior; indeed, some parents accuse them of this. Others step into the role of custodian (or "**parentified child**"), caring for the ill parent and fulfilling that person's household responsibilities. Children may be afraid of a parent who threatens or who is violent or unpredictable.

Children in families with a parent or sibling with a mental disorder may take on roles of custodian, bystander, or adversary (59). The *custodian* serves as a mini-parent, is overly responsible, and fills in for the ill or preoccupied parent. The *bystander* is more detached; less central to meeting the needs of the family, they can coolly analyze the situation or may just try to stay out of the way. The *adversary* acts out the unexpressed tensions of the family; those in this role may be seen as troublemakers. It is not surprising that the adversary may be the one to bring the family to the attention of those who can help; by getting in trouble in school or with the law, adversaries attract intervention.

Case **Study – Attention Problems and Oppositional Behavior**

A 12-Year-Old Boy With ADHD and ODD[2]

Danny B.
Case #38-499

Danny is a 12-year-old boy who is in the fifth grade. He is currently being homeschooled by his father, who is a freelance web designer. His parents started homeschooling this school year because they feel that he is too distracted by peers to function in a school setting because of his behavioral problems (see "Diagnosis at Admission"). His academic history shows below-average academic achievement (he repeated the fourth grade) despite average scores for the verbal comprehension scale and fluid reasoning scale with the *Wechsler Intelligence Scale for Children*, 5th ed. (WISC-V) (75). Since entering school, he has had difficulty getting along with other children and has been picked on and ostracized. In kindergarten, he threw a chair across the classroom. Teachers in the second and third grades restrained him several times when he struck out at classmates. He has been tested for learning disabilities, but none were found. Danny is being medicated with divalproex (Depakote), methylphenidate (Ritalin), and bupropion (Wellbutrin).

---

[2]Composite based on several clinical cases.

DSM-5-TR Diagnosis at Admission
F90.2 Attention-deficit/hyperactivity disorder combined presentation
F91.3 Oppositional defiant disorder

Z codes
Z62.29 Sibling relational problem
Z60.4 Social exclusion or rejection

Danny is the oldest of four children, with a younger sister aged 9 and twin brothers aged 18 months. He was a full-term baby, delivered by cesarean section after unsuccessful attempts to move him from a breech presentation. Mother recalls that as an infant, Danny was fussy and cried a lot in comparison with her other children. Developmental milestones were within normal limits. At age 2, Danny began to have intense temper tantrums. He seemed easily frustrated according to his parents. His parents assumed he would outgrow it, but the behavior continued. He would, for example, refuse to join in family activities, causing the entire family to miss planned events because he would kick anyone who attempted to drag him along. Parents and teachers have described Danny as absent-minded and inattentive, demanding, argumentative, disruptive, loud, stubborn, withdrawn, suspicious, and moody.

Danny has no current peer friendships and has had no sustained peer relationships in the past. Teachers and parents describe his behavior with peers as bullying and unaware, insensitive to context, intense and needy, and in the words of one teacher, "clueless about how to be a member of a group." Relationships with siblings are stormy, but Danny relies on his 9-year-old sister to be a friend and companion. He is jealous of his sister's friends; when friends visit his sister, Danny often disrupts their play, sometimes destroying toys and drawings.

Danny has few chores but does them if reminded several times. He enjoys taking in the mail and sorting it. He takes out the trash sometimes. His mother complains that he dawdles and takes forever to finish some chores, such as setting the table and taking out the trash. He feeds the two cats and the rabbits and likes to pet the animals. The cats have scratched when he has been too rough while playing with the cats. Danny's mother says she does not make him do too many chores because he is impatient and has broken too many things.

Danny has been homeschooled for the past year. On a typical day, he and his father work on the lessons for 2 hours, and then Danny has 4 to 6 hours of independent work. Danny's father says that Danny focuses well on his schoolwork and seems in particular to enjoy math and reading. However, Danny's father has to work longer hours to generate more income and would like to have Danny back in school.

Danny has had 3 years of psychotherapy with a psychologist; his parents say they see little change. They feel the medications have helped somewhat in curbing Danny's impulsivity and oppositional behaviors. The psychologist suggested occupational therapy for evaluation of social skills and for interventions to enable him to develop relationships with other children and to function in a public school classroom.

OT HACKS SUMMARY

O: Occupation as a means and an end

Table 5.1 summarizes occupational performance and occupational participation over the life span

T: Theoretical concepts, values, and principles, or historical foundations

Theoretical concepts from Developmental theory we embrace as occupations and skills impacted by mental health problems and mental disorder difficulties

Adolescence: career role and choices determined via activities in tentative period and then in realistic period; moving toward competency by refining skills associated with structured peer activities; sportsmanship and craftsmanship used with activity; self-identity; experimentation with sexual activity and substance use; body image

Adulthood: providing financially for self and family; leisure participation; preparing for retirement from vocational pursuits

Early Adulthood: symptom management with new mental disorder diagnosis; parenting; intimate partner relationship building; substance use disorders; vocational skills

Infancy and Early Childhood: intellectual functioning; social communication and interaction; development of trusting relationships with others; developmental delays

Later Adulthood: change of role from one who is always producing to one who is focused on role of helper or participator; stress associated with having to care for grandchildren or spouse; ability to accept life's activities and experience; stress associated with primary aging, change of roles, new onset of mental disorders such as depression or substance misuse

Middle Adulthood: reassessment of one's goals and plans for life; managing the beginning of physical loss because of primary aging; acceptance of shrinking family; caring for aging parents; movement toward retirement

Middle Childhood: social awareness; awareness of others' needs; intellectual ability and executive functioning to complete schoolwork and make age-appropriate decisions; attempting new challenges in safe environment, attention, concentration, self-acceptance, respect for others, awareness of social expectations, emotional regulation needed for age-appropriate social situations

H: How can we Help? OT's role in serving clients with mental illness or mental health needs

How occupational therapy can impact the changes that occur over the life span.

Adolescence: self-awareness and self-identity despite peer and family pressures; set limits for unacceptable behaviors; awareness of risks with social media; coping emotional regulation; executive functioning

Adulthood: substance use and abuse: readjustment of goals, work situation, and leisure time pursuits; adjustment disorder: crisis intervention approach; eating disorders: change self-assessment of body image, nutrition education; in early adulthood need to finalize career path, structure of future intimate relationships and family (based in values and beliefs); adult student role for GED completion, advanced

degree obtainment; adjustment to midlife crises; neurocognitive disorders: early stages of changes related to executive function and memory; service members returning home reacclimate to civilian life

Change: People progress through Exploration (discover of new roles and social expectations), Competency (grow in ability to complete tasks and role expectations in new ways), and Achievement (integration of ability to adjust and adapt established roles and abilities into new environments and situations).

Co-occupations include family members assisting and participating with family members with mental health problems and mental disorders; educate family members about the disease process and train family members to use techniques that help the client remain as independent as possible.

Infancy and Early Childhood: sensory processing needs; behavioral approach can be used for self-care activities; trusting relationship building; environmental modifications, increase gross and fine motor associated with developmental delays; improve cognitive performance to prepare child for school activities

Later Adulthood: coping with primary aging changes and chronic conditions, acceptance of assistance now required; renewed focus on leisure skills; cognitive disabilities compensation techniques and caregiver training

Middle Childhood: anger management; social skills; empathy building; self-awareness and self-acceptance; self-esteem; antisocial behaviors; emotional regulation; self-control; executive functioning training

A: Adaptations

Adaptations to support occupational performance.

Adolescence: for those with a new mental disorder diagnosis and the need to manage deficits associated with completing occupational tasks, adjustments to school activities such as smaller classrooms, one-on-one tutoring, a later start time for school attendance, and a distraction-free study area

Adulthood: for those with neurocognitive disorders, add supervision to complex tasks, provide cues for completing complicated many-step tasks (written cues, use of templates, lists)

Infancy and Early Childhood: environmental modifications for sensory processing needs; limit social interactions until emotional regulation abilities allow child to maintain emotional control

Later Adulthood: adaptations for physical impairments that are associated with primary aging and chronic physical and medical conditions; referrals to community agencies that can provide various levels of care and assistance; changes in how self-cares are performed, because of cognitive disabilities, including additional cuing and removal of objects that now present a safety hazard

Middle Childhood: modify environment at home to improve concentration and attention to homework and household chores; alterations in physical spaces made to match the sensory needs of the child; use of "smart" technology devices to identify and provide modifications to help the child maintain emotional regulation

C: Case study includes

Case study of a child with ADHD and ODD. Areas addressed: social interactions with family members and peers, maladaptive behaviors, attention/concentration, and academic performance

K: Knowledge: keeping mental health OT practice grounded in evidence, in occupational science, and in research

Knowledge gained from Evidence-Based Practice. Environmental factors and personal factors associated with outside lighting at night can impact adolescent sleep patterns.

S: Some terms that may be new to you

Accumbens: reward anticipator

Amygdala: associated with emotions

Anterior cingulate cortex: tracks behavior and monitors environment

Athleticism: having the qualities that are characteristic of athletes

Co-occupation: occupation completed between and with two or more people; considerations of these occupations include: physical space, emotions, intentions, time, social influences, and social support.

Environmental factors: determinants of mental health that impact occupational performance; can include areas such as environment, social situations, living and working context

Hippocampus: assists with memory

Parentified child: a child taking on the role of custodian (typically to a parent or sibling)

Prefrontal cortex: manages executive functions and self-regulating behavior

Realistic period: time when adolescent considers career choices based on achievements, satisfaction, status, and economic security

Splitting: a kind of thinking that is "all or nothing," or a way of thinking that is "all good or all bad"

Tentative period: time when adolescent considers possible adult vocation within their interests and abilities

Triangulation: occurs when the person will not communicate directly with one person (the "bad one") but only with someone who is viewed as "good"

Reflection Questions

1. Complete the questions in the *What's the Evidence?* box.
2. What is an example of the Habituation associated with childhood?
3. How is Competency seen during the adolescent years?
4. The occupational therapy professional is working with a 35-year-old client who has a substance use problem. What are the main focuses on occupational therapy intervention?
5. Based on the model of the "ocean therapy" group, what would a "rock climbing therapy" group look like?
6. Based on the following curriculum of a community-based residential care facility trained caregiver educational program (42), what occupational therapy services would be appropriate to add to the services provided to a resident with a neurocognitive disorder?
   Curriculum: fire safety, medication administration and management, standard precautions, first aid and choking, residents' rights, challenging behaviors

REFERENCES

1. Alexander, C. (2015). The invisible war on the brain. *National Geographic, 227*(2), 30–53.
2. American Psychiatric Association. (2022). *Diagnostic and statistical manual of mental disorders* (5th ed., text rev.). https://doi.org/10.1176/appi.books.9780890425787
3. Angier, N. (1992, October 20). The purpose of playful frolics: Training for adulthood. *The New York Times*. https://www.nytimes.com/1992/10/20/science/the-purpose-of-playful-frolics-training-for-adulthood.html
4. Arbesman, M., Bayzk, S., & Nochajski, S. M. (2013). Systematic review of occupational therapy and mental health promotion, prevention, and intervention for children and youth. *American Journal of Occupational Therapy, 67*(6), e120–e130.
5. Associated Press. (2021, September 13). *Oldest US veteran of WWII celebrates his 112th birthday*. https://apnews.com/article/oldest-world-war-ii-veteran-lawrence-brooks-c52e4957963103a906ffcae5519d70b3
6. Baron, K. B. (1987). The model of human occupation: A newspaper treatment group for adolescents with a diagnosis of conduct disorder. *Occupational Therapy in Mental Health, 7*(2), 89–104.
7. Baron, K. B. (1991). The use of play in child psychiatry: Reframing the therapeutic environment. *Occupational Therapy in Mental Health, 11*(2–3), 37–56.
8. Bazyk, S. (2006). Creating occupation-based social skills groups in after-school care. *OT Practice, 11*(17), 13–18.
9. Behnke, C. J., & Fetkovich, M. M. (1984). Examining the reliability and validity of the play history. *American Journal of Occupational Therapy, 38*(2), 94–100.
10. Black, M. M. (1976). Adolescent role assessment. *American Journal of Occupational Therapy, 30*(2), 73–79.
11. Chandler, B. E. (2007). Hidden in plain sight—Working with students with emotional disturbance in the schools. *OT Practice, 12*(1), CE1–CE8.
12. Cogan, A. M. (2014). Supporting our military families: A case for a larger role for occupational therapy in prevention and mental health care. *American Journal of Occupational Therapy, 68*(4), 478–483.
13. Coster, W. (1998). Occupation-centered assessment of children. *American Journal of Occupational Therapy, 52*(5), 337–344.
14. Cramm, H., Krupa, T., Missiuna, C., Lysaght, R. M., & Parker, K. C. H. (2013). Broadening the occupational therapy toolkit: An executive functioning lens for occupational therapy with children and youth. *American Journal of Occupational Therapy, 67*(6), e139–e147.
15. DeLany, J. V. (2009). Children and adolescents with psychosocial and emotional challenges. In J. V. DeLany & M. J. Pendzick (Eds.), *Working with children and adolescents—A guide for the occupational therapy assistant* (Chapter 17). Pearson Prentice Hall.
16. Dickerson, A. E., & Oakley, F. (1995). Comparing the roles of community-living persons and patient populations. *American Journal of Occupational Therapy, 49*(3), 221–228.
17. Dirette, D., & Kolak, L. (2004). Occupational performance needs of adolescents in alternative education programs. *American Journal of Occupational Therapy, 58*(3), 337–341.
18. Downing, D. T. (2006). The impact of early psychosis on learning. *OT Practice, 11*(12), 7–10.
19. Easton, L., & Herge, E. A. (2011). Adult day care: Promoting meaningful and purposeful leisure. *OT Practice, 16*(1), 20–23, 26.
20. Erikson, E. (1963). *Childhood and society*. Norton.
21. Fiorillo, A., Pompili, M., Luciano, M., & Sartorius, N. (2019). Reducing the mortality gap in people with serious mental disorders: The role of lifestyle psychosocial interventions. *Frontiers in Psychiatry, 9*(463), 1–4.

22. Franklin, D. A. (1986). Comparison of the effectiveness of values clarification presented as a personal computer program versus a traditional therapy group: A pilot study. *Occupational Therapy in Mental Health, 6*(3), 39–52.

23. Ginzburg, E. (1971). Toward a theory of occupational choice. In H. C. Peters & J. C. Hansen (Eds.), *Vocational guidance and career development*. Macmillan.

24. Gray, K. (2005). Mental illness in children and adolescents: A place for occupational therapy. *Mental Health Special Interest Section Quarterly, 28*(2), 1–3.

25. Gurley, S. K. (2021, October 18). *Depression across the lifespan: Depression—And its treatments—Are different for each life stage.* Anxiety & Depression Association of America. https://adaa.org/learn-from-us/from-the-experts/blog-posts/consumer-professional/depression-across-lifespan

26. Harris, J. R. (1998). *The nurture assumption: Why children turn out the way they do.* Free Press.

27. Horowitz, B. P. (2002). Occupational therapy home assessments: Supporting community living through client-center practice. *Occupational Therapy in Mental Health, 18*(1), 1–17.

28. Howie, L., Coulter, M., & Feldman, S. (2004). Crafting the self: Older person's narratives of occupational identity. *American Journal of Occupational Therapy, 58*(4), 446–454.

29. Jones, P. B. (2013). Adult mental health disorders and their age at onset. *The British Journal of Psychiatry, 202*(s54), s5–s10.

30. Jonsson, H., Kielhofner, G., & Borell, L. (1997). Anticipating retirement: The formation of narratives concerning an occupational transition. *American Journal of Occupational Therapy, 51*(1), 49–56.

31. Keller, J. *Helping families to help their loved ones with serious mental illness: A white paper of the National Alliance on Mental Illness of New York State.* Retrieved February 2, 2007, from www.naminys.org/famserwp.pdf

32. Kimball-Carpenter, A., & Smith, M. (2013). An occupational therapist's interdisciplinary approach to a geriatric psychiatry activity group: A case study. *Occupational Therapy in Mental Health, 29*(3), 293–298.

33. Kramer, L. A., Deitz, J. C., & Crowe, T. K. (1988). A comparison of motor performance of preschoolers enrolled in mental health programs and non-mental health programs. *American Journal of Occupational Therapy, 42*(8), 520–525.

34. Larson, E. A. (2004). Children's work: The less considered childhood occupation. *American Journal of Occupational Therapy, 58*(4), 369–379.

35. Lawlor, M. C., & Mattingly, C. F. (1998). The complexities embedded in family-centered care. *American Journal of Occupational Therapy, 52*(4), 259–267.

36. Levy, L. L. (2001). Memory processing and the older adult: What practitioners need to know. *OT Practice, 6*(7), CE1–CE8.

37. Liu, L., Gauthier, L., & Gauthier, S. (1991). Spatial disorientation in persons with early senile dementia of the Alzheimer type. *American Journal of Occupational Therapy, 45*(1), 67–74.

38. Menks, F. (1980). Challenges of mid life: An occupational therapy conflict resolution model. *Occupational Therapy in Mental Health, 1*(4), 23–32.

39. National Scientific Council on the Developing Child. (2018). *Understanding motivation: Building the brain architecture that supports learning, health, and community participation* (Working Paper No. 14). https://developingchild.harvard.edu/resources/understanding-motivation-building-the-brain-architecture-that-supports-learning-health-and-community-participation/

40. Nave, J., Helfrich, C. A., & Aviles, A. (2001). Child witnesses of domestic violence: A case study using the OT PAL. *Occupational Therapy in Mental Health, 16*(3–4), 127–135.

41. Norman, A. N., & Crosby, P. M. (1990). Meeting the challenge: Role of occupational therapy in a geriatric day hospital. *Occupational Therapy in Mental Health, 10*(3), 65–78.

42. Northwood Technical College. (n.d.). *Community-based residential facility (CBRF) caregiver curriculum.* Retrieved December 20, 2021, from https://www.northwoodtech.edu/academic-programs/degree-programs-and-certificates/community-based-residential-facility-caregiver/curriculum

43. Olson, L. (1992). Parent–child activity-based therapy. *Mental Health Special Interest Section Quarterly, 15*(3), 3–4.

44. Olson, L. (2006). Activity groups in family-centered treatment: Psychiatric occupational therapy approaches for parents and children. *Occupational Therapy in Mental Health, 22*(3–4), 1–156.

45. Olson, M. R. (2012). Tech support for the emotional regulation needs of children and adolescents with autism. *OT Practice, 17*(21), 20–21.

46. Oxer, S. S., & Miller, B. K. (2001). Effects of choice in an art occupation with adolescents living in residential treatment facilities. *Occupational Therapy in Mental Health, 17*(1), 39–49.

47. Perlmutter, M. S., Bhorade, A., Gordon, M., Hollingsworth, H. H., & Baum, M. C. (2010). Cognitive, visual, auditory, and emotional factors that affect participation in older adults. *American Journal of Occupational Therapy, 64*(4), 570–579.

48. Philipps, D. (2015, February 5). A veteran works to break the "broken hero" stereotype. *The New York Times.* http://www.nytimes.com/2015/02/06/us/a-veteran-works-to-break-the-broken-hero-stereotype.html

49. Pickens, N. D., & Pizur-Barnekow, K. (2009). Co-occupation: Extending the dialogue. *Journal of Occupational Science, 16*(3), 151–156.

50. Pierce, D. (2009). Co-occupation: The challenges of defining concepts original to occupational science. *Journal of Occupational Science, 16*(3), 203–207.

51. Pizur-Barnekow, K., & Knutson, J. (2009). A comparison of the personality dimensions and behavior changes that occur during solitary and co-occupation. *Journal of Occupational Science, 16*(3), 157–162.

52. Plach, H. L., & Sells, C. H. (2013). Occupational performance needs of young veterans. *American Journal of Occupational Therapy, 67*(1), 73–81.

53. Ramchand, R. (2021). *Suicide among veterans.* RAND Corporation. Retrieved December 2, 2021, from https://www.rand.org/pubs/perspectives/PEA1363-1.html

54. Reilly, M. (1974). *Play as exploratory learning.* Sage.

55. Robinson, A. L. (1977). Play: The area for acquisition of rules for competent behavior. *American Journal of Occupational Therapy, 31*(4), 248–253.

56. Rogers, C. M., Mallinson, T., & Peppers, D. (2014). High-intensity sports for posttraumatic stress disorder and depression: Feasibility study of ocean therapy with veterans of Operation Enduring Freedom and Operation Iraqi Freedom. *American Journal of Occupational Therapy, 68*(4), 395–404.

57. Salls, J., & Bucey, J. C. (2003). Self-regulation strategies for middle school students. *OT Practice, 5*(8), 11–16.

58. Schultz, S. (2003). Psychosocial occupational therapy in schools—Identify challenges and clarify the role of occupational therapy in promoting adaptive functioning. *OT Practice, 8*(17), CE1–CE8.

59. Secunda, V. (1997). *When madness comes home.* Hyperion.

60. Segal, R., & Hinojosa, J. (2006). The activity setting of homework: An analysis of three cases and implications for occupational therapy. *American Journal of Occupational Therapy, 60*(1), 50–59.

61. Sheets, J. L., Prevost, J. A., & Reihman, J. (1983). Young adult chronic patients: Three hypothesized subgroups. In *Hospital and community psychiatry service of the American Psychiatric Association. The young adult chronic patient: Collected articles from H&CP.* American Psychiatric Association.

62. Shimp, S. (1990). Debunking the myths of aging. *Occupational Therapy in Mental Health, 10*(3), 101–111.

63. Speicher, S. M., Walter, K. H., & Chard, K. M. (2014). Interdisciplinary residential treatment of posttraumatic stress disorder and traumatic brain injury: Effects on symptom severity and occupational performance. *American Journal of Occupational Therapy, 68*(4), 412–421.

64. Substance Abuse and Mental Health Services Administration. (2020). *2020 National Survey of Drug Use and Health (NSDUH) release: Table 5.1A—Substance use disorder for specific substances in past year: Among people aged 12 or older; by age group, numbers in thousands, 2019 and 2020.* https://www.samhsa.gov/data/sites/default/files/reports/rpt35323/NSDUHDetailedTabs2020/NSDUHDetailedTabs2020/NSDUHDetTabsSect5pe2020.htm

65. Sullivan, A., Dowdy, T., Haddad, J., Hussain, S., Patel, A., & Smyth, K. (2013). Occupational therapy interventions in adult mental health across settings: A literature review. *Mental Health Special Interest Section Quarterly, 36*(1), 1–3.

66. Takata, N. (1969). The play history. *American Journal of Occupational Therapy*, 23(3), 314–318.
67. Taylor, R. R. (2017). *Kielhofner's model of human occupation* (5th ed.). Wolters Kluwer.
68. Toglia, J., & Berg, C. (2013). Performance-based measure of executive function: Comparison of community and at-risk youth. *American Journal of Occupational Therapy*, 67(5), 515–523.
69. Townsend, S., Carey, P., Hollins, N., Helfrich, C., Blondis, M., Hoffman, A., Collins, L., Knudson, J., & Blackwell, A. (1999). *The occupational therapy psychosocial assessment of learning*. Model of Human Occupation Clearinghouse.
70. Tryssenaar, J., Tremblay, M., Handy, I., & Kochanoff, A. (2002). Aging with a serious mental illness: Family members' experience. *Occupational Therapy in Mental Health*, 18(1), 19–42.
71. U.S. Department of Health and Human Services (Administration for Community Living [Administration on Aging]). (2021, May). *2020 profile of older Americans*. https://acl.gov/aging-and-disability-in-america/data-and-research/profile-older-americans
72. Vaillant, G. E., & Vaillant, C. O. (1981). Natural history of male psychological health, X: Work as a predictor of positive mental health. *American Journal of Psychiatry*, 138(11), 1433–1440.
73. Wagenfeld, A. (2013). Nature—An environment for health. *OT Practice*, 18(15), 15–18.
74. Watling, R. L., Deitz, J., & White, O. (2001). Comparison of sensory profile scores of young children with and without autism spectrum disorders. *American Journal of Occupational Therapy*, 55(40), 416–423.
75. Wechsler, D. (2019). *Wechsler intelligence scale for children* (5th ed.). Pearson.
76. Winkler, R. (2021, September 21). Apple is working on iPhone features to help detect depression, cognitive decline. *Wall Street Journal*. https://www.wsj.com/articles/apple-wants-iphones-to-help-detect-depression-cognitive-decline-sources-say-11632216601
77. World Health Organization. (2017, December 12). *Mental health of older adults*. https://www.who.int/news-room/fact-sheets/detail/mental-health-of-older-adults
78. Yu, M.-L., Desha, L., & Ziviani, J. (2013). Aspects of activity participation as risk factors for conduct problems in children and adolescents: A literature review using ecological systems theory. *Occupational Therapy in Mental Health*, 29(4), 395–415.
79. Zemke, R., & Clark, F. (1996). *Occupational science: An evolving discipline*. F.A. Davis.

SUGGESTED RESOURCES

Children

Arbesman, M., Bayzk, S., & Nochajski, S. M. (2013). Systematic review of occupational therapy and mental health promotion, prevention, and intervention for children and youth. *American Journal of Occupational Therapy*, 67(6), e120–e130.
Center on the Social and Emotional Foundations for Early Learning. http://csefel.vanderbilt.edu/index.html
Champagne, T. (2012). Creating occupational therapy groups for children and youth in community-based mental health practice. *OT Practice*, 17(14), 13–18.
Chandler, B. E. (2007). Hidden in plain sight: Working with students with emotional disturbance in the schools. *OT Practice*, 12(1), CE1–CE8.
Cramm, H., Krupa, T., Missiuna, C., Lysaght, R. M., & Parker, K. C. H. (2013). Broadening the occupational therapy toolkit: An executive functioning lens for occupational therapy with children and youth. *American Journal of Occupational Therapy*, 67(6), e139–e147.
Every Moment Counts. https://everymomentcounts.org/
Fazio, L. S. (1992). Tell me a story: The therapeutic metaphor in the practice of pediatric occupational therapy. *American Journal of Occupational Therapy*, 46(2), 112–119.

Generation Mindful. https://genmindful.com/
Larson, E. A. (2004). Children's work: The less considered childhood occupation. *American Journal of Occupational Therapy*, 58(4), 369–379.
Lutman, A., & Funkhouser, E. (2020). Group discussions: Helping kids plan their transition to middle school. *OT Practice*, 25(9), 24–26.
Olson, M. R. (2012). Tech support for the emotional regulation needs of children and adolescents with autism. *OT Practice*, 17(21), 20–21.
Schmelzer, L. (2006). An occupation-based camp for healthier children. *OT Practice*, 11(16), 18–23.
Sepulveda, A., Barlow, K., Benen Demchick, B., & Flanagan, J. E. (2020). Children's mental health: Promoting mental health through early screening and detection. *OT Practice*, 25(4), 26–28.
Social Emotional Developmental Checklists for Kids and Teens from Kiddie Matters. https://www.kiddiematters.com/social-emotional-development-checklists-for-kids-and-teens/

Adolescents

Arbesman, M., Bayzk, S., & Nochajski, S. M. (2013). Systematic review of occupational therapy and mental health promotion, prevention, and intervention for children and youth. *American Journal of Occupational Therapy*, 67(6), e120–e130.
Downing, D. T. (2006). The impact of early psychosis on learning. *OT Practice*, 11(12), 7–10.
Gray, K. (2005). Mental illness in children and adolescents: A place for occupational therapy. *Mental Health Special Interest Section Quarterly*, 28(2), 1–3.
Mental Health Literacy. https://teenmentalhealth.org/
Olson, L. (2006). Engaging psychiatrically hospitalized teens with their parents through a parent–adolescent activity group. *Occupational Therapy in Mental Health*, 22(3–4), 121–133.

Adults

Cahill, S. M. (2020). College students' mental health: Creating supporting learning environments. *OT Practice*, 25(13), 22–24.
Maloney, S. M. (2011). College student high-risk drinking as a maladaptive serious leisure hobby. *Occupational Therapy in Mental Health*, 27(2), 155–177.
Sullivan, A., Dowdy, T., Haddad, J., Hussain, S., Patel, A., & Smyth, K. (2013). Occupational therapy interventions in adult mental health across settings: A literature review. *Mental Health Special Interest Section Quarterly*, 36(1), 1–3.

Older Adults

Bonder, B., & Gurley, D. (2005). Culture and aging—Working with older adults from diverse backgrounds. *OT Practice*, 4(7), CE1–CE8.
Chabot, M., & Galaton, J. (2020). Quiet books: Engaging the interests of people with late-state dementia. *OT Practice*, 25(10), 25–27.
Easton, L., & Herge, E. A. (2011). Adult day care: Promoting meaningful and purposeful leisure. *OT Practice*, 16(1), 20–23, 26.
Glogoski-Williams, C. (2000). Recognition of depression in the older adult. *Occupational Therapy in Mental Health*, 15(2), 17–34.
Jackson, J., Carlson, M., Mandel, D., Zemke, R., & Clark, F. (1998). Occupation in lifestyle redesign: The well elderly study occupational therapy program. *American Journal of Occupational Therapy*, 52(5), 326–344.
Levy, L. L. (2001). Memory processing and the older adult: What practitioners need to know. *OT Practice*, 6(7), CE1–CE8.

Veterans

Paralyzed Veterans of America. https://www.pva.org/publications
Plach, H. L., & Sells, C. H. (2013). Occupational performance needs of young veterans. *American Journal of Occupational Therapy*, 67(1), 73–81.
Rogers, C. M., Mallinson, T., & Peppers, D. (2014). High-intensity sports for posttraumatic stress disorder and depression: Feasibility study of ocean therapy with veterans of Operation Enduring Freedom and

Operation Iraqi Freedom. *American Journal of Occupational Therapy, 68*(4), 395–404.

Stinogel, A. K. (2020). Using positive psychology in occupational therapy: Veterans with post-traumatic stress disorder. *OT Practice, 25*(1), 14–15.

U.S. Department of Veterans Affairs. Office of Research & Development. https://www.research.va.gov/topics/mental_health.cfm

Veterans Recovery Resources. *Occupational therapy.* https://vetsrecover.org/services/integrated-mental-physical-health/

Families

Abelenda, J., & Helfrich, C. A. (2003). Family resilience and mental illness: The role of occupational therapy. *Occupational Therapy in Mental Health, 19*(1), 25–39.

Family & Community Resource Centre. http://fcrc.albertahealthservices.ca/

Olson, L. (2006). Activity groups in family-centered treatment: Psychiatric occupational therapy approaches for parents and children. *Occupational Therapy in Mental Health, 22*(3–4), 1–156.

General

Kaysen, S. (1993). *Girl, interrupted.* Vintage.

Levinson, D. J. (1978). *The seasons of a man's life.* Ballantine Books.

Mallinson, T., Kielhofner, G., & Mattingly, C. (1996). Metaphor and meaning in a clinical interview. *American Journal of Occupational Therapy, 50*(5), 338–346.

Sheehy, G. (1978). *Passages: Predictable crises of adult life.* Bantam.

Occupational therapy's role in sleep: Don't sleep on occupational therapy's role in sleep. https://www.myotspot.com/occupational-therapys-role-in-sleep/

Methods and Models of Interaction and Intervention

OT HACKS OVERVIEW

O: Occupation as a means and an end

Occupation with clients is used as a "means" to develop a sense of doing, being, becoming, and belonging. The outcome, or "end," regardless of method or model used, is to enhance occupational performance.

T: Theoretical concepts, values, and principles, or historical foundations

Models, built on the idea of occupation and how we react to occupational circumstances and use occupation to make ourselves whole include: model of human occupation, Kawa model, occupational adaptation, and biopsychosocial model.

H: How can we Help? OT's role in serving clients with mental illness or mental health needs

How do we provide our services to those with mental illness and mental health needs? We consider personal factors such as culture, diversity, equity, inclusion, and justice.

We consider occupational therapy methods regarding population characteristics (caregivers and community-based programs), society as a whole (models of health outside of occupational therapy and social issues), and individual needs (literacy, medical, or physical needs). We also provide services within an interdisciplinary approach by using the models of recovery, wellness, psychiatric rehabilitation, psychoeducation, and psychosocial rehabilitation.

A: Adaptations

Adaptations for those with lifelong mental disorders and mental health needs are done to allow for the greatest level of independence possible. Based on different methods and approaches, emphasis is geared for society, specific populations, groups, and individual needs.

C: Case study includes

Case study of a man with alcohol use disorder.

K: Knowledge: keeping mental health OT practice grounded in evidence, in occupational science, and in research

New terminology and need for more research regarding pain

S: Some terms that may be new to you

ACEs
adaptation gestalt
adaptive capacity
adaptive mastery
consumer movement
fear avoidance
in vivo
intimate partner violence
lifestyle medicine
nuclear task
occupational adaptiveness
occupational injustice
occupational resilience
positive physical approach
psychosocial rehabilitation
remotivating task
resilience
skills and coping tasks
symbolic tasks

OCCUPATION AND THE CLIENT

This chapter is about the methods and models we use when working with our clients. The objective of the chapter is to "bring alive" what we do and how we do it, versus the next chapter that focuses on where we provide, or do, our services. In this respect, we need to start with the concepts of being, doing, becoming, and belonging. These are fundamental thoughts about how we "see" our clients. These ideas drive how we interact with our clients.

To begin, occupational therapist Ann Wilcox described occupation as a coming together of doing, being, and becoming (189). **Doing** is identified as more than just an action of performance; it involves the person and the impact of their actions on those around them (189). This leads to the idea of **being**, which involves the "doing" of the person, along with their distinct ideas and thoughts. To "be," the person must reflect on what they do, consider the outcomes and consequences, and determine how best to continue doing in the future (189), based on how they see their actions and how they feel about what they are doing. As a part of being, there is an understanding on the part of the person as to how they fit with where they are and what is happening around them (147). **Becoming** has a futuristic tone (189). It encompasses what we do and who we are, plus how we want to be identified in times to come. Finally, the concept of **belonging** is about who we are with, how we interact with them, impact them, and are impacted by them. Because relationships are not conducted in isolation, the impact of personal factors and environmental factors also shapes one's sense of belonging (143).

PERSONAL FACTORS

Occupational therapy professionals encounter clients, consumers, families, groups, and populations with a variety of distinct personal factors. The *American Occupational Therapy Association Occupational Therapy Practice Framework: Domain & Process*-4 defines personal factors as "the particular background of a person's life and living and consist of the unique features of the person that are not part of a health condition or health state" (6, p. 40). In our consideration toward our client's personal factors, we think about culture, diversity, equity, inclusion, and justice.

Culture

Culture can be confused with race, ethnicity, religion, and other things but it is none of these. *Culture* is the combination of the learned patterns of interactions and the shared beliefs of a particular group. For example, North Americans, as a group, have a shared belief in personal freedom as a right. Box 6.1 shows examples of culturally derived patterns of interaction shared in the dominant culture of the United States. All these patterns are *learned behaviors* that belong to a particular culture. These behaviors may cause discomfort to persons from other cultures (110).

BOX 6.1 Examples of Cultural Norms for Behavior in the United States

- **Meeting others:** Make eye contact; shake hands firmly and briefly while standing about 2 to 3 feet away (184).
- **Gestures have specific meaning:** beckon with flexed index finger with palm up (supinated) means to "come here," a thumbs-up movement means "good job" (134).
- **General social behavior to strangers:** Smile; be pleasant; engage in small talk with others (134).

Relating effectively to people who have a different set of expectations for social behavior is a skill that can be learned. When a health care practitioner meets with a client of a different culture, the main objectives should be to make the person comfortable, to communicate effectively, and to engage the person in working on a program of care. Yet because of cultural differences, health care practitioners may inadvertently behave in ways that confuse, embarrass, or offend the client. Thus, it is essential for the occupational therapy professional student (like other health care practitioners) to observe carefully, to ask questions tactfully and humbly, and to learn the cultures and customs of their clients and colleagues.

Bonder and Gurley (19) point out that older adults are more likely to retain cultural traditions. Thus, to improve health outcomes, it is important to find out what traditions and values are important to them. Because of differences in the way health and health care are conceptualized in the culture of origin, older adults in particular may not receive optimum care. Furthermore, cultural misunderstandings may interfere with the person following instructions or returning for visits. Bonder and Gurley (19) note that an attitude of "cultural curiosity" is essential and that developing specific expertise regarding cultures in one's community of care is useful.

The Immigration Experience

The population of the United States has increased dramatically through immigration. In 2018, the proportion of foreign-born persons living in New York City was 38% (106). Foreign-born individuals make up almost 14% of the population of the United States (179).

Immigration status (legal or illegal) affects health behavior. Those with no legal status may be cautious of engaging with the health care system or any other organization for fear of being identified and deported. Immigrants who have experienced stress or violence may experience posttraumatic stress disorder (PTSD). As of 2019, 46% of nonelderly immigrants in the United States who were undocumented did not have health insurance, 25% of nonelderly immigrants in the United States who were lawfully present did not have health insurance, and 9% of nonelderly U.S. citizens did not have health insurance (89).

How do immigrants "fit in" with their adopted country? At one extreme, some new immigrants resist assimilation, clinging to their native languages, customs, and cuisines; at the other extreme are those who are eager to become American in every way. Most immigrants seem to tread a middle path. The technology of the information age and the availability of air transportation have made it possible for them to maintain an ongoing relationship with their countries of origin via social media, phone, text message, Facetime, e-mail, international money wiring, and frequent visits.

The immigration of successive generations to the United States may span several decades, with periods of residence alternating between the two countries. It is common for parents to send their children "home" (eg, to India, Trinidad, Mexico) to learn "proper" behavior or for rigorous schooling. Important life events, such as weddings, births, deaths, and burials, may take place in the country of origin. In other words, an ongoing identification with one's native country may coexist with an American lifestyle. Sending remittances (money) to family "at home" in the native country is a common practice.

The children of first-generation immigrants may undergo stress from the conflicting demands of their parents (and the traditions of the original culture) and the expectations of American peers. This stress is compounded in adolescence, a time for questioning and confirming one's identity. Immigrant parents, in reaction to their offspring's interest in and attempts to adopt American culture and behaviors, may also suffer distress. At one extreme of the generations, the oldest members may stubbornly adhere to native traditions; at the other, the youngest are likely to be listening to popular music and wearing the latest fashions.

Blending and adopting dual or multiple cultures is one way some immigrants cope with this. For example, young people from traditional Indian families may tolerate or even seek arranged marriages for themselves, sometimes marrying a person who is still living in India. A young Indian American woman may wear a designer suit to work in an investment firm yet wear a *salwar kameez* (long loose tunic over pants) at home. Furthermore, she may live across the hall from her mother-in-law, for whom she prepares traditional Indian foods and to whom she defers in decisions relating to home and family (156).

Cultural Differences in Diagnosis

Mental disorders (indeed physical disorders also) are not thought of in all cultures in the same way as in the United States. Fadiman (52), in a fascinating and award-winning account, tells the story of a Hmong refugee family, living in central California, with a young child who had epilepsy. Because epilepsy is regarded in the Hmong culture as a mystical and sacred trance state, the family was inconsistent in applying the remedies provided by the doctors, nurses, and health care team. Problems of language translation, cultural mistrust, and other factors (on both sides) resulted in a frustrating experience for the medical team. Although the child eventually sustained severe brain damage from high fevers and prolonged seizures, the family did not seem unhappy with the outcome and continued to dress, bathe, clothe, and feed the child in the highest standard of their culture. The child held a place of honor in the household.

The *Diagnostic and Statistical Manual of Mental Disorders: Fifth Edition Text Revision* (*DSM-5-TR*) contains in *Section III* information about syndromes that occur only in certain cultures (11). For example, in the Latinx cultures of the United States and of Latin America, the term *nervios* is the "general state of vulnerability to stressful life experiences and to difficult life circumstances" (11, p. 877). *Susto* is a term associated with some Latinx cultures from North, Central, and South America. It refers to a frightening event that results in the soul leaving the body and may cause symptoms like those in depressive disorders (11).

The occupational therapy professional working with immigrants should appreciate that there is much to be learned—and that little can be assumed—about the values, customs, and life situations of these clients. In many countries and cultures, the concept of mental disorders as we know it does not exist; therefore, to speak about it with the client and the family as such is counterproductive. Skilled occupational therapy professionals instead learn to phrase their expectations for the client and families in ways that can be understood and appreciated by them. For example, a psychiatrist, himself Chinese, speaking with the parents of a bright Chinese high school student who was hallucinating and punching walls, never mentions the possibility of schizophrenia or antipsychotic medication. He instead directs them to have their son take "these little pills every day for a week to help his motivation" (99).

Diversity

Diversity includes consideration toward one's particular internal thoughts about themselves and their actions, as well as the external qualities and features that are identifiable by others. Diversity can be thought of as the parts of us that make us unique and make us "our own person." By including in our activities those identified as different from us, we expand the diverse perspective that is used to look at the world around us (7). Our clients can be different from us. Their backgrounds, life occupational histories, family units, life activities, and personal factors can all be different from ours. Respect and acceptance are shown to clients when services are done without preconceived ideas or biases. This leads to a wider, or more diverse, view of what occupational therapy can provide.

Gender Diversity and Identity

Within occupational therapy, and especially within occupational therapy mental health practice, there is the opportunity to demonstrate this understanding toward diversity through gender-affirming care. Occupational therapy professionals have a responsibility to consider the personal factors associated with relating to client's gender identity. Gender identification is not identification of biologic sex at birth, but rather the gender construct an individual has identified for themselves (9). When occupational therapy services are provided, there needs to be an awareness of how one's gender identification impacts their occupational processes, participation, and performance. To guide and facilitate occupational therapy interventions, clients need to be addressed as they see themselves. This is the essence of ensuring clients' occupations are meaningful to them (9).

Equity

A foundational aspect of occupational therapy service provision is identifying individual needs and then connecting clients to the specific opportunities they can participate in to meet those needs. The idea of a meaningful occupation is different for each and every person; thus, the mechanisms by which to fulfill those occupations are just as individualized.

The process of providing equity means seeking out how to respond to clients on an individual level. Interactions are specifically designed for each different and individual client seen in occupational therapy practice (8).

An equity-minded view of occupational therapy encourages a provision of care that is nondiscriminatory. When each person's needs and circumstances are used to determine what best fits with and for them, occupational therapy is provided free of biases or prejudices (7). Occupational therapy includes an equitable distribution of skilled knowledge, service provision, resources, and opportunities.

Stigma

The stigma, or discrimination, against those with mental disorders or mental health needs is directly opposite from the concept and actions of equity and diversity. Clients who are stigmatized by others risk losing the occupational therapy and health care opportunities they need to reorganize themselves to achieve their occupational desires. The impact of stigma is lowered for clients when occupational therapy professionals advocate for the resources and opportunities each client needs, as well as when clients are taught the skills of self-advocacy (5).

Inclusion

Inclusion can be seen as a natural partner, or progression, of diverse and equitable interactions and relationships with clients. Occupational therapy professionals strive to view diverse aspects of clients and to consider equitable methods to meet individual client needs. This is turn demonstrates inclusion. Inclusion involves accepting and supporting clients' diverse selves and welcoming the interactions we have by being with and for our clients. Occupational therapy professionals' outward actions of inclusion fulfill an internal drive to treat each individual for who they are and what they are individually experiencing. Inclusion is much more than tolerance, which is only recognition of a difference. Inclusion is an outward activity, based on an emotional response to the desire to be with and for that individual person (7).

Occupational Justice

Finally, there is the concept of justice. Occupational justice encompasses each person's right to complete their occupations and to have equity with their occupational choices for well-being (80). All the concepts associated with diversity, equity, and inclusion are a part of occupational justice. Through non-biased and intentional actions, occupational therapy professionals can advocate to work toward clients' rights to be treated in a just manner.

Throughout the rest of the chapter, various models of occupational therapy practice, models related to the profession of occupation therapy, and methods for intervention are discussed. The initial concepts of this chapter are about how occupation is connected to the client and how personal factors are used in determining occupational therapy services.

This knowledge helps the occupational therapy professional determine how best to teach the client to manage, adapt, and establish their occupational presence.

PRACTICE MODELS IN OCCUPATIONAL THERAPY—INTERVENTION FOCUS

This section focuses on four occupational therapy models. The model of human occupation (MOHO) has been addressed in previous chapters, including the process for how people change and the process of doing. We now expand these thoughts and bring them directly into occupational therapy intervention.

Three other occupational therapy models will be introduced. The Kawa model and the occupational adaptation (OA) model will be described and applied to occupational therapy intervention. The biopsychosocial model is introduced here, and it will be further reviewed regarding occupational therapy intervention in Chapter 17.

Model of Human Occupation

In order for the changes a person makes to be permanent, multiple steps and pieces need to happen. To begin, we know an alteration—internal or external—must occur. As the person attempts new methods of adaptation and acceptance, they gain new abilities, insights, and considerations toward themselves and the world around them. Next, the person experiences these alterations again and again; the volition, habituation, and performance capacity systems come together to help the person form a new internal organization within themselves. Then, as the person performs occupations, over and over, based on these new thoughts and methods, within a stable environment, solid patterns of new occupational participation emerge. As occupational therapy professionals, we foster this growth, facilitate new personal development, and intervene with new ideas for change when this growth and development do not occur (173).

For us to provide this intervention, we need to return to the six dimensions of occupational participation (see Chapter 3) (173).

- **Participation in occupational roles**. This includes short-term and long-term participation in the activities and projects associated with valued roles. These activities and projects hold personal and specialized meaning, are diverse in nature (allowing for total fulfillment), and encompass all participation dimensions.
- **Occupational form** (choosing an activity within a role). The person considers what can be done within their role(s). The different activities that the person could do, or could not do, are identified and assessed.
- **Occupational performance** (participating in the chosen activity). The person acts on their choice, completing what they have chosen to do, and not do.
- **Participating in one or more steps of the activity**. Participation intensity changes, as and when needed to ensure occupational success.

- **Participating in one or more actions of the activity steps.** Consideration is toward the individual performance capacity components. These components can be focused on individually or as a combination of the individual items.
- **Subjective experience and objective appraisal of performance capacity.** This involves reflecting on the subjective feelings of satisfaction with the person's performance, as well as assessing the objective details seen as the outcome of the performance. From this process being completed over and over, change and self-efficacy emerge.

The methods occupational therapy professionals use to facilitate change with a client are interrelated and are integrated in a unique and flexible manner, which is individualized for each specific client. These methods include the therapeutic use of self-actions and behaviors used by the occupational therapy professional directed toward the client and the specific interventions that emphasize the pieces of the MOHO and include performing specific procedures and the use of specific strategies, all grounded within this model (173).

Therapeutic strategies include the following (173):

- *Validating.* This includes demonstrating respect for the client's experiences and perspectives, without any biases or reactions by the occupational therapy professional that would indicate a bias.
- *Identifying.* A client's participation in occupation is enhanced when the occupational therapy professional provides resources and opportunities in various environments for the client to practice various occupations.
- *Giving feedback.* The occupational therapy professional shares their knowledge and professional experience information with the client, to enhance the client's participation in occupation.
- *Advising.* At times the client does not have the performance capacities to identify and determine a course of action. At these times, the occupational therapy professional provides recommendations for possible goals and strategies to complete goals.
- *Negotiating.* This is a give-and-take process. It involves the views of the client and any of their significant others in relationship to what the client will do. Viewpoints of all involved are considered and the end result should be that the client feels empowered to decide and perform beneficial occupations.
- *Structuring.* The occupational therapy professional provides an orderly intervention environment with clear directions and expectations. Alternative options are a part of structuring and are offered as specific avenues for occupational participation and occupational performance.
- *Coaching.* Activity performance support and assistance are provided via education and training. Demonstration and cuing are essential to this method of interaction.
- *Encouraging.* Emotional support is given to the client and reassurance is provided as the client attempts new

methods and strategies to complete occupations. Often in these situations the client is taking a risk and maintaining their efforts, despite a difficult or trying situation.
- *Providing physical support.* This includes the physical assistance given to a client, as needed, during occupational performance. It can also include accompanying a client into a new situation or helping the client be able to "get to" where an occupation needs to be performed.

Specific interventions include the following (173):

- *Assessment combined with intervention.* From the initial time the occupational therapy professional meets with the client, a relationship is formed and built. From the beginning, active exploration is encouraged, and over-time performance capacities are continually assessed.
- *Participation in meaningful occupations.* Occupations that hold meaning are performed by the client and that performance is assessed, with new insight of performance capabilities becoming a part of the next attempt. The occupational therapy professional needs to establish a connection with the client that allows the occupational therapy professional to see and feel occupation from the client's perspective.
- *Facilitation of exploration.* A client's exploration into their capacity for performance, interests, and values is facilitated by the occupational therapy professional. The aim is for the client's decision-making to be supported, regarding their choices of occupation.
- *Occupational counseling.* The occupational therapy professional and client have a space in which they can discuss and share occupational performance and participation activity and consider future needs.
- *Peer support educational groups.* Using social involvement and social learning, for groups of clients with common needs, diverse topics are discussed, leading to enhanced occupational performance.
- *Occupational self-help groups.* These are organized by people with similar wants and needs. There is a sharing of diverse occupational experiences and occupational topics.
- *MOHO-based skills teaching.* Specifics depend on the practice setting, client performance capacities, and client desires and needs. Multiple other intervention strategies can be incorporated into education, training, and activity. Processes are aligned with the MOHO concepts.
- *Social education.* A team-based approach used for education that is active and participatory. There is a goal for client change, which is fostered through activities to increase client's sense of control and client's autonomy. Education is done formally and informally, based on practice setting, environment, and needs of the individuals and the needs of the group.
- *Environmental management.* The occupational environment and setting are adapted or changed to promote greater occupational performance and participation. Considerations include space, objects, occupational

demands, social atmosphere, and opportunities for participation.

- *Occupational role development and habit change.* During the competency stage of change, clients need to confront situations that present challenges and allow room for growth. Clients need to negotiate between their wants and their internal expectations and expectations of the environment and of society. Motivation (volition) must be incorporated into doing, for substantial change to occur. Role performance done over time provides a mechanism to establish and solidify new habits and routines.

Kawa Model[1]

The Kawa model was developed by occupational therapist Michael Iwama and utilizes a Japanese cultural perspective. This model uses the metaphor of a river, using water, rocks, driftwood, the river floor, and river walls, to depict various aspects of life. This model encompasses a collectivist culture. This includes the following items:

- The concept of "group" is embedded in the model along with the concept of having an interdependence with others in society.
- Society places meaning onto human actions.
- The roles and position of a person have meaning inside their society.
- A person's roles and occupations are integral to their society.
- Harmony with the collective (persons and environment together) is the goal, rather than mastery over the environment.
- Wellness is seen as harmony among oneself and others in society, with nature, and within a person's context.
- A person is embedded in the group and with the whole of nature and the environment; this is the decentralized self.
- To have health of the whole one must act within the environment, not on it.
- Belonging first, being next, then doing, rather than doing, then being, then becoming.
- Society bestows a role on a person and from that comes the connection of the person's actions back to society.

In this model, client-centered goals hold meaning in the person having occupations that meet the requirements of the collective group and maintain the person's function within the group. The goal is: belonging. In occupational therapy, assessment needs to start with this concept of belonging, not with idea of goals to establish individualism. The temporal aspect of goal creation rests in the present and the process of activity, not with a view toward the future and not toward achievement in the future or at a later date.

---

[1]Kawa Model information adapted from Turpin, M., & Iwama, M. K. (2011). *Using occupational therapy models in practice: A field guide.* Churchill Livingstone Elsevier.

Flow of the Water

The water in this model represents *life energy* or *life flow.* One's flow or energy of life can be the person, family, or groups. The flow of a person's life starts at birth, and a collection of moisture in a low part of the land. By the end of life, the river flows into a large body of water. The water is always pivoting to a larger collection of water, just as the person is always directed toward a greater connection within their society. The middle of the river includes twists and turns, obstacles, the input of one's character and one's skills. A person can be born into a river with obstacles or born into a river that flows freely and easily.

Occupational therapy intervention facilitates a person's life flow within the context of having a harmonious balance with all aspects of life, or with the river. A person's life history is represented as the river. Different cross-sections of the river are different times in that life history. Different times in one's life can reveal different river elements. The elements represent a person's life circumstances and are the river floor, river walls, driftwood, rocks, and the spaces between each of these items. Channels are created in the river, as they are in life. These channels are formed based on the size of the elements and are relative to the positions of the elements. Change throughout life is done by increasing and decreasing the water flow and also by altering the elements. Size, shape, and position of the elements all impact one's change over the life span.

Water (Mizu)

The water is pure, cleansing, and renewing. It is often associated with one's spirit. There is a fluidity to the water and it flows over, or around, or through obstacles and makes paths. As a fluid, as it flows over or through parts of the river, it is shaped by these experiences. Water also "takes on" the shape of what it flows near to or what it flows through. A person's life reflects the situations and circumstances the person experiences. Water is powerful and can erode away parts of the land that hold the water in place. A river's volume, shape, flow, and rate are impacted by the river elements. These river elements, surroundings, people, and circumstances bounded by land are shaped by the river's life energy and life flow.

Within the collectivism culture, there are mutually influencing relationships with one's surroundings and flow is always occurring, a little, between the elements. The self is embedded inside relationships with others and with the environment. This leads to a sense of belonging, interdependence, and forms and builds the social context. Within occupational therapy, it is important to consider all these interacting aspects of daily life. Occupational therapy professionals facilitate a greater life flow. Disharmony weakens life flow. Occupational therapy professionals use river elements, individually or in combination, to facilitate that life flow.

River Walls (Kawano souk-heki) and River Floor (Kawa no zoko)

The river walls and river floor shape the course, the depth, and the width of the river. Society's social contexts and physical contexts (environmental factors and personal factors) surround the client and determine the experiences of the person and thus of the actions of the person. Social contexts are key and therefore they direct relationships. A person's relationships are with family members, pets, friends, coworkers, classmates, and memories of departed family members.

This view of the entire river area encourages occupational therapy professionals to have a holistic perspective. There is not a particular shape of the river that is "optimal." If the river walls are narrow and floor is shallow, but free of obstacles, that is okay. A deep river with obstacles can cause problems. One's environments can facilitate or inhibit and can be shaped to increase the harmony the person is seeking between themselves and the contexts of life.

Rocks (Iwa)

Rocks are the circumstances of life. They can be problematic and impede life flow. It can be difficult to remove rocks. Rocks disturb water flow because of their shape, size, and placement in relation to the river walls and river floor. They represent challenges the person faces and impairments affecting the person's life.

In occupational therapy it is important to remember that all the river floors and river walls are shaped differently, therefore rocks impact each river differently. In this respect, rocks represent body structures and body functions. Different rocks can appear and happen in each person's life. These rocks could be: decreased motivation to complete occupations, anxiety, depression, history of relapse, physical injuries and illnesses, self-care deficits, financial problems, or relationship problems.

Driftwood (Ryuboku)

There are positive and negative impacts of driftwood. Driftwood affects a person's life circumstances and their life flow. Driftwood represents a person's attributes and their resources. Examples of these include the following:

- values such as honesty and thriftiness
- characteristics such as optimism and stubbornness
- personality traits such as being reserved or being outgoing
- specialized skills such as carpentry or public speaking

Driftwood includes material and immaterial aspects and living situations. These could be friends, siblings, wealth, special equipment or property, rural or urban dwellings, shared or solo accommodations. For example, more financial income can lead to the potential, goal, or dream for a larger home and a bigger family size; more income can also lead to a greater anxiety if the person does not have the skills to maintain a larger home or the parenting ability to manage a larger family size.

Driftwood is less permanent than rocks and more easily moved. It can be carried along with the water's current. It can connect or combine and form a dam, thus restricting

BOX 6.2 Occupational Therapy Focuses Within the Kawa Model

- We can view the river at cross-sections.
- We can work to expand the spaces in the river.
- We can work to reshape the river walls or the river floors.
- We can work to move around or reduce the rocks.
- We can work to use the driftwood to enlarge the spaces.
- We can work to further open up new channels.

the water flow. Water force can dislodge a driftwood dam or carve channels in the river floor. This is an activity the occupational therapy professional can help facilitate.

Spaces (Sukima)

Spaces in the river are between obstacles. Spaces are the person's social roles and the person's occupations. Occupational therapy emphasizes one's strengths; it is a strength-based discipline. The Kawa model emphasizes strength, rather than remediation, as the Kawa model is not a remedial approach. The Kawa model focuses on where life is flowing and strategically works to maximize that flow. For instance, if the person has an onset of a new mental disorder, such as schizophrenia, the idea is not to remediate to do what used to be, but rather to consider the "now" and look at how occupations can now be done in a new or different way. This is building channels around the rocks. The question is how creative the occupational therapy professional can be in helping to facilitate these channels. In occupational therapy, there is a focus on spaces between objects, rather than on the objects themselves. There is an emphasis on how life flow can be facilitated in a range of ways to decrease size or shape. This is done by making channels in the environment surrounding the person and maximizing the power of the person's existing assets and resources. The spaces where the water flow occurs can be increased through friction that can wear away or dislodge the rocks or driftwood that surround or impede the water flow. Box 6.2 states the focuses of occupational therapy. Box 6.3 provides examples for goals using the Kawa model.

BOX 6.3 Kawa Model Intervention Goals

Aim of Intervention

Belonging first, then establishment of individualism.

Meeting the requirements of the collective group.

Maintaining one's functions within the group.

Present temporal considerations and activity process.

Goals

Client will identify personal attributes and personal resources to establish/reestablish occupational activity within societal parameters to have a sense of belonging during occupational activities of _____ with _____* (add needed amount or type of assistance) and _____** within _____***.

BOX 6.3 Kawa Model Intervention Goals (*continued*)

Client will identify influencing relationships with others and within the environment to have a sense of belonging during occupational activities of _____ with _____ * (add needed amount or type of assistance) and _____ ** within _____ ***.

Client will demonstrate ability to maneuver within societal and physical contexts to complete occupational activity of _____ with _____ * (add needed amount or type of assistance) and _____ *^ within _____ ***.

Client will demonstrate ability to maneuver within life circumstances and situations to complete occupational activity of _____ with _____ * (add needed amount or type of assistance) and _____ *^ within _____ ***.

Client will demonstrate a harmonious balance within life expectations to establish/reestablish a sense of group belonging and meet societal needs for success with completing occupational activity/activities of _____ with _____ * (add needed amount or type of assistance) and _____ *^ within _____ ***.

* guidance, written prompt, written directions, cue, direct supervision/contact, indirect supervision/contact

** exploration of current societal role/societal needed capacities/current life flow; identification of life history; identification/understanding/acceptance of elements that influence life occupational activity,

*^altering/removing elements influencing life occupational activity; use of personal, societal, and environmental factors to change occupational activity; use of environment to facilitate or inhibit occupational activity; removal/decrease of barriers/challenges that limit occupational activity; facilitate use of current strengths to manage occupational activity

*** number of attempts, number of sessions, number of weeks

Occupational Adaptation Model[2]

OA is a normative human process and an intervention process that guides how occupational therapy professionals use professional reasoning. There are times in a person's life when *disruption* occurs. Disruptions can be injuries, new onsets of diagnoses, life transitions, or change with typical developmental processes. Occupational therapy professionals aim to help facilitate a person's OA process.

Normative Human Process

OA comes from engagement in and participation with occupation. The person completes a transaction with the environment. The person responds to change, altered situations, and transitions in life. OA is used to form one's identity.

The person wants to have mastery in occupations via the environment. Cognitive, sensorimotor, and psychosocial capacities enable occupational performance and occupational participation. The person's environment is filled with various settings and contexts (environmental factors and personal factors). Circumstances, physical environments, and societal expectations "push" demands on the person to behave, perform, and participate in ways that limit or facilitate the OA process. The environment in which occupations occur *demands mastery* by the person. An environment needs to be a place of order; thus, the person must balance any chaos and equalize the processes within the environment to produce stability. Participating in occupations leads the person to adapt, or change, so that occupations can be completed, regardless of the person being in a "demanding" or "negative" situation. If a person eats at a restaurant, the environment demands the person eat within a timely manner, sit quietly, talk at a respectful level, and pay the bill. In order for someone to meet these environmental demands for mastery, the occupations used by and with the person that foster this adaptation or change must be engaging, hold meaning for the person, and be goal-oriented. The person participates in occupations out of a desire to master the occupational environment. The person experiences the following processes:

- **Occupational roles**: The actions and behaviors associated with meeting society's expectations
- **Occupational challenges**: The person applies the needed amount of skill capacity and motivation to meet challenge. If the challenge is not met, *dysadaptation* can occur (mastery desire is high, mastery demand is high or low, person's skills are low).
- **Role demands or expectations**: The requirements put on the person from internal role demands or external role demands, or both.
- **Occupational Responses**: The person modifies (calibrates) themselves to meet the challenges, roles, and role demands and expectations. The person determines how to respond to the need to participate in occupations. The person configures an *adaptation gestalt*. The adaptation gestalt allows the person to use a previously successful way to overcome and to manage the stressful situation they are now in, create a new method (if the old method is not possible or useful), or adapt a method used in the past.

The *adaptation gestalt* is what allows the person to modify how much skill capacity is needed to master and competently perform occupation. Different occupational situations require different amounts of each skill. A homework assignment for a statistics course requires more cognition. An intimate partner relationship requires more psychosocial skill.

An *adaptive response* comes from how the person modifies themselves during this new and/or stressful situation. The environment presses the person to adapt to it, as the person meets the occupational challenges and occupational roles and meets role demands and expectations. Occupational responses are identified so that the person can master the environment and be competent in their occupations. Adaptation to the situation occurs as the person tries new approaches, reflects on the outcome and tries again, as needed at the appropriate level (trial-and-error approach).

[2]Occupational Adaptation Model information adapted from Grajo, L. C. (2019). Occupational adaptation as a normative and intervention process: New perspectives on Schkade and Shultz's professional legacy. In L. C. Grajo & A. K. Boisselle (Eds.), *Adaptation through occupation: Multidimensional perspectives* (pp. 83–104). SLACK.

This involves modifying and integrating occupational responses so that challenges are solved and future occupational participation is secured. These are adaptive responses. *Dysadaptive responses* occur when occupational challenges are not overcome. The person's ability to calibrate skills, use of trial-and-error attempts, and occupational participation that balances internal demands and external demands, the person's level of desire for participation, and the demand for mastery are what makes the OA process a normative and internal process.

A person's OA is measured to determine if the person is successfully adapting to the occupational situation. Success is seen when the person manages all that is part of daily life. Actions and behaviors used to achieve this success are seen in the following:

- occupational roles and responsibilities
- occupational challenges
- expectations the person sets and environmental expectations

This success can occur because of strategies the person was successful at using previously. At times a person fails, but is able to move forward without detrimental consequences. It is when the person is unable to move forward that occupational dysadaptation occurs. To determine if the person is in a state of OA, there must be a measurement of *relative mastery* and of *adaptive capacity*.

Relative mastery includes effective participation (how well occupational goals are met), efficiency (good use of resources to meet occupational demands), and satisfaction (feeling of contentment with occupational performance and participation based on oneself and satisfaction of others the person finds important). Adaptive capacity is the ability to realize and understand the need for the adaptation to occur and to make that adaptation happen, in essence, meeting the occupational challenges within the environment. Here the questions are as follows:

- Does the person have the capabilities and strategies to make the adaptation?
- Can the person pick out the needed capabilities and strategies?
- If needed, can the person design and establish the needed capabilities and strategies?
- Can the person modify previously used capabilities and strategies?

Occupational Adaptation as Intervention

It is when the person is in a state of dysadaptation that occupational therapy intervention is appropriate. The person has been unable to manage, or adapt, to the life occurrences, or the changes that happen in life. The person does not have the relative mastery and/or adaptive capacity to be successful with occupational performance and occupational participation. The person's occupational roles can be affected and become too demanding to complete, occupational performance can be diminished, occupational challenges are overwhelming to the point of not being overcome, and/or the person does not have the ability to apply the capabilities or strategies needed to provide an adaptive response.

As a conceptual model, OA is a flexible way of thinking and approaching each client at their individual place (based on time, space, and environment) and within their specific level of capability. The model of OA can be varied and altered to meet each individual's person factors. The elements of occupational intervention are as follows:

1. **Holistic assessment.** An occupational profile is completed through analyzing the person's relative mastery and adaptive capacity.
2. **Reestablishment of occupational roles.** Role performance and capacity is the main emphasis of occupational therapy intervention. One role at a time is considered. Within occupational therapy intervention the client prioritizes their meaningful roles and learns, through a process of graded occupational activity, how to adapt to the changes in their life. Key areas of consideration are habits, routines, and occupational identity.
3. **Client is the agent of change.** The adaptation, or change, the person goes through is guided by the person's understanding of what is meaningful, choices of what to perform and participate in, and initiation of occupational activity.
4. **Occupations bring about adaptive responses.** *Occupational readiness* is meant to prepare the capacity skills needed and *occupational activities* are connected to the environmental factors and personal factors held meaningful by the client.
5. **Occupational Environment.** The person's environment can be modified by removing barriers and installing supports. Role demands can be initiated or changed to start performance or encourage participation.
6. **Relative mastery and adaptive capacity.** These are sought to be increased or improved. Measurement of the person's increased occupational adaptiveness can be seen by asking the following questions:
   - Is there effective participation in occupational goals?
   - Is there efficiency while participating in occupation?
   - Do the client and those meaningful to the client state satisfaction with the occupational performance and occupational participation?
   - Is there variety in the occupational capabilities and strategies used?
   - Are the occupational capacities and strategies used independently?
   - Is there transfer of capacity use and strategies used to new and different occupational situations?
   - Are new capacities and strategies identified and used, as well as old capacities and strategies modified as needed?

The point at which the person demonstrates competency during OA, with or without occupational therapy intervention, is when the person achieves **occupational adaptiveness**. The OA model is shown in Figure 6.1. Box 6.4 provides examples of goals based on OA.

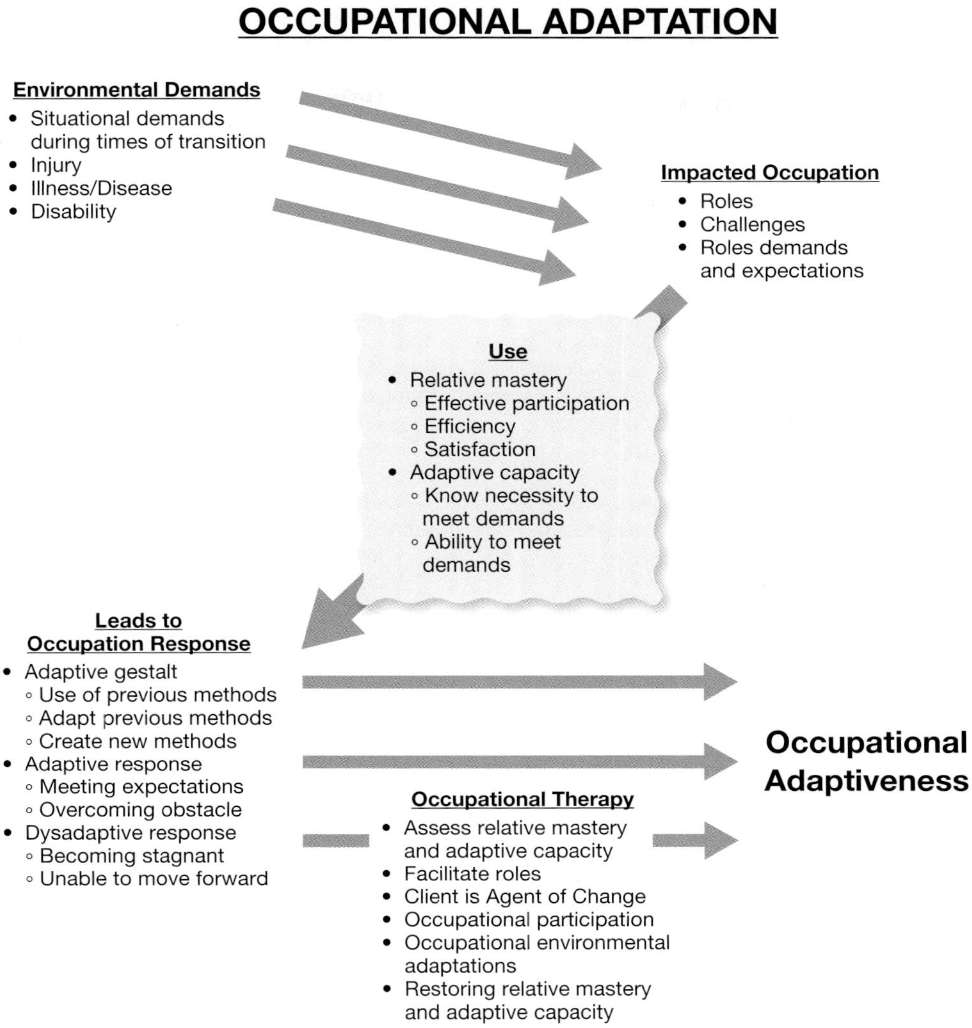

OCCUPATIONAL ADAPTATION

Environmental Demands
- Situational demands during times of transition
- Injury
- Illness/Disease
- Disability

Impacted Occupation
- Roles
- Challenges
- Roles demands and expectations

Use
- Relative mastery
  ◦ Effective participation
  ◦ Efficiency
  ◦ Satisfaction
- Adaptive capacity
  ◦ Know necessity to meet demands
  ◦ Ability to meet demands

Leads to Occupation Response
- Adaptive gestalt
  ◦ Use of previous methods
  ◦ Adapt previous methods
  ◦ Create new methods
- Adaptive response
  ◦ Meeting expectations
  ◦ Overcoming obstacle
- Dysadaptive response
  ◦ Becoming stagnant
  ◦ Unable to move forward

Occupational Adaptiveness

Occupational Therapy
- Assess relative mastery and adaptive capacity
- Facilitate roles
- Client is Agent of Change
- Occupational participation
- Occupational environmental adaptations
- Restoring relative mastery and adaptive capacity

Figure 6.1. Occupational Adaptation (OA). (Adapted from Grajo, L. C. (2019). Occupational adaptation as a normative and intervention process: New perspectives on Schkade and Shultz's professional legacy. In L. C. Grajo & A. K. Boisselle (Eds.), *Adaptation through occupation: Multidimensional perspectives* (pp. 83–104). SLACK.)

Biopsychosocial Model

The biopsychosocial model provides occupational therapy professionals a method to consider and address all aspects of the person. The medical model brings the occupational therapy professional's attention to the biologic, or physical, aspect of client intervention. The medical model is a large component of occupational therapy service delivery. Along with the biologic, or physical, aspect of the client are the aspects of psychological and social. This model puts all three aspects, biologic, psychological, and social, together (Engel, 1977, as cited in 39).

Gentry and colleagues' (58) description[3] of **psychological factors** include items such as cognitive-based abilities, personality aspects of the individual, and internal processes such as values, motivation, and goals. **Social factors** include areas such as personal factors, life situations, and occupation and activity demands.

Psychological factors and social factors directly impact the biologic factors addressed by occupational therapy professionals. Success with improvement for **biologic factors**, or physical disabilities, or physical dysfunction, is intricately connected to how a person manages their psychological factors and meets the demands put on them by their social factors. Although psychological factors and social factors play this important role in the improvement of biologic-based deficits, improvements following physical injuries and illness (such as: biomechanical components, decrease in physical symptoms, improvement in self-care or instrumental activities of daily living, adaptations to task, occupation, and environment, and resource education) are only part of the outcome[3] sought to be achieved with the person.

---

[3]Gentry's (2018) descriptions of biopsychosocial model are adapted from Brewer, B. W., Andersen, M. B., & Van Raalte, J. L. (2002). A biopsychosocial model of sports injury rehabilitation. In D. I. Mostofsky & L. D. Zaichkowsky (Eds.), *Medical and psychological aspects of sport and exercise* (p. 48). Fitness Information Technology.

BOX 6.4 Occupational Adaptation Intervention Goals

Aim of Intervention

Change person's state of dysadaptation.

Adaptation, and management, of life occurrences.

Relative mastery and adaptive capacity for successful occupation.

Completion of occupational roles.

Goals

Client will identify aspects of/reasons for dysadaptation to complete occupation of _____ with _____* (add needed amount or type of assistance) and _____** within _____***.

Client will identify occupational roles/occupational challenges/occupational role demands/occupational role expectations to complete occupation of _____ with _____* (add needed amount or type of assistance) and _____** within _____***.

Client will identify adaptive responses needed to complete occupation of _____ with _____* (add needed amount or type of assistance) and _____** within _____***.

** structured environment, everyday environment of _____, self-awareness, use of inventory checklist tool, self-reporting assessment tool, self-reflection, identifying new/needed roles/habits/routines, participation with occupational profile

Client will improve ability to self-advocate and produce change to complete occupation of _____ with _____* (add needed amount or type of assistance) and _____*^ within _____***.

Client will improve occupational readiness/relative mastery/adaptive capacity to complete occupation of _____ with _____* (add needed amount or type of assistance) and _____*^ within _____***.

Client will reestablish/complete occupational role demands/expectations to complete occupation of _____ with _____* (add needed amount or type of assistance) and _____*^ within _____***.

Client will improve ability with occupational roles/occupational challenges to complete occupation of _____ with _____* (add needed amount or type of assistance) and _____*^ within _____***.

Client will improve occupational responses to complete occupation of _____ with _____* (add needed amount or type of assistance) and _____*^ within _____***.

Client will increase relative mastery/adaptive capacity to complete occupation of _____ with _____* (add needed amount or type of assistance) and _____*^ within _____***.

Client will improve state of occupational adaptiveness to complete occupation of _____ with _____* (add needed amount or type of assistance) and _____*^ within _____***.

*^ structured environment, everyday environment of _____, use of adapted environment, setup of activity, participation of a peer, no peer involvement, no direct involvement from practitioner, assistive technology device, self-monitoring and reflection, mindfulness, stress management techniques, completing new project of _____, establishing new habit of _____, establish new routine for _____, effective participation, efficient participation, self-reflection to identification of satisfaction or performance/participation, prioritizing role/performance needs, ability to transfer new learning to new situations, use of new strategies/capacities, modification of previous/current strategies/capacities, performing occupations in various environments, performing occupations for various roles, grading _____/adapting_____ intervention for client factor need (physical, cognitive, sensory, perceptual, emotional, communication interaction, social [specify areas of need])

* guidance, written prompt, written directions, cue, direct supervision/contact, indirect supervision/contact, physical assistance, no practitioner interaction

*** number of attempts, number of sessions, number of weeks

Adapted from Grajo, L. C. (2019). Occupational adaptation as a normative and intervention process: New perspectives on Schkade and Shultz's professional legacy. In L. C. Grajo & A. K. Boisselle (Eds.), *Adaptation through occupation: Multidimensional perspectives* (pp. 83–104). SLACK.

To bring occupational therapy service delivery back to the consideration of the whole person (39), the interplay among all three factors, biologic, psychological, and social, is needed. When all three aspects are working and fully integrated, occupational therapy outcomes are completely addressed. These outcomes include aspects such as satisfaction, quality of life, perceived decreased occupational performance with disability, increased engagement with participation of meaningful occupation, and decreased risk factors for further deficits and additional diagnoses. Thus, the biopsychosocial model is a holistic approach, surpassing the singular concept of a bottom-up approach focusing on remediation or a top-down approach focusing on compensation and adaptation. Rather, it opens the possibilities to use a variety of approaches and intermingle various practice models and frames of reference, attaching the useful aspects of multiple concepts to the vast needs and values of clients, allowing for occupational performance and participation through numerous media, modalities, and methods (58).

PUBLIC HEALTH, POPULATION HEALTH, COMMUNITY HEALTH

Models of health and models for health practices include the areas of public health, population health, and community health. Although occupational therapy has roles within these models, these are established models, outside the profession of occupational therapy. This section discusses what each of these are and what the role of occupational therapy can be. Table 6.1 provides a summary of each model.

Public Health

Public health has a wide focus on "all people" (145). The goal is to promote health and protect the health of people where they live and complete their daily activities. The health focus of public health is changing the quality of life for all people and toward well-being for the public, which is achieved by living healthy lives. The work of public health revolves around policy and law making, government regulations and standards, education to prevent bad habits (137), training of workers to be safe and healthy, and research. The work of public health activities is tied to the practice of medicine and is not focused on the health care delivery system (45).

Occupational therapy can be thought of as a means to protect health and well-being. An example of this is participation in a national campaign to encourage youth participation in structured extracurricular activities. Participation in such activities can have a significant impact on behavior, health, and well-being. Such participation has been shown to decrease delinquent behavior and decrease substance use.

Table 6.1. Elements of Public Health, Population Health, and Community Health

Elements	Public Health	Population Health	Community Health	Community Health—Mental Health Centers
Who services are intended to serve	Everyone	Population defined by location, health condition, health care situation, or service Individual, as associated with a given population	People within a specific geographic region	Those with mental illness and behavioral health needs
Goal	Promote health Protect people	Prevent disease Promote healthy lifestyles Minimize health disparities	Improve and maintain individual physical and mental health and well-being while improving community health and wellness Prevent spreading of infectious disease Help preparation for a natural disaster Lower people's medical costs	Intervention that is comprehensive, ongoing, and community-based
Health focus	Changing quality of life Well-being through living a healthy lifestyle	Medical outcomes Understanding health conditions and their causes and risk factors	Identifying barriers to health care Improve access to health care Uncover health risks	Provide ongoing intervention for chronic illness in the community setting
Work	Policymakers Government regulations and standards Education for prevention Worker training Research	Measure patterns of health problem occurrences Policymaking for overall societal health and well-being Increase health opportunities Cost-effect strategies for health care	Establish community agency partnerships Build strong relationships with members Reduce health care service inequalities by closing service availability gaps	Provide community-based crisis, screening, and intervention services for people with substance use problems and for people with chronic mental illness
Service provision	Not toward health care system Tied to practice of medicine	Turn health determinant and science-based data into strategies used directly with clients and for care coordination	Connect members to health care services for primary, secondary, and tertiary prevention	Individual or group community-based health care services

From: Brooks, A. (2019, March 4). *What is community health and why is it important?* Rasmussen University: Health Science Blog. Retrieved January 9, 2022, from https://www.rasmussen.edu/degrees/health-sciences/blog/what-is-community-health/; Diez Roux, A. V. (2016). On the distinction—or lack of distinction—between population health and public health. *American Journal of Public Health, 106*(4), 619–620; *Population health vs. public health.* (n.d.). MPHonline. Retrieved January 9, 2022, from https://www.mphonline.org/population-health-vs-public-health/; Rosario, C. (2016, April 25). *The difference between population health & public health.* https://www.adsc.com/blog/the-difference-between-population-health-public-health; Substance Abuse and Mental Health Services Administration (SAMHSA). (2020, April 16). *Community mental health services block grant.* Retrieved January 9, 2022, from https://www.samhsa.gov/grants/block-grants/mhbg; Tulane University: School of Public Health and Tropical Medicine. (2020, May 21). *Why community health is important for public health.* Retrieved January 9, 2022, from https://publichealth.tulane.edu/blog/why-community-health-is-important-for-public-health/

In addition, school attendance has been shown to increase, as well as family and community relationships (Center for Excellence in Youth Engagement, 2003, as cited in 118).

Numerous mental factors that are associated with the stress immigrants experience when reestablishing themselves in a new country can be addressed by occupational therapy. These include the following items (59):

- nutritional imbalance resulting from no longer having access to foods they are accustomed to eating
- social competence with peers at school
- unemployment and poverty
- lack of recognition and acceptance of previous educational degree or background
- discrimination based on appearance can distort previous view of body image
- lack of social support

Being part of a trauma-informed care-based interdisciplinary team during times of war or disaster can be a way occupational therapy professionals provide mental health services. Occupational therapy professionals use therapeutic use of self-techniques to encourage people to tell the story of their experience. These stories can include details of being displaced from their homes and workplaces, loss of physical possessions, and loss of friends and family members. Specific interventions used with these victims and survivors include the following (129):

- mental hygiene recommendations such as: adequate sleep, relaxation techniques, eating proper amounts and types of foods, limiting caffeine intake, fitness, participating in the give-and-take of social relationships, giving oneself permission to take time to take care of themselves
- new role identification and competence
- role acceptance
- learning new routines
- topographical interventions because of new living environment

Population Health

Population health defines populations of people based on location, health condition, and health care plan or services. Individual person outcomes are considered based on their association with, or existence in, a population (45). The goal is to prevent disease, promote healthy lifestyles, and minimize health disparities (137). The health focus is about medical outcomes and understanding health conditions, based on causes and risk factors (137, 145). Those working in population health measure patterns of occurrences associated with health problems, assist with policymaking for overall health and well-being of society, increase health for those with limited resources, and create cost-effective strategies for those with health disparities (137). The work of those in public health is to turn science-based information and data regarding health determinants found outside the biomedical model into strategies health care professionals and physicians can use specifically with a client, as well as toward coordination of care (45).

Working in primary care is considered a part of population health. Within the practice of mental health occupational therapy in the primary care practice setting, areas of mental health intervention include substance use screenings, sleep hygiene, and the Lifestyle Redesign program. This program is an intervention approach that focuses on health and wellness improvement through prevention and management of chronic conditions (123, 182). More information about this program can be found at: https://chan.usc.edu/about-us/lifestyle-redesign.

Working with pediatric clients in a childhood obesity program can help with risk factors associated with their social and emotional mental health. By encouraging joint mobility, and thus addressing a lack of physical activity, there is a greater likelihood the child will be involved in social activities with a physical component, such as sports participation. Also, programs like this help with the risk factors associated with depression and behavior problems (123).

Community Health

Community health is the part of public health that focuses on physical and mental well-being of people within a specific geographic region. The goal of work with community members is to improve and maintain individual health while improving the health and wellness of the community, prevent infectious disease spread, help people prepare for natural disasters (22), and lower people's medical costs (176). The health focus is about improving individual health and wellness by identifying barriers to health care, improving access to health care, and uncovering health risks particular to a geographic region. Community health workers increase availability of resources by establishing partnerships with community agencies, build strong relationships with individual members, and reduce health care service inequalities by closing gaps in service availability (22, 176). The work of community health involves individual member interactions to connect members to available health care services for primary, secondary, and tertiary prevention needs (176).

Community Mental Health Centers

Community mental health centers (CMHCs) are a part of community health. CMHCs provide services to those with mental disorders and behavioral health needs, are located where they live, and are outpatient-based. The goal is to provide comprehensive, ongoing, community-based intervention services (160, 176). Health services provided through CMHCs include 24-hour emergency crisis assistance, screening, substance use treatment, psychological therapy, rehabilitation, and day treatment programming (176). This is often the setting where occupational therapy professionals work to provide occupational therapy services in the community. Occupational therapy services can be provided on site, or at other locations in the community, as an "extended" service provided by the CMHC.

A review of occupational therapy mental health services in the community found the average length of service was 2.5

months, and most of the intervention was provided on an individual basis, rather than in groups or with the community as a whole. Interventions were identified to address areas such as quality of life, mood, and general health. Specific intervention activities included addressing the occupation of basic self-care tasks, community independence, social participation, and decreasing substance addiction relapse and caregiver burden (51).

An example of a program that was done in conjunction with CMHC staff is a *Positive Youth Development* series provided after a cluster of youth suicides occurred. As part of a local suicide prevention initiative, an occupational therapy professional provided intervention activities that involved the participants identifying and exploring their strengths and participating in effective communication sessions (177).

Occupational therapy activities, as presented here, may appear to be identified with the incorrect model, or may seem to be applicable to multiple models. It is difficult to definitively state occupational therapy service provision is solidly attached to only one of these models, or completely encompasses all the aspects of a model. Often occupational therapy "in the community" is used as a descriptor for any interactions occupational therapy professionals undertake outside the traditional, insurance-based reimbursement clinic setting. This can be confusing. Consider the use of school-based Response to Intervention Tier 1 activities that appear as public health because they involve education for prevention without specific consideration to a health condition, and as population health because they target the population of school-aged children. Regardless of the "name" of the model used, occupational therapy professionals align the importance and use of occupation to fit the service agency or system where they are providing their services. They adapt their work into the working environment, no matter if they are interacting with the consumer or the staff, and no matter if they are working with individuals, groups, populations, or entire national or global markets.

SOCIETAL ISSUES

The next section is about mental disorders and mental health–related problems that can be viewed through a societal lens. Occupational therapy professionals' knowledge of public health, population health, and community health can be wrapped into how societal problems are addressed for those with mental disorders and mental health problems. Environmental factors of services, systems, and policies are used throughout the occupational therapy process when addressing these concerns on a global, national, populational, group, and individual level.

Populations in Economic Distress

Too often ignored are the effects of low socioeconomic status and limited financial means. People who do not have much money or have a limited education have a different experience and view of the world from those of the more privileged. This difference in experience and perspective affects their participation in occupational therapy.

Economic Marginalization and Poverty

Health care practitioners may have difficulty appreciating the role of economics in the health care of those who live in poverty. This is true even for practitioners who share a racial or ethnic identification with their clients; differences in social class and economic power inevitably lead to disparities in services (18). Not having enough money may mean any or all the following:

- missing appointments when there is not enough money for transportation
- not making telephone calls as requested because of not having a phone or phone service
- living in a place where it is not safe to be out after dark
- using a single sink for both kitchen tasks and personal bathing
- doing laundry infrequently and by hand
- eating based on the cost of food, rather than on the nutritional value of food

Occupational therapy professionals working with people who live in or near poverty should carefully consider the effects of limited financial means on the client's and family's response to occupational therapy intervention. What may look like uncooperative behavior is instead a combination of inability to follow through for financial reasons and a reluctance to ask for help.

Frequently, families with a low income depend on extended family members to assist with typical parenting duties (95).

Yet another effect of poverty, especially long-term poverty over more than one generation of the family, is a pervasive sense of helplessness and the expectation that things will never change. Fatalism of this sort causes clients to find it unimportant to set future-oriented goals. In this situation, the occupational therapy professional must carefully observe the client's circumstances and encourage the person to participate in setting goals; even so, the person may continue to feel like an outsider to the situation and may fail to connect to the idea of making a change or an improvement (91).

Adults Experiencing No Permanent Living Arrangements

Those who are without permanent housing experience an extreme form of economic marginalization. Living without a permanent home is the way of life for many persons with chronic mental disorders. In the past, those with chronic mental disorders would have been confined to public psychiatric institutions. In 1963, the federal policy of deinstitutionalization released psychiatric clients from the restrictive environment of the state mental hospital without providing appropriate community supports. Immediately after deinstitutionalization, many clients moved into the least desirable community housing. Because of gentrification, older low-cost housing is replaced by more profitable, more expensive homes. Lacking both financial resources and cognitive skills, displaced persons with mental disorders have difficulty finding affordable housing. Thus, though those with mental disorders are no longer in restrictive long-term hospital environments, they are materially worse off in the community, where they lack shelter and structure (see Figure 6.2).

Many other factors compound the lack of housing: unemployment, poverty, limited education, spotty work history, inadequate or discontinuous health care, and a history of domestic violence (121). Having no stable base or environment, persons who are without permanent housing experience multiple barriers to occupational performance. Establishing habits and routine in the absence of a secure environment is challenging. The fact that the person has no stable, nurturing environment cannot be ignored or wished away.

Many of those who are houseless and have a mental disorder are considered *dual-diagnosis* clients, having both psychiatric and substance use disorders. In occupational therapy, it is not unusual to work with a veteran who is homeless and has multiple comorbid conditions (a combination of diagnoses such as of personality disorder, PTSD, human immunodeficiency virus [HIV] infection, hepatitis C, and substance use problems). In a phenomenological study conducted with veterans who were without permanent homes, themes that emerged regarding their lived experience included not only living with substance use, psychiatric disorder, and a chronic illness but also living with anger and regret (154). A subtheme found in this study was the concept of self-medication through substance use to provide relief for diagnoses such as anxiety, depression, and sleep disorders and for symptoms associated with PTSD (154).

Compounding their multiple diagnoses and lack of permanent housing, many in this population have serious physical problems such as diabetes, have been convicted of crimes, or have spent time in jail when no other placement was available. Depending on state and local laws, the person who is without permanent housing who resists assistance and refuses shelter may "have the right" to remain on the streets even in freezing and inclement weather.

A lifestyle that includes living in a nonpermanent residence requires ingenuity. Finding shelter in woods or culverts or overhangs of buildings, scavenging for aluminum cans,

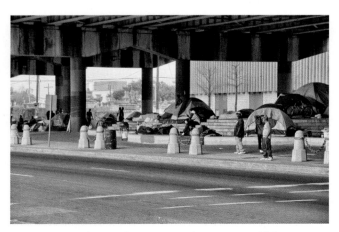

Figure 6.2. Those Who Are Homeless May Establish Encampments Under Highway Overpasses. (Image from Shutterstock.)

asking others for money, and busking (playing music for tips) can all be occupations for those who are experiencing homelessness. Those who have had some success at these occupations may find it difficult to accept health care interventions, preferring life on the streets to the unpredictable expectations from mental health providers. The person who is homeless understands and has adjusted to street life. Getting involved with the mental health system risks disruption of established patterns without providing anything better in the long term.

Obtaining housing usually requires that the person maintain sobriety and abstain from substance use. However, one approach has been to provide supported housing without necessarily requiring abstinence from substances (109). The aim is to reduce client stress while providing stable housing and allowing for increased participation in normal daily occupations. In such a setting, the occupational therapy professional can provide information and training in practical skills based on client priorities. Muñoz et al (121) recommend the *Canadian Occupational Performance Measure* (*COPM*) be used in a culturally responsive way to elicit client preferences. With the *COPM*, those who are homeless may self-identify problems in self-care, such as dressing, grooming, and hygiene, and obstacles to achieving and maintaining productive roles (121).

The *Practical Skills Test* (*PST*) is an assessment developed specifically for the population in economic distress. It measures knowledge of basic life skills required to live independently in the community. Four areas are assessed via a written test, which has true–false, multiple choice, and open-ended short answer questions. The four areas are food management, money management, home and self-care, and safe community participation (35).

Programs and settings designed to serve these clients include drop-in centers, emergency housing programs (EHP), shelters, and single room occupancy hotels (SRO). Occupational therapy services do not exist everywhere and vary by setting and program. Topics covered in one drop-in center occupational therapy program might include diabetes management, life skills, exercise, and relaxation (36). Occupational therapy professionals might use activity analysis and task breakdown to facilitate development of specific life skills. For example, breaking grocery shopping down into its embedded activities (making a list, using coupons and advertisements to comparison shop, money management skills) is necessary for someone who has never done this occupation (36).

Pritchett (141) believes that the success of interventions for those who are homeless depends on tapping into the values of the clients, many of whom would like to perform vocational work, have a home, and be considered a "regular" person with a social life and a family. Viewed from MOHO, many of those are without permanent housing or shelter, have a mental disorder, and have developed a work identity as entrepreneurs, with a focus on begging, collecting and redeeming aluminum cans, and other marginal but materially productive activities. To attract such clients, the outreach program must offer something that meets the same esteem needs.

Another factor in providing interventions to those in economic distress is the question of cognitive level and executive functions. Persons scoring at lower levels on the *Allen Cognitive Level Screen* (*ACLS*) might be predicted to have more difficulty learning new life skills or be unable to do so. However, it is possible that the stresses associated with not having stable housing interfere with executive functions and that even those who score at lower *ACLS* levels benefit from group education and individual training in areas such as those shown in Box 6.5. Although information can be provided in a group psychoeducational format, each client will need individual instruction and hands-on practice (74).

The occupational therapy professional must be focused on the concerns and perceptions of their client to learn how the client sees the world and to understand what the client feels is important. Issues of particular importance are how the person feels about medication; which ones are working, and which are not; whether the person has or is using substances, and if so, what it does for them; and what the person is afraid of and hopes for. Obtaining answers to such questions requires listening. Often, the truth is revealed only after the occupational therapy professional establishes a solid relationship with the person.

As occupational therapy professionals, our goal is to help people achieve and maintain the highest level of occupational functioning possible for them. Thus, we must be creative, compassionate, and flexible in our understanding of the customs and culture of those who are homeless, and we must adapt our interventions to address the occupational skills they find most useful. A major role for occupational therapy with this population comprises helping them recognize

---

BOX 6.5 Persons Without Permanent Housing: Goals and Areas of Intervention

- Stable housing situation and skills needed to maintain housing

- Management of substance use problems, medication management

- Activities of Daily Living (ADLs): personal hygiene and grooming, health, food safety, nutrition

- Instrumental ADLs: money management, budgeting, shopping, home cleaning, garbage and sanitation, obtaining clothing, laundry and clothing care, appointments and calendars

- Education: basic literacy and numeracy, computer and digital literacy

- Work and productivity: possibilities for supported employment, temporary employment, volunteer work

- Personal and public safety: money, first aid, consumer protection

From Helfrich, C. A., Chan, D. V., & Sabol, P. (2011). Cognitive predictors of life skill intervention outcomes for adults with mental illness at risk for homelessness. *American Journal of Occupational Therapy*, 65(3), 277–286.

---

and resolve problems of everyday living, such as obtaining and taking prescription medications, finding and caring for clothing, and managing money. In every case, the skills taught must be targeted to the specific person's situation (66).

For example, skills related to safety, problem-solving, and obtaining food are valued by clients who are homeless, whereas instruction in doing laundry using a domestic washer and dryer may seem irrelevant. Barth (15) described her work with a group of clients who were homeless and had substance use problems in a men's shelter in New York City. One activity especially valued by those in the group was the preparation in the shelter kitchen of simple food for an Alcoholics Anonymous (AA) meeting. The AA group, in which these men previously felt inadequate, welcomed their contribution, and the result for these men was an instant increase in status and recognition. Another opportunity for status is provided through access to computers and information technology, using guided learning to encourage participants to engage with devices that may seem difficult and intimidating (117).

Families Who Are Without Permanent Shelter

Families without permanent shelter or houses experience extreme disruption of routines and patterns (151). Relations between parents and children are strained when the parent is powerless to provide basic shelter, food, and clothing. Children may attend school sporadically or move from school to school as shelter residence changes. Women heads of household may have limited skills and lack resources for obtaining work and childcare, for parenting their children, and simply for understanding how to think about goals for themselves (81).

The context of a homeless shelter is challenging for the occupational therapy professional. It is common for residents to have multiple medical and sensory problems that have not been previously addressed. Physical disabilities may be present. Illiteracy may be a problem. Dental, optical, and audiology care may be needed. In addition, the staff of the shelter need to maintain order and safety; thus, many rules exist that interfere with spontaneity and family authority. Children may be required to be much quieter than they would be in a home environment. Timing of meals and of lights out is institutionalized and not under the family's control (54).

Some occupational therapy interventions offered to families who are without permanent shelter include parenting skills training, parenting skills discussion groups, organizational skills, journaling and self-expression activities, sensory soothing techniques for children who are upset or disruptive, volunteer and paid jobs with part-time and flexible hours, and youth development programs (66, 81, 131).

Adolescents in families who are homeless miss the opportunities to learn life skills typically taught within the home structure. An occupational therapy intervention program designed for youth who were experiencing homelessness included the independent living skills of health management completed through meal preparation and handling food safely, home management activities of securing an apartment, and financial management tasks of budgeting and banking. The participants in the occupational therapy program worked within a group structure sharing in completing the activities and then individually reflecting on the meaning of the occupational performance (17).

People who have been through a natural or other disaster may find themselves without a permanent home. Survivors of disasters experience anxiety and extreme emotional distress while struggling to resume a normal life. Appropriate roles for occupational therapy with this population include (171):

- assisting with housing transition and daily living needs such as clothing, sanitation, food and nutrition,
- providing children and families opportunities to engage in recreation and play, and
- involving people in problem-solving, active doing, and encouraging engagement in daily routines.

Ending the Cycle of Violence

News reports and social media posts all too frequently remind us of the daily violence occurring around us. To imagine a more peaceful world, free of shootings, bombings, beatings, and war, is a beginning. But we can also work for peace in many ways through our practice of occupational therapy.

There are several different types of violence that clients may have experienced. The *Centers for Disease Control and Prevention* focuses on violence prevention efforts in the following areas (29):

- Adverse childhood experiences (ACEs)
- Child abuse and neglect
- Child sexual abuse
- Community violence
- Elder abuse
- Firearm violence
- Intimate partner violence (IPV)
- Sexual violence
- Youth violence
- Coping with stress

Domestic Violence

Domestic violence is a complex social problem involving women, men, and families. The *Centers for Disease Control and Prevention* identifies the forms of domestic violence, or IPV, as physical violence, sexual violence, stalking, and psychological aggression (31). This violence occurs both within and outside of a marriage. It includes dating for both adults and teenagers (30). Domestic violence impacts occupations such as living in a stable environment, vocational jobs, and attending school. Figure 6.3 shows the percentage of women and men who experienced occupational loss because of contact sexual violence, physical violence, and/or stalking by an intimate partner (46). People who have limited occupational participation because of IPV can experience an occupational imbalance and occupational deprivation because of power and control exerted by the perpetrator within the intimate

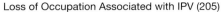
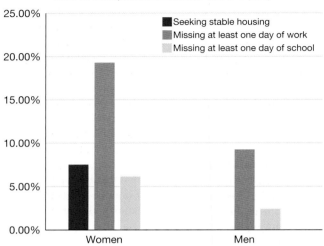

Figure 6.3. Percentage of Lifetime IPV-Related Impacts Among Women and Men of Contact Sexual Violence, Physical Violence, and/or Stalking Actions and Occupational Loss Data Not Reported for Men Seeking Stable Housing. IPV, intimate partner violence. (From D'Inverno, A. S., Smith, S. G., Zhang, X., & Chen, J. (2019, August). *The impact of intimate partner violence: A 2015 NISVS research-in-brief.* National Center for Injury Prevention and Control Centers for Disease Control and Prevention.)

partner relationship. Thus, there is occupational injustice—not being able to engage and participate in the occupations they desire (4).

Addressing domestic violence demands persistent and skillful attention to the dynamics that perpetuate violence.

The American Occupational Therapy Association prefers the word "survivor" to the word "victim" to identify persons who have been or who currently are in abusive relationships, because "it is more empowering and denotes the strength and courage needed to endure as well as leave the abusive relationship" (4, p. 2). In this section, we will use both terms, because a person cannot become a survivor without having first been a victim. Women are most often the victims of abuse, but men may also be victims. Violence may occur between same-sex partners and between different generations. The victim, the abuser, and the witnesses (often children) are all affected (127). Contrary to popular belief, domestic violence is not restricted to persons of lower socioeconomic status or lower educational levels. When the abuser is the caregiver of a dependent, other situations, such as child abuse (including sexual) and neglect (29), can occur.

The cycle of violence consists of the following repeated six phases. Throughout the cycle, the abuser is working to control and isolate the other person. The cycle is committed over and over again. Escalation of violence with each successive cycle is likely, unless the victim receives appropriate intervention, which almost always involves separation from the abuser, at least for a period of time (33).

1. **Violence**. This can take any form of domestic violence.
2. **Guilt**. Self-directed guilt is about the abuser's fear they will be held accountable for their actions and will face consequences for their deeds. There is no guilt over hurting the other person. The underlying goal is for the abuser to reassure themselves they will not be caught or will not face consequences.
3. **Rationalization**. Abuser makes excuses (such as being intoxicated or having been abused as a child) and blames the other person for making the abuser perpetrate the abuse ("If you would have not done _____, I would not have had to hit you"). The underlying goal is for the abuser to push responsibility for their behavior onto the other person.
4. **Normal behavior**. To regain power over the other person, the abuser may act as if nothing happened, or that everything is normal. The abuser may demonstrate charming, loyal, and thoughtful behaviors that are an incentive for the other person to remain or return to the abuser. The underlying goal is to keep the relationship intact and have it appear "normal" to others.
5. **Fantasy and planning**. The abuser has a mental picture of what the next abusive situation will look like. The abuser experiences power once they can initiate the abusive experience. The abuser develops this mental picture and includes what the other person has done "wrong" and, for the abuser, justifies their actions. A scenario is devised in which the abuser controls the narrative, and the other person cannot prove or explain their actions.
6. **Setup**. The plan is put into place and the abuser sets up the other person for the violent act the abuser has planned against the other person (33).

Victims of violence are vulnerable to depression and PTSD. The victim is likely to feel terrorized and hypervigilant, always alert to the possibility of another attack. It is quite common for the victim to identify with the abuser or to blame themselves. Self-help groups are effective for opening discussions, for understanding the abusers' actions, and for building a sense of community.

Occupational therapy interventions should begin with client-centered and occupation-based assessment by the occupational therapist. Assessments may focus on roles and habits, safety and support in the environment, the person's sense of volition, and specific skills (17, 73, 86, 90). Interventions may address life skills, daily routines and organization, goal setting and task management, budgeting, parenting, assertiveness, anger management, emotion identification, and many other aspects of occupational functioning (75, 90).

IPV causes long-lasting emotional effects (82, 83). Survivors of IPV need to acquire skills that will allow them to be employed and self-sufficient and thus able to move themselves and their children into a safe and productive environment. They may identify challenges with daily routines, self-care, parenting, financial management, and obtaining and maintaining employment. Interventions include specific skills training and assistance with supported and competitive employment (76).

A study of occupational therapy interventions considered programming for women victims of domestic violence who possibly had brain injury (67). The program addressed the areas of safety planning, community safety, safe sex practices, assertiveness and advocacy training, anger management, stress management, boundary establishment and limit setting, vocational/educational skills, money management, housing application, leisure exploration, hygiene, medication routine, and nutrition. Practical daily living skills such as banking, driving a car, using public transportation, using a budget, or finding leisure opportunities are also important (86).

Frequently, victims of abuse will not come forward unless asked specifically about such abuse. If the occupational therapy professional suspects that a client is a victim of violence, based on physical injury or other evidence, the client should be asked. Proper and complete documentation of the situation is essential, as is referral to a supervisor or other mental health professional. Victims should be provided with information about local and national hotlines and about shelters. State laws require occupational therapy professionals to act on reported abuse (4, 73).

WHAT'S THE EVIDENCE?

The attention to women victims of domestic and family violence: Care technologies of occupational therapy in basic health care.

This qualitative study used semi-structured interviews with occupational therapists who worked with women victims of domestic violence. The interviews focused on the core application of occupational therapy during interventions with their clients. The care technologies of the occupational therapists included using their knowledge and therapeutic techniques during both individual and group sessions. The occupational therapy intervention practices identified by the research participants included the following:

- Using activities for expressing, identifying, and elaborating about violence-based experiences
- Identifying occupational roles and daily interactions and activities that maintained domestic and family violence
- Strategy construction for coping with the violent situations the women experienced
- Forming other social participation situations to improve self-perception, self-sufficiency, and autonomy

Which of these interventions would be best suited for individual sessions and which would be best suited for group activities? Why?

de Oliveira, M. T., & Ferigato, S. H. (2019). The attention to women victims of domestic and family violence: Care technologies of occupational therapy in basic health care, *Cadernos De Terapia Ocupacional Da UFSCar, 27*(3), 508–521.

Youth and School Violence

In 2020, 4,931 youth aged between 9 and 24 years were murdered. This age group made up 27% of the overall number of murders in the United States in 2020. The number of murders for those aged between 20 and 24 years made up the highest overall percentage, per age group, of murders in the United States in 2020—16% (157). In 2019, homicide was the leading cause of death for Black youth ages 15 to 24 years, and the third leading cause of death for both American Indian/Alaskan Native and Hispanic youth ages 15 to 24 years (32). Males more often than females die from unintentional injuries, homicides, or suicides (32). Youth and school violence may be connected to domestic violence. Children who act violently may have witnessed violence in the home. Other factors have been implicated, including authoritarian child rearing, peer associations, and community factors. Programs for prevention of school violence use techniques of peer mediation and conflict resolution, attempting to reduce risk by increasing respect and facilitating communication. Occupational therapy can be a very effective addition to youth violence prevention, by introducing alternative healthy occupations for leisure time and by assessing for individual factors (such as sensory or cognitive problems or impaired volition) that may predispose youth to violence. Another emphasis might involve teaching emotion identification, assertiveness, anger management, and other specific coping skills.

Champagne (34) reported on an occupational therapy group program for children and youth in a CMHC. The children experienced mental health problems, some because of bullying and others as a result of child maltreatment. Groups were divided by age: 4 to 6 years old, 7 to 12 years old, and 13 to 18 years old. The program focused on strength and resiliency development and on fostering a sense of safety. Groups aimed to develop emotion regulation and social skills. Sensory and motor activities were included to help the children acquire the ability to recognize and control reactions to sensation.

A study providing occupation-based interventions was completed with youths between the ages of 11 and 21 years, several with poor mental health and who were at risk to experience factors that could prevent successful transition into adulthood. It was found these interventions were engaging and meaningful, valuable for the future, valuable for social interaction skills, and helpful toward developing self-regulation skills. The youth participated in games, gross motor activities, scrapbooking, tie-dying, gardening, social media, cooking, and group discussions about emotions. These group interactions allowed for opportunities to improve problem-solving, decision-making, confidence reflection (152).

Cyberbullying is a form of violence that is carried out through technology, such as social media, texting, electronic applications, and online gaming. Examples of this behavior include sending harmful, false, or mean content about someone and sharing someone else's personal information with the intent to cause embarrassment or humiliation. Cyberbullying can be persistent, permanent, and hard to notice by adults (180). Adolescents benefit from education about how to recognize, prevent, and report cyberbullying (3). Unreported cyberbullying can lead to suicide (88).

Trauma-Informed Care and Trauma-Informed Approach

Trauma-informed care comes from using a trauma-informed approach. This approach includes both organizational and clinical practices. An organizational approach includes an atmosphere of recognizing the potential impact trauma has on people, including employees and clients. It is helpful for an organization to transform into a trauma-informed format and then provide individual client trauma-informed care (112). Six guiding principles to providing a trauma-informed approach include the following (28, 112):

- **safety**: provision of treatment and surroundings that consider physical needs and emotional needs
- **trustworthiness and transparency**: clearly stating expectations, treatment details and procedures, and provider information
- **peer support**: assist others through the process of finding their inner strength used toward personal growth, rather than "fixing" someone (77)
- **collaboration and mutuality**: combining work of and ensuring interactions among clients, families, and staff
- **empowerment and choice**: using individuals' strengths in their treatment development and informing them of treatment options
- **cultural, historical, and gender issues**: continual caring awareness and sensitivity to individuals

Underlying themes to being trauma-informed include recognizing the prevalence of trauma among all people, including ACEs; that trauma causes many behaviors and symptoms; and that key components of recovery include being empowered to make one's own decisions regarding treatment and interacting with others with respect and kindness. The overall goal of using a trauma-informed approach is to not retraumatize someone (92).

Trauma-informed care includes asking clients "what happened to you?" versus "what is wrong with you?" (92). Working with those who have experienced trauma helps them participate in the following (92):

- finding purpose and meaning in life
- fulfilling roles
- engaging in life and community as they choose
- seeing themselves as more than victims of trauma
- reducing distress
- practicing autonomy and self-determination with making life choices

Specific components of trauma-informed care are listed in Box 6.6.

Trauma experiences include ACEs. These are childhood experiences that are potentially traumatic. They can include situations of violence and growing up with a family member with a mental disorder and/or substance use problem. ACEs have been identified in 61% of adults, and females are at greater risk for experiencing ACEs. The toxic stress from the ACE can impact brain development and the body's reaction

- Engagement of clients through motivational interviewing
- High-risk client screening
- Matching clients to most beneficial interventions via triage
- Tailoring interventions for individual needs, strengths, situations, and desires through assessment, care conceptualization, and intervention planning
- Ensuring needed treatment frequency and duration is achievable by removing barriers to obtaining services
- Strengthening coping skills through psychoeducation and teaching emotional-regulation skills
- Promoting positive home and school adjustment through maintenance of adaptive routines
- Improvement of parent–child relationships and of child behavior through parenting skills teaching and behavior management training
- Reducing posttraumatic stress reactions by constructing trauma narratives
- Promoting safety by teaching safety skills
- Improving client support and functioning in various environments through advocacy efforts
- Maintaining treatment gains through teaching relapse prevention skills
- Detecting and correcting insufficient therapeutic gains by monitoring progress and treatment responses
- Ensuring productive and meaningful treatment initiatives by assessing treatment effectiveness

Adapted from The National Child Traumatic Stress Network. (n.d.). *Overview: Trauma treatments*. Retrieved January 16, 2022, from https://www.nctsn.org/treatments-and-practices/trauma-treatments/overview

to stress. ACEs can contribute to adulthood chronic health conditions (including heart disease, chronic obstructive pulmonary disorder, kidney disease, and obesity), mental disorders (such as depression), and substance use (including smoking and heavy drinking). ACEs can also lead to future unemployment, not completing a high school education, and not having health insurance. Decreasing the impact of ACEs can be done through health care providers anticipating and recognizing ACE risks for children and signs of ACEs, referring clients to supportive services, and including family-centered intervention that includes substance use treatment and parenting practices (27).

Human Trafficking

Human trafficking is when the trafficker uses methods such as force, fraud, or coercion to exert control over another person. The person, against their will, engages in sexual acts, labor, or services. If the person is under 18 years old and engaging in commercial sex, force, fraud, or coercion does not

need to occur (126). Traffickers identify those who are vulnerable and take advantage of people who, for instance, live in unstable housing, have previously experienced violence and/or trauma, are involved in the juvenile justice system, are immigrants with an undocumented status, are living in poverty, or have substance use problems. Human traffickers can be anyone—a stranger, an acquaintance, a romantic partner, or a family member (125).

Occupational therapy professionals working with victims of human trafficking can use a trauma-informed approach. Both emotional well-being and cognitive impairments, which can occur because of trauma, are appropriate intervention areas within occupational therapy (21). Using results from an evidence-based review of the current research, occupational therapy professionals can provide survivors of human trafficking interventions focused on occupational engagement, social support, community reintegration, and mental disorder identification and symptom management (14). Other possible areas of intervention include sensory modulation to increase self-regulation, decrease anxiety, and improve sleep performance; independent life skills training for the occupations of driving and community mobility, child rearing, house management, financial management, employment, education, social participation and leisure; performance skill intervention for decision-making and assertiveness training; performance pattern intervention for healthy role identification, development, and maintenance (62, 105).

CAREGIVERS

The caregiver is the person in the home who provides physical and emotional care to the person identified as ill or disabled. The person may be a family member, someone from an agency, or a community resident who enjoys this work. Typically, the caregiver is female—based on the general social expectation of the nurturing role of women—but men also serve as caregivers, typically for spouses or partners with neurocognitive disorders. Perceived value of caregiving as a role varies by culture. There may be more than one caregiver, with responsibilities shared by a split schedule or by a division of responsibilities. The health professional cannot assume that someone within the family wants to take on this job, which carries significant stresses and requires great personal sacrifice. Caregivers can feel neglected and burdened; with limited skills and energy, the caregiver can feel overwhelmed. Other family members may resent the caregiver's control of the situation or may expect the caregiver will remain in the role willingly and indefinitely. On the other hand, many caregivers take on their responsibilities gradually, without relinquishing other roles within the family and the community; they may not even consciously label themselves as caregivers (119).

The occupational therapy professional can offer the caregiver information, support, and advice. Occupational therapy professionals can acknowledge the importance of the caregiver role; encourage caregivers to take care of themselves via support groups, outside activities, and respite care; and assist in finding resources to help with some tasks (119). To do this effectively, the occupational therapy professional must learn from the caregiver what the family and the client consider important and what compensatory strategies the caregiver has already attempted. Too often, families reject recommendations from rehabilitation personnel because the recommendations do not address what the family considers important (61). Box 6.7 contains questions that may be useful in revealing how the family views the situation.

Four primary types of interactions engaged in by occupational therapy professionals with caregivers are caring, partnering, informing, and directing (37).

- *Caring* demonstrates friendliness and support for the caregiver and interest in the caregiver's well-being.
- *Partnering* engages caregivers in decision-making; this includes seeking input from the caregiver and

acknowledging and praising independent problem-solving by the caregiver.

- *Informing* focuses on giving, obtaining, or clarifying information.
- *Directing* aims to engage the caregiver in carrying out the treatment; this may include giving instruction or advice.

Box 6.8 provides examples for each type of caregiver interaction. Caregivers may perceive directing and informing as bossy; this is most likely when the health care practitioner comes from or uses a medical model (37). Each type of interaction has its place in occupational therapy professional–caregiver relationship, and each is made more effective when the practitioner aims for collaborative interactions that acknowledge and embrace the commitment, expertise, and skills of the caregiver.

One role of the occupational therapy professional is to educate the caregiver. Thinnes and Padilla (174) state that responding to a specific concern voiced by the caregiver (of a person with a neurocognitive disorder) is more likely to

---

BOX 6.7 Questions for Effective Communications With Caregivers

To **learn** what is meaningful, ask the caregiver the following:

- What is a typical day like for you?
- What most worries or concerns you?
- How is it now vs. before?
- How do you manage your day?
- What are your feelings about the future?
- What are some of your successes here?

To **verify** what is meaningful, ask or say to the caregiver the following:

- Is this how you see it?
- So you are saying that when [_____] happens, you get frustrated.
- It sounds as though that really upset you.

To **think reflectively**, ask yourself the following:

- What do I see happening in this home?
- Do I understand the perspective of the family members?
- Are my views the same as those of the family caregiver(s)?
- In what way are my values in this care situation the same or different from those of the family caregiver(s)?

To **plan intervention,** ask yourself the following:

- What does the disability or impairment mean to the client and family member?
- How does the family member experience the caregiving activity?
- On the basis of an understanding of meaning, what is an appropriate treatment strategy to support the efforts of this family?

Adapted with permission from Gitlin, L. N., Corcoran, M., & Leinmiller-Eckhardt, S. (1995). Understanding the family perspective: An ethnographic framework for providing occupational therapy in the home. *American Journal of Occupational Therapy, 49*(8), 802–809.

BOX 6.8 Four Types of Interactions With Caregivers

Caring: building rapport and alliance with the caregiver

- You are putting a lot of effort into making this work.
- I like the way you have arranged the living room.
- It is a lot of work to care for someone like [_____].

Partnering: involving caregivers in decision-making

- What would you like [_____] to be able to do for themselves?
- I notice that today you have really solved a lot of problems so that [_____] can be safe here while you are at work. That is really good.

Informing: gathering information, explaining rationales or treatment procedures, and clarifying information

- In what ways does [_____] contribute to chores around the house?
- Have you considered taking the knobs off the stove burners when you are not using the stove? This will help keep [_____] from trying to use the stove.
- They might accidentally start a fire or burn themselves.

Directing: instructing and advising the caregiver

- I think they can dress themselves: if you lay out the clothes and remind them to put each item on. Just saying the name of the garment, like "socks," can remind them. Would you like to try that?
- If you ask them to do their chores sometimes, but let them not do the chores at other times, it will be hard to get them to do chores when you are pressed for time and really need them to. Do you see why?

Adapted with permission from Gitlin, L. N., Corcoran, M., & Leinmiller-Eckhardt, S. (1995). Understanding the family perspective: An ethnographic framework for providing occupational therapy in the home. *American Journal of Occupational Therapy, 49*(8), 802–809.

be effective than a more general approach. The occupational therapy professional may provide support in various ways: suggesting home modifications, explaining difficult behaviors of the person and offering behavior management information, providing specific strategies based on cognitive level, and problem-solving how to complete daily activities. The occupational therapy professional can also help caregivers identify ways to engage the client in co-occupations such as doing laundry, carrying out personal hygiene, etc.

Another approach to educating family caregivers is to provide formal instruction in what to expect from the disease process (of neurocognitive disorders). The occupational therapy professional can provide training on how to simplify communication, break down a task, create a safer environment, and engage the person in activities (47, 135). Caregivers especially value hands-on training and practical advice on how to respond to specific problems (135).

Regarding communication, McKay and Hanzaker (111) suggest that caregivers learn to maximize the effectiveness of cues they use when interacting with the client. They advocate a *Positive Physical Approach* (PPA), which follows a three-step sequence: a visual cue, a short verbal cue, and a touch cue (given in that order). Detailed instructions can be found in the reference.

Corcoran (60) has developed an online resource called C-TIPS (Customized Toolkits of Information and Practical Solutions), where caregivers can access a wide range of information through online learning modules to help caregivers individualize care for persons with neurocognitive disorders. The website is listed in the *Suggested Resources* at the end of the chapter.

Many of these recommendations apply also to hired caregivers, who may or may not have received training specific to their responsibilities (135, 187). Some home health aides and other paid caregivers are eager to learn new skills and are very receptive to direction from the family, the client, and the occupational therapy professional. Others may be more resistant to training. It is generally the family's choice as to whether to seek another occupational therapy professional who can support the family by providing a realistic outside appraisal. This would include finding ways to work more collaboratively with a caregiver who is resistant.

LITERACY

Literacy is a concern both when working with clients and with caregivers. Understanding information presented by occupational therapy professionals is difficult if the person's literacy ability is limited, and even more difficult if cognitive loss or mental disorders are involved. Literacy includes the areas of health literacy, functional literacy, financial literacy, digital literacy, and mental health literacy.

Health Literacy

Health literacy is identified as "the degree to which individuals have the capacity to obtain, process, and understand basic health information needed to make appropriate health decisions" (71, para. 1). The language of health care is complex and involves terms not typically used in everyday conversation. Those who are English Language Learners may have an even harder time understanding what a health care professional is talking about. Box 6.9 further describes actions people may perform that demonstrate difficulties with health literacy (102). Health literacy is needed for clients and their families to locate health care services, complete medical forms, discuss health problems with their providers, and understand directions on medication (71).

As occupational therapy professionals we consider education and training as a primary intervention type (6). Both when we educate and train, we provide written information to clients, families, significant others, caregivers, group home managers, teachers, and other professionals. We need to consider the terminology we use and the presentation of that material on the written page.

In a three-part study looking at health literacy of occupational therapy clients, it was found 38% of the participants had less than adequate health literacy, which indicated a reading level below the 10th grade. An analysis of the materials presented to the clients determined 89% were written at an eighth-grade reading level or higher. Occupational therapists interviewed in the study indicated they frequently needed to explain medical information previously provided to the client by a different professional. Situations the occupational therapists encountered included having to repeat information the person had already heard when they might have been sleepy or medicated, finding the person feeling overwhelmed by their health care situation, and the person having a different primary language than that of the occupational therapist. Health literacy strategies determined to use with clients included assessing literacy skills, using the teach-back method, using photographs, reassuring people about the need to ask questions, and providing writing tools to the person when the occupational therapy professional is giving verbal instruction (23).

BOX 6.9 Actions That May Indicate Difficulty With Health Literacy

- Bringing another person to an appointment and indicating that the health professional should address that person
- When being given verbal instructions or information, asking for written or illustrated instructions to take home
- Forgetting eyeglasses or hearing aids and then stating the person needs to take the information home for a family member to read
- Not following home exercise program or other recommended intervention
- Looking around for cues and clues in the environment
- Watching and copying others

Adapted from Luedtke, T., Goldammer, K., & Fox, L. (2012). Overcoming communication barriers—Navigating client linguistic, literacy, and cultural differences. *OT Practice, 17*(4), 15–18.

Functional Literacy

Functional literacy can be considered as the capacity for reading, writing, and calculation needed to effectively engage in personal, group, and community activities (178). As a component of communication management, occupational therapy professionals consider a person's ability to interpret information (6). The role of occupational therapy in functional literacy has been identified as a means toward greater occupational justice; better health, well-being, and adaptive capacity; and belonging and social participation (63).

Two occupational therapy-based assessments of reading are the adult and pediatric version of *The Inventory of Reading Occupations*. The pediatric version is used to develop a profile of the child's *Reading Participation* and identifies the types of materials the child reads. The adult version is used to develop a profile of the adult's *Functional Literacy* and identifies the types of materials the adult reads in occupational participation during daily life situations (40).

Financial Literacy

Occupational therapy professionals provide therapeutic intervention for financial management. Financial management includes the financial activities of using financial resources, performing transactions, and determining goals for both long-term and short-term planning (6). The federal Financial Literacy and Education Commission (53) was created to provide education to improve people's financial literacy (181). Financial literacy includes buying and purchasing practices, personal financial information management, and investment knowledge (183).

Financial literacy intervention in an occupational therapy program with teenagers who were homeless has shown to substantially improve financial literacy skills. This was done through development of individual financial goals and participation in weekly leisure-based activities in which the teenagers first used financial literacy skills to identify low-cost items and then participation in the activity with those items (153).

Another financial literacy intervention program was provided for several weeks as part of a one-semester college readiness course with twelfth-grade students who had diagnoses such as autism spectrum disorder, emotional disturbances, and learning disabilities. Pre- and postsurveys for the budgeting portion of the program showed a strong increased knowledge in areas of understanding personal wants versus needs, regular money saving, and understanding a budget and how to use it. Areas with some increase in knowledge included calculating costs for living expenses and making both monthly and yearly budgets. Responses from the participants included requests for more time to work on activities (20). This study demonstrates a connection between the performance skill needs of those with mental disorders and the therapeutic grading of financial literacy activities to allow for more time to process the information and for active learning participation.

Digital Literacy

Digital literacy encompasses all aspects of using electronic devices to find information, complete electronic transactions, perform vocational duties, and participate in leisure activities such as reading or visiting with family and friends. Activities of digital literacy include the following (24):

- learning keyboarding skills
- engaging in social media (both written interactions as well as taking and posting pictures)
- reading medical charts online

Performance skills included in occupational therapy interventions that are a part of digital literacy include attention span and critical thinking. *The Inventory of Reading Occupations* assessment is one way to help identify reading-based materials (24) for which a person may need to improve their digital literacy skills so they can complete online versions of the material for electronic manipulation or submission.

Mental Health Literacy

Mental health literacy focuses on understanding mental disorders and mental health needs (113). This includes learning and understanding strategies for stress management, sleep preparation and participation, calming anxious feelings, and self-regulation. For children and adolescents, mental health literacy includes learning about mental disorders and substance use problems of parents or other caregivers (115). Language used by occupational therapy professionals teaches clients and families about the language they should use to describe their mental health and/or mental disorders. It is important that words and language are used correctly and appropriately (114). Consider the examples in Table 6.2.

In a study with middle school students who had a primary diagnosis of autism spectrum disorder and a history of trauma, and some students with a secondary diagnosis of anxiety disorder or oppositional defiant disorder, a mental health literacy curriculum was introduced into an established science curriculum. Topics of the mental health literacy curriculum included brain anatomy and function; the brain's role in thoughts, feelings, behavior, and daily functioning; terminology information (such as mental health, mental distress, and mental illness); body and brain stress response; impact of stress responses on well-being and daily functions; stress reduction techniques; and positive stress response plan components used in positive mental health and positive physical health. Participants in the study identified they had learned new calming and coping skills, new information about school mental health, and better comprehension of the material because it was taught through the lens of everyday feelings and behaviors (64).

UNDERSTANDING AND SUPPORTING RECOVERY

A shift of perspective about psychiatric illness has occurred since 1990, with consumers increasingly embracing a view

Table 6.2. The Language of Mental Health		
Depression	is not	"having a bad day"
Obsessive Compulsive Disorder	is not	"being organized"
Attention Deficit Hyperactivity Disorder	is not	"being hyper"
Anxiety Disorder	is not	"feeling stressed before _____"
Posttraumatic Stress Disorder	is not	"feeling upset"
Schizophrenia	is not	"split personality"
Panic Disorder	is not	"feeling afraid"
Bipolar Disorder	is not	"being moody"

Adapted from Mental Health Literacy. (n.d.). *Language matters: The importance of using the right words when we're talking about mental health.* Retrieved January 17, 2022, from https://mentalhealthliteracy.org/schoolmhl/wp-content/uploads/2019/01/final-using-the-right-words.pdf

of themselves as in recovery (not sick, but in recovery from a serious illness). Recovery is a way of life that acknowledges the reality of illness and disability while maintaining hope and working toward meaningful realistic goals and a satisfying life (136). Important to recovery are stable housing, supported education, and employment (68, 163, 166).

Recovery is a person-centered, person-directed perspective that demands that occupational therapy professionals take a back seat and allow the individual to direct and manage their own recovery (164). SAMHSA, the Substance Abuse and Mental Health Services Administration, recognizes "four major dimensions that support recovery" (161).

- **Health**—overcoming/managing disease(s) or symptoms; informed, healthy choices to support physical and emotional well-being
- **Home**—stable and safe living spaces
- **Purpose**—meaningful daily activities; independence, income, resources for societal participation
- **Community**—relationships and social networks for support, friendship, love, and hope

Further, SAMHSA recognizes ten guiding principles of recovery, shown in Box 6.10 (159). Occupational therapy professionals working in recovery-oriented programs employ these principles as a foundation of their work. Pitts (136) suggests that occupational therapy professionals employ specific strategies to support clients in recovery (Box 6.11).

Clients may benefit from concrete help in setting goals, taking control of their health matters, accessing community services, and recognizing their own strengths (172). Decision-making within the recovery movement takes many forms. Olson (130) discusses four major types of decision-making within health care, the implications of each, and the best options for the occupational therapy professional using a client-centered approach.

1. Physician decision (medical model)—the physician makes all decisions about the person's health care.
2. Informed choice—the physician offers choices and provides information but does not recommend a particular choice. The person chooses.
3. Shared decision-making—both the physician and the person share information and discuss possible courses of action.
4. Refusal of care under a psychiatric advance directive (PAD). Similar to other medical advance directives, the

---

BOX 6.10 Ten Guiding Principles of Recovery

1. Hope—people are motivated to face obstacles and overcome them when they are hopeful they can recover, and when those around them also express hope.
2. Person-driven—recovery is self-directed and self-determined. Autonomy and independence are valued and fostered.
3. Many pathways—more than one way exists to reach recovery. Recovery is an individual process, is not linear, and is different for each person.
4. Holistic—all are included; nothing is left out. Body, mind, spirit, housing, education, employment, clinical services, social networks, the environment, and the community are all needed for recovery.
5. Peer support—sharing of knowledge and skills among peers increases support. Peers "have been there." Professionals may contribute by connecting peers together, as, for example, parents of children with behavior problems.
6. Relational—social involvement and participation with others increases a feeling of having support and provides opportunities to develop social interaction skills.
7. Culture—the individual's culture and cultural background are part of the unique nature of that person. Culturally sensitive care is essential.
8. Addresses trauma—services should be "trauma-informed" so that the underlying events and circumstances that contributed to the illness can be understood.
9. Strengths/responsibility—both individuals and communities have strengths and responsibilities.
10. Respect—recognizing the courage required to pursue recovery provides the person with a sense of being valued and increases confidence.

Condensed and adapted from Substance Abuse and Mental Health Services Administration. (2012). *Working definition of recovery: 10 guiding principles of recovery.* Retrieved January 17, 2022, from https://store.samhsa.gov/sites/default/files/d7/priv/pep12-recdef.pdf

- Maintain a hopeful perspective, believing in the possibility of recovery for every client.
- Tolerate uncertainty about the future.
- Tolerate slow movement toward goals.
- Remember and take note of successes.
- Understand that courage and risk-taking are required for growth.
- See the client as a survivor or hero, not as a victim.

Pitts, D. B. (2004). Understanding the experience of recovery for persons labeled with psychiatric disabilities. *OT Practice, 9*(5), CE1–CE8.

person develops a plan to communicate their wishes in the event that they become too incapacitated to voice them directly. The person may also use the PAD to designate a family member or friend to make decisions for them.

Self-determination for persons with major mental disorders is complicated by the varying course of the illness and by cognitive or other impairments that alter executive functions. A person may be quite psychotic at one time and at another time (when using medication) show no signs of the illness. Self-determination requires that the person be able to understand and retain information related to health care, and some individuals with mental disorders seem unable to do so. Olson suggests that the appropriate model for occupational therapy intervention is shared decision-making, because it is collaborative and client-centered (130).

Within the recovery process, experts in psychiatric rehabilitation (PsyR) recognize that medical model decision-making is essential in times of crisis and when someone is first ill (139). Later, when the person is recovering, a gradual movement to greater self-determination would be appropriate.

Occupational therapy has much to offer within a recovery-oriented context. All the guiding principles of recovery are consistent with occupational therapy concepts and processes (38). Occupational therapy professionals promote recovery and a sense of identity by engaging consumers in individually determined purposeful activity and helping them to acquire routines and structure (38). Life skills such as medication management, laundry and clothing care, cleaning and household management, meal preparation, and grocery shopping all increase confidence and self-respect (170). Encouraging the client and stimulating dialogue and self-reflection help the person become more self-aware, confident, and empowered (38, 188). Consistent with the MOHO, the person's sense of personal agency is increased by repeated experiences of using self-help strategies, problem-solving, and decision-making (170).

Resilience

Resilience is defined by the American Psychological Association as "the process and outcomes of successfully adapting to difficult or challenging life experiences, especially through mental, emotional, and behavioral flexibility and adjustment to external and internal demands" (12, para. 1). Factors that contribute to how well people adapt when confronted with an adverse situation include:

- the way a person engages and views the world,
- social resource quality and availability, and
- coping strategies designed to increase one's positive adaptive response to adversity (12).

Resilience is fostered and developed when the person has had, and is in, relationships that provide care and support, has learned to manage emotions and feelings, and demonstrates the skills of problem-solving and communication (124). Resilience can be difficult for those who have experienced trauma, have mental health problems, or a mental disorder.

Benefits of being resilient include a greater balance with life activities and situations, having a sense of adaptability, increased longevity, more satisfaction with life, and fewer mental health issues (2). Occupational therapy interventions designed to build resilience include the following (2):

- Analyze daily routines and consider rearrangements to balance active activities, social participation, and sleep. These changes can help increase resiliency to stress, thus increasing the feeling of alertness, feeling present, and being productive.
- Identify patterns of thinking that are unhelpful and negatively impact behavior. Then, problem-solve ways to increase coping during times of difficulty, thus increasing confidence with coping ability.
- Promote engagement with others and building capacity for relationships with others leading to greater satisfaction in life, increasing feelings of confidence, self-worth, and belonging. Relationships are enhanced through better communication skills, understanding body language, interpreting cues from others, and emotional management.
- Use a strength-based approach. Focus on the person's capabilities and abilities they use to lead and direct one's life activities.

The concept and term *occupational resilience* is a relatively new consideration within the field of occupational science. A recent phenomenological study examined musicians who were forcibly displaced from their homeland and their persistence with music performance. Despite barriers such as adjustment to performing a new type of music, cost for equipment, personal values that differed from their new home, and changing from music performance as a primary vocational role to a secondary vocation role, the participants continued with their music performance activities. The participants sought ways to adapt to their new circumstances with the hope of returning to music performance careers, identifying a strong sense of emotional health, spiritual health, and well-being as being a driving force for their continued musical activities. Continued conversation and research regarding the use of the term *occupational resilience* is encouraged (122).

Wellness Model

Within the recovery model (165, 167, 168) there is a psycho-educational wellness model to promote self-management of illness and a positive attitude toward health among persons with mental disorders. Clients learn self-management skills in groups. The presentation of information is designed to compensate for cognitive deficits; environmental distractors are controlled. Clients direct the selection of content, ensuring relevance and increasing participation. Specific topics include smoking cessation, acquired immunodeficiency syndrome education, substance use awareness, nutrition, and coping with stress and boredom. Individual direction is fostered by programs that encourage clients to create their own definitions of wellness and to identify personal barriers to wellness (146). Other wellness models include aromatherapy, gentle yoga, addictions counseling, Reiki, and tai chi (107).

Psychiatric Rehabilitation

Previously addressed in Chapter 2, PsyR is an approach that is compatible with recovery. It affirms the collaboration between the identified client and the various health care providers. It is client-centered, based on an atmosphere of hope, and uses an individualized approach (139). The PsyR model endorses the use of hospitalization and medication to stabilize individuals in crisis, particularly in the early stages of illness (139). The PsyR model views recovery as an individual process. However, PsyR recognizes the serious nature of the major mental disorders and assumes that medical/psychiatric services are necessary at times.

Psychoeducation

Psychoeducation is not, strictly speaking, an occupational therapy practice model. Rather, it is an educational approach used by many service providers to improve the skills of persons with mental disorders. The PsyR model (138) regularly employs psychoeducation. PsyR and psychoeducation both affirm that problem behaviors shown by persons with chronic mental disorders reflect deficient living skills. Psychoeducation aims to remedy such skill deficits by direct teaching and training. The occupational therapy professional acts as an educator, providing lessons similar to classroom courses, with objectives, learning activities, and homework. Behavioral techniques such as reinforcement are also sometimes used.

Psychoeducation applies the use of homework and educational activities. Its primary focuses are on training and development of skills and functional performance of everyday activities. Psychoeducation draws on the social learning theories of Bandura (see "Cognitive–Behavioral Theoretical Continuum" in Chapter 2). The techniques and general form of psychoeducation come more directly from educational theory. Psychoeducation also shares an emphasis with role acquisition and social skills training, in that it has similar goals. The difference in psychoeducation is in the emphasis on the *educational* nature of behavioral change.

A psychoeducation setting is viewed as an educational environment, a place for learning; it is not a clinic or a place for healing or treatment. For the provision of a psychoeducation course, the occupational therapy professional typically prepares a syllabus containing the course description, rationale, goals, objectives, methods, daily lesson plans, homework assignments, and evaluation or assessment methods (98). The clients are called students, and they are encouraged to adopt this role, take notes in notebooks, keep and use handouts, and do homework. Students who would benefit from increased concentration on a given topic may be directed to use an individualized study method.

Lillie and Armstrong (98) were among the first to apply the psychoeducational model in occupational therapy in their life skills program. They used a hierarchical model of skill development adapted from Hewett (78). Educational goals increase at each level, reflecting that skill development at earlier levels must be achieved before success can occur at higher levels. A task checklist (TCL) highlights the key behaviors pertaining to each level. Figure 6.4 shows a TCL for a middle-aged woman in her first psychiatric hospitalization for bipolar disorder. The client, who previously functioned normally in the community, felt unsure of herself. It was difficult for her to explore new situations and make decisions. The occupational therapist enrolled her in the exploring community course, which required her to call businesses and transportation companies for information, arrange an outing to an unfamiliar site, and so on. This and other psychoeducation experiences increased her confidence to the point that she eventually obtained a volunteer job and moved into her own apartment.

Evaluation of outcome is important in psychoeducation. To what extent do clients actually learn new skills, and, more important, to what extent do they generalize or carry them over into other environments and situations? Hayes and Halford (70), in a review of the literature, noted that many of the techniques (eg, homework assignments) used in psychoeducation are useful for generalization. However, generalization is usually not stated as a goal and is rarely evaluated. Any psychoeducation program should, therefore, include a postprogram assessment (*posttest*) to measure the extent to which students learn and then apply the newly learned concepts in their everyday environments.

The psychoeducational model has been applied in the rehabilitation of adults with multiple disabilities. Courses have focused on functional life skills (cooking, shopping) and appropriate role acquisition (self-advocacy, participation in community recreation). Classroom teaching, homework assignments, quizzes, and examinations involved the clients in their roles as students. Praise and other social reinforcers were used in responses by classroom teachers and in feedback on homework. Outcome was evaluated by pretest and posttest scores and by successful placements in community living.

Occupational therapy professionals have also used the psychoeducation approach to improve skills of persons with codependency problems (128), to teach life skills to persons with chronic mental disorders in a university setting (43),

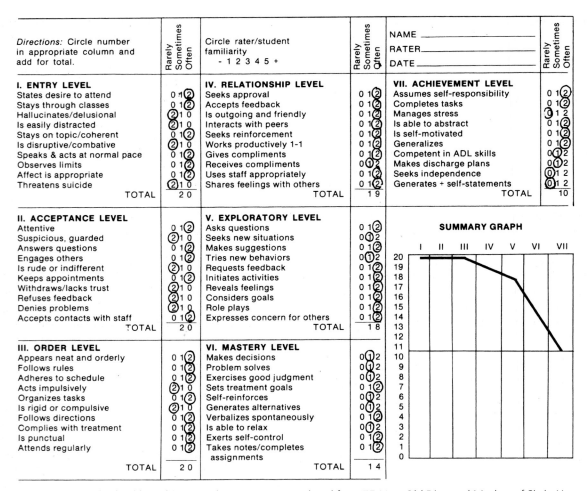

Figure 6.4. Task Checklist. This Example Has Been Completed for a 55-Year-Old Divorced Mother of Six in Her First Psychiatric Hospitalization for Bipolar Disease. (Reprinted with permission from Lillie, M. D., & Armstrong, H. E. (1982). Contributions to the development of psychoeducational approaches to mental health service. *American Journal of Occupational Therapy, 36*(7), 438–443. Used with permission of the American Occupational Therapy Association.)

and to instruct psychiatric clients in a maximum-security forensic hospital about HIV and high-risk behaviors (150). Steed (158) developed a client-centered model for psychoeducation interventions in occupational therapy. This is a more individualized approach that considers the person and the environment. The psychoeducation approach has also been shown effective for those with psychiatric disabilities to return to work or education, through improved academic skills, social skills, and professional behaviors (68).

Typically, the psychoeducation setting is multidisciplinary. Working in a role similar to that of other professionals but using unique occupational therapy skills and perspectives, the occupational therapy professional may serve as case manager or as educator. In this role, the occupational therapy professional is responsible for assisting the learner in planning a program of study. This includes evaluation, identification of goals, selection of learning opportunities, and measurement of outcomes.

The occupational therapy professional within the role of educator may teach individuals or groups. Padilla (132) elaborates on the many activities of an educator: lecturing; guiding role-playing, discussions, and other in-class activities; one-on-one instruction; social modeling; designing and responding to homework assignments; and creating, administering, and evaluating various outcome measures such as pretests and posttests. Pretests and posttests, which document the effects of interventions, may be used in outcome studies and are helpful in research activities.

The focus of evaluation is identification of deficient skill and functional activity areas and of goals that are important to the student. The student is seen as a consumer of an educational service and is expected to participate in self-evaluation and goal setting. The following are some of the methods that have been used for evaluation within this model.

- **Semi-structured interview**. With a focus on occupational performance, this identifies areas in which occupational therapist and student may jointly establish initial goals (128).
- **Task checklist**. Developed by Lillie and Armstrong (98), this is a checklist for assessing student competencies and setting intervention goals.

- *Kohlman Evaluation of Living Skills*. This instrument, which takes only a short time to administer, measures basic skills in functional literacy, financial management, self-care, safety awareness, community mobility, telephone use, and employment (175).
- **Pretest and posttest**. These may be used to assess the student's mastery of various learning module content, both before and after educational instruction.

In this approach, goals for intervention are jointly identified by the case manager and the student–client (101). Goals should focus on specific behavioral objectives or outcomes. The primary environment for psychoeducation is a classroom setting, with educational courses or modules about various life skills. These may include activities of daily living (medication management, shopping, meal preparation), play and leisure, education- and work-related activities, coping skills and management of feelings, relapse prevention and symptom management, decision-making and problem-solving, public speaking, use of the library, digital literacy, time management, and community exploration. Methods of instruction include classroom lectures, guest lectures by experts, video presentations, role-playing and group exercises, recording of student performance to provide feedback, hands-on activities, assigned reading, homework assignments, and individual study. Social modeling by the occupational therapy professional–educator or a peer is often used. Separate one-on-one instruction may focus on needs of individuals.

Psychoeducation makes use of both **in vivo** or naturalistic (real-life) and **simulated** training environments. Students may take a trip to a museum or shopping mall (in vivo). Or, they may simulate a community environment using props in the classroom, where they can role-play experiences and interactions before risking themselves in vivo.

Consumer-Operated Programs

Persons diagnosed with mental disorders have founded organizations and programs for their own advocacy and self-help. The *consumer movement* advocates for consumer involvement in decision-making and program development. In historical terms, this is a natural outcome of consumer dissatisfaction with the stigma attached to medical-based programs and the poor level of community services following deinstitutionalization.

Consumer organizations may provide a range of services, possibly including employment services, case management, crisis counseling, drop-in or self-help centers, peer counseling, financial services, consumer-run business, and subsidized housing (169). Swarbrick and Duffy (169) describe occupational therapy involvement in a consumer-operated self-help center. The self-help center provides a place for consumers to help themselves and each other through peer counseling, to socialize and enjoy leisure activities, to learn about mental health issues, and to plan and engage in advocacy and networking activities. The occupational therapy professional serves as a consultant and collaborator.

Rebeiro (142), a Canadian occupational therapist, gives advice for occupational therapy professionals considering partnering with consumer-operated programs and organizations, identifying specific qualities that are helpful in establishing effective relationships.

- *Advocacy:* including advocating for individual clients, advocating for groups of clients, and teaching clients to advocate for themselves
- *Client centeredness:* placing the needs and goals of the clients first
- *Risk-taking:* being willing to expand into uncharted territory and to give up the unequal power relationship of therapist and client
- *Establishing common ground:* finding ways to make connections and help clients see their goals as shared ones rather than individual ones
- *Nontraditional:* accepting the absence of the kinds of structure found in medical settings and understanding that documentation may mean keeping research notes or writing advocacy letters (rather than progress notes)
- *Redefining professional:* keeping to the values and ethics of the profession while relating on a human-to-human level

Psychosocial Rehabilitation

Psychosocial rehabilitation, which began in 1948 with the founding of Fountain House, is an environmental approach designed to improve the ability of persons with severe and persistent mental disorders to maintain themselves in the community. This is done by providing support, meaningful work experience, and the opportunity to associate with others. Psychosocial rehabilitation focuses on "improving emotional, social, and intellectual skills needed to live, learn, and work in the community with the least amount of professional support" (148, p. 892).

Psychosocial Clubhouse Model

In keeping with the philosophy that people with chronic mental disorders can direct their own affairs, the persons who attend these programs are called "members." Members participate equally with staff in running essential functions such as meal preparation and culinary arts, education, communication, horticulture, and other areas. A multidisciplinary approach may involve professionals as well as paraprofessionals trained on the job, peer mentors (members), and volunteers. Because of the similarity of terms, psychosocial rehabilitation may be confused with *psychiatric rehabilitation*. Although some overlap exists, these are separate movements that are sometimes conflated (blended or mixed together), as discussed previously in Chapter 2. Psychosocial rehabilitation in its original form has more in common with consumer-operated organizations and the recovery movement than with the medical model or psychiatry. Box 6.12 provides the focus of clubhouse settings.

This model focuses on the social rather than medical aspects of mental disorders. Thus, although psychotropic medications and consultation with the psychiatrist may be

- Strong recovery orientation
- Clients called "members"
- Empowering social atmosphere (members and staff are equals)
- Staff as resources rather than authorities
- Peer counseling and mentoring
- Client-directed goals and plans
- Individual programming: mix of group activities and individual activities
- Activities of daily living: personal hygiene and grooming, dressing, sexual activity
- Instrumental activities of daily living: communication management, driving and community mobility, home establishment and management, financial management, shopping, meal preparation, safety and emergency maintenance
- Health management: nutrition management, physical activity, communication with the health care system, medication management
- Leisure: exploration and participation
- Work: employment interests and pursuits, employment seeking and acquisition, job performance and maintenance
- Social participation: participation in community and with peers and family, friendships, intimate partner relationships
- Stress management
- Other age-related and/or gender-specific support groups

available, these are seen as adjunctive rather than essential services. Fountain House in New York City is a comprehensive center and provides services such as employment, relationship building, education, health and wellness, assistance with locating housing, farming and gardening, older adult programming and services, digital literacy, arts-based gallery, college reentry, and care management (55).

Socialization programs are at the heart of this model. By participating in organized activities and casual lounge programs, members acquire and maintain social and leisure skills and meet others with similar needs and interests. Informal activities such as playing pool or cards, watching television, reading, and chatting are typical of lounge programs. Organized activities may include cooking, sewing, home repair, crafts, and theater trips. Depending on facilities and funding, other activities such as swimming, skiing, camping, farming, animal husbandry, and hiking may be available.

Daily living skills programs may include opportunities for self-assessment, counseling with particular problems, and training in desired skills. After many years of illness, with several hospitalizations, the person with a serious mental disorder may have no habits or routines for performing the daily tasks the rest of us take for granted. By providing information, advice, and opportunities to learn and practice new skills, the daily living skills therapeutic professional enables members to acquire such skills as using public transportation, maintaining an apartment, shopping for and caring for clothing, and shopping for and cooking food.

Prevocational rehabilitation, transitional employment, and supported employment (SE) are services aimed at helping members acquire job-related skills and obtain jobs in the community. Prevocational rehabilitation helps members become acculturated to basic work habits and the social rules typical of community work settings. Members attend work groups where they perform jobs needed by the center or contracted for by the center with businesses in the community. They are expected to behave in a businesslike, productive, work-oriented manner and are counseled about behaviors they could change. Clerical groups, janitorial and maintenance groups, thrift shops, art and photo galleries (56), food preparation and service, and simple assembly line work are typical activities. After successful performance in a prevocational program, members may seek entry-level jobs in the community through the transitional employment program (TEP). These jobs give members a chance to be productive in a real-life setting; they are not usually meant to become full-time jobs but are seen rather as stepping stones to other permanent vocational positions. The occupational therapy professional's strong background in task analysis is well suited to preparing members for these transitional employment placements.

Transitional Housing

Transitional living encompasses a range of supervised residential arrangements. The quarter-way or halfway house or supervised community residence may be the first step; here members can receive room and board and round-the-clock supervision from trained staff, often paraprofessional *house parents* or *residential counselors*. Members are expected to be out of the house during the day, working, looking for work, or attending a day treatment program. During the evening and on weekends, they may be supervised as they help prepare their own meals; do the shopping, laundry, housecleaning, and other home tasks; and organize and carry out leisure and social activities. Supervised apartment programs are the next step; the apartments are usually leased or, less commonly, owned by the program, which sublets them to members. Several members live together in an apartment, sharing housework and other responsibilities. Staff visit periodically to provide counseling and support and to oversee cleanliness and other basic issues.

Occupational therapy professionals may notice a role blurring among staff in these settings. They may be concerned their professional identity will be lost as they take on responsibilities like case management, which are typically part of other disciplines, and as members of other disciplines become leaders of activity groups. To work successfully in these settings, occupational therapy professionals must be firmly grounded in the core of our profession and be flexible in applying occupational therapy skills to individuals, groups, and populations.

Psychosocial rehabilitation embodies concepts from *moral treatment* (see Chapter 1) that guided the early development of occupational therapy. Occupational therapy professionals may find the model a natural fit for their skills. Although other professionals and nonprofessionals may lead activities and programs that meet the interests of the members, occupational therapy professionals possess unique training and skills in task analysis, adaptation, and environmental management. The occupational therapy professional can, therefore, serve in a consulting role to assist others in increasing the effectiveness of their groups and interventions.

COMMUNITY-BASED INTERVENTION

Various programs in the community are administered by private nonprofit agencies. They have been developed with the aim of helping persons with serious mental disorders survive and succeed in the community after discharge from the hospital. Programs administered by independent agencies may concentrate on just one aspect of continuing care, such as leisure and recreation or vocational rehabilitation. Others, as seen previously under the topic of psychosocial rehabilitation, provide rehabilitative living arrangements, including supportive housing through halfway houses and supervised apartments; members gradually learn the skills, habits, and attitudes they need to live on their own in the community by practicing them under the supervision and direction of staff. The specific job functions of occupational therapy professionals employed by these independent agencies vary.

Program for Assertive Community Treatment

The Program for Assertive Community Treatment (PACT) serves persons with severe mental disorders within the community. PACT began in Wisconsin and has functioned continuously since 1972. Round-the-clock services are provided in the person's natural living environment (at home, school, or work) as needed by a team of mental health care providers. Services include *treatment* (eg, medication, psychotherapy, crisis intervention), *rehabilitation* (eg, skill teaching in areas such as daily living skills and SE), and *support services* (eg, education of family members, assistance with housing and legal problems) (190). Thus, the client remains in the least restrictive environment, preferably the client's environment of choice.

Ideally, within the PACT model, the clients are equal members of the team, and they direct and coordinate their own care. As discussed previously, several forms of decision-making permit varying levels of self-determination. PACT offers an opportunity for occupational therapy professionals to make a significant contribution in both rehabilitation and support services.

Prevention and Relapse Prevention Programs

A major emphasis in work with those who have mental disorders is relapse prevention. Prevention programs have been described in the occupational therapy literature. For example, Knis-Matthews (93) designed and operated a parenting program for women with substance use dependence. The program taught basic and traditional games, ways to play with children, ways to match the game or activity to the child, and how to use community resources such as parks effectively.

Copeland (41) provides suggestions for helping consumers develop a personal action guide to help identify uncomfortable physical sensations and emotional states that might trigger a relapse. Precin (140) gives exercises and worksheets that could be used in relapse prevention programs to identify stressors and acquire coping skills.

Additional models in prevention are in employee assistance programs (EAPs), smoking cessation, and diabetes prevention. Use of cigarettes and other tobacco products has reached epidemic levels among persons with severe and persistent mental disorders. Besides endangering the health and welfare of the smoker, this habit pollutes the therapeutic environment and creates a health hazard for nonsmoking clients, staff, and family members. Affirming a positive health attitude by enabling clients to reduce, limit, or eliminate smoking can be one facet of a wellness program. Certain psychotropic medications (see Chapter 8) predispose the consumer to gain weight and to be at risk for metabolic syndrome, a condition that can lead to diabetes. Thus, diet and nutrition and exercise are included in a wellness program.

Lifestyle Medicine

The field of lifestyle medicine uses lifestyle to change health outcomes. Using the lifestyle medicine model, the occupational therapy professional engages the client in considering the effects of lifestyle on health and on ability to participate in desired occupations. Figure 6.5 is a drawing made by a client who was morbidly obese. The drawing, which reflects the symbols of the Kawa model (85), meant to illustrate one's journey through life, shows a river with two boulders in it, with the river flowing freely around it. Through discussion with the occupational therapy professional, the client came to recognize that his life was not flowing smoothly and that the two boulders represented his obesity and his pain (104).

Working in prevention programs requires a tolerance for role blurring and an appreciation of the diffuse structure of community programs. Successful workers must be able to create their own programs, sometimes despite community indifference, and provide services flexibly, adapting to the wishes of the people in the community. Hildenbrand and Lamb (79) state that occupational therapy professionals should

- recognize a larger role in promoting health in individuals and populations,
- be creative about funding sources for prevention programming,
- collaborate with other professional groups and with service users, and
- participate in health care policy discussions.

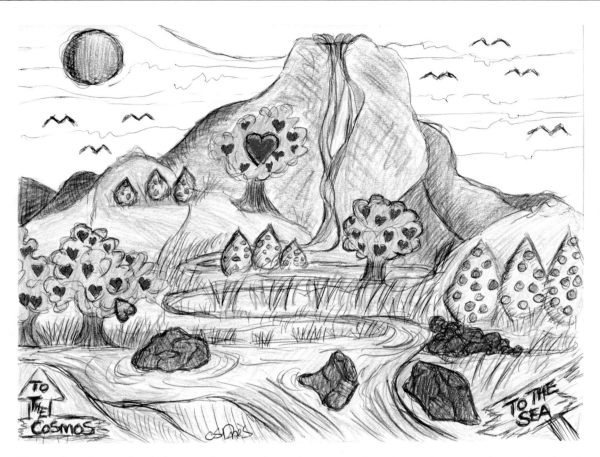

Figure 6.5. Occupational Therapy Client Drawing Reflecting on Obstacles to Changing Behavior. (Used with permission from Mann, D. P., Javaherian-Dysinger, H., & Hewitt, L. (2013). Ounce of prevention—Using the power of lifestyle to improve health outcomes. *OT Practice, 18*(7), 16–21.e19.)

Employment

TEPs and SE are designed to move clients into the work world at a pace that can be matched to their own rate of progress. TEP provides temporary part-time paid jobs with counselors and job coaches who help clients adjust to jobs and may also help adjust job factors to fit individual clients. The goal is to provide a successful experience of work and to prepare the person to move into community employment as early as possible. Research evidence shows that SE is highly effective for persons with serious mental disorders, and employment is an important factor in recovery (13). Many models of SE exist, but the common elements are individualized placement and support from coaches and other professionals (65).

In the past, persons with intellectual disabilities were thought to be unable to enter competitive employment and therefore were placed in sheltered workshops. Sheltered workshops employed persons whose rate of production was low; they were often paid based on how much work (how many pieces) they produced. Tasks one might have seen in a sheltered workshop included sorting, counting, and bagging plastic tableware; assembling ballpoint pens; and counting and packaging envelopes. The present trend is to assist every person with a disability to enter the workforce through SE or job coaching.

Work-related and SE programs may be found in both inpatient and outpatient settings and as independent community programs. Often, these programs are staffed by paraprofessionals and by certified rehabilitation counselors. Occupational therapy professionals may administer such programs or serve as consultants or group leaders. The abilities to evaluate an individual's occupational performance and to analyze, grade, and adapt activities to enable performance are essential skills provided by occupational therapy professionals.

Crisis Intervention

Crisis intervention is a practice model that aims to help people cope during crisis. The client can walk in during clinic hours and receive advice, support, and resources to solve the immediate problem. Alternately, the person can telephone or text. People in crisis tend to be overwhelmed by feelings and sometimes are confused, passive, and unable to act. They may abandon their usual activities and develop maladaptive behaviors such as denying reality, complaining rather than acting, or giving up entirely.

Rosenfeld (146) developed an approach using nuclear tasks and a cognitive–behavioral model to help people in crisis; his approach includes the steps shown in Box 6.13. This model seeks to restore normal occupational behavior patterns by engaging the client in nuclear tasks. A *nuclear task* is a purposeful activity that requires the person in crisis to marshal their resources and get on with life. Rosenfeld identified three types of nuclear task: remotivating tasks, skills and coping tasks, and symbolic tasks. *Remotivating tasks* help the person get started doing something; doing something lets the person move beyond feeling helpless. An example is a person cleaning out a part of their home, even though they are preoccupied about having lost their job. *Skills and coping tasks* help the person acquire the skills needed to resolve or work on the crisis—for instance, the person may need to practice interviewing skills or work on their professional appearance and presentation before looking for another job. *Symbolic tasks* are activities, usually chosen by the person, that show resolution of the crisis—for example, a couple whose infant died suddenly might, after some time, decide to have a party and include friends who have young children.

Whereas the nuclear task approach is an occupational therapy practice model, other crisis intervention methods are used by other mental health professionals in psychiatric emergency rooms, in hospitals and community mental health clinics, in satellite and aftercare clinics, and in some home health programs and community agencies. Examples include calling a crisis hotline or using crisis texting line model. Using a crisis texting line involves inputting an easy six-digit number into a smartphone. Counselors review messages and respond within 5 minutes (42).

PSYCHOSOCIAL ASPECT OF MEDICAL PROBLEMS, PHYSICAL DISABILITIES, AND PAIN MANAGEMENT

There are several reasons physical disabilities are included in a text on mental health. First, psychosocial factors may be contributing factors in physical disabilities. Second, some physical conditions such as traumatic brain injury (TBI) result in behavioral symptoms. Third, *any* physical disability or disease changes a person's life and requires coping. Because occupational therapy professionals are concerned with the occupational life of the person, we take a holistic view, accounting for psychosocial and cognitive responses even when the major presenting problems appear to be physical.

Psychosocial Factors

As stated earlier, psychosocial factors may contribute to disability. This occurs in cases of substance use that leads to physical trauma and prolonged disability (eg, falls, automobile accidents, and chronic health conditions). Consumers benefit from attention to their substance use problems and from open discussions about the risks associated with continued use. Because the substance may be central to the person's coping behaviors, resistance to this message is expected. Underlying psychosocial problems (including severe mental disorders for which the person was self-medicating) may also be present. See Chapter 4 for more discussion of substance use.

Inadequate psychosocial skills, limited awareness or insight, or poor judgment may contribute to disability. For example, Aja (1) described a case of overuse syndrome in which the worker continued to injure herself because she lacked the coping skills to negotiate a better situation for herself. The client was lonely and perceived her only social support to be at her part-time job in a print shop. From her perspective, she *had* to continue her self-injurious work because otherwise she would lose her friends. This is a case in which the major intervention for a physical disability was instructing the person in coping skills, a psychosocial component.

Psychosocial Consequences

The second reason for the inclusion of physical disabilities is that some of these disabilities have associated psychosocial consequences. The most prominent such diagnosis is TBI, in which behavioral problems frequently result. Depending on the area or areas of the brain affected, the person with TBI may be aggressive or demanding; seductive; inappropriate in communications; impulsive; or inattentive to grooming, hygiene, and basic good manners. The Allen cognitive disabilities model can be employed to assess functional level. The occupational

---

BOX 6.13 The Nuclear Task Approach to Crisis Intervention

To identify nuclear tasks through evaluation

- Use expressive activities when indicated to promote expression of affect.
- Seek evidence of task failures and functional deficits that contribute to the crisis.
- Identify uncompleted tasks that disturb and/or motivate the client. Assess the symbolic and realistic value of these tasks for resolving the crisis.
- Assess the client's functional resources. Identify patterns of attribution and activity that tend to promote or diminish effective coping responses.

To promote performance of nuclear tasks in treatment

- Help the client see and accept the challenge inherent in the crisis.
- Promote reasonable attributions to counteract the client's negative, harsh, and hopeless self-estimates.
- Undertake graded remotivating activities designed to yield rapid success in affecting uncompleted task elements of the crisis.
- Teach new functional skills and coping behaviors necessary to surmount the crisis.
- Discuss and implement activities that test or signify progress toward recovery.
- Plan daily activity routines that promote a sense of order, control, and certainty, thereby creating islands of comfort and enjoyment in the client's sea of troubles.

Reprinted with permission from Rosenfeld, M. S. (1984). Crisis intervention: The nuclear task approach. *American Journal of Occupational Therapy, 38*(6), 382–385.

therapist must try to determine which of the client's behaviors are likely to be changed and which ones are relatively fixed and require compensation. Compensatory strategies are used to limit confusing or irrelevant environmental stimuli and to focus the client on the desired task or goal. The neurobehavioral approach can be used to change behavior; positive behavior is reinforced and negative behavior is ignored so long as it is not a danger to the client or to others (155).

Memory impairment can interfere with the person's ability to benefit from a behavioral approach if the person cannot recognize that a specific behavior led to specific consequences. Alternative techniques such as *antecedent management*, in which a consistent sequence of environmental events or cues is used to initiate and shape behavior, are described by Yuen (191).

Depression and anxiety are common reactions to many physical conditions. Motivation can be reduced, and quality of life impaired. Ikiugu (84) cites the example of a corn farmer who was depressed and feeling without value following a heart attack. Helping the farmer explore how his various occupations could be approached differently through environmental modification, time management, and delegation to others is a way to address the negative feelings and sense of worthlessness.

Transformative Life Challenges

The third reason for considering psychosocial aspects of physical disability is that the knowledge of illness and physical disability changes a person's life. The first reaction may be denial, with more complex and intense feelings following. The emotional response to disability and the process of adjustment are described well in other texts (26, 49, 149). In addition to the psychological adjustment, the person experiences grief with the loss of function and faces an adjustment in occupational roles. Sanford (149) writes eloquently of the internal transformations that lead to acceptance and movement toward a new sense of self.

POINT-OF-VIEW

Then there are the quiet deaths. How about the day you realized that you were not going to be an astronaut or the queen of Sheba? Feel the silent distance between yourself and how you felt as a child, between yourself and those feelings of wonder and splendor and trust. Feel your mature fondness for who you once were, and your current need to protect innocence wherever you might find it. The silence that surrounds the loss of innocence is a most serious death, and yet it is necessary for the onset of maturity.

—Matthew Sanford (149), yoga teacher, paraplegic since age 13

- What does Matthew's story say about loss and resilience?
- Does knowing his story change your view of what is possible for people with disabilities?
- If his disability were psychiatric, would you have a different opinion of his job as a yoga teacher?

Reading Sanford's words, and learning his history, one is struck by the power of the lived body and the mind to create a future that to many may seem impractical or fantastic. As occupational therapy professionals, we must remember that we can serve best as partners and collaborators on our clients' journeys to wholeness and that we must encourage and help them to lead the way.

Mental Health–Based Occupational Therapy for Clients With Primary Medical Diagnoses

Mental health–based occupational therapy has much to offer clients with primary medical diagnoses. Cognitive–behavioral strategies and cognitive pain control techniques may help clients with low back pain or with burns (13). Other appropriate interventions for clients with general medical diagnoses may include use of expressive activities such as collage (particularly useful for clients who cannot speak and for those experiencing emotional reactions to their conditions) and production of small craft items as gifts. Activities chosen should be appropriate for bedside and not create a housekeeping problem for other staff. When possible, occupational therapy staff should help clients renew connections to valued life occupations and roles (or explore new ones). Leslie (96) reported on an opera singer, hospitalized for a liver transplant, who found his way back to health and to his career. The occupational therapist brought a recording of the client's favorite opera to his room. This led to spontaneous singing (at first very weak and with lots of coughing) but ultimately led to requests from nursing staff for songs. Other occupational therapy for the client included cognitive activities, memory training, and crafts.

Multiple sclerosis (MS) is a chronic disease of the central nervous system that causes gradual physical impairment as well as mental health problems such as depression, mood changes, and cognitive impairment. Interventions to support the mental health of persons with MS and other chronic and degenerative diseases of the central nervous system may focus on education about the disease process, fatigue management, support for appropriate social engagement and emotion regulation, and learning new strategies to cope with a progressive condition (116).

Occupational therapy for persons living with chronic disease may provide good outcomes and needs continued research (69). Working with survivors in groups should be balanced with client-centered goals and should provide strategies for following through when not in the occupational therapy setting. Occupational therapy may promote exercise as well as train the person in coping strategies such as meditation, stress management, and relaxation (69).

Physical disability may mean a change in social roles and difficulties with social and community integration. A disfiguring condition involving the face may lead to social isolation. More than anything, the person with a physical disability desires to be accepted and to be a member of the community, treated as normally as possible. But the stigma and associated compensations by others may become tiresome. As one adolescent with a spinal cord injury said, "It sounds so simple, but just have a place for them in the class. It makes it easier to just have a place to go and sit like a normal person, and even aisles, where you can go up and bring your paper up to the desk. It sounds little, but it's not" (120, p. 311).

Community integration is even more difficult for persons with behavioral and cognitive deficits. For example, persons with TBI are often poorly accepted by the community because of their disinhibited sexual behavior, odd manners, and difficulty controlling and expressing emotions appropriately. Poor social skills may prevent the development of new relationships, and the person can become increasingly isolated and more prone to depression. This trend typically becomes more pronounced over time (25). These clients could benefit from increased rehabilitation efforts in cognitive and social skills.

Coping Strategies for Persons With Physical Disabilities

How does a person respond to and cope with a physical disability? And how can coping be improved? Gage (57) described the *appraisal method of coping*, or how the person appraises and evaluates the experience. Appraisal consists of evaluating first the event or experience in terms of whether it is positive or negative (primary appraisal). The next step is evaluating the resources available for coping with the event (secondary appraisal). Resources may be personal, social, financial, or environmental.

Coping response may be emotion focused, problem focused, and/or perception focused.

- **Emotion-focused** responses are used to control the emotional reaction.
- **Problem-focused** responses emphasize changing the environment or the interaction with the environment to reduce stress.
- **Perception-focused** responses work on changing the person's perception of the event.

This cognitive–behavioral analysis (see Chapter 2) is useful for understanding how clients respond to occupational therapy and for predicting how well they will carry over or generalize skills to the community. For example, avoidant emotion-focused responses, such as denial, wishful thinking, and self-blaming, are associated with high levels of stress and poor adjustment (57). This suggests a role for occupational therapy professionals in training the person coping strategies that facilitate generalization of skills and community adjustment for persons with physical disabilities and/or chronic disease.

A related concern is the client's motivation toward intervention; with current health care expectations to reduce costs yet increase quality of care, occupational therapists must quickly evaluate the rehabilitation potential of a person with a physical disability and estimate achievable functional outcomes. The client's goals must be considered a priority. Interviewing the client about goals or conducting a client-centered assessment such as the *COPM* can yield this information; the occupational therapy assistant can be asked to assist with this type of assessment. In addition, occupational therapy professionals should cultivate an ongoing dialogue in which the client can be heard. The therapeutic relationship can be enhanced when using a lifestyle-based approach where the client directs the plan and the occupational therapy professional provides guidance. Using this approach involves the client identifying meaningful and purposeful goals and the occupational therapy professional providing intervention ideas to facilitate goal achievement (97).

Pain Management

Occupational therapy has a particular place in pain management. In 2018, the *Substance Use Disorder Prevention that Promotes Opioid Recovery and Treatment (SUPPORT) for Patients and Communities Act* (HR6) (162) was signed into law. It included occupational therapy as a nonpharmacologic pain management treatment. This law promotes development of best practices in acute care settings for nonpharmacologic evidence-based strategies for pain management and opioid use disorder prevention. Occupational therapy professionals can add to the development of these practices. The law requires Medicare Advantage plans to include nonpharmacologic therapies, such as occupational therapy, and requires the Centers for Medicare and Medicaid Services to provide states with guidance on using non-opioid treatments for pain management, again, such as occupational therapy. An additional requirement of the law is training of health professionals in nonpharmacologic pain management treatments. Finally, the law expands National Institutes of Health research on nonpharmacologic treatments for pain (133).

Long-term pain, which may last for decades and vary in intensity, is associated with a range of diagnoses, including birth defects, back injury, spinal cord injury, arthritis, fibromyalgia, and cancer. Pain can be undermedicated; clients could be more comfortable if appropriate doses of pain medication were given at closer intervals (87). A different consideration is those who may reject pain medication, such as those recovering from substance misuse and others who avoid drugs and alcohol, for instance, because of religious reasons (100). From a psychosocial perspective, chronic pain may lead to depression, fatigue, inactivity, isolation, loss of valued occupations, failure to participate in daily life, and a sense of helplessness.

The experience of pain is subjective and individualized. Spiritual beliefs and emotional temperament seem to affect pain perception (100). Research and personal reports have suggested that involvement in valued purposeful activity related to chosen life roles or hobbies may make pain easier to endure (72, 103, 108, 149). However, long-term pain may cause the person to believe that occupational performance and participation will be painful and impractical.

People who experience chronic pain distinguish between usual or expected pain and unexpected pain (48). It is possible to plan activities around expected pain, because it is predictable. Unexpected pain, on the other hand, comes without warning and disrupts planned activities. People who have ongoing pain problems develop strategies to deal with the two types of pain (48). For usual pain, the common strategies are prevention, planning, and making practical decisions with activity. For unexpected pain, the strategies are mind–body dissociation (focusing one's mind elsewhere), relief safety nets (medication and social supports), and reviewing priorities and being persistent. Use of relapse prevention techniques to identify increasing pain symptoms and then completing strategies to address plan flares can be useful as can the use of adaptive patterns of thinking for occupational participation (10).

Having clients monitor their pain levels at specific intervals and write down what they are doing at that time may help create an awareness that activity is possible and may be beneficial. A smartphone alarm beeper can be used to signal the intervals at which to record these perceptions (87). Perhaps the simplest method is a visual analog scale (Figure 6.6); clients are asked to mark the line at the point corresponding to their perception of the pain at that moment.

Occupational therapy professionals can use the biopsychosocial model as a method to address pain. Use of this model "evaluates the integrated 'whole person', with both the mind and the body together as interconnected entities, recognizing biological, psychological, and social components of pain and illness" (16, p. 99). Evaluation then uses an occupational profile that collects information about the person's occupational participation, performance patterns, and client factors. This information is intertwined with their contexts of personal factors and environmental factors. In addition, an analysis of occupational performance addresses performance skill abilities. By synthesizing this information, the occupational therapist identifies supports and barriers the client has and how all these items impact the client's perception and experience of their pain (10, 97).

Engel (50) suggested that occupational therapy professionals could intervene with the client who has pain by using the following methods:

- Teaching and reinforcing socially appropriate pain expressions (eg, speaking with involved health care practitioners rather than to anyone who will listen)
- Praising and reinforcing social interaction about issues other than pain
- Encouraging appropriate physical activity
- Introducing the client to support groups
- Teaching distraction as a method of pain management

Using distraction, the client in pain may focus within the self (eg, meditation, memory) or on a diverting activity (reading, doing a puzzle). Cognitive restructuring, a cognitive–behavioral method for challenging negative automatic thoughts (see Chapter 2), is also recommended.

Occupations are the primary intervention strategy used by occupational therapy professionals. Other intervention techniques include physical agent and mechanical modalities, assistive technology, environmental modifications, activity modifications, self-regulation, self-management techniques, medication management, advocacy, self-advocacy, group interventions, energy conservation, and virtual interventions (10).

Work simplification, education for performing correct body mechanics, positioning, activity pacing, ergonomics, compensatory techniques, and environmental adaptations may also help (97). A needed aspect of energy conservation is the person's ongoing reflection on how much energy they have at a given time or on a given day, as this can vary greatly. With practice, a person gains awareness to what extent energy levels vary and becomes attuned to sensing how much energy is available at a given time. Accurate assessment of one's energy level helps in planning what one might accomplish on a particular day. Performance patterns such as daily routines can then be changed or adapted to allow for greater occupational performance and participation (97).

Fear or expectation of pain may become an impediment to engaging in occupation. This is termed **fear avoidance**. As an example, fear of falling may lead to reduced activity, which then reduces balance and strength, thereby increasing the risks associated with falling. And fear of upper extremity

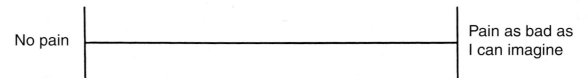

No pain | Pain as bad as I can imagine

Figure 6.6. Visual Analog Scale. (Reprinted with permission from Engel, J. (1998). Treatment for psychosocial components: Pain management. In: M. E. Neistadt & E. B. Crepeau (Eds.), *Willard and Spackman's occupational therapy* (9th ed., pp. 454–458). Lippincott Williams & Wilkins.)

pain following trauma may interfere with return to work and to valued occupations. Fear avoidance can be assessed through tools such as the *Fear-Avoidance Beliefs Questionnaire*. This tool helps identify the relationship between a client's fear-avoidance beliefs about how work and physical activity can impact and contribute to low back pain and the resulting disability (186). Only by engaging in the feared activity in a thoughtful way can the person explore to what extent the fear is realistic. Graded exposure to the feared situation, along with systematic appraisal at each step, is a cognitive–behavioral approach that may allow a person to resume real-life activities (144). Participation in new or familiar occupations may result in a decrease in perceived pain (185).

Pain Neuroscience Education (PNE) is a technique using storytelling and metaphors to educate people on the biologic and neurophysiologic perspectives of pain, along with the psychosocial factors associated with the pain experience. This technique helps people to understand the reason for the pain and learn about the output of pain and appropriate responses and actions to a situation. For instance, if a person is beginning to experience chest pains, the person can identify the need to seek medical treatment to either stop a heart attack or to limit the ramifications of a heart attack (44). This technique can be useful in teaching children about pain. By using a social environment, occupational therapy professionals can better encourage discussion and questioning to deepen learning about the complexities of pain. Connecting the biologic and psychosocial information to daily life activities and environments can aid with understanding (44).

Case Study – A 37-Year-Old Man With Alcohol Use Disorder[4]

B. Jebson Case #038947

Mr Jebson is a 37-year-old married Caucasian man admitted to the detox unit after his employer confronted him about poor job performance and absenteeism owing to persistent and heavy alcohol use (see later). Client reported that his wife has been threatening to leave him over the past year. Client was transferred to inpatient substance use rehabilitation after 3 days in detoxification.

DSM-5-TR Diagnosis at Admission

F10.20 Alcohol Use Disorder, Severe

Z Codes

Z63.0 Relationship distress with spouse or intimate partner
Z56.6 Other physical and mental strain related to work

Client began drinking alcohol at age 15 and stated that it has been a problem in his life for at least the past 5 years. He has been fired from two jobs during that time and is having difficulty at a local factory job in which he has been employed for almost 18 months. Client was able to maintain one job for 11 years, but that ended 5 years ago. He and his wife have been married for 10 years and have an 8-year-old daughter and a 5-year-old son. Client denied any marital problems other than drinking.

Mr Jebson has two brothers and one sister and was raised by his parents on a farm. He stated that he is the only one in his immediate family who drinks, but he has heard that his maternal great-grandfather was alcoholic. Client completed high school and vocational technical training, acquiring a welding certificate. He stated his pattern is to drink at least six to eight beers after work, and on weekends in excess of a case of beer plus several half-pints of whiskey. Client says he has mainly drunk alone at home in his tool shop. He does very little individual or family leisure activity. He stated that he has difficulty expressing his feelings and drinks especially when he feels angry. Client admitted to being violent when drunk, throwing things and punching the wall on several occasions. He denies ever hitting his wife or children. Client said that he used to go to the local Baptist church with his family but quit because of his drinking. He had one DUI charge approximately 2 years ago and after that quit going to bars to drink.

Client identified his strengths as loving his family, being a skilled welder, and caring about people. He named his weaknesses as drinking and holding in his feelings. He identified his family and his job as most important to him. Client was verbal but tearful at times during the interview. He appears motivated to get sober because of pressure from employer and wife.

Goals, objectives, and intervention are shown in the treatment summary for this case (Table 6.3).

Occupational Therapy Discharge Summary (3 Weeks After Admission)

Mr Jebson has been a model client, following through on all planned activities and interventions. He made several projects in occupational therapy for his family and identified woodcraft as a hobby he could pursue and teach to his children. He named the following as family activities he would like to develop: cookouts, camping, movies, vacations, and community park excursions. He named additional activities for himself as hunting, fishing, boating, flea markets, and AA retreats. He has met several men from his community through AA and has asked two of them to be his sponsors in the program. Client had difficulty labeling his feelings in the log initially and was given a chart with facial expressions (94) to use as a guide. He began identifying feelings of anger and fear as dominant in his experience. In assertiveness group, he identified himself as passive unless intoxicated, when he would become aggressive. He talked openly about things he has stuffed his anger over and role-played effective expression. He reported using assertion in a marital session with his wife with positive results. Client asked about becoming a volunteer after a year of sobriety. He identified this as a long-term goal for aftercare. Family and employer are expected to support and encourage client after discharge.

[4]Adapted from a case contributed by Susan Voorhies, COTA/CAADAC, of HCA Regional Hospital Rediscovery Unit, Jackson, TN, in consultation with Anne Brown, OTR, MS.

Table 6.3. Occupational Therapy Treatment Summary

Goals	Objectives	Occupational Therapy (OT) Intervention Given
1. To improve leisure and social involvement	1a. Client will identify at least five leisure activities to provide socialization and support for his recovery (by 2 wk) 1b. Client will identify a variety of leisure activities to pursue with his family (by 2 wk) 1c. Client will introduce himself to at least one male peer at nightly 12-step meetings and will inquire about the group's recreational activities (by 3 wk)	1a. Leisure education 1 × wk; community out-trips 1 × wk 1b. Leisure education 1 × wk; community out-trips 1 × wk; family recreation night biweekly; OT clinic 4 × wk 1c. 12-step meetings nightly; individual leisure assignment
2. To improve assertive behavior and expression of feelings	2a. Client will begin keeping a daily feeling log (within 3 d) 2b. Client will identify situations in which he has withheld angry feelings (by 2 wk) 2c. Client will role-play specific situations in which he has been angry using assertive techniques to express his anger (by 3 wk)	2a. Individual OT assignment 2b. Assertiveness training 2 × wk 2c. Assertiveness training 2 × wk

OT HACKS SUMMARY

O: **Occupation as a means and an end**

Becoming includes what we do and who we are, plus looks to the future about how we are identified in times to come.

Being includes doing, and the person's distinct ideas and thoughts.

Belonging is about who we are with the interactions and relationships we have with others.

Doing includes the action, the person, and the impact of that action on others.

T: **Theoretical concepts, values, and principles, or historical foundations**

The change people do to resolve problems or to compensate for difficulties is grounded in occupational participation with consideration toward the person's roles, occupational form and performance, participation in activity, and reflection on occupation. Occupational therapy professionals use specific therapeutic strategies (validating, identifying, giving feedback, advising, negotiating, structuring, coaching, encouraging, and providing physical support) and specific methods of intervention (assessment combined with intervention, participation in meaningful occupation, facilitation of exploration, occupational counseling, peer support educational groups, occupational self-help groups, skill teaching based on the MOHO, social education, environmental management, and occupational role development and habit change).

Biopsychosocial model: Combining of biologic, or physical factors, with social factors, and psychological factors so that the occupational therapy professional views the client holistically.

Kawa model: By using the metaphor of a river (water flow, water, rocks, driftwood, the river floor, river walls, and spaces in the river) to depict various aspects of life, the occupational therapy professional uses a Japanese cultural perspective and encompasses a collectivist cultural view to aid clients in occupational performance.

Occupational adaptation model: Disruptions that occur in one's life bring about a need to adapt to the new circumstance and regain stability in occupational actions.

Considerations include a person's occupational roles, occupational challenges, role demands or expectations, and occupational responses. Occupational therapy is provided to enhance adaptation and intervene in situations of dysadaptation. Through a person using their adaptation gestalt and adaptive responses, OA occurs. OA is measured through a person's relative mastery and adaptive capacity.

H: **How can we Help? OT's role in serving clients with mental illness or mental health needs**

How we provide interventions to our clients is influenced by the following personal factors.

Culture: how a client and their family view mental illness can be different than how those from American culture view it; factors such as immigration status can impact availability of health insurance; when someone is an immigrant, social expectations are new and the person may not know how to "fit it," especially in light of a need or desire to stay strongly connected to their country of origin

Diversity: an individual's thoughts about who they are and what they do; a person's external qualities and features that are observed by others

Equity: providing specifically what each individual needs, rather than equal distribution across all people

Inclusion: acceptance and supporting of client's diverse selves

Occupational Justice: a person's right to complete desired occupations and have equity with occupational choices for well-being

We consider occupational therapy methods regarding:

Population Characteristics

Caregivers: supporting their mental health needs, considering family dynamics, communication designed to understand them and include them in decision-making; building rapport and strengthening relationships with them

Community-based programs: focus on housing and community living skills

Program for Assertive Community Treatment offers services where the person lives providing medical-based treatment, rehabilitation, and support services

Prevention programs are geared for coping skills training and trigger relapse identification; can be for substance use, mental disorders, and mental health needs

Employment programs support clients with job coaches and counselors; some programs work to transition clients to full community-based employment

Crisis interventions include use of the Nuclear Task Approach, inpatient and outpatient emergency services, crisis hotlines, and crisis text lines

Society

Community health: specific region; improve maintain individual and community, prevent, prepare; identify barriers, improve access, uncover risks; partnerships, relationships, service; connect member to service

Community mental health centers: clients; intervention; chronic care; provision of services; individual or group

Population health: location, condition, situation; individual inside population; prevent promote, decrease disparities; outcomes and health information; data, societal-based, health opportunities, costs; strategies based on science

Public health: for all; promote protect; quality of life and well-being; policymakers, government-based, education, training, research; practice of medicine not health care system

Social Issues

Domestic violence and working with victim or survivors to cope with their experiences within the cycle of violence and forming new coping strategies

Populations in economic distress working to provide support, resources, and opportunities for those with lower incomes; working with those who do not have permanent housing, with particular focus on the multiple needs of veterans, support needs of adults, and teaching daily life skills to adolescents

Trauma-informed care starts with a trauma-informed approach that includes all members of an organization and focuses on recognizing trauma in any client and providing an atmosphere of respect and empowerment; human trafficking interventions for community reintegration, home management, education, employment, leisure, social participation, emotional regulation, executive functions, and performance patterns

Youth violence work to include interventions for bullying behavior and for transitioning into adulthood

Individual Needs

Literacy: health, functional, financial, digital, and mental health

Medical or physical needs: psychosocial factors contribute to disability; psychosocial consequences to physical disabilities; transformative life changes; coping response; mental health–based interventions—cognitive–behavioral strategies, expressive activities, education about disease process, stress management, coping strategies, motivation via client-centered care; pain management—SUPPORT Act, medication use, relapse prevention, monitoring pain levels, occupational profile during evaluation, compensatory and adaptive strategies, fear avoidance, Pain Neuroscience Education

Provision of services within an interdisciplinary approach:

Psychiatric rehabilitation: more medically aligned in that medication and hospitalization encouraged during crisis; collaboration with provider; atmosphere of hope

Psychoeducation: a life skills educational approach; occupational therapy professional functions educator; clients are identified as students; goal is for generalization of new learning to be used with everyday activities

Recovery: the view of having a psychiatric illness not as a situation of being "sick," but as a time of "recovery"; person-centered and person-directed; focus on health, home, purpose, and community

Wellness: within recovery, used to promote self-management of illness and increase a positive attitude toward health

Psychosocial rehabilitation:

Psychosocial rehabilitation: focus is community living with limited support

Clubhouse model offers a wide variety of services for improving all occupations

Transitional housing provides some supervision and has a group atmosphere

A: **Adaptations**

Adaptation considerations identified in this chapter include the following:

Adapting to a time of change. Both the MOHO and the model of OA specifically address the importance of a person adapting to new situations.

Adaptive response. Occupational readiness prepares the person's capacity skills and occupational activities are connected to the environmental factors and personal factors held meaningful by the person.

Environmental management. Adapting the world around someone, including the social atmosphere, to promote greater participation. Barriers are removed and supports are installed within the occupational environment.

Literacy. Adapting education and training materials to match the various literacy skills of clients and caregivers.

Neurocognitive disorders. Clients with these disorders can benefit from caregivers being taught home modifications, behavior management, and occupational specific strategies for revising how the person completes occupations (such as grading the activity steps of an occupation and using co-occupations).

Occupational adaptation. During dysadaptation, the occupational therapy professional facilitates the client being an agent of change. The person's understanding of what is meaningful, their choices, and initiation of occupational activity guide the person's adaptation, or change.

Populations in economic distress. Occupational therapy professionals must adapt their intervention approach for those without permanent housing. Consideration must be given to limited daily life resources and space used to perform many typical daily occupations.

Resiliency. Being resilient means being able to quickly adapt to new life circumstances. Managing emotions and feelings, as well as having problem-solving and communication skills are all a part of being resilient. Part of the adaptation associated with resiliency is the hope that the person will be able to return to their desired occupations.

Self-advocacy. One adapts to a new situation by asking for, seeking, and working toward needed changes in the environment (physical or social) the person needs to be successful with occupations.

C: **Case study includes**

Case study of a man with alcohol use disorder. Areas addressed: leisure occupations, social participation, assertiveness, and self-expression.

K: **Knowledge: keeping mental health OT practice grounded in evidence, in occupational science, and in research**

Occupational science is researching what constitutes occupational resilience.

More current evidence is needed for pain interventions. We can add this body of knowledge through the new initiative from the SUPPORT Act for research regarding nonpharmacologic treatment methods for opioid and other substance use problems.

S: **Some terms that may be new to you**

ACEs: adverse childhood experiences that are potentially traumatic

Adaptation gestalt: allows person to modify how much skill capacity is needed to master and competently perform occupation

Adaptive capacity: realization and understanding of the need for adaptation and being able to make that adaptation happen

Adaptive mastery: effective participation, efficiency, and satisfaction with occupational performance and participation based on oneself and satisfaction of others who are important to the person

Consumer movement: consumer involvement in care decision-making and programming development

Fear avoidance: when fear or the expectation of pain becomes an impediment to occupational engagement

In vivo: naturalistic or real life

Intimate partner violence: includes physical violence, sexual violence, stalking, and psychological aggression

Lifestyle medicine: using lifestyle to change health outcomes

Nuclear task: purposeful activity requiring a person in crisis to marshal their resources and get on with life

Occupational adaptiveness: point at which the person demonstrates competency during OA

Occupational injustice: not being able to engage and participate in desired occupations

Occupational resilience: having the personal resolve to make the needed adjustments to ensure desired occupations are completed, regardless of barriers presented

Positive Physical Approach: three-step sequence of giving cues: visual, short verbal, and touch

Psychosocial rehabilitation: using emotional, social, and intellectual skills to live, learn, and work in the community with as little support as possible

Remotivating tasks: help a person get started "doing"

Resilience: ability to adapt to a difficult situation through skills such as flexibility and adjustment to demands

Skills and coping tasks: help a person acquire skills needed to resolve a problematic situation

Symbolic tasks: activities used to show resolution to a crisis

Reflection Questions

1. When thinking about health equity in the context of occupational therapy services, discuss what the following statement means and what implications it might have for everyday OT practice: "Occupational therapy includes an equitable distribution of skilled knowledge, service provision, resources, and opportunities."
2. Discuss the therapeutic strategies that occupational therapy professionals use to help the client facilitate change. Apply the Kawa model to explain how therapeutic change occurs according to that model of practice.
3. When considering the OA model of practice, why are role performance and role capacity considered critical aspects of intervention planning?
4. In what ways does population health inform day-to-day occupational therapy practice? Which common OT settings do you think are rooted in population health? Please provide your rationale.
5. Describe the overarching goals of public health, population health, and community health/mental health centers.
6. List and describe some of the occupational barriers for those experiencing homelessness.
7. Reflect upon and explain how culture can influence the varied roles of the caregiver of a person with physical, social, or emotional mental health problems. Discuss how the roles of the caregiver have changed over the last several decades.
8. Summarize the essential components of mental health literacy.
9. Compare and contrast the Psychosocial Clubhouse Model and transitional housing models and discuss how these models reflect shared characteristics with the core values of occupational therapy practice.
10. How could principles of the Nuclear Task Approach to Crisis Intervention be applied to the client case study included in this chapter (Mr Jebson)?

References

1. Aja, D. (1991). Occupational therapy intervention for overuse syndrome. *American Journal of Occupational Therapy, 45*(8), 746–750.
2. Allay Occupational Therapy. (2020, October 22). *Boosting your resilience through occupational therapy*. Retrieved January 17, 2022, from https://www.allayoccupationaltherapy.com.au/boosting-your-resilience-through-occupational-therapy/

3. American Occupational Therapy Association. (2013). *Bullying prevention and friendship promotion*. Retrieved January 06, 2022, from https://www.aota.org/~/media/Corporate/Files/Practice/Children/SchoolMHToolkit/BullyingPreventionInfoSheet.pdf

4. American Occupational Therapy Association. (2017). Occupational therapy services for individuals who have experienced domestic violence. *American Journal of Occupational Therapy, 71*(Suppl. 2), 1–13.

5. American Occupational Therapy Association. (2020). *AOTA's guide to acknowledging the impact of discrimination, stigma, and implicit bias on provision of service*. Retrieved January 08, 2021, from https://www.aota.org/-/media/corporate/files/aboutot/dei/guide-racial-discrimination.pdf

6. American Occupational Therapy Association. (2020). Occupational therapy practice framework: Domain and process—Fourth edition. *American Journal of Occupational Therapy, 74*(Suppl. 2), 1–87.

7. American Occupational Therapy Association. (2020). Occupational therapy's commitment to diversity, equity, and inclusion. *American Journal of Occupational Therapy, 74*(Suppl. 3), 1–6.

8. American Occupational Therapy Association. (2021). *Diversity, equity, and inclusion word bank*. Retrieved January 08, 2022, from https://www.aota.org/practice/practice-essentials/dei/dei-toolkit-word-bank

9. American Occupational Therapy Association. (2021). *Draft: American Occupational Therapy Association Policy E: Affirming gender diversity and identify*. Retrieved January 08, 2022, from https://www.aota.org/-/media/corporate/files/aboutaota/officialdocs/policies/policy-e15-20211115.pdf

10. American Occupational Therapy Association. (2021). Role of occupational therapy in pain management. *American Journal of Occupational Therapy, 75*(Suppl. 3), 1–29.

11. American Psychiatric Association. (2022). *Diagnostic and statistical manual of mental disorders* (5th ed., text rev.). American Psychiatric Association. https://doi.org/10.1176/appi.books.9780890425787

12. American Psychological Association. (2020). *APA Dictionary of Psychology: Resilience*. Retrieved January 17, 2022, from https://dictionary.apa.org/resilience

13. Arbesman, M., & Logsdon, D. W. (2011). Occupational therapy interventions for employment and education for adults with serious mental illness: A systematic review. *American Journal of Occupational Therapy, 65*(3), 238–246.

14. Bahn, L., Wells, S., & Wisniewski, S. (2020, April 20). *Occupational therapy: Breaking the barriers with survivors of human trafficking*. [Masters Capstone Project, Thomas Jefferson University]. Jefferson Digital Commons.

15. Barth, T. (1994). Occupational therapy interventions at a shelter for homeless, addicted adults with mental illness. *Mental Health Special Interest Section Quarterly, 17*(1), 7–8.

16. Bevers, K., Watts, L., Kishino, N. D., & Gachtel, R. J. (2016). The biopsychosocial model of the assessment, prevention, and treatment of chronic pain. *US Neurology, 12*(2), 98–104.

17. Black, M., & Campbell, A. (2019). *Life skills program for youth who have experienced homelessness*. [Master Capstone, University of North Dakota]. UND Scholarly Commons.

18. Blanche, E. I. (1996). Alma: Coping with culture, poverty, and disability. *American Journal of Occupational Therapy, 50*(4), 265–276.

19. Bonder, B., & Gurley, D. (2005). Culture and aging—Working with older adults from diverse backgrounds. *OT Practice, 4*(7), CE1–CE8.

20. Borillo, R. M. (2019). *Development of a financial literacy component for a comprehensive secondary transition program for diploma-based students with learning disabilities*. [Doctoral project, University of St. Augustine for Health Sciences]. Student Open Access Repository @ USA: Student Capstone Projects Collection.

21. Boyanapalli, A. A. (n.d.). *Occupational therapy for human trafficking*. Retrieved January 16, 2022, from https://www.aota.org/Education-Careers/Students/Pulse/Archive/career-advice/Human-Trafficking.aspx

22. Brooks, A. (2019, March 4). *What is community health and why is it important?* Rasmussen University: Health Science Blog. Retrieved on January 9, 2022, from https://www.rasmussen.edu/degrees/health-sciences/blog/what-is-community-health/

23. Brown, F. K. (2016). *Integrating health literacy into occupational therapy*. [Doctoral dissertation]. Texas Woman's University–Denton, TX.

24. Bruegger, T., Henderson, D., Garfinkel, M., & Costello, P. (2020). *The role of occupational therapy in supporting literacy across the lifespan* [presentation]. American Occupational Therapy Association. https://www.aota.org/Conference-Events/member-appreciation/webinar-library/Practice.aspx

25. Burleigh, S. A., Farber, R. S., & Gillard, M. (1998). Community integration and life satisfaction after traumatic brain injury: Long-term findings. *American Journal of Occupational Therapy, 52*(1), 45–52.

26. Burnett, S. B. (2018). Personal and social contexts of disability: Implications for occupational therapists. In H. M. Pendleton & W. Schultz-Krohn (Eds.), *Pedretti's occupational therapy practice skills for physical dysfunction* (8th ed., pp. 71–91). Elsevier.

27. Centers for Disease Control and Prevention. (2019, November). *Adverse childhood experiences (ACEs): Preventing early trauma to improve adult health*. https://www.cdc.gov/vitalsigns/aces/pdf/vs-1105-aces-H.pdf

28. Centers for Disease Control and Prevention. (2020, September 17). *6 guiding principles to a trauma-informed approach*. Retrieved January 16, 2022, from https://www.cdc.gov/cpr/infographics/6_principles_trauma_info.htm

29. Centers for Disease Control and Prevention. (2021, September 28). *Violence prevention*. Retrieved January 13, 2022, from https://www.cdc.gov/violenceprevention/

30. Centers for Disease Control and Prevention. (2021, October 9). *Intimate partner violence*. Retrieved January 14, 2022, from https://www.cdc.gov/violenceprevention/intimatepartnerviolence/index.html

31. Centers for Disease Control and Prevention. (2021, November 2). *Fast facts: Preventing intimate partner violence*. Retrieved January 14, 2022, from https://www.cdc.gov/violenceprevention/intimatepartnerviolence/fastfact.html

32. Centers for Disease Control and Prevention. (2021, December 2). *Injury prevention and control: Fatal injury and violence data*. Retrieved January 16, 2022, from https://www.cdc.gov/injury/wisqars/fatal.html

33. Center for Hope & Safety. (n.d.). *The cycle of domestic violence*. Retrieved January 14, 2022, from https://hopeandsafety.org/learn-more/the-cycle-of-domestic-violence/

34. Champagne, T. (2012). Creating occupational therapy groups for children and youth in community-based mental health practice. *OT Practice, 17*(14), 13–18.

35. Chang, F.-H., Helfrich, C. A., & Coster, W. J. (2013). Psychometric properties of the Practical Skills Test (PST). *American Journal of Occupational Therapy, 67*(2), 246–253.

36. Chapleau, A., Seroczynski, A. D., Meyers, S., Lamb, K., & Buchino, S. (2012). The effectiveness of a consultation model in community mental health. *Occupational Therapy in Mental Health, 28*(4), 379–395.

37. Clark, C. A., Corcoran, M., & Gitlin, L. N. (1995). An exploratory study of how occupational therapists develop therapeutic relationships with family caregivers. *American Journal of Occupational Therapy, 49*(7), 587–593.

38. Clay, P. (2013). Shared principles: The recovery model and occupational therapy. *Mental Health Special Interest Section Quarterly, 36*(4), 1–3.

39. Cole, M. B., & Tufano, R. (2020). *Applied theories in occupational therapy: A practical approach* (2nd ed.). SLACK.

40. Columbia University. (n.d.). *OT for literacy*. Retrieved January 17, 2022, from https://www.vagelos.columbia.edu/education/academic-programs/programs-occupational-therapy/faculty-innovations/ot-literacy

41. Copeland, M. E. (2000). Wellness recovery action plan: A system for monitoring, reducing and eliminating uncomfortable dangerous physical symptoms and emotional feelings. *Occupational Therapy in Mental Health, 17*(3–4), 127–150.

42. Crisis Text Line. (n.d.). *Text HOME to 741741 to reach a crisis counselor*. Retrieved January 17, 2022, from https://www.crisistextline.org/text-us/

43. Crist, P. H. (1986). Community living skills: A psychoeducational community-based program. *Occupational Therapy in Mental Health, 6*(2), 51–64.

44. Davis, C., & Pololak, J. (2018, December 7). *Kids in pain: Educating kids about pain and promoting health, from childhood through adulthood.*

American Occupational Therapy Association. https://www.aota.org/Publications-News/otp/Archive/2018/kids-in-pain.aspx

45. Diez Roux, A. V. (2016). On the distinction—or lack of distinction—between population health and public health. *American Journal of Public Health, 106*(4), 619–620.

46. D'Inverno, A. S., Smith, S. G., Zhang, X., & Chen, J. (2019, August). *The impact of intimate partner violence: A 2015 NISVS research-in-brief.* National Center for Injury Prevention and Control Centers for Disease Control and Prevention. https://www.cdc.gov/violenceprevention/pdf/nisvs/nisvs-impactbrief-508.pdf

47. DiZazzo-Miller, R,. Samuel, P. S., Barnas, J. M., & Welker, K. M. (2014). Addressing everyday challenges: Feasibility of a family caregiver training program for people with dementia. *American Journal of Occupational Therapy, 68*(2), 212–220.

48. Dudgeon, B. J., Tyler, E. J., Rhodes, L. A., & Jensen, M. P. (2006). Managing usual and unexpected pain with physical disability: A qualitative analysis. *American Journal of Occupational Therapy, 60*(1), 92–103.

49. Early, M. B. (2013). The disability experience and the therapeutic process. In M. B. Early (Ed.), *Physical dysfunction practice skills for the occupational therapy assistant* (3rd ed., pp. 17–40). Elsevier.

50. Engel, J. (1998). Treatment for psychosocial components: Pain management. In M. E. Neistadt & E. B. Crepeau (Eds.), *Willard and Spackman's occupational therapy* (9th ed., pp. 454–458). Lippincott Williams & Wilkins.

51. Estrany-Munar, M.-F., Talavera-Valverde, M.-Á., Souto-Gómez, A.-L., Màrquez-Álvarez, L.-J., & Moruno-Miralles, P. (2021). The effectiveness of community occupational therapy interventions: A scoping review. *International Journal of Environmental Research and Public Health, 18*(6), 1–16.

52. Fadiman, A. (1998). *The spirit catches you and you fall down.* Farrar Straus & Giroux.

53. Financial Literacy and Education Improvement Act. *Section 513 of Public Law No. 108–159, as amended through Public Law 111-203. 20 U.S.C. Section 511 § 9701.* (2010). https://www.govinfo.gov/content/pkg/COMPS-11864/pdf/COMPS-11864.pdf

54. Finlayson, M., Baker, M., Rodman, L., & Herzberg, G. (2002). The process and outcomes of a multimethod needs assessment at a homeless shelter. *American Journal of Occupational Therapy, 56*(3), 313–321.

55. Fountain House. (n.d.). *Our services.* Retrieved January 17, 2022, from https://www.fountainhouse.org/services

56. Fountain House Gallery. (n.d.). *Gallery talk.* Retrieved January 17, 2022, from https://www.fountainhousegallery.org/

57. Gage, M. (1992). The appraisal model of coping: An assessment and intervention model for occupational therapy. *American Journal of Occupational Therapy, 46*(4), 353–362.

58. Gentry, K., Snyder, K., Barstow, B., & Hamson-Utley, J. (2018). The biopsychosocial model: Application to occupational therapy practice. *The Open Journal of Occupational Therapy, 6*(4), 1–19.

59. George, U., Thomson, M. S., Chaze, F., & Guruge, S. (2015). Immigrant mental health, a public health issue: Looking back and moving forward. *International Journal of Environmental Research and Public Health, 12*(10), 13624–13648.

60. George Washington School of Medicine & Health Sciences. (n.d.). *Customized Toolkit of Information & Practical Solutions (C-TIPS).* Retrieved January 16, 2022, from https://cme.smhs.gwu.edu/course-catalog-table#:~:text=C%2DTIPS%20is%20the%20Customized,negative%20consequences%20of%20providing%20care

61. Gitlin, L. N., Corcoran, M., & Leinmiller-Eckhardt, S. (1995). Understanding the family perspective: An ethnographic framework for providing occupational therapy in the home. *American Journal of Occupational Therapy, 49*(8), 802–809.

62. Gorman, K. W., & Hatkevich, B. A. (2016). The role of occupational therapy in combating human trafficking. *American Journal of Occupational Therapy, 70*(6), 1–6.

63. Grajo, L. C., & Gutman, S. A. (2019). The role of occupational therapy in functional literacy. *The Open Journal of Occupational Therapy, 7*(1), 1–7.

64. Gray, E. (2020). *Mental health literacy for adolescents with special needs: A pilot occupational therapy curriculum in a middle school.* [Doctoral project, St. Catherine University]. SOPHIA: An e-community of scholarship & creativity.

65. Gray, K. (2005). Evidenced-based employment services for persons with serious mental illness. *Mental Health Special Interest Section Quarterly, 28*(3), 1–2.

66. Griner, K. R. (2006). Helping the homeless: An occupational therapy perspective. *Occupational Therapy in Mental Health, 22*(1), 49–61.

67. Gutman, S. A., Diamond, H., Holness-Parchment, S. A., Brandofino, D. N., Pacheco, D. G., Jolly-Edouard, M., & Jean-Charles, S. (2004). Enhancing independence in women experiencing domestic violence and possible brain injury: An assessment of an occupational therapy intervention. *Occupational Therapy in Mental Health, 20*(1), 49–79.

68. Gutman, S. A., Kerner, R., Zombek, I., Dulek, J., & Ramsey, C. A. (2009). Supported education for adults with psychiatric disabilities: Effectiveness of an occupational therapy program. *American Journal of Occupational Therapy, 63*(3), 245–254.

69. Hand, C., Law, M., & McColl, M. A. (2011). Occupational therapy interventions for chronic diseases: A scoping review. *American Journal of Occupational Therapy, 65*(4), 428–436.

70. Hayes, R. L., & Halford, W. K. (1993). Generalization of occupational therapy effects in psychiatric rehabilitation. *American Journal of Occupational Therapy, 47*(2), 161–167.

71. Health Resources & Services Administration. (2019, August). *Health literacy.* Retrieved January 16, 2022, from https://www.hrsa.gov/about/organization/bureaus/ohe/health-literacy/index.html

72. Heck, S. A. (1998). The effect of purposeful activity on pain tolerance. *American Journal of Occupational Therapy, 42*(9), 577–581.

73. Helfrich, C. A., & Aviles, A. (2001). Occupational therapy's role with victims of domestic violence: Assessment and intervention. *Occupational Therapy in Mental Health, 16*(3–4), 53–70.

74. Helfrich, C. A., Chan, D. V., & Sabol, P. (2011). Cognitive predictors of life skill intervention outcomes for adults with mental illness at risk for homelessness. *American Journal of Occupational Therapy, 65*(3), 277–286.

75. Helfrich, C. A., Lafata, M. J., MacDonald, S. L., & Aviles, A. (2001). Domestic abuse across the lifespan: Definitions, identification and risk factors for occupational therapists. *Occupational Therapy in Mental Health, 16*(3–4), 5–34.

76. Helfrich, C. A., & Rivera, Y. (2006). Employment skills and domestic violence survivors: A shelter-based intervention. *Occupational Therapy in Mental Health, 22*(1), 33–48.

77. Henry, P. (n.d.). *Trauma-informed peer support.* Mental Health America. Retrieved January 16, 2022, from https://www.mhanational.org/cps-blog-trauma-informed-peer-support

78. Hewett, F. M. (1964). A hierarchy of educational tasks for children with learning disorders. *Exceptional Children, 34*(4),459–467.

79. Hildenbrand, W. C., & Lamb, A. J. (2013). Occupational therapy in prevention and wellness: Retaining relevance in a new health care world. *American Journal of Occupational Therapy, 67*(3), 266–271.

80. Hocking, C. (2017). Occupational justice as social justice: The moral claim for inclusion. *Journal of Occupational Science, 24*(1), 29–42.

81. Hotchkiss, A., & Fisher, G. S. (2004). Community practice for the homeless—OT education at the Mercy Center for Women. *OT Practice, 14*(7), 17–21.

82. Humbert, T. K., Bess, J. L., & Mowery, A. M. (2013). Exploring women's perspectives of overcoming intimate partner violence: A phenomenological study. *Occupational Therapy in Mental Health, 29*(3), 358–380.

83. Humbert, T. K., Engleman, K., & Miller, C. E., (2014). Exploring women's expectations of recovery from intimate partner violence: A phenomenological study. *Occupational Therapy in Mental Health, 30*(4), 358–380.

84. Ikiugu, M. N. (2010). The new occupational therapy paradigm: Implications for integration of the psychosocial core of occupational therapy in all disciplines. *Occupational Therapy in Mental Health, 26*(4), 343–353.

85. Iwama, M. K. (2006). *The Kawa model: Culturally relevant occupational therapy.* Elsevier.

86. Javaherian, H. (2006). Helping survivors of domestic violence. *OT Practice, 11*(10), 12–16.

87. Joe, B. E. (1998, July 16). Managing chronic pain and fatigue. *OT Week*, 12–13.

88. John, A., Glendenning, A. C., Marchant, A., Montgomery, P., Stewart, A., Wood, S., Lloyd, K., & Hawton, K. (2018). Self-harm, suicidal behaviors, and cyberbullying in children and young people: Systematic review. *Journal of Medical Internet Research, 20*(4), 1–15.

89. Kaiser Family Foundation. (2021, July 15). *Health coverage and care of immigrants.* Retrieved January 08, 2022, from https://www.kff.org/racial-equity-and-health-policy/fact-sheet/health-coverage-of-immigrants/

90. Kessler, A. (2012). Addressing the consequences of domestic violence. *OT Practice, 17*(3), 6.

91. Kielhofner, G., & Barrett, L. (1998). Meaning and misunderstanding in occupational forms: A study of therapeutic goal setting. *American Journal of Occupational Therapy, 52*(5), 345–353.

92. Khan, S. (2020, August 12). *What does it mean to be trauma-informed?* American Psychiatric Association. Retrieved January 16, 2022, from https://smiadviser.org/knowledge_post/what-does-it-mean-to-be-trauma-informed

93. Knis-Matthews, L. (2003). A parenting program for women who are substance dependent. *Mental Health Special Interest Section Quarterly, 26*(1), 1–4.

94. Korb, K. L., Azok, A. D., & Leutenberg, E. A. (1989). *Life management skills: Reproducible activity handouts created for facilitators.* Wellness Reproductions.

95. Lawlor, M.C., & Mattingly, C.F. (1998). The complexities embedded in family-centered care. *American Journal of Occupational Therapy, 52*(4), 259–267.

96. Leslie, C. A. (2001). Psychiatric occupational therapy—Finding a place in the medical/surgical arena. *OT Practice, 6*(7), 10–14.

97. Lieb, L. C. (2019, October 22). *Occupational therapy, chronic pain, and lifestyle-based treatment.* American Occupational Therapy Association. https://www.aota.org/publications/ot-practice/ot-practice-issues/2019/chronic-pain-lfestyle

98. Lillie, M. D., & Armstrong, H. E. (1982). Contributions to the development of psychoeducational approaches to mental health service. *American Journal of Occupational Therapy, 36*(7), 438–443.

99. Lipsyte, R. (1998, August 30). Coping: The two ways of Dr Hu. *New York Times.* https://www.nytimes.com/1998/08/30/nyregion/coping-the-two-ways-of-dr-hu.html

100. Low, J. F. (1997). Religious orientation and pain management. *American Journal of Occupational Therapy, 51*(3), 215–219.

101. Luboshitzky, D., & Gaber, L. B. (2000). Collaborative therapeutic homework model in occupational therapy. *Occupational Therapy in Mental Health, 15*(1), 43–60.

102. Luedtke, T., Goldammer, K., & Fox, L. (2012). Overcoming communication barriers—Navigating client linguistic, literacy, and cultural differences. *OT Practice, 17*(4), 15–18.

103. Lyons, M., Orozovic, N., Davis, J., & Newman, J. (2002). Doing-being-becoming: Occupational experiences of persons with life-threatening illnesses. *American Journal of Occupational Therapy, 56*(3), 285–295.

104. Mann, D. P., Javaherian-Dysinger, H., & Hewitt, L. (2013). Ounce of prevention—Using the power of lifestyle to improve health outcomes. *OT Practice, 18*(7), 16–21.

105. Mariano, R. (2019). *The role of occupational therapy for survivors of human trafficking* [Doctoral project, University of St. Augustine for Health Sciences]. Scholarship and Open Access Repository @ USA: Student Capstone Projects Collection.

106. Mayor's Office of Immigrant Affairs. (2018, March). *State of our immigrant city: Annual report March 2018.* https://www1.nyc.gov/assets/immigrants/downloads/pdf/moia_annual_report_2018_final.pdf

107. McClintock, A. M. (2001). An OT's venture into wellness practice. *Mental Health Special Interest Section Quarterly, 24*(2), 1–3.

108. McCormack, G. (1988). Pain management by occupational therapists. *American Journal of Occupational Therapy, 42*(9), 577–581.

109. McElroy, A. (2012). Housing first meets harm reduction—Adapting existing social services models to help people with addictions. *OT Practice, 17*(15), 6–8.

110. McGruder, J. (1998). Culture and other forms of human diversity in occupational therapy. In M. E. Neistadt, & E. B. Crepeau (Eds.), *Willard and Spackman's occupational therapy* (9th ed., pp. 54–66). Lippincott Williams & Wilkins.

111. McKay, H., & Hanzaker, M. M. (2013). Dementia care communication: A toolbox for professionals and families. *OT Practice, 18*(3), CE1–CE8.

112. Menschner, C., & Maul, A. (2016, April). *Key ingredients for successful trauma-informed care implementation.* Center for Health Care Strategies, Inc. Retrieved January 16, 2022, from https://www.samhsa.gov/sites/default/files/programs_campaigns/childrens_mental_health/atc-whitepaper-040616.pdf

113. Mental Health Literacy. (n.d.). *Get literate.* Retrieved January 17, 2022, from https://mentalhealthliteracy.org/

114. Mental Health Literacy. (n.d.). *Language matters: The importance of using the right words when we're talking about mental health.* Retrieved January 17, 2022, from https://mentalhealthliteracy.org/schoolmhl/wp-content/uploads/2019/01/final-using-the-right-words.pdf

115. Mental Health Literacy. (n.d.). *What is stress? Mental health literacy resource.* Retrieved January 17, 2022, from https://mentalhealthliteracy.org/product/what-is-stress-mental-health-literacy-resource/

116. Mesa, A., Hoehn Anderson, K., Askey-Jones, S., Gray, R., & Silber, E. (2012). The mental health needs of individuals with multiple sclerosis: Implications for occupational therapy practice and research. *Mental Health Special Interest Section Quarterly, 35*(2), 1–4.

117. Miller, K. S., Bunch-Harrison, S., Brumbaugh, B., Sankaran Kutty, R., & FitzGerald, K. (2005). The meaning of computers to a group of men who are homeless. *American Journal of Occupational Therapy, 59*(2), 191–197.

118. Moll, S. E., Gewurtz, R. E., Krupa, T. M., & Law, M. C. (2013). Promoting an occupational perspective in public health. *Canadian Journal of Occupational Therapy, 80*(2), 11–119.

119. Morris, A. L., & Gainer, F. (1997). Helping the caregiver: Occupational therapy opportunities. *OT Practice, 2*(1), 36–40.

120. Mulcahey, M. J. (1992). Returning to school after a spinal cord injury: Perspectives from four adolescents. *American Journal of Occupational Therapy, 46*(4), 305–312.

121. Muñoz, J. P., Garcia, T., Lisak, J., & Reichenbach, D. (2006). Assessing the occupational performance priorities of people who are homeless. *Occupational Therapy in Health Care, 20*(3/4), 135–146.

122. Muriithi, B., & Muriithi, J.(2020). Occupational resilience: A new concept in occupational science. *American Journal of Occupational Therapy, 74*(4, Suppl. 1).7411505137p1.

123. Myers, C. (2020, July 1). *Population health: Implications for occupational therapists.* Elite Learning. Retrieved January 09, 2022, from https://www.elitelearning.com/resource-center/rehabilitation-therapy/population-health-implications-for-occupational-therapists/

124. National Council for Mental Wellbeing. (n.d.). *Fostering resilience and recovery: A change package: Advancing trauma-informed primary care.* Retrieved January 17, 2022, from https://www.thenationalcouncil.org/fostering-resilience-and-recovery-a-change-package/

125. National Human Trafficking Hotline. (n.d.). *Recognizing the signs.* Retrieved January 16, 2022, from https://humantraffickinghotline.org/human-trafficking/recognizing-signs

126. National Human Trafficking Hotline. (n.d.). *What is human trafficking?* Retrieved January 16, 2022, from https://humantraffickinghotline.org/

127. Nave, J., Helfrich, C. A., & Aviles, A. (2001). Child witnesses of domestic violence: A case study using the OT PAL. *Occupational Therapy in Mental Health, 16*(3–4), 127–135.

128. Neville-Jan, A., Bradley, M., Bunn, C., & Gehri, B. (1991). The model of human occupation and individuals with co-dependency problems. *Occupational Therapy in Mental Health, 11*(2–3), 73–97.

129. Oakley, F., Caswell, S., & Parks, R. (2008). Occupational therapist's role on U.S. Army and U.S. Public Health Service Commissioned Corps disaster mental health teams. *American Journal of Occupational Therapy, 62*(3), 361–364.

130. Olson, L. M. (2012). Self-determination and mental illness. *Mental Health Special Interest Section Quarterly, 35*(1), 1–4.

131. Oxer, S. S., & Miller, B. K. (2001). Effects of choice in an art occupation with adolescents living in residential treatment facilities. *Occupational Therapy in Mental Health, 17*(1), 39–49.

132. Padilla, R. (2001). Teaching approaches and occupational therapy psychoeducation. *Occupational Therapy in Mental Health, 17*(3–4). 81–95.

133. Parsons, H. (2018, October 8). *OT services for pain management included in the SUPPORT for Patients and Communities Act.* American Occupational Therapy Association. https://communot.aota.org/blogs/heather-parsons/2018/10/11/ot-services-for-pain-management-included-in-suppor

134. Penn State Harrisburg. (n.d.). *Guide to American culture and etiquette.* Retrieved January 8, 2022, from https://harrisburg.psu.edu/international-student-support-services/guide-american-culture-etiquette

135. Piersol, C. V., Earland, T. V., & Herge, E. A. (2012). Meeting the needs of caregivers of persons with dementia. *OT Practice, 17*(5), 8–12.

136. Pitts, D. B. (2004). Understanding the experience of recovery for persons labeled with psychiatric disabilities. *OT Practice, 9*(5), CE1–CE8.

137. *Population health vs. public health.* (n.d.). MPHonline. Retrieved January 9, 2022, from https://www.mphonline.org/population-health-vs-public-health/

138. Pratt, C. W., Gill, K. J., Barrett, N. M., & Roberts, M. (2006). *Psychiatric rehabilitation* (2nd ed.). Elsevier.

139. Pratt, C. W., Gill, K. J., Barrett, N. M., & Roberts, M. (2013). *Psychiatric rehabilitation* (3rd ed.). Elsevier.

140. Precin, P. (2015). *Living skills recovery workbook.* Echo Point Books and Media.

141. Pritchett, J. (1992, December 9). *Address given to the Mental Health Special Interest Group of the Metropolitan New York Occupational Therapy Association* [Presentation].

142. Rebeiro, K. L. (2002). Partnerships for participation in occupation. *Mental Health Special Interest Section Quarterly, 25*(3), 1–3.

143. Rebeiro, K. L., Day, D., Semeniuk, B., O'Brien, M., & Wilson, B. (2001). Northern initiative for social action: An occupation-based mental health program. *American Journal of Occupational Therapy, 55*(5), 493–500.

144. Robinson, K., Kennedy, N., & Harmon, D. (2011). Is occupational therapy adequately meeting the needs of people with chronic pain? *American Journal of Occupational Therapy, 65*(1), 106–113.

145. Rosario, C. (2016, April 25). *The difference between population health & public health.* https://www.adsc.com/blog/the-difference-between-population-health-public-health

146. Rosenfeld, M. S. (1984). Crisis intervention: The nuclear task approach. *American Journal of Occupational Therapy, 38*(6), 382–385.

147. Rowles, G. D. (1991). Beyond performance: Being in place as a component of occupational therapy. *American Journal of Occupational Therapy, 45*(3), 265–271.

148. Saha, S., Chauhan, A., Buch, B., Makwana, S., Vikar, S., Kotwani, P., & Pandya, A. (2020). Psychosocial rehabilitation of people living with mental illness: Lessons learned from community-based psychiatric rehabilitation centers in Gujarat. *Journal of Family Medicine and Primary Care, 9*(2), 892–897.

149. Sanford, M. (2006). *Waking: A memoir of trauma and transcendence.* Rodale.

150. Schindler, V. P., & Ferguson, S. (1995). An education program on acquired immunodeficiency syndrome for patients with mental illness. *American Journal of Occupational Therapy, 49*(4), 359–361.

151. Schultz-Krohn, W. (2004). The meaning of family routines in a homeless shelter. *American Journal of Occupational Therapy, 58*(5), 531–542.

152. Shahin, J. (2021). *Occupational therapy in youth violence: An occupation-based program for at-risk youth.* [Doctoral project, University of St. Augustine for Health Sciences]. Scholarship and Open Access Repository @ USA: Student Capstone Projects Collection.

153. Shaver, A., Abrahamian, A., Baskovich, K., Li, C., Russ, E., & Schultz-Krohn, W. (2019). Promoting financial literacy for homeless teens through a leisure-based OT program. *American Journal of Occupational Therapy, 73*(4, Suppl. 1). 7311520389p1.

154. Sipe, J. L. (2021). *The lived experience of homeless veterans* [Doctoral dissertation, University of the Sciences in Philadelphia]. Pepperdine Digital Commons. https://www.proquest.com/openview/2263621e8d16d4d7775ff-b4a55a46e60/1.pdf?pq-origsite=gscholar&cbl=18750&diss=y

155. Sladyk, K. (1992). Traumatic brain injury, behavioral disorder, and group treatment. *American Journal of Occupational Therapy, 46*(3), 267–269.

156. Sontag, D., & Dugger, C. W. (1998, July 19). The new immigrant tide: A shuttle between two worlds. *New York Times.* A1, A28–30. https://www.nytimes.com/1998/07/19/nyregion/the-new-immigrant-tide-a-shuttle-between-worlds.html

157. Statista. (2021, October 7). *Number of murder victims in the United States in 2020, by age.* Retrieved January 15, 2022, from https://www.statista.com/statistics/251878/murder-victims-in-the-us-by-age/

158. Steed, R. (2014). A client-centered model of instructional design for psychoeducation interventions in occupational therapy. *Occupational Therapy in Mental Health, 30*(2), 126–143.

159. Substance Abuse and Mental Health Services Administration. (2012). *Working definition of recovery: 10 guiding principles of recovery.* Retrieved January 17, 2022, from https://store.samhsa.gov/sites/default/files/d7/priv/pep12-recdef.pdf

160. Substance Abuse and Mental Health Services Administration. (2020, April 16). *Community mental health services block grant.* Retrieved January 09, 2022, from https://www.samhsa.gov/grants/block-grants/mhbg

161. Substance Abuse and Mental Health Services Administration. (2020, April 23). *Recovery and recovery support.* Retrieved January 17, 2022, from https://www.samhsa.gov/find-help/recovery

162. *Substance use-disorder prevention that promotes opioid recovery and treatment (SUPPORT) for patients and Communities Act.* Public Law No. 115-271. (2018). https://www.congress.gov/115/plaws/publ271/PLAW-115publ271.pdf

163. Swarbrick, M. (2009). Does supportive housing impact quality of life? *Occupational Therapy in Mental Health, 25*(3–4), 352–366.

164. Swarbrick, M. (2009). Historical perspective—From institution to community. *Occupational Therapy in Mental Health, 25*(3–4), 201–223.

165. Swarbrick, M. (2010). Occupation-focused community health and wellness programs. In M. K. Scheinholtz (Ed.), *Occupational therapy in mental health: Considerations for advanced practice* (pp. 27–43). AOTA Press.

166. Swarbrick, M., Bates, F., & Roberts, M. (2009). Peer Employment Support (PES): A model created through collaboration between a peer-operated service and university. *Occupational Therapy in Mental Health, 25*(3–4), 325–334.

167. Swarbrick, M., Roe, D., Yudof, J., & Zisman, Y. (2006). Participant perceptions of a peer wellness and recovery education program. *Occupational Therapy in Mental Health, 25*(3–4), 312–324.

168. Swarbrick, P. (1997). Wellness model for clients. *Mental Health Special Interest Section Quarterly, 20*(1), 1–4.

169. Swarbrick, P., & Duffy, M. (2000). Consumer-operated organization and programs: A role for occupational therapy practitioners. *Mental Health Special Interest Section Quarterly, 23*(1), 1–4.

170. Synovec, C. (2014). Utilizing the recovery model in occupational therapy practice. *Mental Health Special Interest Section Quarterly, 37*(3), 1–3.

171. Taylor, E., Jacobs, R., & Marsh, E. D. (2011). First year post-Katrina: Changes in occupational performance and emotional responses. *Occupational Therapy in Mental Health, 27*(1), 3–25.

172. Taylor, R. R. (2003). Extending client-centered practice: The use of participatory methods to empower clients. *Occupational Therapy in Mental Health, 19*(2), 57–75.

173. Taylor, R. R. (Ed.). (2017). *Kielhofner's model of human occupation* (5th ed.). Wolters Kluwer.

174. Thinnes, A., & Padilla, R. (2011). Effect of educational and supportive strategies on the ability of caregivers of people with dementia to maintain participation in that role. *American Journal of Occupational Therapy, 65*(5), 541–549.

175. Thomson, L. K., & Robnett, R. (2016). *Kohlman evaluation of living skills* (4th ed.). AOTA Press.

176. Tulane University: School of Public Health and Tropical Medicine. (2020, May 21). *Why community health is important for public health.* Retrieved January 09, 2022, from https://publichealth.tulane.edu/blog/why-community-health-is-important-for-public-health/

177. Tyminski, Q., Bates, M., & Fette, C. (2019). Building community capacity for mental health program development in underserved populations. *SIS Quarterly Practice Connections, 4*(1), 20–22.

178. UNESCO Institute for Statistics. (n.d.). *Functional literacy.* Retrieved January 17, 2022, from http://uis.unesco.org/en/glossary-term/functional-literacy

179. United States Census Bureau. (2019). *Selected social characteristics in the United States.* Retrieved January 08, 2021, from https://data.census.gov/cedsci/table?q=immigrant&tid=ACSDP1Y2019.DP02

180. United States Department of Health and Human Services. (2021, November 2). *What is cyberbullying.* Retrieved January 16, 2021, from https://www.stopbullying.gov/cyberbullying/what-is-it

181. United Stated Department of the Treasury. (2009, August 31). *Financial Literacy and Education Commission.* Office of Domestic Finance. https://web.archive.org/web/20090903055303/http://www.treas.gov/offices/domestic-finance/financial-institution/fin-education/commission/

182. USC Chan Division of Occupational Science and Occupational Therapy. (n.d.). *Lifestyle Redesign®.* Retrieved January 09, 2022, from https://chan.usc.edu/about-us/lifestyle-redesign

183. U.S. Financial Literacy and Education Commission. (n.d.). *Do you want to learn how to save, invest, and manage your money better?* Retrieved January 17, 2022, from https://web.archive.org/web/20090903075446/http://www.mymoney.gov/

184. Valparaiso University. (n.d.). *American culture & culture shock.* Retrieved January 8, 2022, from https://www.valpo.edu/international/living-in-valpo/u-s-culture/american-culture-culture-shock/

185. Vaughn, P. (2014). Chronic pain. In B. A. B. Schell, G. Gillen, & M. E. Scaffa (Eds.), *Willard and Spackman's occupational therapy* (12th ed., pp. 1135–1137). Lippincott Williams & Wilkins.

186. Waddell, G., Newton, M., Henderson, I., Somerville, D., & Main, C. J. (1993). A Fear-Avoidance Beliefs Questionnaire (FABQ) and the role of fear-avoidance beliefs in chronic low back pain and disability. *Pain, 52*(2), 157–168.

187. Waite, A. (2012). Helping the helpers—Caregiver training and occupational therapy. *OT Practice, 17*(5), 14–17.

188. Werner, J. (2012). Occupation and recovery: Identity, routines, and social support. *Mental Health Special Interest Section Quarterly, 35*(4), 1–3.

189. Wilcox, A. A. (1998). Reflections on doing, being, and becoming. *Canadian Journal of Occupational Therapy, 65*(5), 248–256.

190. Wisconsin Department of Health Services. (2020, August 31). *Mendota Mental Health Institute: Program of assertive community treatment.* https://www.dhs.wisconsin.gov/mmhi/pact.htm

191. Yuen, H. K. (1994). Neurofunctional approach to improve self-care skills in adults with brain damage. *Occupational Therapy in Mental Health, 12*(2), 31–45.

SUGGESTED RESOURCES

Caregivers

Customized Toolkits of Information and Practical Solutions (C-TIPS). https://smhs.gwu.edu/academics/health-sciences/research/research-initiatives/customized-toolkit-information-practical

Family Caregiver Alliance. (2012). *Alzheimer's disease and caregiving.* https://www.caregiver.org/alzheimers-disease-caregiving

McKay, H., & Hanzaker, M. M. (2013). Dementia care communication: A toolbox for professionals and families. *OT Practice, 18*(3), CE1–CE8.

National Alliance for Caregiving. *Guidebooks.* https://www.caregiving.org/guidebooks/

Piersol, C. V., Earland, T. V., & Herge, E. A. (2012). Meeting the needs of caregivers of persons with dementia. *OT Practice, 17*(5), 8–12.

Community-Based

Fazio, L. S. (2007). *Developing occupation-centered programs for the community: A workbook for students and professionals* (2nd ed.). Prentice Hall.

To Know Us Is to Like Us. https://www.facebook.com/knowuslikeus

Human Trafficking

National Human Trafficking Hotline. https://humantraffickinghotline.org/

Literacy

Agency for Healthcare Research and Quality. (2019). *Personal health literacy measurement tools (Revised).* https://www.ahrq.gov/health-literacy/research/tools/index.html

Always Use Teach-back! http://www.teachbacktraining.org/home

Centers for Disease Control and Prevention. *Health literacy: Find training.* https://www.cdc.gov/healthliteracy/gettraining.html

The role of OT in supporting literacy through the lifespan. https://www.youtube.com/watch?v=48E6n09N9oc

Medical Problems, Physical Disabilities, and Pain Management

American Occupational Therapy Association. *Pain management.* https://www.aota.org/practice/clinical-topics/pain-management

Fine, S. B. (1991). Resilience and human adaptability: Who rises above adversity? 1990 Eleanor Clarke Slagle Lecture. *American Journal of Occupational Therapy, 45*(6), 493–503.

Ikiugu, M. N. (2010). The new occupational therapy paradigm: Implications for integration of the psychosocial core of occupational therapy in all disciplines. *Occupational Therapy in Mental Health, 26*(4):343–353.

Mills, M. D., & Lehman, R. M. (2021). Exploring perspectives on illness and disability throughout the continuum of care: A case-based client centered approach. In M. E. Patnaude (Ed.), *Early's physical dysfunction practice skills for the occupational therapy assistant* (4th ed., pp. 14–26). Elsevier.

Neville-Jan, A. (2003). Encounters in a world of pain: An autoethnography. *American Journal of Occupational Therapy, 57*:88–98.

Robinson, K., Kennedy, N., & Harmon, D. (2011). Is occupational therapy adequately meeting the needs of people with chronic pain? *American Journal of Occupational Therapy, 65*(1), 106–113.

Personal Factors

American Occupational Therapy Association. *Diversity, equity, and inclusion word bank.* https://www.aota.org/practice/practice-essentials/dei/dei-toolkit-word-bank

Black, R. M. (2018). Culture, diversity, and culturally effective care. In B. A. B. Schell, & G. Gillen, (Eds.), *Willard and Spackman's occupational therapy* (13th ed., pp. 223–239). Wolters Kluwer.

Bonder, B., & Gurley, D. (2005). Culture and aging—Working with older adults from diverse backgrounds. *OT Practice, 4*(7), CE1–CE8.

DeVol, P. E., Payne, R. K. Dreussi Smith, T. (2014). *Bridges out of poverty* (5th ed). aha! Process.

Fadiman, A. (1998). *The spirit catches you and you fall down.* Farrar Straus & Giroux.

Luedtke, T., Goldammer, K., & Fox, L. (2012). Overcoming communication barriers—Navigating client linguistic, literacy, and cultural differences. *OT Practice, 17*(4),15–18.

Populations in Economic Distress

Helfrich, C. A., Chan, D. V., & Sabol, P. (2011). Cognitive predictors of life skill intervention outcomes for adults with mental illness at risk for homelessness. *American Journal of Occupational Therapy, 65*(3), 277–286.

McElroy, A. (2012). Housing first meets harm reduction—Adapting existing social services models to help people with addictions. *OT Practice, 17*(15), 6–8.

Muñoz, J. P., Garcia, T., Lisak, J., & Reichenbach, D. (2006). Assessing the occupational performance priorities of people who are homeless. *Occupational Therapy in Health Care, 20*(3/4), 135–146.

Schultz-Krohn, W. (2009). Working with homeless families. *OT Practice, 14*(5), 19–20.

Swarbrick, M. (2009). Does supportive housing impact quality of life? *Occupational Therapy in Mental Health, 25*(3–4), 352–366.

Psychiatric Rehabilitation and Psychoeducation

Gutman, S. A., Kerner, R., Zombek, I., Dulek, J., & Ramsey, C. A. (2009). Supported education for adults with psychiatric disabilities: Effectiveness of an occupational therapy program. *American Journal of Occupational Therapy, 63*(3), 245–254.

Luboshitzky, D., & Gaber, L. B. (2000). Collaborative therapeutic homework model in occupational therapy. *Occupational Therapy in Mental Health, 15*(1), 43–60.

Sarkhel, S., Singh, O. P., & Arora, M. (2020). Clinical practice guidelines for psychoeducation in psychiatric disorders general principles of psychoeducation. *Indian Journal of Psychiatry, 62*(8), 319–323.

Therapy Worksheets. https://therapyworksheets.blogspot.com/search/label/Workbooks

Torrey, E. F. (1997). *Out of the shadows: Confronting America's mental illness crisis.* Wiley.

Total Ability. *Free ebooks.* https://totalability.ca/free-ebooks/

Psychosocial Rehabilitation

Daily Living Skills Worksheets. http://dailylivingskills.com/

Swarbrick, P., & Duffy, M. (2002). Consumer-operated organization and programs: A role for occupational therapy practitioners. *Mental Health Special Interest Section Quarterly, 23*(1), 1–4.

Public Health

Minnesota Department of Health. *Resource library for advancing health equity in public health.* https://www.health.state.mn.us/communities/practice/resources/equitylibrary/index.html#all

Recovery

Clay, P. (2013). Shared principles: The recovery model and occupational therapy. *Mental Health Special Interest Section Quarterly, 36*(4), 1–3.

Expressive Therapist. (n.d.). http://www.expressivetherapist.com/group-activities.html?fbclid=IwAR1NnyZw3hKNV5x8_sEphSqtfaLgb0jO6myr1xFgAyKroyGjAEr1GhfyvGM

IROC Wellbeing. *Mental health recovery—Evidence-based recovery tools.* https://irocwellbeing.com/?fbclid=IwAR3HrNOT9tBqMRSjeLTdhQURLfS0_HRYQF0yep0isAIY9KFNlOQYt1X6N8g

NHS Foundation Trust. *Mental health self help guides.* https://web.ntw.nhs.uk/selfhelp/

Pitts, D. B. (2004). Understanding the experience of recovery for persons labeled with psychiatric disabilities. *OT Practice, 9,* CE1–CE8.

Recovery Assessment Scale: Domains and Stages (RAS-DS). https://ses.library.usyd.edu.au/handle/2123/9317

Rethink Mental Illness. https://www.rethink.org/

Rethink Mental Illness. *100 ways to support recovery.* https://www.rethink.org/advice-and-information/living-with-mental-illness/treatment-and-support/100-ways-to-support-recovery/

Substance Abuse and Mental Health Services Administration. *Motivational interviewing: An effective technique in recovery support.* https://www.samhsa.gov/homelessness-programs-resources/hpr-resources/motivational-interviewing-recovery

Substance Abuse and Mental Health Services Administration. *Staying connected is important: Virtual recovery resources.* https://www.samhsa.gov/sites/default/files/virtual-recovery-resources.pdf

Synovec, C. (2014). Utilizing the recovery model in occupational therapy practice. *Mental Health Special Interest Section Quarterly, 37*(3), 1–3.

Werner, J. (2012). Occupation and recovery: Identity, routines, and social support. *Mental Health Special Interest Section Quarterly, 35*(4), 1–3.

Wollenberg, J. L. (2001). Recovery and occupational therapy in the community mental health setting. *Occupational Therapy in Mental Health, 17*(3–4), 97–114.

Violence and Trauma Issues

Basile, K. C., Clayton, H. B., DeGue, S., Gilford, J. W., Vagi, K. J., Suarez, N. A., Zwald, M. L., & Lowry, R. (2020, August 21). Interpersonal violence victimization among high school students—Youth risk behavior survey, United States, 2019. *Morbidity and Mortality Weekly Report, 69*(1), 28–37.

Beacon House. *Resources. Developmental trauma.* https://beaconhouse.org.uk/resources/?fbclid=IwAR2GG6VHQgXcqxUbXZAtHMUFHuvwGfTfYdUJQ-sBGii1CNkEpCRZtVHchok

Bent, M. A. (2003, September 22). An occupational-based approach to crisis debriefing. *OT Practice, 8,* 13–17.

Champagne, T. (2012). Creating occupational therapy groups for children and youth in community-based mental health practice. *OT Practice, 17*(14), 13–18.

HelpGuide.org. *Emotional and psychological trauma.* https://www.helpguide.org/articles/ptsd-trauma/coping-with-emotional-and-psychological-trauma.htm

Humbert, T. K., Engleman, K., & Miller, C. E. (2014). Exploring women's expectations of recovery from intimate partner violence: A phenomenological study. *Occupational Therapy in Mental Health, 30*(4), 358–380.

Kimberg, I. (2003). The downtown therapists' assistance project. *Occupational Therapy in Mental Health, 19*(3–4), 125–127.

National Domestic Violence Hotline. *800-799-SAFE (800-799-7233) or TTY 1-800-787-3224.* http://www.thehotline.org

Sanford, M. (2006). *Waking: A memoir of trauma and transcendence.* Rodale.

Substance Abuse and Mental Health Services Administration. (2017). *Tips for health care practitioners and responders: Helping survivors cope with grief after a disaster or traumatic event.* https://store.samhsa.gov/product/Tips-for-Health-Care-Practitioners-and-Responders-/SMA17-5036

Wellness

Alberta Family Wellness Initiative. *The resilience scale: A tool for change.* https://www.albertafamilywellness.org/

Center for Workplace Mental Health. https://www.workplacementalhealth.org/?DID=70

Center on Integrated Health Care and Self-Directed Recover. *Nutrition and exercise for wellness and recovery.* https://www.center4healthandsdc.org/new-r.html?fbclid=IwAR1aK1I5fqHiC6wgdugzXq_1hSYb6ZidYzbRBrszTjyB_wj6R33ZXsKQgGg

Centers for Disease Control and Prevention. *Tools and resources.* https://www.cdc.gov/mentalhealth/tools-resources/index.htm

Crisis Prevention Institute. (2021, February 24). *How to avoid power struggles.* https://www.crisisprevention.com/Blog/How-to-Avoid-Power-Struggles

World Health Organization. (2020, April 29). *Doing what matters in times of stress.* https://www.who.int/publications/i/item/9789240003927

Service Areas, Environments, and Focuses

OT HACKS OVERVIEW

O: Occupation as a means and an end

Occupations used in different practice settings are aligned with the focus of that setting and the physical space of that setting. Occupations can be used to improve performance skills so that the person can return to the community. Occupations are the typical interventions used in community settings. Finally, when long-term living is done within a facility (institutional living), meaningful occupations become what the client identifies as their day-to-day activities within the institution.

T: Theoretical concepts, values, and principles, or historical foundations

Theoretical concepts from occupational therapy include the impact the environment has on one's occupations. Thus, the environment of the practice setting impacts the client, the occupational therapy professional, and the occupational therapy services provided.

H: How can we Help? OT's role in serving clients with mental illness or mental health needs

How is the role of occupational therapy professional depicted in various settings?

A: Adaptations

Adaptations are done for daily life occupations, while managing symptoms of a mental disorder, and the focus of intervention varies based on the practice setting.

C: Case study includes

Not applicable for this chapter.

K: Knowledge: keeping mental health OT practice grounded in evidence, in occupational science, and in research

Not applicable for this chapter.

S: Some terms that may be new to you

care
care recipient
chronosystem
consumer
environmental constraints
environmental demands
environmental impact
Epidemiology
exosystem
forensic care
health determinants
macrosystem
mesosystem
microsystem
psychiatric survivor
service
social determinants of health
Welfare of a population

INTRODUCTION

Occupational therapy professionals work with people diagnosed with mental disorders in numerous settings, each with its own mission, intervention philosophy, funding pattern, and population. Some settings, such as the locked unit, are highly restrictive, aiming to reduce the risk of harm to the client, other clients, and staff. Although such units still exist, the standard today is that persons with mental disorders receive services in the least restrictive environment, such as community housing and community mental health centers (CMHCs). Individuals whose first diagnosis is other than psychiatric and who experience psychosocial problems receive services in still other settings. Each setting or environment influences the behavior of its occupants, be they consumers of mental health services or the professionals that provide these services. The roles of occupational therapy professionals and the ranges of services provided vary accordingly.

THE SCOPE OF WHERE OCCUPATIONAL THERAPY SERVICES ARE PROVIDED

A Picture of Those Who Participate With Occupational Therapy

As discussed in Chapter 4, mental health problems range from transient situational disturbances to severe and persistent disorders. For mild depression and anxiety brought on by life circumstances, people typically seek help from their family physicians in the primary care setting and may be referred to treatment with a psychiatrist, psychologist, or professional counselor. People with mild problems are rarely seen by occupational therapy professionals, except in cases of sustained difficulty in carrying out daily life activities; even then, verbal consultation with another mental health professional may be the only occupational therapy provided. Most mild mental health problems resolve themselves satisfactorily as the person learns to cope or when life circumstances change. Depending on the funding and programs available in a local area, some occupational therapy services may be available to people with mild mental health problems through CMHCs, home health services, and prevention programs.

People with more serious and persistent mental disorders do not always seek treatment and may resist it; in many states, they cannot be forced to accept treatment unless they are a danger to themselves or to others. Because public psychiatric beds have been in short supply since deinstitutionalization in 1963 and because some people with serious mental disorders may create a public nuisance, they may be taken by the police to the local jail or may be sentenced to long prison terms. Approximately one in seven state and federal prisoners have reported experiences that meet the threshold for serious psychological distress (50). Children with mental disorders, particularly males, are especially likely to be housed in the prison system. It is estimated that as many as 90% of children and youth in the criminal justice system in the United States have at least one mental health diagnosis (14). In general, psychiatric services in prison settings are minimal; inmates may experience physical and sexual abuse and receive only limited psychiatric care. Only a handful of occupational therapy professionals work in such settings, although interesting program ideas have been and continue to be reported (19, 43, 45, 47, 52).

Persons with severe mental disorders may be hospitalized or referred to an outpatient department, day hospital, partial hospitalization program, or CMHC where occupational therapy personnel work with them as part of a team of professionals. Some of the people seen in these settings, such as victims or survivors of abuse, children with mental disorders, persons without permanent housing, and the frail elderly, must cope with social and economic problems as well as mental disorders. Persons with substance use–related disorders, persons with personality disorders and eating disorders, and persons with mild intellectual disorders may also be seen.

Occupational therapy professionals who work in psychiatric hospitals and mental health community settings most often provide services to persons with severely disabling psychiatric disorders (eg, schizophrenia, bipolar disorder). Serious mental health problems are often first recognized when the person becomes so symptomatic or disorganized as to require hospitalization or, in the case of substance-related disorder, admission for detoxification. Often, but not always, this initial hospitalization is the first of many.

Schizophrenia and bipolar disorder (see Chapter 4) may be severe and progressive, with an expectation the client will have decreased ability to function in the community and, in some cases, there is a lifelong association with the mental health system. Increasingly, professionals have come to understand that many persons with these serious mental disorders are interested in and capable of engaging in a program of recovery. Advances in medication and improved understanding of effective interventions and supports have made it possible for many to function well enough to attend school and hold jobs.

Many labels (*patient*, *client*, *consumer*, *inmate*, *resident*, *care recipient*, and *psychiatric survivor*) are applied to the people served in mental health programs. What do these terms mean, and which ones are appropriate in which situations? Box 7.1 gives terms in use at this writing. Terms

---

BOX 7.1 The Person Who Receives Mental Health Services: What's in a Name?

patient Suggests a dependent relationship to professional staff; services are compulsory, done for safety, or the person is part of the criminal system.[a]

care recipient Someone who is receiving support or assistance from another person.[a]

client A person who is an active participant in the therapeutic process.[b]

consumer Someone who has experienced a mental disorder, has received, is receiving, or is seeking treatment and support.[a]

inmate A person confined in a correctional facility.[c]

resident A person who lives somewhere permanently and for the long term.[d]

psychiatric survivor Individuals who are out of the health care system and feel a sense of survival regarding the system.[e]

Definitions taken from the following:

[a]Victoria State Government Health and Human Services. (2019, June). *Mental health lived experience engagement framework.* https://www.health.vic.gov.au/publications/mental-health-lived-experience-engagement-framework

[b]American Occupational Therapy Association. (2020). Occupational therapy practice framework: Domain and Process—Fourth edition. *American Journal of Occupational Therapy, 74*(Suppl. 2), 1–87.

[c]Merriam-Webster. (n.d.). *Inmate.* Retrieved January 23, 2022, from https://www.merriam-webster.com/dictionary/inmate

[d]Google Dictionary. (n.d.). *Resident.* Retrieved January 23, 2022, from https://www.google.com/search?channel=cus5&client=firefox-b-1-d&q=resident

[e]Camhpra. (n.d.). *Mental health consumer movement 101: The story of a social change movement.* Retrieved January 23, 2022, from https://camhpro.files.wordpress.com/2016/03/outreach-materials-mh-movement.pdf

change with time and customs. Stigma is attached to labels of any kind; the effective and compassionate practitioner is alert and attuned to the preferences and sensitivities of the recipient of services, regardless of the setting.

Social Determinants of Health and Epidemiology Factors

Before looking at the places where occupational therapy professionals work, it is important to look at "why" they work there. In this respect, we will review the concepts of social determinants of health and epidemiology in relation to public health and welfare of populations. This review will be done through the lens of mental health and mental disorders.

There are numerous **social determinants of health**. Compton and Shim identify the following as social determinants of health (15, p. 421):

- racial discrimination and social exclusion;
- adverse early life experiences;
- poor education;
- unemployment, underemployment, and job insecurity;
- poverty, income inequality, and neighborhood deprivation;
- poor access to sufficient healthy food;
- poor housing quality and housing instability;
- adverse features of the built environment; and
- poor access to health care.

Other issues that impact social health include limited or inadequate community mobility; living in situations of violence; incarceration of segments of a population and limited relations with local law enforcement personnel; natural environmental pollution; poor outlook for climate sustainability; discrimination based on biologic sex, gender, age, religion, and other non–race-based discrimination; and negative and unsupportive work environments (15).

Healthy People 2030 identifies five social determinants of health (49). They are:

- economic stability,
- education access and quality,
- health care access and quantity,
- neighborhood and built environment, and
- social and community context.

Figure 7.1 is a picture of these social determinants of health from *Healthy People 2030* (49). Social determinants of health are tracked by their International Classification of Diseases (ICD)-10-CM codes, which are the *Z codes* that identify reasons for encounters in the health care system. These codes allow for identification of social determinants or socially related reasons for health-related problems. They include problems related to, for instance, education, literacy, employment, occupational exposures, housing, social environment, family circumstances for minors, health care, and various psychosocial circumstances. By tracking this information, health care organizations can create strategies to specifically target social needs of the populations they serve (1, 12, 22).

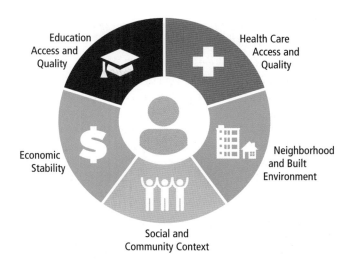

Figure 7.1. Social Determinants of Health. (U.S. Department of Health and Human Services. (n.d.). *Social determinants of health*. Retrieved January 26, 2022, from https://health.gov/healthypeople/objectives-and-data/social-determinants-health)

Epidemiology is the study of what happens to a population. This includes focusing on how health-related events and situations are distributed in a population, as well as the health determinants found in a population. This information is then used to control health problems within that population (9–11). Health determinants include social determinants, as well as a person's individual traits and actions (54).

As identified in Chapter 6, public health encompasses health promotion and protection for "all people" (41). Protection can be framed as a preventative measure, thus protecting the population from a future deficit. Beyond our consideration for public health issues is our consideration toward the welfare of populations. This involves the impact of various health factors and environmental factors. These factors impact not only individuals but also populations. A population's welfare is impacted when individuals within that population are affected by health and environmental concerns (36).

The use of social determinants of health and epidemiology factors within mental health occupational therapy follows a systematic process. The flow chart in Figure 7.2 explains this process.

Environmental Factors and Personal Factors Associated With Occupational Therapy Service Provision

The relationship between the organism and its environment fascinates scholars in the life sciences and social sciences. Basic questions of evolution and development and health and disease may be answered in part by environmental influences. What is the effect of the environment on the human engaged in occupation?

Concepts From Occupational Therapy

The model of human occupation (MOHO) and other occupational therapy practice models propose that all human

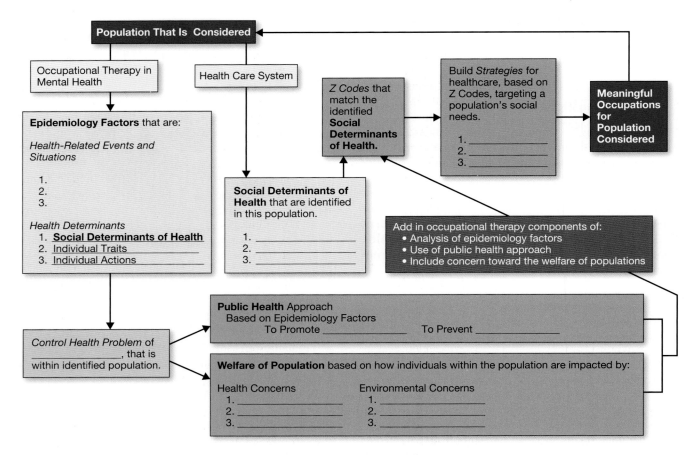

Figure 7.2. Systematic Process for Use of Social Determinants of Health and Epidemiology Factors.

activity arises from the human being's basic urge to explore and master the environment. Contexts of intervention and service are different from the natural and human-made environments in which most people spend their time and hence have different effects on the occupations of the people who inhabit them. Before we discuss these effects, it is important to review some of the basic concepts of person–environment interaction from occupational therapy models.

All occupational performance and occupational participation occur in the context of environment. The person intends to act within the environment. In general, the more complexity and novelty in the environment, the greater the person's urge to explore it. However, if there are too many new, different, and complicated things in the environment, the person may feel overwhelmed and become unable to act purposefully.

The occupational therapy practice framework: domain and process—fourth edition (OTPF-4) identifies different environmental factors. They include natural environment; human-made changes to the environment; products and technology; support and relationships; attitudes; and services, systems, and policies (4). Environmental factors "are the aspects of the physical, social, and attitudinal surroundings in which people live and conduct their lives" (4, p. 36). The person–environment–occupation model (PEO; see

Chapter 3) similarly views the environment as a context in which occupational performance happens.

The MOHO recognizes that the environment places **demands** and **constraints** on the individual. **Demands** elicit behaviors by asking the person to act, as, for example, the sight of bread and other ingredients might provoke a person to begin making a sandwich. **Constraints** limit behavior, by sending a message that certain actions are permitted, and others are not. Kielhofner uses the example of a security line at an airport (46). The MOHO also recognizes that because of individual differences, not everyone reacts in the same way to a given environment. **Environmental impact**, in the MOHO, "refers to the opportunity, support, demand, and constraint that the environment has on a particular individual" (46, pp. 97–98).

Consistent with Eastern traditions such as Zen Buddhism, the Kawa model sees the person as inseparable from the environment. It is not so much that the person acts within or on the environment, but rather that the person and the environment act together (21, 48). Harmony and balance are achieved when the person acts in a manner consistent with and respectful of the environment.

Let us consider health care environments and their effects on occupational performance. Inpatient and residential settings seem remarkably dull compared with typical home, work, and leisure settings. The space typically has fewer interesting objects in it; because of safety precautions, the setting may seem bare. Curtains, carpets, and stuffed furniture may be absent, which creates an atmosphere more like an airport lounge than like a living room, kitchen, or bedroom inside of a home. Clients or residents may be prohibited from placing decorations on the walls. The lighting is likely to come from fluorescent ceiling fixtures rather than incandescent floor and table lamps. Overall, the space may feel barren, sterile, and somewhat depressing—even to staff members.

Although there are usually a lot of people around, many of these are staff. It is clear to everyone that the staff intends to perform almost all the necessary tasks in the setting, including preparing and serving meals, caring for laundry and housekeeping, and preparing and cleaning up after activities. Clients or residents may be involved to a limited extent in any or all these tasks, but usually under the supervision of staff.

The environmental characteristics of inpatient settings communicate an expectation that clients need to do very little and that they probably will not be able to do even that very well. Many outpatient settings also fail to communicate an expectation that the client can perform anything like a typical level of ability.

To help the person with a mental disorder develop and maintain the skills and behaviors needed to function independently, the occupational therapy professional may alter some features of the environment. Furniture can be rearranged, folding screens placed to eliminate distractions, and walls painted or wall coverings added to the extent permitted. Clients should participate in these decisions and do the work when practical. The occupational therapy professional can control the effect of social participation by modifying the role of group leader and the roles of volunteers and students in groups. The less the staff does, the more clients will do themselves. Making tasks available to clients often requires working with administrators to change policies; there is no reason clients should not be allowed or required to do their own laundry, but administrators may feel that this would be inconvenient or inefficient or interfere with routine.

Seeing clients in their homes presents different opportunities to apply environmental concepts. A person's home or any environment (eg, office) that they create for themselves communicates their interests and habits. The objects present, the care given to different rooms or parts of rooms, the age of the furnishings, and the amount of use they seem to have received all indicate their relative importance to the individual. For example, Levine (24) describes a home in which the furniture in all the rooms, but the kitchen, was 40 years old and quite worn, but the kitchen was freshly painted and had new appliances. Levine inferred that the kitchen was the center of the family's activities.

Usually, a person has more control of the environment at home than in a hospital or long-term care facility; this increases the sense of personal causation. The occupational therapy professional is the guest and relinquishes control naturally to the client, supporting the person's motivation to control and master the environment.

Another situation that may call for a different application of environmental concepts occurs when the client travels with the occupational therapy professional out into the community.

Observing how the person reacts to the different stimulation presented by stores, bus stops, and public agencies may reveal skills the client has or does not have. This information may help the occupational therapy professional identify what kinds of environmental changes will facilitate independent occupational participation.

In summary, demands and opportunities in the environment have a profound effect on human occupational participation. Inpatient units and many outpatient programs convey only limited expectations for clients to participate and to be competent in daily life tasks and occupational roles; occupational therapy professionals may increase performance expectations for persons with mental disorders by selectively altering features of the environment. Working with clients in their homes or in various community environments may provide information about which environmental features best facilitate independent functioning for a particular person.

Many Roles for Those Who Participate With Occupational Therapy Services

Considering the many environments through which clients move, it is not surprising that they acquire strategies and roles particular to each. For example, in an in-patient setting, the person is often referred to as a 'patient' and is expected to be dependent and compliant, to accept a schedule set by others, to take medications, and to perform tasks such as personal hygiene and grooming on demand. The person may use coping strategies such as isolation, triangulation (pitting staff members against each other), and overcompliance to maintain a sense of self-direction within a controlling environment.

Once discharged to home, the same person as "family member" is expected to be the spouse, child, sibling, or parent, with all the history and attendant feelings, modified somewhat by an expectation that the person is not quite well. Many behaviors that appear dysfunctional, such as getting a spouse to make excuses for the nonperformance of the sick person to reduce demands by others, may instead be survival strategies.

As an "inmate" in a correctional facility, the same person might be expected to stand at attention for guards, to respond quickly and accurately to directives from persons in authority, and to accede to the bullying of more powerful inmates; in addition, the person must maintain an attitude of alertness and vigilance to avoid victimization. The prisoner with a mental disorder may forge alliances with stronger inmates, curry favor with guards, or submit to sexual abuse to avoid painful experiences.

The person experiencing homelessness on the street or in a shelter exposes themselves to the risk of violence (including sexual assault), disease (such as hepatitis or a sexually transmitted infection), theft, malnutrition, or hypothermia.

Survival strategies include wearing multiple layers of clothing (to stay warm, to guard one's belongings, and to prevent sexual assault), carrying weapons, eating from bulk trash containers and trash barrels, and sleeping in storm sewers.

These are only a few of the environments in which clients live and survive. The roles and strategies they adopt are specialized to these environments. Because cognitive deficits often accompany severe and persistent mental disorders, clients may not recognize which behaviors or roles pertain to a particular environment or may have difficulty responding to unfamiliar environmental demands, such as may occur in a progressive treatment environment (eg, demands to set their own goals, to dress and behave in ways that are closer to the social norm). As rehabilitation specialists, we must be sensitive to the occupational histories of our clients and appreciate their considerable skills and life experience. When we engage them in intervention and ask them to function in community programs and housing, we are at the same time asking them to abandon roles that have served them well. Listening carefully to the person's experiences and dreams should be the starting point for setting small mutual goals toward greater community integration.

Promoting Change at Many Environmental System Levels

Bronfenbrenner's Bioecological Model, as presented by Rigby et al (39), has five environmental systems. The person is continually receiving input from the levels of the environmental systems (strongest input coming from level closest to the person) and simultaneously producing behaviors and actions that are received by the environment (again, the person most strongly influences the level closest to them). The system levels are as follows:

- Microsystem. Includes the person's interactions with the entities nearest to the person and thus provides the most influence toward the person. Examples include family, home, educational facility, religious facility, and neighborhood.
- Mesosystem. In this system are the interactions between the various entities that are a part of the person's microsystem. Examples include family members' interactions with the person's teachers or people within the neighborhood interacting with the local clergy.
- Exosystem. This system involves entities that happen beyond the person, yet involve other persons or entities that impact the individual. Examples include a family member's interactions (based on role and assigned tasks) at work, the health care services offered in the person's community, and government policies that identify the criteria for funding various health care and social services initiatives.
- Macrosystem. This includes the cultural identification, cultural attitudes, values, and social conditions of the cultural group the person resides within. Examples are Western culture, Latin American culture, Western

European culture, and Eastern culture. A person's culture helps to shape and form their identity. Because culture involves generations of people, the macrosystem exists across a continuum of time.
- Chronosystem. This includes all the environmental influences and activities that occur over time, impacting the person's roles and occupations throughout their life span. Consider how the dominant culture the person lives in influences government policies and laws, which in turn impacts the roles of the person's family members and neighbors, and then finally the direct impact on the person, influencing how the person changes and develops.

Figure 7.3 demonstrates the intermeshed nature of these five environmental system levels. Notice how the first four levels are interconnected, meaning they influence and depend on each other. This interconnectedness means what is happening in one level is based on and includes what is happening on all levels that come before it, or that are closer to the person. Appreciation for and the ability to act within all five levels are essential for occupational therapy professionals. Table 7.1 gives examples of occupational therapy service provision throughout the levels that surround the person.

Focus of Occupational Therapy Services

It is helpful to see "where" occupational therapy is offered based on the purpose of the facility and the services offered. As the title of this chapter indicates, the information presented here is about environments, areas, and focuses. It is difficult to pin down an exact term for what we offer and where we offer it.

A term not used in the title of this chapter, but just as applicable and important, is **practice setting**. Practice setting can imply an identification of occupational therapy services based on the specific criteria.

- General age of the clients seen in that setting (pediatrics, geriatrics)
- One diagnosis/condition, or a similar group of diagnoses/conditions, which most or all the clients in the setting have (work hardening, day treatment for those with mental disorders, neuro-rehabilitation)
- What else is going on at the facility (general hospital, school system, long-term acute care)

Terminology describing our profession, who we work with, where we work, and even what we do, changes over time and differs depending on cultural, societal, and political systems of a particular country or geographic region. Before we specifically address places where mental health, or psychiatric, occupational therapy is provided, it is important to provide a review of typical and often heard terms regarding what we provide.

Treatment is generally considered to refer to medical care for disease, injury, or other medically treatable condition. Treatment generally is thought of as something "done to" a client, or "given to" a client. On the client's part it is a passive acceptance of the service provided. This term does

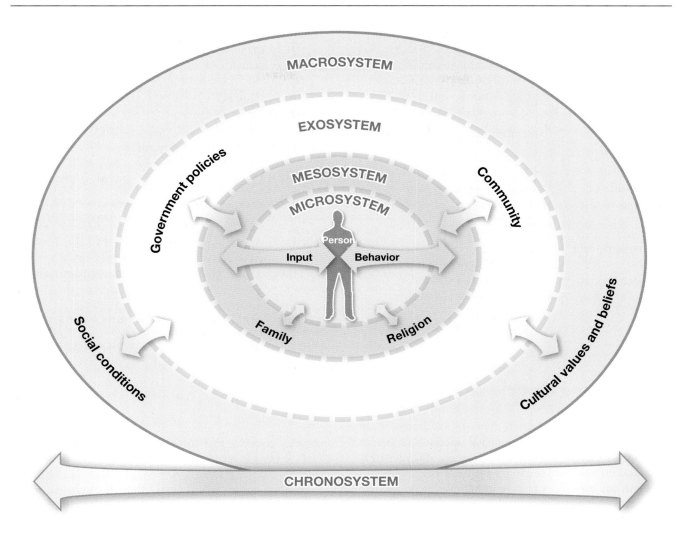

Figure 7.3. Five Environmental System Levels. (Reprinted with permission from Rigby, P. J., Trentham, B., & Letts, L. (2018). Modifying performance contexts. In B. A. B. Schell & G. Gillen (Eds.), *Willard and Spackman's occupational therapy* (13th ed., pp. 460–479). Wolters Kluwer.)

not accurately describe services given in community settings and those that are related to housing, employment, or engagement in occupation. It does make sense when the person is ill and is receiving services designed to heal.

Intervention is a broad term. In mental health or psychiatric settings, it can describe actions taken on behalf of another and has come to suggest the prevention of undesirable outcomes (such as in substance use intervention by a family). The term *intervention* also includes many of the services occupational therapy professionals provide and involves participation by the client in the intervention action. It is about the client "doing" with the service provided, versus passively accepting the provision of services offered.

Service refers to what is provided. This term suggests that the person receiving the service has some control over what is being provided. Service is a useful term to describe the interactions that clients and professionals mutually decide will be beneficial for the client. Clients may decide to refer to themselves as service users.

Care is a term that suggests "tending to" or "supervising" someone, as in childcare and eldercare. The implication is that the person needs the ministrations and supervision of one or more other persons. This term makes sense when applied to settings serving those with advanced neurocognitive disorders, severe intellectual disabilities, and similarly disabling conditions.

FACILITIES BASED ON PAYMENT

Facilities can be funded by public monies, private corporations, or through the Veterans Administration. Services provided vary by type, environment, and intensity.

Large State or County Hospitals and Other Public Facilities

Public institutions include federal, municipal, state, and county hospitals. Funding comes from local, state, and federal governments. Most such facilities have inpatient and

Table 7.1. Focus and Examples of Occupational Therapy at Five System Levels of the Environment

Level of Intervention	Focus	Examples Seen in Occupational Therapy
Microsystem	Client	Teach compensatory techniques for use in the home or educational setting. Early intervention for children under 5 yr old
Mesosystem	Members of microsystem	Educate and train caregiver, peer, teacher, or significant other. Work with client and client's friend at local playground. Assist with neighborhood fundraiser for client.
Exosystem	Entities outside the mesosystem that influence the microsystem and mesosystem	Caregiver support so they can seek assistance under the Family Medical Leave Act Occupational therapy services being offered in local area. Advocacy by occupational therapy professional for local, state, or federal health care coverage.
Macroenvironment	Cultural and societal influences	Infusing societal and cultural expectations of daily weekday school attendance into an afterschool program that is offered. Consideration toward timing for afterschool extracurricular activities, evening activities at home, and weekday school schedules.
Chronosystem	Environment and change across the life span	Treatment planning with an adolescent and including an adverse childhood experience as well as their hopes and dreams for future intimate relationships and raising a family of their own Completing an occupational history with an older client and concentrating on how they view their current capabilities and achieving self-actualization or generativity

Information adapted from Rigby, P. J., Trentham, B., & Letts, L. (2018). Modifying performance contexts. In B. A. B. Schell & G. Gillen (Eds.), *Willard and Spackman's occupational therapy* (13th ed., pp. 460–479). Wolters Kluwer.

outpatient services, and many have specialized forensic (criminal) units, alcohol and substance use disorder treatment, and for specific age ranges such as older adults, children, and adolescents. A few are in urban centers. Most are very large, consisting of several buildings on a sprawling campus, often in rural areas. Inconvenient locations may make it difficult for family members to visit.

The deinstitutionalization of psychiatric clients, compelled by the *Community Mental Health Act of 1963* (PL 88–164), resulted in the discharge of many persons who previously lived in locked facilities such as large state psychiatric hospitals. The original mission of deinstitutionalization (to liberate people from confinement and enable them to integrate into community housing and employment) has not been realized; many of those discharged or not hospitalized today are found in correctional facilities, in shelters for the homeless, or on the street. An estimated 52.9 million U.S. residents have mental disorders, emotional disorders, or behavioral disorders (28). In 2016 there were just over 37,500 inpatient psychiatric beds available in the United States, which is about 11.5% fewer psychiatric beds than were available in the United States in 2010 (31).

At this time, the inpatient population of public psychiatric centers consists of three main categories: those who are too violent or suicidal to be released, those who have intact families or social support systems but who are so severely impaired and disorganized that they cannot live in the community even with this support, and those who find it difficult to integrate into individual living places and have shown repeated hospitalizations. Political pressure and limitations on

insurance coverage may force premature discharge of these clients, leading to repeated readmission and a revolving-door pattern.

Yet another group of clients, although competent to remain for long periods in the community, may be admitted for occasional brief hospitalization, often precipitated by stressful life events.

Public hospitals receive admissions on a geographical location; the person is admitted to the state, county, or municipal hospital within their place of residence. Large public institutions can be understaffed, not only in occupational therapy and other activity programs but also in medical and nursing services. Funding is erratic and hiring freezes and supply shortages are common. Cyclical fluctuations in budget and staff follow election of liberal or conservative politicians.

Despite these drawbacks, such facilities provide many opportunities and challenges for occupational therapy professionals. Clients with a variety of diagnoses are seen and the possibilities for working with individuals of different ages and severity of disorder are challenging. Also, because clients tend to remain for long periods or are frequently readmitted, occupational therapy professionals can develop long-term therapeutic relationships, can observe the progression of the disorder, can participate in the person's recovery process, and can watch the effect of intervention over time.

Occupational therapy professionals focus on rehabilitation with the aim of independent living; appropriate practice models for these settings and populations include the MOHO and the psychiatric rehabilitation (PsyR) model

(16, 35). Because of the emphasis on returning persons with serious mental disorders to community living wherever possible, occupational therapy for inpatient settings emphasizes assessment of and training in occupational life skills. Ideally, as a component of transition away from the inpatient setting, the client is directed to a CMHC or satellite hospital clinic to obtain continuing services.

Proprietary Hospitals

Proprietary hospitals are private hospitals run for profit; because of their profit orientation, these hospitals may exclude those who do not belong to their sponsoring insurance group or who do not have private insurance and adequate funds. Because most of these inpatient stays are paid for through insurance coverage, the stays are short, somewhere between 1 and 4 weeks. Often, only the private clients of doctors on staff are admitted; sometimes these doctors are themselves part owners of the hospital. The team approach, as described in "Acute Care Inpatient Units" section in this chapter, is less often used in proprietary hospitals; instead, the individual physicians write orders for their own clients, which they intend other staff to carry out. Clients may be treated with a combination of psychotropic medication, electroconvulsive therapy, and various verbal therapies. Physicians' attitudes toward occupational therapy vary from indifferent to enthusiastic. Departments may provide a range of diversional and therapeutic activities, including discussion groups, games, sports, gardening, task groups, and leisure and socialization experiences. Work-oriented and rehabilitative services may be included if the physicians understand and endorse this approach.

Veterans Administration Hospitals and Services

The *U.S. Department of Veterans Affairs* (*VA*) offers mental health services to veterans and their family members (51). Settings include residential programs, inpatient hospitalization, outpatient care, and specialized services for specific problems such as substance use, services for those without permanent housing, suicide prevention, and geriatric psychiatric disorders. Occupational therapy professionals work within the *VA* in a variety of mental health settings as well as in physical rehabilitation and medicine. Working with military veterans is discussed in more detail in Chapter 6.

INPATIENT SETTINGS

Inpatient settings, such as hospital and skilled nursing facilities, provide nursing and medical care around the clock. Persons who need supervision because they are violent or so disorganized that they cannot meet their own needs for food, clothing, and shelter can be protected only in this type of setting.

Inpatient settings are generally divided into two subcategories: short term (sometimes termed *acute*) and long term (sometimes termed *chronic*).

Acute Care Inpatient Units

Short-term care inpatient units offer a secure environment in which persons who are seriously ill can be evaluated and treated for a short time; typically, this means stabilization and reduction of positive symptoms by medication. Suicide attempts or threats of suicide are a common reason for admission. Clients are then discharged with or without an outpatient service plan or may be transferred to a long-term care unit or other facility such as a state hospital. Short-term care units may be housed in a general hospital, a large private hospital, or a public institution; they are usually locked for the protection of the clients and the general population. Goals in the short-term care setting include observing and reporting clients' performance and response to medication, improving clients' occupational performance in preparation for return to the community, assisting in discharge and transition planning, and helping stabilize behavior.

To aid in returning to the community, the emphasis is on assessments and discharge or transition planning. Assessment may focus on cognitive level, self-care skills, and independent living skills. A lengthy evaluation process is impractical when quick results are needed for discharge and transition planning.

Note writing and documentation require a great deal of staff time. Initial and intervention session notes must be completed for every client; with 10 to 20 new client admissions a week (in some acute care settings), this means that 20 to 40 notes are completed every week. Meetings to communicate observations and findings about clients and plans for transition or discharge occur daily; up to half of the staff's time may be given to these types of meetings. Occupational therapy professionals are sometimes frustrated when clients are not able to attend therapeutic intervention groups or must leave in the middle of a group to attend an interview or have a test done.

Many short-term, acute care settings are locked, so that clients are prevented from leaving and harming themselves or others. Clients are discharged as soon as they are medically stable, usually 3 to 21 days after admission. Unfortunately, the recidivism rate is high, with many clients becoming very ill again and returning multiple times, usually because of difficulty with medication management and incorporating appointments in their scheduled routines. Insurance benefits may restrict length of stay or frequency of admission. Box 7.2 outlines the focus of intervention in short-term inpatient settings.

Long-Term Care Inpatient Units

Long-term inpatient settings (such as large state or country psychiatric hospitals, nonprofit voluntary psychiatric hospitals, or proprietary hospitals) provide supervision and services for persons who have severe and persistent mental disorders and serious disabilities that impair community living (generally clients have diagnoses such as schizophrenia, bipolar disorder, or neurocognitive disorder). Long-term

---

BOX 7.2 Acute Care Inpatient Programs: Focus of Intervention

- Rapid individual functional assessment, mutual collaborative goal setting
- Group programming necessitated by short stay and rapid turnover
- Mixed level occupational therapy groups focused on assessment and monitoring of change
- Normal daily routine: mix of activities of daily living, instrumental activities of daily living, work, and leisure or play occupations
- Social participation: social skills, interaction with community and family
- Self-awareness and self-expression activities
- Psychosocial skills: stress management, coping skills, problem-solving, mindfulness
- Discharge and transition planning: relapse prevention, symptom identification and reduction, medication management, community reintegration

BOX 7.3 Long-Term Inpatient Programs: Focus of Intervention

- Protective environment
- Individual client functional assessment and mutual collaborative goal setting
- Individual programming (mix of group activities and individual activities)
- Emphasis on establishing and maintaining habits and routines
- Behavior management
- Compensatory techniques and adapted environments for those with cognitive deficits
- Activities of daily living occupations such as showering, dressing, personal hygiene and grooming, and education about safe sexual activity practices
- Instrumental activities of daily living occupations such as communication management and religious and spiritual expression
- Health management occupations such as social and emotional health maintenance, symptom and condition management, physical activity, and nutrition management
- Rest and sleep occupations such as sleep preparation and sleep participation
- Work occupations such as employment seeking (for transitional and supported employment), volunteer exploration, and volunteer participation
- Leisure and play occupations such as for exploration and participation
- Social participation occupations such as family participation, friendships, intimate partner relationships, and peer group participation
- Age-related and/or gender-specific support groups, parenting skills, and so on

care settings for clients with highly disorganized thinking are usually locked.

Most long-term inpatient psychiatric settings have some occupational therapy professionals on staff. Older adults and those with neurocognitive disorders may live in long-term care settings such as skilled nursing facilities, assisted living environments, community-based residential facilities (CBRF), and the person's home. People who have been convicted of violent crimes but found to be not guilty by reason of mental disease or defect may live in forensic units of large state hospitals.

Occupational therapy professionals in inpatient settings may also work with special groups, such as victims of domestic violence, sex offenders, parents convicted of child abuse, persons with substance use disorders, and persons with selected personality disorders or eating disorders. It is believed that the special needs of these groups are best met when peers with similar problems receive care together. Separate units exist also for substance detoxification, geriatric psychiatry, and research into the effectiveness of medications and other treatments for persons with a particular diagnosis (eg, schizophrenia, eating disorders, borderline personality disorder).

Box 7.3 outlines the focus of intervention for long-term inpatient settings.

Behavioral Units

Hays and Baxley (18) describe a special unit for clients who have persistent behavioral deficits. Diagnoses of the clients seen on these units may be schizophrenia, other psychoses, and traumatic brain injury (TBI). Behavioral or cognitive–behavioral intervention aims to reduce problem behaviors and enhance coping strategies. Thus, for example, the person who constantly makes inappropriate sexual advances is helped to curb the behavior, understand the feelings that precipitate the impulse, learn appropriate boundaries for sexual expression, and substitute coping strategies such as distraction or deep breathing.

Forensic Settings

Working in a **forensic setting** means providing occupational therapy within the criminal justice system. Although this system is focused on deprivation of certain occupations, it is important for the occupational therapy professional to remain client-centered and use a holistic view of the client, incorporating into occupational therapy intervention as much of their wishes as possible. Safety is a primary objective. The occupational therapy professional in this setting will have limited equipment and supplies both to use with the client during intervention sessions, as well as to provide the client to use on their own. Typical adaptive equipment items, such as a button hook, cannot be used. In addition, items such as scissors, wood working tool, and crochet hooks or knitting needles cannot be a part of the chosen intervention (34).

When working within the forensic setting, the actual physical facility can be a federal prison, a military prison, a state corrections facility, a county jail, or a forensic unit within a general or psychiatric hospital.

For those clients who remain incarcerated for many years, identified occupations will involve the physical environment of the prison system and primary role of inmate. Some occupations may involve their family, such as writing letters or talking on the phone with them, or even virtual chats with an electronic tablet. Many of the client's occupations will be strictly limited by the small world in which they live. Certainly, self-cares are still a necessary occupation, but after that, other daily life occupations will vary greatly depending on the client's privileges and level of needed security. Relatively simple occupations such as reading may still require adaptation.

There are numerous programs and activities that occur within a prison that the client may be able to participate in, for instance, work duties such as working in a kitchen, laundry, library, garment shop, or machine shop. Horticulture tasks and agriculture activities may be possible. Programs connected to those outside the prison facility may also be available. An example of such a program is the Paws in Prison program. Dogs rescued from the community are placed with an inmate. The inmate and dog live together, for several weeks, with the inmate training and teaching the dog obedience skills and how to properly socialize with people (5, 8).

The occupation of education is another common area addressed within the corrections system. Clients may study for a general education development (GED) diploma, or a certificate of high school equivalency. Clients may also seek to earn higher education degrees. Occupational therapy considerations for the occupation of education can include frustration tolerance and attention deficit/hyperactivity disorder symptoms.

Community reintegration is addressed with those being released from the facility. Initially, the client needs to acclimate, or adjust to new social norms and customs, technology, and laws associated with living outside the facility. This prepares the client to assimilate into their near-future surroundings, fully understand societal expectations, and become a part of society beyond prison. These processes may be done in a progressive manner, with the client newly released from prison first living in transitional housing that provides some support and structure. Returning to live in the community may also involve some new learning. The client may not have previously been responsible for occupations such as meal preparation, financial management, and home establishment or management. Performance skills may need to be taught and performance patterns established or adjusted to include new instrumental activities of daily living (ADLs).

A part of community reintegration can include education and training for roles the client will find themselves in upon release from the facility. Part of their parole may require them to live with parents or they may be returning home to a partner and children. Parents who are older adults may personally benefit from having the client live with them. Over time, these parents may have developed medical conditions that necessitate physical or cognitive assistance and support. Education about chronic conditions and training in how to help those with chronic conditions can help the client be better prepared to live within that home environment. Clients who are parents may be coming home to children who have aged several years since the client was last living in the family home. The client may have gone into the correctional facility as only a spouse or partner but is leaving as also a parent. Parenting skills, for children of all ages, can help ease the transition back into family life. General education about all aspects of development over the life span can also be beneficial (34).

The occupation of work is another area to be addressed in occupational therapy. Employment for those who have a criminal record often means finding work in places different from where they worked prior to their conviction. Initial employment pursuits involve the occupational therapist assessing work skills and abilities. Acquiring employment may require the client to submit a resume or complete an interview. These activities can be practiced inside the facility, prior to the client having to perform them independently once they live outside of the prison. Normally expected job performance components, such as arriving at a certain time to start a work shift, working as part of a team, and being able to follow multiple requests or demands from a supervisor, are areas for which the occupational therapy professional can provide guidance and practice.

Some who have been incarcerated have substance use disorders or problems. Occupational therapy professionals can help the client establish 12-step group resources in the community. Specific interventions can be done to build self-efficacy toward the client "working their 12-step program" while managing a different lifestyle, both from what they are doing now inside the facility and prior to their incarceration.

Consideration must also be given to the mental disorder diagnosis. The structure, or living environment, the client may have grown extremely accustomed to, and knew how to live in and manage their symptoms, is now gone. Learning a new system of day-to-day living and coping with the symptoms of a mental disorder can be overwhelming. The client may suffer psychotic episodes more quickly or detach from the situation and become despondent. Addressing the new life circumstances the client finds themselves now in is a priority for the occupational therapy professional working in this setting. Helping the client become aware of new triggers and learning to cope without people, objects, or places the client has been used to when managing their disorder are all aspects to address in occupational therapy sessions (34).

Transitional Services

Transitional services prepare clients to move from the hospital to the community. Some state psychiatric hospitals have transitional houses on or near the hospital grounds. These live-in settings allow residents to explore the experience of more freedom in the community while receiving direct supervision from trained staff. Once they have demonstrated that they can function under these conditions, residents are discharged to independent community living. Regardless of inpatient setting, clients that can return to community living are helped to transition into that environment. Community reintegration intervention begins in acute care or inpatient settings and continues through various outpatient and community-based services and programs.

OUTPATIENT AND COMMUNITY PROGRAMS

Outpatient programing is vast both in types and environments where it is provided. Many traditional outpatient services are provided in a "clinic" setting. These types of services may be provided 1 to 2 hours a day a few days a week or for most of the day for several days a week. Some services encompass occupations done both at home and throughout the person's community environments. Many are an extension of inpatient services the person received, whereas some are completely independent of an inpatient connection.

Various outpatient and community settings include the following:

- satellite clinics and aftercare clinics that are affiliated with large hospital systems
- day hospitals or partial hospitalization programs that are an extension of inpatient services
- walk-in services provided through CMHCs
- psychosocial clubhouses (discussed in Chapter 6)
- supported and transitional employment programs (discussed in Chapter 6)
- schools and afterschool programs
- private counselor and psychologist offices
- special programming at community centers, public libraries, or community-based fitness or civic centers
- intensive services provided both in the home and community environments

All share a philosophical orientation that the person can get better faster and stay out of the hospital longer while living as independently as possible in the community.

Community settings match well with occupational therapy's focus on natural and normal engagement in occupation and are compatible with recovery principles. Box 7.4 summarizes the focus of community settings. To be effective in community settings, the occupational therapy professional must be attuned to political and economic events affecting funding and the direction of services provided to these clients. Careful attention to systemwide factors (eg, reimbursement shifts, grant application deadlines, and legislative constraints and mandates) helps identify forthcoming changes and opportunities for program improvements and new programming development.

BOX 7.4 Community Programs: Focus of Intervention

- Careful individual functional assessment, mutual collaborative goal setting
- Individual programming: mix of group activities and individual activities
- Activities of daily living occupations such as: bathing and showering, personal hygiene and grooming, and sexual activity
- Instrumental activities of daily living occupations such as: care of pets and animals, child rearing, communication management, driving and community mobility, financial management, home establishment and management, meal preparation and cleanup, religious and spiritual expression, safety and emergency maintenance, and shopping
- Health management occupations such as: social and emotional health promotion and maintenance, symptom and condition management, communication with the health care system, medication management, physical activity, and nutrition management
- Rest and sleep occupations such as: rest, sleep preparation, and sleep participation
- Education occupations such as: formal educational participation, informal personal education needs or interests exploration, and informal educational participation
- Work occupations such as: employment interests and pursuits, employment seeking and acquisition, job performance and maintenance, retirement preparation and adjustment
- Leisure and play occupations for: exploration and participation
- Social participation: community participation, family participation, friendships, intimate partner relationships, and peer group participation
- Age-related and/or gender-specific support groups, parenting skills, retirement preparation and adjustment

Partial Hospitalization, Day Hospitals, and Day Programs

Partial hospitalization provides a less costly alternative to inpatient treatment and a transition to community life. Rather than living day and night in a hospital, the client resides in the community and visits the hospital to receive services. Day treatment allows clients to receive training in daily living skills and to develop social interaction skills while they remain in the community where they will ultimately need these skills. This approach is cost-effective and less restrictive than an overnight stay hospital. Day hospitals may be designed to serve specific populations, such as older people (geriatric) or adolescents.

Depending on local practices, clients may be referred to day treatment directly from inpatient settings or by counselors or outpatient centers as an alternative to hospitalization.

The goals of partial hospitalization include management of short-term problems, rehabilitation for independent living, and support services. The staff is interdisciplinary but varies tremendously with availability of trained personnel. The roles and scope of practice of occupational therapy within a partial hospitalization program depend on the mix of professional staff. For example, although a nurse may be better trained to provide information on the uses and effects of medication, the occupational therapy professional may lead a group about medication management and side effects. Other roles include provision of rehabilitation groups and individual programming for independent living skills and teaching of problem-solving skills, symptom management, stress management, and coping skills.

The therapeutic program within a day hospital may consist of a mix of community meetings, small group learning sessions, and individual case management. Community meetings encourage clients to take an active voice in deciding program policies, field trips, and other special activities and thus promote leadership and self-assertion. Small group sessions facilitate the development of skills such as fiscal management, basic hygiene, work habits, health and safety, nutrition and basic cooking, home management, communication, and self-expression. Clients' group schedules are made according to need and whether they possess prerequisite skills. Groups may be performed by occupational therapy professionals, other activity therapists, social workers, or nurses.

Case management is a method of tracking each client's progress by assigning specific staff members to be responsible for the overall program of a few clients. Thus, every staff member from the psychologist to the mental health therapy aide may coordinate the services provided for one to five clients; this includes setting goals and identifying methods for collaboration with the client to complete various administrative duties such as making sure the client has enough medication, attends medical appointments, and applies for and receives appropriate public assistance.

A typical focus for occupational therapy is vocational services. One such program described by Richert and Merryman (38) was organized around Mosey's levels of group interaction skills (see Chapter 3) and Allen's cognitive levels (see Chapter 3). The authors reported that approximately 90% of the recipients of these services were functioning at cognitive levels 4 to 6. This program provided actual work experience within the hospital setting, often performed within a sheltered workshop (a form of supported employment). Level 4 clients were found to function at the prevocational level, needing structured, concrete, well-supervised assignments. Level 5 clients were in general more capable of independent functioning, with 24% engaged in volunteer work. Volunteer work was used extensively in this program for several reasons. It met the self-esteem needs of those who previously worked at jobs with high levels of responsibility, and it offered a gradual transition to paid employment. Volunteer work also safeguards the clients' social security and Medicaid benefits, which may terminate if the person works too many hours of paid employment.

A day program may fit well within the recovery model. Such a program keeps the client at home and in a community environment, while encouraging gradual development of life skills.

Intensive Psychiatric Rehabilitation Services Units

Intensive psychiatric rehabilitation treatment (IPRT) outpatient programs provide clients who are medically stable services in their home and community for up to 24 months. Occupational therapy professionals may manage rehabilitation programs or may provide direct services under this model. Interventions focus on developing specific skills needed for the person's target environments (at home and within the community), identifying and supplying environmental supports, and providing social supports, such as supervised housing and supported employment (40).

Community Rehabilitation Programs

Community rehabilitation programs (CRPs) offer life skills training and supported employment (vocational skills training) in daytime programs. Clients seen in CRPs transition from inpatient units and may have difficulty changing from the dependent role of inpatient to the more independent role of member of the community. Repeated rehospitalization is a frequent result. The occupational therapy professional can help ease the transition by analyzing and breaking down tasks, training staff, and making the expectations and demands of this new setting explicit to clients. Individualizing the program to meet needs and interests of individual clients is essential. By serving in the role of consultant, liaison, or case manager, the occupational therapy professional can ensure that clients receive services appropriate to their individual needs and abilities.

Community Mental Health Centers

CMHCs are large agencies that provide a wide range of services within residential communities; some have inpatient services for brief hospitalization. Occupational therapy professionals may be employed by the agencies themselves or by specific programs or services within these agencies, such as vocational rehabilitation, transitional living programs, PsyR programs, and day treatment centers.

Occupational therapy professionals may work with clients who have been released from the facility within the criminal justice system and clients recovering from substance use disorders (37). Educational materials may be created, and training completed on topics such as parenting, employment, financial management, sleep preparation and participation, leisure participation for those with limited income, preparing for work interviews, and shopping for clothing on a budget (37).

CMHCs traditionally have been and continue to be dependent on public funding. The Community Mental Health Act of 1963 spurred widespread development of CMHCs. CMHCs were intended to provide for the treatment and rehabilitation of the seriously mentally ill within the community. Under amendments passed between 1965 and 1979, the centers were expected to provide inpatient and outpatient services, partial hospitalization, round-the-clock emergency services, and consultation as well as services to children, the elderly, and alcohol and drug users. During those years, federal funding was allotted by service categories, ensuring that a variety of services were available and that special groups such as the elderly and children received attention. In 2014, the Centers for Medicare & Medicaid Services included occupational therapy as a service that must be available to all clients (26).

Community Behavioral Health Centers

A community behavioral health center (CBHC) provides integrated care and coordinated comprehensive services. The goal is to achieve "whole health" for the client (2). The comprehensive services include substance use services, mental health services, risk assessments, crisis planning, targeted case management, peer support and family support services, PsyR, and 24/7 crisis response (27, 29). Integration of services is completed through partnerships with law enforcement, schools, and hospitals (27). Services at a CBHC must be offered when those in the community need the service, which might be evenings or weekends. Based on state law, services can be in-home, telehealth, and/or on-site at the center. Care coordination must occur, thus there must be a sharing of the client's information with providers of care, including the client's needs and preferences concerning care offered (44).

The role of occupational therapy at a CBHC is to work with clients with cognitive impairments and mental disorders. Cognitive limitations addressed in occupational therapy include executive functioning tasks and performance pattern problems. Occupational therapy professionals can provide services for employment, education, and community integration (2). Assessment for clients seen at a CBHC should include daily activity ability, housing needs, vocational ability, educational needs, leisure needs, family and caregiver support, cognitive ability, client strengths, and resource availability (3).

School Systems

In the schools, interventions must be "educationally relevant"; occupational therapy is but one of several disciplines working together with a special educator to develop a complete individualized education program (IEP) for each child. In the schools, occupational therapy can support the child's performance in the student role by providing environmental modifications and supports, by providing opportunities for gross motor play and release of energy, by improving sensory modulation, and by working with teachers and parents.

Schools are oriented to providing education to large numbers of children. The child with a mental disorder will have an IEP, like other children designated in need of special services. The child will be seen either in the classroom *(push-in model)* or in a separate therapy area *(pull-out model)*. The push-in model is more common than the pull-out model. Goals may be educational (such as improving handwriting or keyboarding skills) or cognitive (such as improving focus, attention, organization). Additional goals could address peer group relationships and improving skills for identifying feelings and managing emotional distress. Classroom modification strategies to promote better self-regulation can be as simple as altering the level of lighting and reducing sound by using insulating materials (23). Noise-cancelling headphones are another option. Privacy shields can reduce or block distractions. Children with a high energy level may benefit from movement breaks to work off excess energy and improve ability to concentrate.

Emotional regulation programs aim to help children who are prone to angry outbursts. The goals are to help children recognize and identify their feelings, to educate them about the body's response to anger, and to teach them coping skills and sensory strategies (13, 25). See Figure 7.4.

Another sensory-based intervention is the Alert Program (42, 53), in which students are taught to identify their level of excitement or arousal and to manipulate it through sensory input. This is especially important for middle school students who are sometimes in trouble in school because

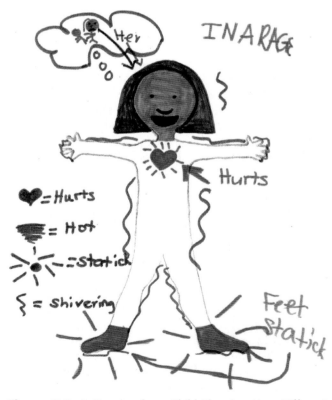

Figure 7.4. A Drawing by a Child Showing How Different Body Parts Feel When They Are Angry. (Reprinted with permission from Maas, C., Mason, R., & Candler, C. (2008). When I get mad. *OT Practice, 13*(19), 9–14.)

they are either inattentive or so keyed up that they are disruptive to the class. A poster with a thermometer measuring level of excitement can be used as a visual aid, and the child is asked to point to where they are on the scale at that moment.

The role of occupational therapy services in the schools has expanded as the number of children diagnosed with autism spectrum disorders has increased (17). Occupational therapy professionals have used sensory strategies and vigorous motor activities to increase focus and attention. They also consult with teachers, collaborating on how best to meet the child's needs within the classroom and other school environments such as the lunchroom or play area.

Summer Camp

Summer camp provides an exciting context for occupational therapy intervention because it represents a vacation from the routines of the school year and an opportunity for the child to explore and reinvent themselves. Camp is a time off from ordinary life and provides opportunities to experiment with new activities, friendships, and experiences.

Many excellent pediatric reference texts exist for occupational therapy, and the reader is encouraged to consult these if working with children.

SERVICES PROVIDED IN CLIENT'S COMMUNITY RESIDENCES

Home Health Care

Once a person transitions away from inpatient care and is discharged, the person may receive services in their home. Although most of those receiving home health services have disabilities that are primarily physical, secondary psychiatric disabilities are quite common, especially when the first diagnosis is neurologic. Clients functioning at Allen cognitive level 4 need assistance to transfer skills from one environment (hospital) to another (home) and to solve routine problems and thus can benefit from occupational therapy intervention.

Within home health care programs, the occupational therapist may "open a case" and begin completion of a transdisciplinary client assessment. The occupational therapy assistant would follow the intervention plan designed by the occupational therapist.

Typical interventions provided in the home include memory aids; training in coping mechanisms and crisis management; educating and training caregivers with supervision of hygiene, grooming; and nutrition management. In addition, the occupational therapy professionals could supervise home modifications and educate the client and caregivers about safety (7). Depending on state licensing laws, the occupational therapy professional may need a certain number of years of experience providing occupational therapy services before being allowed to work in home health care. Supervision requirements of the occupational therapy assistant in home health care often include a visit by the occupational therapist in the home with the client approximately every 2 weeks.

Psychiatric home care provides a natural environment for occupation-based intervention and involves the client and family as coequals with occupational therapy professionals (Box 7.5). The client's ability to fit into the home and community is the ultimate test of functional outcomes.

Adult Foster Homes

Adult foster homes provide room and board for a small number of residents. There are varying levels of supervision provided. Any specific self-care or home maintenance assistance may be provided by the owner of the home or may be provided through a community-based support service.

Group Homes

Group homes provide a place for residents to live together in a long-term residence in the community, with varying levels of supervision from staff. Sometimes each resident has their own room and bathroom; in other facilities, residents may have their own bedrooms but share all other living areas.

BOX 7.5 Psychiatric Home Health Care: Focus of Intervention

- Client-directed, caregiver-directed goals and plans
- Education and training of caregiver in co-occupation strategies to optimize client engagement
- Naturally occurring occupations (eg, unloading groceries, opening the mail) in the client's regular environment
- Education of family and caregivers about the person's occupational performance abilities (especially for clients with dementia or Alzheimer disease)
- Activities of daily living occupations such as: bathing and showering, toileting and toilet hygiene, dressing, eating and swallowing, feeding, functional mobility, personal hygiene and grooming, and sexual activity
- Instrumental activities of daily living occupations such as: care of others, care of pets and animals, child rearing, communication management, home establishment and management, meal preparation and cleanup, religious and spiritual expression, and safety and emergency maintenance
- Health management occupations such as: social and emotional health promotion and maintenance, symptom and condition management, communication with the health care system, medication management, physical activity, and nutrition management
- Rest and sleep occupations such as: rest, sleep preparation, and sleep participation
- Work occupations such as: retirement preparation and adjustment
- Leisure and play occupations for: exploration and participation
- Social participation: family participation, friendships, intimate partner relationships, and peer group participation

Some group homes have live-in managers or house parents, and many provide other services through their affiliation with hospitals or CMHCs.

Assisted Living

Assisted living is a residence designed for those who need help with instrumental ADLs (clothing care, housekeeping, transportation) but who do not require skilled nursing in a 24-hour setting. Residents who require assistance with basic ADLs (dressing, bathing, grooming) may contract to pay for those services. The primary population for assisted living is older adults with physical and/or cognitive impairments. The largest assisted living environments have round-the-clock staffing and on-site nursing. Most assisted living residents reside in large buildings (or groups of buildings on a single campus) with a hotel or apartment atmosphere. Many assisted living facilities offer continuum of care, with the option for the resident to move to a more care-intensive part of the facility as required.

Community-Based Residential Facility—Memory Care

These are licensed facilities that must follow state requirements. These facilities may be small, having only a few residents, or large, having 20 to 30 residents. Often, they are part of a health system's continuum of care. The memory care (MC) aspect includes providing services for those with various dementia diagnoses, such as Alzheimer disease, Parkinson disease, and vascular dementia. A CBRF may have a MC unit, or the whole facility can be designated as a CBRF-MC, admitting only those with MC problems. Those that live in a CBRF-MC need 24/7 supervision and monitoring, and typically need more physical assistance with self-care than do those who live in an assisted living facility (6, 20, 32, 33). Direct care staff are required to have training in managing difficult behaviors, dietary needs, fire safety, first aid, cardiopulmonary resuscitation, choking, medication administration, resident's rights, standard precautions, and infection control (30).

The environment of the CBRF-MC is designed to provide social participation and leisure activities. These activities include small and large group participation, individual activities, and visits to community events. The occupational therapy professional may fill the role as consultant, establishing activity plans for residents and teaching direct care staff how best to interact with residents. Occupational therapy professionals may also work full- or part-time in the CBRF-MC, providing both activity of daily living sessions and leisure-based sessions.

OT HACKS SUMMARY

O: Occupation as a means and an end

Occupational focus in the community: instrumental ADLs, health management, rest and sleep, education, work, play, leisure, social participation

Occupational focus during long-term facility living: ADLs, rest and sleep, leisure, social participation

T: Theoretical concepts, values, and principles, or historical foundations

According to person–environment models of practice, the environment influences occupational performance and occupational participation. The person is striving to achieve mastery over the environmental challenges presented to them.

Environmental influences must be novel enough to create an urge to explore, but not so new and different that the environment becomes overwhelming.

The environment places demands on the person as well as constraints.

H: How can we Help? OT's role in serving clients with mental illness or mental health needs

How is the role of occupational therapy professional depicted in various settings?

Community residences: focus of intervention is ADLs, leisure, and social participation. Caregivers are trained on how best clients perform occupations.

Inpatient acute care: observe and evaluate behaviors during occupation and report findings to medical staff. Focus on community reintegration.

Inpatient long-term care: assist with establishing new habits and routines within a protective environment.

Outpatient settings: community living needs are the primary aspect of intervention. Instrumental ADLs, work, education, and social participation are key focuses of individual and group activities.

A: Adaptations

Adaptations are done for daily life occupations, while managing symptoms of a mental disorder, and the focus of intervention varies based on the practice setting.

Inpatient acute care: coping with daily stressors, self-regulation and self-management for success with social participation.

Inpatient long-term care: adapt environment for success with new habits and routines and behavior management.

Outpatient settings: focus of occupational therapy is how to "manage" symptoms and behaviors and how to cope through self-regulation and self-management skills. Routines may need alteration to allow for extra time for completing daily life tasks.

Community residences: environments and routines may need changes to allow for greatest independence that is possible with ADLs, leisure activities, and social participation.

C: Case study includes

Not applicable for this chapter.

K: Knowledge: keeping mental health OT practice grounded in evidence, in occupational science, and in research

Not applicable for this chapter.

S: Some terms that may be new to you

Care: "tending to" someone or supervising someone

Care recipient: someone who is receiving support or assistance from another person

Chronosystem: This system includes all the environmental influences and activities that occur over time, impacting the person's roles and occupations throughout their life span. There is consideration of how the dominant culture the person lives in influences government policies and laws, which in turn impacts the roles of the person's family members and neighbors, and then finally the direct impact to the person, influencing how the person changes and develops.

Consumer: someone who has experienced a mental disorder, has received, is receiving, or is seeking treatment and support

Environmental constraints: aspects of environment that limit behavior

Environmental demands: aspects of environment that elicit behaviors by asking the person to act

Environmental impact: "the opportunity, support, demand, and constraints that the environment has on a particular individual" (49, pp. 97–98)

Epidemiology: study of what happens to a population

Exosystem: system involves entities that happen beyond the person, yet involve other persons or entities that impact the individual

Forensic care: services provided to those within the criminal justice system

Health determinants: social determinants, a person's individual traits, and a person's actions

Macrosystem: includes the cultural identification, cultural attitudes, values, and social conditions of the cultural group the person resides within

Mesosystem: in this system are the interactions between the various entities that are a part of the person's microsystem

Microsystem: person's interactions with the entities nearest to the person and thus provide the most influence toward the person

Psychiatric survivor: individual who is out of the health care system and feels a sense of survival regarding the system

Service: what is provided to the client

Social determinants of health: socially based reasons for health-related problems

Welfare of a population: involves impact of various health factors and environmental factors

Reflection Questions

1. What are some of the reasons why people with serious mental illness or chronic mental health problems are not identified earlier, or provided with intervention and supports to help manage their health?

2. Describe the process used to identify and document social determinants of health. Which aspects of the occupational therapy process do you believe best captures the documentation of socially related health factors in clients who receive occupational therapy services? Please explain your answer.

3. Describe how the application of environmental concepts can positively (or negatively) impact occupational therapy evaluation and intervention.

4. Compare and contrast the following ideas: defense mechanisms, survival strategies, coping strategies, and protective factors. Defend the importance of understanding a client's occupational history and clarifying how the client applied such strategies throughout past experiences, to provide the most authentic client-centered occupational therapy services.

5. Describe the different uses and interpretations of the term *intervention.*

6. How does the environment and context of the acute care inpatient unit impact the provision of occupational therapy services? Discuss some of the challenges of working as an occupational therapy professional in an acute care inpatient setting.

7. Apply the constructs of Bronfenbrenner's Bioecological Model to help explain the relationship between a person, their occupations, and occupational engagement. What aspects of the model align with the occupational therapy domain and process?

8. According to the primary goal or anticipated outcomes for each setting, summarize the typical role(s) and responsibilities of an occupational therapy professional who works within: a CMHC, a CBHC, the school system, or within the psychiatric home health arena.

REFERENCES

1. American Hospital Association. (2021, October 07). *Medicare releases data on Z code use to document social determinants of health.* Retrieved January 26, 2022, from https://www.aha.org/news/headline/2021-10-07-medicare-releases-data-z-code-use-document-social-determinants-health

2. American Occupational Therapy Association. (n.d.). *Occupational therapy practitioners: A key member of the Community Behavioral Health team.* Retrieved January 23, 2022, from https://www.aota.org/-/media/Corporate/Files/Advocacy/Federal/Overview-of-OT-in-Community-Behavioral-Health.pdf

3. American Occupational Therapy Association. (2016). *Occupational therapy service outcome measures for Certified Community Behavioral Health Centers (CCBHCs): Framework for occupational therapy service with rationale for outcome measures selection and listing of occupational therapy outcome measure tools.* https://www.aota.org/-/media/Corporate/Files/Practice/MentalHealth/occupational-therapy-outcome-measures-community-mental-health-services.pdf

4. American Occupational Therapy Association. (2020). Occupational therapy practice framework: Domain and process—Fourth Edition. *American Journal of Occupational Therapy, 74*(Suppl. 2), 1–87.

5. Arkansas Department of Corrections. (n.d.). *Paws in prison.* Retrieved January 30, 2022, from https://doc.arkansas.gov/correction/paws-in-prison/

6. Azura Memory Care. (n.d.). *What's the difference: Assisted living—RCAC, CBRF and MC.* Retrieved January 31, 2022, from https://www.inclusa.org/wp-content/uploads/Scope-of-Service-CBRF.pdf

7. Bridges, A. E., Szanton, S. L., Evelyn-Gustave, A. I., Smith, F. R., & Gitlin, L. N. (2013). Home sweet home—Interprofessional team helps older adults age in place safely. *OT Practice, 18*(16), 9–13.

8. Care for Animals. (n.d.). *Paws in prison.* Retrieved January 30, 2022, from https://www.careforanimals.org/paws-in-prison

9. Centers for Disease Control and Prevention. (2018, May 18). *Introduction to epidemiology. Section 1: Definition of epidemiology.* Retrieved January 26, 2022, from https://www.cdc.gov/training/publichealth101/epidemiology.html#:~:text=Epidemiology%20is%20the%20%E2%80%9Cstudy%20of,.%E2%80%9D%20%E2%80%94%20A%20Dictionary%20of%20Epidemiology

10. Centers for Disease Control and Prevention. (2016, June 17). *Introduction to public health. Public health 101 series.* Retrieved January 26, 2021, from https://www.cdc.gov/training/publichealth101/public-health.html

11. Centers for Disease Control and Prevention. (2018, November 15). *Introduction to epidemiology.* Retrieved January 26, 2022, from https://www.cdc.gov/training/publichealth101/epidemiology.html

12. Centers for Medicare & Medicaid Services. (2021, September). *Utilization of Z codes for social determinants of health among Medicare fee-for-service beneficiaries, 2019.* Retrieved January 26, 2022, from https://www.cms.gov/files/document/z-codes-data-highlight.pdf

13. Chandler, B. E. (2007). Hidden in plain sight: Working with students with emotional disturbance in the schools. *OT Practice, 12*(1), CE1–CE8.

14. Children and Family Justice Center. (2020, March). *Harm instead of health: Imprisoning youth with mental illness.* Retrieved January 23, 2022, from https://wwws.law.northwestern.edu/legalclinic/cfjc/documents/communitysafetymentalhealthfinal.pdf

15. Compton, M. T., & Shim, R. S. (2015). The social determinants of mental health. *Focus, 13*(4), 419–425.

16. De las Heras, C. G., Dion, G. L., & Walsh, D. (1993). Application of rehabilitation models in a state psychiatric hospital. *Occupational Therapy in Mental Health, 12*(3), 1–32.

17. Harris, E. A. (2015, February 17). Sharp rise in occupational therapy cases at New York's Schools. *The New York Times.* https://www.nytimes.com/2015/02/18/nyregion/new-york-city-schools-see-a-sharp-increase-in-occupational-therapy-cases.html

18. Hays, C., & Baxley, S. (1998). The roles of the state psychiatric hospital and the occupational therapy practitioner. *Mental Health Special Interest Section Quarterly, 21*(1), 3–4.

19. Herlache-Pretzer, E., & Jacob, J. (2018, April 23). From prison to the community: Programs for developing life skills. *OT Practice, 23*(7), 9–12.

20. Inclusa. (2019, October 02). *Scope of service: Community Based Residential Facility (CBRF).* https://www.inclusa.org/wp-content/uploads/Scope-of-Service-CBRF.pdf

21. Iwama, M. K. (2006). *The Kawa model: Culturally relevant occupational therapy.* Elsevier.

22. John Hopkins Medicine. (2020, February). *ICD-10 Codes to identify social determinants of health.* https://www.hopkinsmedicine.org/johns_hopkins_healthcare/providers/physicians/resources_guidelines/provider_communications/2021/PRUP135_ICD10-km.pdf

23. Kinnealey, M., Pfeiffer, B., Miller, J., Roan, C., Shoener, R., & Ellner, M. L. (2012). Effect of classroom modification on attention and engagement of students with autism or dyspraxia. *American Journal of Occupational Therapy, 66*(5), 511–519.

24. Levine, R. (1984). The cultural aspects of home delivery. *American Journal of Occupational Therapy, 38*(11), 734–735.

25. Maas, C., Mason, R., & Candler, C. (2008). When I get mad. *OT Practice, 13*(19), 9–14.

26. *Medicare program: Conditions of participation (CoPs) for community mental health centers.* 78 F.R. 64635 (proposed October 29, 2013) (to be codified at 42 C.F.R. §. 485). https://www.federalregister.gov/documents/2013/10/29/2013-24056/medicare-program-conditions-of-participation-cops-for-community-mental-health-centers

27. National Council for Mental Wellbeing. (n.d.). *Overview: Home.* Retrieved January 23, 2022, from https://www.thenationalcouncil.org/ccbhc-success-center/ccbhcta-overview/

28. National Institute of Health. (2022, January). *Mental illness.* https://www.nimh.nih.gov/health/statistics/mental-illness

29. New York State Office of Mental Health. (n.d.). *Certified Community Behavioral Health Clinics (CCBHC).* Retrieved January 23, 2022, from https://omh.ny.gov/omhweb/bho/ccbhc.html

30. Northwood Technical College. (2021). *Community based residential facility.* Retrieved January 31, 2022, from https://www.northwoodtech.edu/continuing-education-and-training/professional-development/cbrf

31. Ollove, M. (2016, August 2). Amid shortage of psychiatric beds, mentally ill face long waits for treatment. *Stateline.* https://www.pewtrusts.org/en/research-and-analysis/blogs/stateline/2016/08/02/amid-shortage-of-psychiatric-beds-mentally-ill-face-long-waits-for-treatment

32. Oregon Department of Human Services. (2020, June 24). *Endorsed memory care communities.* https://www.oregon.gov/DHS/SENIORS-DISABILITIES/SPPD/APDRules/2020-01-01%20Temp%20411-057.pdf

33. Oregon Department of Human Services. (2022, January 1). *Residential care and assisted living facilities.* https://www.dhs.state.or.us/policy/spd/rules/411_054.pdf

34. Ozkan, E., Belhan, S., Yaran, M., & Zarif, M. (2018). *Occupational therapy in forensic settings.* IntechOpen.

35. Pratt, C. W., Gill, K. J., Barrett, N. M., & Roberts, M. (2013). *Psychiatric rehabilitation* (3rd ed.). Elsevier.

36. Public Health Ontario. (2012, April). *A framework for the ethical conduct of public health initiatives.* Retrieved January 26, 2022, from https://jcb.utoronto.ca/wp-content/uploads/2021/03/framework-ethical-conduct.pdf

37. Quake-Rapp, C., Schluter Strickland, L., Cecil, A. M., & Story, S. (2014). Mental health in underserved communities—Engaging students to promote the value of occupational therapy. *OT Practice, 19*(18), 18–20.

38. Richert, G. Z., & Merryman, M. B. (1987). The vocational continuum: A model for providing vocational services in a partial hospitalization program. *Occupational Therapy in Mental Health, 7*(3), 1–20.

39. Rigby, P. J., Trentham, B., & Letts, L. (2018). Modifying performance contexts. In B. A. B. Schell, & G. Gillen, (Eds.), *Willard and Spackman's occupational therapy* (13th ed., pp. 460–479). Wolters Kluwer.

40. Rochester Regional Health. (n.d.). *Behavioral health.* Retrieved February 5, 2022, from https://www.rochesterregional.org/services/behavioral-health/mental-health-and-emergency-inpatient-services/psychiatric-rehabilitation-services/intensive-psychiatric-rehabilitation-services

41. Rosario, C. (2016, April 25). *The difference between population health & public health.* https://www.adsc.com/blog/the-difference-between-population-health-public-health

42. Salls, J., & Bucey, J. C. (2003). Self-regulation strategies for middle school students. *OT Practice, 5*(8), 11–16.

43. Shea, C.-K., & Wu, R. (2013). Finding the key—Sensory profiles of youths involved in the justice system. *OT Practice, 18*(18), 9–13.

44. Substance Abuse and Mental Health Services Administration. (2016, May). *Criteria for the demonstration program to improve community mental health centers and to establish certified community behavioral health clinics.* Retrieved January 23, 2022, from https://www.samhsa.gov/sites/default/files/programs_campaigns/ccbhc-criteria.pdf

45. Tan, B. L., Kumar, V. R., & Devaraj, P. (2015). Development of a new occupational therapy service in a Singapore prison. *British Journal of Occupational Therapy, 78*(8), 525–529.

46. Taylor, R. (2017). *Kielhofner's model of human occupation* (5th ed.). Wolters Kluwer.

47. Thiel, A., Alexander, M., Gerig, L., Short, N., & Henton, P. (2019, October 22). *Restoration through occupation: Participating with prison inmates to refurbish seating and mobility equipment.* https://www.aota.org/Publications-News/otp/Archive/2019/refurbished-seating.aspx

48. Turpin, M., & Iwama, M. K. (2011). *Using occupational therapy models in practice: A field guide.* Churchill Livingstone Elsevier.

49. U.S. Department of Health and Human Services. (n.d.). *Social determinants of health.* Retrieved January 26, 2022, from https://health.gov/healthypeople/objectives-and-data/social-determinants-health

50. U.S. Department of Justice. (2017, June). *Indicators of mental health problems reported by prisoners and jail inmates, 2011–2012.* Retrieved January 23, 2022, from https://bjs.ojp.gov/content/pub/pdf/imhprpji1112.pdf

51. U.S. Department of Veterans Affairs. (2015, June 3). *Mental health care.* http://www.va.gov/healthbenefits/access/mental_health_care.as

52. Waite, A. (2012). Researchers in action: John A White. *OT Practice, 17*(3), 14–17.

53. Williams, M. S., & Shellenberger, S. (1996). *How does your engine run? A leader's guide to the alert program for self-regulation.* Therapy Works.

54. World Health Organization. (2017, February 3). *Determinants of health.* Retrieved January 26, 2022, from https://www.who.int/news-room/questions-and-answers/item/determinants-of-health

SUGGESTED RESOURCES

Articles

Anderson, M., & Grinder, S. (2020). Occupational therapy's role in social-emotional development throughout childhood. *OT Practice, 25*(7), CE1–CE8.

Cahill, S. M., & Egan, B. E. (2020). Identifying youth with mental health conditions at school. *OT Practice, 25*(5), 12–16.

Champagne, T. (2012). Creating occupational therapy groups for children and youth in community-based mental health practice. *OT Practice, 17*(14), 13–18.

Chandler, B. E. (2007). Hidden in plain sight: Working with students with emotional disturbance in the schools. *OT Practice, 12*(1), CE1–CE8.

Eggers, M., Sciulli, J., Gaguzis, K., & Muñoz, J. P. (2003). Enrichment through occupation: The Allegheny County jail project. *Mental Health Special Interest Section Quarterly, 26*(2), 1–4.

Knis-Matthews, L. (2003). A parenting program for women who are substance dependent. *Mental Health Special Interest Section Quarterly, 26*(1), 1–4.

Mehrich, K. D., & Wasmuth, S. (2020). Tell my story: Narrative medicine as a unique approach to forensic mental health intervention. *OT Practice, 25*(1), 17–19.

Sheehan, S. (1982). *Is there no place on Earth for me?* Houghton Mifflin.

Websites

American Residential Treatment Association. https://artausa.org/
Every Moment Counts. https://everymomentcounts.org/

<table>
<tr><td>CHAPTER
8</td><td>Medications, Medication Considerations
and Concerns, Medical-Based Treatments,
Complementary Practices, and Detoxification</td></tr>
</table>

OT HACKS OVERVIEW

O: Occupation as a means and an end

Occupational performance is affected by diagnoses symptoms that can be changed through medication.

T: Theoretical concepts, values, and principles, or historical foundations

The medical model is of primary consideration in this chapter. Other models may be utilized during occupational therapy intervention.

H: How can we Help? OT's role in serving clients with mental illness or mental health needs

NA for this chapter.

A: Adaptations

NA for this chapter.

C: Case study includes

Not applicable for this chapter.

K: Knowledge: keeping mental health OT practice grounded in evidence, in occupational science, and in research

Medical knowledge is the primary focus for this chapter.

S: Some terms that may be new to you

Akathisia
Detoxification
Dystonia
Medication adherence
Mental obtundation
Metabolic syndrome
Neuroleptic malignant syndrome
Neuroleptics
Parkinsonism
Psychotropic
Serotonin syndrome
Tardive dyskinesia

INTRODUCTION

Until the middle of the 20th century, severe mental disorders could not be effectively treated in a medical sense. The introduction in the 1950s of drugs that could control hallucinations and other symptoms of psychosis brought new hope. Suddenly, clients who had been unapproachable because they could not cope and manage their psychiatric symptoms could engage in occupational therapy and other rehabilitative treatments. In the decades since, many more psychotropic (mind-changing) drugs have been discovered and introduced. These drugs are effective in reducing symptoms and returning people to their premorbid level of functioning.

This chapter presents information on the major types or classes of drugs used in psychiatric practice today, their therapeutic uses, and their side effects. Specific considerations and concerns for the client in occupational therapy and for the occupational therapy professional are described. Nonpharmacologic medical-based treatment and complementary medicine practices are presented. Because the detoxification

process involves many of the items already identified in this chapter (medication use, side effects, and complementary practices), detoxification is also addressed here.

It should be noted that information provided about side effects includes both signs and symptoms. Signs are observable. They are seen by the occupational therapy professional (or by other professionals) and/or measured through an assessment (such as degrees of body temperature, pounds of weight gain or loss, or blood pressure [BP] readings). Symptoms are "felt" or "experienced" by the client. The client provides a self-report of symptoms that are both physical and psychological (11).

PSYCHOTROPIC MEDICATIONS

Psychotropic means "mind changing." Thus, psychotropic medications are drugs that alter, or change, the way the brain works. Many drugs have psychotropic qualities. These include medications prescribed for mental disorders, medications that are prescribed for physical disorders but that produce mind-altering side effects, and other mind-changing but illegal drugs (eg, phencyclidine [PCP] and lysergic acid diethylamide [LSD]).

This chapter considers only the first of these three groups: the psychotropic medications that physicians prescribe to treat the symptoms of mental illness. Occupational therapy professionals must know about these drugs because they work directly with clients and are in a position to observe the effects of medications on the person's symptoms, occupational performance, and occupational participation. Occupational therapy professionals can see firsthand whether a person is able to function better today than yesterday or whether side effects such as tremors are interfering with the ability to perform routine tasks. The physician relies on observations made by occupational therapy professionals and nursing staff and from clients' self-reports to monitor how well a medication is working, whether it should be changed, and whether the dosage should be increased or reduced. In addition, physicians rely on staff to support their medical decisions, to encourage clients to comply with taking the medication, and to help clients understand that some side effects are temporary. For these reasons, it is important for the occupational therapy professional to know the classes of drugs, the problems for which they are prescribed, and the side effects.

Research and development of psychotropic medication is ongoing. New medication is continually available. New research identifies medicine that is more effective and efficient. This also means older medications are removed from the market. Therefore, this chapter provides a foundation for approaching the subject and is not an exhaustive guide. The reader must take responsibility for keeping themselves informed about changes in medications, to provide appropriate support to clients. Additional references and suggestions for staying current with medicine information are provided at the end of the chapter.

How Psychotropic Drugs Work

Psychotropic drugs affect neurotransmitters in the brain, altering levels of key brain chemicals (dopamine, norepinephrine, serotonin). Drugs for schizophrenia (sometimes called *neuroleptics*) work primarily on the dopamine system (Table 8.1),[1] and different antipsychotic medications target specific dopamine receptors (eg, D_2, D_3, D_4). The newer medications (termed *second-generation* and also "atypical antipsychotic") have selective effects restricted to parts of the brain (eg, the frontal lobes and the limbic system) and fewer side effects from unwanted actions on other parts of the brain. Antidepressants work by altering levels of serotonin and other neurotransmitters; each antidepressant has a slightly different action.

Most psychotropic drugs are manufactured for oral administration via tablets (some of which are *disintegrating*, which is helpful for those with swallowing difficulties or who "cheek" [hide] their medication) (17), capsules,

or extended-release capsules. Some are available in liquid form, and some can be given by injection. Some injectable drugs come in a depot formulation, which is long lasting; the client is administered the medication only every few weeks. This helps with **adherence** (following the plan) in patients who have trouble remembering to take oral medications.

The Psychotropic Drugs and Their Side Effects

Tables 8.1 through 8.6 summarize six major categories of drugs: antipsychotic drugs, antiparkinsonian drugs, antidepressant drugs, antimanic drugs, antianxiety drugs, and psychostimulants. For each category, the generic name and some of the brand names of individual drugs are listed in the tables. Drugs in Tables 8.1, 8.3, and 8.6 are grouped by class. The last column in each table lists some of the side effects. Side effects shown in **boldface type** are medically dangerous, either life threatening or indicators of possible permanent damage. These side effects *must* be reported to the nurse or doctor immediately, *and* the occupational therapy professional must also record in the client's chart the symptom and the person to whom it was reported. As medications begin to take effect, the occupational therapy professional will notice a gradual increase in the person's ability to perform occupations. The physician will be interested in reports about functional level, because this indicates whether a given medication is effective.

The authors have attempted to provide accurate and useful information, based on the sources referenced. The reader is cautioned that this chapter was written at a given time and that information changes as time moves forward. It is always advisable to consult current sources, including trustworthy internet sites and the prescribing physician, to verify accuracy and to obtain current information.

Antipsychotic Drugs

Antipsychotic drugs are prescribed most often for persons with schizophrenia and other psychotic disorders (Table 8.1). These drugs control psychotic symptoms, such as hallucinations and delusions, and generally bring the person into better contact with reality. These medications are also used to reduce violent or possibly dangerous behaviors in persons having manic episodes and in drug abusers. Some of the second-generation antipsychotics are useful in mood disorders, even when no psychotic symptoms are present.

The first-generation antipsychotics, or dopamine receptor antagonists, have no beneficial effect on the negative symptoms of schizophrenia (apathy, lack of interest in other people and one's environment, self-absorption, and lack of motivation). Examples of these first-generation medications are chlorpromazine (Thorazine), trifluoperazine (Stelazine), and haloperidol (Haldol). The second-generation antipsychotics are just as effective as the first-generation antipsychotics in reducing positive symptoms and far

---

[1] All tables appear at the end of this chapter.

Table 8.1. Therapeutic and Adverse Effects of Antipsychotic Drugs

Class	Generic Name (Trade Name)	Selected Therapeutic Effects (Vary Based on Drug)	Selected Side Effects (Vary Based on Drug)
First-generation antipsychotics	Chlorpromazine (Thorazine) Haloperidol (Haldol) Loxapine (Loxitane) Mesoridazine (Serentil) Molindone (Moban; no longer available in the United States) Perphenazine (Trilafon) Trifluoperazine (Stelazine) Thioridazine (Mellaril) Thiothixene (Navane)	Decrease in psychotic symptoms (reduction in hallucinations, delusions, psychomotor agitation) Sedation	Orthostatic hypotension, dry mouth and nose, blurred vision, constipation, urinary retention, allergic dermatitis, photosensitivity Signs of **TD: involuntary movements of the face, trunk, extremities;** signs of **NMS: severe muscle rigidity and dystonia, akinesia, mutism, confusion, agitation, increased pulse rate, increased blood pressure, extreme hyperthermia** EPS with abnormal movements addressed with antiparkinsonian drugs (Table 8.2)
Second-generation antipsychotics	Aripiprazole (Abilify) Asenapine (Saphris) Cariprazine (Vraylar) Clozapine (Clozaril) Iloperidone (Fanapt) Lurasidone (Latuda) Olanzapine (Zyprexa) Paliperidone (Invega) Quetiapine (Seroquel) Risperidone (Risperdal) Ziprasidone (Geodon)	Decrease in psychotic symptoms (reduction in hallucinations, delusions, psychomotor agitation) More effective than traditional antipsychotics in reducing negative symptoms of schizophrenia Improvement in depressive symptoms Improvement in irritability associated with autism spectrum disorder (aripiprazole) Low or no motor impairment effect (aripiprazole)[a]	Dry mouth, dizziness, constipation, orthostatic hypotension, seizures, insomnia, akathisia, weight gain Possible **metabolic syndrome** and type 2 diabetes **Agranulocytosis,** fatal unless caught early, occurs in about 1% of patients taking clozapine, which hence necessitates blood monitoring Olanzapine may **elevate liver enzymes,** cause significant weight gain, elevate cholesterol and blood sugar

EPS, extrapyramidal syndrome; NMS, neuroleptic malignant syndrome; TD, tardive dyskinesia.
[a]Data from Viana, T. G., Almeida-Santos, A. F., Aguiar, D. C., & Moreira, F. A. (2013). Effects of Aripiprazole, an atypical antipsychotic, on the motor alterations induced by acute ethanol administration in mice. *Basic & Clinical Pharmacology & Toxicology, 112*(5), 319–324.
Data, unless noted otherwise, from Sadock, B. J., Sussman, N., & Sadock, V. A. (2019). *Kaplan & Sadock's pocket handbook of psychiatric drug treatment* (7th ed.). Wolters Kluwer.

better at reducing negative symptoms. The side effects of second-generation antipsychotics, in general, are more easily tolerated. Among these atypical or second-generation drugs are clozapine (Clozaril), risperidone (Risperdal), olanzapine (Zyprexa), and aripiprazole (Abilify). Among the side effects of some of the second-generation drugs is the stimulation of lactation (galactorrhea) and breast development in males (gynecomastia) (17).

Atypical antipsychotics have some disadvantages. They are more expensive, and some are not available in generic form. Some require frequent blood monitoring to detect potentially fatal side effects. Weight gain is common. A frequent dangerous side effect of many atypicals is **metabolic syndrome**, which increases the risk of heart disease, diabetes, and stroke. Because of the side effects of the atypicals, persons diagnosed with mental disorders may still be prescribed one of the older medications such as Haldol. Individuals receiving any antipsychotic medication are very much in need of occupational therapy and other rehabilitative services to help them function better in daily life. Even with the second-generation medications, the person who has had a major mental disorder for several years may be at a disadvantage in performing occupations, including areas such as activities of daily living and social participation.

POINT-OF-VIEW

I am happy with this medication now. It allows me to be creative and do more, and to take more on board. It keeps me stable.

—Mark, diagnosed with bipolar depression, commenting on the switch to olanzapine (1, p. 160).

All medications have some adverse effects, side effects that are undesirable. Some of those that may occur with antipsychotic medications are movement disorders (extrapyramidal side effects [EPS]), a tendency to sunburn very easily (photosensitivity), dry mouth, and blurred vision.

The EPS are of four types: parkinsonian movements, dystonia, akathisia, and **tardive dyskinesia** (TD). Signs and symptoms of **Parkinsonism** include tremor, slowed movement, muscular rigidity, and impaired balance (among others). **Dystonia** is manifested in painful muscle spasms, often of the face, neck, and jaw. **Akathisia** shows itself as extreme motor restlessness, the need to move around, and inability to sit still. TD is described separately later. Akathisia and dystonia should be reported to the physician, because they are very distressing, and treatable. While they persist, the occupational therapy professional can help the client with managing the effects (see Table 8.7).

The second-generation drugs have a lower incidence of motor side effects. Postural hypotension may also occur; the person's BP drops on rising—from lying to sitting or from sitting to standing—causing dizziness or fainting. Side effects are most unpleasant during the first 10 days of treatment. After this time, movement disorders tend to diminish, although the cholinergic effects (dry mouth and blurred vision) may remain. The general public has a low opinion of antipsychotic medication and its side effects; this may cause problems for clients who listen to friends or family and who then stop taking their medication. Thus, the occupational therapy professional and all other staff need to support the client in maintaining medication adherence.

TD is the most serious side effect of the antipsychotic drugs and is primarily (but not exclusively) associated with the older, first-generation, drugs. TD does not happen right away; it may occur after a person has been taking an antipsychotic for a long time, often for years. It is a movement disorder that may become permanent unless the client stops taking the medication. The initial signs include facial movements, writhing motions of the tongue, and small writhing motions of the fingers. Any suspected signs of TD should be reported to the physician immediately. Some persons develop permanent TD if their medication is not discontinued soon enough. This movement disorder is disfiguring and embarrassing, and may cause social rejection, impairments at work, and feelings of depression. Despite this, some persons may be quite unconcerned. On noticing that someone who is receiving antipsychotic medication is displaying any behaviors that seem similar to those described here, the physician or nurse should be contacted immediately and the report documented in the chart.

Neuroleptic malignant syndrome (NMS) is a rare but life-threatening effect of first-generation antipsychotic medication. Symptoms include extreme hyperthermia, severe muscular rigidity and dystonia, akinesia, mutism, confusion, agitation, and increased pulse rate and BP (17, p. 113). Any client taking these antipsychotics who suddenly becomes rigid or unresponsive requires medical evaluation for NMS.

Currently, there are clinical trials for a third-generation antipsychotic drug (2). This drug is called SEP-363856. Whereas first- and second-generation antipsychotics work as antagonists, blocking certain neurotransmitter receptors, SEP-363856 works as an agonist to certain neurotransmitter receptors (10). In a clinical trial study with adults who were experiencing an acute schizophrenia exacerbation, those who were given SEP-363856 experienced a significant decrease in both positive and negative symptoms. Further clinical trials and research need to be conducted to determine the full potential of this drug.

Antiparkinsonian Drugs

Because EPS is a frequent but unwelcome side effect of antipsychotic medication, antiparkinsonian drugs are often prescribed along with first-generation drugs (Table 8.2). Examples of drugs to treat medication-related movement disorders are benztropine (Cogentin), biperiden (Akineton), and amantadine (Symmetrel). These drugs reduce the EPS, enabling the person to engage more easily in activities in which physical coordination is a factor. Unfortunately, these drugs may exacerbate dry mouth, blurred vision, dizziness, and nausea.

Antidepressant Drugs

The major therapeutic value of antidepressant drugs is relief from depression and the risk of suicide and social withdrawal associated with it (Table 8.3). However, because of an increased risk of suicide in persons under age 25, the Food and Drug Administration (FDA) requires a black-box warning for all antidepressants (5). Often, the physician prescribes brief trials of different drugs before the one that produces the desired effect for a particular person is identified. Unfortunately, no one has yet found a way to predict which drug will be effective for a given person. In addition, an antidepressant that is effective initially may become less effective over time. Again, the reasons for this are unknown. The physician may recommend a larger dose or a switch to another medication.

Chemically, antidepressants can be classified by their effects on neurotransmitters. Five classes are recognized by their actions (17):

1. Blocking reuptake (presynaptic nerve ending absorbing its secreted neurotransmitter) of norepinephrine and serotonin. These are the **tricyclics** and **tetracyclics**.

Table 8.2. Therapeutic and Adverse Effects of Antiparkinsonian Medications

Generic Name (Trade Name)	Selected Therapeutic Effects (Vary Based on Drug)	Selected Side Effects (Vary Based on Drug)
Amantadine (Symmetrel) Benztropine (Cogentin) Biperiden (Akineton) Diphenhydramine (Benadryl) Orphenadrine (Norflex, Disipal) Ethopropazine (Parsitan) Procyclidine (Kemadrin) Propranolol (Inderal) Trihexyphenidyl (Artane)	Control of EPS caused by the use of antipsychotic medications (relief from or reduction of akathisia, akinesia, dystonic reactions, etc.)	Dry mouth, blurred vision, dizziness, nausea, fatigue, weakness Propranolol may cause life-threatening **cardiac symptoms**

EPS, extrapyramidal symptoms.
Data from Sadock, B. J., Sussman, N., & Sadock, V. A. (2019). *Kaplan & Sadock's pocket handbook of psychiatric `drug treatment* (7th ed.). Wolters Kluwer.

Table 8.3. Therapeutic and Adverse Effects of Antidepressant Drugs

Class	Generic Name (Trade Name)	Selected Therapeutic Effects (Vary Based on Drug)	Selected Side Effects (Vary Based on Drug)
Tricyclics and tetracyclics	Amitriptyline (Elavil) Amoxapine (Asendin) Clomipramine (Anafranil) Desipramine (Norpramin, Pertofrane) Doxepin (Sinequan) Imipramine (Tofranil) Maprotiline (Ludiomil) Nortriptyline (Pamelor, Aventyl) Trimipramine (Surmontil)	Relief from depression Reduction in suicidal ideation and risk of suicide Increased activity Normalization of sleep, appetite	Drowsiness, nausea, blurred vision, weight gain, dry mouth, tremors, delirium, sedation, light-headedness, increased blood pressure, constipation **Arrhythmia, seizures, urinary retention, orthostatic hypotension, narrow-angle glaucoma** Potentiate effects of alcohol Suicidal patients may try to overdose; large quantities can be fatal
Selective serotonin reuptake inhibitors (SSRIs)	Citalopram (Celexa) Escitalopram (Lexapro) Fluvoxamine (Luvox; not approved in United States] Fluoxetine (Prozac) Sertraline (Zoloft) Paroxetine (Paxil) Vilazodone (Viibryd)	Relief from depression Reduction in suicidal ideation and risk of suicide Increased activity Normalization of sleep	Fewer side effects than other antidepressants, but does include: sexual dysfunction, anxiety, nausea, headaches possible, long-term weight gain, sleep disturbances, sweating, constipation, subtle cognitive deficits, decreased blood sodium concentration, fatigue, emotional blunting, may cause an acute decrease in glucose concentration Signs of **serotonin syndrome: diarrhea, restlessness, agitation, hyperreflexia, autonomic instability, myoclonus, seizures, hyperthermia, uncontrollable shivering, rigidity, delirium** **Increased risk of suicidal tendencies**[a]
Norepinephrine and dopamine reuptake inhibitor	Bupropion (Wellbutrin)	Relief from depression Reduction in suicidal ideation and risk of suicide Treatment for Seasonal Affective Disorder Increased activity Normalization of sleep, appetite Less likely to provoke a switch to manic state May have less negative effect on libido	Insomnia, seizures, orthostatic hypotension, dry mouth, memory impairment, headache, tremor, restlessness **Psychotic symptoms: hallucinations, delusions, catatonia, delirium**
SNRIs	Duloxetine (Cymbalta) Levomilnacipran (Fetzima) Venlafaxine (Effexor)	Relief from depression Reduction in suicidal ideation and risk of suicide Increased activity Normalization of sleep May work more quickly than some other antidepressants	Increased suicidal thinking[a] Sleepiness or insomnia, headache, nervousness, dry mouth, increased blood pressure, decreased libido, nausea
Serotonin antagonists/ reuptake inhibitors (SA/RI)b	Nefazodone (Serzone) Trazodone (Desyrel)	Relief from depression Normalization of sleep	Orthostatic hypotension, nausea, dry mouth, dizziness, sleepiness, cardiac arrhythmias **Priapism (painful, long-lasting erection)**
Noradrenergic and specific serotonergic inhibitor	Mirtazapine (Remeron)	Relief from depression Helps reduce anxiety, agitation, nausea, and diarrhea Increases appetite May have faster onset of effects than other antidepressants	Fatigue, sleepiness, impaired psychomotor functioning, dry mouth, constipation, myalgia, weight gain, dizziness

Table 8.3. Therapeutic and Adverse Effects of Antidepressant Drugs (*continued*)			
Class	**Generic Name (Trade Name)**	**Selected Therapeutic Effects (Vary Based on Drug)**	**Selected Side Effects (Vary Based on Drug)**
Monoamine oxidase inhibitors (MAOIs)	Irreversible non-selective: Isocarboxazid (Marplan) Phenelzine (Nardil) Tranylcypromine (Parnate) Irreversible selective: Selegiline (Eldepryl) Reversible selective: Moclobemide (Manerix; not approved in United States]	Relief from depression Reduction in suicidal ideation and risk of suicide Increased activity Normalization of sleep, appetite May be effective in ADHD Treatment for atypical depression[d]	Paresthesias, myoclonus, muscle pain, orthostatic hypotension, nausea, weight gain, edema, insomnia, dizziness, sexual dysfunction, restricted diet, induction of mania for those in depressed phase of bipolar I, psychotic decomposition in those with schizophrenia **Tyramine-induced hypertensive crisis: sweating, myocardial injury,[c] headache, stiff neck, severe hypertension Serotonin syndrome: tremor, hypertonicity, myoclonus, autonomic signs**

ADHD, attention-deficit/hyperactivity disorder; SNRIs, serotonin and norepinephrine reuptake inhibitors.
[a]Data from Bielefeldt, A. Ø., Danbort, P. B., & Gøtzsche, P. C. (2016). Precursors to suicidality and violence on antidepressants: Systematic review of trials in adult healthy volunteers. *Journal of the Royal Society of Medicine, 109*(10), 381–392.
[b]Data from Chang, J. P.-C., Zamparelli, A., Nettis, M. A., & Pariante, C. M. (2021). Antidepressant drugs: Mechanisms of action and side effects. In S. D. Sala (Ed.), *Encyclopedia of behavioral neuroscience* (pp. 613–626). Elsevier.
[c]Data from Salter, M., & Kenny, A. (2018). Myocardial injury from tranylcypromine-induced hypertensive crisis secondary to excessive tyramine intake. *Cardiovascular Toxicology, 18*(6), 583–586.
[d]Atypical depression includes: mood reactivity, extreme sensitivity to interpersonal loss or rejection, hyperphagia, hypersomnia, prominent anergia.
Data, unless noted otherwise, from Sadock, B. J., Sussman, N., & Sadock, V. A. (2019). *Kaplan & Sadock's pocket handbook of psychiatric drug treatment* (7th ed.). Wolters Kluwer.

2. Blocking monoamine oxidase's (enzyme on mitochondria) removal of norepinephrine, serotonin, and dopamine. These are the **monoamine oxidase inhibitors** (MAOIs).
3. Blocking reuptake of norepinephrine and possibly dopamine. This is a **norepinephrine and dopamine reuptake inhibitor**.
4. Blocking presynaptic receptors for norepinephrine and serotonin. This is a **noradrenergic and specific serotonergic** inhibitor.
5. Blocking the reuptake of serotonin alone are SSRIs or **selective serotonin reuptake inhibitors**. Or blocking the reuptake of both serotonin and norepinephrine are **serotonin and norepinephrine reuptake inhibitors** (SNRIs).

The tricyclics and the MAOIs are older medications and are used less often today but may still be prescribed. Common side effects of tricyclic antidepressants include dry mouth, blurred vision, and constipation (these can be relieved with lemon drops, magnifying glasses, and bran, respectively). **Epileptic seizures** may also be precipitated in susceptible individuals. When stopped, all antidepressants produce withdrawal symptoms; therefore, the drug should be tapered off gradually under physician supervision. The tricyclics were the first antidepressants to be prescribed for most cases (17). However, a significant danger of overdose exists, because taking a large quantity at one time may be fatal. Also, they create a feeling of being drugged or sleepy.

MAOIs produce an antidepressant effect by interfering with the breakdown of certain brain chemicals. These drugs may be prescribed for people who have shown a poor response to SSRIs (17). MAOIs also take up to 3 weeks to reach their full effect (12), and they are appropriate only for those who are willing to follow a strict dietary regimen (17). The amino acid tyramine interacts with MAOIs to cause a **tyramine-induced hypertensive crisis**. Signs and symptoms of this crisis include severe paroxysmal hypertension, severe headache, stiff neck, pallor, excessive sweating, nausea, vomiting, extreme prostration, which may lead to intracerebral hemorrhage, hypertensive encephalopathy, or acute hypertensive heart failure (17, 20). When working with clients who are using MAOIs, occupational therapy intervention that involves meal preparation or consumption of foods or beverages should be modified to avoid foods and beverages that contain tyramine. Alcoholic beverages such as liqueurs and cocktails can cause orthostasis, when mixed with MAOIs, and should thus also be avoided. Box 8.1 lists several food and beverages that should not be consumed (17). When persons taking MAOIs are participating in occupational therapy, a complete list of unsafe foods and beverages should be obtained from a physician, nurse, or clinical dietician.

Bupropion (Wellbutrin) increases the transmission of norepinephrine and possibly dopamine. It has advantages in that it can be used to treat seasonal affective disorder and does not cause sexual side effects (as some other antidepressants do). In addition, it has an alerting quality, whereas most of the other antidepressants are sedating. This may interfere with sleep and may cause agitation in susceptible individuals (17).

Remeron (mirtazapine) acts by increasing the release of serotonin and norepinephrine in the presynaptic gap. As in the case of bupropion, its sexual side effects are minimal. It may cause weight gain, sedation, and dizziness. It may be prescribed with other antidepressants to assist with counteracting other drugs' side effects of nausea, agitation, and insomnia (17).

increases and becomes toxic. Signs and symptoms of this syndrome appear in an ever-worsening order (17):

1. diarrhea;
2. restlessness;
3. extreme agitation, hyperreflexia, and autonomic instability with possible rapid fluctuations in vital signs;
4. myoclonus, seizures, hyperthermia, uncontrollable shivering, and rigidity; and
5. delirium, coma, status epilepticus, cardiovascular collapse, and death (17, p. 203).

The SNRIs are thought by some to be more effective in achieving remission of depression, as opposed to just relief of depressive symptoms. They may cause high BP and have sexual side effects similar to those associated with the SSRIs (17).

All antidepressants take time to become effective; most do not begin to take effect until at least 7 to 10 days after they are first ingested, and they reach full effectiveness only after 3 weeks.

Mood Stabilizers

Mood-stabilizing drugs reduce intensity of mood swings and control the symptoms of mania (Table 8.4). They are prescribed for bipolar and related disorders. Lithium drugs (Table 8.4) contain lithium carbonate, a common metal salt. Lithium is toxic, and, therefore, frequent blood tests (~ every 2–6 months) are performed to ascertain the level of lithium in the blood. Side effects of lithium include thirst, diarrhea, frequent urination, fatigue, hand tremor, impaired memory, and worsening psoriasis.

The SSRIs produce fewer side effects than do the tricyclics or MAOIs. However, sexual dysfunction (decreased libido and inhibited orgasm) commonly affects people taking these drugs. Furthermore, sometimes the SSRIs become less effective over time, and the person again becomes depressed, requiring a switch to a different medication (17).

One very serious side effect of the SSRIs is **serotonin syndrome**. It can occur when the person is taking an SSRI and another medication such as an MAOI or lithium. In serotonin syndrome, the plasma serotonin concentration

Table 8.4. Therapeutic and Adverse Effects of Mood-Stabilizing Drugs

Class	Generic Name (Trade Name)	Selected Therapeutic Effects (Vary Based on Drug)	Selected Side Effects (Vary Based on Drug)
Antimania	Lithium carbonate (Eskalith, Lithotabs, Lithonate) Lithium citrate[a] (Lithobid)	Treatment for acute manic episodes of bipolar I and for maintenance of bipolar I Treatment of mixed episodes of mania and depression Treatment for severe cyclothymic disorder Treatment of rapid cycling bipolar disorder Treatment of depression associated with bipolar I Prophylactic effect for mania, more so than for depression, in bipolar I Help reduce incidence of suicide for those with bipolar I	80% of clients using lithium experience side effects Bradycardia, cardiac arrhythmias, weight gain, fatigue, thirst, nausea, decreased appetite, vomiting, diarrhea, tremor (if person has hypokalemia, supplements of potassium may help improve tremor), dysphoria, decreased spontaneity, decreased reaction time, impaired memory, mild Parkinsonism, ataxia, dysarthria, polyuria with secondary polydipsia, imbalance of circulating thyroid hormones, worsening psoriasis, acne resembling papules and pustules, leukocytosis that is benign and reversible Changes in body's water and salt can affect lithium amount excreted by the body, causing changes for lithium concentrations in the body. Excessive sodium intake causes decrease in lithium concentration. Too little sodium intake can cause possible toxic levels of lithium in the body. A decrease in body fluids (such as through perspiration) can cause dehydration and lithium intoxication. **Lithium toxicity: coarse tremor, dysarthria, ataxia, gastrointestinal problems, cardiac and renal dysfunction, impaired consciousness, muscular fasciculations, myoclonus, seizures, coma**

Table 8.4. Therapeutic and Adverse Effects of Mood-Stabilizing Drugs (*continued*)

Class	Generic Name (Trade Name)	Selected Therapeutic Effects (Vary Based on Drug)	Selected Side Effects (Vary Based on Drug)
Anticonvulsants	Carbamazepine (Tegretol)	Acute antimanic effects Prevention of relapses with bipolar II, schizoaffective disorder, and dysphoric mania Does not cause weight gain Increased tolerance to side effects, over time	Mild gastrointestinal symptoms and central nervous system symptoms (ataxia, drowsiness), double or blurred vision, vertigo, benign maculopapular rash, hyponatremia, water intoxication May cause birth defects, liver damage, and heart damage Life-threatening dermatologic syndromes: **exfoliative dermatitis, erythema multiforme, Stevens–Johnson syndrome, toxic epidermal necrolysis** **Blood dyscrasias (aplastic anemia, agranulocytosis); symptoms to be aware of that can precede condition are: fever, sore throat, rash, petechiae, bruising, easy bleeding** (condition is rare but dangerous)
	Valproate (Depakote, Depakene)	Manic episodes associated with bipolar I Some response to bipolar I depressive episodes (more so for agitation than for dysphoria) May be beneficial as a prophylactic for bipolar I Rapid onset of medication's action Well tolerated	Nausea, vomiting, indigestion, diarrhea, sedation, ataxia, dysarthria, tremor, weight gain Neural tube defects **Liver toxicity (includes symptoms of lethargy, malaise, anorexia, nausea, vomiting, edema, abdominal pain); pancreatitis; hyperammonemia-induced encephalopathy; thrombocytopenia**
	Lamotrigine (Lamictal)	Maintenance treatment for bipolar I (more so to extend time between depressive episodes than between manic episodes) Well tolerated	Dizziness, ataxia, headache, drowsiness, diplopia, blurred vision, nausea, cognitive impairment, joint or back pain **Initial benign maculopapular rash that develops into Stevens–Johnson syndrome or toxic epidermal necrolysis**

[a]Data from Tucker, R. G. (2022). *2022 Lippincott pocket drug guide for nurses.* Wolters Kluwer.
Data, unless noted otherwise, from Sadock, B. J., Sussman, N., & Sadock, V. A. (2019). *Kaplan & Sadock's pocket handbook of psychiatric drug treatment* (7th ed.). Wolters Kluwer.

Lithium toxicity can occur for a variety of reasons. Risk factors for lithium toxicity include taking more of the medication than what is prescribed; renal dysfunction, a diet low in sodium; dehydration; and interactions with certain other drugs. There are early signs and symptoms of lithium toxicity as well as later signs and symptoms.

- The early signs and symptoms of lithium toxicity include neurologic symptoms, such as coarse tremor, dysarthria, and ataxia; GI symptoms; cardiovascular changes; and renal dysfunction.
- The later signs and symptoms include impaired consciousness, muscular fasciculations, myoclonus, seizures, and coma (17, p. 137).

The other major group of medications used for bipolar disorder are the anticonvulsants, also shown in Table 8.4. The mechanism by which anticonvulsants control moods is not clear. Lithium and an anticonvulsant can be prescribed to be taken at the same time.

Anxiolytic Drugs

Anxiolytic drugs are antianxiety and antipanic drugs with a hypnotic or sleep-inducing effect. Some of the drugs have also been identified to help with agitation, insomnia, muscle spasms, and symptoms of alcohol withdrawal (Table 8.5). There are a variety of classes of drugs that are considered anxiolytic drugs (17).

- Benzodiazepines: affect benzodiazepine receptors
- Nonbenzodiazepine Z drugs: bind to receptors close to benzodiazepine receptors
- Antihistamine (hydroxyzine): target the H_1 receptors
- Azapirone (buspirone): affinity for serotonin receptors and dopamine receptors
- Orexin receptor antagonist (suvorexant): blocks chemical function of orexin (which works to keep person awake and alert) (17)

A concern with all anxiolytic drugs is using them concurrently with alcohol (17). This combination can intensify the sedating effect and increase risk of injury or harm when driving or using tools.

The drug flumazenil (Romazicon) is a benzodiazepine receptor antagonist. It is used to reverse the sedating, psychomotor, and amnestic benzodiazepine-induced effects present in a benzodiazepine overdose. The side effects of flumazenil include nausea, vomiting, dizziness, agitation, emotional lability, increased blood flow to the skin, fatigue, impaired vision, headache, and **seizures**.

Table 8.5. Therapeutic and Adverse Effects of Anxiolytic Drugs

Class	Generic Name (Trade Name)	Selected Therapeutic Effects (Vary Based on Drug)	Selected Side Effects (Vary Based on Drug)
Benzodiazepines	Alprazolam (Xanax) Clonazepam (Klonopin) Clorazepate (Tranxene) Chlordiazepoxide (Librium) Diazepam (Valium) Estazolam (ProSom) Flurazepam (Dalmane) Lorazepam (Ativan) Midazolam (Versed) Oxazepam (Serax) Temazepam (Restoril) Triazolam (Halcion) Quazepam (Doral)	Reduction of anxiety, agitation Panic reduction (alprazolam, clonazepam, clorazepate) Reduction of social phobia (clonazepam) Reduction of symptoms of alcohol withdrawal (chlordiazepoxide, clorazepate) Relief from muscle spasm Relief from insomnia (flurazepam, temazepam, triazolam) Reduce akathisia (a feeling of inner restlessness, mental distress, and inability to sit still)[a]	Dizziness, drowsiness, mild cognitive impairment, daytime residual sedation, rapid onset of sleep, ataxia, weight gain and appetite stimulant (alprazolam) When used concurrently with alcohol: marked drowsiness, disinhibition, respiratory depression Manifestation of serious aggressive behavior (triazolam) **benzodiazepine intoxication includes confusion, slurred speech, ataxia, drowsiness, dyspnea, and hyporeflexia** (p. 68) **Benzodiazepine withdrawal syndrome consists of anxiety, nervousness, diaphoresis, restlessness, irritability, fatigue, light-headedness, tremor, insomnia, and weakness** (p. 69)
Nonbenzodiazepine Z drugs	Eszopiclone (Lunesta) Zaleplon (Sonata) Zolpidem (Ambien)	Reduce insomnia	Zolpidem: automatic behavior, amnesia, hallucinations zolpidem and zaleplon: dizziness, drowsiness, diarrhea, indigestion eszopiclone: in those who are elderly: pain, dry mouth, unpleasant taste
Antihistamine	Hydroxyzine (Atarax)	Short-term use Sedative effect Reduction of anxiety	Sedation, dizziness, hypotension, decreased motor coordination, gastrointestinal problems, dry mouth, urinary retention, blurred vision
Azapirone	Buspirone (BuSpar)	Treatment for generalized anxiety disorder May be more effective than benzodiazepines for anger and hostility management Does not: sedate, have a potential for dependence or abuse, adverse cognitive and psychomotor effects, typically cause weight gain or cause sexual dysfunction	Headache, nausea, dizziness, insomnia (rare), minor restlessness Does not have muscle relaxant effects Delayed initial effect of 2–4 wk
Orexin receptor antagonist	Suvorexant (Belsomra)	Keep person awake and alert	Residual daytime sedation

[a]Data from American Psychological Association. (n.d.). *APA Dictionary of Psychology: Akathisia.* Retrieved April 24, 2022, from https://dictionary.apa.org/akathisia
Data, unless noted otherwise, from Sadock, B. J., Sussman, N., & Sadock, V. A. (2019). *Kaplan & Sadock's pocket handbook of psychiatric drug treatment* (7th ed.). Wolters Kluwer.

Drugs for Attention-Deficit/Hyperactivity Disorder (ADHD)

Medications prescribed for ADHD are shown in Table 8.6. The use of both stimulants and norepinephrine reuptake inhibitors (NRIs) is indicated to reduce symptoms of ADHD. Side effects can include impaired growth, tics, insomnia, dysphoria, and Raynaud Phenomenon (5, 7, 17, 18). Serious adverse effects can include the possible **increase in suicidal thoughts and actions** during the first few months the person is taking the medication (18).

Stimulant use must be monitored because those who use them can be at risk for abuse or dependency of the drug (5, 17). Serdexmethylphenidate/dexmethylphenidate (Azstarys) is a stimulant that blocks the reuptake of norepinephrine and dopamine (5). It is the first medication for ADHD to combine the use of serdexmethylphenidate and dexmethylphenidate. The dexmethylphenidate is released on entering the body, and the serdexmethylphenidate is absorbed by the body over several hours. This combination means the drug begins to work quickly as well as continues to work for an extended number of hours (7).

Table 8.6. Therapeutic and Adverse Effects of Medications for Attention-Deficit Disorders

Class	Generic Name (Trade Name)	Selected Therapeutic Effects (Vary Based on Drug)	Selected Side Effects (Vary Based on Drug)
Stimulant	Methylphenidate (Ritalin) Dextroamphetamine (Dexedrine) Dextroamphetamine and mixed amphetamine salts (Adderall) serdexmethylphenidate/dexmethyl-phenidate (Azstarys)[a]	Reduces hyperactivity Improves attention span Reduces Impulsivity Reduces symptoms of ADHD[a]	Anxiety, irritability, insomnia, tachycardia, stomach irritation, cardiac arrhythmias, dysphoria, decreased appetite (tolerance to this typically develops), increased heart rate, tics Increased blood pressure and heart rate, cause manic symptoms in persons without prior history, **priapism**, Raynaud Phenomenon, long-term growth suppression, risk of abuse and dependence[a]
NRI	Atomoxetine (Strattera) Viloxazine[c] (Qelbree)	Treatment of symptoms for ADHD Less likely to provoke excited mood or euphoria (atomoxetine) Not a controlled substance, therefore limiting abuse potential[b] (sad)	Atomoxetine: insomnia, dizziness, nausea and abdominal pain, anxiety, blood pressure irregularities[c] Viloxazine: sleepiness, decreased appetite, nausea, vomiting, difficulty sleeping, irritability[d] **May increase suicidal thoughts and actions, especially in first few months of treatment (viloxazine)[d]**

ADHD, attention-deficit/hyperactivity disorder; NRI, norepinephrine reuptake inhibitor.

[a]Data from Food and Drug Administration. (2021, March). *Azstarys*. Reference ID: 4755866. Retrieved April 24, 2022, from https://www.accessdata.fda.gov/drugsatfda_docs/label/2021/212994s000lbl.pdf

[b]Data from Yu, C., Garcia-Olivares, J., Candler, S., Schwabe, S., & Maletic, V. (2020). New insights into the mechanism of action of viloxazine: Serotonin and norepinephrine modulating properties. *Journal of Experimental Pharmacology, 12*, 285–300.

[c]Data from National Alliance on Mental Illness. (2021). *Atomoxetine (Strattera)*. Retrieved April 24, 2022, from https://www.nami.org/About-Mental-Illness/Treatments/Mental-Health-Medications/Types-of-Medication/Atomoxetine-(Strattera)

[d]Data from Supernus Pharmaceuticals. (2021). *Qelbree: Discover an ADHD treatment that helps make symptoms manageable*. Retrieved April 24, 2022, from https://www.qelbree.com/pediatrics

Data, unless noted otherwise, from Sadock, B. J., Sussman, N., & Sadock, V. A. (2019). *Kaplan & Sadock's pocket handbook of psychiatric drug treatment* (7th ed.). Wolters Kluwer.

CONSUMER CONCERNS RELATED TO MEDICATIONS

It is common to experience problems with medication. These are complex chemicals that affect the brain and the body. Generic forms may not be as effective as brand name versions. The consumer may not tolerate some inactive ingredients used to aid in absorption of the medication or improve taste or appearance (15). Time-release versions of medication will not be absorbed by the digestive system in the same way in different individuals (4).

Adherence (taking medications as prescribed) can be difficult to achieve for several reasons. Taking medication feels unnatural; it is inconvenient. Consumers may complain that the medication is toxic or that it makes them less healthy (6). Side effects are unpleasant. Often, the side effects are obviously long before any therapeutic effect is achieved. Medications may not reach effective levels for some time, up to several weeks. Complicated dosing regimens that involve taking pills at different times of the day are hard to follow. Taking several medications, some to counteract the effects of others, may feel overwhelming. The cost of medication or the insurance co-pays may be an unacceptable financial burden. The person may decide to buy the drugs at a lower cost over the internet and then receive something other than what was prescribed (4). The person may be taking other substances (including street drugs) and prefer those. The person may be feeling better (because the drug is working) and decide it is not needed. The rate of **nonadherence** (not taking prescribed medication) is estimated at more than 50% within 1 year, which is similar to what happens with medications prescribed for physical conditions such as high BP (3, 6, 14).

The prescribing physician may require some time and a few attempts to determine the best medication(s) for an individual. Not everyone responds in the same way. And the initial diagnosis may prove incorrect. Some medications may require 6 weeks to become effective (or to be shown as ineffective). And the **half-life** (amount of time for the drug to fall to one half of its initial level) may be prolonged. A person may be coming off one medication, and starting another, or waiting until one gets out of the body before beginning something else. A medication at a given dosage level may be effective for a period of time, and then stop working, or may need to be increased in dosage to regain the same effect. This can feel tiresome, and the person may begin to think there is no hope.

Adherence to a medication schedule may fail for reasons related to client factors, such as physical or cognitive deficits. Older persons, those with arthritis, and those with sensory deficits or problems with fingertip dexterity may find it difficult to open or close the containers. Deficits in fingertip dexterity or sensation can interfere with handling the pills (Figure 8.1). Swallowing may be a problem. Vision deficits may cause the person to take the wrong medicine by accident. The prescribing pharmacy may switch to a different generic that has a different color than the one the person was used to. The person may not remember to take the medication at the correct time, and then compensate for a missed dose, or may not recall which medication is which. Some individuals may mix several different kinds of medication together in one container and then not recall which one is to be taken at what time (Figure 8.2).

Family and caregivers may deliberately or inadvertently undermine the medication plan. A spouse whose partner has lost interest in sex because of a medication may advise the person to stop taking it. Families may feel that the person is too medicated. Caregivers may change the time the medication is given because the dosing schedule is inconvenient for them (4). Families and caregivers need education and support to guide them in following the plan.

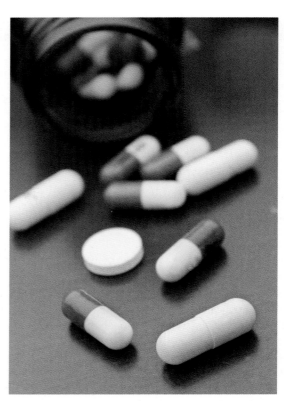

Figure 8.2. Storing Several Medications in the Same Container Makes It Difficult to Remember the Name, Purpose, Dosage, and Schedule for Each One. (Image from Shutterstock.)

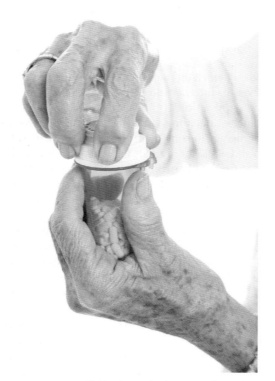

Figure 8.1. Aging Individuals and Those With Arthritis or Diminished Sensation Will Have Difficulty Opening Medication Containers. (Image from Shutterstock.)

Nonadherence used to be called **noncompliance**, which suggested that the patient was being uncooperative by refusing to comply with medical orders. The recovery movement has brought about a new understanding in which the consumer is more involved and is empowered to ask questions, to state preferences, and to share in decision-making. Collaboration between consumers and their physicians is a better starting place for achieving adherence than is a top-down medical model. In an inpatient setting, and in times of crises, consumer participation in making decisions about medication may not be possible or advisable. Equally, children and persons with neurocognitive disorders will have less ability to participate in making decisions.

POINT-OF-VIEW

Reasons for adherence:

- "I started to get my life back and have some degree of normality."
- "Meds keep my head just above water."
- "My psychiatrist is fantastic with e-mail access and I have her mobile number."

Selected service user comments concerning reasons for adherence to medication plan (6).

Reasons for nonadherence

- "Didn't like the sedative side effects."
- "I was working nights and needed to feel alert during the night."
- "I had a meeting at work the next day, so I skipped my evening dose."
- "I was once very active and went to the gym 4 times a week; now I have become lethargic and fatigued from my medication."

Selected service user comments concerning reasons for nonadherence (6).

The Roles of the Occupational Therapy Professionals

Since occupational therapy professionals do not themselves prescribe medication, how can they be helpful to the client and to the physician? Occupational therapy professionals may interact regularly with the client or consumer, in contrast to the psychiatrist who sees the person once a week or less frequently. Thus, occupational therapy professionals may become aware of information and behavioral change, of which the psychiatrist may be unaware.

Observing and Reporting Functional Level

Psychotropic medications affect the client's occupational performance and functional skills. By providing a baseline evaluation of the person's functional skills before the medication is started, the occupational therapist establishes a point for comparison. The occupational therapy professional can follow the patient's progress and report improvements or problems to the physician. This is helpful in determining whether a medication is likely to be beneficial. When medication is working as it is intended, the client should be more able to engage in daily life routines and avoid episodes that may lead to hospitalization or crisis. Sometimes, clients do not focus on the positive effects, and it helps to remind them of how well they are doing now, in contrast to before taking medication.

Issues Related to Adherence and to Use of Other Medications and Substances

Clients may stray from their treatment plans to achieve balance and manage side effects in relation to the demands of everyday life. It is not uncommon for someone to take a little more medication, or a little less, or at a different time of day. Individuals may or may not communicate these changes to the physician. The occupational therapy professional should coach the person to report these changes to the doctor. If the person will not, the occupational therapy professional should reach out to the doctor.

Negative effects contribute to nonadherence and place the person at risk of relapse. Among the adverse effects are tremors, mental slowing, diminished alertness, excessive sedation, weight gain, and lethargy. Clients diagnosed with bipolar disorder who previously enjoyed high energy levels during manic episodes may feel diminished and unable to be productive and creative. People may also get busy and forget to take a medication at the scheduled time. People who have been physically active may stop going to the gym and working out because they feel fatigued or sedated (6). Motor and vision effects such as incoordination or blurred vision may interfere with the use of machines and tools, as well as with driving (8). The occupational therapy professional can be helpful to the client by observing medication-related changes that affect functional skills and by inviting the client to discuss them. In addition, the occupational therapy professional should communicate these changes to the physician.

Another area in which an occupational therapy professional can be helpful is in detecting and reporting the use of other medications or substances. Clients are often prescribed more than one type of medication. For example, an antipsychotic may be used with lithium to reduce acute psychotic symptoms of mania. Not only are different psychotropic drugs used in combination with each other but also clients who have medical problems are generally taking other medications as well, including perhaps over-the-counter (OTC) drugs and herbal preparations. Because drugs interact with each other, the physician is especially careful to prescribe only medications that are compatible with the ones the person is already taking. Use of drugs that are not prescribed or not documented in the medical record (eg, street drugs or drugs prescribed by the family physician for a medical problem or herbal supplements such as St. John's wort and valerian) should be reported to the psychiatrist in charge of the case. Ideally, the occupational therapy professional would encourage the client to report this, as it is much more empowering for the person to self-manage medication as much as possible.

Management of Side Effects

Although occupational therapy professionals cannot prescribe medications or reduce their undesirable side effects, they can help clients learn to identify, tolerate, and adapt to the way their bodies respond to these side effects. Table 8.7 lists selected side effects and provides strategies the occupational therapy professional can employ to help clients deal with them and function better.

Like anyone prescribed a drug with unwelcome effects, the person with a mental disorder may find the cure worse than the disease. Feeling like a zombie, feeling restless and wound up, or having no sex life is not pleasant. Even though a medication may be controlling the symptoms of a mental disorder, the person may consider the overall effect not worth it. Furthermore, as discussed previously, family members may be opposed to the person's taking medication. The occupational therapy professional can help by gently guiding the client and by engaging them in discussion and reflection about the day-to-day benefits of the drug and the dangers of relapse and what that would be like. The person who complains about side effects deserves a listening ear and a sympathetic response.

Table 8.7. Drug Side Effects and Recommended Occupational Therapy Adaptations and Interventions

Side Effect	Adaptations and Interventions
Extrapyramidal syndrome	In general, report all symptoms to physician or nurse when first observed and then report changes as they occur
Parkinsonism: muscular rigidity, tremors, drooling, shuffling gait, mask-like face	1. Use gross motor activities that involve rotation of head and trunk 2. Avoid activities that require the patient to work against resistance
Akathisia: restlessness, muscular tension (often worse in the legs than the arms)	1. Help the patient select activities that allow for movement, getting up and down, and so on 2. Avoid activities that require prolonged sitting or standing still 3. Put the patient at a separate table if persistent movement is disruptive to others
Dystonia: painful, sudden muscle spasms, often localized to neck, jaw, eyes, or back; the patient may arch back, roll eyes, and so on	1. The physician should be notified by you or by the patient. 2. Help the patient engage in activities that do not require fine coordination or attention to detail 3. Avoid use of power tools, sharps, and so on
Akinesia: muscular weakness and fatigue, reduction of movement	1. The physician should be notified by you or by the patient 2. Permit breaks in activity 3. Avoid activities in which the patient must work against resistance or for a long time
Tardive dyskinesia (movement disorder thought to be caused by prolonged use of antipsychotics): movement patterns may be choreiform (jerky, twitching) or athetoid (writhing); often include facial distortions such as tongue thrust, lip smacking, tics, and chewing; early signs include facial tics, slight but definitely abnormal eye or lip movements, rocking, swaying	1. *If new,* notify the physician at once; side effects can be reversed if caught early but, if neglected, may become permanent 2. *If chronic* and if the patient is aware and concerned, provide support and encouragement; allow the patient to verbalize embarrassment and discomfort
Postural hypotension: the patient feels faint or blacks out when rising from lying to sitting or from sitting to standing; caused by effect of gravity	1. Notify the physician 2. Teach the patient to sit up slowly, stand up slowly; stand close and be prepared to support the patient at the waist; do not try to support the patient by grabbing the arm 3. Encourage the patient to use furniture and other supports to maintain balance 4. Avoid activities that involve sudden postural changes 5. Avoid gross motor activities to reduce sudden movements
Dry mouth: the patient feels thirsty	1. Allow the patient to get water whenever thirsty 2. Have hard (sucking) candies available; lemon drops are best; some people prefer sugar-free breath mints 3. Teach the patient about dehydrating effect of caffeinated drinks and alcohol
Blurred vision: vision may be blurry or double vision may occur	1. Help the patient select activities that do not involve fine visual attention 2. In gross motor activities, use mats and soft equipment to avoid injury 3. In crafts, use large pieces that are easily seen (eg, 1-inch mosaic tiles) 4. Provide magnified reading glasses (several levels of magnification) to be used in OT clinic
Hand tremors: rhythmic involuntary hand movements (see also *ataxia*)	1. If the patient is on a new trial of a lithium-based mood stabilizing medication and tremor is gross, notify physician; gross bilateral hand tremor may be a sign of drug toxicity 2. Fine hand tremors are common in patients taking lithium for a month or more; help the patient learn to compensate by stabilizing elbow or arm to prevent tremor 3. If the patient is taking an antipsychotic and the tremor has a writhing or wormlike appearance, notify physician; these movements may indicate tardive dyskinesia
Ataxia: failure of muscle coordination, manifested as clumsiness when a motor action is attempted (eg, walking or doing a craft)	1. If the patient is on a new trial of lithium-based antimanic medication, notify the physician immediately, because this may be a sign of drug toxicity 2. Prepare to provide support when the patient gets up out of a chair or turns corners while walking 3. Help the patient select and engage in activities in which incoordination will not interfere with success
Nausea	1. Have soda crackers, graham crackers, and bread available 2. Over-the-counter antacids are sometimes recommended by physician; because these preparations may interfere with action of some antipsychotic and other medications, physicians' approval is required
Photosensitivity: the patient is extremely sensitive to effects of sun and will sunburn after brief exposure; most commonly seen in patients who are taking certain antipsychotics	1. Teach the patient about photosensitizing effect of medications 2. Have the patient wear sunscreen, long sleeves, hat, and sunglasses; be sure the patient applies sunscreen to the tops of feet, backs of hands, earlobes, top of head (bald men) 3. Keep time in sun as brief as possible 4. Observe the patient closely for signs of sunburn

WHAT'S THE EVIDENCE?

Improving medication adherence through different intervention techniques.

These two research studies indicated a significant increase in the mean score for pre- and post administration of the Medication Adherence Rating Scale (MARS) for adults with schizophrenia.

The MARS is a 10-question self-reporting measure that indicates medication adherence, attitudes toward taking medications and the negative side effects associated with taking medications, and attitudes toward taking psychotropic medications (13). Answers demonstrating adherence are scored one point and answers demonstrating nonadherence are scored zero point.

The intervention in the study by Ibeh was an 8-week period of using the Medisafe Reminder App. This device provided notifications when it was time to take medication and tracked both doses taken and doses missed. The average MARS mean score increase from pre- to posttesting was 3.3 points (9).

In the study by Gebreamlak, completion of the MARS was done pre- and post intervention of two sessions of motivational interviewing. The areas addressed during the sessions were identifying difficulties in obtaining medication adherence and motivation toward changing behaviors so that medication adherence could be increased. The average MARS mean score increase from pre- to post testing was 1.7 points (9).

In the study by Gebreamlak, participants were excluded if their past medication adherence was greater than 50%. Why would this be important?

What would be the benefit of using both motivational interviewing and the Medisafe Reminder App together?

Gebreamlak, M. (2019). *The use of motivational interviewing to improve medication adherence among mentally ill patients with schizophrenia* (Order No. 27735863) [Clinical scholarly project, Brandman University]. ProQuest Dissertation Publishing; Ibeh, J. (2021) *Increasing adherence to antipsychotic medication in patients with schizophrenia using mobile app reminder* (Order No. 28549010) [Clinical scholarly project, Brandman University]. ProQuest Dissertation Publishing.

Driving and Other Safety Concerns

Because psychotropic medications can be sedating, it is important to consider the effect on driving. Rouleau and colleagues (16) conducted a survey of mental health therapists in Canada and learned that driving-related services were offered to only 30% of consumers they surveyed. Some people stop driving voluntarily, but others who continue to drive may need assessment and interventions related to driving fitness and behaviors.

Medication Education and Management

In a recovery model, the aim is for the client or consumer to oversee his or her own recovery. Knowledge of medication is part of this. Integrating medication habits into daily routines is another. Being able to talk to one's doctor about medication and finding a doctor who is willing to collaborate in such discussion is yet another. Psychoeducation groups on medication management may cover topics such as the names of medications and their side effects, how to respond to problems in obtaining medication, when to take medication and how to remember to do so, and so on. Important life skills include maintaining a record of drugs taken (including OTC) and reasons for each; reading prescription labels and understanding information; informing physicians when multiple pharmacies are used; and informing the pharmacies about drugs dispensed elsewhere.

Keeping drugs out of the reach of children is critical, as is remembering to take the medications as directed. A variety of pill sorting boxes can be found in drug stores. Automated pill dispensing systems are also available. Many apps exist for smartphones, tablets, and wearable technology such as watches that can help the consumer with medication-related issues.

The occupational therapy professional must support consumers by encouraging them to communicate directly with their doctors, to ask questions, to voice concerns, and to share in decision-making as much as possible.

OTHER BIOLOGIC TREATMENTS

Biologic, or somatic, treatments are those that act on the body to produce an effect on the mind. These include electroconvulsive therapy (ECT) and psychosurgery. ECT is sometimes incorrectly called "shock therapy." The person is given general anesthesia, after which an electrical current is briefly applied to the temples, causing a convulsion. Some medical risk exists owing to the anesthesia. No one is certain why this treatment is effective, but it does relieve severe depression and reduce the risk of suicide in 80% to 90% of depressed individuals who fail to respond to drug therapies. Usually, 8 to 12 ECT treatments are given every other day over several weeks. The only side effects are occasional headaches immediately after a treatment and short-term memory loss lasting a few weeks. Typically, the person does not remember the treatment at all, and the only permanent memory loss may be of events in the few days before the treatment. Clients receiving ECT are often confused and may not remember (for example) who the occupational therapy professional is or that they were working on a particular project in occupational therapy.

Psychosurgery was a common treatment in previous decades,[2] when it was erroneously believed that surgically cutting the connections between the prefrontal cortex and the hypothalamic area of the brain would relieve mental symptoms. This procedure, called a prefrontal lobotomy, often left the client with impaired judgment and a complete lack of motivation. Psychosurgical techniques are occasionally practiced today for relief of seizures and of intractable depression or violence. Gamma radiation surgery is being considered as a treatment for symptoms of obsessive–compulsive disorder (OCD) and is currently in development.

Recent additions to somatic therapies for mental disorders include vagus nerve stimulation (VNS), transcranial magnetic stimulation (TMS), and magnetic seizure therapy. VNS was originally approved to treat seizures. A stimulator is implanted in the chest to stimulate the vagus nerve, a

---

[2]For a detailed and sobering discussion of the history of psychosurgery, see reference (19).

part of the autonomic nervous system. In TMS, an electrical magnetic impulse is applied in short bursts to the client's forehead or scalp; this is considered a milder form of ECT. The same apparatus is used for magnetic seizure therapy, but higher frequencies are used to cause seizures.

Bright light therapy (BLT) uses timed exposure to ultraviolet filtered light (similar to sunlight) to treat depression. The client sits in front of a light box at a specific time of day for 30 to 45 minutes. Eye irritation and skin irritation may occur if the light is not filtered. Clients cannot use this therapy if they are taking medications that make them photosensitive.

HERBAL AND ALTERNATIVE THERAPIES

A variety of herbs, vitamins, and other naturally occurring substances have been used to treat mental disorders. Kava kava (a root from the Pacific Islands) may have some effects in reducing anxiety. St. John's wort (an herb) has been used in Europe for depression. A compound called S-adenosylmethionine (SAMe), a substance that occurs naturally in the brain, also seems to be effective in relieving depression. Valerian (an herb) shows positive effects in patients with insomnia. These and other substances should be used cautiously because dosage and quality control vary by manufacturer and batch. Consumers who are interested in using alternative therapies should be advised to consult with their physician and to follow medical advice.

CONCERNS RELATED TO THE INTERNET

You, as a trained health care provider or student, should be highly skilled at using the internet to obtain information. Some of the consumers you work with may be just as skilled, or more so. However, some clients or service users are not. Erroneous information and marketing may cause consumers to abandon their medication regimens in favor of some other remedy, to order medications from external sources that may not be legitimate, or to try out herbs and vitamins that are advertised as helpful for their symptoms. Be attentive to consumer comments about what they find on the internet, and encourage them to report their concerns or changes to their physician. In medication management psychoeducation groups, a session or two on how to evaluate internet sources can be helpful to those consumers who do not already have this skill (Box 8.2).

DETOXIFICATION[3]

The detoxification (detox) process is often the first phase of the client's recovery from substance misuse or substance abuse. This is the time when the person initially stops using one or more substances and these substances are cleared out of the body. The occupational therapy profession works as a partner, working with the client in a supportive manner and without making judgments about the client or their current situation. Another partner in this collaborative team is the client's social support network. This can include family and

---

[3]All information for detoxification is taken from Substance Abuse and Mental Health Services Administration. (2015, October). *TIP 45: Detoxification and substance abuse treatment*. https://store.samhsa.gov/product/TIP-45-Detoxification-and-Substance-Abuse-Treatment/SMA15-4131

> ### BOX 8.2 Recommended Internet Sources for Drug Information
>
> National Institutes of Health—http://www.nimh.nih.gov/health/publications/mental-health-medications/index.shtml
>
> Physicians' Desk Reference—http://www.pdrhealth.com/drugs

friends who are encouraged to be actively involved with the client in this process.

Professional Qualities

The occupational therapy professional working with someone in active detox must demonstrate specific qualities. When working with the client, the occupational therapy professional should do so in a supportive and nonjudgmental manner, showing empathy and humbleness. When talking with the client, the occupational therapy professional should remain calm and have their own emotions in check. Part of therapeutic use of self is being able to set limits with the client, without enacting a struggle for power. Interactions with the client should be done to demonstrate trust, and they should thus be done on a consistent and reliable basis. When speaking with the client, the occupational therapy professional should present themselves confidently and knowledgeably, showing that they know how to engage with the client during this process as well as when a referral to another mental health care professional is required. The occupational therapy professional should encourage the client to practice self-expression. They should discuss the difficulties the client will face on the path toward recovery and acknowledge the progress the client is making toward their recovery goals. Box 8.3 offers suggestions for how to de-escalate a situation where the client is displaying aggressive behaviors.

Signs and Symptoms of Withdrawal and Medical Treatment

The medical team members (physician, nurse, physical assistant) will identify the detox situation based on medical tests

> ### BOX 8.3 De-Escalation Suggestions for a Client Who Is Displaying Aggressive Actions
>
> - Talk with, not **to** or **at,** the client, using a soft and neutral tone.
> - Remove excessive sensory stimulation from the environment (such as loud conversations, video watching, harsh lighting).
> - Reassure the client of your care and concern.
> - Ask other clients to leave the physical environment.
> - Enlist other staff help as necessary with assisting other clients away from the area, and ask staff to provide additional support if situation escalates.
>
> Adapted from Substance Abuse and Mental Health Services Administration. (2015, October). *TIP 45: Detoxification and substance abuse treatment*. https://store.samhsa.gov/product/TIP-45-Detoxification-and-Substance-Abuse-Treatment/SMA15-4131

to detect the substance (from blood, urine, or breath). They can use subjective reporting instruments with questions about what the client is experiencing, as well as objective assessments to document what actions and behaviors the medical personnel are observing from the client.

The occupational therapy professional, during ongoing intervention throughout the period of detox, will observe signs of withdrawal and hear client's state symptoms they are experiencing. Table 8.8 shows some withdrawal signs and symptoms of alcohol, opioids, sedatives, and stimulants. It should be noted that not all signs and symptoms are listed in Table 8.8 and that each person is different and, therefore, not all signs and symptoms will be seen in all individuals.

Medical treatments will be determined by the medical staff. During the detoxification period from alcohol, the client may be at risk for seizures or delirium tremens (DTs) (a particular state of delirium with severe tremors that can result in death). For those with a history of severe withdrawal symptoms, there is a greater risk of seizures or DTs. Withdrawal from sedatives can also carry the risk of seizures and DTs. Seizures can occur before other withdrawal signs are

Table 8.8. Withdrawal Signs and Symptoms

Sign or Symptom	Alcohol Withdrawal	Opioid Withdrawal	Sedative Withdrawal	Stimulant Withdrawal
Restless or irritable behavior	✔			✔
Insomnia	✔	✔	✔	✔
Decreased energy, sleepiness, or fatigue			✔	✔
Lack of appetite	✔			
Increase in appetite				✔
Tremors	✔		✔	
Muscle spasms		✔		
Bony and/or muscle pain	✔	✔	✔	
Ataxia and incoordination			✔	
Psychomotor retardation				✔
Slurred speech			✔	
Seizure	✔		✔	
Delirium tremens	✔			
Abdominal cramps or Digestive complications	✔	✔	✔	
Anterior chest or cardiac symptoms				✔
Increased heart rate	✔	✔	✔	
Increased blood pressure	✔	✔	✔	
Increased body temperature	✔	✔	✔	
Increased sweating		✔	✔	
Increased respiratory rate		✔		
Decreased attention, concentration, or memory	✔			✔
Increased sensory sensitivity	✔			
Hallucinations (sensory distortion)	✔		✔	
Delusions (false belief or thought process)	✔			
Anxiety	✔	✔	✔	✔
Delirium	✔		✔	
Dysphoria				✔
Depression				✔
Suicide ideation				✔

Adapted from Ackermann, K. (2022, April 4). *Ambien withdrawal: Symptoms, timeline, & detox treatment*. American Addiction Centers. https://americanaddictioncenters.org/withdrawal-timelines-treatments/ambien; American Addiction Centers. (2022, March 15). *Adderall withdrawal symptoms & detox treatment near you*. https://americanaddictioncenters.org/adderall/how-to-quit; Crane, M. (2022, January 7). *Alcohol & benzo detox at home: How to, risks & alternatives*. American Addiction Centers. https://americanaddictioncenters.org/withdrawal-timelines-treatments/alcohol-benzos-at-home; Substance Abuse and Mental Health Services Administration. (2015, October). *TIP 45: Detoxification and substance abuse treatment*. https://store.samhsa.gov/product/TIP-45-Detoxification-and-Substance-Abuse-Treatment/SMA15-4131 identified. During withdrawal from opioids, there is a chance that the client will experience severe gastrointestinal (GI) symptoms, causing vomiting or diarrhea, thus resulting in dehydration or an electrolyte imbalance. If the person has cardiac disease, the increased BP, pulse, and sweating (autonomic arousal) associated with opioid withdrawal can worsen the cardiac problems. Cocaine (stimulant) withdrawal can also produce cardiac problems, including arrhythmia and myocardial infarction.

A mental disorder may be a comorbidity in the person withdrawing from alcohol or other drug substances. The medical team will determine continued use of medications needed for the mental disorder and assess treatment of psychiatric symptoms during the withdrawal period. The occupational therapy professional should be astutely aware and observant of decomposition, or deterioration, associated with the mental disorder and report their findings to the nursing staff.

Assessment

Assessment of the person seeking treatment for substance withdrawal will initially be performed by the medical staff. Medical information available about the client should be reviewed by the occupational therapist prior to an occupational therapy assessment. Medical information important to the assessment process includes overall health history, current mental status, neurologic findings, vital signs, history of substance abuse and admissions for detoxification treatment, and toxicology report. Owing to the medical condition of the client on admission, some psychological aspects of the assessment may be only marginally addressed. Any information available should be reviewed, but these are areas the occupational therapist may specifically assess and in turn be able to add valuable assessment data to the client record. These areas include demographic items such as cultural habits and educational history, current living environment, access to various types of community mobility, financial status, family member information, and performance skill abilities (motor, process, and social interaction).

Assessment of vital signs should be a regular occurrence with each occupational therapy session.

Intervention Considerations During Detoxification

Detoxification is a time for change. The person experiencing detoxification needs to shift from ingesting harmful substances to bringing healthy substances into their body. Occupational therapy professionals view eating as a primary occupation, as well as health management. To this end, occupational therapy should include introducing healthy food choices that are so presented as to encourage the client to try healthy food choices. Reestablishing routine mealtimes is a performance pattern consideration.

During the initial phase of detoxification, owing to withdrawal effects such as GI problems, the person may only be able to digest clear liquids. With increasing tolerance of solid foods, low fat foods, fresh fruits and vegetables, complex carbohydrates such as whole grain breads, protein, and foods with dietary fiber should be suggested. By utilizing the pleasing sensory components of food (visual, olfactory, and gustatory), the occupational therapy professional can aid in promoting consumption of foods not tried before or not eaten while the person was misusing harmful substances. Because the olfactory and gustatory senses are interconnected, the use of enticing aromas can stimulate a desire to partake of meals with new foods. Consideration should also be given to how foods are arranged on the plate and the use of healthy food items with vibrant and pleasing colors.

The client in the detoxification phase can be filled with a wide breadth of emotions. There can be fear, ambivalence, expectations of success with the recovery process, joy, sadness, as well as pain and newly identified needs and wants. Occupational therapy professionals must support the client's recovery attempts and provide hope for success. The environment needs to consider the client's needs for comfort, relaxation, and security. This is a time to engage the client and offer guidance and support for what will be a long-term (truly a life-long) process of change.

The occupational therapy professional needs to motivate the client to seek more and continued recovery services. Some of the continued recovery efforts should be connected to social supports. This can be done through an appropriate 12-step program for substance misuse or abuse recovery. The occupational therapy professional needs to provide therapeutic use of self (addressed in Chapter 15) that demonstrates respect, care, and concern through use of person-first language, collaboration during intervention, and actively listening to the client's questions and concerns.

There are several areas to approach through education. To begin with, the withdrawal process and its impact on the client's mind and body need to be explained. Reassurance that what the client is experiencing is typical can be provided by educating the client about the sequence of the detoxification process. A cognitive–behavioral approach can be used to help the client learn to self-identify and cope with urges to misuse or abuse a substance. In occupational therapy, a plan can be established for ways to manage urges, looking at environmental factors and personal factors. Performance patterns can also be addressed by reviewing what activities the client associates with an urge to use the substance. Therapeutic intervention can be done to reorganize the spatial and temporal aspects of where and when the client's occupations can be completed while decreasing occupational participation with or near use of a substance. The client can also be alerted to the negative consequences of choosing to misuse or abuse a substance in the future.

Transition

Time for the detoxification phase of recovery is short. The occupational therapist, with input from the occupational therapy professional, should be considering transition from detox treatment to further inpatient or outpatient treatment. The occupational therapist will need to design a transition plan based on community supports, family supports, and vocational or educational interests. There must always be a dual thought process occurring—will the person have their next medical services inpatient or outpatient? Because that information may not be known yet, be dependent on how medically well the person presents at the end of the detox period or can simply change throughout the detox period, the occupational therapy team must always decide on how to best meet the needs of the client in both inpatient and outpatient settings.

SUMMARY

Psychotropic medications affect the way the mind works. Physicians prescribe these drugs and other somatic treatments, such as ECT, for people with mental disorders. Although psychotropic medications have great value in reducing or controlling symptoms, unpleasant side effects may also occur. For many persons with mental disorders, the choice is between side effects, on the one hand, and symptoms of a mental disorder, on the other. Either may interfere with their ability to carry out everyday activities. The occupational therapy professional must be aware of the different kinds of medication and their effects, both therapeutic and adverse. By observing the client closely day after day, the occupational therapy professional can notice the effects of medication on a functional level; this information, when communicated to the physician, aids in the proper adjustment of the dosage level. In addition, the occupational therapy professional can adapt activities to enable clients to succeed despite side effects, can educate clients about the effects of medications, can listen sympathetically to complaints about side effects while encouraging adherence to drug regimens, and can provide recommendations for adjustments in daily routine and environment.

Any information on psychotropic medications may rapidly become obsolete. New drugs are under development, and unsuspected adverse effects of drugs recently released to the market are sometimes reported. Keeping current with psychopharmacology requires regular review of the literature and use of research and internet sources to obtain current information.

OT HACKS SUMMARY

O: Occupation as a means and an end

Occupational performance can be more organized when medications are used to stabilize psychotic symptoms. Medications can assist with stabilizing moods, allowing clients time with clear cognitive abilities, thus improving occupational participation. Unfortunately, medication side effects can cause decreases in fine motor ability that can limit physical ability and thereby limit success with occupation. Medication side effects can also cause changes in outward appearance, thus limiting the desire to participate in social occupations.

T: Theoretical concepts, values, and principles, or historical foundations

The medical model is foundational to decision-making regarding medication use (completely directed by the medical team). Occupational therapy professionals must understand what, and how, occupations are impacted by medication effects and be able to relay their observations of clients' behaviors and actions to the medical team so that medication effects can be considered as the physician adjusts medication dosage.

A cognitive–behavioral theoretical approach can be used to help with client self-awareness and self-identification feelings related to substance misuse and abuse and how to manage those urges.

H: How can we Help? OT's role in serving clients with mental illness or mental health needs

NA for this chapter.

A: Adaptations

NA in this chapter.

C: Case study includes

NA for this chapter.

K: Knowledge: keeping mental health OT practice grounded in evidence, in occupational science, and in research

Medical knowledge in this chapter was addressed in the following items.

Psychotropic Medication:
- Alter levels of dopamine, norepinephrine, serotonin.
- Block the reuptake of chemical.
- Block removal of chemical.
- Block presynaptic receptor action.
- Side effects can be common or cause severe or adverse reactions that can ultimately be life threatening. Such side effects include metabolic syndrome, TD, Parkinsonism, dystonia, akathisia, NMS, serotonin syndrome, and lithium toxicity.
- Several food and beverage restrictions when taking MAOIs
- Use of alcohol with use of psychotropic medication can be contraindicated.
- Risk of addiction with use of a stimulant

Detoxification:
- Signs and Symptoms of substance withdrawal
- Medical treatments for substance withdrawal
- Assessment of vital signs
- Nutrition considerations during detoxification

S: Some terms that may be new to you

Akathisia: extreme motor restlessness, a need to move around, and inability to sit still

Detoxification: time when person initially stops using one or more substances and the substance is cleared out of the body

Dystonia: painful muscle spasms, often of face, neck, and jaw

Medication adherence: following prescription for taking medication

Mental obtundation: mental blurring, reduced alertness, diminished reaction to pain

Metabolic syndrome: can be caused by atypical medicines for schizophrenia and increases risk of heart disease, diabetes, and stroke

Neuroleptic malignant syndrome: extreme rigidity, fever around 104°F and higher, and mental obtundation

Neuroleptics: medications for schizophrenia

Parkinsonism: tremor, slowed movement, muscular rigidity, impaired balance

Psychotropic: mind changing

Serotonin syndrome: plasma serotonin concentration increases and becomes toxic with use of medications such as SSRIs, MAOIs, and lithium

Tardive dyskinesia: movement disorder that includes unwanted facial movements, writhing motions of the tongue, small writhing motions of the fingers

Reflection Questions

1. Complete the questions in the *What's the Evidence?* box.
2. What are the major categories of medications used to treat mental disorders?
3. For each major category of psychotropic medication, what are the common side effects?
4. For each side effect listed in Table 8.7, what is an appropriate response or therapeutic intervention consideration?
5. What are the somatic therapies, and what is a brief description of each?
6. What are the organic substances that clients may use, and why is each used?
7. What are the responsibilities of occupational therapy professionals regarding clients and their medications.
8. What are the areas the occupational therapist should assess for the client undergoing the detoxification phase of recovery? What should be assessed with each occupational therapy visit?

REFERENCES

1. Clewes, J., Shivamurthy, S., & Wrigley, S. (2013). Brightening his days: A reflective single case-study of social integration and recovery. *Occupational Therapy in Mental Health, 29*(2), 159–180.
2. Davenport, L. (2021, April 27). Potential first-in-class schizophrenia drug cuts negative symptoms. *Medscape.* https://www.medscape.com/viewarticle/950059#vp_1
3. Diamond, R. J. (2009). *Instant psychopharmacology: A guide for the nonmedical mental health professional* (3rd ed.). Norton.
4. Dziegielewski, S. F. (2006). *Psychopharmacology handbook for the non-medically trained.* Norton.
5. Food and Drug Administration. (2021, March). *Azstarys.* Reference ID: 4755866. Retrieved April 24, 2022, from https://www.accessdata.fda.gov/drugsatfda_docs/label/2021/212994s000lbl.pdf
6. Gibson, S., Brand, S. L., Burt, S., Boden, Z. V. R., & Benson, O. (2013) Understanding treatment non-adherence in schizophrenia and bipolar disorder—A survey of what service users do and why. *BMC Psychiatry, 13*(153), 1–12.
7. Gragnolati, A. B. (2021, March 31). *FDA approves Azstarys, a once-daily stimulant for ADHD.* Good Rx Health. Retrieved April 24, 2022, from https://www.goodrx.com/conditions/adhd/azstarys-approved-for-adhd-treatment
8. Howland, R. H. (2010). Psychopharmacology. In B. R. Bonder (Ed.), *Psychopathology and function* (4th ed.). SLACK.
9. Ibeh, J. (2021). *Increasing adherence to antipsychotic medication in patients with schizophrenia using mobile app reminder* (Order No. 28549010) [Clinical scholarly project, Brandman University]. ProQuest Dissertation Publishing.
10. Koblan, K. S., Kent, J., Hopkins, S. C., Krystal, J. H., Cheng, H., Goldman, R., & Loebel, A. (2020). A non-D2-receptor-binding drug for the treatment of schizophrenia. *The New England Journal of Medicine, 382*(16), 1497–1506.
11. Kraft, N. H., & Keeley, J. W. (2015, January 23). *Sign versus symptom.* Wiley Online Library. Retrieved April 24, 2022, from https://onlinelibrary.wiley.com/doi/abs/10.1002/9781118625392.wbecp145
12. Laban, T. S., & Saadabadi, A. (2021, August 6). *Monoamine Oxidase Inhibitors (MAOI): Continuing education activity.* National Library of Medicine: National Center for Biotechnology Information. https://www.ncbi.nlm.nih.gov/books/NBK539848/
13. Owie, G. O., Olotu, S. O., & James, B. O. (2018). Reliability and validity of the Medication Adherence Rating Scale in a cohort of patients with schizophrenia from Nigeria. *Trends in Psychiatry and Psychotherapy, 40*(2), 85–92.
14. Rappa, L., & Viola, J. (2012). *Condensed psychopharmacology 2013: A pocket reference for psychiatry and psychotropic medications.* RXPSYCH LLC.
15. Reker, D., Blum, S. M., Steiger, C., Anger, K. E., Sommer, J. M., Fanikos, J., & Traverso, G. (2019, March 13). 'Inactive' ingredients in oral medications. *Science Translational Medicine, 11*(483), 1–14.
16. Rouleau, S., Mazer, B., Ménard, I., & Gautier, M. (2010). A survey on driving in clients with mental disorders. *Occupational Therapy in Mental Health, 26*(1), 85–95.
17. Sadock, B. J., Sussman, N., & Sadock, V. A. (2019). *Kaplan & Sadock's pocket handbook of psychiatric drug treatment* (7th ed.). Wolters Kluwer.
18. Supernus Pharmaceuticals. (2021). *Qelbree: Discover an ADHD treatment that helps make symptoms manageable.* Retrieved April 24, 2022, from https://www.qelbree.com/pediatrics
19. Valenstein, E. S. (1986). *Great and desperate cures.* Basic Books.
20. Wilcox, C. S. (2009). Hypertensive crises. In R. W. Schrier (Ed.), *Atlas of disease of the kidney* (Vol. 3). NKF Cyber Nephrology.

SUGGESTED RESOURCES

Website

Substance Abuse and Mental Health Services Administration. (2021, July). *TIP 63: Medications for opioid use disorder—Full document.* https://store.samhsa.gov/product/TIP-63-Medications-for-Opioid-Use-Disorder-Full-Document/PEP21-02-01-002?referer=from_search_result

CHAPTER 9

Safety Considerations and Techniques

OT HACKS OVERVIEW

O: Occupation as a means and an end

Not applicable in this chapter.

T: Theoretical concepts, values, and principles, or historical foundations

Nonmaleficence is a core ethical standard in occupational therapy.

H: How can we Help? OT's role in serving clients with mental illness or mental health needs

4 Key Points About Safety

1. Safety precautions and procedures are meant to decrease the risk of injury and harm to the client, colleagues, and the occupational therapy professional.
2. Including safety as a main component of service delivery within the occupational therapy process and in the occupational therapy work environment.
3. Risks associated with psychiatric emergencies.
4. Considerations toward safe occupational performance at home and in the community.

A: Adaptations

Design of therapeutic environment is done purposefully and intentionally to compensate for decreased client safety awareness.

C: Case study includes

Case Study: Addressing safety in transition.

K: Knowledge: keeping mental health OT practice grounded in evidence, in occupational science, and in research

Following industry standards to maintain a safe environment and to ensure safe practices in the workplace.

S: Some terms that may be new to you

Emergency hold
Nonmaleficence
Photosensitivity
Prudence
Psychiatric elopement
RICE
Safety Data Sheets
Standard precautions
Transmission-based precautions

INTRODUCTION

Occupational therapy professionals must put safety first so that they can protect clients, colleagues, and themselves. Some people with mental disorders are at risk of harming themselves, either by accident or on purpose. Some are suicidal or self-mutilating; others have histories of violence; and others are confused or inattentive and are likely to get lost, have accidents, or expose themselves to infection or environmental dangers. It is important to recognize that suicide is a risk for clients whose diagnoses are other than psychiatric. A person may think of suicide after sustaining a spinal cord injury or head injury or after being diagnosed with a chronic or terminal disease. Thus, the safety considerations and techniques in this chapter are applicable beyond the practice setting of mental health.

Persons hospitalized for psychiatric reasons often require the protection of physical boundaries (locked doors) and attentive staff. Locked units restrict the use of sharps and other objects that can be used self-destructively or violently, and some have padded seclusion rooms for individual treatment of clients who cannot independently manage their behaviors and actions. When clients leave a locked inpatient unit to come to occupational therapy or when occupational therapy is conducted on such a unit, special precautions are needed to reduce the risk of harm. Occupational therapy professionals have a legal and ethical duty to refrain from actions that could cause harm. This is the principle of nonmaleficence and is a key component of the occupational therapy profession's ethical standards. Occupational therapy professionals practice within the core value of prudence, or the idea of using reason to make solid judgments about how occupational therapy should be delivered and to be vigilant during all occupational therapy–based interactions with others (2).

Clients may also be seen in their own homes, in an outpatient clinic, in a clubhouse, or in transitional housing. Safety education and training in responding to emergencies can improve a client's functional independence in the community. No matter what the setting, it is sensible to follow standard general safety, public health, and fire code regulations and to teach clients about them so that they too can follow them at home and in the community.

This chapter addressed safety in four ways.

- Safety precautions and procedures are meant to decrease the risk of injury and harm to the client, colleagues, and the occupational therapy professional.
- The inclusion of safety as a main component of service delivery within the occupational therapy process and in the occupational therapy work environment.
- Risks associated with psychiatric emergencies, such as elopement, assault, or suicide.
- Considerations toward safe client occupational performance at home and in the community.

This chapter is not meant to substitute for training in current disease-specific safety-related prevention methods or as a substitute for basic first aid training. The authors assume that the reader will maintain certification in standard first aid and cardiopulmonary resuscitation (CPR), including training for an automatic electronic defibrillator (AED). These types of certifications must be renewed regularly, and occupational therapy professionals need to remain cognizant of currently accepted personal safety techniques.

PRECAUTIONS AND PROCEDURES TO CONTROL INFECTION AND REDUCE ACCIDENTAL INJURY AND HARM

Precautions and infection controlling procedures are identified by agencies such as the Centers for Disease Control and Prevention (CDC) and the World Health Organization (WHO). These precautions and procedures target infections that are caused by disease agents that may be found in blood and other bodily fluids.

Health care students and workers should be aware that it is possible to contract an infection or other disease from those in their care. For occupational therapy professionals, the risk is often smaller than for members of some other professions more likely to come in contact with bodily fluids. Many disease-causing agents can be transmitted from person to person, whether through direct contact or through the spread of germs in the environment. Remember that infection can travel both ways: the client can contract a disease from the health care worker as well. For these reasons, it is important that health care workers always observe basic infection control procedures and precautions and do so with *all* persons in the work environment.

Since 1992, employers (eg, hospitals) have been required to have an exposure control plan and to provide adequate handwashing facilities (including single-use towels or hot-air blowers) and protective barriers such as gloves for the use of employees who may come in contact with blood or other bodily fluids (25). Because many individuals are allergic to latex or to the talc used with some gloves, nonlatex gloves should be made available.

Standard Precautions

Standard precautions are infection control techniques to be used when working with all clients. They involve practice procedures and use of personal protective equipment (PPE). The goals are to protect health care providers from contracting an infection and to prevent an infection from spreading from one client to another. Activities specifically addressed as a part of standard precautions include the following (8):

- hand hygiene
- use of PPE
- respiratory hygiene and cough etiquette
- client care equipment and instruments disinfection
- environment disinfection
- textile and laundry disinfection
- safe injection practices
- safe handling of needles and other sharps
- advancing to transmission-based precautions when needed

Transmission-Based Precautions

Along with standard precautions, transmission-based precautions are used when a client could be infected or colonized with an infectious agent that requires more advanced care. Precautions associated with this level of infection control include the following (9):

- Contact
- Droplet
- Airborne

Handwashing

The first and most effective method of disease prevention is regular and thorough handwashing. Box 9.1 provides details about when and how hands should be washed.

The key points of any handwashing sequence are to clean all hand surfaces and crevices, use soap and water, avoid recontamination from sink or faucets or other surfaces, and use clean disposable towels or hot air to dry the hands.

Protective Barriers

At times, the occupational therapy professional will encounter bodily fluids. This may be caused by interventions that include activities of daily living such as bathing, showering, toileting, oral care, or feeding. Thus, protective barriers (primarily gloves) must be worn when working with the client

---

BOX 9.1 Handwashing: The First Defense Against Infection

When to Wash

- Before starting work
- Before and after treating clients if physical contact is involved
- Before donning and after removing gloves
- During performance of normal duties
- Before and after handling or preparing food
- After personal use of the toilet or toileting with a client
- After sneezing, coughing, or contact with oral and nasal areas
- Before eating or preparing food
- On completion of duty

Sequence for handwashing. Process should take 40 to 60 seconds.

1. Have paper towel available.
2. Remove hand jewelry, including watch. Secure items.
3. Turn on water, creating a solid stream of water.
4. Apply enough soap to cover all surfaces of the hand.
5. Rub palms together.
6. Rub posterior of each hand and finger surfaces by lacing fingers of one hand over the posterior of the other hand.
7. Place palms together and interlace fingers, rubbing all finger surfaces of both hands.
8. Cup hands together by flexing fingers and placing dorsum of fingers next to the other hand's palm. Rub surfaces together.
9. Grasp each thumb in opposite fisted hand and rub thumb by rotating opposite hand.
10. Flex fingers of hand and rub in rotational direction (and then opposite rotational direction) over palm of opposite hand.
11. Rinse hands with water.
12. Dry hands thoroughly with a one-time only use paper towel.
13. Use towel to turn off water.
14. Dispose of paper towel.

World Health Organization. (2009). *WHO guidelines on hand hygiene in health care.* Author. Retrieved April 01, 2022, from https://apps.who .int/iris/bitstream/handle/10665/44102/9789241597906_eng.pdf

---

as well as when cleaning areas that have been or *may have been* contaminated. Proper techniques for donning and doffing PPE is available from the CDC at: https://www.cdc.gov/hai/pdfs/ppe/ppe-sequence.pdf. Adhesive bandages should always be used to cover tiny cuts and even hangnails and should be changed whenever hands are washed.

Medical Emergencies and First Aid

Occupational therapy professionals need to know how to respond to medical emergencies. Fainting, seizures, minor cuts, burns, and contusions are the most common medical emergencies. Serious burns and wounds, fractures, poisoning, choking, cardiac arrest, and strokes are less common but still occur. In addition, occupational therapy professionals need to be aware of items that can cause allergic reactions. The outcome of these serious conditions depends heavily on the ability of the person nearest the scene to respond quickly and correctly. The general rules for responding to a medical emergency are covered in a basic first aid course.

Seizures

Some of the medications used to treat psychiatric disorders are associated with an increased risk of seizures. The occupational therapy professional should know what a seizure looks like and what to do if a client has one. The usual pattern in a seizure is for the person to become rigid and statue-like for a few seconds and then begin to move with an all-over jerking motion. The person may void urine or feces or stop breathing and will probably turn bluish. The procedure for responding if someone starts having a seizure is covered in first aid courses.

Bleeding

Bleeding can range in severity from relatively minor to quite serious and even fatal. Because sharp objects and power tools are used in occupational therapy, it is important for all occupational therapy staff to know how to respond to a bleeding emergency. The first goal is to stop the bleeding; it may be necessary to send someone else for help, and sometimes the only person available will be another client. Be sure the person summoning help knows whom to contact and what to say. It is also important to avoid contaminating the wound. Again, basic first aid courses cover this information.

Burns

Most of the burns that occur in occupational therapy are relatively minor, superficial burns and can be treated with basic first aid. Partial thickness and full thickness burns require immediate medical attention. Because these types of burns are each treated differently, and it can be difficult to tell one from the other, the occupational therapy professional should summon help when the burn has any blistering or when skin is missing or charred.

Scalding with boiling water is a hazard in the kitchen. If boiling water is poured on the person's clothes, the first step is to remove the clothing. If boiling water has gotten into the shoes, remove them first.

Sunburn

Photosensitivity, or increased sensitivity to the sun's rays, is a side effect of some medications used to treat psychiatric disorders and of some other common prescription medications (eg, tetracycline). Because occupational therapy activities may be conducted out of doors, the occupational therapy professional must know what medications clients are taking. Sunburn can be prevented. Make sure that the person wears an effective sunblock, a hat, and (if necessary) long pants and long sleeves. Be sure the person applies sunblock to all exposed surfaces, especially to the shoulders, neck, ears, the top of the head (if skin is directly exposed), and the tops of the feet and backs of the hands if these are bare. Sunglasses are recommended because the eyes are also affected by the medications.

Strains, Sprains, Bruises, and Contusions

Strains, sprains, bruises, and contusions are common types of soft tissue damage; blood vessels under the skin are broken and bleed into surrounding areas, but there is no external bleeding. Pain, discoloration, and swelling result if these injuries are not treated promptly. The protocol is RICE (rest, ice, compression, elevation), which is explained in basic first aid courses.

Allergic Reactions

Clients and occupational therapy staff can have allergic reactions to common items found in the work and home environment. Medical charts or client history and informational records should be reviewed so that known allergic reactions can be prevented. A client may have medication they carry with them to counteract the allergen. If this is the case, the occupational therapy professional should speak with medical and administrative staff of their facility to learn the procedures the occupational therapy staff are expected and required to follow regarding the medication. Allergies most often seen in occupational therapy departments would be associated with food items, insect bites or stings, or latex.

Because meal preparation and community outings to restaurants are common occupational therapy intervention activities, care should be taken to be aware of any known food allergies. When a client is allergic to a certain food or beverage, food substitutions will need to be made. Food allergies include not only the final food product that is consumed (eg, strawberries or shell fish), but also ingredients used to make the food, such as peanuts. Occupational therapy professionals need to be aware of how the allergic reaction is caused, such as ingestion of the item, touching the item, breathing in the fumes or vapor of the item, or simply being near the item.

Beyond food allergies, occupational therapy professionals need to be aware of digestive conditions and disorders that limit the intake of certain foods or ingredients, such as milk products for those who are lactose intolerant and gluten for those who have celiac disease.

Latex allergic reactions occur when the person is exposed to an item with latex. Symptoms can be mild, such as a skin rash, sneezing, itchiness, or mild nausea. Symptoms can also be severe and life threatening such as difficulty breathing or an inability to breathe. Beyond gloves, latex can be found in a variety of items, such as some contraceptive devices, female sanitary items, balloons, rubber toys, rubber bands, and computer mouse pads (19).

It should be noted that a person could be allergic to almost anything; that includes, but is not limited to, items such as cleaning or other chemical products, nail care or hair care items, animals, and plants or plant products (such as wood used in craft kits).

One other consideration is observing the client for a medical alert pendant. This may be on jewelry such as a bracelet or necklace. If the client does not have such an item and has an allergy, occupational therapy intervention can include the person working to secure such an item.

CONTROLLING THE CLINIC ENVIRONMENT

In addition to standards and recommendations set by the CDC, agencies such as the Occupational Safety and Health Administration (OSHA) and Food and Drug Administration (FDA) provide standards and guidelines for occupational therapy professionals to follow regarding safety and infection control in the clinic environment and with occupational therapy service delivery.

Infection Control in Common Areas

The occupational therapy clinic in mental health settings typically appears less medical than the physical disabilities clinic. A home-like appearance and informal atmosphere should not be taken as an opportunity to relax and ignore proper infection control. Tables, counters, and other surfaces should be washed and disinfected daily and anytime contamination is suspected. Adequate supplies of cleaning materials such as hand soap, paper towels, trash bins, janitorial items, detergents, and disinfectants should be maintained. Disposable gloves, utility gloves, adhesive bandages, and a first aid kit should be kept in each occupational therapy area.

Cleaning must be performed per facility and government regulations. For instance, if blood is found on the floor, it cannot be left unattended (you must call for help), and it must be cleaned up with a blood spill kit. Blood spill kits can be commercially purchased or made at the facility per government regulations (6).

Linens used in homemaking groups should be replaced or laundered after each use. Cosmetics and personal hygiene items (combs, toothbrushes) should never be shared. For personal hygiene sessions, consumers should bring their own supplies, or the occupational therapy professional should provide brand new items for each person. Some cosmetic companies provide samples on request for this purpose. All personal items should be labeled with the individual client's name.

Under federal regulations, eating, drinking, smoking, applying cosmetics or lip balm, and handling contact lenses are prohibited when there is a likelihood of occupational exposure to blood or bodily fluids (25).

Infection Control and Safety for Specific Situations

Clients often say that they enjoy coming to occupational therapy because the clinic has many interesting things in it. Unfortunately, some of these "interesting things" are not very safe unless handled properly. The safety of clients and staff can largely be protected by organizing the occupational therapy clinic properly and by having all staff follow certain procedures.

1. *Keep track of your keys.* In some settings, occupational therapy professionals attach their keys to their clothing with a clip. Do not set keys down and turn around to do something else. Remember that even in community settings, staff members have keys to areas from which clients are restricted. When using keypad entry codes, be alert to the presence of others, and make sure they are not able to view the code.

2. *Make sure restricted items are not taken onto inpatient units.* Depending on the setting, clients may not be permitted to have certain objects on the unit. Some examples are razors, belts, anything in a glass container, hair lifts, hair picks or rattail combs, plastic bags that are head size or larger, wire hangers, and anything breakable (3). In practical terms, this means that a client may not be able to take some finished projects and supplies to their room. Examples are ceramic pieces, leather lace, yarn and cord, macramé, and cosmetics in glass containers. Any questionable items should be discussed with nursing staff *before* they are brought onto the unit.

3. *Have everything ready before patients arrive in the clinic or intervention area.* The occupational therapy professional who needs to move around finding supplies and tools and getting people started cannot at the same time pay attention to where all clients are and what they are doing. For the same reason, any tools or supplies that may be needed during the group should be available in the same room, in neat and accessible storage. If staff is busy rummaging through the supply cabinet, clients may misuse items or attempt to remove items from the occupational therapy area. *Never* leave clients from a locked unit alone and unattended.

4. *Use shatterproof mirrors.* This solves the problem of anyone being harmed by pieces of a broken mirror, but this precaution may not be needed in every setting, depending on the population.

5. *Use good judgment about who comes to occupational therapy.* Clients on an inpatient unit on suicidal or elopement observation may not be permitted to leave the unit. Even if they are allowed to come to occupational therapy, the occupational therapy professional providing the intervention activity should carefully consider the risks before permitting the person to attend the group. Is this person going to take so much energy and attention that others will be neglected? Is this a safe activity for this person? Will other staff be close by in case there is a problem?

6. *Organize tool and supply cabinets to permit a fast, accurate count of all potentially dangerous items.* There are several ways to achieve this. Many clinics use a shadow board, in which every tool has a shadow or outline marking its place. Any tool that is missing can be identified immediately. The shadows can be cut out from brightly colored contact paper or painted on. Having clients return tools to the rack at the end of the session helps them develop good work habits and feel responsible and in control (21). Tools can also be counted at the end of the session to ensure they have all been returned. Allen (1) recommended using transparent plastic containers for small items; these containers are available as flat, compartmentalized boxes or as small standing chests of drawers. Knives and other sharp objects must be kept in locked storage.

7. *Alert clients to potential dangers in activities.* You should inform them about any materials that may cause injury and teach them how to prevent it. Safety information for tools, supplies, and procedures used in occupational therapy activities should be posted for easy reference. For example, paper, foil, glazed ceramics, and even sandpaper may cut. A reed, dowel, or wire can cause eye injuries. Wood has splinters.

8. *Follow safety precautions for toxins.* Some of the substances used in occupational therapy activities can be harmful or fatal if ingested. The occupational therapy professional should read the label of every spray can and every bottle and jar in the clinic and follow the precautions indicated. Breathing even small amounts of mist from hair spray, silicone spray used on tiles, and spray paint or lacquer is harmful. The fumes from color markers can cause dizziness. Some leather dyes and wood finishes are toxic. Exposure to wood dust can cause allergic reactions, and prolonged or repeated exposure is associated with increased incidence of nasal cancer.[1] Some glues and their vapors are toxic. Nothing containing lead should be used in occupational therapy. Anything that might irritate the eyes or lungs (eg, grout powder) should be used cautiously. Provide adequate ventilation whenever solvents or aerosol sprays are used.

9. All users, clients and staff alike, should wash their hands thoroughly after handling toxic materials; the room should be damp mopped rather than swept to avoid sending particles into the air (1). Do not transfer dangerous materials to unmarked containers. Keep them in their original containers wherever possible. If a small amount is poured out for clients to use, it should be put in an appropriate container, not paper, plastic, or foam plastic, and should be discarded correctly after the session. ***Never use any container that might be mistaken for a food or drink or medication container.*** Place jars and containers of all liquids near the center of the table, where they are less likely to be knocked over. Because of the danger from accidental ingestion of toxins, eating, drinking, and smoking must be prohibited in areas where these supplies are used.

Safety Data Sheets (SDSs) should be made available for every chemical used in the occupational therapy department. This includes items such as markers, ink pens, glue, hand soap, and dish soap. SDSs provide information about the chemical properties and how to treat inhalation or ingestion of the chemical. These sheets should be immediately available in case of emergency (24).

---

[1] A summary of the health effects of common wood finishes and solvents is presented in Mustoe (22).

10. *Know and use proper safety equipment.*[2] Safety goggles, appropriate clothing, and sometimes dust masks should be worn by clients and staff using any power tool. Long hair and long sleeves should be fastened back so that they do not drop into tools, fluids, or heat sources. Shirts should be tucked in. No jewelry should be worn when using power tools. Neoprene gloves should be worn when handling alcohol and solvents. Vapor masks should be worn when solvents are used in large quantities or for a long time, as in furniture stripping and refinishing. Eyewash kits should be available. Earplugs can be worn, if desired.

11. Those who are in a hurry may be tempted to do without safety equipment "just this once." Just this once, for instance, may be the time that a tool breaks, and if safety precautions are appropriately taken, risk of personal injury is decreased. Besides an allergy to wood, a client may have an allergy to animal fibers (such as wool). Finally, dust from plaster and clay can be very irritating to the lungs, skin, and eyes.

12. *Observe the local fire code.* Flammables should be kept in a separate cabinet designed for that purpose. Fire extinguishers and fire blankets should be mounted in easily accessible places wherever fire or flammables are used. The occupational therapy professional should know how to use them. "No Smoking" and "No Eating and Drinking" signs and signs indicating the location of safety equipment should be clearly visible.[3] Doorways and fire exits should be kept clear, unlocked, and unobstructed. Fire drills should be scheduled regularly to acquaint staff and clients with evacuation routes and procedures. Clients should not be permitted near the ceramic kiln when it is operating. The door to the kiln should be locked so that no one opens it while it is on. Remember to use a stairway (not an elevator) during a fire (Figure 9.1).

13. *Pay attention to the condition of the floor.* Clean up spills immediately. Highly waxed floors are slippery and dangerous for shop and kitchen areas. Sweep up sawdust and debris in the workshop frequently; this means every half hour or even more often, depending on level of use.

14. *Eliminate electrical hazards.* Be sure that the current is sufficient for the demand; do not overload a circuit or use multiple plugs with a single socket. Appliances with a three-prong plug must be grounded; if there is no three-prong outlet available, do not use the appliance unless the green grounding wire is screwed into the switch plate. Make sure that electricity and water cannot come in contact with each other in the clinic. Have electrical outlets near sinks or other water sources

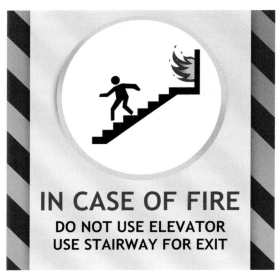

Figure 9.1. Always Use a Stairway to Evacuate During a Fire or Smoke Condition.

disconnected if necessary. Arrange for damaged cords and plugs (including those that get hot) to be repaired or replaced immediately. The facility's maintenance department should annually inspect all electrical equipment and cords to ensure they are intact. Be sure that electrical equipment is unplugged or switched off before you leave the clinic. This is especially important for devices that have a heating element (irons and curling irons, copper enameling kilns, and coffee makers). It is often a good idea to have a central power cutoff installed for shop areas or kitchens.

15. *Observe food safety guidelines and fire safety precautions in the kitchen.* The occupational therapy kitchen may be used by many staff and clients; things can quickly become disorganized and hazardous unless all involved take responsibility for keeping it clean and safe. Generally, one person is designated to have final responsibility. The refrigerator and freezer should be kept at the proper temperatures. The refrigerator should be at 40 °F or below and the freezer at 0 °F (15). Leftover canned food should be transferred to another storage container that is labeled with the name of the food product. All food and beverages, perishable and nonperishable, should be marked with the date they entered the storage area. The refrigerator should be cleaned out once a week to discard items at risk for spoiling. The occupational therapy kitchen should be equipped with good, thick potholders and oven mitts. The oven should be well insulated to prevent accidental burns. Clients and staff must tie back long hair, roll up shirt sleeves, and wear aprons while working at the stove and oven or with small appliances. Handles of pots should be turned so that they do not stick out past the edge of the stove.

16. Clients need to be observed closely; it is not unusual for a person with a mild cognitive impairment to try to pick up something hot with a bare hand or reach into boiling

---

[2]Safety equipment appropriate for shops in which solvents, carcinogens, and flammables are used can be obtained from Lab Safety Supply, Janesville, WI 53567-1368.
[3]These fire safety items are available from Lab Safety Supply, Janesville, WI 53567-1368.

water. Because medication may cause poor coordination, have clients set containers away from the edge on a firm surface before pouring liquids into them. This is most important when the liquids are hot.

17. *Apply techniques for proper positioning, body mechanics, energy conservation, and work simplification, and teach these to clients.* Occupational therapy professionals generally learn these techniques in relation to persons with physical disabilities, but they apply to everyone. Observe and correct the consumer's body and hand position to prevent repetitive strain injuries; teach the person positioning to prevent deformity and reduce strain. Provide rest breaks and explain their importance. Teach clients how to be organized in their approach to a task. Refer to physical disabilities texts for particulars.

18. *Provide increased structure for those functioning at lower cognitive levels.* Be alert to varying functional levels, especially in persons undergoing changes in medications. A client may approach a familiar task with confidence and yet be a danger to self because of a cognitive impairment.

PSYCHIATRIC EMERGENCIES

Psychiatric emergencies can occur in any setting. We tend to associate them with inpatient environments because locked units and hospitalization suggest that the clients are more impaired. But with shorter hospital stays and more rigorous admissions criteria, seriously ill clients are now seen in outpatient and community settings. Furthermore, suicide is a risk also for persons who are seen in outpatient physical medicine settings and who have no acknowledged mental health problems. It is important for the occupational therapy professional to be able to recognize and respond to the suicidal client.

At times, a client may be perceived as a danger to themselves or others. In these cases, the person needs emergency hospitalization for evaluation. Terminology examples for this include the following:

- emergency hold
- psychiatric hold
- detention or being detained
- provisional hospitalization
- 72-hour emergency hold or admission

The official terminology and length of time the person is legally required to remain at the facility is determined by individual state statutes (29).

Such a hospitalization is different from what is termed an "*inpatient commitment.*" Several components must be in place for an inpatient commitment. These items include:

- having a diagnosis of a serious mental disorder (usually does not include a substance use disorder, intellectual disability, or dementia),
- posing a danger to themselves or others,
- being unable to meet their basic personal care needs,
- demonstrating a need for treatment, and
- being deemed incompetent.

Typically, inpatient commitment is considered only if the needed level of care and treatment cannot be provided in a less restrictive environment (such as in an outpatient or community setting) (27).

Suicide

Some of the basic precautions for dealing with suicidal persons are covered in the section on depression in Chapter 16. In inpatient settings, the occupational therapy professional must be alert to the possibility that the depressed and suicidal individual will try to elope from the treatment facility or to remove objects from the occupational therapy clinic to use them in a later suicide attempt.

Suicidal persons who succeed in eloping from a locked inpatient unit may try to commit suicide immediately by the first means possible (jumping in front of a moving car or train, off the roof, or out of a high window) (3). Therefore, the occupational therapy professional should take precautions to prevent the client from eloping. The client will most likely not be allowed to leave the unit and must thus have occupational therapy services on the unit. The occupational therapy professional should report any suspicion that the person may be suicidal to the physician or charge nurse, including any risk-taking behaviors or actions observed by the occupational therapy professional.

The occupational therapy professional needs to be especially alert to ways in which tools and supplies can be used in a suicide attempt. The list of dangers is extensive: toxins (leather dyes), flammables (turpentine), sharps (needles, pins, scissors, knives), matches, objects that can be used in hanging (belts, yarn, leather, lace), and so forth. The person who is intent on suicide will use anything at hand: break a mirror or a light bulb, stick a fork in an electrical socket, or try to drown in the toilet (3). The fact that suicide can be achieved with objects that appear to be harmless poses a real problem in occupational therapy. Inpatient clients who are intensely suicidal should not be permitted off the unit or admitted to the occupational therapy clinic. But because individuals may be more impulsive and suicidal than they appear, precautions should be taken with any person who has a history of suicidal ideation or actual suicide attempts. Clients who are receiving antidepressant medications and who show an increase in activity level may be at risk, as explained in Chapter 8.

In locked inpatient settings, all supplies and tools should be kept under lock and key; tools (and needles, pins, matches, flammables and toxins, and items in glass containers) should be counted before clients enter the clinic and before any of them leave. When clients must leave the room to go to the bathroom or get a drink of water, a staff member must accompany them; likewise, any sharps should be accounted for because with some wounds it takes only a few minutes to bleed to death.

In outpatient settings, the occupational therapy professional needs to be aware of the potential for suicide. Box 9.2 lists some of the factors that may increase the risk of suicide. The occupational therapy professional, although not

---

BOX 9.2 Some Risk Factors for Suicide

- Current diagnosis of major mental disorder
- Past suicide attempts
- Access to firearms or other lethal means (such as prescription medication, knives, or poisons)
- Comorbidity with other disorders
- Recent diagnoses of a mental disorder
- Family history of suicide
- Adverse childhood experiences (loss of parents, abuse)
- Past physical or sexual abuse
- Unemployment or recent loss of income
- Poor physical health
- Alcohol- or substance-related disorder
- Sudden life changes or changes in mental health treatment
- Physical illness or impairment
- Living alone
- Belonging to a particular group of people:
  - Non-Hispanic American Indian/Alaska Native and Non-Hispanic White
  - Men (middle-aged and older adult)
  - Veterans and those actively in the Armed Forces
  - Those who live in rural areas
  - Those who work in mining and construction
  - Those who identify as lesbian, gay, bisexual, or transgender
  - Psychosocial problems (family tension, school problems, breakup with girlfriend or boyfriend, or separation or divorce from spouse)
  - Those who lack plans or goals for the future

Adapted from Centers for Disease Control and Prevention. (2022, March 22). *Preventing suicide.* https://www.cdc.gov/suicide/resources/publications.html#Fact-Sheets-Definitions; Substance Abuse and Mental Health Service Administration. (2009, September). *SAFE-T pocket card: Suicide assessment five-step evaluation and triage for clinicians.* https://store.samhsa.gov/product/SAFE-T-Pocket-Card-Suicide-Assessment-Five-Step-Evaluation-and-Triage-for-Clinicians/sma09-4432; Substance Abuse and Mental Health Service Administration. (2012, September). *How you can play a role in preventing suicide.* https://store.samhsa.gov/product/national-strategy-suicide-prevention-2012-how-you-can-play-role-preventing-suicide?referer=from_search_result; Substance Abuse and Mental Health Service Administration. (2021, May). *Helping your loved one who is suicidal: A guide for family and friends.* https://store.samhsa.gov/product/helping-your-loved-one-suicidal-guide-family-friends/PEP20-01-03-001?referer=from_search_result

---

BOX 9.3 Warning Signs of Suicidal Intent

- Talking about killing oneself or wanting to die.
- Talking about being a burden to others.
- Recent acquisition of the means to die (eg, stockpiling medication, buying a gun).
- Making a will or taking out life insurance.
- Giving away personal belongings.
- Demonstrating rage toward others or talking about wanting to take revenge.
- Placing distressing messages on their social media.
- Passive suicidal behavior (not eating, drinking too much, engaging in unsafe behaviors).

Adapted from Arshad, M. K. (2016). Elder suicide intervention: Learning to identify patient profiles at greatest risk can position providers to save lives. *Today's Geriatric Medicine, 9*(5), 24–27. National Institute of Mental Health. (n.d.). *Warning signs of suicide.* Retrieved April 03, 2022, from https://www.nimh.nih.gov/health/publications/warning-signs-of-suicide; Substance Abuse and Mental Health Service Administration. (2012, September). *How you can play a role in preventing suicide.* https://store.samhsa.gov/product/national-strategy-suicide-prevention-2012-how-you-can-play-role-preventing-suicide?referer=from_search_result; Substance Abuse and Mental Health Service Administration. (2021, May). *Helping your loved one who is suicidal: A guide for family and friends.* https://store.samhsa.gov/product/helping-your-loved-one-suicidal-guide-family-friends/PEP20-01-03-001?referer=from_search_result

Assault

In the hospital setting, individuals who have assaulted another person should not be seen in occupational therapy until they are stabilized through proper medications; there is simply no reason to risk the safety of others. However, occasionally, a person becomes assaultive while in occupational therapy. Often, this is an escalation of general anger or hostility; sometimes, the assaultive behavior could have been contained if the behavior had been identified earlier and the situation responded to more quickly (see "Anger, Hostility, and Aggression" in Chapter 22). At other times, the assault occurs without warning, seemingly unprovoked, and the person may have no memory of the incident after it occurs; clients who have abused phencyclidine (PCP) are especially prone to this (1).

The occupational therapy professional should consider what may have caused the onset of the agitation and aggression. If underlying causes can be identified, such situations have a greater chance of being avoided in the future. Questions to consider when trying to determine a causative agent, or trigger, include the following:

- What was occurring immediately before the behavior began? What occurred in the past hour to two?
- What physical location had the person been coming from?
- What were the expectations put on the person before they came to the new area?
- What was occurring in the environment during the transition to the new area?

trained to assess suicidal intent, should be alert to possible signs (Box 9.3). The occupational therapy professional must use good judgment, discretion, and speed in seeking psychiatric evaluation of any person who expresses suicidal intent or who shows other signs that they may be considering or planning suicide (18).

- What might someone have suggested the person was going to be expected to do during the new situation?
- What self-management or self-regulation skills is the person lacking?
- What did the person need from you? Why did they want your attention? What were they trying to communicate? Why was it important to the client?

If the situation does get out of control and the person strikes out or appears ready to do so, the occupational therapy professional should take the following steps, in order:

1. Call for more staff.
2. Remove other clients from the area.
3. Attempt to calm the client.

If you need more staff, yell or scream if you must. Ask a higher-functioning client to telephone or go for help. Similarly, a relatively competent client can oversee escorting the others to a safe area.

Talking to the aggressive person in a calm, soothing tone may help him or her de-escalate; if you can get the person to talk, he or she will usually feel more comfortable and make the situation more manageable. Be mindful of your body language, keeping your nonverbal actions neutral and nonthreatening. Speak in simple terms associated with everyday language. Avoid the use of medical terminology. Ask questions that use your words but reflect the client's statements. Give the client extra time to respond, do not rush them to answer you (14).

More staff members will be needed to calm and subdue the person who gets out of control. Under no circumstances should the occupational therapy professional attempt to overpower the person by physical force. Someone in a psychotic rage is extremely strong; all energy is channeled into striking out. A small person who is having a violent episode may require as many as six strong individuals to restrain them effectively and safely. If the occupational therapy professional has undertaken advanced training in safe restraint maneuvers, they may assist with such actions, per their facility guidelines. The use of restraint and force is a last resort; every attempt to calm the person by other means should be exhausted first.

In an outpatient setting or in the community, incidents of personal violence usually necessitate calling the police or ambulance service. Assaultive persons should not be allowed to remain in the community because they are likely to commit further violent acts. If a violent incident occurs, the occupational therapy professional should follow their employer's procedure for reporting and documenting such incidents. Once the incident is over and the person is calmed or removed from the scene, the occupational therapy professional can encourage other clients who were present to express their feelings about what has happened. This should be done through an interdisciplinary approach, with the occupational therapy professional working with a psychologist, licensed counselor, or social worker on staff.

Elopement

Psychiatric elopement refers to leaving an inpatient (mental health) treatment facility without being discharged in the customary way. Clients may elope for many reasons: because of concerns about their own homes and belongings, because they just do not want to be in the hospital, because they do not want to receive medication or treatment, or because they have something specific they want to do—like use drugs or alcohol, commit suicide, or hurt someone else. A hospital and its staff may be sued for consequences that occur after a client elopes.

Preventing elopement starts with securing doors and windows. Doors should be locked except when in use. Keys should never be left unattended. Windows should be kept closed or, if opened, should have gates or window guards. Some window locks that use a circular key can be opened with another object that matches the size of the circle (such as caps of some color markers); occupational therapy staff should be alert to this possibility when ordering supplies.

When escorting clients to and from a locked unit, the occupational therapy professional should be especially careful; it is easy for a client to walk away if your back is turned. Similarly, clients who want to escape from a locked unit may loiter by the door, waiting for an unsuspecting staff member to unlock it. Sometimes, these clients are disoriented and confused and will not know where to go once they do get out; others have a definite plan. Always look behind you to see who is nearby when you are opening a locked door; and continue to watch the door until it closes behind you. Always notify nursing staff when you take clients off a locked unit.

Trips from a locked unit into the community present special concerns. Sometimes, it is hard to determine in advance just who is likely to try to run away during a trip. Two staff members should always accompany clients when they leave the facility grounds; it is important to have two staff members available because one can stay with the group if the other must go after someone who is running away. If you are alone with a group and a client elopes, return the other clients to the unit or to the care of a responsible staff member before attempting to reach the one who ran away.

Elopement may be prevented or reduced by reducing conflict between clients and staff and by careful analysis of which clients are likely to elope and why (5).

ADDRESSING SAFETY IN THE COMMUNITY

Beyond inpatient and outpatient clinical facilities, clients are provided services in their homes or in community settings. The following section will highlight some issues of concern regarding safety. Some examples of programming for safety education and injury prevention will be described. These are only examples. The occupational therapy professional must use professional and clinical judgment as well as supervision and networking with other mental health practitioners to determine best practices for a given situation.

Home and Personal Safety

Independent living in the community requires knowledge and application of household and personal safety precautions, personal hygiene, basic first aid, and emergency procedures. The occupational therapy professional can help clients improve occupational performance in these areas. The occupations of health management and of safety and emergency management require education and training for community living. Examples of knowledge related to these occupations include emergency phone numbers, simple first aid, household safety hazards, and how and where to obtain medical care (26). In addition, clients should receive instruction in personal safety (use of locks, how to manage interactions with strangers) and weather-related and natural disaster procedures (such as tornados and earthquakes). Education and training for home and community living can include methods such as using written materials with photographs or cartoons of common safety hazards, having small groups of clients hear from guest speakers from fire or police departments or from a hospital or the Red Cross, and having clients create a list of emergency numbers that can be kept in a visible and typically used space in their home (20). Education about safe sex practices and techniques must also be addressed with clients.

Materials used for education and training with clients include workbooks, worksheets, small activity booklets, and informational pamphlets. These can be utilized both in one-on-one sessions with a client or with a small group of clients. Topics consistent with this type of intervention include the following (12, 13):

- emergency planning for sheltering in place
- healthy home environment
- identity and financial theft
- money management
- pet ownership preparedness
- preventing crime
- safe community mobility
- sexual health and safe sexual practices
- sleep
- staying safe online
- violent neighborhood environment

Medication safety has been discussed in Chapter 8. Those with poor impulse control or poor judgment may leave prescription medications out in plain view, on a kitchen or bathroom counter, or in an unlocked area accessible to children and visitors. The occupational therapy professional working in the home with the client should make note of this and provide safety information to the client. If the occupational therapy professional is unsure about the safety of a home situation, they should consult their supervisor or another health professional involved with the case.

Regarding use of electronics, the following additional ideas apply:

- Store important phone numbers on the phone itself, or on a computer or tablet.
- Avoid unsecured browsing and online purchasing to decrease the risk of identity theft.
- Observe internet safety precautions regarding password creation and storage.
- Do not text when driving or in other situations where multitasking creates a risk (eg, when crossing the street).
- Avoid conducting personal conversations in hearing range of others.

The occupational therapy professional cannot anticipate every emergency or odd situation that someone may encounter in the community. Rote learning of specific safety procedures is not sufficient preparation for safe independent living (30). Safety training must also incorporate activities that require the person to critically think through safety situations and use executive functioning skills. The client should identify problems and generate alternative responses to multiple safety-related scenarios. The occupational therapy professional should develop the habit of collecting examples of stories and anecdotes about health and safety situations a client might encounter. These can be turned into interactive learning sessions or discussion topics. Videos from YouTube and internet news outlets are also useful.

Modifying Environments to Enhance Safety

Particularly as clients age, they are at risk from unsafe conditions in their homes and communities. Psychiatric medication-related obesity, diabetes, chronic cardiac and pulmonary conditions, and activities such as smoking can increase safety risks (4). Some clients have cognitive impairments, some have vision impairments, and some have mobility and strength impairments that further compromise their safety. Clients may be resistant to changes in their home environments. As with any other intervention, home safety modifications should represent a collaboration between the occupational therapy professional and client. Recommended home modifications are shown in Box 9.4.

BOX 9.4 Recommended Home Modifications for Consumer Safety

- Provide railings for balance.
- Remove throw rugs to decrease tripping hazards.
- Arrange furniture for easy movement, especially in small or tight areas.
- Reduce clutter.
- Use a single key for multiple door locks use or an electronic security (can be connected to cell phone).
- Replace switched lights with motion-sensitive lighting.
- Provide task lighting under cabinets, shelves, in drawers, and in other dark spots.
- Organize storage and match to client's cognitive level.
- Consider safety and storage of sharps, tools, and potentially harmful objects.
- Use transparent storage boxes if client can tolerate this much stimulation.
- Remove nonessential items from areas next to cooktops and sinks.
- Install ground fault interrupter (GFI) switches for all outlets near water.
- Install temperature guard for tub, shower, and water heater.
- Replace oven-top tea kettle with automatic-shutoff electric appliance.

BOX 9.4 Recommended Home Modifications for Consumer Safety (*continued*)

- Purchase auto shutoff versions of other appliances such as electric irons.

- Replace batteries on smoke alarms and carbon monoxide detectors twice yearly; have these checked regularly by someone other than the consumer if cognitive deficits or physical limitations cause difficulty with maintenance of these items.

- Check that the client has sufficient strength and mobility to use bathroom equipment, small tools, and other items in the home; if indicated, replace with modified versions.

- Provide adequate storage space so that clients do not store items on the back of the toilet (where they may fall in).

- Provide grab bars for clients who may otherwise reach for a less sturdy support like a towel rod, toilet paper holder, or doorknob.

- Insulate exposed pipes.

- Label liquids clearly to avoid misuse (eg, drain cleaner and cleaning products vs. shampoo and personal hygiene products).

Adapted with permission from Barrows, C. (2006). Home adaptations—Creating safe environments for individuals with psychiatric disabilities. *OT Practice, 11*(18), 12–16.

Firearms

Firearm safety is extremely important in preventing death and accidental injury. Based on varying state regulations, the occupational therapy professional may wish to consider firearm safety as an issue for community-living consumers. In addition, the occupational therapy professional might assess any personal risk to self if the client seems impaired by drugs or alcohol or an untreated mental or disorder.

Suicide is a primary risk for someone with a mental disorder who possesses or has access to firearms. According to the CDC, more than half of all suicides in the United States in 2020 involved firearms (10, 11). In 2020, 55% of gun-related deaths in the United States were from suicide (11). Firearm suicides consistently outnumber firearm homicides (7).

The presence of firearms in the home is a safety risk, even for persons with no history of a mental disorder. Adults with cognitive disorders and children may unintentionally cause accidental death or injury by mishandling a firearm or by gaining access to a locked weapon. In some homes, weapons may be out in the open, loaded, and accessible.

United States federal law states: "It shall be unlawful for any person to sell or otherwise dispose of firearms or ammunition to any person knowing or having reasonable cause to believe that such person—has been adjudicated as a mental defective or has been committed to any mental institution" (17).

Further restrictions on gun ownership vary by state or jurisdiction. The following are examples of different state gun laws (16):

- Those who have completed a voluntary mental health hospitalization can be prohibited from gun ownership for a certain length of time.
  - Connecticut for 6 months
  - District of Columbia for 5 years
  - Illinois until the person is certified as not being a danger to themselves or others
- Maryland law does not allow those with a mental condition and who have a history of violent behavior to own a gun, unless the person has had their eligibility restored through a certification process by the Maryland Health Department.
- Hawaii prohibits gun ownership for those with mental disorders until the person is no longer affected by the mental disorder.

The National Alliance on Mental Illness (NAMI) has taken a policy position that people with mental illness, when there is not an evident risk of danger, should not be treated differently regarding guns because of their diagnosis or condition (see Box 9.5) (23).

What is the role of the occupational therapy professional? The first rule is to use common sense and avoid being in unsafe situations. If the occupational therapy professional enters a home and sees a weapon out in the open, this might be reason for concern. But in many jurisdictions, it is perfectly legal.

BOX 9.5 NAMI's Policy Platform on Violence and Guns

NAMI recognizes that when dangerous or violent acts are committed by persons with serious mental illnesses, it is too often the result of neglect or ineffective treatment. Mental health authorities must implement and sustain policies, practices, and programs that provide access to early diagnosis, crisis intervention, appropriate treatment (including integrated treatment when there is co-occurring substance abuse) and support that saves lives. NAMI strongly advocates that people with mental illnesses not be stigmatized and subjected to discrimination by being labeled "criminal" or "violent." Very rarely is there correlation between mental illness and violent behavior, and mental illness must not be confused with sociopathic behavior.

NAMI recognizes that epidemic gun violence is a public health crisis that extenuates risks of lethal harm by others, self-harm, and harm to others for people with mental illnesses. Gun violence is overwhelmingly committed by people without mental illness. NAMI believes that firearms and ammunition should not be easier to obtain than mental health care. NAMI supports reasonable, effective, consistently, and fairly applied firearms regulation and safety as well as widespread availability of mental health crisis intervention, assistance, and appropriate treatment. In the absence of demonstrated risk, people should not be treated differently with respect to firearms regulation because of their lived experience with mental illness. (p. 71)

National Alliance on Mental Illness. (2016, December). *Public policy platform*. https://www.nami.org/Advocacy/Policy-Platform

If it appears the client has been drinking alcohol or using drugs, there is more reason for concern. To protect oneself, the occupational therapy professional may need to ask if the weapon is loaded and then explain that it is unsafe for their personal safety to provide occupational therapy services to the client at this time in this environment, owing to the presence of a loaded weapon. In all such situations, the occupational therapy professional must report and seek guidance from a supervisor or manager. It is best to discuss the possibility of such a situation with the facility or agency administration prior to initiating home or community service visits with clients.

A primary responsibility is to promote gun safety. Another responsibility is to be aware of and sensitive to statements from clients that may indicate suicidal intention. To be clear, clients who intend and commit suicide are found across practice settings. A person with a spinal cord injury may have suicidal intent but no psychiatric diagnosis. The obvious victim of a suicide is the person who dies. But the survivors often suffer intense guilt and in that sense are also victims.

If the occupational therapy professional becomes aware that a client possesses a weapon, and the occupational therapy professional feels there is a question of safety or risk of violence, they should contact their supervisor or manager. In case of an actual emergency and imminent danger, the occupational therapy professional should first call 9-1-1 and then contact their facility or agency.

Since laws vary by state, the occupational therapy professional must be culturally sensitive and seek information applicable to the individual state and jurisdiction. Weapons used for hunting or personal protection will be found in many areas. Encourage the consumer to protect themselves, and others by following gun safety rules.

The occupational therapy professional is neither promoting nor discouraging gun ownership but rather helping to make sure that safety guidelines are followed.

Case Study – Safety With Transition

Charlie is 53 years old and within the past month was diagnosed with Anxiety Disorder Due to Another Medical Condition. Approximately 6 months ago, Charlie was diagnosed with atrial fibrillation (a-fib) and early-stage chronic obstructive pulmonary disease (COPD). He was referred to a biweekly outpatient occupational therapy group to better manage his anxiety and be able to complete daily occupations without limitations resulting from his anxiety.

DSM-5-TR and ICD-10 Diagnoses at Admission

F06.4 Anxiety Disorder Attributable to Another Medical Condition

Z72.9 Problem related to lifestyle

I48.20 Atrial Fibrillation

J44.9 Chronic Obstructive Pulmonary Disease

Charlie lives in a two-story home with his wife. Both bedrooms and the master bathroom are located upstairs. There is a half-bath located on the first floor of the home. There is a den at the rear of the home.

Charlie works as an independent insurance agent. He has owned this small business for the past 20 years. He works out of his home. He travels to his customer's homes throughout the week. Prior to this career, he taught economics at a community college. He has a master's degree in business and bachelor's degree in sociology. His wife works at the local high school as a biology instructor.

The occupational therapist completed an intake assessment during Charlie's first session of occupational therapy. It was noted he had a slightly elevated heart rate, was moderately overweight, demonstrated anxious behaviors (such as constant movement in his lower extremity), and had a gentle demeanor. A Kohlman Evaluation of Living Skills (KELS) assessment (28) indicated a need for assistance with the following:

- Awareness of dangerous household situations

- Plans for future employment

- Leisure activity involvement

Charlie stated he was unsure he could continue working a job that included so much travel throughout the week and indicated he was too tired to do anything "fun." During the *Safety and Health* section of the KELS he was noted to glance quickly at the picture and not scan the complete picture but rather to comment about one section of the picture and then move the picture out of his working area.

The occupational therapist spoke with the occupational therapy assistant about adding Charlie to their caseload. The occupational therapy assistant leads a group on relaxation techniques and a group on career change. The occupational therapist also asked the occupational therapy assistant to work one-to-one with Charlie on safety. These were the goals the occupational therapist identified for Charlie.

The occupational therapy assistant began by having a conversation with Charlie and going through the binder the department keeps, listing and describing various relaxing activities such as yoga, tai chi, visualization activities, progressive muscle relaxation, and meditation. Charlie identified tai chi and visualization activities as items of interest. Next, the occupational therapy assistant asked Charlie about specific concerns with various aspects of his job, what he feels he can do regarding vocation, and why he made his previous job change from a teacher to an insurance agent. Finally, the occupational therapy assistant expressed a need for Charlie to work on increasing his safety awareness and discussed physical consequences to an injury caused by missing a safety concern in his environment.

Charlie agreed to attend occupational therapy for 1 to 2 months and then assess his progress. The occupational therapy assistant went through the objectives of occupational therapy service delivery plan with the occupational therapist. These objectives included the following:

- Complete tai chi and visualization activities to decrease anxiety and fatigue.

- Complete a career interest assessment and follow up with options based on preferences.

- Begin mindfulness to increase sensory awareness of surroundings.

It was decided that the occupational therapy assistant would meet with the occupational therapist in 2 to 3 weeks to discuss Charlie's progress. Charlie's intervention plan included the possible transition to services once a week for 2 to 3 weeks prior to discharge from occupational therapy services in the outpatient department. It was also indicated Charlie may benefit from a transition plan including two to three visits in his home, with one visit occurring just prior to discharge from the outpatient services.

OT HACKS SUMMARY

O: **Occupation as a means and an end**

Not applicable in this chapter.

T: **Theoretical concepts, values, and principles, or historical foundations**

Nonmaleficence is a core ethical standard in occupational therapy.

Grounded in the core value of prudence.

The occupational therapy professional refrains from doing harm to others and uses prudence and acts with vigilance when making judgments about how to safely provide occupational therapy services.

H: **How can we Help? OT's role in serving clients with mental illness or mental health needs**

4 Key Points About Safety

1. Safety precautions and procedures are meant to decrease the risk of injury and harm to the client, colleagues, and the occupational therapy professional.
   - standard and transmission-based precautions
   - handwashing and PPE use
   - first aid needed for seizures, bleeding, burns, sunburn, and strains, sprains, bruises, and contusions
   - allergic reactions to items such as food products and latex

2. Including safety as a main component of service delivery within the occupational therapy process and in the occupational therapy work environment.
   - disinfection and infection control in clinic areas
   - cleaning clinic areas
   - washing linens
   - not sharing personal items
   - proper use of blood spill kit
   - minding one's keys and ensuring sharps are accounted for after client use
   - preparing items before clients arrive
   - not using breakable objects
   - making available medical treatment information for toxin exposure
   - clients who attend occupational therapy must have medical clearance to do so
   - provide training for use of tools and safety equipment to prevent injury

- keep electrical items maintained
- know fire code regulations
- store food in proper containers and at required temperatures
- keep personal items away from hot areas in the kitchen
- use and teach proper body mechanics and energy conservation
- modify tasks for those with decreased cognition

3. Risks associated with psychiatric emergencies.
   - Emergency hospitalization may be needed for the person who is a danger to themselves or to others.
   - Those who are suicidal should not leave the unit, and risk-taking actions should be reported.
   - Items that could be used to harm oneself or others should be kept locked away.
   - When clients become agitated or aggressive, it is important to try and de-escalate the situation. If the person becomes violent, or if it appears they will, other staff should be called to assist, and other clients should be removed from the area.
   - Psychiatric elopement should be guarded against. Care should be taken to keep areas locked and to maintain therapeutic relationships to reduce the chance of power struggles between staff and clients.

4. Considerations toward safe occupational performance at home and in the community.
   - Household safety includes a variety of health management, activities of daily living, and instrumental activities of daily living occupations. Education and training are provided for these areas, including demonstration and written information.
   - Physical aspects of the environment are modified for physical, mental, and cognitive limitations.
   - Firearms are a specific concern for those who have expressed suicidal ideation or suicidal intent, or who have threatened violence against others. State laws vary regarding reporting requirements.

A: **Adaptations**

Therapeutic environment is arranged purposefully and intentionally to compensate for decreased client safety awareness.

- objects such as glass containers, belts, pointed hygiene items, plastic bags that are head size or larger, and wire hangers are not used with clients
- all needed items are set up and made available before clients enter the service area so that the occupational therapy professional does not have to leave clients to retrieve needed items and does not have to divert attention away from clients to prepare assessment or intervention items
- sharp items are only used with clients who do not pose a threat to themselves or others and are collected and counted before clients leave the occupational therapy area
- some clients can have decreased cognitive abilities, so occupational task directions must be simplified as needed

C: Case study includes

Case Study: Addressing safety in transition.

K: Knowledge: keeping mental health OT practice grounded in evidence, in occupational science, and in research

Following industry standards to maintain a safe environment and to ensure safe practices in the workplace. Government entities provide recommendations, guidance, and rules concerning items such as

- handwashing
- exposure control plan
- standard precautions
- transmission-based precautions
- PPE
- blood spills
- food storage
- toxins (Safety Data Sheets)
- fire code compliance

S: Some terms that may be new to you

Emergency hold: inpatient hospitalization required of someone in danger of hurting themselves or someone else.

Nonmaleficence: principle of doing no harm.

Photosensitivity: increased sensitivity to the sun's rays.

Prudence: idea of using reason to make solid judgments.

Psychiatric elopement: leaving an inpatient (mental health) treatment facility without being discharged in the customary way.

RICE: rest, ice, compression, elevation

Safety Data Sheets: provide information about a chemical's properties and how to treat inhalation or ingestion of the chemical.

Standard precautions: infection control techniques to be used when working with all clients.

Transmission-based precautions: used when a client could be infected with an infectious agent that requires more advanced care.

Reflection Questions

1. Why is safety a particular concern when working with persons with mental disorders?
2. What are the reasons for standard precautions?
3. What typical occupational therapy items are unsafe for the client to have on the inpatient unit?
4. What are the types of safety information that should be shared with the client regarding danger in activities?
5. What types of containers should not be used with clients in occupational therapy?
6. What are warning signs of suicidal intent?
7. What are precautions the occupational therapy professional should take to decrease the opportunity for someone to commit suicide?
8. What should the occupational therapy professional do if a client becomes aggressive toward another person?
9. What is psychiatric *elopement*? How can the occupational therapy professional decrease the risk of elopement?
10. Why is it important for clients to know about safety?
11. Why are persons with psychiatric disorders possibly at risk for injury in their homes? For each reason, what is an example that is not listed in the last section of this chapter?
12. What are the legal considerations associated with firearm safety?

References

1. Allen, C. K. (1985). *Cognitive disabilities: Part one: Measurement and management* [Workshop]. Advanced Rehabilitation Institutes.
2. American Occupational Therapy Association. (2020). AOTA 2020 occupational therapy code of ethics. *American Journal of Occupational Therapy, 74*(Suppl. 3), 1–13.
3. Bailey, D. S., & Bailey, D. R. (1997). *Therapeutic approaches to the care of the mentally ill* (4th ed.). F.A. Davis.
4. Barrows, C. (2006). Home adaptations—Creating safe environments for individuals with psychiatric disabilities. *OT Practice, 11*(18), 12–16.
5. Brumbles, D., & Meister, A. (2013). Psychiatric elopement: Using evidence to examine causative factors and preventative measures. *Archives of Psychiatric Nursing, 27*(1), 3–9.
6. Cardinal Health. (n.d.). *Spill kits and cleaning*. Retrieved April 02, 2022, from https://www.cardinalhealth.com/en/product-solutions/medical/infection-control/hazardous-drug-protection/spill-kits-cleaning/kendall-spill-kit-for-blood-body-fluids.html
7. Centers for Disease Control and Prevention. (n.d.). *10 Leading causes of violence-related deaths, United States: 2017–2020, all races, both sexes.* Retrieved April 09, 2022, from https://wisqars.cdc.gov/data/lcd/home?lcd=eyJjYXVzZXMiOlsiVklPIl0sInN0YXRlcyI6WyIwMSISIjAyIiwiMDQiLCIwNSIsIjA2IiwiMDgiLCIwOSIsIjEwIiwiMTEiLCIxMiIsIjEzIiwiMTUiLCIxNiIsIjE3IiwiMTgiLCIxOSIsIjIwIiwiMjEiLCIyMiIsIjIzIiwiMjQiLCIyNSIsIjI2IiwiMjciLCIyOCIsIjI5IiwiMzAiLCIzMSIsIjMyIiwiMzMiLCIzNCIsIjM1IiwiMzYiLCIzNyIsIjM4IiwiMzkiLCI0MCISIjQxIiwiNDIiLCI0NCIsIjQ1IiwiNDYiLCI0NyIsIjQ4IiwiNDkiLCI1MCIsIjUxIiwiNTMiLCI1NCIsIjU1IiwiNTYiXSwicmFjZSI6WyIxIiwiMiIsIjMiLCI0Il0sImV0aG5pY2l0eSI6WyIxIiwiMiIsIjMiXSwic2V4IjpbIjEiLCIyIl0sImZyb21ZZWFyIjpbIjIwMjAiXSwidG9ZZWFyIjpbIjIwMjAiXSwibnVtYmVyX29mX2NhdXNlcyI6WyIxMCJdLCJhZ2VZZ3JvdXBBfm9ybWF0dGluZyI6WyJsY2QYWdllI0sImN1c3RvbUFnZXNNaW4iOlsiMCJdLCJjdXN0b21BZ2VzTWF4IjpbIjE5OSJdLCJ5cGxvYWdlcyI6WyI2NSJdfQ%3D%3D
8. Centers for Disease Control and Prevention. (2016). *Standard precautions for all patient care*. Retrieved April 01, 2022, from https://www.cdc.gov/infectioncontrol/basics/standard-precautions.html
9. Centers for Disease Control and Prevention. (2016). *Transmission-based precautions*. Retrieved April 01, 2022, from https://www.cdc.gov/infectioncontrol/basics/transmission-based-precautions.html
10. Centers for Disease Control and Prevention. (2022, January 5). *Assault or homicide*. Retrieved April 09, 2022, from https://www.cdc.gov/nchs/fastats/homicide.htm
11. Centers for Disease Control and Prevention. (2022, March 25). *Suicide and self-harm injury*. Retrieved April 09, 2022, from https://www.cdc.gov/nchs/fastats/suicide.htm
12. Channing Bete. (n.d.). *Products*. Retrieved April 08, 2022, from https://www.channingbete.com/
13. Courage to Change. (n.d.). *Life skills*. Retrieved April 08, 2022, from https://www.couragetochange.com/Life-Skills/
14. Crisis Prevention Institute. (2021). *Seven verbal strategies for health care professionals*. Retrieved April 03, 2022, from https://institute.crisisprevention.com/Refresh-Seven-VI-Strategies-for-Health-Care.html
15. Food and Drug Administration. (2021, February 9). *Are you storing food safely?* https://www.fda.gov/consumers/consumer-updates/are-you-storing-food-safely

16. Giffords Law Center. (n.d.). *Who can have a gun: Firearm prohibitions.* Retrieved April 10, 2022, from https://giffords.org/lawcenter/gun-laws/policy-areas/who-can-have-a-gun/firearm-prohibitions/#footnote_29_5595

17. *Gun Control Act of 1968*, 18, U.S.C. § 922 (d) (4). (1968).

18. Gutman, S. A. (2005). Understanding suicide: What therapists should know. *Occupational Therapy in Mental Health, 21*(2), 55–77.

19. Healthwise. (2021, February 10). *Latex allergy: Care instructions.* The Ohio State University Wexner Medical Center. https://www.healthwise.net/osumychart/Content/StdDocument.aspx?DOCHWID=abq0133

20. Kartin, N. J., & Van Schroeder, C. (1982). *Adult psychiatric living skills manual.* Schroeder.

21. Kidner, T. B. (1982). The hospital pre-industrial shop. *Occupational Therapy Mental Health, 2*(4), 63–69.

22. Mustoe, G. (1983). Respiratory hazards: Choosing the right protection. *Fine Woodworking, 41*, 36–39.

23. National Alliance on Mental Illness. (2016, December). *Public policy platform.* https://www.nami.org/Advocacy/Policy-Platform

24. Occupational Safety and Health Administration. (2012). *OSHA brief: Hazard communication standard: Safety data sheets.* Retrieved April 02, 2022, from https://www.osha.gov/publications/OSHA3514.html

25. Occupational Safety and Health Administration. (2019). *Standard number 1910.1030—Bloodborne pathogens.* Retrieved April 01, 2022, from https://www.osha.gov/laws-regs/regulations/standardnumber/1910/1910.1030

26. Ogren, K. (1983). A living skills program in an acute psychiatric setting. *Mental Health Special Interest Section Quarterly, 6*(4), 1–2.

27. Substance Abuse and Mental Health Services Administration. (2019). *Civil commitment and the mental health care continuum: Historical trends and principles for law and practice.* https://www.samhsa.gov/resource/ebp/civil-commitment-mental-health-care-continuum-historical-trends-principles-law

28. Thomson, L. K., & Robnett, R. (2016). *Kohlman evaluation of living skills* (4th ed.). AOTA Press.

29. Treatment Advocacy Center. (2018). *Emergency hospitalization for evaluation.* Retrieved April 03, 2022, from https://www.treatmentadvocacycenter.org/component/content/article/180-fixing-the-system/2275-emergency-hospitalization-for-evaluation#top

30. Willson, M. (1983). *Occupational therapy in long-term psychiatry.* Churchill Livingstone.

SUGGESTED RESOURCES

Articles

Novalis, S. D. (2017). Suicide awareness and occupational therapy for suicide survivors. *OT Practice, 23*(21), CE1–CE8.

Rivard, N., Steinbeisser, K., & Nielsen, S. (2020). Saving lives through suicide prevention and intervention. *OT Practice, 25*(5), 28–30.

Weaver, L. L. (2015). Effectiveness of work, activities of daily living, education, and sleep interventions for people with autism spectrum disorder: A systematic review. *American Journal of Occupational Therapy, 69*(5), 1–11.

Websites

Centers for Disease Control and Prevention. *Sequence for putting on personal protective equipment.* https://www.cdc.gov/hai/pdfs/ppe/ppe-sequence.pdf

Channing Bete. *Products.* www.channingbete.com

Courage to Change. *Life skills.* www.couragetochange.com/Life-Skills/

Crisis Prevention Institute. https://www.crisisprevention.com/

Focus Therapy. *ABA, Occupational therapy helps address safety concerns for Florida children with autism.* https://focusflorida.com/occupational-therapy/aba-occupational-therapy-helps-address-safety-concerns-for-florida-children-with-autism/

National Self Harm Network. *Downloads.* http://www.nshn.co.uk/downloads.html

National Self Harm Network. *What is self-harm?* http://www.nshn.co.uk/whatis.html

Occupational Safety and Health Administration. *Construction industry: Preventing suicides.* https://www.osha.gov/preventingsuicides

Substance Abuse and Mental Health Services Administration. *Treatment for suicidal ideation, self-harm, and suicide attempts among youth.* https://store.samhsa.gov/sites/default/files/SAMHSA_Digital_Download/PEP20-06-01-002.pdf

CHAPTER 10

Using Evidence

OT HACKS OVERVIEW

O: Occupation as a means and an end

Research for mental health and mental disorders often is focused on how those in the study view an aspect of occupation or how a specific skill enhances a particular occupation.

T: Theoretical concepts, values, and principles, or historical foundations

Research includes the use of theories and conceptual frameworks.

H: How can we Help? OT's role in serving clients with mental illness or mental health needs

Evidence-based practice and the translation of knowledge give occupational therapy professionals the tools to provide occupational therapy grounded in best practices.

A: Adaptations

Not applicable in this chapter

C: Case study includes

Four Learning Activities are presented based on different types of evidence.

K: Knowledge: keeping mental health OT practice grounded in evidence, in occupational science, and in research

Knowledge is EVIDENCE that is:

Provided for various purposes

Completed through different designs and methods

Used in various ways

Presented in different possibilities in the professional health care arena

S: Some terms that may be new to you

This chapter continually presents terms associated with research and evidence-based practice. In the summary is a list of the terms presented in the chapter.

INTRODUCTION

Occupational therapy professionals formulate evidence for the purpose of strengthening occupational therapy practice approaches and activities. Evidence is developed through various research designs and methods. Evidence is used when occupational therapy professionals review research studies and when they perform evidence-based practice. Finally, knowledge is shared through different activities associated with the translation of knowledge with various audiences.

Figure 10.1 provides a pictorial display of each of these components of evidence.

WHAT IS IT?

There are several purposes for the research activities used to develop the evidence occupational therapy professionals use in everyday practice.

- **Basic**. Basic research is based on scientific principles and is investigative in nature. It is completed within a controlled setting. The aim of basic research is to provide an understanding of a phenomenon and generate new knowledge to a profession (32).
- **Applied**. Applied research is done to solve practical problems. It investigates the psychometrics of assessment tools. The goal of applied research is to generate information specifically to inform practice (32).
- **Transformative**. Transformative research is an inquiry undertaken to bring about a change in a practical situation or within a specific context. It embeds stakeholders' views and is embedded within a practice setting (32).
- **Action**. Action research focuses on the quality of functions within a particular context. It encompasses the cycle of identifying a problem, planning for action, working with coparticipants of the situation, assessing the completed action, reflecting on the outcome of the action, and revising future action as needed (10).

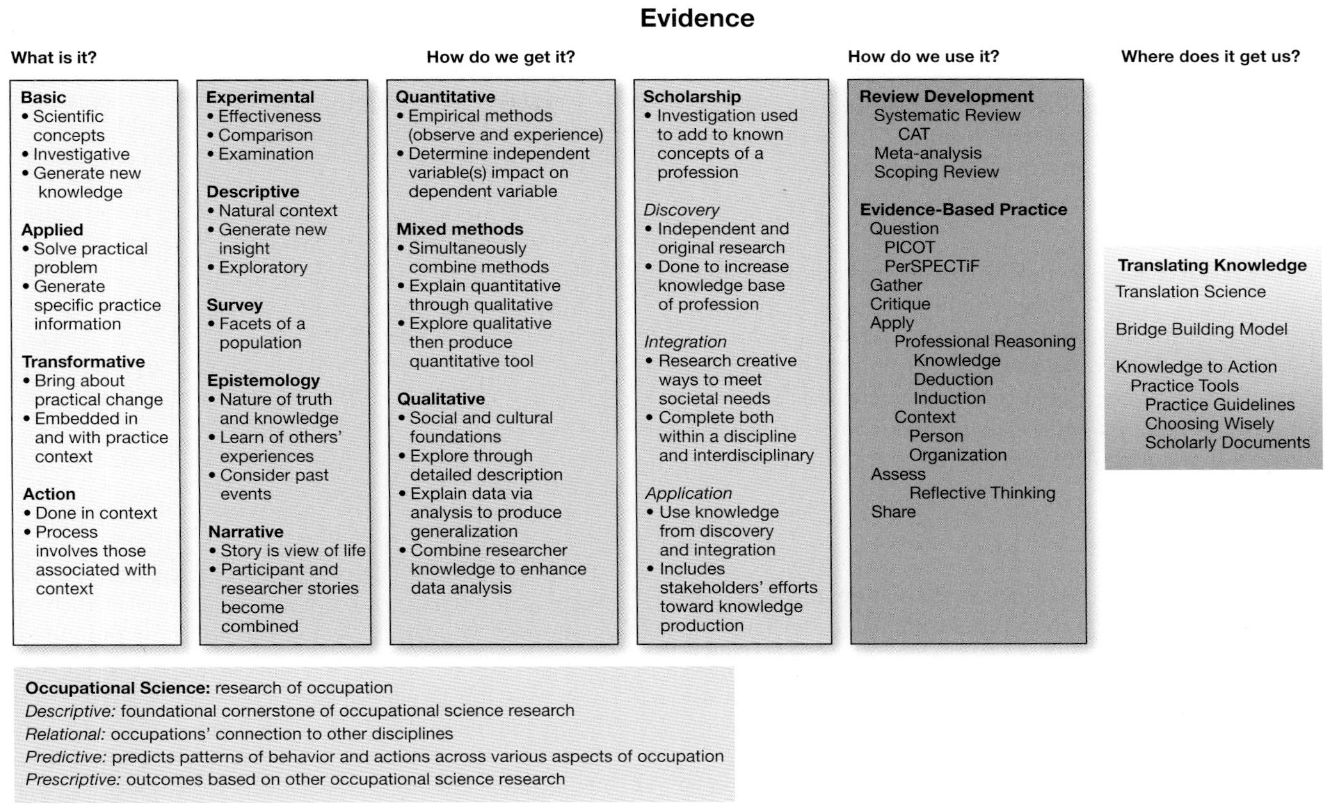

Evidence

What is it?		How do we get it?		How do we use it?	Where does it get us?
Basic • Scientific concepts • Investigative • Generate new knowledge **Applied** • Solve practical problem • Generate specific practice information **Transformative** • Bring about practical change • Embedded in and with practice context **Action** • Done in context • Process involves those associated with context	**Experimental** • Effectiveness • Comparison • Examination **Descriptive** • Natural context • Generate new insight • Exploratory **Survey** • Facets of a population **Epistemology** • Nature of truth and knowledge • Learn of others' experiences • Consider past events **Narrative** • Story is view of life • Participant and researcher stories become combined	**Quantitative** • Empirical methods (observe and experience) • Determine independent variable(s) impact on dependent variable **Mixed methods** • Simultaneously combine methods • Explain quantitative through qualitative • Explore qualitative then produce quantitative tool **Qualitative** • Social and cultural foundations • Explore through detailed description • Explain data via analysis to produce generalization • Combine researcher knowledge to enhance data analysis	**Scholarship** • Investigation used to add to known concepts of a profession *Discovery* • Independent and original research • Done to increase knowledge base of profession *Integration* • Research creative ways to meet societal needs • Complete both within a discipline and interdisciplinary *Application* • Use knowledge from discovery and integration • Includes stakeholders' efforts toward knowledge production	**Review Development** Systematic Review 　CAT Meta-analysis Scoping Review **Evidence-Based Practice** Question 　PICOT 　PerSPECTiF Gather Critique Apply 　Professional Reasoning 　　Knowledge 　　Deduction 　　Induction 　Context 　　Person 　　Organization Assess 　　Reflective Thinking Share	**Translating Knowledge** Translation Science Bridge Building Model Knowledge to Action 　Practice Tools 　　Practice Guidelines 　　Choosing Wisely 　　Scholarly Documents

Occupational Science: research of occupation
Descriptive: foundational cornerstone of occupational science research
Relational: occupations' connection to other disciplines
Predictive: predicts patterns of behavior and actions across various aspects of occupation
Prescriptive: outcomes based on other occupational science research

Figure 10.1. Evidence.

HOW DO WE GET IT?

Evidence is gathered and produced in numerous ways. These ways include research designs and methods, as well as the action of scholarship.

Designs

Research designs include experimental, descriptive, survey, epistemology, and narrative.

Experimental

Experimental research includes data that are collected during experimental activities in which variables are manipulated and observations are made (26). Some often-used experimental designs include the following (32):

- Random control trials. Participants are identified for the study through randomization and the dependent variable is the outcome.
- Quasi-experimental. Randomization or nonrandomization of participants in a convenience sample. Typically, a posttest only or pretest/posttest design is utilized.
- Comparison. Two groups are exposed to a different variable and the outcomes are compared.
- Single subject. Examine an experimental variable on a single subject.

Descriptive

In descriptive research designs, the work is done within the participants' naturally occurring context. It is exploratory and is done to generate new insights (32).

- Normative. This type of research often describes the characteristics of a problem or how something is performed (32).
- Developmental. Patterns of growth or change over a period of time are identified and described, particular to a group of people (32).
- Cohort. A type of developmental research focused on a cohort, or group of participants, over a time period and outcome measurements are assessed at specific time intervals (32).
- Cross-sectional. A type of developmental research where outcomes are measured at stratified levels throughout a group (such as with people who are of different ages but all in the same sample group) (32).
- Correlational. Demonstrates a relationship between the studied variables. There is a relationship or association between the variables (32).
- Methodological review. This type of research considers multiple specifics about a context, with the aim of describing a situation, identifying the needs of the population, identifying similarities between the

studied population and other populations, and identifying the mechanics of how best to work with the study's population (26).

- Evaluative. Research using an evaluative design aims to identify programming effectiveness. The entire organization and its activities are considered (26).

Survey

Survey research is performed with a cross-section of a population and is longitudinal in nature. Its aim is to quantify trends, attitudes, and opinions of a given population (12, 26). A population is examined regarding its defining characteristics or the extent to which a particular situation defines a population (32). Data gained from a survey can assist with planning activities and programming for an organization (26).

Epistemology

Epistemological research looks at the nature and scope of knowledge. It considers concepts of truth (such as what truth is and what the nature of truth is) and what can be learned. This type of research asks questions about what knowledge can be believed in, beyond what can be observed. It focuses on the lived experiences of others and considers past events. It includes the idea that a person's foundation of thinking is the person's philosophies (32). Some often-used epistemological designs are as follows:

- Participatory Action. Participatory action research addresses social problems. Active interventions are a part of the research efforts. The participants are cocreators with shaping research questions, methods, and outcomes.
- Ethnography. This research design is used to describe the inside view of the participants. Those participating in the research direct and interpret the data. The focus of ethnography is on a specific group of people in a particular place and at a specific time. There is also emphasis placed on the group's social and cultural connection to their larger society.
- Grounded Theory. In this type of research, the focus is the theory that emerges from the data. From the collected data, a theory unfolds, is generalized, and is constructed. The interpretation of the data occurs as data are gathered. As new data enter the study, it is considered "in light of" or "in reference to" the already gathered data. Similar pieces of data are collected into categories, which leads to a generalization about the specifically studied phenomenon. Box 10.1 explains a grounded theory study.
- Critical Theory. This type of research focuses on a small group, not on individuals. The focus is on social injustices those in the small group can suffer. Thus, the aim of critical theory design is to bring to light, to mainstream society, the uniqueness of the small group's reality and the challenges and barriers associated with the small group's activities that occur because of societal structures.

BOX 10.1 Learning From the Evidence—e-Mental Health Resources

Williams, A., Fossey, El, Farhall, J., Foley, F., & Thomas, N. (2021). Impact of jointly using an e-mental health resource (self-management and recovery technology) on interactions between service users experiencing severe mental illness and community mental health workers: Grounded theory study. *Journal of Medicine Internet Research Mental Health, 8*(6), 1–13.

In this grounded theory study, service users' and mental health workers' perceptions of using electronic mental health resources were explored. A key outcome of this study was how freedom of choice can improve the therapeutic relationship.

The questions for this learning activity will be provided by the instructor.

- Phenomenology. The phenomenological research design is about everyday living experiences, which are described in detail and are based on how individuals perceive these experiences and use them to perform everyday life activities. Through the narrative process, people share how their life experiences are defined and how they think of these life experiences. People's lived experience includes their aspects of temporal, spatial, living within the parameters of one's body and relation to others. There is an analysis of the consciousness of others, which leads to a greater understanding of others' experiences. Themes of others' expressed experiences emerge from the multiple detailed interpretations provided by the participants. This forms an "essential central meaning" (32, p. 191).

Narrative

Narrative research is based on life stories. These stories are about the participant's view of their life. The research outcome is a combination of the participant's telling of their story and the researcher's retelling and *restorying* of the participant's story (12).

Methods

Research methods include quantitative, mixed methods, and qualitative.

Quantitative

Quantitative methods use empirical research, research based on measurement and observation of the researcher about the phenomena being studied, to determine relationships between and among various independent and dependent variables. This type of research starts with a hypothesis about the dependent variable and its proposed relationship to the independent variable(s). The outcome, or dependent variable, can be identified as significant, as influenced by the independent variable(s) (26).

Mixed Methods

Mixed methods research uses components of quantitative methods and components of qualitative methods. The following are three often-used mixed methods (12):

- Convergent. This type of research merges quantitative method activities with qualitative method activities. The quantitative and qualitative data are collected at the same time. The collected data are integrated to interpret the results.
- Explanatory Sequential. In this method, the quantitative research is completed first. Next, the qualitative research is completed to explain the quantitative results.
- Exploratory Sequential. For this method, the qualitative research is completed first to gather the participants' view on the research study topic. The qualitative analyzed data are then used to build a quantitative research tool to provide outcome data. Finally, additional quantitative research is completed to validate the new research tool. This research can be for an evaluation tool or used to measure outcomes for intervention.

Qualitative

Qualitative methods are focused on the connectiveness, both in research processes and in the structure of the research study. Participants' cultural underpinnings are mixed with the perspectives of the researcher. The collected data are gestalt in nature, the shape of life is formed through the whole of the lived experience. Interactions during the research and interpretation of the data collected are through a social lens. There is an extensive amount of data gathered through detailed observation and interactions with the participants. Constructs are developed through exploration of the descriptive data that are collected. New ideas and theories are introduced through explaining the subjective experiences, thoughts, and occupations of the participants. These new ideas help to explain the social constructs the participants live in. Data analysis produces generalizations that can benefit further study and interactions with others. Existing knowledge and experiences complement the data analysis process (32). Box 10.2 explains a qualitative study.

BOX 10.2 Learning From the Evidence—Digital Health Competence

Jarva, E., Oikarinen, A., Andersson, J., Tuomikoski, A.-M., Kääriäinen, Meriläinen, M., & Mikkonen, K. (2022). Health-care professionals' perceptions of digital health competence: A qualitative descriptive study. *Nursing Open*, 1379–1393.

In this qualitative study, health care professionals from various disciplines provided their perspectives on digital health competencies needed from both the client and the professional. This information can lead to a targeted professional development plan for professional competencies.

The questions for this learning activity will be provided by the instructor.

Scholarship

Scholarship is the investigation of data and using the research results to increase the body of scientific knowledge and recognized knowledge of a profession. Scholarship work is reviewed by others and disseminated publicly to others. Three different types of scholarship that occupational therapy professionals participate in are listed as follows (5):

- Discovery. This is independent and original research. Scholarship of this type is done to broaden and to deepen a profession's theoretical base. Work of this type is typically undertaken inside an academic institution.
- Integration. Scholarship of this type is a creative endeavor completed within a professional discipline and is completed interprofessionally. It is done to identify new perspectives and to build new theories. The goal is to research outcomes to identify meaningful individual pieces of information that can be integrated with knowledge both from the original discipline and with other disciplines. It is completed to provide a collective group of professionals' new methods of meeting the needs of society.
- Application. Application scholarship is completed to apply knowledge gained from discovery or integration research. Theoretical information is applied to occupational therapy service delivery. It includes engagement of others and adds stakeholders' interactive participation to the activity being studied.

Occupational Science[1]

Occupational science research and knowledge come from the field of occupational science and are applied within the profession of occupational therapy. Also, there are occupational therapy professionals who complete original basic research within the profession of occupational science. For this text, occupational science is placed within the section of how we receive evidence, so that the different types of occupational science research can be explained.

Occupation

To begin, occupation, as described by Pierce, is "a subjective event in perceived temporal, spatial, and sociocultural conditions that are unique ... has a shape" (22, p. 139). As occupational therapy professionals examine occupation, they align their thinking with these aspects of doing and completing occupation. They can see the shape or form that the occupational performance takes on by the person completing it, and how the person achieves success in the occupational process.

---

[1]Occupational science information is adapted from the academic paper: Meyer, C. (Spring 2017). *The co-occupation of teaching and learning with a special emphasis on the profession of occupational therapy.* Eastern Kentucky University. Course: OTS 882 Advanced Occupational Science.

Descriptive Occupational Science Research

Descriptive research in the profession of occupational science is the foundational cornerstone on which occupational science knowledge and understanding is built. This research provides rich details about occupations and describes occupations within their contexts (23). Descriptive research is the substructure of occupational science that sets the stage, allowing the other types of research to achieve the delicate balance of interacting with occupational science and coming forth from occupational science (11, 23).

It is research from the perspective of the participant of the occupation. It is the experience of an individual person. It is occupation as it occurs in the typical individual. Results or outcomes of this research are typically used with the profession of occupational therapy or occupational science.

Relational Occupational Science Research

Relational occupational science research considers the relationship occupational science has with the main concepts of other disciplines (24). The concepts from more mature disciplines, which have been deeply researched, help move occupational science forward (23). Relational research branches from topics that are fully developed as descriptive occupational science research (23). Topics of consideration within relational research include items such as cultural awareness within a specific occupation, consideration of cultures across an occupation, disabilities or illness associated with an occupation, occupation and its impact on a gender identity, health and quality of life regarding occupation, and the role of occupational justice to people meeting their occupational needs (23, 24).

In this type of research, occupation is related to another concept such as a disability, gender, or another diversity issue. It looks at how occupation is related to, impacts, or is impacted by the other concept.

Predictive Occupational Science Research

Predictive research in occupational science strives to predict patterns of behavior and actions across various aspects of occupation. The goal is to have a broader view of the occupation and its effects, to or within, different contexts or environments (23). These concentrations can include specific populations of people, time particular to an age range or amount of time spent in an occupation, space demands or the spatial environment in which the occupation takes place, and social conditions surrounding the occupation (23). Of importance to understanding occupation on a grander scale is the impact occupation has to development, and especially across the transitional periods of development through which people pass (23). In addition, the use of assessment instrumentation, particularly in the occupation's naturally occurring environment, is of great value to occupational therapy (23).

Assessments focused on the occupation one is studying are considered occupation-focused assessments. They assess patterns of occupations, such as occupation across development, across the globe, across cultures, across seasons, across times of day, or around the clock. Predictive research, being predictive in nature, also looks at large sample sizes.

Prescriptive Occupational Science Research

Prescriptive research focuses on being the outcome to the first three types of occupational science research (23). It is important to align how effective and occupation focused the research activities of both occupational therapy and occupational science are regarding the service occupational therapy professionals perform with clients (23). Prescriptive research is designed to further develop the occupation as an end or to substantiate the occupation as a means toward greater fulfillment for the client. Prescriptive research focuses on occupation in the natural environment for the client and the natural practice setting for occupational therapy service delivery (23). Finally, prescriptive research tends to focus on the most used interventions in occupational therapy practice and considers the role of occupational justice within the delivery of occupational therapy (23).

This type of research includes studies that use the occupation as a means (use the occupation to improve something else) or use the targeted occupation as an outcome, or as an end (use of something else to improve the occupation).

HOW DO WE USE IT?

Evidence is used in various ways. It can be used to create large-scale reviews, to answer institution-wide concerns, and individual client clinical questions. Occupational therapy professionals critique research evidence to find best practices to provide during occupational therapy service delivery. Various methods to use evidence are as follows:

- Systematic Reviews. In a systematic review, a specific topic is identified, and individual research studies are collected and analyzed. These reviews are developed by at least two people. First, a problem is determined, and then specific criteria are identified as to what type of research evidence will be considered. Database searches are done to collect the data that will be critiqued. The type and number of studies to be considered are done by narrowing the inclusion criteria and exclusion criteria for the participants in the research. Evaluation of the research quality is completed, and the findings are published (19).
- Critically Appraised Topic (CAT). A CAT is completed from an individual research study. The study is reviewed by an individual occupational therapy professional. It is based around a client-based scenario (25).
- Meta-analysis. This is a synthesis of research studies' outcomes. The results gained are used to represent a large, targeted population. The outcomes of several research studies are pooled, thus increasing the power and generalization of the analyzed results (25).

BOX 10.3 Learning From the Evidence—Use of Apps With Caregivers

Désormeaux-Moreau, M., Michel, C.-M., Vallières, M., Racine, M., Poulin-Paquet, M., Lacasse, D., Gionet, P., Genereux, M., Lachiheb, W., & Provenecher, V. (2021). Mobile apps to support family caregivers of people with Alzheimer disease and related dementias in managing disruptive behavior: Qualitative study with users embedded in a scoping review. *Journal of Medical Internet Research Aging, 4*(2), 1–10.

In this scoping review, apps for use by caregivers for managing disruptive behaviors by those with Alzheimer disease and related dementias were reviewed. A focus group was performed, and app relevance and usefulness were considered. Several areas were noted to be further reviewed.

The questions for this learning activity will be provided by the instructor.

- Scoping Review. A scoping review is used to explore a topic's scope of practice. It identifies any lack of depth and breadth of research evidence pertaining to the given topic. Diverse sources are gathered, including but not limited to research studies, gray literature (these are nonacademic research items such as official documents, executive reports, white papers or working papers, policy literature, and government statements), and clinical trials. Stakeholders involved in various institutions and environments impacted by the topic include experts in the topic, or related fields, consumers, policymakers, organization administrators, and service providers. These people all contribute by clarifying information, suggesting options for the format of future research activities, and assisting with prioritizing research focuses. Box 10.3 explains a scoping review (25).

Evidence-Based Practice

Evidence-based practice means using current scientific evidence by integrating it into practice situations. It also involves using one's clinical expertise and reasoning. In addition, the client's values and preferences drive practice decisions. Finally, the clinical circumstances involved play a part in how practice decisions are made and how practice is performed (25). There are several steps in evidence-based practice. They are as follows (36):

1. Asking a question
2. Acquire current evidence
3. Critique
4. Apply
5. Assess
6. Share

Step 1: Asking a Question

- When seeking quantitative data, ask a PICOT question (20):
  - P: patient or population
  - I: intervention or indicator
  - C: comparison or control
  - O: outcome
  - T: time or type of study or type of question
- Sample quantitative PICOT questions for intervention or therapy are as follows (20):
  - In ___ (P), how does ___ (I) compared to ___ (C) impact ___ (O) within ___ (T)?
  - In ___ (P), what is the impact of ___ (I) on ___ (O) compared with ___ (C) within ___ (T)?
  - What is the ___ (O) for ___ (P) who did/experienced ___ (I) as opposed to ___ (C) within ___ (T)?
- When seeking qualitative data, ask a PerSPECTiF question (9).
  - Per: perspective
  - S: setting
  - P: phenomenon of interest/problem
  - E: environment
  - C: comparison (optional)
  - Ti: time or timing
  - F: findings
- Sample qualitative PerSPECTiF question is as follows:
  - From the perspective of ___ (Per), in the ___ setting (S), how does the phenomenon of ___(P), within the environment of ___ (E), compare with ___ (C), in the time period of ___ (Ti), in relation to the "population's" ___ perceptions and experiences (F)?

Step 2: Acquire Current Evidence

This is accomplished by searching databases and websites based on a disease process, setting, or population. These websites can be considered "alerting" or "pushing." This means one can sign up for alerts or notices; when evidence that meets the parameters the person sets in the website's electronic system is identified by the system, an alert or notice is e-mailed to the professional. Another avenue by which to find evidence is through a higher education library system. Membership is often required to utilize this type of source. Table 10.1 provides various evidence databases and websites.

Step 3: Critique

The occupational therapy professional or professionals seeking evidence will select criteria by which to include items of evidence. Once the initial criteria are met, the entire research study or article will need to be critiqued. Individual research studies are critiqued, as are systematic reviews (which encompass several pieces of evidence). Table 10.2 explains the differences in critiquing individual qualitative versus quantitative research studies (14, 17), and Table 10.3 explains the difference in critiquing qualitative systematic reviews versus quantitative systematic reviews (18, 31).

As a part of the critique process, the *level of evidence* for each research study must be established.

A model for quantitative research studies is derived from evidence-based medicine and focuses on numerical data and statistical methods. This model excludes studies that are

Table 10.1. Evidence Databases and Websites

Database or Website	Information
Amedeo Medical Literature Guide. http://www.amedeo.com/	Alerting service of scientific publications for health professionals
American Psychiatric Association Directories and Databases. https://www.psychiatry.org/psychiatrists/search-directories-databases	Resources such as Diagnostic and Statistical Manual of Mental Disorders (DSM) updates, clinical practice guidelines, electronic applications information, and diversity initiatives
American Psychological Association PsychInfo. https://www.apa.org/pubs/databases/psycinfo	Databases available for psychological-based resources for areas such as research journals, books, videos, and factsheets
CanChild Resources. https://www.canchild.ca/en/resources/newsletters	Newsletter with research developments for those with cerebral palsy
DynaMed. https://www.dynamed.com/	Alerting service evidence-based medicine category for psychiatry
Evidence Alerts from McMaster PLUS. https://www.evidencealerts.com/	Alerting service for clinical studies
MedWorm. https://medworm.com/occupational-therapy/news/	RSS (Really Simple Syndication) feed provider—this link is for the subspecialty of occupational therapy
National Institutes of Health: NIH Library. https://www.nihlibrary.nih.gov/resources	Resources, including database information
PubCrawler. http://pubcrawler.gen.tcd.ie/about.html	Alerting service that scans PubMed and GenBank

Table 10.2. Research Study Critique of Adequacy of Research Components for Individual Research Study Articles

	Single Qualitative Study	Single Quantitative Study
Participants	• Themselves and their voices represented	• Sample size • Response rate large enough • Population choice bias free • In comparative study: Randomization Baseline comparison done or incomparability addressed
Methodology Congruent with	• Stated philosophical perspective • Research question or objectives • Methods used • Representation of data • Analysis of data • Interpretation of data	• Methods clear for data collection • Appropriate type utilized • Clearly stated for replication purposes
Data Collection	See Methodology	• Valid instrument • At appropriate time • Relationship to outcomes clear
Results/conclusion	• Flow from analysis or interpretation of data	• Confounding variables accounted for • Accurately reflect analysis • Subsequent analysis a minor focus • Suggestions for further research
Researcher considerations	• Own influence on the research addressed	• If survey completed face-to-face, was bias reduced • Population choice bias free • Statistics free from subjectivity • Data collector and intervention provider different persons
Psychometrics	NA	• Instrument validated • Face validity with design • External validity
Ethical	• Internal Review Board (IRB) • Based on current criteria, or for recent studies	• IRB

Adapted from: Glynn, L. (n.d.). *EBLIP critical appraisal checklist*. Memorial University of Newfoundland. Retrieved February 18, 2022, from http://ebltoolkit.pbworks.com/f/EBLCriticalAppraisalChecklist.pdf; Joanna Briggs Institute. (2020). *Critical appraisal checklist for qualitative research*. https://jbi.global/critical-appraisal-tools

Table 10.3. Research Study Critique of Adequacy of Research Components for Systematic Reviews

	Qualitative Systematic Review	Quantitative Systematic Review
Research question	• Clearly stated	• Clearly stated
Inclusion criteria	• Clearly described	• Appropriate
Search/screening	• Strategy appropriate for question • Relevant literature sufficiently captured	• Strategy appropriate for question • Adequate sources and resources used
Appraisal	• Appropriate criteria to assess risk of bias • Appropriate criteria to assess quality of methodology • Completed independently • Completed by more than one reviewer • Consensus met	• Assessment of possible publication bias • Appropriate criteria used • Completed independently • Completed by more than one reviewer
Synthesis	• Appropriate for research question • Appropriately conducted • Adequate competence by needed number of researchers	• Combination methods appropriate • Errors in data extraction minimized
Findings	• Primary studies used demonstrate clear connection to synthesized findings • Moved beyond a "results summary"	• Publication bias possibility assessed • Policy and practice recommendations supported by data • New research directives appropriate

Adapted from: Swedish Agency for Health Technology Assessment and Assessment of Social Services. (n.d.). *Tool to assess methodological limitations of qualitative evidence synthesis*. Retrieved February 18, 2022, from https://www.sbu.se/contentassets/14570b8112c5464cbb2c256c11674025/methodological_limitations_qualitative_evidence_synthesis.pdf; Joanna Briggs Institute. (2020). *Critical appraisal checklist for systematic reviews and research synthesis*. https://jbi.global/critical-appraisal-tools

qualitative. Table 10.4 shows the kinds of evidence and their rankings, in the traditional evidence-based practice model. Level 1 is the highest level and Level 5 is the lowest (8, 15, 27).

Qualitative levels of evidence allow for subjective data analysis, yet still consider quality of evidence based on the breadth and depth of evidence information and practices. Table 10.5 compares the different levels of qualitative evidence, based on various aspects of the research process. The four different qualitative levels of evidence are as follows (13):

- Level I: Generalizable Studies. These studies build on previous research work. There is a conceptual framework identified for data collection that is provided

Table 10.4. Levels of Evidence in an Evidence-Based Practice Model Derived From Evidence-Based Medicine

Level	Type of Evidence
1	Systematic reviews, meta-analyses, and randomized controlled trials (RCTs)
2	Strong evidence from at least one RCT of sufficient size and statistical power
3	Well-designed trials, not randomized, or single group—measured pre- and postintervention
4	Descriptive studies with outcomes analysis (single subject or case series)
5	Case reports and expert opinion from respected authorities, reports of expert committees, and consensus of experts

through an extensive literature review. (A conceptual framework uses concepts and perceptions gathered from various sources. It includes an integration of situational views, concept explanations, theories, and predictions. There is a joining of individual pieces of information and concepts that are used to explain relationships within a topic. The population group is extended when conceptual categories are called for in the study. The full amount of collected data is clearly reported (16).) The results are analyzed via diverse categorization and saturation of the data. Generalization of the results is compared to the relevant literature for application to other populations.
- Level II: Conceptual Studies. In these types of studies, significant conceptual categories of earlier research are understood through the selected population. A conceptual framework is used to select the population being addressed. The sample population is not diversified. Analysis is solely connected to the depth of comprehension provided by the original conceptual framework. The focus of the study is to develop the overall participants' view on the topic. Conclusions from the results are appropriately drawn.
- Level III: Descriptive Studies. For these studies, there is not often identification of a theoretical connection. The population in the study is used from a specific group or setting. The objective is to describe the views or the experiences of those in the study population. The research is done to present additional support of current research. Within the results, there is a greater use of quotes to illustrate views of the population, rather than data being used to explain the view of the population.

Table 10.5. Qualitative Levels of Evidence

	Level I: Generalizable Studies	Level II: Conceptual Studies	Level III: Descriptive Studies	Level IV: Single Case Studies
Earlier Studies	Foundation research is built from	Used to better understand conceptual categories	x	x
Conceptual Framework	Used for data collection Comes from extensive literature review	Used to select population	Lacks theoretical connection	x
Population	Expanded as new conceptual categories identified	Not diversified during research	Specified group	Single subject or limited number of participants
Data Collection	Clearly reported from full sample Saturation achieved	Not expanded past initial population	Describes view or experience of group Use of illustrative quotes	Emotional accounts
Analysis	Category diversification	Based on comprehensive depth of original conceptual framework	Supports concurrent research	Insight to new situation
Results	Results compared to relevant literature to provide generalization	Focused on current population's view	Not explanatory of group	Can generate future research hypothesis

Adapted from Daly, J., Willis, K., Small, R., Green, J., Welch, N., Kealy, M., & Hughes, E. (2007). A hierarchy of evidence for assessing qualitative health research. *Journal of Clinical Epidemiology, 60*(1), 43–49.

- Level IV: Single Case Study. A single case study has a single subject or a limited number of subjects' interviews. It can offer insight into previously unexplored situations. Often it includes emotional accounts that increase the reader's empathetic response. It can assist in generating future research hypotheses.

Although single case studies are identified at the lowest end of the qualitative evidence level scale, just as they are for quantitative levels of evidence, the single case design can still provide evidence-based practice. Often, single case studies are extremely descriptive, because they are only focused on one individual or one situation. Not only is the situation heavily described, but so is the assessment or intervention process. This type of study may be seen as more closely associated with a "real-time" clinical problem. They may provide details on the use of an adaptive technique or describe how to use a new technology. They can also spur the lone occupational therapy professional into beginning the professional work of evidence collection, which can increase the evidence base for the profession.

Step 4: Apply

When evidence is applied, it is combined with professional reasoning. Professional reasoning is based on clinical knowledge and experience. It combines medical information and the occupational aspects of the person, the experience, and the knowledge of the occupational therapy professional. The knowledge brought to the situation by the occupational therapy professional includes but is not limited to medical information, client information, context considerations, and situational information (6).

Deductive-Based Professional Reasoning

Deductive professional reasoning is mainly focused on quantitative evidence. The reasoning moves general information into being used in a specific situation. It is usually centered about experimentation and seeks to move theoretical concepts and knowledge into active engagement.

The idea is often to test variables within a theory, to determine if the variables are "correct." Generalization is connected to the observable phenomena (32). The research is done to test a hypothesis or to test variables—to determine if they hold true (12). Types of professional reasoning that are more often seen in quantitative evidence are as follows (28):

- Scientific. Here the focus is on the research hypothesis. It involves testing of the client, use of evidence in decision-making, consideration of a diagnosis or condition, and on the *typical* client presentation.
- Diagnostic. This can be viewed as a subset of scientific reasoning. It uses scientific and personal information to discover "why" a situation is occurring and "why" problems are being experienced.
- Procedural. Typically used routines in practice are based on science or on situational factors.
- Pragmatic. This is practical based and focused on nonclient contextual factors.
- Ethical. This type of reasoning is based on an analysis of an ethical-based situation. The focus is on what is the "right" or "correct" action.
- Conditional. There is a combination of multiple types of professional reasoning.

Inductive-Based Professional Reasoning

Inductive professional reasoning is mainly focused on qualitative evidence. The reasoning moves specific information into being used in a general nature.

Inductive professional reasoning combines information to generate a theory. There is identification of individual pieces of data or observations. These pieces are identified as belonging to a larger class or phenomena. The pieces indicate an underlying pattern or meaning (32). Specific observations lead to generalization and to constructing theories. Data analysis leads to broad themes that are generalized into theories or models (12). Types of professional reasoning that are more often seen in qualitative evidence are as follows (28):

- Narrative. This can help to explain a person's medical and occupational history, as well as their current and future occupational situations. It demonstrates an appreciation of the client's personal factors.
- Interactive. A collaborative process used to build a relationship with a client and improve client cooperation. It is based on the client's values and interests. It is problem-solving in nature.

Step 5: Assess

The outcomes need to be reviewed and documented, and the findings need to be summarized. Reflective thinking is used when considering the outcomes associated with the application of the evidence. The reason for what was planned and completed is considered.

Through the writing process, the occupational therapy professional can gain a clearer understanding of actions, people, and situation. Areas to be investigated include what was learned, how all the parties felt during the application, and the responses by all the parties involved. This can lead to a better understanding of the consequences of people's actions and behaviors. Reflective thinking can assist with purging detrimental or anxious thoughts about the application of the evidence (35).

Step 6: Share

Finally, details of the evidence-based practice activities are provided, or disseminated, to others.

WHERE DOES IT GET US?

Evidence is meant to be identified, reviewed, used, and shared. All these actions translate knowledge and are often collectively known as *knowledge translation.*

The Science

The theoretical base to translating knowledge is known as **translational science** (34) or **implementation science** (33). Scientific medical information is connected to practical medical and health activities with client and within populations. This work is done to benefit the client and the greater public (population, public health, and policymaking) (33, 34).

Models

Bridge Building (21) is a model of knowledge translation that combines evidence-based practice, evidence-based research, public involvement, and needs-led research. Evidence-based practice means research studies are critiqued for the best practice application with clients. Evidence-based research includes a systematic process of research that builds on previously completed research. Involving the public includes research and health care professionals partnering with several different stakeholders to determine research questions. Stakeholders include researchers, public and private institutions, payers, and policymakers. Needs-led research fills the gaps identified by systematic reviews, while meeting the needs and priorities of the users and of a society.

Knowledge to Action (29) is another model of knowledge translation. It includes an action cycle, which is how knowledge is utilized. It involves two processes happening simultaneously. Both processes are dependent on each other and drive the activity of the other process. (Bolded items in the next subsection are specific items within the knowledge to action model.)

Action Phases

Action phases (29) bring knowledge to the public and maintain its use. Through an identified **gap in evidence** needed to complete health care–related work, a **problem** is identified, and available **information sources** are identified and reviewed. Available evidence is then **adapted** to the local context and environment in which it will be used. **Barriers and facilitators** to using the knowledge are identified and assessed. Interventions that are appropriate for the situation are **selected**, **modified** as needed for the situation, and **implemented**. Knowledge used is **monitored** and **evaluated** for effectiveness of outcomes. Knowledge use is designed to be **sustained.**

Knowledge Creation Funnel (30)

The knowledge creation funnel brings research information into easily accessible and comprehensible formats to the end users of the information. Health care areas identified as lacking evidence are made a part of **research activities**. Knowledge gained from research is synthesized into **topic-specific review documents—practice tools.**

Practice Tools

Practice tools are developed and targeted for various end users (30).

Practice Guidelines (25) include various documents designed to provide health care workers with information that can be used for immediate client needs. Four different types are described as follows:

- Clinical: based on systematic review providing evidence-based assessments and interventions (2). Examples include practice guidelines from the American Occupational Therapy Association, such as:
  - *Adults Living With Serious Mental Illness*

- *Adults with Alzheimer Disease and Related Major*
- *Neurocognitive Disorders*
- *Individuals With Autism Spectrum Disorder*
- *Children and Youth With Challenges in Sensory Integration and Sensory Processing*
- Outcome-based: evidence-based information with measurement for guideline's impact toward quality care
- Preference-based: evidence-based information with client preferences identified
- Expert-based: provides expert professional's opinion (may not have evidence-based component)

Choosing Wisely (1) is a national campaign meant to alert clients and families to necessary and unnecessary medical and rehabilitation activities. The questions, created by different professional organizations, are designed to encourage conversations between clients and health care providers (4). For instance, as part of the *Choosing Wisely* campaign by the American Occupational Therapy Association, one item discusses working with those on the autism spectrum. It states the following information:

> Don't provide interventions for autistic persons to reduce or eliminate 'restricted and repetitive patterns of behavior, activities, or interests' without evaluating and understanding the meaning of the behavior to the person, as well as personal and environmental factors. (1, para. 7)

Scholarly Documents (26) provide policymaking information and a description of the current scope of practice within a health care field (3). Decision guides help occupational therapy professionals practice decision and answer questions such as: When should services be offered? How should services be provided? What specific concerns are associated with working with this population (such as ethical considerations, documentation needs, or payer requirements)? Box 10.4 explains a decision for working with those who are without permanent housing (7). Other scholarly documents include items such as guidance document, position statements, professional standards, societal statements, and professional policies.

BOX 10.4 Learning From the Evidence—Deciding on Intervention Use

American Occupational Therapy Association (2021). *AOTA decision guide: Working with adults experiencing homelessness (across practice settings)*. https://www.aota.org/practice/practice-settings/working-with-adults-experiencing-homelessness

This decision guide provides resources and information to assist the occupational therapy professional with determining the "best practice" assessment and intervention strategies while working with those who are experiencing homelessness.

The questions for this learning activity will be provided by the instructor.

OT HACKS SUMMARY

O: Occupation as a means and an end

Qualitative methods and mixed methods often are used in research for mental health and mental disorders. Descriptive and epistemological designs typically are used, as are open-ended surveys and narrative studies.

T: Theoretical concepts, values, and principles, or historical foundations

Theories are the foundation in which ideas are developed for research activities. Theories are developed from certain types of research (such as grounded theory research).

Conceptual frameworks are designed through extensive literature review and are used to identify appropriate populations from which study participants are selected. Conceptual frameworks join individual pieces of information and concepts together to explain topic relationships.

H: How can we Help? OT's role in serving clients with mental illness or mental health needs

Through evidence-based practice occupational therapy professionals can individually, or with colleagues, review appropriate studies and develop systematic reviews, CAT papers, meta-analyses, and scoping reviews. Through the steps of evidence-based practice occupational therapy professionals develop client-based questions to study, gather appropriate evidence, critiqued for its value (through use of *levels of evidence*) and usefulness, apply gained knowledge (in conjunction with professional reasoning), assess outcomes through reflective practice, and share new insights and knowledge with others. Translation of knowledge is grounded in translation science and performed through models such as the bridge building model and knowledge to action model. Shared knowledge is used in practice tools such as practice guidelines, public health documents, and scholarly documents (decision guides, guidance documents, position statements, professional standards, societal statements, professional policies).

A: Adaptations

Not applicable in this chapter

C: Case study includes

Four Learning Activity cases:
Box 10.1: e-Mental Health Resources
Box 10.2: Digital Health Competence
Box 10.3: Use of Apps with Caregivers
Box 10.4: Deciding on Intervention Use

K: Knowledge: keeping mental health OT practice grounded in evidence, in occupational science, and in research

Knowledge is evidence that is provided for the research purposes of basic experimentation, applied study, transformative activity, action research completed through different designs and methods:

- **designs**: experimental (random control trials, quasi-experimental, comparison, single subject), descriptive (explorative, normative, developmental, cohort, cross-sectional, correlational, methodological, evaluative), survey (cross-sectional, longitudinal), epistemological (participatory action, ethnography, grounded theory, critical theory, phenomenology), and narrative

- **methods**: quantitative, mixed methods, qualitative
- **occupational science**: this discipline provides occupational therapy professionals a theoretical view of occupation
- **scholarship**: discovery, integration, application

Evidence is used in various ways:

- **evidence-based practice**: question, gather, critique, apply, assess, share
- **presents different possibilities in the professional health care arena**: translating knowledge (translation science, bridge building model, knowledge to action [knowledge creation—practice tools])
- **review development**: systematic review, CAT, meta-analysis, scoping review

S: Some terms that may be new to you

Action research: focuses on the quality of functions within a particular context including: identifying a problem, planning for action, working with coparticipants of the situation, assessing the completed action, reflecting on the outcome of the action, and revising future action as needed

Application scholarship: scholarship that is completed to apply knowledge gained from discovery or integration research

Applied research: generates information specifically to inform practice

Basic research: provides an understanding of a phenomenon and generates new knowledge to a profession

Bridge building model: a model of knowledge translation that combines evidence-based practice, evidence-based research, public involvement, and needs-based research

Cohort research: A type of developmental research focused on a cohort, or group of participants, over a time period and outcome measurements are assessed at specific time intervals

Comparison research: two groups are exposed to different variables, and the outcomes are compared

Conditional reasoning: a type of professional reasoning often associated with interactions involving quantitative evidence and based upon application of a combination of various types of reasoning that are dependent upon existing conditions (of the situation, context, environment, diagnosis/illness, and client)

Convergent research: a type of mixed methods research that merges quantitative and qualitative activities by collecting the quantitative and qualitative data simultaneously and further integrating the data to interpret the results

Correlational research: a descriptive research design that demonstrates a relationship or association between the studied variables

Critical theory research: epistemological research design that focuses on social injustices within a particular group (ie, the focus is not on individuals); its primary aim is to enlighten

mainstream society of the challenges, barriers, and realities of the small group's life activities as they have been impacted or are the result of societal structures

Critically appraised topic (CAT): completed from the review of an individual research study; the study is reviewed by an occupational therapy professional and is based upon a client scenario resulting in a "clinical bottom line" for OT professionals.

Cross-sectional research: a type of developmental research where outcomes are measured at stratified levels throughout a group (such as with people who are of different ages but all in the same sample group)

Deductive reasoning: a type of professional reasoning that is generally applied to analysis of quantitative evidence, moving from general to specific use of information, and usually involving experimentation, with the goal of moving theoretical concepts and knowledge to active engagement

Descriptive research: research that is exploratory and carried out to generate new insights; descriptive research designs primarily occur within the participants' naturally occurring context(s).

Developmental research: a descriptive research design that identifies and describes patterns of growth or change over a period of time, and that are particular to a specific group of people

Diagnostic reasoning: a type of professional reasoning often associated with interactions involving quantitative evidence, can be viewed as a subcategory of scientific reasoning, and uses both scientific and personal information to investigate the "Why" aspects of a situation—Why is this occurring? Why are the problems being experienced?

Discovery scholarship: independent and original research that is undertaken to broaden and deepen a profession's theoretical base

Empirical methods: any research methodologies where conclusions of the study are stringently drawn from authentic (usually experimental) evidence and are therefore considered "verifiable" evidence

Epistemological research: looks at the nature and scope of knowledge, considers concepts of truth, and what can be learned by asking questions about what knowledge can be believed in (accepted as true), beyond what can be observed; includes the idea that a person's foundation of thinking is their personal philosophies, also considers people's past and present lived experiences

Ethical reasoning: a type of professional reasoning often associated with interactions involving quantitative evidence and based on an analysis of the ethics of a situation; the focus is on what is the "right" or "correct" action

Ethnography research: epistemological research design used to describe an insider's perspective of a specific group of people, in a particular place, at a specific time, and emphasizing the group's social and culture connections to larger society; research participants direct and interpret the data.

Evaluative research: research that uses an evaluative design aimed to identify program effectiveness and typically involving consideration of an entire organization and its activities

Experimental research: characterized by data that are collected during experimental activities in which variables are manipulated and observations are made, and then compared to an initial hypothesis

Explanatory sequential: a type of mixed methods research that completes the quantitative research first, and the qualitative research second, to explain the quantitative results

Exploratory sequential: a type of mixed methods research that completes the qualitative research first to gather the participants' perspectives on the study topic; the qualitative data are analyzed and then used to build a quantitative research tool to provide outcome data. Further quantitative research is conducted to validate the new research tool.

Gestalt: a concept that embraces the idea that the product, final overall result, or organized whole of a person, process, or thing is seen as more than the sum of its parts

Grounded theory research: epistemological research design that focuses on theory that continually emerges from the data as they are collected; as theory unfolds, it is generalized and continually constructed while the interpretation of the data simultaneously occurs; similar pieces of data are categorized, and a generalization is then made regarding the studied phenomenon.

Inductive reasoning: a type of professional reasoning that mainly focuses on interactions involving qualitative data and evidence, moving from specific information to use of the information in a more general way, such as when combining information to generate a theory

Integration scholarship: scholarship completed within a professional discipline, and interprofessionally, to identify new perspectives and theories with the goal of providing a collective group of professionals' new methods of meeting the needs of society

Interactive reasoning: a type of professional reasoning often associated with interactions involving qualitative evidence and focused on the collaborative process of considering a client's values and interests, and problem-solving with the client using a relational approach

Knowledge to Action model: a model of knowledge translation that includes the simultaneous and interdependent processes of an action cycle (how knowledge is utilized, brought to the public, and maintained) and a knowledge creation funnel (which brings research information into easily accessible and comprehensible formats to the end uses of the information) for the purposes of driving action and synthesizing research and knowledge gains into topic-specific documents

Knowledge translation: actions that translate knowledge including the processes of identifying, reviewing, using, and sharing evidence, data, information, research, and scholarly endeavors

Levels of evidence: hierarchical approaches resulting in various models (for quantitative research and/or qualitative research) that classify and rank research evidence from strongest to weakest

Longitudinal research: research that takes place over time; studies where data are collected over a minimum of two points in time (typically over extended time as in years, or decades), for the purposes of studying change in the subjects over time

Meta-analysis: a synthesis of research studies' outcomes where multiple research studies are pooled, thus increasing the power and generalization of the analyzed results

Methodological review: research that considers multiple specifics about a context, with the aim of describing a situation, identifying the needs of the population, identifying similarities between the studied population and other populations, and identifying the mechanics of how best to work with the study's population

Mixed methods research: research that uses components of quantitative and qualitative methods within the research design

Narrative reasoning: a type of professional reasoning often associated with interactions involving qualitative evidence; narrative reasoning synthesizes an appreciation of the client's personal factors with their medical and occupational history, and their current situation and future occupational aspirations, to help explain or tell the client's "story."

Narrative research: research based on participants' telling of life stories, with outcomes that combine the participant's telling of their story, and the researcher's retelling of the story, thus creating a narrative

Normative research: a type of research that often describes the characteristics of a problem or how something is performed

Participatory action research: epistemological research design where the participants are cocreators in shaping research questions, methods, and outcomes—usually to address social problems

PerSPECTiF: An acronym that supports the initial step in the application of evidence-based practice, *asking a question*, used when seeking qualitative data; Per: perspective, S: setting, P: phenomenon of interest/problem, E: environment, C: comparison (optional), Ti: time or timing, F: findings

Phenomenological research: epistemological research design focused on understanding the experiences (or phenomena) of others from their perspective

PICOT: An acronym that supports the initial step in the application of evidence-based practice, *asking a question*, used when seeking quantitative data; P: patient or population, I: intervention or indicator, C: comparison or control, O: outcome, T: time, type of study, or type of question

Practice tools: topic-specific review documents

Pragmatic reasoning: a type of professional reasoning often associated with interactions involving quantitative evidence that are based on practicality and are focused on nonclient contextual factors

Procedural reasoning: a type of professional reasoning often associated with interactions involving quantitative evidence, procedural reasoning is based on typically used routines from OT practice and are derived from and developed based on scientific data or situational factors.

Qualitative research: a type of research that focuses on participants' meaning and experiences; data are often collected and interpreted through a social lens, and constructs are developed through exploration of the descriptive data that are collected.

Quantitative research: a type of research that employs empirical analysis using statistical procedures based on measurement and observation about the phenomena being studied to determine relationships between and among various independent and dependent variables; the outcome, or dependent variable, can be identified as significant, as influenced by the independent variable(s).

Quasi-experimental research: an experimental research design characterized by randomization or nonrandomization of participants in a convenience sample; typically, within a posttest only or pretest/posttest design

Random control trial: an experimental research design characterized by participants being identified for the study through randomization, and where the dependent variable is the outcome

Reflective thinking: a way of thinking that is used when considering the outcomes associated with the application of the evidence and when considering the reasons for what was planned and how a process was completed

Scholarship: the investigation of data and information, and the use of research that results in increasing the body of scientific knowledge and recognized knowledge of a profession; scholarship work is typically reviewed by others and disseminated publicly

Scientific reasoning: a type of professional reasoning often associated with interactions involving quantitative evidence; focused on the research hypothesis, testing of the client, use of evidence in decision-making, consideration of diagnosis, and the *typical* client presentation

Scoping review: a review that includes use of diverse sources such as research studies, gray literature, and clinical trials to explore a subject's scope of practice and identify any lack of depth and breadth of research evidence pertaining to the given topic

Single-subject research: an experimental research design that examines an experimental variable on a single subject

Survey research: research that is performed with a cross-section of a population, often longitudinal in nature with an aim of quantifying trends, attitudes, and opinions of the given population

Systematic review: a methodological review in which a specific topic is identified, and individual research studies are collected, analyzed, and synthesized

Transformative research: an inquiry undertaken to bring about a change in a practical situation or within a specific context

Translational science: the theoretical base to translating knowledge, also known as implementation science

Reflection Questions

1. Summarize and discuss the steps associated with implementation of evidence-based practice.
2. Highlight the essential purpose of evidence development research activities used in everyday OT practice for basic, applied, transformative, and action research.
3. Compare and contrast experimental and descriptive research designs. Which research design do you believe would be the most productive in a community-based setting?
4. Describe the Scholarship of Integration. How could Scholarship of Integration be applied and carried out in a behavioral health setting?
5. Discuss the relationship between occupational science research and occupational therapy.
6. How does prescriptive occupational science research incorporate occupation as a means and as an end within its process?
7. Differentiate PICOT questions from PerSPECTiF questions.
8. Although single case studies are considered to be low-level evidence, these studies do have potential benefits. List and describe some of the potential contributions that single case studies have.
9. What factors distinguish qualitative research from quantitative research?

REFERENCES

1. American Board of Internal Medicine. (n.d.). *Choosing Wisely®: Promoting conversations between patients and clinicians*. Retrieved March 06, 2022, from https://www.choosingwisely.org/
2. American Occupational Therapy Association. (n.d.). *AOTA store*. Retrieved March 06, 2022, from https://myaota.aota.org/shop_aota/search.aspx#q=guideline&sort=relevancy
3. American Occupational Therapy Association. (n.d.). *Scope of practice: Decision guides*. Retrieved March 19, 2022, from https://www.aota.org/practice/practice-essentials/scope-of-practice/scope-of-practice-questions-answers
4. American Occupational Therapy Association. (n.d.). *Evidence-based practice: Choosing Wisely*. Retrieved March 06, 2022, from https://www.aota.org/practice/practice-essentials/evidencebased-practiceknowledge-translation/aotas-top-10-choosing-wisely-recommendations
5. American Occupational Therapy Association. (2016). Scholarship in occupational therapy. *American Journal of Occupational Therapy, 70*(Suppl. 2), 1–6.
6. American Occupational Therapy Association. (2020). Occupational therapy practice framework: Domain and process—Fourth edition. *American Journal of Occupational Therapy, 74*(Suppl. 2), 1–87.
7. American Occupational Therapy Association. (2021). *AOTA decision guide: Working with adults experiencing homelessness (across practice settings)*. https://www.aota.org/practice/practice-settings/working-with-adults-experiencing-homelessness
8. Arbesman, M., Scheer, J., & Lieberman, D. (2008). Using AOTA's critically appraised topic (CAT) and critically appraised paper (CAP) series to link evidence to practice. *OT Practice, 12*(15), 18–22.
9. Booth, A., Noyes, J., Flemming, K., Moore, G., Tunçalp, Ö., & Shakibazadah, E. (2019). Formulating questions to explore complex interventions within qualitative evidence synthesis. *BMJ Global Health, 4*, 1–7.
10. Burns, A. (2015). Action research. In J. D. Brown & C. Coombe (Eds.), *The Cambridge guide to research in language teaching and learning* (pp. 99–104). Cambridge University Press.
11. Clark, F. A., Parham, D., Carlson, M. E., Frank, G., Jackson, J., Pierce, D., Wolfe, R. J., & Zemke, R. (1991). Occupational science: Academic innovation in the service of occupational therapy's future. *American Journal of Occupational Therapy, 45*(4), 300–310.
12. Creswell, J. W., & Creswell, J. D. (2018). *Research design: Qualitative, quantitative, and mixed methods approaches* (5th ed.). Sage.
13. Daly, J., Willis, K., Small, R., Green, J., Welch, N., Kealy, M., & Hughes, E. (2007). A hierarchy of evidence for assessing qualitative health research. *Journal of Clinical Epidemiology, 60*(1), 43–49.

14. Glynn, L. (n.d.). *EBLIP critical appraisal checklist*. Memorial University of Newfoundland. Retrieved February 18, 2022, from http://ebltoolkit.pbworks.com/f/EBLCriticalAppraisalChecklist.pdf

15. Holm, M. B. (2000). Our mandate for the new millennium: Evidence-based practice. *American Journal of Occupational Therapy, 54*(6), 575–585.

16. Imenda, S. (2014). Is there a conceptual difference between theoretical and conceptual frameworks? *Journal of Social Science, 38*(2), 185–195.

17. Joanna Briggs Institute. (2020). *Critical appraisal checklist for qualitative research*. https://jbi.global/critical-appraisal-tools

18. Joanna Briggs Institute. (2020). *Critical appraisal checklist for systematic reviews and research synthesis*. https://jbi.global/critical-appraisal-tools

19. Kuehn, J. (2020). *Understanding the systematic review process*. American Occupational Therapy Association. Retrieved February 18, 2022, from https://www.aota.org/practice/practice-essentials/evidencebased-practiceknowledge-translation

20. Northern Arizona University. (n.d.). *Evidence based practice*. Retrieved February 18, 2022, from https://libraryguides.nau.edu/c.php?g=665927&p=4682772

21. Ormstad, H., Jamtvedt, G., Svege, I., & Crowe, S. (2021). The bridge building model: Connecting evidence-based practice, evidence-based research, public involvement and needs led research. *Research Involvement and Engagement, 7*, 77.

22. Pierce, D. (2001). Untangling occupation and activity. *American Journal of Occupational Therapy, 55*(2), 138–146.

23. Pierce, D. (2012). Promise. *Journal of Occupational Science, 19*(4), 298–311.

24. Pierce, D. (2014). Relational research in occupational science. In D. Pierce (Ed.), *Occupational science for occupational therapy* (pp. 81–89). SLACK.

25. Portney, L. G. (2020). *Foundations of clinical research: Applications to evidence-based practice*. F.A. Davis.

26. Rice, M. S., Stein, F., & Tomlin, G. (2019). *Clinical research in occupational therapy* (6th ed.). SLACK.

27. Sackett, D. L. (1986). Rules of evidence and clinical recommendations on use of antithrombotic agents. *Chest, 89*(Suppl. 2), 2S–3S.

28. Schell, B. A. B. (2018). Professional reasoning in practice. In B. A. B. Schell & G. Gillen (Eds.), *Willard and Spackman's occupational therapy* (13th ed., pp. 482–497). Wolters Kluwer.

29. Straus, S. E. (2013). The action cycle. In S. E. Straus, J. Tetroe, & I. D. Graham (Eds.), *Knowledge translation in health care: Moving from evidence to practice* (2nd ed.). Wiley Blackwell.

30. Straus, S. E. (2013). The K in KT: Knowledge creation. In S. E. Straus, J. Tetroe, & I. D. Graham (Eds.), *Knowledge translation in health care: Moving from evidence to practice* (2nd ed.). Wiley Blackwell.

31. Swedish Agency for Health Technology Assessment and Assessment of Social Services. (n.d.). *Tool to assess methodological limitations of qualitative evidence synthesis*. Retrieved February 18, 2022, from https://www.sbu.se/contentassets/14570b8112c5464cbb2c256c11674025/methodological_limitations_qualitative_evidence_synthesis.pdf

32. Taylor, R. R. (2017). *Kielhofner's research in occupational therapy: Methods of inquiry for enhancing practice*. F.A. Davis.

33. Titler, M. G. (2018). Translation research in practice: An introduction. *OJIN: The Online Journal of Issues in Nursing, 23*(2), 1.

34. Tufts. (n.d.). *What is translational science?* Tufts Clinical and Translational Science Institute. Retrieved March 5, 2022, from https://www.tuftsctsi.org/about-us/what-is-translational-science/

35. UM RhetLab. (n.d.). *What is reflective thinking?* Retrieved February 18, 2022, from https://courses.lumenlearning.com/olemiss-writing100/chapter/what-is-reflection/

36. Wilson, B., & Austria, M.-J. (2021, February 26). *What is evidence-based practice?* https://accelerate.uofuhealth.utah.edu/improvement/what-is-evidence-based-practice

Suggested Resources

Evidence-Based Practice

EBP Society (professionals using evidence-based information). https://www.ebpsociety.org/

Free Mobile Apps for evidence based practice. East Tennessee State University. https://www.etsu.edu/medlib/documents/ebm-resources.pdf

McMaster Online Rating of Evidence (MORE). http://hiru.mcmaster.ca/more/index.html

Knowledge Translation

A guide for developing health research Knowledge Translation (KT) plans. https://ictr.wiscweb.wisc.edu/wp-content/uploads/sites/163/2016/10/SickKidsGuideKnowledgeTranslationPlans.pdf

American Occupational Therapy Association. (n.d.). *Evidence-based practice: Choosing Wisely*®. Retrieved March 06, 2022, from https://www.aota.org/practice/practice-essentials/evidencebased-practice knowledge-translation/aotas-top-10-choosing-wisely-recommendations

Innovation to implementation: A practical guide to knowledge translation in healthcare. Mental Health Commission of Canada. https://www.mentalhealthcommission.ca/sites/default/files/2016-06/innovation_to_implementation_guide_eng_2016_0.pdf

Knowledge translation: A cornerstone of youth engagement work. https://www.camh.ca/en/camh-news-and-stories/knowledge-translation-a-cornerstone-of-youth-engagement-work

Knowledge translation planning tools for addiction and mental health research. https://www.albertahealthservices.ca/assets/info/res/mhr/if-res-mhr-kt-planning-tools.pdf

CHAPTER

11

Gina Baker

Professional Issues: Supervision, Professional Teams, Varied Roles, Managing Yourself and Your Practice

OT HACKS OVERVIEW

O: Occupation as a means and an end

This chapter focuses on how understanding the nuances of mental health occupational therapy practice can promote optimal performance of the occupational therapy student and the professional.

T: Theoretical concepts, values, and principles, or historical foundations

Professional reasoning can guide how occupational therapists think through practice in mental health scenarios.

H: How can we Help? OT's role in serving clients with mental illness or mental health needs

How do occupational therapy professionals (OTPs) think through and react to complex situations that can occur in mental health practice?

How do OTPs ensure they are serving themselves to best serve clients living with mental health needs?

A: Adaptations

OTPs (and students) often have to adapt practice methods such as critical thinking, therapeutic use of self, and clinical skills when working in mental health settings.

C: Case study includes

Case studies include real-life examples of professional issues that have occurred within mental health practice scenarios.

K: Knowledge: keeping mental health OT practice grounded in evidence, in occupational science, and in research

Knowledge of team members and their roles and responsibilities, best practices for managing professional issues, managing oneself as a professional, and best practice for supervision are areas of focus within this chapter.

S: Some terms that may be new to you

Mindful self-care
Professional reasoning
Trauma stewardship

INTRODUCTION

The American Occupational Therapy Association (AOTA) (1) clearly outlines that occupational therapy has a "distinct value [to] improve health and quality of life through facilitating participation and engagement in occupations" (para. 1). This value certainly extends into mental health occupational therapy practice. However, with few OTPs working in mental health practice settings as of 2023 (3), fewer models and examples of professional practice in mental health exist to guide students and professionals. This said, professional issues related to supervision requirements, role distinction, and managing oneself and one's practice can arise. This chapter aims to provide a guide to professional competence for mental health occupational therapy practice through the theory of professional reasoning so that the occupational therapy profession can continue to work toward our professional vision:

As an inclusive profession, occupational therapy maximizes health, well-being, and quality of life for all people, populations, and communities through effective solutions that facilitate participation in everyday living (6, para. 3)

PROFESSIONAL REASONING

Boyt Schell (11) defines **professional reasoning** as "the process that professionals use to plan, direct, perform, and reflect on client care" (p. 482). Because OTPs work with human beings who can display unexpected behaviors, we oftentimes must think and react quickly, yet skillfully, to situations. Situations across practice settings and across clients can vary immensely. So, having a theory such as professional reasoning to guide thinking and decision-making can be incredibly valuable.

Professional reasoning, much like cognitive interventions that OTPs use in practice, offers an opportunity for

OTPs to take a complex problem and work through it using "chunking" by examining aspects of the situation: scientific, narrative, interactive, pragmatic, and ethical aspects. For example, imagine the following scenario.

Case Example

You are a level II fieldwork student within a community mental health organization that supports adults living with mental health conditions. A client comes to you and expresses that they are feeling out of control and overwhelmed because they have been experiencing what seems to be a domestic violence situation. The client does not feel safe in their home or community and they don't know what to do.

You have gotten to know this client well during your fieldwork rotation and care deeply about their health, well-being, and safety. You even notice in your body that you're feeling emotions of anger and fear for this individual. You have also never supported someone in this specific situation before. How does an OTP even support someone in this specific situation?

Practice scenarios such as the one described can and do happen in mental health settings and even in settings that one would not consider to be a mental health setting (eg, an outpatient hand therapy clinic). Knowing what to do in such a situation can be challenging. Emotions can and do come up. It is the responsibility of the OTP, though, to think critically and within our occupational therapy scope of practice and ask ourselves questions such as the following:

- What more do I need to know from the client about this situation? (Narrative reasoning)
- How can I regulate my emotions and simultaneously use therapeutic use of self to support this human in front of me? (Interactive reasoning)
- Is there anything about the person's medical and occupational performance history that is important to consider in this situation (eg, trauma history, environmental factors, personal skills and abilities, etc)? Are there any theories, practice models, frames of reference, or pieces of evidence that can support me in supporting this person? (Scientific reasoning)
- What resources do I have available to me? What resources does this person have available to them? What resources are there in our community? (Pragmatic reasoning)
- What am I allowed to do based on my organization's policies and procedures? What am I allowed to do based on local and federal laws? Am I obligated to report this as a mandated reporter? (Ethical reasoning)

No matter one's experience in a mental health setting or with individuals experiencing mental health needs, professional reasoning can serve as a go-to tool to manage professional issues in the moment. However, OTPs and students do have the capability to build professional

reasoning skills for certain situations and practice scenarios before they arise through building their knowledge base. This chapter aims to contribute to the occupational therapy student and professional's knowledge base for professional practice in mental health occupational therapy and uses professional reasoning as a guide to build that knowledge base. Scientific reasoning is not a focus of this discussion as other chapters of this textbook focus on mental health conditions and diagnoses, occupational performance problems, and psychological and social theories. Current evidence is dispersed throughout the chapter.

PRAGMATIC REASONING: "WHAT" AND "WHO" DO I HAVE AVAILABLE TO ME AS A RESOURCE?

A primary difference in mental health occupational therapy practice are the places in which OTPs can work and the team members with whom the OTP will work and collaborate. Understanding the "what" and "who" is essential to making quick and skillful decisions when professional issues arise.

The "What" of Mental Health Practice

The "What" of mental health occupational therapy practice obviously includes much of what is discussed in other chapters of this textbook, so in this chapter, the focus is on the mental health system and the continuum of care in which individuals can receive care, as well as those in which OTPs can work. Frameworks that can assist in understanding this complex system include the following:

- Low-severity mental health concern versus high-severity mental health concern
- Acute versus postacute versus long-term settings
- Medical versus community settings

These frameworks of understanding are further displayed in Figure 11.1.

As shown in Figure 11.1, mental health needs can occur everywhere from the community to medical to education systems. The place in which care occurs often depends on the intensity or severity of the need and what type of care—promotion, prevention, or intervention—the system or setting can provide. Implicitly shown in this figure is that mental health need also occurs across the lifespan, from infancy to elder years. Of additional note is that this figure displays a visual of the United States mental health system, which, of course, is quite different from that of other countries throughout the world. The United States' mental health system is in development as we speak and has potential to change and develop over the coming years. That said, this information is not inclusive of *all* spaces and places in which mental health care occurs but it does provide a focused overview.

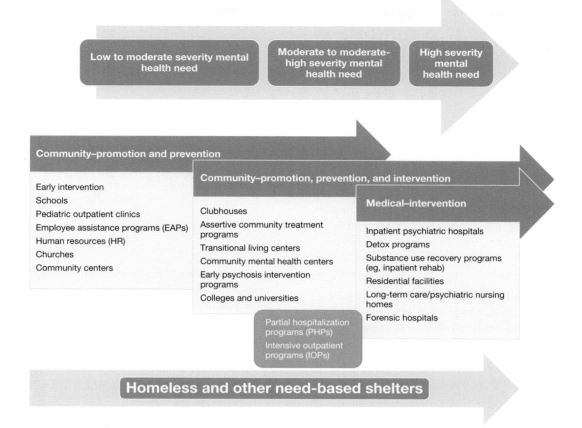

Figure 11.1. Mental Health Continuum of Care: A Complex System in the United States.

WHAT'S THE EVIDENCE?

Mental Health Promotion, Prevention, and Intervention in Occupational Therapy Practice

The AOTA published a position paper in 2017 to make a statement on how OTPs have the knowledge and ability to promote mental health and prevent and intervene when mental health conditions can and do impact occupational performance, participation, and engagement across the lifespan. Within this statement, the AOTA incorporated evidence of occupational therapy serving children, adults, and older adults; individuals with "mental health needs" and those with "serious mental illness" (1, p. 14); and within community programs, schools, and forensic settings. Outcomes ranged from improved sense of belonging to improved activity engagement to improved socialization.

American Occupational Therapy Association. (2017). Mental health promotion, prevention, and intervention in occupational therapy practice. *American Journal of Occupational Therapy, 71*(Suppl. 2), 7112410035p1–7112410035p19.

Within these settings, OTPs can engage in meaningful occupational therapy practice through direct service, program development, and consultation services. Table 11.1 provides some examples of what service delivery could look like as an OTP.

The "Who" of Mental Health Practice

As an OTP demonstrates familiarity with mental health settings and service delivery models, they can begin to understand supports they have among other professionals within these settings. To best be able to collaborate with and utilize such supports, it is essential to be able to distinguish between the variety of professionals in mental health practice and their roles and responsibilities. Again, this can help significantly with making quick, skillful decisions when professional issues arise.

Professionals and Their Roles and Responsibilities in Mental Health

Within the wide array of settings where mental health needs can occur and can be addressed, there can be several professionals to make up the care teams, such as psychiatrists, case managers, clinical social workers (CSWs), expressive therapists, nurses, peer support specialists, mental health therapists, counselors, and, of course, the individual needing service, as well as their significant others/family, as applicable. Presence of individual team members will vary across settings but this text aims to give a general overview, as well as distinguish some team members specific to medical, community, and education systems.

Table 11.1. Occupational Therapy Practice Across Service Delivery Models

Type of OT Service	Direct	Program Development	Consultation
Example of OT practice within a setting	**Inpatient Psychiatric Hospital:** An OTA works on the geriatric unit serving adults who are older than 65 years (as well as those with significant limitations impacting mobility and self-care). They consider the person's psychiatric diagnosis and how that affects what the person wants, needs, and has to do. They implement the treatment plan developed in collaboration with the OT. The OTA and OT are in constant communication about the client's progress and any barriers impacting ability or safety to discharge.	**Community Exercise and Wellness Program:** A need to address social and emotional well-being of adults with Parkinson disease (a progressive disorder) attending a community boxing gym was identified. An OTA and an OT work together to develop a class within their program that uses drama therapy to promote sense of belonging and quality of life among these individuals.	**Clubhouse:** A psychosocial clubhouse is looking to develop sensory rooms within their space to support emotional regulation and participation of their members (ie, adults living with mental health conditions). They recognize the skill of OTPs in sensory processing and environmental adaptations. The OTP works with the members to gather their interests for such spaces and provides recommendations to the clubhouse organization for design of the sensory rooms.

Psychiatrist

Psychiatrists are most seen within medical systems, such as inpatient hospitals or community practice settings. On an interprofessional team, the psychiatrist often serves as the team lead, making final decisions regarding admission, medical treatment, and discharge. The psychiatrist will have qualification as a doctor of medicine (MD) or doctor of osteopathic medicine (DO). They must be licensed in the state within which they provide service (12), which is particularly important in cases of telehealth service, a commonly used practice within psychiatry, even before the COVID-19 pandemic. Psychiatrists use their expertise in psychiatric medicine by prescribing and monitoring effectiveness of psychiatric medications, assessing for and assigning diagnoses per the *Diagnostic and Statistical Manual of Mental Disorders, Fifth Edition, Text Revision* (*DSM-5-TR*) (7), and assessing for risk of harm to self or others, a skill that demands considerable responsibility.

Outside of medical hospitals or institutions, psychiatrists' roles remain important but are often less intensive. Individuals may meet with their psychiatrist once every 3, 6, or even 12 months to ensure effectiveness of medications and other treatment regimens or to assess and diagnose for newly presenting mental health conditions. In the education system, a clinical psychologist might take on roles similar to that of the psychiatrist for students and their families but would not prescribe and manage medications.

Clinical Social Worker

Clinical social workers have obtained a social work master's or doctoral degree and hold the credentials of CSW (12). The role of the CSW in mental health practice is broad and can vary depending on the individual setting and the specialty of the CSW. A CSW's role can include assessment, diagnosis, and treatment of mental and behavioral health conditions. They might employ individual therapy, group therapy, or crisis intervention as treatment modalities (8, 12). Crossover with other disciplines can occur as CSWs serve in a variety of roles including counseling, disaster relief, case management, direct services, advocacy, community mental health, and care coordination (8). Social workers often have a great understanding of community resources.

Case Manager

As with social workers, case managers often are great resources for understanding the client's current and potential resources. The Commission for Case Management Certification (CCM) states that "case management is a dynamic process that assesses, plans, implements, coordinates, monitors, and evaluates to improve outcomes, experiences, and value" (13, para. 1). In the medical setting, the case manager most often acts as liaison to other services such as to the psychiatrist or CSW, helping with community transitions and bureaucratic issues (eg, insurance benefits). As do OTPs and social workers, case managers often function under a strengths-based model (2). A Midwest community mental health organization indicates that the role of their case managers is to "directly assist people to access helpful community resources, teach daily living skills in each person's living/working environment, as well as observe and assist people in learning coping skills and skills and social skills needed to develop healthy relationships within their communities" (10, para. 3). The AOTA asserts that OTPs have a unique value and the capabilities to even serve in the role of case manager on mental health teams (2).

Nurse

Within medical settings, the clinical nurse specialist (CNS), registered nurse (RN), and licensed practical nurse/licensed vocational nurse (LPN/LVN) are often the face of the care team. The nurse provides services in collaboration with the psychiatrist, including administering and supervising diagnostic psychological and neuropsychological testing as needed (12), administering medications and other treatment regimens, practicing crisis intervention and stabilization, assisting with self-care activities, educating clients and families, and coordinating care (8). Nurses also manage other care team members such as technicians and aids.

Mental Health Technician

Mental health technicians (MHTs) work in psychiatric hospitals and parallel to personal care assistants (PCAs) or certified nursing assistants (CNAs) within physical medicine settings such as medical hospitals, inpatient rehab, or skilled nursing facilities. Contrary to CNAs, though, MHTs do not require certification for their role. One can obtain a position as an MHT as an entry-level position. MHTs report to a CNS, RN, or LPN/LVN within their day-to-day work responsibilities, which can include taking vitals, assisting with personal care, providing supervision for safety needs, managing the therapeutic milieu on a unit, and even leading therapeutic groups. Despite differences in educational preparation, MHTs serve an integral role on the care team and often know clients better than anyone else on the team.

Expressive Therapists/Recreation Therapists

Within mental health systems, "expressive therapy" is often used as a term to encompass a range of therapies including recreation therapy (RT), theater or drama therapy, music therapy, or even occupational therapy. Professionals on the expressive therapy team use their area of expertise to assess and provide intervention to individuals and groups, as well as to make recommendations to the care team. For example, recreation therapists use recreation (ie, leisure and play) as a lens to assess gaps in recreation participation and provide opportunities for meaningful recreation to promote mental health and well-being. RT sessions might include use of art, physical activity, games, or any other mode of recreation. Similarly, music therapists use music, and theater/drama therapists use theater as their mode to therapy and eliciting therapeutic benefits. These professionals often have advanced degrees in which they have formally learned their trade and are required to be licensed per state regulations. Therapists within this category can be found across medical, community, and education systems but are not guaranteed across these systems.

Peer Support Specialist

Peer support specialists can be found in psychiatric hospitals and community settings for adults. According to the Substance Abuse and Mental Health Services Administration (SAMHSA):

> Peer support workers are people who have been successful in the recovery process who help others experiencing similar situations. Through shared understanding, respect, and mutual empowerment, peer support workers help people become and stay engaged in the recovery process and reduce the likelihood of relapse. Peer support services can effectively extend the reach of treatment beyond the clinical setting into the everyday environment of those seeking a successful, sustained recovery process (23, para. 1)

Peer support can occur informally and formally. When occurring formally, the peer support worker is referred to as a peer support specialist (or something similar) and receives the "specialist" title through engaging in training and certification as required by the state in which they provide peer services. A common role of a peer support specialist is to use their lived experience to support someone with a mental health or substance use condition to walk through their recovery journey as they so choose.

Mental Health Therapist/Counselor

Many individuals who have accessed mental health services are familiar with the title of "therapist" and use the title to refer to an individual with whom they engage in talk therapy. However, there are several professionals who can fill this role including counselors, licensed therapists, social workers, and psychologists. Some of these professionals have been discussed previously, so this section aims to focus on those most specifically referred to as therapists as well as counselors (20).

In the community, a person with a mental health condition or need often seeks out a "therapist," or a professional might provide a person with a referral to a therapist. Sometimes these therapists are employed by an organization or function as self-employed clinicians. Therapists can range from clinical psychologists to licensed clinical social workers (LCSWs) to licensed professional counselors (LPCs; ie, mental health counselors) to licensed marriage and family therapists (LMFTs). Each of these professionals has training in their specific line of practice and individuals seek out and refer to them for specific reasons (20).

Resources such as Psychology Today's "Find a Therapist" search tool (https://www.psychologytoday.com/us/therapists) can be particularly helpful for piecing through the differences among psychologists, therapists, and counselors and to find the right professional for one's needs. It can also be a great occupation-based tool to use within interventions focusing on mental health management (ie, a client wants to start seeing a therapist but does not know how to go about finding one).

School Counselors

Moving into the education system, school counselors differ from mental health counselors/therapists in terms of their backgrounds, education, and roles and responsibilities. According to the American School Counselor Association (9), the school counselor's qualifications include a master's degree in school counseling at minimum and certification and/or licensure as required by their state. School counselors are present within schools to serve individual students by counseling on academic achievement strategies, managing emotions, applying interpersonal skills, and planning for the future. Mental health–related counseling can be provided in the short-term but referrals to mental health therapists should occur if needs expand beyond the academic setting and beyond short-term need. Contrary to mental health therapists, mental health counselors work at the school organization level serving *all* students, which can look like an ideal caseload of 250:1 (9).

Clinical Psychologist

Continuing to consider the education system, a clinical psychologist's role is often within the special education section of the school. Their role is to conduct special education evaluations when classroom teachers, school counselors, parents, or others working with a student might suspect a disability. From the evaluation, the clinical psychologist would determine whether the evaluation results indicated criteria for the student to receive special education services (M. Schoen Fritsche, personal communication, October 30, 2022).

Clinical psychologists can work across other sectors of the mental health system including medical and community sectors. Just like other professionals, their role will look different depending on the setting in which and the population with whom they work.

Classroom Teachers (and Other Professionals in the Classroom)

Within the education system, classroom teachers, along with other professionals working in the classroom, such as behavioral aides and paraprofessionals, support students in the context of the classroom with their mental health needs (Box 11.1). For example, many classroom teachers are taking to social media these days to share what they are doing at a mental health promotion level to support all students' emotional and mental well-being through activities such as positive affirmations, emotional regulation activities, and psychosocial skill building. Other teachers are working to prevent mental health barriers through educational activities such as writing assignments that target emotional expression. From this author's perspective, more classroom teachers are not only implementing these approaches but are *sharing* these approaches on social media platforms following the fallout of the COVID-19 pandemic. Classroom teachers have always had a tall task to

support large numbers of students amid the demands of their role within the educational system. However, the COVID-19 pandemic has obviously created additional challenges related to student mental health, learning, and teaching.

This section has outlined myriad professionals that an OTP could encounter across mental health practice scenarios; however, OTPs know that the most important part of any interprofessional team is the client and, if applicable, their significant other and/or family. The next section examines these important individuals' roles through the lens of narrative reasoning.

NARRATIVE REASONING: "WHAT IS THE STORY OF THE PERSON AND THEIR SIGNIFICANT OTHER/FAMILY?"

Boyt Schell (11) describes narrative reasoning in a powerful manner: "Understanding the meaning that a disease, illness, or disability has to an individual is a task that goes beyond scientific understanding of disease process and organ systems. Rather, it requires that professionals find a way to understand the meaning of this experience from the client's perspective" (11, p. 489).

If the professional issue we encounter as an OTP has to do directly with a client, the first question we must ask ourselves is: "Do I know the full story of the situation from the client's perspective?" If the answer to that question is "no," then it is the responsibility of the OTP to use narrative reasoning and to gather the story from them as you are able and as the client is willing to share. Consider the following practice example to solidify this idea.

BOX 11.1 Stop, Think, and Apply

Classroom teachers can be a school OTP's greatest resource and partner when mental health is impacting a student's occupational performance. Consider stopping and taking a moment to jump on a social media platform. Go to the search engine on the social media platform and search terms such as the following:

• Mental health classroom

• Teacher mental health

• Mental health classroom management

• Any other search terms that spark your interest on this topic!

Think about how teachers are promoting mental health in their classrooms.

Apply this information by examining shared approaches between occupational therapy and classroom teachers such as those you found from your social media search. In addition, ask yourself "What could an OTP add to the picture to support these teachers and their students?"

Case Example

I'm Gina Baker, the author of this chapter and a mental health occupational therapist, OT professor, and fieldwork educator. At the time of this story, I had been practicing for about 4 to 5 years and was working per diem at a psychiatric hospital, a job that propelled me into full-time education and focus on mental health OT practice.

Within this position, my main role was to implement OT groups, and I did so for a variety of individuals with a variety of mental health conditions and needs. One group that I worked with often was a group that I would see on the unit. The group members consisted of adults who were in the hospital for such experiences as suicidal ideation, depression, anxiety, and substance use. This was one of my favorite groups to work with because I could often engage in rich dialogue with the group members through education and therapeutic activities. A group that I most enjoyed facilitating was a sensory processing and modulation education and exploration group.

One day after running this group on this unit, a group participant who had recently been admitted to the hospital approached me before I left the unit. She mentioned that she had been struggling with anxiety and obsessive compulsive disorder (OCD) and she was wondering what sensory strategies would specifically help her to manage. Because this was the end of the group, I had places to be and things to do, and I was not sure if I would even see this client again because of the short length of stay and my per diem schedule, I could have rattled off some suggestions and been on my way. Instead, I considered my schedule for the day, and asked if I could come back later to ask her some more questions (ie, gather an occupational profile). She said, "yes," and so I came back in the afternoon with the AOTA's *Occupational Profile* in hand.

Through the questions of the *Occupational Profile*, I spent somewhere around 45 minutes to an hour with this client in her hospital room gathering her story, a story that was nowhere to be found within her medical chart. From her narrative, I learned that she had experienced sexual abuse as a child and that compulsions for cleanliness started around this same time. I learned that her parents and family have never understood her compulsions and family relationships were a source of immense pain for her. I learned that she had a love for art that she formally pursued as a teen and younger adult but that OCD and other life factors created such large barriers that she had not touched anything art related in years. I learned that she had a boyfriend whom she regarded as the most supportive person in her life, especially when it came to her OCD, and that the two of them had just moved into a new apartment that they had not yet settled into. I learned her goals for her current stage of recovery (ie, being admitted to the inpatient psychiatric hospital), but more importantly her dreams for her future.

Within this time with this individual, I was able to think like an OTP and put together a picture of the person, environment, occupation, and occupational performance. And from there, I could start to put together some ideas to her original question: *"Are there any sensory strategies that can help with my anxiety and OCD?"*

Fortunately for her need, she ended up staying in the hospital for about 3 weeks (the normal hospital stay in the United States is 3–5 days), so during my initial meeting with her and every time after, I was able to make plans for the next time I would see her. Over a handful of sessions, we addressed her sensory preferences, how she could manage her anxiety within her current context that was the psychiatric hospital, her environment and her routines within her daily life living in her apartment with her boyfriend, and ways she could start getting back to art, an occupation that had brought a lot of meaning to her life previously.

In just a handful of sessions together, this client and I built a strong professional and therapeutic relationship, and progress was made. I think it is best, though, that I let her share that part of the story with you in her own words.

Given here is part of a note she wrote to me on her discharge day:

You've helped me see I can do this and helped me blossom in having hope I can be independent. You've helped avert my attention with the fidget objects when I've felt like my chest would explode. Your time you have put aside to help me make a plan to not be so anxious and assisted me in knowing I can change/do the things I love slowly but surely . . . I am so grateful and honored to have had your expertise and have met you.

This note was written on the back of the colored mandala shown in Figure 11.2.

This story demonstrates that if you do not know what to do in the moment for a client, gather their story, and let that guide you to the next step.

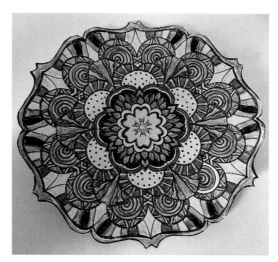

Figure 11.2. A Client Colored This Mandala Over Several Days, Demonstrating a Step Back to Engaging in Art.

In cases that our clients cannot speak for themselves, choose to allow us to speak to another party, or the age of the client requires we speak with a parent or guardian, other stakeholder's stories can provide us with rich information to guide our thinking and our actions. Do not hesitate to take the time in practice for gathering such stories.

INTERACTIVE REASONING: "HOW CAN I REGULATE MY EMOTIONS AND SIMULTANEOUSLY USE THERAPEUTIC USE OF SELF TO SUPPORT THIS HUMAN IN FRONT OF ME?"

Within mental health occupational therapy practice, the OTPs' use of narrative reasoning (ie, gathering the person's occupational story) can lead to hearing scenarios and situations that are not always easy to hear. In these situations, OTPs can experience a professional issue of needing to demonstrate professional competence in performance skills (eg, gathering an occupational profile) and interpersonal skills (eg, listening and responding to the person) while simultaneously managing their own human emotions. If OTPs are not aware of this potential professional issue, then they might avoid challenging conversations, incorporate biases and personal feelings into the therapy session, or risk experiences of burnout or secondary trauma. To avoid such professional issues, OTPs can work toward developing a professional practice called "trauma stewardship."

Trauma Stewardship

Researchers and health professionals have described **trauma stewardship** as the practice of caring for the client without taking on their trauma as your own (15, 21). The need for such practice can seem obvious but the practicality of implementing such practice can seem complex, especially to those who might be new to the concepts of trauma or trauma-informed care. Fortunately, though, there are some clear steps to practicing trauma stewardship (21).

1. **OTPs need to understand their own history of trauma as applicable.** This practice can include understanding current definitions of trauma and reflecting on what trauma has looked like in your own life. A way to do this could be through reading about adverse childhood experiences (ACEs) and take the *ACE Quiz* (18); however, one should do so cautiously and with supports set up around them as exploring one's trauma can be triggering. If you hesitate to examine your own trauma because you suspect trauma in your own life, or even for unexplainable reasons, you might do so with support from a professional, such as a mental health therapist.

2. **OTPs need to know how their trauma can influence reactions with clients.** Trauma can cause individuals to react with agitation, mentally or emotionally shutting down, avoiding conflict, and other behaviors. Such reactions are normal and natural; however, if a professional is unaware of such reactions and where they come from, these reactions can impact the way in which the professional engages with the client. In some instances, the impact of a professional's reactions could be causing traumatization or retraumatization of the client (22).

3. **OTPs need to know the signs of burnout.** According to the Mayo Clinic (16), signs of burnout within work include the following:
   - Cynicism related to or within work
   - Irritability or impatience with others at work
   - Extreme difficulty getting yourself to work or getting started with work
   - Lack of energy
   - Difficulty with concentration
   - Lack of satisfaction within your work
   - Feeling disillusioned about your job
   - Using food, drugs, or alcohol to feel better or to not feel
   - Changed sleep habits—more or less than usual
   - Unexplained headaches, stomach or bowel problems, or other physical complaints that are troubling to you

4. **OTPs must prioritize mindful self-care.** Mindful self-care in this context means attending to both your physical and emotional needs within your daily routines, relationships, and environment. It involves practicing relaxation, mindfulness, physical care, self-compassion, purpose, supportive relationships, supportive structure, and mindfulness (14). Reflection on these practices or formal assessment measures such as the *Mindful Self-Care Scale (MSCS)* (14) can be useful for professionals to understand their own performance issues with practicing self-care as well as to develop plans to improve your self-care.

Recent literature related to burnout supports self-care practices and mindfulness as intervention methods directed at the person; however, it also highlights a great need for better and more supports within workers'

environments, and that sometimes a person can change and become more mindful but still experience burnout due to the impact of the workplace (17, 19). From this angle, this research also highlights the need for advocacy for oneself and one's needs as well as overall needs for all workers within a work setting. One way that OTPs can advocate for themselves is through requesting reasonable accommodations. Many individuals with more "invisible" conditions such as mental health conditions and trauma do not receive or seek out reasonable accommodations. However, places of employment are required by law to provide such accommodations. These accommodations can put necessary supports in place at work to prevent burnout or to address signs and symptoms of burnout. For more information or to see if you would qualify for workplace accommodations, use the following link to the Job Accommodation Network's web page that provides an *Employers' Practice Guide to Reasonable Accommodation Under the Americans with Disabilities Act (ADA)*: https://askjan.org/publications/employers/employers-guide.cfm.

ETHICAL REASONING: "WHAT IS EXPECTED AND REQUIRED OF ME WITHIN THIS SETTING OR SITUATION?"

Up to this point, we have discussed professional aspects of OT practice within mental health settings from the lens of pragmatic reasoning, narrative reasoning, and interactive reasoning: what resources are available to the OTP, the importance of the client and their story to mental health practice, and the practice of managing oneself within mental health practice. Another important, and arguably the most important lens for practice, is ethical reasoning. Boyt Schell states that "ethical reasoning goes one step further [than the other lens of reasoning] and asks: What should be done?" (11, p. 490). As demonstrated in the case example about the fieldwork student, ethical dilemmas can and do come up in mental health practice. Ethical dilemmas can and do come up in *any* practice setting. However, there are certain specific challenges to ethical reasoning in the mental health setting that are addressed within this section.

As previously mentioned, there are fewer OTPs working in mental health practice settings compared to other practice settings. For example, as of 2023, 3.1% of OTPs work in mental health (3). Comparatively, 12.6% of OTPs work in long-term care/skilled nursing facilities and 20.8% of OTPs work in hospitals (other than mental health) as of 2023 (3). The only settings with lower statistics as to mental health practice were those related to innovative or emerging settings, ranking in at 1.5% (3). What this means for supervision in mental health practice is that supervision and mentorship might be harder to come by when pursuing practice, working, or placing fieldwork students in mental health settings. This information is not meant to be a deterrent to practicing in mental health but rather to set up realistic expectations and to examine how ethical reasoning can guide students and OTPs in successful, ethical practice within mental health.

The AOTA (23) defines supervision as "a cooperative process in which two or more people participate in a joint effort to establish, maintain, and/or elevate competence and performance" (23, p. 1) and states the following about supervision and the relationship between the supervisor and supervisee:

- It is "based on mutual understanding between the supervisor and supervisee about each other's education, experience, credentials, and competence" (23, p. 1).
- The process between the supervisor and supervisee should "provide education and support, foster growth and development, promote effective utilization of resources, and encourage creativity and innovation" (23, p. 1).

On the basis of these guidelines from our national association, there is a broadness to what supervision can look like, and this can be gray to students and entry-level OTPs. In mental health settings, then, a supervisee to supervisor relationship could look something like the following:

- OTA fieldwork student to OT professional
- OT fieldwork student (level II) to occupational therapist
- OTA or OT fieldwork student to a supervisor of another discipline (alongside the appropriate OT professional)
- Entry-level OTA or OT to seasoned OTA or OT
- Entry-level or seasoned OTA or OT to a seasoned mental health clinician or other non-OT professional
- Formal supervision between an OTA and OT

Specific supervision needs depend significantly on the type of setting and the experience of the clinician, and understanding these differences is a part of ethical reasoning. Consider the following case example of Jaeda and Clark.

Case Example

Situation 1

Jaeda (she/her) has just accepted her first position as an OTA at a psychiatric hospital where occupational therapy services are covered under the daily lump sum for the client's hospital stay. Therefore, no billing is required in this setting. Her formal supervisor will be the manager of the OT/RT department who is an LCSW. There are three OTs who work in the OT/RT department.

Situation 2

Clark (they/them) has been working as an OT in skilled nursing/long-term care for a few years now but has decided to take a new opportunity as a wellness coordinator at a psychosocial clubhouse. The clubhouse does not bill for occupational therapy services and Clark will not be working in a "traditional" occupational therapy role. Clark has also never worked in this practice setting. Clark's supervisor will be the program manager who has a long history of working in community mental health. There will be no other OTPs at this site.

In both situations, the system in which the OTP will be working does not require the OTP to bill for their services, which means that the OTP will be functioning in somewhat

of a "nontraditional" role, making supervisory needs and requirements less clear. So, let us break down what is expected and required of Jaeda and Clark within their specific situations.

First, let us start with what we *know* about Jaeda's situation.

- Jaeda is an entry-level OTP.
- She is an OTA.
- She will be employed as an OTA.
- She will be working in a setting where billing is not required.
- She will be working within the medical system (ie, inpatient psychiatric hospital).
- She has formal supervision from another professional, her manager, an LCSW.
- She has opportunities for formal and informal supervision from OTs within the OT/RT department.

Next, let us examine what is *required* of Jaeda in this setting.

According to the AOTA's (4) *Guidelines for Supervision, Roles, and Responsibilities During the Delivery of Occupational Therapy Services*, an OTA is required to "receive supervision from an occupational therapist when delivering occupational therapy services" (4, p. 2). Even though Jaeda will not be billing for occupational therapy services, she is working in a setting where she will be "delivering occupational therapy services" (4, p. 2). This means that Jaeda is required to designate a supervisory relationship with at least one of the three OTs who work in the OT/RT department, even though her direct supervisor within this context is her manager who is an LCSW. Depending on the knowledge of the department manager and the department or organization's experience with OTAs, Jaeda might have to educate and advocate for this need within this setting.

Finally, let us examine what's *expected* of Jaeda within this setting.

As previously mentioned, supervision should include the following:

- Educating and supporting
- Fostering growth and development
- Promoting effective resource utilization
- Encouraging creativity and innovation (4)

Ideally, this process should occur dynamically across the supervisor and supervisee relationship, meaning that there should be discussion and collaboration as well as growth and development on both sides of the partnership. This is a reasonable expectation to have within an OTA/OT supervisory relationship; however, it might be less reasonable within a manager/OTP relationship where more of a system hierarchy exists. With this said, though, there are many managers who approach the manager/supervisee relationship in a collaborative manner. It is up to the OTP, though, to discern what exactly are the expectations of their manager/supervisor who might or might not be an OTP.

Within Jaeda's situation where she has a manager and should have an OT supervision relationship, she can expect that formal evaluation should be a part of the process and will likely look different across both relationships. Within her OTA/OT supervisory relationship, she and her OT collaborate might use formal OT documents or informal conversation to evaluate Jaeda's skills and abilities and how Jaeda can continue developing professionally as an OTP, whereas evaluation with her manager might occur in a broader way where her manager evaluates her on her skills as an employee and professional within the hospital system. This situation can require that Jaeda takes on a strong sense of responsibility for the full scope of her role as an OTP within an inpatient psychiatric hospital. Understanding supervision guidelines is essential to Jaeda's success as well as professional and personal wellness as an entry-level professional.

Now, let us turn to the situation of Clark.

We *know* the following about Clark:

- Clark has been working as an OTP for a few years.
- Clark is an OT.
- They have experience in skilled nursing/long-term care.
- Community mental health is a new setting to Clark.
- They will be functioning in the role of "wellness coordinator" (not occupational therapist) in this new position.
- They will be working within a psychosocial clubhouse.
- There is no billing in this setting.
- They will have formal supervision from a non-OTP, their manager.
- They will be the only professional at the site with an occupational therapy background.
- They will likely be using their occupational therapy lens to guide their role as wellness coordinator.

Now, let us examine what is *required* of Clark within this setting that is different from Jaeda's.

According to the AOTA's (4) *Guidelines for Supervision, Roles, and Responsibilities During the Delivery of Occupational Therapy Services*, an occupational therapist is considered to be an "autonomous practitioner" who is able to "deliver occupational therapy services independently" (4, p. 1); however, this depends on their education and training and assumes they have met initial certification, state licensure, and governmental requirements as needed. Within Clark's role as a "wellness coordinator," they technically are not "delivering occupational therapy services" (4, p. 1). So, do they require any supervision? Do they even require the education and training, certification, state licensure, or governmental requirements required of those OTs who are "delivering occupational therapy services?" This can be a gray area for both OTs and OTAs working in nontraditional settings and roles. So, let us break these questions down.

Q: *Does Clark require any supervision?*

A: General Principle 2 within the AOTA's *Guidelines for Supervision, Roles, and Responsibilities During the Delivery of Occupational Therapy Services* (4) provides clarity to this gray area in stating: "to ensure safe and effective occupational therapy services, it is the responsibility of occupational therapy practitioners to recognize when they require peer supervision or mentoring that supports current and advancing levels of competence and professional development" (4, p. 2). In Clark's situation, they have likely received at least the minimum requirements of occupational therapy education related to mental health and community practice; however, Clark is moving into an area of practice that they have never worked in before. It is a professional and ethical responsibility of anyone who will be using an occupational therapy lens to ensure they are equipped to serve the public. Seeking out peer supervision or mentorship in this situation might not be the "required" thing to do but it is certainly *expected*. Because Clark will have a manager within this setting with years of experience in mental health, it would be the right thing to do to seek out both formal and informal supervision and/or mentorship from this individual. They could also seek out mentorship from another professional within the clubhouse. In addition, it would be advantageous for Clark to seek out mentorship from an OTP who has experience in mental health, community practice, health and wellness, and/or psychosocial clubhouses.

As previously mentioned, mentorship within mental health occupational therapy practice can be more challenging than other areas of practice because of the fewer number of OTPs in mental health. In these cases, the AOTA's online communities through *CommunOT* can be an excellent resource for OTPs seeking out informal, or even formal, mentorship from OTPs with experience. There is even a mental health–specific community for those OTPs interested in working or currently working in mental health practice. Individuals with an AOTA membership can access this resource at this web link https://communot.aota.org/communities/communityhome?CommunityKey=85426443-ea20-4df1-b0db-5d4b-f719ea41

Q: *Do they even require the education and training, certification, state licensure, or governmental requirements required of those OTs who are "delivering occupational therapy services?"*

A: Again, the AOTA's *Guidelines for Supervision, Roles, and Responsibilities During the Delivery of Occupational Therapy Services* (4) provides guidance to this gray area (see a theme here?). The AOTA states: "the occupational therapist and occupational therapy assistant should obtain and use credentials or job titles commensurate with their roles in these employment arenas" (4, p. 4). In addition, they should continue to defer to sources such as state practice acts, regulatory agency standards and rules, the *AOTA Occupational Therapy Practice Framework: Domain & Process, 4th Edition* OTPF, 4th edition (5), and other AOTA official documents regarding education, training, licensure, and governmental requirements for these questions. The time and work to review such resources can be dry as well as daunting; however, this is *essential* to maintaining our occupational therapy code of ethics, particularly within emerging/reemerging practice areas such as mental health.

In the case of Clark, what was *required* of them in their site overlapped significantly with what was *expected*, which can be common within community mental health settings where service delivery can occur outside of stereotypical occupational therapy practice. With this in mind, a student or OTP assigned to or working in mental health practice should have the AOTA's *Guidelines for Supervision, Roles, and Responsibilities During the Delivery of Occupational Therapy Services* (4) at the ready to reference in preparation for and when ethical dilemmas may arrive. This resource can be accessed at https://research.aota.org/ajot/article/74/Supplement_3/7413410020p1/6690/Guidelines-for-Supervision-Roles-and

OT HACKS SUMMARY

O: Occupation as a means and an end

Occupational therapy practitioners can engage in meaningful practice within mental health settings and with individuals living with mental health conditions. To perform optimally as a professional in these spaces, OTPs must demonstrate familiarity with unique aspects of the mental health environment that might differ from other practice environments.

T: Theoretical concepts, values, and principles, or historical foundations

Professional reasoning is a valuable tool to guide OTPs in thinking and decision-making within mental health occupational therapy practice.

H: How can we Help? OT's role in serving clients with mental illness or mental health needs

To be able to help clients experiencing mental health needs, OTPs must know the following:

- Their professional team
- Their client and their loved ones as applicable
- How to help and manage themselves
- Supervision expectations and requirements

A: Adaptations

Occupational therapy students and practitioners assigned to, working, or interested in practice in mental health settings can utilize common frameworks and practice guidelines, such as professional reasoning and AOTA documents, to support professional practice in mental health. They might just have to adapt their thinking to apply such foundational concepts to the mental health setting.

C: Case study includes

- Case example of fieldwork student
- Case example of Jaeda and Clark
- Case example story of an OTP and a client in the inpatient psychiatric hospital

K: Knowledge: Keeping mental health OT practice grounded in evidence, in occupational science, and in research

The occupational therapy profession is currently in a place where we are advocating for our role in mental health promotion, prevention, and intervention. It is essential for OT students and professionals to understand our role in these areas with individuals across the lifespan so that we can (i) delineate our role from other professionals and (ii) continue to advance practice. There is current evidence of occupational therapy demonstrating positive outcomes within promotion, prevention, and intervention across a variety of practice settings and across the lifespan.

Today in 2024, researchers are continually producing evidence related to professionals' well-being. At this time, students and OTPs within mental health practice settings can support their well-being by practicing mindful self-care, making conscious choices of where and how they work, and advocating for worker needs for oneself and for all.

S: Some terms that may be new to you

Mindful self-care attending to both your physical and emotional needs within your daily routines, relationships, and environment

Professional reasoning "the process that practitioners use to plan, direct, perform, and reflect on client care" (11, p. 482)

Trauma stewardship the practice of caring for the client without taking on their trauma as your own

Reflection Questions
Describe the mental health continuum in the United States.

1. Identify a practice setting within Figure 11.1, research it online, and describe what OT could look like in this setting through direct service delivery, program development, or consultation.
2. Identify a professional that an OTP could work with in a mental health setting and create a Venn diagram that illustrates the overlap and differences in the two roles.
3. Reflect on the importance of the client's story within mental health OT practice. How will you ensure you gather the person's story within the demands of your role as an OTP?
4. What challenges might you personally encounter in hearing stories from individuals with mental health conditions and/or trauma? How might mindful self-care practices support you to hear these stories and be there for the client?
5. Continuing from Question 4: What additional supports might you need in a work environment within mental health OT work?
6. As an entry-level OTP, what supervision needs, formal and informal, might you need within mental health occupational therapy practice? What supervision needs would be required?

REFERENCES

1. American Occupational Therapy Association. (2016). *Mental health promotion, prevention, and intervention: Across the lifespan.* https://www.aota.org/-/media/corporate/files/practice/mentalhealth/distinct-value-mental-health.pdf

2. American Occupational Therapy Association. (2018). Occupational therapy's role in case management. *American Journal of Occupational Therapy, 72*(Suppl. 2), 7212410050p1–7212410050p12.

3. American Occupational Therapy Association. (2023). AOTA 2023 workforce and compensation survey premium report. https://www.aota.org/career/state-of-the-profession/what-do-practitioners-earn/workforce-and-compensation-survey-premium-report

4. American Occupational Therapy Association. (2020). Guidelines for supervision, roles, and responsibilities during the delivery of occupational therapy services. *American Journal of Occupational Therapy, 74*(Suppl. 3), 7413410020p1–7413410020p6.

5. American Occupational Therapy Association. (2020). Occupational therapy practice framework: Domain and process—Fourth edition. *American Journal of Occupational Therapy, 74*(Suppl. 2), 1–87.

6. American Occupational Therapy Association. (n.d.). *About AOTA: Mission and vision.* https://www.aota.org/about/mission-vision

7. American Psychiatric Association. (2022). *Diagnostic and statistical manual of mental disorders* (5th ed., text rev.). https://doi.org/10.1176/appi.books.9780890425787

8. American Psychiatric Nurses Association. (2022). *About psychiatric-mental health nursing.* https://www.apna.org/about-psychiatric-nursing/#:~:text=Nurses%20in%20psychiatric%2Dmental%20health%3A&text=Provide%20Case%20management,Practice%20crisis%20intervention%20and%20stabilization

9. American School Counselor Association. (2022). *The role of the school counselor.* School Counselor Roles & Ratios—American School Counselor Association (ASCA).

10. Johnson County Kansas. (2023). *Adult services. Johnson County Mental Health.* https://www.jocogov.org/department/mental-health/our-services/mental-health-services/adult-services

11. Boyt Schell, B. A. (2019). Professional reasoning in practice. In B. A. Boyt Schell & G. Gillen (Eds.), *Willard and Spackman's occupational therapy* (13th ed., pp. 482–497). Wolters Kluwer.

12. Center for Medicare and Medicaid Services. (2021). *Medicare & mental health coverage.* https://www.cms.gov/files/document/mln1986542-medicare-mental-health.pdf

13. Commission for Case Manager Certification. (2022). *Definition and philosophy of case management.* https://ccmcertification.org/about-ccmc/about-case-management/definition-and-philosophy-case-management#

14. Cook-Cottone, C. P., & Guyker, W. M. (2017). The development and validation of the Mindful Self-Care Scale (MSCS): An assessment of practices that support positive embodiment. *Mindfulness, 9*, 161–175.

15. Fette, C., Lambdin-Pattavina, C., & Weaver, L. L. (2019). *Understanding and applying trauma-informed approaches across occupational therapy settings.* American Occupational Therapy Association Continuing Education.

16. Mayo Clinic Staff. (2021, June 5). *Job burnout: How to spot it and take action.* Mayo Clinic. https://www.mayoclinic.org/healthy-lifestyle/adult-health/in-depth/burnout/art-20046642

17. National Academies of Sciences, Engineering, and Medicine. (2019). *Taking action against clinician burnout: A systems approach to professional well-being.* The National Academies Press.

18. Aces aware. (2020, May 5). *Screening tools.* https://www.acesaware.org/wp-content/uploads/2022/07/ACE-Questionnaire-for-Adults-Identified-English-rev.7.26.22.pdf

19. Popova, E. S., Hahn, B. J., Morris, H., Loomis, K., Shy, E., Andrews, J., Iacullo, M., & Peters, A. (2023). Exploring well-being: Resilience, stress, and self-care in occupational therapy practitioners and students. *OTJR: Occupation, Participation, and Health, 43*(2), 159–169.

20. Psychology.org. (2022, August 17). *Counseling, therapy, and psychology: What's the difference?* https://www.psychology.org/resources/counseling-therapy-psychology-differences/

21. Raja, S., Hasnain, M., Hoersch, M., Gove-Yin, S., & Rajagopalan, C. (2015). Trauma-informed care in medicine: Current knowledge and future research directions. *Family and Community Health, 38*, 216–226.

22. Substance Abuse and Mental Health Services Administration. (2014). *SAMHSA's concept of trauma and guidance for a trauma-informed approach.* https://store.samhsa.gov/sites/default/files/d7/priv/sma14-4884.pdf

23. Substance Abuse and Mental Health Services Administration. (2022, September 27). *Peer support workers for those in recovery.* https://www.samhsa.gov/brss-tacs/recovery-support-tools/peers

The Occupational Therapy Domain and Process in Mental Health

In *Section One* of this text, the primary focus throughout many of the chapters emphasized occupational therapy's philosophy and historical context. Frames of reference and models of practice were introduced to reexamine how theoretical approaches help navigate our collaborative work with clients. The authors have emphasized connections that help to define service provision and professional practice considerations for occupational therapy professionals working in behavioral mental health settings. A foundation was built throughout the first part of the book that aimed to situate the unique aspects of psychosocial occupational therapy practice together with a more comprehensive understanding of psychiatric diagnoses, while taking into consideration the publication of an updated version of the *Diagnostic and Statistical Manual of Mental Disorders*, Fifth Edition, Text Revision (*DSM-5-TR*) (2).

In *Section Two* of this text, the reader will be introduced to the occupational therapy domain and process and, using the *Domain*, or *Home Metaphor*, journey through learning more about the nuts and bolts of an occupational therapy professional's role in psychosocial settings. We will take a "house tour," one might say, to learn **what we DO** as an occupational therapy professional when we collaborate with our clients to help them optimize their occupational participation.

THIS IS WHAT WE DO . . . OT'S DOMAIN

The word **domain** is a Scottish word meaning "landed property," written as *desme*. Desme was borrowed from Middle French as *domaine* and is a derivative of several Latin words, including *dominion*—meaning property—and *domus*—meaning house (3). Understanding the origin of the word domain provides a good structure for a metaphor to help guide occupational therapy professionals through the OT Domain and Process guided by The American Occupational Therapy Association (AOTA) *Occupational Therapy Practice Framework: Domain and Process, Fourth Edition* (*OTPF-4*) (1).

THIS IS HOW WE DO IT . . . OT'S PROCESS

Evaluation: We can imagine the occupational therapy evaluation process as supporting each of our clients in constructing the optimal "home." These are all the places, spaces, and dimensions that we must collaborate with the client to evaluate.

Intervention: The intervention phase of the occupational therapy process can be imagined as collaborating with our client to do maintenance, or remodeling, repairing, and, in some cases, rebuilding, to improve the value and quality of their home.

Outcomes: During the outcomes part of the occupational therapy process, our role can be compared to that of a property or real-estate appraiser. Our job is to appraise the "home" to help determine what the homeowner should do next.

REFERENCES

1. American Occupational Therapy Association. (2020). Occupational therapy practice framework: Domain and process—Fourth edition. *American Journal of Occupational Therapy, 74*(Suppl. 2), 1–87.
2. American Psychiatric Association. (2022). *Diagnostic and statistical manual of mental disorders* (5th ed., text rev.). https://doi.org/10.1176/appi.books.9780890425787
3. Barnhart, R. K. (1995). *The Barnhart concise dictionary of etymology: The origins of American English words.* Harper Collins Publishing.

Occupational Therapy Domain and Process

WHAT we do = OT's Domain
HOW we do it = OT's Process
- **Evaluation**—constructing the optimal "home"
- **Intervention**—doing home maintenance, or remodeling, repairing, or rebuilding
- **Outcomes**—home appraisal

Context: Personal Factors: "Personal factors are the particular background of a person's life and living and consist of the unique features of the person that are not part of a health condition or health state." (OTPF-4, p. 40)

Imagine a portrait that hangs on a prominent wall of each person's home. Our client Alex's portrait is below. Personal factors make up the background of the client's life.

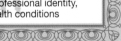

Age, sexual orientation, gender identity, race and ethnicity, cultural identification and cultural attitudes, social background, social status, socioeconomic status, upbringing and life experiences, habits and behavioral patterns, individual psychological assets, education, profession and professional identity, lifestyle, other health conditions

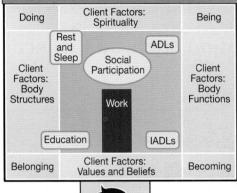

Health Management

Doing | Being

Client Factors: Spirituality

Rest and Sleep | ADLs

Client Factors: Body Structures | Social Participation | Client Factors: Body Functions

Work

Education | IADLs

Belonging | Client Factors: Values and Beliefs | Becoming

This is Alex.
Alex lives here.
This is Alex's domain.

Context: Environmental Factors
"Environmental factors are the aspects of the physical, social, and attitudinal surroundings in which people live and conduct their lives." (OTPF-4, p. 36)

- Natural environment and human-made changes to environment
- Products and technology
- Support and relationships
- Attitudes
- Services, systems, and policies

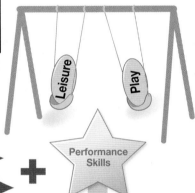
Leisure Play

Performance Skills

Activity Demands: What is required to climb the steps?

Occupation Demands: What is required for ALEX to climb the steps?

+

- **"Motor skills** refer to how effectively a person moves self or interacts with objects, including positioning the body, obtaining and holding objects, moving self and objects, and sustaining performance." (OTPF-4, 2020, p. 13)

- **"Process skills** refer to how effectively a person organizes objects, time, and space, including sustaining performance, applying knowledge, organizing timing, organizing space and objects, and adapting performance." (OTPF-4, 2020, p. 13)

- **"Social interaction skills** refer to how effectively a person uses both verbal and nonverbal skills to communicate, including initiating and terminating, producing, physically supporting, shaping content of, maintaining flow of, verbally supporting, and adapting social interaction." (OTPF-4, 2020, p. 13)

Performance Skills
Performance skills may be thought of as the degree to which a person has the observable abilities and skills that contribute to satisfying, safe, desired, and effective participation in occupations of their priority.

Performance skills are categorized as: Motor Skills, Process Skills, and Social Interaction Skills.

Performance Patterns

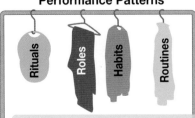

Rituals | Roles | Habits | Routines

In every person's home there is a closet which holds four items of clothing that can be worn in a variety of ways to create innumerable outfits. The "outfits" that a client wears can either support or hinder occupational engagement. The outfit might be imagined as performance patterns.

Performance Patterns
"Performance patterns are the habits, routines, roles, and rituals that may be associated with different lifestyles and used in the process of engaging in occupations or activities. These patterns are influenced by context and time use and can support or hinder occupational performance." (OTPF-4, 2020, p. 41)

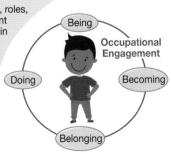

Being
Occupational Engagement
Doing   Becoming
Belonging

Infographic created by Courtney S. Sasse, PhD, MA EDL, MS OTR/L, MA DPS

CHAPTER

12

Evaluation and Data Collection

OT HACKS OVERVIEW

O: Occupation as a means and an end

Many times, because of the transactional nature of occupation, interactions between situational aspects of the client's daily life (ie, contexts: environmental factors and personal factors) and occupation can be supported or improved to benefit or improve the client's overall health, wellness, and quality of life. This is how **occupation** is utilized **as a *means*** (occupational engagement on the journey toward optimal occupational participation) and **as an *end*** (occupational outcomes: better overall health, wellness, and quality of life).

T: Theoretical concepts, values, and principles or historical foundations

The word ***domain*** is derived from the word(s) that mean "home." Understanding the origin of the word domain allows us to use metaphor where home might be thought of as a client's occupational life, which is the center of our profession's focus. Occupational therapy professionals collaborate with clients to move through the Occupational Therapy Process: evaluation, intervention, and outcomes. This process begins with a client-centered, collaborative, occupation-centered evaluation, which will be further discussed in this chapter.

H: How can we Help? OT's role in serving clients with mental illness or mental health needs

The Occupational Therapy Priority Checklist Guidelines was developed by colleagues S. Cratchley, S. Parkinson, S. Town, S. Watling, of the Derbyshire Mental Health Services NHS Trust, U.K. (2004). It is available for download in the Free Resources (with the establishment of an account) from the MOHO-IRM Clearinghouse, University of Illinois Chicago (UIC) (https://moho-irm.uic.edu/products.aspx?type=free).

The form was designed to provide a starting point for screening, discussion about potential intervention, and determining whether occupational therapy services would best support the wellness and recovery priorities of the client. It is particularly helpful for discussions with colleagues in other disciplines (and client and caregivers), because the developers paid particular attention to choosing easily understandable language that still maintains an occupational focus.

A: Adaptations

According to the ***Occupational Therapy Intervention Process Model*** *(OTIPM)* (35) introduced in this chapter, during the evaluation and goal-setting phase that leads up to the intervention phase of the occupational therapy process, the occupational therapy professional (in collaboration with their client) has three main objectives:

1. **Gather initial information:** "Understand the complex relationship between the client's occupations and situational contexts" (35, p. 50). **Develop therapeutic rapport and relationship! Create the Occupational Profile!**
2. **Implement performance analyses.**
3. **Finalize evaluation:** "Synthesize the findings of the performance analysis. . . . Finalize the client's occupation-focused goals. Speculate about the reasons for the client's occupational challenges" (35, p. 50).

C: Case study includes

A 27-year-old male with Bipolar I Disorder with Psychotic Features

D. Kennedy, Case# 291083

Mr Kennedy is a 27-year-old Caucasian male who has a diagnosis of Bipolar I Disorder with Psychotic Features (F31.9). He was referred to occupational therapy for evaluation to assess the need to develop or reestablish skills necessary to resume community living with his wife of 1 year. The client was admitted to the emergency room (ER) of a general hospital following an incident on Valentine's Day a little more than a year ago in which he stabbed and enucleated his right eye. Mr Kennedy cited a biblical passage as the reason for this self-mutilation.[1] The client was subsequently transferred to an outpatient mental health clinic, but 4 months later, he could not be maintained in the community and was admitted to a state psychiatric facility. This was his first psychiatric hospitalization, although he had a history of psychiatric consultations dating from adolescence; and since age 23, he has had difficulty maintaining employment secondary to his reports of having trouble "handling his emotions." Medical history indicates that Mr Kennedy had a provisional diagnosis of schizophrenia, paranoid type in the past. The client has no history of drug or alcohol abuse.

---

[1]Matthew 5:28–30.

Evidence-based practice has become the standard expectation in the modern health care landscape. For occupational therapy professionals' understanding, incorporating into occupational therapy practice, and utilizing evidence-based strategies to make well-reasoned decisions throughout the occupational therapy process is essential. However, two important pieces of the evidence-based practice process appear to be neglected by busy occupational therapy professionals in daily practice; *knowledge translation* and *research capacity*. **Knowledge translation** is the process that moves research from the clinical lab settings, the scholarly research databases, and academic conferences into the hands of occupational therapy professionals and communities of practice who can apply the evidence to provide the highest quality of occupational therapy services for their clients. **Research capacity** is the availability of the resources and structures necessary for an occupational therapy professional to be able to develop, manage, or participate in scholarly activities or research.

Read the following study (accessed from the following link) and reflect on the connection between knowledge translation, research capacity, and occupational therapy evaluations that are anchored by evidence. Follow-up reflection and discussion questions related to the research study can be found in the *Knowledge* section of the *OT HACKS Summary* at the close of the chapter.

Hitch, D., Lhuede, K., Vernon, L., Pepin, G., & Stagnitti, K. (2019). Longitudinal evaluation of a knowledge translation role in occupational therapy. *BMC Health Services Research,* *19*(1), 154.

Link to the Article: https://rdcu.be/cWbnv

S:	Some terms that may be new to you

Assessment

Barrier

Bottom-up evaluation

Construct validity

Context

Criterion-referenced assessment

Environment-first evaluation

Evaluation

Expected environment

Face validity

Health disparities

Health equity (inequity)

Interrater reliability

Normative data

Norm-referenced assessment

Occupational engagement

Occupational experience

Occupational participation

Occupational performance

Performance measures

Personal factors

Reliability

Service competency

Standardization

Strength

Test–retest reliability

Top-down evaluation

Validity

INTRODUCTION

The evaluation process is the foundation for designing intervention plans that emphasize the central client desires. This process helps the occupational therapy professional and the client identify barriers and supports to overall health, well-being, and optimal occupational participation. Essentially, the evaluation supplies the information on which the intervention plan is built and establishes client-centered outcomes that are determined by what the client wants and needs to be able to do. Furthermore, evaluation serves as the initiation point for developing the therapeutic relationship and rapport that is required for client-centered care and optimal therapeutic outcomes. Occupational therapy professionals evaluate occupational performance and consider how situational elements and occupation dynamically and perpetually inform one another (21). At the heart of occupational therapy is the desire to provide services that have a positive impact on the quality of the client's occupational engagement and on how the client experiences their occupation. Many

times, because of the transactional nature of occupation, interactions between situational aspects of the client's daily life and occupation can be supported or improved to benefit or improve the client's overall health, wellness, and quality of life (8). This is how occupation is utilized as a means (the journey toward optimal occupational participation) and as an end (better overall health, wellness, and quality of life).

Occupational therapy professionals are concerned with how clients are functioning now and how they have functioned in the past. They are interested in what the client wants to do, or is motivated by, but is having trouble with performing. Only after gathering this information, establishing a therapeutic rapport with the client, performing a realistic performance analysis, and reflecting on the data, can the practitioner begin to consider how to support or positively impact improvements in the client's future occupational function. If we are to provide truly client-centered care, to identify and understand the problems that our clients are facing, the occupational goals they envision for themselves, and the resources they possess that might help them, we must consistently reflect on the inseparable transactional relationship between occupation and context (9, 34, 35). Finally, consideration of aspects of the client and the occupation, which cannot be separated from each other, and which mutually inform and shape one another, make the occupational therapy professional uniquely qualified to evaluate the constraints and opportunities afforded in everyday life activities that impact client health. Our clients are our partners throughout the occupational therapy process. This begins during the evaluation and goal-setting phase, and the collaboration continues during therapeutic intervention and reevaluation phases. Occupation-centered evaluation and goal setting must be a starting point (9, 33).

This chapter describes the kinds of information that occupational therapy professionals collect with consumers (clients) to compose an occupational profile and determine what is further needed to conduct an analysis of a client's

occupational performance. The American Occupational Therapy Association (AOTA) created the AOTA Occupational Profile Template (2017) to assist practitioners in gathering this essential client information. The *AOTA Occupational Profile Template* is presented in Table 12.1. The multidimensional nature of occupational therapy evaluation is rooted in our core values and beliefs, our expertise in the therapeutic value of occupation, and our therapeutic use of self (23, 36, 73). Whether guided by a theoretical orientation, or by a process-driven model of practice, the occupational therapist uses evidence and expertise to help guide and organize the information that will be collected and reviewed in collaboration with the client.

The roles of the occupational therapy professionals, including the occupational therapist and the occupational therapy assistant, both of whom make unique contributions to the evaluation process, are briefly outlined and contrasted here. A thorough explanation of how an occupational

Table 12.1. AOTA Occupational Profile Template

Occupational Profile

Client Report	**Reason the client is seeking service and concerns related to engagement in occupations (9, p. 16)**	Why is the client seeking services, and what are the client's current concerns relative to engaging in occupations and in daily life activities? (This may include the client's general health status.)
	Occupations in which the client is successful and barriers impacting success (9, p. 16)	In what occupations does the client feel successful, and what barriers are affecting their success in desired occupations?
	Occupational history (9, p. 16)	What is the client's occupational history (ie, life experiences)?
	Personal interests and values (9, p. 16)	What are the client's values and interests?
Contexts		What aspects of their contexts (environmental and personal factors) does the client see as supporting engagement in desired occupations, and what aspects are inhibiting engagement?
	Environment (9, p. 36) (eg, natural environment and human-made changes, products and technology, support and relationships, attitudes, services, systems and policies)	Supporting engagement Inhibiting engagement
	Personal (9, p. 40) (eg, age, sexual orientation, gender identity, race and ethnicity, cultural identification, social background, upbringing, psychological assets, education, lifestyle)	Supporting engagement Inhibiting engagement
Performance Patterns	**Performance patterns (9, p. 41) (eg, habits, routines, roles, rituals)**	What are the client's patterns of engagement in occupations, and how have they changed over time? What are the client's daily life roles? (Patterns can support or hinder occupational performance.)
Client Factors		What client factors does the client see as supporting engagement in desired occupations, and what aspects are inhibiting engagement (eg, pain, active symptoms)?
	Values, beliefs, spirituality (9, p. 51)	Supporting engagement Inhibiting engagement
	Body functions (9, p. 51) (eg, mental, sensory, neuromusculosketal and movement-related, cardiovascular functions)	Supporting engagement Inhibiting engagement
	Body structures (9, p. 54) (eg, structures of the nervous system, eyes and ears, related to movement)	Supporting engagement Inhibiting engagement

Table 12.1. AOTA Occupational Profile Template (*continued*)	
Occupational Profile	
Client Goals — Client's priorities and desired targeted outcomes (9, p. 65)	What are the client's priorities and desired targeted outcomes related to the items below? Occupational performance Prevention Health and wellness Quality of life Participation Role competence Well-being Occupational justice

Reprinted with permission from American Occupational Therapy Association. (2020). Occupational therapy practice framework: Domain and process—Fourth edition. *American Journal of Occupational Therapy, 74*(Suppl. 2), 1–87. ©2020 by the American Occupational Therapy Association.

therapy professional might collect data for analysis, by looking at medical records, observing clients, administering assessments, and interviewing clients and family members, is included. Finally, methods for recording and reporting information are also discussed. Although not an exhaustive list, a sample of some of the widely used, current, evidence-based, psychosocial occupational therapy interviews and assessments are described. The purpose of each assessment is followed by a brief discussion of the client or population for whom the assessment might be useful. Some standardized tests and other commonly used assessments are also described (37, 50). Although it is beyond the scope of this text to comprehensively cover the wide variety of assessments utilized during the evaluation process with clients who experience mental illness, the selected assessments that follow are considered valid and reliable tools that support best practices in occupational therapy.

A HOLISTIC PERSPECTIVE: A DYNAMIC PROCESS

The stages in the occupational therapy process form a unified whole. Although evaluation is discussed here as a separate topic, in the mind of the experienced occupational therapist, all stages of the occupational therapy process, from screening and evaluation, intervention planning and implementation, to measuring outcomes, are inherently linked. From the moment the referral is received, the occupational therapist accepts the client or patient as a partner in therapy and begins to sort and analyze information and ideas and to weigh alternative plans for intervention and continuity of care. This is the beginning of professional reasoning. For example, an occupational therapy professional in an acute care setting will often prioritize transition options on first meeting the client simply because clients' stays are so short in such settings. The client will most likely be concerned about whether and when they can return home. Thus, screening and evaluation in this scenario would focus on transition planning and readiness to

return to home or community, rather than on more lengthy intervention planning. In some settings, evaluation may be ongoing; the occupational therapist in a long-term setting may identify a need for further evaluation of a client as new information comes to light over a longer period of time, such as when the client's health status changes in response to intervention or deteriorates as a result of the disease process.

The occupational therapy process, comprising evaluation, intervention, and outcome deliberation, or the conclusion of occupational therapy services, should, according to best practices, be client centered, occupation centered, outcome oriented, and evidence based (9). Occupational therapy evaluation is *holistic* in that all aspects of the client are contemplated, whether the client is an individual, a group, or a population. It is *contextual* because elements of the client's contexts and environments are considered, with the understanding that in occupational participation, everything is related to everything else. It is *dynamic* in that plans are adjusted as new information comes to light, as the client's ability to perform in occupation evolves, and as environmental circumstances change. For example, a thorough evaluation may be deferred so that immediate medical needs, including psychiatric crisis, can be addressed (9). Also, at any point during intervention, the need for an evaluation of a new area may be recognized.

What we understand as occupational therapy professionals is that whenever one situation or aspect of a client's life changes, there will always be a shift in all the other aspects of the client's life. This is an important philosophical principle to thoroughly understand because from this holistic perspective, and with occupation enmeshed centrally to every other part of a client's life, we can begin to conceptualize the depth and the breadth of what it means to perform, in collaboration with the client, a truly occupation-centered evaluation (41). In other words, when we evaluate a client from an occupational perspective, we are attempting to understand the person and all person's intricate connections, seen and unseen, that impact their participation and engagement in life (35).

It is also important to recall that from a transactional perspective on occupation, a perspective embraced by occupational scientists and occupational therapists alike, situational aspects of the client, including contextual elements, sociocultural aspects, and past or present experiences, among other things, cannot be separated from occupation, or occupational elements (26, 35). For this reason, if the occupational therapy professional views occupation as inextricably linked to other situational aspects of the client, as suggested theoretically by the *Transactional Model of Occupation*, and by the associated and integrated occupation-centered reasoning model, the *OTIPM* (32, 35), then an occupational therapy evaluation must be reliably able to assess three interwoven essential elements: the **occupational performance**, which is the "doing" of the occupation; the **occupational experience**, which is how the "doing" is experienced by the client; and **occupational participation or occupational engagement**, which are used in this text interchangeably to mean that a person is engaged in doing something and they experience it as valuable (1, 21, 25, 35). For our clients who are experiencing mental and behavioral health challenges or persistent mental illness, the focus during the evaluation will often be not only on the client's functional ability to perform a task but at times even more so about understanding the occupational experience of the client. As occupational therapists, we want to know more about how a person's occupational experiences may be hindering them from optimally participating in recovery and in life in general.

Client-Centered Evaluation

Evaluation focuses on what is currently important and meaningful to the client (9). Evaluation also considers the client's past experiences, or occupational history, because these may help in understanding the present situation. The client should be involved at every step; involving the client demonstrates respect for the person's priorities and values. Recognizing the client as a partner beginning in the evaluation and goal-setting phase, the therapist uses collaborative communication skills to invite maximum client participation. The client contributes valuable information to authenticate the purposefulness of the data that is collected , because this interaction and communication between the occupational therapy professional and the client is what leads to the creation of meaningful goals that are relevant and important *to the client*. It is through the therapeutic relationship, and the occupational therapy professional's therapeutic use of self, that clients with mental illness or a history of trauma feel safe enough to be encouraged to ask questions and share their thoughts and opinions (73).

Occupation Centeredness

As occupational therapy professionals, we should consistently remind ourselves that we have an ethical obligation to make sure that throughout the evaluation, intervention, and reevaluation process we are keeping all aspects of our service anchored in occupation (6). The purpose of occupational therapy intervention is to support the client's optimal engagement in occupation in accordance with priorities that the client values. Occupational therapy professionals use occupations and occupational tasks, as well as carefully planned therapeutic activities, with the aim of improving or maintaining the client's ability to engage in necessary and valued occupations (10). Although some methods may not be considered explicitly as therapeutic activities or occupations, these methods and tasks (formerly called "preparatory methods") are considered interventions that support optimal occupational engagement, and they are always connected to enhancing and improving occupational function to meet client-driven goals and outcomes (9).

Outcome Oriented

Outcomes describe the ways that a client's occupational engagement or occupational performance has the potential to be impacted as a result of collaborating with the occupational therapy professional in the occupational therapy process. In short, the *Occupational Therapy Practice Framework: Domain & Process, 4th Edition (OTPF-4)* states that "Outcomes are the end result of the occupational therapy process" (9, p. 80, Table 14). Although the most fundamental result or outcome is the improved ability of the client to engage in occupation, measurable outcomes can be determined and used in a variety of ways. The intervention may be developed for a client who is an individual, a group, or a population. Some examples of outcomes might include reduced fatigue in clients with multiple sclerosis (as a result of applying energy conservation techniques) which lead the client to more effectively clean up after an evening meal or a child with attention-deficit hyperactivity disorder (ADHD) who completes their homework more efficiently secondary to having increased time on task as a result of sensory training or learning to use self-regulation strategies. Outcomes are categorized by the aspects of the occupational therapy domain of concern that are targeted throughout the occupational therapy process, and particularly when the occupational therapy professional and client collaboratively participate in the initial evaluation and goal-setting phase. The range of potential outcomes includes setting goals that focus on the following:

- Occupational performance
- Prevention
- Health and wellness
- Quality of life
- Participation
- Role competence
- Well-being
- Occupational justice (9)

ROLES AND RESPONSIBILITIES OF OCCUPATIONAL THERAPISTS AND OCCUPATIONAL THERAPY ASSISTANTS

Although the methods, types of supervision, and relationship between an occupational therapist (OT) and an occupational therapy assistant (OTA) may vary, both professionals are equally responsible for developing a collaborative plan for supervision that ensures the safe and effective delivery of occupational therapy services to clients. Of foremost importance is that the OT and the OTA abide by obligatory facility, state, or jurisdictional, and payer requirements regarding the supervisory relationship, as well as the documentation of the supervision plan. The roles of the OT and the OTA during evaluation are interrelated and complementary. The OT manages, directs, and documents the evaluation process. Throughout the initial evaluation phase and on an ongoing basis during the entire occupational therapy process, because of the collaborative relationship between the OT and the OTA, the OT can delegate aspects of service to the OTA as appropriate. The AOTA defines the role of the OTA in the evaluation process as follows: "The occupational therapy assistant contributes to the evaluation process by implementing delegated assessments and by providing verbal and written reports of assessments, analysis of performance, and client capacities to the occupational therapist" (7, p. 3). The OT takes the information that the OTA provides and utilizes it to inform the overall evaluation and therapeutic process.

The OT may conduct the assessment(s) in their entirety or delegate relevant tasks to the OTA. Before assigning any part of the evaluation to the OTA, the OT must feel confident that the OTA has the skills to administer the particular assessment and that they would obtain the same or very similar results to what the OT would obtain when using that same instrument. This is known as *establishing service competency* (7). **Service competency** can be established using standardized or criterion-referenced tests to compare results obtained by the OTA with those obtained by the OT. Another way to establish service competency is to have raters view, and rate for similarities, a video of the OT and the OTA each performing a particular task. The OT is, nevertheless, responsible for selecting the appropriate assessment tool or method for each client and for assisting the OTA to develop service competency in areas that will be delegated. The OTA is responsible for acquiring service competency with a given instrument before undertaking independent use of the instrument. The OTA may help the OT to identify instruments that are needed in specific client situations and for which they would like to develop service competency (7). The description and comparison of the roles of the OT and the OTA during the intervention phase will be discussed in Chapter 14.

Finally, the OT has the primary responsibility for selecting and determining the outcomes of intervention and for measuring and interpreting them. The outcome measures should accurately identify and assess the client's engagement in occupations. The OT evaluates changes in the client's performance and capacities to determine whether a change in the type or level of therapy or a discontinuation of services is necessary. The OTA is responsible for implementing delegated responsibilities and tasks related to outcome measures, as well as for collecting and documenting outcomes data and reporting outcome measures to the OT. "An occupational therapy assistant contributes to the transition or discontinuation plan by providing information and documentation to the OT related to the client's progress toward goals, needs, performance, and appropriate follow-up resources" (11, p. 5).

DEFINITION AND PURPOSE OF EVALUATION

In some ways, the **evaluation** can be thought of as the overall comprehensive process of beginning with the end in mind; it is very important to work with the client to select intended or hoped for outcomes, even as early as the initial screening. Sometimes, this occurs when information is collected prior to the official evaluation. Various methods may be employed during evaluation, including observation, interview, review of medical records, and formal or informal testing. The word **assessment** is used to identify specific tests, instruments, interviews, and other measures used to learn about and evaluate holistic aspects of the client and their contextual connections (11, 39). Regardless of the setting, the occupational therapy evaluation should seek to investigate factors that impact client participation in the dynamic aspects and areas of our domain, with a particular focus on engagement in meaningful occupations, including activities of daily living (ADLs), instrumental activities of daily living (IADLs), health management, rest and sleep, education, work, play, leisure, and social participation (10).

The World Health Organization (WHO) with its publication of *The International Classification of Functioning, Disability, and Health (ICF)* has triggered a shift in paradigm regarding how health, disability, and well-being are understood and addressed (76). Occupational therapy perspective and practice has consistently grown and flourished, in part because of its alignment with the principles and the scope of work related to public health contributed by the WHO. The *ICF* introduced a focus on client health and quality of life that can be achieved despite the presence of disease or disability. It emphasized how supports could be put into action that would remove barriers to engaging in and living a meaningful life. Importantly, the ideas introduced in the *ICF* align with several of the cornerstones of occupational therapy practice. Our profession finds value and therapeutic potential in helping clients to successfully participate in the meaningful occupations of life (9, 10).

Furthermore, the *ICF* initiated a change in perspective that "puts all disease and health conditions on an equal footing irrespective of their cause. A person may not be able to attend work because of a cold or angina, but also because of depression. This neutral approach puts mental disorders on a par with physical illness and [for example] has contributed to the recognition and documentation of the world-wide burden of depressive disorders, which is currently the leading cause, world-wide, of life years lost due to disability" (14, para. 6). This shift in perspective has helped highlight and reclaim the roles that occupational therapy professionals have historically played in providing client-centered care for people with mental health disorders. In 2021, WHO published the *Comprehensive Mental Health Action Plan 2013–2030,* an ambitious global plan that recognizes the crucial role of mental health in achieving overall health for every individual (77).

The occupational profile is one way to initiate evaluation; its purpose is to summarize a person's occupational experiences to present a client profile that explores their daily life and history, thus synthesizing client perspective and priorities with an occupational perspective. As mentioned previously, the AOTA has developed *The Occupational Profile Template* (shown in Table 12.1) to encourage practitioners to use the profile to demonstrate what occupational therapy professionals do differently than the other health care providers and to measure, document, and advocate for the value of occupational therapy services to consumers, reviewers, and payers. In addition, in 2017, occupational therapy evaluation and reevaluation codes from the American Medical Association's *Current Procedures Terminology, CPT* (5), began requiring the inclusion of an occupational profile as a part of every OT evaluation.

Through client-centered collaborative evaluation, establishment of the occupational profile, and occupation-centered performance analysis, the occupational therapy professional hopes to identify client goals and priorities. Together, the client and the occupational therapy professional discuss strengths, supports, resources, and barriers that impact, and are impacted by, the client's occupations and occupational participation. In other words, the initiation of a therapeutic relationship during this phase encourages the client to tell a part of their story. If the right questions are asked, and as the client–therapist relationship develops, details of the client's experiences and other situational aspects are often revealed. The OT learns more about what makes life meaningful and valuable that is unique to the individual within the safe and trusting context of this relationship. Therapeutic use of self, which is an integral part of the provision of occupational therapy services, is introduced and discussed further in Chapter 15.

To review, the primary purposes of occupational therapy evaluation are to identify clients' goals and priorities (what they want and need to be able to do) and to analyze their occupational performance. Occupational performance analysis should include an assessment of how the client experienced the occupational performance and should also assess the quality of the occupational performance. Occupational performance analysis that takes place within the client's natural environment, or in an environment that is as contextually and ecologically relevant as possible, will yield the most valid and reliable data (35). If a client cannot do the things that they need and want to do, the OT wants to know why not? Furthermore, the occupational therapy professional, in collaboration and through relationship with the client, hopes to identify changes or interventions that might make the "doing" of a task more possible. Although procedures will vary with the context of the setting and the myriad of other situational aspects unique to each client, in general, evaluation seeks to answer questions such as the following:

- Why is the client seeking occupational therapy services?
- Does the client know what occupational therapy is or how occupational therapy might be able to help them?

- What activities and occupational roles does the person identify as important?
- What is interfering with the client's engagement in these activities and roles?
- To what extent is it possible for this person to develop new skills or redevelop past skills?
- What aspects of the client or their situation facilitate or interfere with the person's ability to function?
- What modifications, resources, or supports can improve this person's ability to function?
- What has been the effect of the person's illness on engagement in occupation? What is the person's view of the illness and the medications as they affect ability to function? What is the prognosis?

UNDERSTANDING BEHAVIORAL STRENGTHS AND BARRIERS IN THE CONTEXT OF OCCUPATIONAL ENGAGEMENT

It can be difficult to decide whether a given behavior is a strength or a barrier until we know more about the situational aspects and contexts of a person's life or history, and this is especially true when working with a person who is experiencing mental health problems. A **strength** is a useful, adaptive behavior, one that helps the client get what they need. Strengths can help clients carry out daily life activities. A **barrier** is anything that interferes with the client's occupational performance, hence impacting their overall participation. According to the *Transactional Model of Occupation*, clients cannot be separated from their context, their occupations, or their situational elements (32, 34, 35). A behavioral barrier might be created as a result of a poor fit between the person's occupational performance and the physical environmental elements, which prohibits an adaptive response, or it may be that a set of behaviors creates a barrier and interferes with the client meeting their needs and doing the things that they are expected to do (ie, sociocultural expectations). Regardless of what strengths or barriers a client possesses, exploring these elements is a fundamental goal of the evaluation phase. To appreciate the enormous importance of reflecting on the client to context relationship in evaluating strengths and barriers, while also taking behaviors or observations into consideration, look at the following descriptions of behavior. Try to decide whether each behavior could be analyzed as a strength or as a barrier.

1. They did not listen to the directions. They just went ahead on their own.
2. They stared out the window during the lecture.
3. They always make sure that their child has a healthy dinner every night.
4. They praised each child who finished the block design puzzles.

How did you classify these behaviors—as strengths or as barriers? At first consideration, many people would say that the first two are barriers and the second two are strengths. But is this always true?

In the first example, the person may have already known the directions; in that case, did it not show initiative for them to proceed on their own? In the second example, is it not possible that the person already knew the information in the lecture or that they were thinking over a point the lecturer had made? Parents who make sure that their child has a healthy meal every night (the third example) would seem to be very appropriate, unless their children were adults with families of their own who lived some distance away. Similarly, praising a child who has done something well (the fourth example) encourages the child to keep trying and to do new things, which develops resiliency. This is a useful behavior in a teacher or occupational therapy professional. However, when administering a standardized test, an occupational therapy professional is supposed to follow the test instructions exactly and should not add to them or alter them. Praising the child may change the results of a standardized test.

As all these examples illustrate, a given behavior may be a strength or a barrier, depending on the details of the person's life situations and occupational and social roles. Of course, some behaviors are almost always barriers, regardless of context. Very poor hygiene and grooming can only interfere with getting along with other people socially and on the job. Other behaviors are almost always strengths—for example, cooperating with others. In general, however, occupational therapy professionals need additional information about the person and the context of their situation before determining which behaviors are strengths and which are barriers. Some other elements to consider that can help us understand whether a behavior is a strength or a barrier and to conceptualize how occupations, the contexts, and the client are dynamically shaped within each transaction can include consideration of: geopolitical elements, social environmental elements, physical environmental elements, task elements, client elements (including personal factors and body functions), temporal elements, and sociocultural elements (9, 35).

CONCEPTS CENTRAL TO THE OT EVALUATION PROCESS

The exploratory work of evaluation is to determine what a person wants and needs to do and what is helping them or hindering them. Client strengths and barriers to occupational engagement can be analyzed by considering the transactional relationships between the following: **Situational Contexts**, valued **Occupations**, **Performance Patterns**, and what we refer to here as the client's **Expected Environment**. A simple acronym, *SCOPE,* can serve as a reminder to focus on these transactional relationships when evaluating clients with mental health dysfunction. Table 12.2 uses the SCOPE acronym to suggest "plain language," simplified questions that occupational therapy professionals can use in initial client screening or informal interviews, and in interprofessional communications, to underscore the unique scope of occupational therapy services. The following sections further describe the relevance and importance of taking into

Table 12.2. The SCOPE of an OT Evaluation in the Psychosocial Practice Arena

The Golden Rules of an OT Evaluation	Questions for Client Interview
Client factors, including (1) values, beliefs, and spirituality, (2) isolated body functions, and (3) isolated body structures; as well as **specific isolated performance skills** (including motor, process, and social interaction skills), **are *not*** the focus of occupational therapy services unless these factors or skills are impacting the ability, quality, safety, or experience of the client to engage in valued occupations! These example questions are presented only as springboards to launch rich occupation-centered discussions about the connections between situational contexts and occupational engagement.	These can be used to gather information for the occupational profile and to encourage further practitioner reflection, client-centered services, and a focus on occupations. ✓ Always begin with a greeting and introduction of yourself. ✓ Always provide a simple explanation of what occupational therapy is and what services we can offer. ✓ We (the authors) understand the practical realities of the modern health care landscape and would not expect that for the sake of time, all of these questions would be able to be asked. Let the *context* and the *client* help you reason through your information seeking. Even the response to one of the following questions can help a client begin to tell their story.
Situational Contexts 1. **Sociocultural Elements** 2. **Temporal Elements** 3. **Client Elements** 4. **Task Elements** 5. **Geopolitical Elements** 6. **Environmental Elements: Social** 7. **Environmental Elements: Physical**	***Questions Related to Sociocultural Elements*** 1. How do you celebrate special occasions? 2. Who makes the rules in the place where you live? How much do you get to help make the rules in the places where you spend time, school, home, at work? ***Questions Related to Temporal Elements*** 1. Do you have certain prayers, sayings (quotes), chants, or songs you have been taught that make you feel better during hard times? 2. What were some of the most important turning points in your life, things that changed you or your life?

(continued)

Table 12.2. The SCOPE of an OT Evaluation in the Psychosocial Practice Arena (*continued*)

	Questions Related to Client Elements
	1. Can you finish this sentence? I think that most people are influenced by _____.
	2. What are three things that you think that you need to be happy?
	3. What is the most difficult habit you have ever tried to get rid of?
	4. What are the first thoughts that go through your mind when you wake up in the morning?
	5. What are some things that you are good at, either now or in the past? How do you know that you are good at those things?
	Questions Related to Task Elements
	1. Can you think of a task that you do every day, and tell me about the items you need to have to get the job done? Are there items that you do not have to have but that would sure make the task easier?
	Questions Related to Geopolitical Elements
	1. Who is a world leader that you admire? (Can be from the past or present)
	2. If you heard different stories on the news, which source would you be most likely to believe: the radio news, the television news, magazines, newspapers, or the internet. Or are you the most likely to believe the "news" that is shared with you by a family member or friend whom you trust?
	3. What was the biggest news event during your life so far?
	Questions Related to Environmental Elements: Social Environment
	1. Where are places that you like to go for entertainment or fun, and whom do you like to go there with?
	Questions Related to Environmental Elements: Physical Environment
	1. Is there anything about the places where you live now or have lived before that you wish you could change about the physical spaces or structure?
	2. What about at your school or work space; is there anything about the space you wish you could change?
	3. What is a task, activity, or job that you think is completely different if you do it in person versus online? Which format do you prefer?
Valued Occupations	1. What are some things that you really like to do?
	2. What are some things that you might not want to do but that you know are important?
	3. What are some things that you wish you could do or want to do a little bit better?
	4. Are there things that you need to do but that you are having trouble with?
	5. Is (name of challenging occupation) something you would like someone to help you with (maybe even something we could work on together during OT)?
Performance Patterns *What are the person's habits, routines, roles, and rituals? How does the client budget or use their time among different activities?*	1. Can you tell me about the things that you do every day? What does a normal day look like for you?
	2. Who or what is important to you?
	3. Do you have responsibility to take care of anyone else besides taking care of yourself? (Ask about humans and nonhumans, that is, pets, plants in a garden, coworkers, children, parents)
Expected Environments **(primarily for inpatient clients)** *Where will the client be going after discharge? (if known) … and Where does the client prefer to go after discharge? (if the client can express this)*	

consideration for reflection the SCOPE elements: situational contexts, valued occupations, performance patterns, and expected environments, during psychosocial occupational therapy evaluation and throughout the intervention and re-evaluation process.

Initiating every occupational therapy evaluation with information gathering that contributes to forming an occupational profile helps explain what occupational therapy is and what kinds of things the client can achieve with support from occupational therapy services. It also highlights and further communicates our main priority and areas of expertise, the client's successful, efficient, safe, and positive occupational function and participation.

As mentioned throughout *Section One* of this text, although occupational therapy has roots in mental health and psychiatry, it is not uncommon to hear students, and even experienced occupational therapy professionals, struggle to clearly or confidently communicate what exactly an occupational therapy professionals generally does in the context of behavioral mental health practice settings. What is our unique identity and contribution in this arena (23)? To communicate what an occupational therapy professional does in a behavioral mental health setting, to express how exactly we do what we do, presents quite a challenge. According to Fisher and Marterella, the authors of *Powerful Practice: A Model for Authentic Occupational Therapy,* and their *Transactional Model of Occupation* (35), "Moreover, they [occupational therapy practitioners] often use evaluation and intervention methods that are so similar to those of their colleagues in physical therapy, psychology, speech-language pathology, education, social work, and nursing, that any distinctions between occupational therapy and these professions become blurred, and even abolished. . . . our unique focus on occupation is not always obvious in practice" (35, p. 94). For this reason, it is extremely important for occupational therapy practitioners to be mindful that a focus on occupation should always be made apparent. Maintaining an evaluation process that consistently includes an occupational profile; utilizing appropriate, evidence-based formal and informal assessments; and analyzing occupational performance are critical ways to make sure that occupation is apparent, regardless of the practice setting or the diagnosis of the client.

Contexts: Environmental and Personal Factors

Context or **contexts** are broad constructs that describe the conditions and situations that are intimately bound to occupation and that give meaning to occupational performance, hence influencing and being influenced by one another in a persistent, multidimensional dynamic. Two aspects of context are recognized within the *OTPF-4* and as elements of the AOTA's *Occupational Profile Template*: Environmental Factors and Personal Factors. The contextual factors of the environment are further broken into the categories of the physical environment and the social environment. The

contextual reference to personal factors are further divided into four aspects: cultural, personal, temporal, and virtual. **Personal factors** are defined by the *OTPF-4* as "the particular background of a person's life and living, and consist of the unique features of the person that are not part of a health condition, or a health state" (9, p. 40). Although the contexts named in the *OTPF-4* have been categorized as separate from each other, in reality, they overlap and intermix. All aspects of the client's situational context(s) and the psychosocial implications that arise from their constant interactions and transactions are to be considered in an occupational therapy evaluation. This includes *all* various aspects the client encounters in daily life. It can feel quite overwhelming to try to take so many things into account in an evaluation, especially for a new occupational therapy professional. Even for an experienced occupational therapy professional who is working with a client who has mental illness, or for an occupational therapy professional on a behavioral mental health team for the first time, thinking about these dynamics can feel daunting, particularly with the common time constraints and practical realities at work in our health care system today (35).

Understanding and Applying Contexts

The effects of context on ability to function or engage in occupation cannot be overstated. One way to understand this is to reflect on how your own life has changed over different phases of your life, as you grew up; experiences that you remember from your youth; and the people, places, and things (contexts and personal factors) that shaped you in ways both positively and, yes, sometimes had negative impacts. How would the situational contexts of your life change the way you engage in life if, in the future, you changed jobs or moved to a new country where a language that you did not yet understand was spoken or perhaps found out that you were going to be a new parent or grandparent? Life would be different if your situations and contexts changed.

So, how can an occupational therapy professional possibly consider all of these factors in relationship to occupation with a client during the evaluation phase? An informal interview or conversational discussion (if the setting allows time) can often initiate reflection on the multifaceted aspects of your client. As with so many other information-seeking tasks, a good place to start gathering information is by asking thoughtful questions. The questions in Table 12.2 offer a few suggestions as starting points. Often, allowing the client a safe and welcoming space to answer questions leads to hearing from the client what aspects of their narrative are the most meaningful and important.

Understanding the sociocultural features of the client's life is essential. Each group has unique sets of norms, values, and expectations for what "typical" behaviors are, and these affect the quality and experience of what and how occupation occurs. A person's interests and values may reflect the cultural group, and often, especially for clients with mental illness, their interests, values, and behaviors conflict with the cultural norms and expectations of the larger group. Sometimes, the person's family or cultural group pressures them into abandoning personal interests and values. Although sometimes the unacceptable or inappropriate choices and behaviors that result from, or are symptoms associated with a person's mental illness, have so disrupted family or community dynamics, that the individual is no longer a welcomed member.

Occupational therapy professionals consider how contexts affect functional performance in terms of the opportunities they provide *and* the demands or constraints that they place on the person. For example, a family caregiver may help the person function by setting up a cold meal to be eaten at midday or may interfere by limiting opportunities for the person to perform that same task independently. Geopolitical factors can constrain a person's efforts to function if, for example, eligibility for medical benefits end because a person has lost employment secondary to the impacts of their mental illness. Geopolitical factors heavily impact marginalized populations, creating enormous health disparities (63).

Patterns

Along with the performance context, occupational therapy professionals are interested in the person's *performance patterns*. What are the person's habits, routines, roles, and rituals? How does the person budget time among different activities? How much do they sleep or watch television? Do they schedule time for leisure and play activities? How much time do they spend on self-care and care of their living environment, their home, or their workspace? The way that time is allocated among activities is only one aspect of patterns. How and why the person pursues each activity are equally important temporal aspects of patterns, as are habits, roles, and routines that have become pervasive or overly repetitive over time and that then interfere with occupational engagement. One example of the ways that these aspects of occupational engagement and situational aspects of the client (client factors, personal factors) are inextricably linked can be seen by observing the interconnected relationships between **Adverse Childhood Experiences** (ACEs), long-standing **health disparities**, and the predicted long-term impacts of the Coronavirus Disease of 2019 (70). The COVID-19 pandemic has highlighted preexisting health disparities and created a new increased risk for occupational dysfunction and occupational injustice for clients who are likely to suffer long-term negative effects from conditions like depression, ADHD, anxiety, Posttraumatic stress disorder (PTSD), and suicidality, all of which are predicted to continue to impact already marginalized communities. The ripples of these transactional relationships, in turn, impact other sociocultural and geopolitical elements, especially in terms of food insecurities, housing instability or homelessness, and household poverty characteristics (70).

Habits, described by Matuska and Barrett (2019) as "Specific, automatic behaviors performed repeatedly, relatively automatically, and with little variation" (55, p. 214), can be classified as useful, impoverished, or dominating. Persons with severe or chronic mental illness generally have some habits that are impoverished, often in the areas of completion of necessary ADLs and time use, which then further impact their routines and roles. Insufficient and unsafe living conditions and limited resources contribute further to the impoverishment of habits. Since occupational therapy's intended targeted outcomes include, among other things, supporting the client's optimal occupational participation, improved quality of life, and role competence, evaluation of these factors (situational contexts, performance patterns, habits, roles, and routines) is especially important with regard to clients who have mental health needs.

Expected Environment

In addition to general background information, occupational roles, performance context, and performance patterns, it is very important to know where a client will be going after discharge from occupational therapy services (if inpatient), or about their postrehabilitation environment at home, work, or school. This is sometimes called the **expected environment**, or discharge environment (56). Relatively few clients who are admitted to acute hospitals are transferred to another like facility. Clients typically go home or to partial hospitalization programs, board and care homes, single-room occupancy hotels, community-based temporary shelters, or supervised group homes, and semi-independent living communities. When the expected environment is different from the most recent previous environment, the contexts for occupational performance will be different. For this reason, the person may need to develop new skills or refine or modify the way everyday activities are completed. Someone who will be living independently for the first time, even in a supervised apartment, will need to be able to care for clothing, budget money, and manage other self-care and independent living tasks. To summarize, the main purpose of evaluation is to determine what a person needs and wants to do and what is helping and hindering them. Remember that strengths, resources, supports, and barriers can be determined only in relation to valued occupations, situational contexts, performance patterns, and expected environment.

THE EVALUATION PROCESS

The *OTPF-4* (9) suggests that evaluation should begin with the **occupational profile** and the **analysis of occupational performance**; however, in many psychosocial settings, especially if the OT is a member of a multidisciplinary team, and working on goals that are transdisciplinary in nature, the OT may need to rearrange the components of the occupational therapy evaluation process, but it is nevertheless important that occupation should be the central focus of the evaluation. In the United States, constantly changing regulations from government agencies and insurers are external factors that will always impact the way in which occupational therapy professionals approach evaluation. It is also true that time-based or setting-based constrictions often necessitate changes in the evaluation approach that is utilized. In a long-standing debate, several occupational therapy scholars have argued that a bottom-up or environment-first evaluation is appropriate in many situations (17, 38).

This contrasts with beginning with the occupational profile and analysis of contextually accurate occupational performance, which are inherently top-down approaches. What do these terms mean, you may be wondering? Which approach is correct? **Top-down evaluation** begins with exploring the client's overall occupational goals. No other data is collected, and no assessments or techniques that isolate specific body structures or functions, or isolated client factors, are administered until the client's perspective and occupational outcomes are understood and made clear. The occupational profile exemplifies this principle. **Bottom-up evaluation** begins with the factors that appear to impede occupational engagement. An example in a burn unit is the assessment of wounds and the need for specific splinting to prevent contractures. In this case, the medical necessity cannot wait for an interview to learn the client's goals. In a psychiatric setting, prioritizing the assessment of cognitive level would represent a bottom-up approach to evaluation. **Environment-first evaluation** is appropriate when safety is a factor, as, for example, when assessing the home environment for an elderly client to reduce the risk of falls.

The OT using a top-down approach will first obtain information to complete the occupational profile. Interviews, questionnaires, and casual conversation can provide background on the person's occupational history and interests, experiences, goals, and priorities. The **analysis of occupational performance** would be done once the OT has a sense of the person's goals and problems. Analysis of occupational performance may require the OT to observe the client repeatedly, or to use one or more assessments or methods, and to observe the client in a variety of social and environmental contexts to capture information about the true nature of the client's occupational engagement. This can provide assurance to both the client and the occupational therapy professional that the occupational performance is as ecologically relevant as possible.

The top-down approach would then proceed to assessment of performance skills, performance patterns, and contexts and environments, as well as potentially evaluating particular client factors. Although a top-down approach is often characterized as one that begins with an occupational profile, and also includes an analysis of occupational performance, if the process continues by evaluating body functions, environmental factors, and/or other contextual factors in isolation, to speculate about which of those factors are impacting the occupational performance problems, then the therapist risks placing body structures, body functions, or other client factors or contexts at the heart of function (32).

According to Dr Fisher and colleagues, in a true top-down approach, the occupational therapy professional will focus on the client's occupational engagement by gathering the information for an occupational profile, determining the client's priorities, analyzing occupational performance and the quality of the occupational performance, all while reflecting on the transactional nature of occupation and its inseparable relationship to all other situational elements, including specific client factors (35).

Nevertheless, evidence does suggest that some specific performance skills are particularly relevant to assess in psychiatric occupational therapy practice; these are process skills and social interaction skills (SIS), two skill sets often found to be among the primary barriers prohibiting a return to optimal occupational participation for people with psychiatric conditions. Adverse effects of medications may also impair particular motor skills, cognitive, or SIS. Therefore, in some cases, the OT would have substantial reason to more closely assess particular client factors. This is sometimes the case when there is a need to further assess isolated cognitive functions that are commonly associated with characteristic symptomology of psychiatric diagnoses like depression, substance use disorders, and dementia. In these cases, the occupational therapy professional will use professional reasoning to determine which client factor is most important to assess more closely, that is, which factor is hindering occupational participation the most.

Factors such as attention span, memory, task initiation, sequencing, emotional regulation, sensory or motor functions can be intervention targets that help clients reach their occupational performance goals and significantly improve the quality of their overall occupational engagement. Other areas may be assessed, depending on the reference to a theoretical perspective or practice model. In the end, the most important responsibility, regardless of the evaluation approach, is that the evaluation is occupation-centered and rooted in the analysis of occupational performance. Further, the evaluation should be measured using assessments that are reliable and valid (37, 50).

Although the OT chooses the methods and approach to be used in evaluation, part of the collaborative process demands that the occupational therapy team thoroughly summarize and explain the evaluation plan to the client, to the family (when relevant and with adherence to privacy laws), and to other health professionals involved in caring for the client. In short-term acute settings (and in many community settings), only a short time is available for evaluation. Caseloads may be so high that extensive evaluation is not possible in the time frame of the initial evaluation. Thus, the evaluation may be brief, but it is essential that it remain comprehensive. During later sessions, and on an ongoing basis, the occupational therapy professionals may determine the need for additional information. When the initial evaluation is complete, the OT organizes, analyzes, and interprets the information, summarizing the person's occupational performance goals and priorities and making note of particular strengths, supports, and barriers that were derived from completing the occupational profile with the client. Finally, the OT writes an initial occupational therapy evaluation note, which becomes part of the medical record (17).

CONCEPTS RELATED TO ASSESSMENT AND MEASUREMENT

The overarching purpose of assessment is to measure the qualities or characteristics of something or someone so that a baseline can be determined by which progress or lack of progress toward goals can be documented. In this section, we will look briefly at some important measurement-related factors that must be considered when selecting specific assessment tools. In the final part of the chapter, we will introduce four assessment administration methods associated with evidence-based, occupation-focused practice and utilized by occupational therapy professionals in mental health or psychosocial settings: **self-report**; **interview**; **performance or observation**, and **mixed methods assessments or approaches** (37). Lastly, we will concisely review several existing assessment tools or processes from each of the four evaluation methods. The assessment methods and the corresponding examples of selected assessment tools each have unique functions in the professionals' evaluation process. For example, self-report tools and interviews are most useful for collecting information relevant to putting together an occupational history and an occupational profile. Observation-based tests are helpful for administering an ecologically and contextually appropriate occupational performance analysis, and some tests, if they are deemed reliable and valid, can assist occupational therapy professionals in further evaluating, when necessary, isolated performance skills or client factors in the context of a specific area of occupational engagement.

The first important concept with regard to assessment and measurement is standardization. **Standardization** is a way of ensuring the accuracy and consistency of an assessment method or tool. Regarding assessments, standardization is generally achieved in relationship to normative data or to specific criteria. **Normative data** are collected from many administrations of the test or assessment. This means that many people (individuals, groups, or populations) have been given the assessment and their scores recorded. Working from the scores of this larger sample group, the developers of the assessment predict what the normal range of scores is likely to be. Once the normal range has been identified, the score of a particular individual can be compared with it. A **norm-referenced assessment** will provide tables of normative data. These data are sometimes skewed by cultural or other forms of bias. For example, if the test has been administered only in English, or a translated version contains concepts that have not been shown to carry similar meanings after translation, or the assessment has only been administered to a group with particular characteristics (eg, males versus females, certain diagnostic groups, or people of a certain socioeconomic status), this will impact the overall utility

of the assessment. Normative populations that are dissimilar to the person being assessed may be a poor standard against which to compare that client's results (50).

The other common method of standardization is by **criteria**. **Criterion measures**, sometimes called **performance measures,** are standards by which an individual's performance is measured. Performance or **criterion-referenced assessments** are particularly important for occupational therapy practitioners because they give us information and evidence about the influence of particular interventions or performance skill development on a client's overall quality and efficiency during occupational engagement. When selecting the criterion for particular occupation-centered assessments, occupational therapy professionals need to consider five critical aspects, including the importance or relevance of the criteria to the client's life, comparisons to external standards, consideration and use of formal evidence criteria, an assessment tool's sensitivity to changes, and what degree of changes in occupational engagement are most highly prioritized as being meaningful to the client, including consideration of both the quality and the experience of the performance (from the client's perspective) (28). To appreciate the differences between norm-referenced and criterion-referenced measures, the reader might consider the way grades are awarded in a course. If the course is graded on a curve, then the professor has used a norm-referenced standard, aiming to distribute the scores in a normal distribution. If the professor grades students on their achievement of specific competencies, this is a criterion-referenced standard.

Perhaps the two most important concepts in measurement for the occupational therapy professional to understand when selecting an assessment tool, or tools for a particular client, are reliability and validity. **Reliability** represents the consistency of the results when the test is repeated. **Test–retest reliability** shows the degree of sameness of scores when a test is repeated. **Interrater reliability** shows the degree to which two people giving the test will obtain similar results. Both are important to consider. Test–retest reliability shows that the test is stable, that what it is measuring, and the way in which it is measuring, can be trusted to some extent. Interrater reliability allows different evaluators to use the same test and compare results, combine data, and so on. According to Magasi et al (2017), "Reliability is a necessary prerequisite for validity because validity implies that an instrument is relatively free from error. A score derived from an unreliable measure cannot be considered valid" (54, p. 33).

Validity or **content validity** shows the degree to which the test measures what it says it is measuring. Some tests have obvious validity, known as **face validity**—for example, a test of range of motion seems to be a valid measure of the degree to which motion occurs at different joints in an individual. Other tests, however, claim to measure something that is not so obvious, in this situation, and particularly if criterion-referenced assessment is not possible, such as when there is not an agreed upon gold standard by which comparisons can be made; in these situations, construct validity can be considered. **Construct validity** is the degree to which the scores of an instrument are internally consistent according to hypothesized internal relationships, or how the assessment measures concepts it claims to measure when compared with other tools that also measure similar concepts. Lastly, construct validity can be used to consider how an assessment measures differences between two groups or populations (54). What remains a priority is that "Assessments... utilized during the evaluation process should be valid and reliable, and should illuminate the areas of occupational performance in which the patient has limitations" (37, p. 16). These assessment principles are also critical because following evaluation and assessment, intervention planning and goal setting occurs, largely drawing from the expectation that the assessments or assessment process was evidence-based and utilized reliable and valid methods and tools that included an occupational focus.

A BRIEF REVIEW OF OCCUPATIONAL THERAPY ASSESSMENT METHODS AND TESTS USED IN MENTAL HEALTH SETTINGS

Although there are many valid and reliable assessments that can be utilized throughout occupational therapy practice, it is beyond the scope of this textbook to adequately cover the range. Our goal for this textbook is to provide a glimpse of selected evidence-based tools or processes that will help the reader recognize assessments that exemplify the various assessment approaches. As the reader begins to recognize particular approaches to evaluation and develops an awareness of the types of assessments, the client-centered and holistic nature of the evaluation process will come into focus, highlighting occupational therapy's unique contribution in psychosocial and behavioral mental health settings. Our contribution is to place emphasis on the client's optimal occupational participation.

Generally, each assessment will include a procedural manual with a detailed guide as to how the test is to be administered. Frequently, the test also includes materials, scoring sheets, and any additional items. The occupational therapy professional is encouraged to study the administration guidelines and the protocols thoroughly well in advance of using it, especially if this is a tool that the practitioner has not previously administered. Also, before each use of an assessment, it is prudent to check that no parts are missing and that all forms and other items are ready to use. Finally, keep in mind that with many assessments, specialized training is required to be able to administer them. This means that in adherence to The *AOTA Code of Ethics* (6), the professional has the responsibility to make sure that they can ethically administer the evaluation.

Having everything prepared and organized before the client arrives conveys to the client confidence and professionalism, which are standards of occupational therapy. Additionally, if there are particular portions of the test record that can be completed in advance such as completing any necessary identifying information or historical data that can be obtained from the client's chart or records, ensure that it is complete. Finally, make note of any data that you and/or the client will need to complete or sign on their arrival.

INTERVIEW AND SELF-REPORT METHODS AND ASSESSMENTS

As previously mentioned, there are a variety of ways to collect evaluative information about the client. The approach and strategy that the OT chooses to engage with the client is related directly to the type of information that one is looking for and what the intended use of, or outcome, will be for the information gathered. Interview-based assessments and techniques are typically classified as either formal or informal and can be considered either structured, semistructured, or unstructured. Typically, the more formal an interview is considered to be, the higher the degree of structure or more rigid the protocol of the assessment will be, sometimes with fewer options for expanding the questions. Nevertheless, the use of a structured interview allows the practitioner to collect objective data that can be used to compare across similar diagnostic groups or with clients who share similar personal and contextual characteristics. Less formal or unstructured interviews are generally based on conversations shared between the OT and the client.

Somewhere in the middle of structured and unstructured assessments exist the semistructured interviews. Semistructured interviews are considered more formalized because they are typically comprised of a set of primary questions but also offer secondary questions that are considered optional and can be chosen according to the dynamics of the interview in context. Semistructured interviews can be quantified through the use of rating scales, but the unique pattern of questions selected for each interview, and the subjective nature of each individual's response, does not lend itself to utilizing these types of assessments for quantitative analysis. Nevertheless, the use of semistructured interviews has been substantially noted in the literature and evidence to be associated with the provision of authentic client-centered care (17, 37). In the following section, we will briefly review several commonly used assessment tools that utilize the interview and self-report approaches during occupational therapy evaluation.

Interviews: *World Health Organization Disability Assessment Schedule 2.0 (WHODAS 2.0)*

The WHO created the *WHODAS 2.0* as an attempt to measure health and disability at the population level and to make it easier to administer these assessment measures in everyday practice situations (78). A client's functional levels are measured in six domains of life that were selected after extensive surveys and research. The functional domains are loosely based on the *International Classification of Function and Disability (ICF)* and provide a generic means to compare the impact of differing health conditions relative to function and disability. The Domains of the *WHODAS 2.0* are:

Domain 1: Cognition—understanding and communicating
Domain 2: Mobility—moving and getting around
Domain 3: Self-care—attending to one's hygiene, dressing, eating, and staying alone

Domain 4: Getting along—interacting with other people

Domain 5: Life activities—domestic responsibilities, leisure, work, and school

Domain 6: Participation—joining in community activities, participating in society. A profile and a summary measure of functioning and disability are provided relative to each domain (78).

The *WHODAS 2.0* does not target a specific disease, and many occupational therapy practitioners will appreciate the similarities between the *OTPF-4* (the domain of occupational therapy) and the domains assessed by the *WHODAS 2.0*. Additionally, just as occupational therapy professionals do not assess or make intervention plans based on diagnosis, the *WHODAS 2.0* was designed to assess disability to support the design of interventions that focus on participation, which cannot usually be initiated based on diagnosis or disease type alone. Disability assessment supports identification of client needs, which promotes client-centered care. It allows interdisciplinary health teams to match treatments and interventions and determine the best role for each caregiver, which in turn allows appropriate allocation of time, energy, priorities, and resources (78).

There are several different versions of *WHODAS 2.0*—the full version has 36 questions, and the *WHODAS 2.0* short version has 12 questions. These questions relate to functioning difficulties experienced by the respondent in the six domains of life during the previous 30 days. Self-guided training is available so that the assessment can be administered by a lay interviewer, as a self-report, or through interview by a caregiver or proxy (ie, family member or friend). All versions of the *WHODAS 2.0* have been shown to be reliable, and norms for the general population are also available. Please see the link to download the *WHODAS 2.0*, as well as the information and training materials in the *End of Chapter Resources* (78).

Interviews: *Occupational Performance History Interview II (OPHI-II), Version 2.1*

One of the semistructured interviews that both the OT and the OTA might collaboratively conduct is the *Occupational Performance History Interview, Version 2.1*, known as the *OPHI-II* (46). It is used to obtain an occupational history, determine how well the person is functioning in occupational roles, and estimate the balance between occupational and leisure activities. The *OPHI-II* has three parts: a semistructured interview about the client's occupational history, rating scales, and a life history narrative (43, 46). The interview itself has five sections: *Occupational Roles, Daily Routine, Occupational Settings, Activity/Occupational Choices,* and *Critical Life Events* (46). The *Occupational Roles* section is made up of questions that explore the occupational roles that are significant in a person's everyday life. The *Daily Routine* section asks about how the person uses time. The *Occupational Settings* section asks about the kinds of environments in which occupational participation occurs. The *Activity/Occupational Choices* section asks about how a person chooses the occupations they now do and looks at the person's sense

of control and volition regarding occupation. The *Critical Life Events* section asks about turning points that may have changed the person's life direction. The entire interview takes about an hour and can be divided into two sessions. The OT may delegate portions of the interview to the OTA.

The *OPHI-II* is highly flexible, allowing the interviewer to rephrase questions and probe for more information to obtain sufficiently detailed answers. Flowcharts in the examiner's manual guide the interviewer to move to different sections or questions, depending on how the person answered a previous question (hence its consideration as a semistructured interview tool). For example, if the person says that they have never worked, the questions about work are skipped, and the interviewer asks: "Why do you think it is that you have not worked?" (46). After completing the interview, the interviewer uses a 4-point rating system to rate the person's occupational functioning. Three separate scales are used: *Occupational Identity, Occupational Competence,* and *Occupational Settings.* The reader is referred to the *OPHI-II* manual for the rest of the interview questions, the rating system, and other components (46).

The *OPHI-II* is a well-developed assessment with strong research evidence and an expansive and user-friendly manual (43). Kielhofner (*Personal communication*, March 14, 2007) stated that the *OPHI-II* could be administered by an OTA with established service competency. With careful study of the manual and supervised training with someone who is experienced in administering the *OPHI-II*, the motivated OTA can master this useful interview. It may also prove helpful to have the OT administer this interview as the OTA captures and records the responses, so that the OT can more fully dialogue with the client. This approach sometimes helps alleviate the client's anxiety and builds trust that helps establish therapeutic rapport.

Interviews: *Canadian Occupational Performance Model, 5th Edition (COPM)*

The *Canadian Occupational Performance Measure, 5th Edition (COPM)* is a structured interview that measures a client's own perceptions about his or her own occupational performance (49). This assessment tool provides an excellent foundation for establishing priorities for intervention because it elicits from the client the goals that the client deems most important. In many cases, the OT administers the *COPM* when working with an individual client, but the advanced and experienced occupational therapy professional might find the *COPM* useful in case management in the community, and also for use in research. Use of the *COPM* by the OTA should not be undertaken independently; it requires establishment of service competency and the supervision of an OT.

Interviews: *The Activity Card Sort (ACS), 2nd Edition*

The *Activity Card Sort (ACS), 2nd Edition* developed by Baum and Edwards (16), seeks information on client's instrumental, leisure, and social activities. The assessment has different versions so that information can be obtained at admission, during recovery, or when the client is living in the community. The client sorts 89 photograph cards showing occupations being performed into four categories:

1. Instrumental activities of daily living (IADLs)
2. Leisure activities with low physical demands
3. Leisure activities with high physical demands
4. Social activities

Depending on the version selected, the client is asked to label the activities as to whether they have been performed in the past, are being performed in the present, have been given up owing to illness, are done at a lower level than previously, and so on. Because this is a visual sorting task, it is less reliant on literacy. The photos remind the client of specific activities, and each photograph is labeled with the name of the activity (eg, home maintenance is the label on a card showing exterior household cleaning). When a client does not understand the picture, the examiner explains. The results can be used in many ways. Similar to the *COPM*, the client may be asked to select five high-priority activities. These priorities become a starting point for intervention planning and identifying intervention goals.

Self-Reports: *Role Checklist Version 3 (RCv3)*

The *Role Checklist (RC),* developed by Oakley (57), provides information on occupational roles as perceived by the client. The *RC* is a short, written inventory that can be completed by people who have basic literacy skills and intact cognition. The client is asked to indicate which roles have been performed in the past, are performed in the present, or will be performed in the future. In the second part of the checklist, the client is asked to rate the value attached to each role (43, 57). Published in 2019, Dr Patricia Scott established the most recent version of the *Role Checklist, the Role Checklist Version 3 (RCv3)* (69). The *RCv3* measures client participation and is a single page measure of participation in 10 common roles used to gauge client satisfaction with their participation, and to distinguish their reasons for non-participation (69).

Service competency for administration of the *RC* can easily be developed by an OTA. This checklist is valuable for quickly assessing roles important to the client so that priorities for intervention can be established. Role assessments have been examined by a large number of studies, which increasingly improves their utility, validity, and reliability (66).

Self-Reports: *Occupational Self-Assessment (OSA), Version 2.2*

Person-centered care and occupational therapy's call to collaborate with our clients to acquire the most authentic evaluation information require the occupational therapy professional to more deeply investigate what the client believes about their own occupational performance (what their perception is about their abilities and the qualitative aspects of the experience) when they are engaging in occupations

that are meaningful to them. The following self-report assessments measure how the client's **competence** and the **value** of the occupation to the client impact their performance and participation in the task (72).

The *Occupational Self-Assessment (OSA)* is a self-rating format that is essentially divided into two sections, or in other words, asks the client to rate two aspects of their occupational participation. In the first part, the client responds to a series of statements about how competent they feel doing certain daily tasks (their perception of their ability to perform the task). In the following section, the client rates the importance, or value, of the daily tasks using the same series of statements. Lastly, the client and the occupational therapy professional can revisit the statements, reflecting on both the client's perceived competence and the value ratio to determine priorities for initiating changes that can then be translated into therapeutic goals (15). The *OSA* has good reliability in adults who are 18 years and older. The *OSA* is a good example of an evidence-based assessment that demonstrates good internal validity, and it is a tool that is sensitive enough to differentiate between individuals regarding their Occupational Competence and Values (15, 37).

Occupational Self-Assessment—Short Form (OSA-SF)

The *Occupational Self-Assessment-Short Form (OSA-SF)* is a valid and reliable measure that is based on the concepts of the Model of Human Occupation (MOHO) (15, 60). The shortened version of the *OSA* was derived from the *OSA* to assess occupational competence and value, just as its predecessor does. However, the *OSA-SF* can be administered in 7 to 15 minutes, improving its usefulness with adults in inpatient or acute rehabilitation settings and fast-paced environments (60).

Occupational Self-Assessment—Daily Living Scales (OSA-DLS)

The *Occupational Self-Assessment—Daily Living Scales (OSA-DLS),* another off-shoot of the *OSA,* gathers self-reported data on the performance and importance of 12 ADL and IADL items using the same prompts as the *OSA* (68). This assessment can be administered in 10 to 15 minutes, depending on the context. It is a convenient tool that can be utilized in home health, outpatient rehabilitation clinics, and in behavioral health settings to quickly assess a client's perceptions and priorities about their participation in IADLs. It is particularly helpful to gather information for the client's occupational profile, specifically for IADLs. Occupational therapy professionals often play a large role in collaborating with clients who have been diagnosed with mental illness, as well as with their caregivers, to assess and support improvements in the client's engagement in IADLs. However, there is a paucity of research related to this area of occupation, although that is changing with the recent uptick in smaller mixed methods studies that look more closely at how particular diagnostic groups experience mental illness regarding their perception of the quality of their IADL participation (67, 74). Assessment tools like the *OSA-DLS* make the collection of data for the purposes of research far easier for busy occupational therapy professionals. Furthermore, this scale is available with other valid and reliable tools, free from the UIC *MOHO-IRM Clearinghouse* website. Refer to the link to this website in the Suggested Resources at the end of the chapter. Users must create an account to access the free resources.

Self-Reports: *Medical Outcomes Study: Survey of Social Support (MOS:SOS)*

The *Medical Outcomes Study: Survey of Social Support* (*MOS:SOS*) is a brief, self-administered survey originally developed for use with clients with chronic conditions (62). It takes only a few minutes to administer. Available online (62), it can be given to clients to complete on their own or done in the presence of the occupational therapy professional. There are 19 brief descriptions of different kinds of social support (eg, "someone you can count on to listen to you when you need to talk"). The items are grouped by the type of support:

- Emotional/social support
- Tangible support (eg, help with personal care or food preparation)
- Affectionate support
- Positive social interaction

The person taking the survey rates each item on a 5-point scale ranging from "none of the time" to "all the time." The higher the score, the higher the social support as perceived by the client. The results can be used as a starting point for discussion of how social support or lack thereof may affect engagement in occupation.

Self-Reports: *Multidimensional Scale of Perceived Social Support (MSPSS)*

The *Multidimensional Scale of Perceived Social Support* (*MSPSS*) (50, 79) is shorter than the *MOS Social Support*, with only 12 items. These items are identified in relation to the likely source of social support: SO, family (Fam), or friends (Fri). The items are stated in simple declarative sentences, for example: "There is a special person who is around when I am in need." The person taking the survey rates each item on a 7-point scale from 1 (strongly disagree) to 7 (strongly agree). Higher scores are associated with higher levels of perceived social support. Like the *MOS Social Support*, it can be completed in a short time, about 5 minutes, and can be factored into discussions about support for engaging in desired occupations. The survey is widely available, free, and downloadable online (79).

Self-Reports: *Adolescent and Adult Sensory Profile*

The *Adolescent/Adult Sensory Profile* is a paper and pencil form that asks the client to indicate their reaction to a range of sensory statements, such as "I'm afraid of heights" and "I dislike having my back rubbed" (19). The results from the 60 items are then coded onto a scoring sheet and transferred to a profile page. The profile shows the degree to which the person is similar to "most people" in four aspects of overall sensory function. The results can be shared with the client, and often a sensory regulation intervention plan that can include environmental adaptations can be collaboratively determined. Successful sensory-based interventions can vastly reduce the client's barriers to occupational participation (19). This assessment takes approximately 15 to 20 minutes to administer, not including the time to score it. The examiner's manual gives useful suggestions to help clients manage sensory reactions by modifying the environment, changing activities, and getting support from others. However, to identify how the client is reacting to specific types of sensations, the examiner must carefully reflect on the individual items (50).

PERFORMANCE OR OBSERVATION-BASED METHODS AND ASSESSMENTS

According to Law et al. (50), "Basic to an occupational performance approach are the skills of the therapist to analyze tasks, activities, and occupations and propose and use learning or adaptive strategies to support the individual to perform meaningful occupations" (50, p. 5). As an essential part of the occupational evaluation process, the approach that the occupational therapy professional incorporates into the occupational analysis is influenced by the client information collected for the occupational profile and further defined by the model of practice or theoretical approach engaged. However, regardless of these details, an occupational performance analysis must always include an observation or performance-based assessment tool (6, 10, 11).

Performance or Observation-Based Assessments: *The Comprehensive Occupational Therapy Evaluation (COTE)*

A checklist or other structured format may be used to record observations. Of these, the *Comprehensive Occupational Therapy Evaluation* (*COTE*) scale (4, 18) has been widely used. The *COTE* scale may be used for a single observation or a series of observations of a client performing virtually any occupational task. It lists 26 behaviors and provides a scale for rating them. Behaviors are divided into three general constructs: General Behavior (8 items), Interpersonal Behavior (6 items), and Task Behaviors (12 items). Each can be rated on a scale of 0 (normal) to 4 (extreme or grossly abnormal). Some items, activity level, for example, have two rating scales, reflecting the possibility of abnormal behaviors in either direction. The observer chooses either hyperactive (overactive) or hypoactive (underactive), depending on the client's behavior during the observation.

The *COTE* scale assessment protocol contains 15 columns, so that the client's behavior all through 15 sessions can be noted on the same page; this is helpful in measuring progress and documenting effects of medication or other alternative therapies such as electroconvulsive therapy (ECT) on participation in occupation. Some OTs use the 15 columns in a different way, to rate several clients during the same group session; each person is rated in a different column. The ratings can then be transferred to each client's individual form.

Whether the *COTE* or another observational scale is used, when observing a client for purposes of evaluation, the occupational therapy professional must remain an observer and not interfere with what the client is doing. The OT must not give help, advice, or encouragement; recommend that the client try a different technique; or even smile approvingly. All these behaviors may change what the person does, and what then ends up on the rating form is how the client performs with advice and support rather than how they perform independently. Administering an assessment and providing interventions are different tasks that require different behaviors from the OT or OTA.

Notwithstanding the importance of strictly following the assessment protocol, there are instances when **dynamic assessment** is used. The person giving the assessment adjusts the demands to accommodate the person's perceived difficulties. In this way, one gets a sense of whether compensatory methods may improve occupational performance. Dynamic assessment is an advanced practice skill but is within the OTA scope of practice.

Performance or Observation-Based: *Independent Living Scales (ILS)*

The *Independent Living Scales (ILS)* is a semistructured interview with several performance-based elements. The assessment was designed to assess the likelihood of successful independent community living (52). The *ILS* is an individually administered assessment that evaluates client competency in performing IADLs. The items present situations relevant to independent living and require the client to engage in problem-solving, to demonstrate knowledge, or to perform tasks using skills necessary for safely living independently. The *ILS* is also commonly used to help identify and suggest areas of occupation where the client may need support to be successful in semi-independent living situations. The *ILS* is comprised of five subscales: *Memory/Orientation, Managing Money, Managing Home and Transportation, Health and Safety,* and *Social Adjustment.* The five subscale scores are added to obtain an overall score reflecting the person's ability to function independently. The following list briefly covers the area assessed by each subscale.

- *Memory/Orientation Subscale:* Assesses the individual's general awareness of their surroundings and assesses short-term memory.
- *Managing Money Subscale:* Assesses the individual's ability to count money, do monetary calculations, pay bills, and take precautions with money.
- *Managing Home and Transportation Subscale:* Assesses the individual's ability to use the telephone, utilize public transportation, and maintain a safe home.
- *Health and Safety Subscale:* Assesses the individual's awareness of personal health status and ability to evaluate health problems, handle medical emergencies, and take safety precautions.
- *Social Adjustment Subscale:* Assesses the individual's mood and attitude toward social relations [relationships].

Other aspects of independent living such as problem-solving factors and performance or information factors can be evaluated by combining particular items on the subscales, as defined in the examiner's manual. The *Problem-Solving Factor* assesses the client's knowledge of relevant facts, capabilities in abstract reasoning, and problem-solving. Items that are used in this Factor Score are indicative of the client's level of ability when they must reason through information, apply the knowledge to solve a problem or safely complete a task. The *Performance/Information Factor* combines test items that require general knowledge, short-term memory, and ability to perform uncomplicated daily tasks. Items in this Factor Score are generally skills that can be taught, practiced, or rehearsed over time (52).

Performance or Observation-Based: *Test of Grocery Shopping Skills (TOGSS)*

This test was originally designed by an OT and a nurse (and later joined by a psychologist) specifically for people with schizophrenia. It was developed to assess the person's ability to locate items in a grocery store accurately and efficiently (20). Since its inception, the *TOGSS* has been validated with multiple diagnostic groups. The test takes a little more than 1 hour to administer. This is an assessment that would be appropriate for an OTA with earned service competency to perform. The manual is very clear and user friendly. The procedure is as follows:

1. The client completes a self-evaluation of anxiety level for this task as well as a rating of personal sense of own ability to perform the task.
2. The OT and client visit a grocery store, and the client is given a list of 10 items.
3. The OT observes the client performance and, using a map of the store, marks the route taken by the client. Multiple trips to the same aisle are also noted.
4. Client performance is rated on *redundancy* (excess visits to aisles in relation to aisles in the store).
5. Client performance is rated on accuracy (items obtained correctly).

The OT then interprets the client's scores. Higher accuracy, faster performance, and low redundancy are associated with greater independence. The OT uses the information to develop interventions to improve client performance in the task of grocery shopping and other similar IADL tasks (20, 37, 50).

Performance or Observation-Based: *Allen Cognitive Levels Screen—5 (ACLS-5)*

The Cognitive Disabilities Model (CDM) is a model of practice designed for supporting people whose primary barrier to safe occupational participation is cognitive disability (31). In settings or situations where the CDM is applied, the *Allen Cognitive Levels Screen, 5th Edition (ACLS-5)* the *Large Allen Cognitive Levels Screen, 5th Edition (LACLS-5)*, for individuals who have visual deficits or hand impairments, or the disposable form of the *Large Allen Cognitive Levels Screen, 5th Edition (LACLS-5[D])*, for individuals who require a higher level of infection control, may be utilized as a screening tool to initiate functional cognitive assessment (31). The *ACLS-5* series of screening tools use the client's performance of progressively more difficult leather-lacing stitches to produce an estimation of the client's current functional cognitive capabilities. The test includes a script of verbal cues and, when needed, visual demonstrations of the running stitch, the whip stitch, and the single cordovan stitch (Figure 12.1).

Results of the screening are used to estimate the client's placement on the Allen Cognitive Scale, a 27-point hierarchical, cumulative, and ordinal scale made up of six levels, Level I through Level 6. Each level is then further subdivided into five modes (also hierarchical). These modes are labeled 0.0, 0.2, 0.4, 0.6, and 0.8. According to the Allen and Colleagues, the authors of the *ACLS-5* (2), "The task demands [of the *ACLS-5*] span a range of abilities associated with cognitive levels 3 (running stitch), 4 (whipstitch), and 5 (single cordovan stitch) or modes 3.0 to 5.8 on the Allen scale. . . . Complexity is defined by identifying the elements of each [stitching] task, and comparing them to the [observable] sensory cues, motor actions, and problem solving capabilities described in the hypothesized cognitive levels and modes" (2, p. 9).

Performance or Observation-Based: *Allen Diagnostic Module, 2nd Edition (ADM-2)*

The *Allen Diagnostic Module, 2nd Edition (ADM-2)* (3, 29–31) consists of 35 standardized craft project kits that are used to verify ACL scores from the *ACLS-5* and to monitor progress as medication takes effect or as symptoms diminish

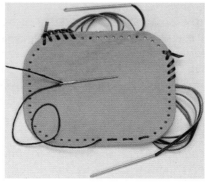

Figure 12.1. The Allen Cognitive Level Screening Test. (Courtesy S&S Worldwide, Colchester, CT.)

and cognitive level improves. Functional cognitive levels may improve as a result of medication changes, clearing of delirium from illness or substance use, and return of memory following a series of ECT treatments. The projects in the *ADM-2* kit are rated in difficulty from level 3.0 to level 5.8. The manual (29) includes the range of ratings for each project according to appropriate functional cognitive level. Craft projects require use of basic activity skills such as drawing a line, placing, gluing, sanding, and sewing (30). Many motor and process performance skills can be observed while the client participates in the craft activity (eg, placing, stabilizing, sequencing, and handling). Client factors such as working memory, short-term memory, attention, and concentration can also be observed. The manual is clear and detailed with introductions to the projects, administration procedures, and hints for what to observe while scoring the *ADM-2* (29). One potential challenge in using the *ADM* kits is that other staff may assume that the craft materials can be used for other purposes, being unaware of their specificity for assessment. It is important for the occupational therapy professional to establish a protocol for securing the materials when not in use and explaining the rationale to other staff. A link to short video clip examples of the administration of the *ACLS-5* Series and instructions for using the *Allen Diagnostic Module, 2nd Edition* as well as many other resources related to the CDM are available in the *End of Chapter Resources*.

Performance or Observation-Based: *Routine Task Inventory-Expanded (RTI-E)*

The *Routine Task Inventory Expanded (RTI-E)* is a measure of cognitive impairment in relationship to the client's performance of daily living activities, and it is another assessment tool associated with the CDM, as are the *Allen Cognitive Level Screen, 5th Edition (ACLS-5* series) and the *Allen Diagnostic Module* mentioned in the preceding section (31, 44, 45). Dr Katz, the author of the *RTI-E*, describes the *RTI-E* as an assessment that is "easy to administer yet provide[s] valid and reliable information that can be easily utilized clinically" (45, p. 211).

Four categories of activities are assessed:

1. Physical ADL
2. Community IADL
3. Communication
4. Work readiness

The *RTI-E* is a paper and pencil questionnaire that is based on a rating scale completed on the observation of a client's participation in 30 tasks in the 4 occupational areas. *RTI-E* may be administered on its own or as part of an overall cognitive functional evaluation. When used with the *CDM*, the *RTI-E* or another general measure of cognitive function can be used to verify an initial cognitive screening (specifically when using the *ACLS-5* as an initial cognitive screening tool) (45). Administration may require as much as 90 minutes, not including the performance of the tasks. The OT may ask the client to complete the *RTI-E*, as a self-report, although people with cognitive impairments may not give accurate information, and so this approach is rarely recommended. Alternately, if the client is not able to fill it out, a family member or caregiver familiar with the client's usual performance of the tasks can do so instead. Here too, a falsely high score may result because those who spend a lot of time with the client may remember better past performance or may overestimate the client's skills. If the client or caregiver does not have sufficient literacy levels to read and understand the *RTI-E*, the occupational therapy professional can read the items and fill out the form according to the person's responses. Katz (44) recommends that an occupational therapy professional complete the *RTI-E* after observing client performance on numerous occasions. The administration manual and protocols are available in PDF form online using the link in the *End of Chapter Resources* (44).

Performance or Observation-Based: *Continuous Performance Test*

The *Continuous Performance Test (CPT)* (22) is a tool associated with The Cognitive Disabilities Reconsidered Model (51). The Cognitive Disabilities Reconsidered Model is, essentially, a reimagined version of the CDM that was developed for clients who have cognitive decline, and, like the CDM, the Cognitive Disabilities Reconsidered Model aims to focus on the client's best ability to function. For the Cognitive Disabilities Reconsidered Model, The Allen Cognitive Levels are described in terms of functional cognitive decline, with the lower levels being unresponsive or automatic and postural actions and the highest levels being planned actions, or normal functioning (51).

As mentioned, the *CPT* (22) was designed to be used with adults with cognitive impairment or suspected dementia. It is also used in the same manner as the *RTI-E*, to verify a person's level of cognitive function on the Allen Cognitive Scale, following use of the *ACLS-5* screening tool (45). The *CPT* requires the client to perform up to seven daily activities, and the occupational therapy professional completes an observation form that measures cognition as it impacts occupational performance. The score from the data collected on the *CPT* can then be converted to a Cognitive Disabilities Reconsidered Model Levels (22, 51). The scores on the Cognitive Disabilities Reconsidered Model Levels combined with the information collected during the gathering of the occupational profile help the client and caregiver to support the client in engaging in ADLs and IADLs to the optimal level of safety and function possible. Recommendations for suggested types of assistance are also available for clients' particular cognitive level (51).

Performance or Observation-Based: *The Performance Assessment of Self-Care Skills*

The *Performance Assessment of Self-Care Skills (PASS), Version 4.1* is a performance-based and observational tool that allows occupational therapy practitioners to assess changes in functional status (64). The instrument is comprised of four functional domains: Functional Mobility (FM), basic activities of daily life (BADLs), instrumental activities of daily life with a cognitive emphasis (CIADLs), and IADLs with a physical emphasis (PIADLs), which consist of 26 core occupations (64). Administration of the *PASS* is especially helpful for intervention and discharge planning because it was designed to analyze the particular elements of a functional task at the point of breakdown, or dysfunction, determine the level and type of assistance that the client may need, and identify the safety risks while engaged in the occupational activity (40).

There are two versions of the *PASS*, The *PASS-Clinic* and the *PASS-Home*. Each of the *PASS* versions measure independence, safety, and adequacy—three aspects of a client's occupational performance. One of the strengths of the *PASS* is that each pass item stands alone, and occupational therapy professionals can, therefore, administer any number of task items. Occupational therapy professionals can also determine which *PASS* tasks are the most appropriate to the particular priorities of each person, because each task is psychometrically sound when considered alone (40). It is important to consider, however, that two of the tasks (*Money Management* and *Meal Preparation*) include elements of dynamic assessment and graduated prompting and are meant to be administered as a series to increase their complexity and challenge (40).

Since the introduction of the original version of the *PASS* in 1984, which was designed for an adult population, the *PASS* has been consistently updated to include additional subtasks and data collection and scoring forms and has been used with a variety of adult and adolescent populations, including adults with depression, bipolar disorder, mild cognitive impairment (MCI), spinal cord injury, schizophrenia, multiple sclerosis, and heart failure, among other diagnostic populations (40). "In addition to the home and clinic performance-based measures, self-report and proxy report versions of the *PASS* address habit and skill for the 26 core occupations." Available at https://www.shrs.pitt.edu/performance-assessment-self-care-skills-pass-materials (40, p. 359).

MIXED METHODS ASSESSMENTS OR APPROACHES

Mixed Methods Assessments or Approaches: *Kohlman Evaluation of Living Skills, 4th Edition*

The *Kohlman Evaluation of Living Skills, 4th Edition (KELS-4E)* (47), assesses several skills in the areas of personal care, safety and health, money management, transportation, use of the telephone, and work and leisure. The client must perform a task or respond to questions from the evaluator (47). As an example, for the occupational task of making change, the evaluator presents the client with an item (a magazine or a bar of soap) marked with a price. The client must pretend to purchase the item with play money and is scored on whether they are able to identify whether the evaluator has given the correct change. The client is rated as "independent" or "needs assistance." There is a brief reading and writing test that is intended to supplement the rest of the assessment. The *KELS-4E* is appropriate for screening; it does not measure skills in the client's natural environment and thus may not accurately indicate the person's likelihood for successful functioning when transitioning into the community (37).

Mixed Methods or Approaches: *Bay Area Functional Performance Evaluation, 2nd Edition (BaFPE-2)*

The *BaFPE-2* (42, 75) is a standardized instrument that assesses some of the general skills needed for independent functioning. Decision-making, motivation, and organization of time and materials are some of the items rated. The evaluator also observes and records perceptual–motor behaviors such as use of both hands in sorting shells. Finally, the way the client relates to other people is rated on a separate Social Interaction Scale (42, 75). It begins with a brief interview to orient the person to the purpose of the assessment and to collect basic information. This is followed by a task-oriented assessment (TOA) consisting of five tasks: sorting shells, a money and marketing task, drawing a house floor plan, constructing nine block designs from memory, and drawing a person. The evaluator rates the person's performance of these tasks using a rating guide included in the assessment. Decision-making, motivation, and organization of time and materials are some of the items rated. The evaluator also observes and records perceptual–motor behaviors such as use of both hands in sorting shells. Finally, the way the client relates to other people is rated on a separate Social Interaction Scale (42, 75).

Normative data are available for the *BaFPE-2,* and research indicates that it is reliable and has good construct validity (42, 75). The *BaFPE-2* has been used in both inpatient and outpatient settings, school-based special education settings, and vocational rehabilitation settings to evaluate the behavioral and functional performance of clients with psychiatric illness, brain injury, developmental or intellectual disabilities in adolescent, adult, and geriatric populations (61).

Mixed Methods Assessments or Approaches: *The St. Louis University Mental Status Exam (SLUMS)*

The *Saint Louis University Mental Status Examination (SLUMS)* is a quick screening assessment of mental functions. It takes about 15 minutes to administer. Some research shows it may be more sensitive to mild neurocognitive impairment (MCI) than older similar assessments such as the *Short Mini–Mental Status Examination 2 (ShortMMSE-2)* (71). The 11 items on the *SLUMS* are designed to test long-term memory, short-term memory, working memory, and other cognitive functions. The maximum score is 30. The test is scored differently depending on the levels of a variety of different social factors, including the person's level of education (71).

Although it is more typical for a psychologist or psychiatrist to administer mental status examinations, cognitive screening tools such as the *SLUMS* and others like it can also be administered by an OT (10). The person giving the *SLUMS* must be trained to administer this assessment. (A version is available online; please see the *End of Chapter Resources* for a link to this assessment.) The *Montreal Cognitive Assessment (MoCA)* is another assessment similar to the *SLUMS* and the *Short MMSE-2* (27). Other examples include the OT conducting functional cognition assessments that require special training, such as the *Assessment of Motor and Process Skills (AMPS)*, Volume 2, which measures a person's motor skills and organizational abilities as revealed in familiar household tasks (34, 35). Generally, these are not appropriate for delegation to the OTA (7). Many other assessments of cognition exist, and this brief introduction is not intended as an exhaustive list but rather a general introduction to several of the assessments an occupational therapy professional may see in psychosocial settings (Table 12.3).

Table 12.3. Evaluation Approaches and Selected Assessment Examples

Interviews	Self-Reports
• *World Health Organization Disability Assessment Schedule 2.0 (WHODAS 2.0)* (78) • *Occupational Performance History Interview II (OPHI-II)*, Version 2.1 (46) • *Canadian Occupational Performance Model, 5th Edition (COPM)* (49) • The *Activity Card Sort (ACS)*, 2nd Edition (16)	• *Role Checklist (RC)* (57) • *Role Checklist Version 3 (RCv3)* (Scott 69) • *Occupational Self-Assessment (OSA)*, Version 2.2 (15, 48 [COSA]) • *Occupational Self-Assessment—Short Form (OSA-SF)* (60) • *Occupational Self-Assessment—Daily Living Scales (OSA-DLS)* (68) • *Medical Outcomes Study: Survey of Social Support (MOS:SSS)* (62) • *Adolescent and Adult Sensory Profile* (19) • *Multidimensional Scale of Perceived Social Support (MSPSS)* (79)
Performance-Based or Observation-Based	**Mixed Methods Assessments/Approaches**
• *Comprehensive Occupational Therapy Evaluation (COTE)* (18) • *Independent Living Scales (ILS)* (52) • *Test of Grocery Shopping Skills (TOGSS)* (20) • *Allen Cognitive Levels Screen-5 (ACLS-5)* (2) • *Allen Diagnostic Module, 2nd Edition (ADM-2)* (29) • *Routine Task Inventory—Expanded (RTI-E)* (44) • *Cognitive Performance Test (CPT)* (22) • *Performance Assessment of Self-Care Skills (PASS)*, Version 4.1 (64)	• *Kohlman Evaluation of Living Skills, 4th Edition (KELS-4E)* (47) • *Bay Area Functional Performance Evaluation, 2nd Edition (BaFPE-2)* (42) • *The St. Louis University Mental Status Exam (SLUMS)* (71) • *Model of Human Occupation Screening Tool 2.0 (MOHOST)* (59)

Mixed Methods Assessments or Approaches: *Model of Human Occupation Screening Tool 2.0 (MOHOST)*

The *MOHOST* was developed by an OT in a psychiatric setting, and with some practice the tool can be administered in 10 to 20 minutes. It is a highly flexible screening instrument that can be used to gather more information about the client's occupational strengths and challenges, but it can also be utilized as an assessment method to illuminate the client's progress toward their occupational therapy goals (43). The examiner's manual for the *MOHOST* additionally includes the instructions and protocol to administer the *MOHOST-SOF*, the *Model of Human Occupation Screening Tool-Single Observation Form*. Using the *MOHOST-SOF*, the OT (and the OTA who has achieved service competency) can observe the client while the client participates in a single activity (occupation). This can be achieved during a single session and takes approximately 15 minutes, depending on the occupation. The ease of use and flexibility of this assessment makes the *MOHOST* or the *MOHOST-SOF* a convenient, valid, and reliable way to measure individual client change in a clinical environment (43, 53).

Importantly, the *MOHOST* was developed using terminology that is familiar and easier to understand to describe the sometimes difficult to understand concepts and terms used in the *Model of Human Occupation Theory* (72). With more accessible language, the occupational therapy professional can more efficiently communicate information about the results of the *MOHOST* to other members of the behavioral health team, but most importantly to provide clear information to the client and family or caregivers. Finally, the *MOHOST* examiner's manual provides guidance for intervention planning, including examples of goals and strategies that are aligned with specific MOHO concepts such as motivation (volition), pattern of occupation (habituation), communication and interaction skills, process skills, motor skills, and environment (58, 59).

SUMMARY

Data gathering and evaluation are the foundation of the occupational therapy treatment process, providing essential information about who clients are, what their lives are like, the kinds of things they want and need to do, and the problems that stand in their way. The ability to observe dispassionately, free from personal bias or preconceived ideas, is essential. The observations and assessments performed by the occupational therapy team and the interdisciplinary team form the foundation of the intervention plan. For evaluation to be ecologically authentic, whenever possible, assessment should be done in the environment that is customary (and preferable) for the individual. Being involved in any part of a client's evaluation is a serious and often complex responsibility, but it is also a wonderful opportunity to explore and better understand the unique and sometimes perplexing world of another human being.

Obviously, because of space limitations, only some of the assessments that may be used in mental health occupational therapy practice are presented here. The occupational therapy professional is encouraged to engage in consistent continuing education and champion work cultures where knowledge translation is apparent. This helps practitioners to remain aware of the ongoing contributions from occupational therapy and occupational science research and evidence as updates and discoveries lead to improvements in the occupational lives of our clients.

Case Study – A 27-Year-Old Man With Bipolar I Disorder With Psychotic Features

D. Kennedy Case #291083

Mr Kennedy is a 27-year-old Caucasian male who has a diagnosis of Bipolar I Disorder with Psychotic Features (F31.9). He was referred to occupational therapy for evaluation to assess the need to develop or reestablish skills necessary to resume community living with his wife of one year. The client was admitted to the ER of a general hospital following an incident on Valentine's Day a little more than a year ago in which he stabbed and enucleated his right eye. Mr Kennedy cited a biblical passage as the reason for this self-mutilation.[2] The client was subsequently transferred to an outpatient mental health clinic, but 4 months later, he could not be maintained in the community and was admitted to a state psychiatric facility. This was his first psychiatric hospitalization, although he had a history of psychiatric consultations dating from adolescence; and since age 23, he has had difficulty maintaining employment secondary to his reports of having trouble "handling his emotions." Medical history indicates that Mr Kennedy had a provisional diagnosis of schizophrenia, paranoid type, in the past. The client has no history of drug or alcohol abuse.

DSM-5-TR Diagnosis at Admission

F31.9	Bipolar I disorder with psychotic features

ICD-10-CM

H54.10	Blindness, one eye, low vision in other eye, not otherwise specified

Z Codes

Z91.52	Personal history of self-harm
Z63.0	Relationship distress with spouse (12)

The client's family background is unclear; his parents separated when he was 6 years old, shortly after a sister, his only sibling, was born. He moved with his mother and sister from Virginia to Maryland and has had no contact with his father since. Per client report, his mother is "rigid, controlling, and very religious." According to his medical records, the emotional problems were recognized during his middle and high school years; he was described as a "very isolated student who has difficulty with interpersonal relationships." Mr Kennedy did earn a high school diploma and then maintained employment for approximately 5 years as a horse trainer and groomer at a racetrack, until he began working at his mother's florist business (for ~5 years.).

---

[2]Matthew 5:28–30.

Around his 24th birthday, the client began experiencing symptoms and could no longer function at work. The precipitating incident occurred when a stranger knocked on the door of his home, asking for a man with the same name as the client; the client then became suspicious and concerned about men following him. He attended Bible-study class regularly with his mother, met his future wife there, and became engaged to her. Subsequently, he became anxious and indecisive about the pending marriage, and it was at this time that he mutilated his eye. After 8 weeks in acute inpatient care in a general hospital, he was discharged and followed up with weekly outpatient visits. He then married his wife. Over the next 10 to 12 months, his symptoms of mania and increasing delusions were considered unmanageable at home by his wife. He was admitted to the state psychiatric hospital 12 months after his marriage. On admission, he was withdrawn, showed blunted affect, exhibited festinating gait, and was actively experiencing delusions claiming that "someone is gripping his mind."

Medical care of the right eye during the client's tenure as an outpatient and during the first month of his inpatient stay was extensive. Chronic infections, stretching of the eye socket, and poor hygiene and grooming resulting from carelessness and poor cooperation by the client made it impossible for him to use a prosthesis. He has been wearing an eye patch.

The rehabilitation team, in its initial treatment planning conference and in collaboration with the client, identified the primary goal as helping the client make an effective adjustment to resume community living with his wife. The client's wife was interested in a possible switching of roles: She would continue her work as a rental agent secretary in an apartment complex, and he would take care of the home. It was not clear initially whether this was the best arrangement or whether Mr Kennedy should return to work.

The initial occupational therapy evaluation included an occupational profile use of the *KELS-4E*. A deficit in the client's standing balance was noted. In addition, the client was unable to perform basic household tasks; was unfamiliar with typical household situations; did not know proper first aid; was unable to identify household safety problems; had poor laundry skills; and was unfamiliar with budgeting, grocery shopping, paying bills, and banking. The client was withdrawn and demonstrated poor social skills throughout the occupational therapy evaluation. He was unable to identify leisure interests and showed no motivation for using leisure time productively. The occupational therapy team and the client established the following priorities as immediate goals:

- Improve standing balance
- Improve grooming, personal hygiene, and self-care
- Assess and develop work skills in preparation for return to full-time employment, or
- Develop independent living IADL and home management skills so that his wife can continue in her job, and, if desired, increase her hours.

The client began participating in a series of one-to-one occupational therapy sessions to improve standing balance and self-care. The occupational therapy team arranged for the client to attend daily IADL and independent living skills occupational therapy groups that focused on topics such as home management and personal finance, as well as helping him join a work adjustment program for a 6-month work skills assessment and program in horticulture. (The area was selected because of the client's previous experience in a florist's shop.) Mr Kennedy's progress was reviewed prior to his completion of this program, at which time it seemed that the client would not be able to return to work because of overwhelming anxiety. Although Mr Kennedy had participated actively in the work skills program, he and his wife agreed that it would be best for him to take over the household responsibilities rather than work full-time. Criteria for Mr Kennedy's release were based on his ability to maintain stability of mood and cooperate with daily treatment programs. The ultimate occupational outcome was to enable Mr Kennedy to function safely in his role as a home manager while living in the community.

The OT and the OTA who cofacilitated the IADL groups, collaboratively administered the *PASS* to obtain more detailed information on the client's skills and needs. The following additional deficits were noted: unstable and unsafe posture; failure to compensate for loss of vision on the right; no knowledge of nutrition, menu planning, meal preparation, or grocery shopping; and a tendency to panic when confronted with stressful decisions. The following additional goals were established by the occupational therapy team and the client.

Increase sense of comfort and confidence in ability to carry out the home management role.

- Improve ability to plan and execute basic household tasks.
- Develop social skills in basic communication, ability to relate to others in small groups, and appropriate self-assertion.
- Teach techniques to compensate for the visual defect; teach hygiene and maintenance for eye socket and patch.
- Teach stress management techniques and establish a habit of using them.
- Explore leisure interests, and develop a habit of participating in leisure on a regular basis.

The schedule included attendance in group and individual occupational therapy sessions for 4 hours a day, 3 times a week for 8 weeks. Mr Kennedy completed a course of instruction in all areas of home management. He became gradually more comfortable in social situations and showed appropriate curiosity and interest in the program and in other clients. He learned stress management techniques using music, progressive relaxation, and imagery, and he became less suspicious and more spontaneous in his interactions with others.

The client was discharged from occupational therapy services in the spring, a little more than 1 year after his admission, following his successful completion of the Independent Living program. He works part-time in a local greenhouse and nursery and takes an active role in managing the home. He appears stable and is managing his role as homemaker and part-time worker very well. Health maintenance checkups in the community behavioral mental health clinic in his neighborhood are ongoing.

OT HACKS SUMMARY

O: Occupation as a means and an end

Recalling the metaphor of the occupational therapy domain as home, occupational therapy professionals might imagine the occupational therapy evaluation process as supporting each of our clients in constructing their personal optimal "home." A client's "home" is inclusive of all places, spaces, and dimensions (transactional relationships (21)) that we must collaborate with the client to evaluate.

T: Theoretical concepts, values, and principles, or historical foundations

In her 2003 *Eleanor Clarke Slagle Lecture* titled Chaotic Occupational Therapy: Collective Wisdom for a Complex Profession, Dr Charlotte Brasic Royeen embraced 15 standards that were developed by an AOTA committee of Physicians chaired by Dr William R. Dunton and finally presented in 1925, although not ever officially adopted. Nevertheless, Dr Royeen adapted the principles as part of her address, "as a focus forward for the year 2025" (65, p. 510).

Take a moment to reflect specifically on two of these principles. Think about how this modern translation of principles of occupational therapy written nearly 100 years ago summarizes what occupational therapy professions *do* as it relates to occupational therapy evaluation.

- "Occupation is a process of participation in meaningful activity to promote quality of life and health" (65, p. 511).
- "All forms of the process of doing with meaning constitute engagement in the process of occupation. Thus, the scope of occupational therapy is holistic, widespread, and integrated into most all human functions as reflected in the *Occupational Therapy Practice Framework*, and is an entitlement of all humans in the form of occupational justice" (65, p. 511).

H: How can we Help? OT's role in serving clients with mental illness or mental health needs

It can be difficult to decide whether a given behavior is a strength or a barrier until we know more about the situational aspects and contexts of a person's life or history, and this is especially true when working with a person who is experiencing mental health problems. A **strength** is a useful, adaptive behavior, one that helps the client get what they need. A **barrier** is anything that interferes with the client's occupational performance, hence impacting their overall participation.

Regardless of what strengths or barriers a client possesses, exploring these elements is a fundamental goal of the evaluation phase.

A: Adaptations

"Basic to an occupational performance approach are the skills of the therapist to analyze tasks, activities, and occupations and propose and use learning or adaptive strategies to support the individual to perform meaningful occupations" (50, p. 5).

C: Case study includes

Can you answer the following questions related to Mr Kennedy's case?

1. The client participated in services in a variety of settings for nearly 12 months, which is highly unusual, particularly considering the health disparities that were likely involved in Mr Kennedy's case. Based on the information provided, what other options could have been explored, considering his recent eye injury and his occupational history?
2. What occupational roles has the client acquired? What additional occupational performance skills can you foresee that he will need in the future?
3. The goals stated in this case are a mix of OT goals (what the OT would do) and client goals (what the client would do). Can you restate the goals so that they make the occupational focus and outcomes more explicit? For the stress management goal, write your methods and approach, and break the goal into smaller behavioral objectives.

K: Knowledge: keeping mental health OT practice grounded in evidence, in occupational science, and in research

Follow-up Reflection and Discussion Questions for:

Hitch, D., Lhuede, K., Vernon, L., Pepin, G., & Stagnitti, K. (2019). Longitudinal evaluation of a knowledge translation role in occupational therapy. *BMC Health Services Research*, *19*(1), 154.

Link to the Article: https://rdcu.be/cWbnv

1. Based on this study, what do the OTs who were surveyed list as factors that motivate them toward a desire to participate in research at work? What were the stressors or barriers against research capacity in daily occupational therapy practice?
2. What was the purpose of this study?
3. When occupational therapy professionals collaborate with the client to perform an occupational therapy evaluation, part of the occupational therapy process is determining what the priorities are for outcomes.
   a. Describe what is meant by *knowledge translation outcomes*?
   b. Compare and contrast knowledge translation outcomes with the outcomes that are the end result of the occupational therapy process.
4. What did this study find regarding the relationship between client-centeredness and knowledge translation?
5. How was social network analysis utilized in this study?

S: Some terms that may be new to you

Assessment: The word used to identify specific tests, instruments, interviews, and other measures of occupational function that make up the overall occupational therapy evaluation.

Barrier: anything that interferes with the client's occupational performance, hence impacting their overall participation

Bottom-up evaluation: Bottom-up evaluation begins with the factors that appear to impede occupational engagement.

Construct validity: the degree to which the scores of an instrument are internally consistent according to hypothesized internal relationships or how the assessment measures concepts it claims to measure when compared to other tools that also measure similar concepts; construct validity can also be used to consider how an assessment measures differences between two groups or populations

Context: "Construct that constitutes the complete makeup of a person's life as well as the common and divergent factors that characterize groups and populations. Context includes environmental factors and personal factors . . ." (9, p. 76).

Criterion-referenced assessment: criterion-referenced tests and assessments are designed to measure performance against a fixed set of predetermined criteria, competency threshold, or learning standards

Environment-first evaluation: Environment-first evaluation approaches are most appropriate when safety is a factor, decreasing clients' potential risk of harm and eliminating hazards are the foremost priorities.

Evaluation: "The comprehensive process of obtaining and interpreting the data necessary to understand the person, system, or situation. . . . Evaluation requires synthesis of all data obtained, analytic interpretation of that data, reflective clinical reasoning, and consideration of occupational performance and contextual factors" (39, p. 3).

Expected environment: The environment where the client will be living following discharge from rehabilitation (especially in inpatient settings).

Face validity: describes assessments, for example, range of motion testing, that have fairly obvious validity

Health disparities: differences in health status between people related to social or demographic factors such as race, gender, income, or geographic region

Health equity (inequity): inequities are created when barriers prevent individuals and communities from accessing these conditions and reaching their full potential

Interrater reliability: shows the degree to which two people giving the test will obtain similar results

Normative data: Normative data are collected from many administrations of a test or assessment method. This means that many people (individuals, groups, or populations) have been given the assessment and have had their scores recorded. From the scores of this larger sample group, the developers of the assessment predict what the normal range of scores is likely to be. Once the normal range has been identified, the score of a particular individual can be compared with it.

Norm-referenced assessment: norm-referenced assessment refers to standardized tests that are designed to compare and rank test takers in relation to one another using normative data

Occupational engagement: used interchangeably in this text with occupational participation; characterized by a person engaging in something that they experience as valuable

Occupational experience: how the "doing" is experienced

Occupational participation: used interchangeably in this text with occupational engagement; characterized by a person engaging in something that they experience as valuable

Occupational performance: the "doing" of the occupation

Performance measures: another way to describe criterion-referenced tests

Personal factors: "Unique features of the person reflecting the particular background of their life and living that are not part of a health condition or health state. Personal factors are generally considered to be enduring, stable attributes of the person, although some personal factors may change over time" (9, p. 81).

Reliability: represents the consistency of the results of an assessment when the test is repeated

Service competency: A method used to ensure that the OTA has the necessary skills and experience to administer aspects of a particular assessment or participate otherwise in an occupational therapy evaluation. In collaboration with an OT, service competency is established when the OTA demonstrates that they would obtain the same or very similar results to what the OT would obtain, when using the same instrument

Standardization: a way of ensuring the accuracy and consistency of an assessment method or tool; standardization is generally achieved in relationship to normative data or to specific criteria

Strength: a useful, adaptive behavior, one that helps the client get what they need

Test–retest reliability: shows the degree of sameness of scores when a test is repeated

Top-down evaluation: Top-down evaluation begins with exploring the client's overall occupational goals. No other data are collected, and no assessments or techniques that isolate specific body structures or functions, or isolated client factors, are administered until the client's perspective and occupational outcomes and priorities are made clear. Completing an occupational profile exemplifies the top-down principle.

Validity or content validity: shows the degree to which the test measures what it says it is measuring

Reflection Questions

1. If a score on an assessment is derived from an unreliable measure, can the score be valid? Why or why not? Please explain your answer.
2. Differentiate between the *occupational profile* and the *assessment of occupational performance* aspects of evaluation.
3. Discuss the ways that the client's goals and priorities can be integrated into the evaluation process.
4. Define *strengths, supports, resources, and barriers* in relationship to occupational performance.
5. Relate *contexts* and *environments* to evaluation of occupational performance.
6. Use the *Transactional Model of Occupation* to describe the relationship between occupation and client engagement in occupation.

7. Differentiate the responsibilities of the OT and OTA in evaluation.
8. Describe ways in which information for the occupational profile and the analysis of occupational performance can be obtained.
9. How do you think health inequities might affect the occupational evaluation process and/or influence the assessment results?

REFERENCES

1. Aldrich, R. M. (2008). From complexity theory to transactionalism: Moving occupational science forward in theorizing the complexities of behavior. *Journal of Occupational Science, 15*(3), 147–156.
2. Allen, C. K., Austin, S. L., David, S. K., Earhart, C. A., McGraith, D. B., & Riska-Williams, L. (2007). *Manual for the Allen Cognitive Level Screen-5 (ACLS-5) and large Allen Cognitive Level Screen-5 (LACLS-5)*. ACLS and LACLS Committee.
3. Allen, C. K., Reyner, A., & Earhart, C. A. (2008). *How to start using the Allen Diagnostic Module* (9th ed.). S&S Worldwide. https://www.ssww.com/senior-activities/allen-diagnostic-module/?fp=CU22
4. Allison, J., & Shotwell, M. P. (2020). The comprehensive occupational therapy evaluation. In B. J. Hemphill & C. J. Urish (Eds.), *Assessments in occupational therapy mental health: An integrative approach* (4th ed., pp. 371–382). SLACK.
5. American Medical Association. (2020). *Current Procedures Terminology (CPT®)*. https://www.ama-assn.org/amaone/cpt-current-procedural-terminology
6. American Occupational Therapy Association. (2020). AOTA 2020 occupational therapy code of ethics. *American Journal of Occupational Therapy, 74*(Suppl. 3), 7413410005.
7. American Occupational Therapy Association. (2020). Guidelines for supervision, roles, and responsibilities during the delivery of occupational therapy services. *American Journal of Occupational Therapy, 74*(Suppl. 3), 7413410020.
8. American Occupational Therapy Association. (2020). Occupational therapy in the promotion of health and well-being. *American Journal of Occupational Therapy, 74*(3), 7403420010.
9. American Occupational Therapy Association. (2020). Occupational therapy practice framework: Domain and process—Fourth edition. *American Journal of Occupational Therapy, 74*(Suppl. 2), 1–87.
10. American Occupational Therapy Association. (2021). Occupational therapy scope of practice. *American Journal of Occupational Therapy, 75*(Suppl. 3), 7513410030.
11. American Occupational Therapy Association. (2021). Standards of practice for occupational therapy. *American Journal of Occupational Therapy, 75*(Suppl. 3), 7513410050.
12. American Psychiatric Association. (2022). *Diagnostic and statistical manual of mental disorders* (5th ed., text rev.). Author. https://doi.org/10.1176/appi.books.9780890425787
13. American Public Health Association. (n.d.). *APHA health equity fact sheets, briefs, reports and infographics.* https://www.apha.org/topics-and-issues/health-equity
14. Bagozzi, D. (2001, November 15). *News release: WHO publishes new guidelines to measure health.* World Health Organization. https://www.who.int/news/item/15-11-2001-who-publishes-new-guidelines-to-measure-health
15. Baron, K., Kielhofner, G., Iyenger, A., Goldhammer, V., & Wolenski, J. (2006). *The occupational self-assessment* (version 2.2). Model of Human Occupation Clearinghouse.
16. Baum, C. M., & Edwards, D. (2008). *Activity card sort* (2nd ed.). AOTA Press.
17. Bonder, B. R. (2022). *Psychopathology and function* (6th ed.). SLACK.
18. Brayman, S. J., Kirby, T. F., Misenheimer, A. M., & Short, M. J. (1976). Comprehensive occupational therapy evaluation scale. *American Journal of Occupational Therapy, 30*(2), 94–100.
19. Brown, C., & Dunn, W. (2002). *Adolescent/adult sensory profile: User's manual.* The Psychological Corporation.
20. Brown, C., Rempfer, M., & Hamera, E. (2009). *Test of grocery shopping skills manual.* AOTA Press.
21. Bunting, K. L. (2016). A transactional perspective on occupation: A critical reflection. *Scandinavian Journal of Occupational Therapy, 23*(5), 327–336.
22. Burns, T. (2006). *The cognitive performance test manual.* Maddak.
23. Cohn, E. S. (2019). Asserting our competence and affirming the value of occupation with confidence. *American Journal of Occupational Therapy, 73*(6), 7036150010.
24. Connor, L. T., & Baum, C. M. (2020). Activity card sort as an essential tool to obtain an occupational history and profile in individuals with mental health challenges. In B. J. Hemphill & C. J. Urish (Eds.), *Assessments in occupational therapy mental health: An integrative approach* (4th ed., pp. 77–90). SLACK.
25. Cutchin, M. P., & Dickie, V. A. (2012). Transactionalism: Occupational science and the pragmatic attitude. In G. E. Whiteford & C. Hocking (Eds.), *Occupational science: Society, inclusion, participation* (pp. 23–37). Wiley-Blackwell.
26. Dickie, V., Cutchin, M. P., & Humphry, R. (2006). Occupation as transactional experience: A critique of individualism in occupational science. *Journal of Occupational Science, 13*(1), 83–93.
27. Douglas, A., Letts, L., Eva, K., & Richardson, J. (2012). Use of the cognitive performance test for identifying deficits in hospitalized older adults. *Rehabilitation Research and Practice, 2012*, 638480.
28. Dunn, W. (2017). Measurement concepts and practices. In M. C. Law, C. M. Baum, & W. Dunn (Eds.), *Measuring occupational performance: Supporting best practice in occupational therapy* (3rd ed., pp. 17–28). SLACK.
29. Earhart, C. A. (2014). *Allen diagnostic module: [Revised] manual* (2nd ed.). S & S Worldwide.
30. Earhart, C. A. (2015). *Using Allen diagnostic module-2nd edition assessments.* S&S Worldwide. http://www.ssww.com/pages/?page_id=227
31. Earhart, C. A., & McCraith, D. B. (2020). Cognitive disabilities model: Allen cognitive level screen-5 and Allen diagnostic module (2nd edition) Assessments. In B. J. Hemphill & C. J. Urish (Eds.), *Assessments in occupational therapy mental health: An integrative approach* (4th ed., pp. 179–210). SLACK.
32. Fisher, A. G. (2009). *Occupational therapy process model: A model for planning and implementing top-down, client-centered, and occupation-based interventions.* Three Star Press.
33. Fisher, A. G. (2013). Occupation-centered, occupation-based, occupation-focused: Same, same or different? *Scandinavian Journal of Occupational Therapy, 20*(3), 162–173.
34. Fisher, A. G., & Jones, K. B. (2017). Occupational therapy intervention process model. In J. Hinojosa, P. Kramer, & C. B. Royeen (Eds.), *Perspectives on human occupation: Theories underlying practice* (2nd ed., pp. 237–286). Wolters Kluwer, Lippincott Williams & Wilkins.
35. Fisher, A. G., & Marterella, A. (2019). *Powerful practice: A model for authentic occupational therapy.* Center for Innovative OT Solutions.
36. Gillen, G., Hunter, E. G., Lieberman, D., & Stutzbach, M. (2019). AOTA's top 5 Choosing Wisely© recommendations. *American Journal of Occupational Therapy, 73*(2), 7302420010.
37. Hemphill, B. J., & Urish, C. K. (Eds.). (2020). *Assessments in occupational therapy mental health: An integrative approach* (4th ed.). SLACK.
38. Hinojosa, J., & Kramer, P. (Eds.). (2014). *Evaluation in occupational therapy* (4th ed.). AOTA Press.
39. Hinojosa, J., Kramer, P., & Crist, P. (2014). Evaluation: Where do we begin? In J. Hinojosa & P. Kramer (Eds.), *Evaluation in occupational therapy: Obtaining and interpreting data* (4th ed., pp. 1–18). AOTA Press.
40. Holm, M. B., & Rogers, J. C. (2020). The performance assessment of self-care skills. In B. J. Hemphill & C. J. Urish (Eds.), *Assessments in occupational therapy mental health: An integrative approach* (4th ed., pp. 359–370). SLACK.
41. Hooper, B., & Wood, W. (2019). The philosophy of occupational therapy: A framework for practice. In B. A. B. Schell & G. Gillen (Eds.),

Willard and Spackman's occupational therapy (13th ed., pp. 43–55). Wolters Kluwer.

42. Houston, D., Williams, S. L., Bloomer, J., & Mann, W. C. (1989). The bay area functional performance evaluation: Development and standardization. *American Journal of Occupational Therapy, 43*(3), 170–183.

43. Januszewski, C., & Mahaffey, L. (2020). Assessments used within the model of human occupation. In B. J. Hemphill & C. J. Urish (Eds.), *Assessments in occupational therapy mental health: An integrative approach* (4th ed., pp. 279–305). SLACK.

44. Katz, N. (2006). *Routine task inventory-expanded (RTI-E)*. https://www.allen-cognitive-network.org/index.php/allen-cognitive-model/routine-task-inventory-expanded-rti-e

45. Katz, N. (2020). Routine task inventory-expanded. In B. J. Hemphill & C. J. Urish (Eds.), *Assessments in occupational therapy mental health: An integrative approach* (4th ed., pp. 211–221). SLACK.

46. Kielhofner, G., Mallinson, T., Crawford, C., Nowak, M., Rigby, M., Henry, A., & Walens, D. (2004). *Occupational performance history interview II (OPHI-II)* (Version 2.1). Model of Human Occupation Clearinghouse.

47. Kohlman Thomson, L., & Robnett, R. H. (2016). *The Kohlman evaluation of living skills* (4th ed.). AOTA Press.

48. Kramer, J., ten Velden, M., Kafkes, A., Basu, S., Federico, J., & Kielhofner, G. (2014). *The user's manual for child occupational self-assessment (COSA) (version 2.2)*. Model of Human Occupation Clearinghouse.

49. Law, M., Baptiste, S., Carswell, A., McColl, M. A., Polatajko, H., & Pollack, N. (2014). *COPM 5th edition: Canadian occupational performance measure manual* (5th ed). CAOT Publications ACE.

50. Law, M. C., Baum, C. M., & Dunn, W. (Eds.). (2017). *Measuring occupational performance: Supporting best practice in occupational therapy* (3rd ed.). SLACK.

51. Levy, L. L., & Burns, T. (2011). The cognitive disabilities reconsidered model: Rehabilitation of adults with dementia. In N. Katz (Ed.), *Cognition, occupation, and participation across the life-span: Neuroscience, neurorehabilitation and models of intervention in occupational therapy* (3rd ed., pp. 407–441). AOTA Press.

52. Loeb, P. A. (1996). *ILS: Independent living scales manual*. The Psychological Corporation.

53. Maciver, D. Morley, M., Forsyth, K., Bertram, N., Edwards, T., Heasman, D., Rennison, J., Rush, R., & Willis, S. (2016). A Rasch analysis of the model of human occupation screening tool single observation tool (MOHOST-SOF) in mental health. *British Journal of Occupational Therapy, 79*(1), 49–56.

54. Magasi, S., Gohil, A., Burghart, M., & Wallisch, A. (2017). Understanding measurement properties. In M. C. Law, C. M. Baum, & W. Dunn (Eds.), *Measuring occupational performance: Supporting best practice in occupational therapy* (3rd ed., pp. 29–41). SLACK.

55. Matuska, K., & Barrett, K. (2019). Patterns of occupations. In B. A. B. Schell & G. Gillen (Eds.), *Willard & Spackman's occupational therapy* (13th ed., pp. 212–220). Wolters Kluwer.

56. Mosey, A. C. (1970). *Three frames of reference for mental health*. C.B. SLACK.

57. Oakley, F. (2006). *The Role Checklist (RC)*. Chicago: *Model of Human Occupation Clearinghouse*.

58. Parkinson, S., Forsyth, K., & Kielhofner, G. (2004). *A user's manual for the model of human occupation screening tool (MOHOST)*. Model of Human Occupation Clearinghouse.

59. Parkinson, S., Forsyth, K., & Kielhofner, G. (2006). *Model of human occupation screening tool (MOHOST) (version 2.0)*. Model of Human Occupation Clearinghouse.

60. Popova, E. S., Ostrowski, R. K., Wescott, J. J., & Taylor, R. R. (2019). Development and evaluation of the occupational self-assessment short form (OSA-SF). *American Journal of Occupational Therapy, 73*(3), 7303205020p1–7303205020p10.

61. Ramano, E. M., & De Beer, M. (2020). The outcome of two occupational therapy group programs on the social functioning of individuals with major depressive disorder. *Occupational Therapy in Mental Health, 36*(1), 29–54.

62. Rand Health. (n.d.). *Medical outcomes study: Social support survey*. 1994–2015.http://www.rand.org/health/surveys_tools/mos/mos_socialsupport_survey.html

63. Reinert, M., Fritze, D., & Nguyen, T. (October, 2021). *The state of mental health in America 2022*. Mental Health America.

64. Rogers, J. C., Holm, M., & Chisolm, D. (2016). *Performance assessment of self-care skills*. (Version 4.1). https://moho-irm.uic.edu/resources/files/#:~:text=The%20Model%20of%20Human%20Occupation%20Clearinghouse%2C%20a%20non%2Dprofit%20organization,and%20development%20of%20these%20resources

65. Royeen, C. B. (2003). Chaotic occupational therapy: Collective wisdom for a complex profession. In R. Padilla & Y. Griffiths (Eds.), *The Eleanor Clarke Slagle lectures in occupational therapy 1955–2016: A professional legacy, Centennial Edition* (pp. 508–527). AOTA Press.

66. Schindler, V. (2020). Role assessments used in mental health. In B. J. Hemphill & C. J. Urish (Eds.), *Assessments in occupational therapy mental health: An integrative approach* (4th ed., pp. 321–339). SLACK.

67. Schwartz, J. K., & Brown, C. (2019). Activities of daily living and instrumental activities of daily living. In C. Brown, V. C. Stoffel, & J. P. Munoz (Eds.), *Occupational therapy in mental health: A vision for participation* (2nd ed.). F.A. Davis.

68. Scott, P. J. (2016). *Occupational self-assessment: Daily Living Scales© Model of Human Occupation Clearinghouse*. Department of Occupational Therapy, University of Illinois at Chicago.

69. Scott, P. J. (2019). *Role Checklist Version 3: Participation and Satisfaction, (RCv3)*. Chicago: Model of Human Occupation Clearinghouse.

70. Sonu, S., Marvin, D., & Moore, C. (2021). The intersection and dynamics between COVID-19, health disparities, and adverse childhood experiences: "Intersection/Dynamics between COVID-19, Health Disparities, and ACEs." *Journal of Child & Adolescent Trauma, 14*, 517–526.

71. Tariq, S. H., Tumosa, N., Chibnall, J. T., Perry, III, H. M., & Morley, J. E. (2006). The Saint Louis University Mental Status (SLUMS) examination for detecting mild cognitive impairment and dementia is more sensitive than the mini-mental status examination (MMSE): A pilot study. *American Journal of Geriatric Psychiatry, 14*(11), 900–910.

72. Taylor, R. R. (Ed.). (2017). *Kielhofner's Model of Human Occupation: Theory and application*. Wolters Kluwer.

73. Taylor, R. R. (2020). *The intentional relationship: Occupational therapy and use of self*. F.A. Davis.

74. Walshaw, C. E. (2020). *Exploring occupational therapy interventions for people with multiple sclerosis within instrumental activities of daily living* [Doctoral dissertation, University of Huddersfield].

75. Williams, S. L., & Bloomer, J. (1987). *Bay-Area functional performance evaluation* (2nd ed.). Consulting Psychologists Press.

76. World Health Organization. (2008). *International classification of functioning, disability, and health: ICF*. WHO Press.

77. World Health Organization. (2021). *Comprehensive mental health action plan 2013–2030*. Author. License: CC BY-NC-SA 3.0 IGO.

78. World Health Organization. (n.d.). *Measuring health and disability: Manual for WHO Disability Assessment Schedule (WHODAS 2.0)*. T. B. Üstün, N. Kostanjsek, S. Chatterji, & J. Rehm (Eds.). Author. https://www.who.int/publications/i/item/measuring-health-and-disability-manual-for-who-disability-assessment-schedule-(-whodas-2.0)

79. Zimet, G. D., Dahlem, N. W., & Zimet, S. G., Farley GK. (1988). The multidimensional scale of perceived social support. *Journal of Personality Assessment, 52*(1), 30–41.

SUGGESTED RESOURCES

Podcast

Public Health on Call is a podcast from The Johns Hopkins Bloomberg School of Public Health. This episode features Dr Lisa Cooper, a leading expert in health equity, discussing the publication of her recent book, *Why Are Health Disparities Everyone's Problem?* (~24 minutes). https://www.youtube.com/watch?v=u14CFKpcuNA

Videos

This brief video, developed by Clinical Scholars and the UNC Center for Health Equity Research (CHER), explains how social determinants of health impact the daily lives and health status of marginalized clients and communities (~7 minutes). https://www.youtube.com/watch?v=oC_MPCXs0Sw

Among other offerings, the Allen Cognitive Group (https://allencognitive.com/free-offerings/) offers brief videos of a simulated *ACLS-5/LACLS-5* (2) Administration, as well as brief videos on topics such as how to set up for administration of the *ACLS-5*, how to insert intentional whipstitch errors (so that the client can identify and attempt to correct an error as a part of the assessment), and multiple videos on how to make and incorporate a test kit using the craft activities that are a part of the Allen Diagnostic Model 2nd ed. Revised (29).

Websites

The website of The American Public Health Association (APHA) offers excellent current data and resources regarding health disparities and health equity in the United States (13). The following are links to examples of some of the available resources. When an OT professional performs an evaluation, it is essential to reflect on how the client's occupational history (their "story") has been influenced by social determinants of health and to consider the ways that the client may be experiencing social or health-related inequities.

COVID-19 vaccination: An equitable response (Fact Sheet)
https://www.apha.org/-/media/Files/PDF/topics/equity/COVID_Vaccine_Equity.ashx

COVID-19's impact on housing instability (Infographic)
https://www.apha.org/News-and-Media/Multimedia/Infographics/Housing-Instability-and-COVID-19

COVID-19's impact on health of the unsheltered (Infographic)
https://www.apha.org/News-and-Media/Multimedia/Infographics/Unsheltered-and-COVID-19

Creating the healthiest nation: Food justice (Fact Sheet)
https://www.apha.org/-/media/Files/PDF/advocacy/CHN_Food_Justice.ashx

Creating the healthiest nation: Health and educational equity (Fact Sheet)
https://www.apha.org/-/media/Files/PDF/factsheets/Health_And_Educational_Equity.ashx

The Model of Human Occupation (MOHO) Clearinghouse at UIC has now merged with The Intentional Relationship Model (IRM) Clearinghouse to form the MOHO-IRM Web and has recently transitioned to an e-store and online database. Many of the assessments and other resources mentioned in this chapter can be purchased here, and many of the resources can be obtained for free by selecting "Free Resources" from the drop-down menu of the products tab.
https://moho-irm.uic.edu/products.aspx

For members of the AOTA, the AOTA website offers *Evaluation & Quality Measures Checklists* for OT practitioners to utilize as a reference for what types of information to collect and what common things may need to be evaluated that are specific to particular client groups or settings. The AOTA suggests that "practitioners . . . [can] use the checklists to help guide client evaluations, as well share with colleagues to provide information about the occupational therapy evaluation process" (retrieved from: https://www.aota.org/practice/domain-and-process/evaluation-and-assessment). At the time of publication of this text, evaluation checklists had been created for: Home Health Evaluation & Quality Measures; Medicare Part B Evaluation & Quality Measures; and Skilled Nursing Evaluation & Quality Measures. Members of AOTA can access these resources by logging in and from the home page of the AOTA website choosing the *Practice* Tab and then selecting *Domain & Process*. The checklists can be found in the Evaluation & Assessment Section.

The Dementia Care Specialists at Crisis Prevention Institute offers excellent and valuable information for incorporating the Allen Cognitive Disabilities Model and its associated assessment tools and resources to support clients with dementia and their caregivers. The blog includes an excellent description of the Allen Cognitive Level Screen (*ACLS/LACLS*) and explains how the test is used and what the assessment tool measures, all without using jargon, making this a wonderful and easy-to-understand resource to share with caregivers. https://www.crisisprevention.com/Blog/Cognitive-Assessment-Tools

The Routine Task Inventory—Expanded (44)
https://www.allen-cognitive-network.org/index.php/allen-cognitive-model/routine-task-inventory-expanded-rti-e

The Performance Assessment of Self-Care Skills—Version 4.1 (65)
https://moho-irm.uic.edu/resources/files/#:~:text=The%20Model%20of%20Human%20Occupation%20Clearinghouse%2C%20a%20non%2Dprofit%20organization,and%20development%20of%20these%20resources

The Saint Louis University Mental Status Examination (71)
https://www.slu.edu/medicine/internal-medicine/geriatric-medicine/aging-successfully/assessment-tools/mental-status-exam.php

Determining the Type and Approach to Intervention

OT HACKS OVERVIEW

O: Occupation as a means and an end

Returning to our Occupational Therapy Domain and Process Metaphor of the Home, in the evaluation phase, the occupational therapy professional is collaborating with the client to construct a "home" that will allow optimal occupational engagement for the client in their daily life. As we move into the intervention planning, the intervention phase of the occupational therapy process can be imagined as collaborating with our client to do maintenance, or remodeling, repairing, and, in some cases, rebuilding, to improve the value and quality of their home (ie, their occupational participation).

T: Theoretical concepts, values, and principles, or historical foundations

While planning interventions, a practice model or theoretical orientation organizes practitioner thinking. The practice model proposes ways for the occupational therapy professional to imagine the client's occupational performance on a continuum of what functional occupational engagement might look like versus what dysfunctional occupational engagement looks like, according to the model, so that the focus of the intervention can remain on occupation, rather than on isolated client factors.

Occupational therapy professionals who work in psychosocial settings often rely heavily on the general constructs of various theories of learning, especially during the intervention planning stages of the occupational therapy process. This is because many of the theories of learning have influenced and provided the foundation for the development of specific occupational therapy theories and models of practice. This chapter revisits some of the underpinnings of behaviorist theory, social learning and social cognitive theory, self-efficacy theory, and motivational theory, some introduced in the first half of the text. The intention of this chapter is to help the reader bring theoretical assumptions to practical interventions that promote positive changes to the client's occupational participation and health.

H: How can we Help? OT's role in serving clients with mental illness or mental health needs

As occupational therapy professionals, we are proficient in analyzing, teaching about, and adapting activities

of daily living (ADLs), and a wide range of work, education, leisure, and social interaction occupations. We know how to break new learning into manageable small steps so that a person can master a complex set of skills one step at a time with the goal of improving some aspect of their occupational engagement. We have many occupation-centered, evidence-based intervention methods, approaches, and types at our disposal. But how do we choose which ones to use? The "choices" that are collaboratively made with the client guide the intervention planning and implementation.

A: Adaptations

Choosing Wisely is an initiative of the American Board of Internal Medicine (ABIM) Foundation. The campaign promotes action-oriented conversations between providers and clients to ensure that safe, effective, and cost-contained quality health care is provided. The American Occupational Therapy Association (AOTA) joined the *Choosing Wisely* initiative in 2016. Championed by Dr Glen Gillen, and with support and input from AOTA members, the Board of Directors, and staff, AOTA implemented a process to develop and publish a list of *Ten Things Patients and Providers Should Question* (2, 22).

The intent of the list was to increase dialogue within the occupational therapy profession about strategies for improving the quality and value of our occupational therapy services. As you read about intervention planning in this chapter, reflect upon how these recommendations may impact occupational interventions in a psychiatric setting.

- Do not provide intervention activities that are nonpurposeful (eg, cones, pegs, shoulder arc, arm bike).
- Do not provide sensory-based interventions to individual children or youth without documented assessment results of difficulties processing or integrating sensory information.
- Do not use physical agent modalities (PAMs) without providing purposeful and occupation-based intervention activities.
- Do not use pulleys for individuals with a hemiplegic shoulder.

- Do not provide cognitive-based interventions (eg, paper-and-pencil tasks, table-top tasks, cognitive training software) without direct application to occupational performance.
- Do not initiate occupational therapy interventions without completion of the client's occupational profile and setting collaborative goals.
- Do not provide interventions for persons with autism to reduce or eliminate "restricted and repetitive patterns of behavior, activities, or interests" without evaluating and understanding the meaning of the behavior to the person, as well as personal and environmental factors.
- Do not use reflex integration programs for individuals with delayed primary motor reflexes without clear links to occupational outcomes.
- Do not use slings for individuals with a hemiplegic arm that place the arm in a flexor pattern for extended periods of time.
- Do not provide ambulation or gait training interventions that do not directly link to functional mobility.

To read more about these AOTA *Choosing Wisely* statements, visit:

- American Occupational Therapy Association (2023). Evidence-Based Practice. *Choosing Wisely: An update on AOTA's best practice recommendations* (formerly Choosing Wisely®). Retrieved from: https://www.aota.org/practice/practice-essentials/evidencebased-practiceknowledge-translation/aotas-top-10-choosing-wisely-recommendations
- Gillen, G., Hunter, E. G., Lieberman, D., & Stutzbach, M. (2019). AOTA's top 5 choosing wisely recommendations. *American Journal of Occupational Therapy, 73*, 7302420010p1–7302420010p9.

C: **Case study includes**

In this chapter, the reader is introduced to the case examples of Mark and Drew. Mark has sustained a physical injury following a car accident. Drew is living with a newly diagnosed mental illness. Although the two clients share many similarities (similar age, similar systems of support, etc), the differences in their conditions, or diagnoses, mean that it is likely that the occupational therapy professional who works with these clients would choose vastly different approaches and employ quite different types of interventions. In this chapter, the reader is introduced to strategies and evidence about how to determine the most efficacious place to begin.

K: **Knowledge: keeping mental health OT practice grounded in evidence, in occupational science, and in research**

Motivational interviewing (MI) is "a collaborative, person-centered form of guiding [the client] to elicit and strengthen [their own] motivation for change" (37, p. 137). MI is introduced with theories of motivation in this chapter to highlight the uses for the method of communication as it pertains to occupational therapy intervention planning.

The need for occupational therapy professionals across a variety of settings to administer screening, brief intervention, and referral for treatment (SBIRT) for clients who have problematic substance use that interferes with their occupations, and who are resistant to change, is increasing. MI is a method of communication, a skill set that can be practiced over time, which can be used as an approach for enhancing a client's intrinsic motivation toward change. The five key communication skills that occupational therapy professionals need to engage with clients in MI are as follows:

1. Asking open-ended questions
2. Affirming client responses
3. Being reflective
4. Summarizing
5. Providing information and advice only with permission and constantly listening for the client's use of "change language" (24)

The following study describes the impact of a training simulation aimed to increase preparedness and confidence of users' strategies in conducting screening and brief intervention (SBI, where some aspects of MI were applied). A computer role-play simulation training in MI strategies was used to measure and detect changes in the confidence and preparedness in selecting appropriate responses during the virtual SBIRT.

Sullivan, A., Albright, G., & Khalid, N. (2021). Impact of a virtual role-play simulation in teaching motivational interviewing communication strategies to occupational therapy students for readiness in conducting screening and brief interventions. *Journal of Higher Education Theory and Practice, 21*(2).

Because MI is a complex art that requires ongoing practice, after reading the study, can you comment on other ways that occupational therapy students and professionals can become more proficient in both improving their competency in administering SBIRTs and in communicating with clients using an MI approach?

S: **Some terms that may be new to you**

Not applicable for this chapter.

INTRODUCTION

There are three parts to the occupational therapy intervention process: intervention planning, intervention implementation, and intervention review. The intervention plan is derived from information collected during the collaborative evaluation between the occupational therapy professional and the client or client proxy. This chapter presents an overview of the intervention planning process with emphasis on the "how-to" of developing an intervention plan. The chapter describes the nature of occupational therapy intervention planning in psychosocial settings, or for clients who have mental or behavioral health problems that interfere with occupational engagement. It begins by discussing some of the problems that occupational therapy professionals encounter in planning intervention for clients with mental disorders, which they may not necessarily encounter as often in planning intervention for those with other diagnoses, or in other settings.

Although it should remain foremost in the occupational therapy professionals' minds that the target of occupational therapy intervention is not related to the diagnoses of our clients, it is worthwhile to note that occupational therapy intervention planning with clients who have psychiatric diagnoses can be complex. These complexities will often require careful consideration of the occupational therapy approach and type of intervention that will most successfully lead to occupation-based outcomes. To accomplish this, the chapter introduces the reader to a variety of intervention types and intervention approaches. The final sections of the chapter describe how evaluation results are used to create client-centered goals and consider several ways to go about writing goals with occupational outcomes. The chapter concludes with a brief discussion on the role of the occupational therapist and the occupational therapy assistant during intervention planning.

OCCUPATIONAL THERAPY INTERVENTION PLANNING IN PSYCHIATRY

Planning intervention for a person with a psychiatric disorder may feel like trying to assemble a complex puzzle without having all the pieces. Our scientific and clinical understanding of mental disorders is progressing rapidly but it is not yet sufficiently well developed enough for us to be certain of the real cause of the person's problems, and because of this, it is often a difficult task to identify the best solution(s). And it can be even more difficult to develop the best route toward recovery and improved occupational function. To appreciate what a serious obstacle this can be, let us look first at the situation of someone with a *physical* disability.

Case Example

Mark is a 17-year-old high school senior who sustained a severe crushing injury to his right (dominant) hand as a result of a car accident. His index, middle, and ring fingers were amputated just distal to the proximal interphalangeal (PIP) joint. Post amputation and during recovery, it was noted that all motions of the thumb and fingers were severely limited. Mark reported severe pain on movement that persisted throughout therapy. Mark has a girlfriend and several close friends. His coursework at school is a part of the Science Technology Engineering and Math (STEM) track. His future plans are to attend college and major in computer engineering and technology. He ran on the cross-country team during his freshman and sophomore years, and still runs for exercise, but stopped running with the team in his junior year to focus on his grades and getting into college.

We believe we know enough about this client to think about what an appropriate plan might be. First, we can anticipate that because of his injury, he will have problems performing bilateral (two-handed) activities such as dressing, grooming, texting on his phone, and using a computer keyboard. We know that the immediate causes of Mark's difficulty are limited motion, weakness, and pain, and we know what caused them—a crushing injury. We can see the effects of the injury physically by examining the client and looking at his records, x-rays, and ultrasounds. We know methods that will increase range of motion and strength in the hand, and we know ways to reduce pain. We can suggest adaptive equipment and adapted methods for performing activities. In short, we know that once Mark tells us what goals are most important to him, occupational therapy interventions can help him learn new ways to do the things he wants and needs to do. We have ways to help him regain his physical functions and previous level of activity.

Contrast Mark's situation with the following case of someone of similar age and background diagnosed with a psychiatric disorder.

Case Example

Drew

Drew is a 19-year-old college freshman, living at home with his parents while attending school. During Thanksgiving weekend, his parents found his room empty one morning and Drew could not be reached on his cell phone. After a frantic 24 hours, his parents notified the police. He was found several days later in a town 15 miles away, wandering on the street, wearing clothing that his parents could not identify as belonging to him. He reported having not eaten "for a while." His parents reported that he had been growing more isolated over the past 18 months, staying in his room for days at a time, and sometimes refusing to come downstairs even for meals. He had been a relatively good student, earning average grades in his courses for the first 3 years of high school, but his grades fell to Cs and Ds in his senior year, which made gaining acceptance into college difficult. He tells the psychiatrist who evaluates him in the aftermath of his initial disappearance that "he just needs to be left alone because voices tell him that he ruins other people's lives." After 6 months, and after ruling out other diagnoses, the psychiatrist diagnoses Drew with schizophrenia as a provisional diagnosis.

What exactly do we know about Drew? We know that he has a diagnosis of schizophrenia and has been having increasing difficulty functioning in his roles as a student, and as a family member, over the past year and a half. His grooming and hygiene habits have deteriorated; his ability to maintain a proper diet seems questionable; and he is socially self-isolating. What can we do to help him? Where should we begin? Unlike physical disabilities, the causes of which can many times be seen upon physical examination, and with laboratory and medical tests, the causes of the psychiatric disability associated with many psychiatric diagnoses such as schizophrenia are elusive and the definitive diagnosis made by a psychiatric professional involves a complex system of ruling out other diseases and conditions. Sophisticated neuroimaging technology and advances in the use of functional magnetic resonance imaging (MRI) and computed tomography (CT) scans, along with improved understanding of neurochemical processes, have helped identify neurologic markers and abnormalities in the brains of individuals with schizophrenia and other mental illnesses but not necessarily the reasons for these anomalies. Psychiatrists can prescribe medications that help relieve the symptoms for some consumers but they are still trying to understand why and how these medications work, and what the impacts are on function (26, 28).

In the meantime, however, how are we to help Drew? How can Drew benefit from participating in occupational therapy? It is not clear what his immediate and long-term goals might be, although we can identify areas that will likely need attention: self-care, other independent daily living skills, nutrition, academic and study skills, leisure, and social skills. But which one shall we work on first, and why? Once the occupational therapy professional and Drew collaborate to prioritize Drew's goals, how do we move forward to address them? As occupational therapy professionals, we are proficient in analyzing, teaching about, and adapting ADLs, and a wide range of work, education, leisure, and social interaction activities. We know how to break new learning into manageable small steps so that a person can master a complex skill one step at a time. We have many evidence-based techniques and methods at our disposal. But how do we choose which ones to use?

Simply put, there are often greater uncertainties surrounding the functional implications of mental illness in the daily lives of people with a mental health diagnosis. Another source of uncertainty for new occupational therapy professionals, whether a newly graduated student or a long-time practitioner who is working for the first time in a primarily psychosocial setting, is inexperience with clients such as the one described in the second example, Drew. When the occupational therapy professional begins working with a client who has an unfamiliar diagnosis, to target function in occupational engagement, intervention planning and implementation must rely on selecting and synthesizing the best available evidence with an occupation-based approach and type of intervention, as defined by the *AOTA Occupational Therapy Practice Framework: Domain and Process, 4th Edition (OTPF-4)* (6). These are times when occupational therapy professionals must rely heavily on our understanding of general physical health, occupational therapy frames of reference and models of practice (discussed in depth in the first part of the textbook), and on our therapeutic reasoning as a bridge between focused clinical inquiry (occupational therapy evaluation) and the development of an intervention plan.

THERAPEUTIC REASONING

Faced with the task of developing an evaluation and intervention plan that the client will find meaningful and empowering, the occupational therapy professional needs a logical approach to gathering information and using it to generate intervention goals and types. Although many approaches to

organizing data and planning intervention have been presented over the years in the occupational therapy literature, until the 1990s, little had been written about how experienced and skillful clinicians approach the process. How does the occupational therapist know which practice model to select, which evaluations to administer, which problems to target, and which approaches to use? And how can the occupational therapy professionals ensure client-centeredness and collaboration?

Asking the Right Questions

Therapeutic reasoning is a complex cognitive and affective process—in other words, a process of analysis using thinking and feeling. The occupational therapist must consider and select theories and methods that best apply to each client's unique situation. At the same time, the occupational therapist must learn and appreciate the client's story, particularly their priorities and values. The occupational therapist must come to understand how the person's life looks from the inside. In her Eleanor Clarke Slagle lecture in 1983, Rogers (44) identified three crucial questions on which the occupational therapist should focus (Box 13.1). These questions form the core concerns of the clinical reasoning process and are still current today.

The first question, "What is the person's status?" is evaluative. Before the occupational therapist begins to think about intervention goals and outcomes, approaches, or types of intervention, they must develop an understanding of who the client is, what the client's problems and strengths are, and how strongly motivated for treatment the person is. The

---

BOX 13.1 The Focus of Clinical Inquiry

First question: What is the client's status?

- What is the client's occupational role status?
- What problems do they have?
- What strengths do they possess?
- What are they motivated to try?

Second question: What are the available options?

- What approaches are available?
- What outcomes are predicted for each of these? What results can we expect?
- How much time is needed to reach the objectives using each of these approaches?

Third question: What ought to be done?

- Which options are consistent with this client's values?
- Has the client been informed of the consequences of different treatment options and been allowed to choose among them?

Adapted from Rogers, J. C. (1983). Clinical reasoning: the ethics, science, and art. In R. Padilla & Y. Griffiths (Eds.), *The Eleanor Clarke Slagle Lectures in occupational therapy 1955–2016: A professional legacy, centennial edition* (pp. 265–280). AOTA Press.

occupational therapist considers the person's engagement in occupation, performance skills and performance patterns, the situational contexts that are dynamically connected to the occupation, and any pertinent client factors that may be obstacles or supports. The occupational therapist manages and coordinates gathering data and asks evaluative questions to create an occupational profile and obtain information to answer questions about the client's occupational performance. The occupational therapist selects from among the many assessments available, the ones most likely to yield useful results (25).

To arrive at an answer to the second question, "What are the available options?" the occupational therapist must search their memory for knowledge and experience that relate in any way to the client's problem. This includes thoughts about occupational therapy theory and techniques acquired through basic or continuing education, in clinical practice, or through appraising the evidence. It may also include talking with or observing other professionals. The occupational therapist thinks about previous clients who were similar to this one, considers the outcome of the interventions they have incorporated into therapy in the past, and tries to imagine how those interventions might work with this person. The occupational therapist also takes into account the person's environmental and social contexts. What supports are available? How might they help or hinder the person's ability to function? Ultimately, the occupational therapist generates an internal list of interventions that might address this client's goals and needs.

The third question, "What ought to be done?" focuses on the ethical aspects of the occupational therapy process (3). As Rogers (44) states: "Simply because a goal appears technically feasible for the patient does not mean that it should be set as a goal." The client has a right to choose. The notion that through human occupation each person becomes what they do, and by doing, shapes their own identity has always been at the core of occupational therapy (27). The client should select their own goals, although these may differ from those the occupational therapist might have chosen. Professional ethics oblige the occupational therapist to try to persuade the client to accept an intervention that the occupational therapist knows or suspects will improve the person's condition, or without which the client's condition is more likely to deteriorate. This does not mean that the client will accept the plan or can be made to do so. Whatever we may feel about society's obligation to persons with mental illness, legal and constitutional protections guarantee them the right to refuse interventions when they are not an immediate danger to themselves or others.

"THERE ISN'T A COOKBOOK . . . ." STEPS IN INTERVENTION PLANNING

Although you may hear seasoned occupational therapy professionals say that there are no cookbooks that contain particular plans for interventions, and especially not interventions that "work every time," for a client simply because they are a

member of a particular diagnostic group, that does not necessarily mean that there are not a variety of evidence-based, tried and true, "recipes" that the occupational therapy professional can consider. However, we have probably all had the experience of having the same recipe, used to make the same dish, but made by two different people, but having one dish, for reasons we cannot always describe, taste subjectively "better." Among other things, such as situational contexts and varying client factors, there are other integral considerations that affect the way a recipe (intervention) turns out, just as there are other integral factors that lead to the outcomes of occupational therapy interventions. Among those considerations are the use of therapeutic reasoning and the experience of the occupational therapy professional, the quality and thorough nature of the evaluation process from which the intervention plan follows, and the quality of the therapeutic relationship and collaboration with the client. Let us break down this clinical reasoning process into discrete steps. Using these steps is one way to help formulate intervention plans that are occupationally focused. Box 13.2 highlights the steps in intervention planning.

Intervention Planning Follows From Evaluation Results

The first step, reviewing the results of the occupational therapy evaluation, should be executed with an open mind but with a clear idea of what kinds of information one is seeking. Intervention planning is based on the results of the evaluation: the occupational profile and analysis of occupational performance. Planning entails identifying the client's strengths and barriers, and personal goals, choosing outcomes, and partnering with the client to establish realistic and reasonable goals. Furthermore, it is essential that the occupational therapy professional has a working knowledge of the various intervention approaches and types that are most likely to help the client achieve their goals. The outcomes and priorities tentatively identified by the client and the occupational therapist are fundamental. The occupational therapist tries to evaluate the person's potential to benefit from intervention based on history (the past), the current condition (the present), and the prognosis. The person's **prognosis** is the degree to which we can predict recovery from disability or dysfunction, and the degree to which we can support the

---

BOX 13.2 Steps in Planning Intervention

1. Review the results of the evaluation and discuss them with the client.
2. Identify problems and, if possible, their causes.
3. Identify the person's strengths and assess/estimate the person's readiness and motivation for intervention.
4. Collaborate with the client to set goals (long and short term, in order of priority).
5. Identify intervention principles using the practice model.
6. Select methods appropriate to the practice model.

client as they return to optimal occupational participation. It is often difficult to judge whether a particular person with a given diagnosis or history is likely to achieve a specific intervention goal. Similarly, it is difficult to estimate time frames for goal achievement, particularly in short-term settings. Occupational therapy professionals in a short-term setting will be more concerned with evaluation and with helping the person make a transition to the next level of care than with long-term planning.

The purpose of reviewing the evaluation is to obtain the answers to the second and third steps and to learn as much as you can about the client's problems (barriers), strengths (and supports and resources), and readiness or motivation for change. This requires combining information from many sources to learn the suspected causes of the client's problems, as well as learning about the problems themselves. An understanding of the causes is often the key to selecting the most effective approach to intervention.

For example, a client may have very poor hygiene—as evidenced by disheveled hair, poor oral hygiene, or noticeable and offending body odor. Nevertheless, poor hygiene may be present for a variety of reasons (or have a variety of causes). Perhaps the client never had an opportunity to develop good hygiene skills, or they may have gotten out of the habit of performing those habits and routines. Maybe their usual environment makes it difficult to perform hygiene and grooming tasks (eg, because of homelessness). There may be cultural reasons as well, daily bathing and frequent shampooing are, in some instances, considered Western values; personal hygiene standards elsewhere vary. There may be reasons for poor hygiene that derive from the disease process: the person may not remember to bathe and care for their body, the sense of time may be distorted, or the person may be so frightened of other people that they subconsciously ignore hygiene, as a self-protective defense mechanism, to drive others away. Sensory processing difficulties may be present as well. You can see that these various root causes for the person's poor hygiene will lead to very different ideas about what kind of intervention is needed and where it should begin. Thinking through the causes in this way helps the occupational therapy professional determine whether a given practice model is appropriate to the client's situation and further helps the practitioner to determine the appropriate intervention approach and type.

Obviously, evaluation results that relate directly to the occupational area in question would be critically important but other information may be equally valuable. For example, the client's relationship with other family members in the household may give some clues about why they show deficits in independent living skills. It is important not to confine your investigation to what you expect to find and to maintain a curious and alert perspective. Try not to be too strongly influenced by the person's diagnosis or by the opinions of other staff. Openness to the person as an individual is the surest route to the development of trust and to learning the client's strengths and potential.

Approaches to Intervention

The AOTA *OTPF-4* (6) describes approaches to intervention as "specific strategies selected to direct the evaluation and intervention processes on the basis of the client's desired outcomes, evaluation data, and research evidence. Approaches inform the selection of practice models, frames of references, and treatment theories" (6, p. 63). Occupational therapy intervention approaches are categorized into five main paths that an OT professional might travel upon to meet a client throughout the occupational therapy process, but especially during goal setting and intervention plan development. When studying the approaches to intervention, it may be helpful to notice that the five paths are titled using the action verbs: **create, promote, establish, restore, maintain, modify** (compensate, adapt), and **prevent**. This serves as a reminder that the approach may be thought of as what the occupational therapy professional and the client collaboratively are going to take action and do. The approach signifies the "doing" aspects of occupational therapy intervention. The five main approaches are **health promotion**, **remediation** or **restoration**, **maintenance of function**, **modification** (further classified as **adaptive strategies** or compensatory, **compensation strategies**), and **prevention** (6). The focus of intervention and the intervention type differ depending on the approach. A brief description of the approaches follows.

Health promotion (create, promote) applies to all populations, including those with no present disability. Its aim is to enrich or enhance occupational engagement for all people within their natural context. Examples might include such things as falls prevention education for older adults who are aging in place or creating resources to support homework management for high school students (6).

Remediation or **restoration (establish, restore)** aims to "change client variables to establish a skill or ability that has not yet developed or to restore a skill or ability that has been impaired" (as cited in 8, p. 63; adapted from [18], p. 533).

Maintenance of function (maintain) is aimed at assisting the person to use their remaining capabilities by providing supports (6). In this approach, the occupational therapy professional works at creating an environment that supports and encourages individuals to care for their own needs and to take charge of their own lives in whatever way they can, for as long as possible. Despite the best efforts of the client and occupational therapist, the long-term outlook for some conditions is that the person will function qualitatively less and less well as time goes by. "The assumption is that without continued maintenance intervention, performance would decrease and occupational needs would not be met, thereby affecting health, well-being, and quality of life" (6, p. 63).

Modification (modify) (6, p. 64) is an "Approach directed at 'finding ways to revise the current context or activity demands to support performance in the natural setting, [including] compensatory techniques ... [such as] enhancing some features to reduce distractibility'" (excerpt from [18], p. 533).

Prevention (prevent) aims to intervene before dysfunction occurs and can target the clients with or without an existing disability. It is usually applied with populations at risk, for whom a future problem is predicted. "This approach is designed to prevent the occurrence or evolution of barriers to performance in context. Interventions may be directed at client, context, or activity variables" (as cited in 8, p. 64; adapted from [18], p. 534).

Partnership With the Client or Consumer

A relationship with the consumer or client should be established before the occupational therapy professional begins to plan intervention. Assessments such as the *Canadian Occupational Performance Measure, 5th Edition (COPM)* (32), discussed in Chapter 12, provide a clear picture of the goals valued by the client and suggest areas for intervention. If the evaluation phase has gone well, the occupational therapy team and the client should be able to use information to collaboratively make a tentative plan to address specific goals that are priorities for the client. The occupational therapist, once the initial plans are deemed satisfactory, formally documents the intervention plan. The occupational therapist continues to adjust the plan as the relationships of the OTA and OT with the client develop, and as the client's goals become better known. Thus, professional reasoning is continually focused and refined through collaboration and therapeutic relationship with the client.

The client can often tell you what is wrong and help define the problem. Involving the client in planning intervention to the extent the person is capable ensures that the client understands and agrees with the plan, a first step in encouraging motivation to make progress on client goals. Even clients who have limited ability to verbalize their concerns can be guided to participate. In such cases, the occupational therapy professional may have to present limited choices from which the client can select. For example, the client might choose which goal or area to tackle first.

The person's strengths must be considered even though the focus of our energies appears to be on finding solutions to the client's problems. The skills and habits the client has developed and maintained, and the client's resolve to work hard and succeed, can only be strengthened by our recognition and support. Furthermore, we should consider the supports and resources present in the environment, such as helpful family members and the social support of friends.

Questions sometimes arise about a client's motivation for change. The person who fails to work toward goals that the occupational therapy professional considers appropriate and necessary may be labeled by other staff members as "unmotivated." This may indicate that the goals do not reflect the person's real concerns. An example is the 27-year-old legal secretary with a diagnosis of bipolar disorder who tells a colleague that they would rather collect public assistance and watch television than go back to work. Rather than forcing this client's acceptance of a work adjustment training program, the occupational therapy professional might have more

success in meeting the client where they are and explore the thoughts and experiences that led to this expression or decision. The intervention cannot succeed unless the client is actively involved in making the plan (if they are capable).

The occupational therapy professional should make a concerted effort to communicate with all people who are involved in the client's care. If other staff members have identified problems that they believe the client should address, the occupational therapy professional can assist with explaining to the client why the suggestion may or may not be considered by the client as a priority for them to work on during occupational therapy. The question to consider with the client is how much the staff-identified problem, or problems, interfere with the client's ability to perform their chosen occupations.

In inpatient settings with acutely ill individuals, it is not always possible to obtain the client's cooperation and participation in planning intervention. Engaging the attention of someone who is experiencing psychotic symptoms or a client who has an inadequate orientation to reality can be very difficult, particularly for a new occupational therapy professional. Therefore, in acute care settings, the behavioral health team (including the occupational therapy professional) may develop an intervention plan on behalf of the client, sometimes in consultation with members of the client's family.

THEORY, PRACTICE MODELS, AND THE OCCUPATIONAL THERAPY PROCESS

Theory can clarify the client's situation. For example, the person with very poor hygiene and grooming, at first glance, seems to need some sort of intervention or support with ADLs, but the skilled occupational therapy professional, for the purposes of developing an intervention plan, will want to know *why* this person's ADLs are so poor. Is it the result of a condition such as dementia or part of a lifelong mental illness? Has there been a sudden and abrupt decompensation after a lifetime of normal functioning? Is substance use involved? Is the person unconsciously using this behavior to avoid a situation that feels psychologically overwhelming? Each of these possibilities suggests a different theoretical model, and each model in turn suggests a line of inquiry and a focus of evaluation and intervention. The occupational therapy professional must have a working knowledge of theories and occupation-centered models of practice that might be appropriate to the setting and the population. Then, through collaboration with the client and by gathering data from multiple sources during the evaluation, the occupational therapy professional can more effectively, and over time, more rapidly, formulate hypotheses to sort and discard potential courses of action before determining where to begin. As the occupational therapy process continues, and the therapeutic relationship grows, the client becomes more deeply known and understood and the occupational therapist may change course, using a model that better fits this new understanding of the person (52, 53).

Using Theory and Practice Models to Guide Intervention Planning

While planning occupational therapy interventions, a practice model organizes practitioner thinking. The practice model will propose ways for the occupational therapy professional to imagine the client's occupational performance on a continuum of what functional occupational engagement might look like, versus what dysfunctional occupational engagement looks like, according to the particular model. Practice models also inform the practitioner of potential sources of problems and suggest certain strategies or approaches for addressing the problem. Best practice in occupational therapy evaluation and intervention can only be achieved by synthesizing theory, evidence-based planning, therapeutic reasoning, and collaboration with the client (12, 22). A brief review follows demonstrating how the constructs or perspectives of several theoretical practice models can be used to create a bridge to drive occupational interventions forward. The questions that the occupational therapy team asks during assessment and intervention planning are determined by the elements and subsystems within the model or theme.

MOTIVATIONAL THEORIES: MODEL OF HUMAN OCCUPATION

Let us look at how an occupational therapy professional might derive the starting place or direction following the evaluation phase if they were employing a theoretical perspective from the *Model of Human Occupation* (MOHO). The MOHO is a broad theory developed in the early 1980s by Dr Gary Kielhofner and colleagues, Burke, and Igi (16, 19). On the basis of the combination of a general systems theory and the human need for achievement and competence, and meant to expand upon Mary Reilly's theory of occupational behavior, today the MOHO is one of the most researched and practiced models of occupational therapy in the world (19, 33, 39). The MOHO proposes that "when individuals maintain patterns of occupational participation within environments that reflect a sense of who they are as occupational beings, the end result is a sense of occupational adaptation which involves the 'construction of a positive occupational identity and achieving occupational competence over time' (30, p. 121)" (as cited in 29, p. 280).

To apply the MOHO to evaluation and intervention, the occupational therapy professional attempts to find out which internal and external subsystems, in concert with the client's interactions within the context and environment, are contributing to or creating barriers to a person's construction of a positive occupational identity. The goal is to help them achieve competence in their preferred occupational tasks (21, 29, 51). There are four principles or themes within the MOHO that a practitioner will need awareness of when choosing this theoretical model to guide intervention planning, the MOHO subsystems of volition, habituation, performance capacity, and environment. During the evaluation

part of the occupational therapy process, while the practitioner is collaborating with the client to create an occupational profile, and then administering assessments, if they are considering the MOHO as a theoretical model to guide them, they should be collecting client data related to these four themes.

One way to do this is to consider guiding questions related to each of the four themes. These guiding questions can be thought of as street signs, which help the occupational therapy professional to map a course. The following questions have been proposed as being helpful in developing reasoning using the MOHO theoretical model (30):

- Does the client anticipate successful outcomes of action?
- Does the client have valued goals?
- Does the client have interests?
- Does the client have primary occupational roles?
- Does the client have organized habit patterns?
- Does the client have performance skills to carry out valued occupations?
- Does the client use performance skills competently and consistently?
- Does physical environment support use of skills?
- Does social environment require roles the client enjoys and performs well?
- Does social environment support successful occupational behavior?

The purpose of the guiding questions is 2-fold because not only will they guide occupational reasoning and help the practitioner and client find a direction but the guiding questions will also help organize the information collected so that it can be more easily analyzed and reflected upon. Analysis of the data collected will help narrow the focus toward the subsystem that interventions can target to best serve the client and the occupational therapy professional in setting realistic and thoughtful goals toward occupational adaptation and occupational competence (21, 30, 51). Readers may refer to Figure 13.1 for a visual reminder of how to apply the MOHO concepts as a "roadmap" to developing occupational reasoning during intervention planning.

MOTIVATIONAL THEORIES AND MOTIVATIONAL INTERVIEWING

Motivational theories emphasize that change comes from within an individual and that individuals are most successful at changing when they are intrinsically motivated to make the change. Theories of motivation suggest that the process of changing is not linear, but rather occurs in a spiral manner. Relapses while a person is learning new behaviors are not uncommon; this can be a place where occupational therapy takes on the role of supporting the client in developing enough resiliency for them to reestablish movement toward their goals. Another core premise of motivational theories is that the more a client is prepared to change (readiness) and wants to change (desire, volition, motivation), the more likely that the intended changes will have positive outcomes (24).

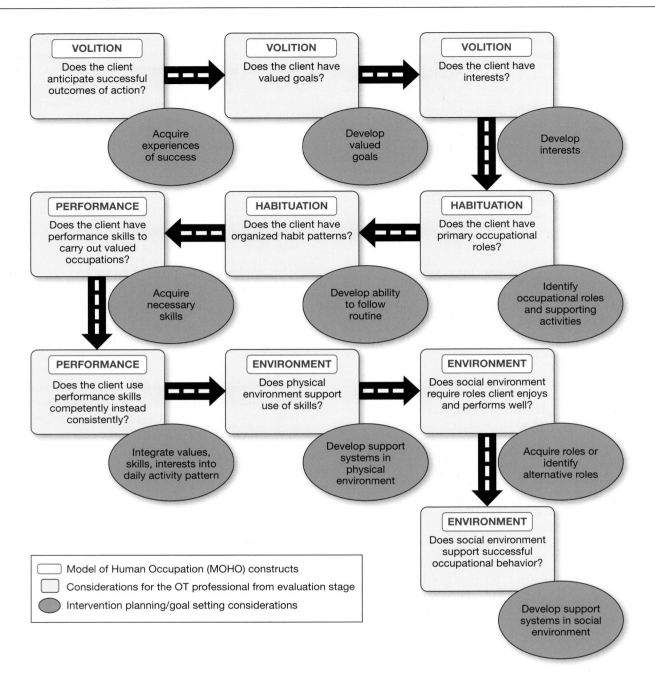

Figure 13.1. Roadmap: Occupational Reasoning Using the *Model of Human Occupation* (MOHO) as a Guide. (Adapted from Kielhofner, G. (2002). *A Model of Human Occupation: Theory and application* (3rd ed.). Lippincott Williams & Wilkins; Taylor, R. R. (Ed.). (2017). *Kielhofner's Model of Human Occupation: Theory and application*. Wolters Kluwer; Forsyth, K., Taylor, R. R., Kramer, J. M., Prior, S., Ritchie, L., & Melton, J. (2019). The Model of Human Occupation. In B. A. B. Schell & G. Gillen (Eds.), *Willard and Spackman's occupational therapy* (13th ed., pp. 601–621). Lippincott Williams & Wilkins.)

Occupational therapy professionals who work in psychosocial settings should be particularly aware that implementation of intervention will be most successful if the intervention closely matches the stage of behavioral change readiness that the client is currently in. Furthermore, sincere efforts should be made to assess how motivated the person is to make positive changes and to encourage discussion about

the positive occupational implications for successfully making behavioral changes.

Motivational theories are sometimes referred to as change theories and are often used by occupational therapy professionals as a theoretical frame of reference when working with clients with mental illness. Motivational theories and change theories are well matched to the recovery approaches; as the interventions progress and the client gains more independence, ideally the intervention processes become more self-directed, the client is increasingly self-motivated, and that leads to higher levels of function. The client's improved ability to self-monitor positively impacts the way that behaviors are regulated, which impacts their participation in occupation (24).

One method of encouraging a client to consider and possibly implement a change is by employing **motivational interviewing (MI)** with the client. MI is particularly helpful during the occupational therapy intervention planning process leading up to selecting an occupational therapy intervention approach and type. Miller and Rollnick, the creators and authors of MI, refer to MI as a specific clinical method that boosts the client's own motivation for change. They further describe it as "a collaborative conversation style for strengthening a person's own motivation and commitment for change" (38, p. 12). Nevertheless, in the more than 25 years since this intervention approach was introduced, the authors have suggested that with its quick dissemination and the popularity and success of the method, professionals who implemented the method over time have not necessarily kept the spirit of the original intent of MI in place. They were concerned that the method may have lost "some critical elements of the innovation, 'active ingredients' in its efficacy" (37, p. 129). In an effort to rearticulate and remind others about what the core components of MI are, "and what components can be altered without disrupting the defining nature of a method" (37, p. 130), Miller and Rollnick penned an article titled *Ten Things That Motivational Interviewing Is Not* (37). A link to this article is included in the "*Knowledge*" section at the end of this chapter, in the *OT HACKS Summary*. The article is included with the hope that it offers a glimpse of the process that sometimes happens as a new methodology is introduced into the health care landscape. In the case of MI, the methodology was developed first (it arose from the intuitive daily practices of one of the creators, Dr Miller), and only later after evidence began mounting that the methodology seemed to be efficacious, did Drs Miller and Rollnick further investigate the method's relationship to various theoretical perspectives.

Nevertheless, MI is considered an evidence-based method and has amassed volumes of research, touting the efficacy of its use in encouraging clients to find their own reasons to motivate changes in their behavior (38). But MI is a complex process and developing MI skills requires a commitment to practicing the method and refining one's skills over time. It is considered an advanced practice skill set for that reason. However, all practitioners can benefit from incorporating aspects of MI into their occupational therapy intervention planning, particularly with clients who are resistant to change or ambivalent about therapy. The four key interpersonal processes involved in MI are as follows:

1. **Engaging:** The occupational therapy professional must establish a trusting and mutual therapeutic rapport and relationship with the client. This encourages therapeutic connection.

2. **Focusing:** The occupational therapy professional consistently guides the conversation toward developing and maintaining a focal point in the conversation around the sometimes-difficult topic of change.

3. **Evoking:** The occupational therapy professional must draw into the conversation the client's own motivation for change.

4. **Planning:** The occupational therapy professional (over time) develops the ability to listen for the client's use of change language. Change language is characterized by the client beginning to identify solutions and strategies that indicate their desire to change. When the occupational therapy professional hears these indications, they collaborate with the client to develop a plan targeting the change that the client desires. Remember that for an occupational therapy professional, the targeted change and outcome should be made explicit as positively impacting *occupation*.

Beyond facilitating the processes of MI (ie, engaging, focusing, evoking, and planning), the other significant factor in using MI with clients is the emphasis on the nature of the therapeutic relationship (52). Best practice in applying MI requires that the spirit of the method be present, meaning that the approach includes (i) a true partnership between the client and the occupational therapy professional; (ii) acceptance of the client, regardless of their readiness or willingness to change, or their present level of motivation; (iii) demonstration of compassion; and (iv) evocation (24, 38).

Motivational Change Theories: The Transtheoretical Model of Change

The Transtheoretical Model of Change, or TTM, is also known as the *Stages of Change Model* (SCM). The TTM was developed in the early 1980s by researchers Prochaska and DiClemente as they explored possible reasons why some clients were more successful at quitting smoking than others (43). Although not directly related, the SCM was developed at approximately the same time that MI methods were articulated by their creators. For this reason, the two methods are often considered together (37). The SCM proposes that there are five stages that a client may go through as they work to change a health-related behavior. The five stages and a brief explanation of each can be found in Table 13.1.

The relevance and indelible mark that the introduction of the TTM/SCM has made not just on the treatment of addiction but on treatments of mental and physical health problems, and on prevention and health promotion sciences, cannot be overstated. The TTM/SCM transformed the treatment of addiction and substance use disorders. Perhaps most importantly, the introduction of the SCM changed the way that behavioral and mental health care providers approach supporting their clients in facilitating changes to health behaviors. Before the development of this model, the assumption was that most people with problematic behaviors were at minimum in the preparation stage. Health professionals

Table 13.1. The Stages of Change Model

Stage of Change	The OT Professional May Hear Statements From the Client Like . . .
Precontemplation People in the precontemplation stage are unmotivated to find solutions to problems typically because they are not aware that a problem exists or they lack insight regarding the potential risks and consequences of their negative behaviors. **Recognize This:** It is important to recognize that a person in this stage is in complete denial and even tends to defend their actions . . .	"I don't see a problem with what I'm doing, so there's no reason to change anything." **Typical Timing:** People in this stage have no intention of making a change in the next 6 mo.
Contemplation This stage is marked by some degree of acknowledgment of the problematic choices or behaviors. There can also be thoughtful consideration of making the change but the person struggles internally about how worthwhile (necessary) the change would be to make. The person becomes stuck in the internal struggle and makes no commitment to taking steps to change.	"I know I have a problem, and I think I should do something about it." **Typical Timing:** Most people in this stage remain stuck in their ambivalence and contemplation for at least 6 mo.
Preparation At this stage of the change process, the pros for changing the problematic behavior outweigh the cons, and the individual acknowledges problem behaviors and commits to correcting the problem. Clients at this stage begin gathering resources, exploring information, and planning to make a change. **Recognize This:** Gathering information and planning is a critical part of the preparation stage. If this is lacking, it is often the case that the person has fully considered the impact that the change will have on their occupational engagement. They may struggle with the challenges and relapse occurs.	"Smoking is such a bad habit. I've been reading about different ways to quit, and even though I haven't totally quit yet, I am smoking less than I did before." **Typical Timing:** If appropriate planning occurs, people tend to initialize action within the next 30 d; many begin to make behavioral changes in that direction over the previous year.
Action CHANGE HAPPENS during the Action stage! In the action stage, people gain confidence and they start to develop hope in the belief that they have the willpower sustain the change. **Recognize This:** People sometimes mistakenly believe that change occurs (or even happens because of) the actions they have taken and they dismiss the critical importance of the planning and preparing stages. As noted, taking action without adequate preparation is a recipe for relapse!	"It's easy to say you'll quit smoking, but I'm doing something about it. I haven't smoked a cigarette in four months." **Typical Timing:** During the action stage, total abstinence of the adverse behavior is the expectation for a period of up to 6 mo.
Maintenance In the maintenance stage, the focus is on the person successfully continuing the new changed behavior.	**Typical Timing:** During the maintenance stage, people have maintained total abstinence of the adverse behavior for more than 6 mo.

Adapted from Raihan, N., & Cogburn, M. (2022, January). Stages of change theory. In *StatPearls* [Internet]. StatPearls Publishing. Retrieved March 9, 2022, from https://www.ncbi.nlm.nih.gov/books/NBK556005/

wrongly assumed that most people arrived at the health care facility in the action stage . . . meaning that people who sought help came prepared to take actions to change their negative health behaviors.

The SCM brought recognition to these erroneous assumptions and instead highlighted the fact that the typical person who struggled with addiction was unlikely to have decided to change and was furthermore very unlikely to be acutely ready to make any level of commitment to change their problematic behaviors. With this new awareness, health care providers began to realize that if an intervention is to be effective, the interventions would need to be adjusted to meet the client where they were, meaning meet them at their current level of readiness for change. "Rather than blaming people for being unmotivated, it became part of the clinician's task to enhance motivation for change" (37, p. 130). It is this idea of meeting a client where they are, at their current level of occupational function and current level of readiness

to change, to support the client in making positive changes in their occupations, that drives much of the occupational therapy process, especially intervention planning and implementation (5, 43).

SOCIAL LEARNING, SOCIAL COGNITIVE THEORIES AND BEHAVIORISM: THE COGNITIVE BEHAVIORAL CONTINUUM

Practitioners using other practice models follow similar processes to generate a series of questions to guide their reasoning based on the design of the chosen model. Tracing the roots of the cognitive behavioral continuum, cognitive theories and frames of reference in occupational therapy mostly came from theories of learning, which in turn came from behaviorism (16). In its earliest iterations, behaviorists applied the scientific method to human behavior and strictly adhered to the notion that human behavior was only what could be observed and measured using the scientific method. Although the principles of behaviorism changed the field of psychology, and many ideas from behaviorism remain useful to occupational therapy interventions today, these theories left no room to consider the client's internal processes, nor was there consideration of the unconscious processes that psychodynamic and psychoanalytic approaches championed (16). The modern cognitive behavioral continuum gives way to frames of reference that combine various principles of learning (cognition) with consideration of human internal and external physiologic and psychological processes, social learning theory, and behavioral concepts (16, 43). In the *Cognitive Behavioral Model*, to take a different example, some of the questions that guide reasoning to direct intervention planning might be like these:

- What are this person's beliefs and assumptions about life?
- What does this person say are the causes of any life problems?
- What errors in thinking are behind the clients beliefs?

The data and information collected in answering these questions would guide the development of an intervention plan to challenge and refute the client's erroneous thinking.

The Cognitive Behavioral Continuum: Cognitive Behavioral Therapy

The reader is likely to recognize cognitive behavioral therapy (CBT) as a well-used intervention in psychosocial settings. The cognitive behavioral continuum of models of practice are widely incorporated in multidisciplinary team-based plans of care for people with a variety of mental health conditions. As part of a team, the occupational therapy professional may reinforce learning from individual and group sessions and can apply the CBT techniques using occupation as the means to helping clients reach their occupational goals. The client's work with an individual psychotherapist or mental health counselor and other members of the team is expanded and enhanced by applications in occupational therapy.

The overarching goal of applying CBT techniques into occupational therapy intervention is to help individuals learn effective coping skills and build their confidence and sense of personal agency to support their recovery process, reduce relapses, and improve their overall occupational engagement and quality of life. As mentioned, CBT was derived from the cognitive model of psychopathology. This model suggests that a person's emotions, their physical responses, and their behaviors are all influenced by their perception of events (10, 19). This model further indicates that situations do not necessarily determine how a person will behave, nor the feelings they will experience. Instead, the person's *perception* of the situation determines how they react and the manner of their response (10, 19). So, according to this model, a context or situation alone is not the source of distress, it is the way that the person interprets the situation that determines the distress (49).

According to the cognitive model of psychopathology, from which CBT techniques are established, in daily experiences people face a variety of situation-specific contexts and events, and in response to those situations they have automatic thoughts about the situation (the "situation" can also be internal or external triggers that bring about automatic thoughts). The automatic thoughts that a person has influence how they feel, how their body responds, and how they behave (49). An additional consideration in this model that is critical to understanding it and applying its principles is that people's perceptions of situations, and so also their automatic thoughts, are shaped by their internal beliefs about themselves, about others, and about the world around them (11). When a person's internal or underlying belief system is heavy with self-doubt, they may form **doubt labels** that bias the way the individual views and perceives situations. "Doubt labels (also known as core beliefs) reflect the negative names we call ourselves when our self-doubt is activated" (49, p. 10).

Applying CBT principles to occupational therapy interventions gives occupational therapy professionals an evidence-based method to help clients understand the connection between their perceptions and their (sometimes) problematic responses and behaviors. Many times, it is these problematic responses and behaviors that are primary barriers to optimal occupational engagement. Initiated by Dr Aaron Beck's work in the 1960s when he created a model to support the general understanding about the role that underlying cognitive beliefs play in depression, today the impact that cognitive beliefs have on a wide variety of diagnostic groups has been widely researched. In addition, research related to the efficacy of using CBT programs and techniques designed for specific diagnostic populations has also grown. Readers can take a closer look at these evidence-based targeted CBT interventions in Section III, with the use of CBT for Anxiety in Chapter 18; for Depression, Self-Harm, and Suicidality in Chapter 19; for Symptoms of Psychosis in Chapter 20; for Anger in Chapter 22; and for Addiction or Substance Use Disorders in Chapter 23.

Dialectical Behavior Therapy

Dialectical behavior therapy (DBT) was originally developed by Dr Marsha Linehan (36, 42) to address the impulse control and emotional dysregulation problems of people with borderline personality disorder (BPD) but has since been extensively expanded, researched, and applied with other populations (41). Linehan's initial *Skills Training Manual* (34) contained structured exercises and homework to support the client's development of four key skills: mindfulness, interpersonal effectiveness, emotion regulation, and distress tolerance. Modern DBT protocols expand the modules. In one example, Dr Lane Pederson, a leading expert on DBT and founder of the Dialectical Behavior Therapy National Certification and Accreditation Association, in her text, incorporates the four original key skills into an expanded set of six modules: *dialectics, cognitive modification, problem-solving, addictions, building a satisfying life,* and *social media* (42). Occupational therapy is an appropriate venue for teaching this set of skills because of its practical orientation to typical daily occupations.

Linehan (34, 35) cites mindfulness skills as a core element of the original DBT protocol. As with the other disorders, where a primary symptom is impulse control, BPD is characterized by acting on uncomfortable feelings without exploring or understanding what the feelings are (the opposite of mindfulness). People with BPD often present with self-injurious behaviors such as cutting; they also are at a greater risk of experiencing suicidal thoughts and attempts (9). Linehan discovered that when a person with BPD develops habits associated with mindfulness or mindfulness practices, they are more equipped to identify their feelings and then to be able to "sit with the feelings," which reduces their likelihood of engaging in self-destructive behavior (34, 35). That same principle has carried over to the DBT protocols used in interventions with other diagnostic populations (41). By understanding the primary mechanisms involved in the DBT methodology, occupational therapy professionals can incorporate aspects of this evidence-based practice into occupational therapy interventions, especially when implementing an education or a training type of occupational therapy intervention, as defined by the *OTPF-4* (6).

INTERACTION, ADEQUACY OF FIT, AND RESPONSE THEORIES: PERSON–ENVIRONMENT–OCCUPATIONAL PERFORMANCE MODEL AND THE OCCUPATIONAL ADAPTATION MODEL

The Person–Environment–Occupational Performance (PEOP) model (15), similar to MOHO, is a systems model concerned with the interactions and fit between the client, the environment, and the client's occupational performance. An occupational therapy professional who applies this model during intervention will be asking questions related to helping the client enhance their skill set or reach their goals, typically through modifying the context, environment, or occupation (13). The Occupational Adaptation (OA) model (23, 46, 47) applied during intervention will pay attention to the client's adaptive responses and the occupational demands and role expectations that lead to the client's effective (or ineffective) adaptive responses. Thus, using a specific theoretical approach, practice model, or frame of reference is helpful in generating assessment questions and obtaining data on which to base the intervention plan.

GENERAL GOALS OF PSYCHIATRIC OCCUPATIONAL THERAPY

Let us start with the understanding that the overall aim of occupational therapy, regardless of the area of specialization, or setting, is to help individuals engage in occupation, to function as independently as possible, with a level of quality of occupational engagement that is satisfying to the individual, or client group, within the limits of their current level of function, and in the contexts of their choice. Thus, whether the occupational therapy professional is helping the person who has arthritis apply energy conservation and joint protection techniques while the client is cooking a meal, or they are providing tactile stimulation to encourage movement, the final purpose is the same, to make it possible for that person to function optimally within their chosen occupations, activities and occupational roles. Thus, all goals should address functional occupation–centered outcomes.

Once the staff and the client or family have agreed upon a general direction for intervention, the next step is to set specific goals. A goal is a statement about what the client will achieve. Goals can be classified as long term or short term. A **long-term goal** states the functional outcome or destination of the intervention; that is the ultimate aim. Examples are, "to get a job," or "to live alone in my own apartment."

Short-term goals can be understood as small steps to achieve a long-term goal. A short-term goal considers the length of time available for treatment as well as the client's sense of time and ability to visualize the future; short-term goals are those that can be accomplished in a few weeks or less. Breaking down long-term goals into a series of short-term goals can make it easier for the client to tackle them. It has become common, particularly in settings that use the psychiatric rehabilitation model, to use the term **objective** when referring to short-term goals. Thus, we advise the reader that the terms **short-term goal** and **short-term objective** for all practical purposes may be synonymous.

Goals should be organized in order of priority. **Priority** means the importance or urgency of the goal to the client. In many cases, especially with persons who have severe and persistent mental illness, it is possible to come up with a list of 5 or 6 long-term goals and 20 or more short-term goals (or objectives). Not all of them will be equally important, however, and the client, together with the occupational therapist, must decide which ones are to be tackled first. Some goals by their nature must be achieved before others; for example, someone who needs to learn basic cooking to live independently must first learn elementary kitchen safety. Usually, only a few (not more than three or four) goals are attempted at one time; sometimes, only one goal is selected at first. The number of goals should be based on the client's ability to divide their energies effectively among the different goals, and on an initial prediction of the amount of effort that will be necessary to reach a particular goal. In choosing short-term objectives, it is important (especially at first) to select specific and objective goals that the client can achieve in a relatively short period of time. Recognizing that a goal has been reached inspires confidence and encourages the person to move forward to gradually more challenging goals.

An overall plan that describes the long-term goals of the client's program should be established. Although it may take months or years to reach some long-term goals, having a clear final aim helps unify the smaller goals. In other words, short-term goals, such as "learning to follow a schedule" or "arriving on time for activity groups," should be part of a larger plan, the ultimate goal of which might be, for example, "to get a job and become more financially independent."

These first steps in intervention planning (identification of problems, discovering strengths, assessing levels of motivation and readiness for change, and setting intervention priorities based on client need and desire) should be done in consultation with other health care professionals who are working with the client. Plans that the client, the family, and the staff agree on have the best chance of success because everyone is clear about the hoped-for outcomes, and generally will work toward supporting them.

HOW TO WRITE AN INTERVENTION GOAL

Goals in an intervention plan should be written so that they describe very clearly what the person will do, and what action the person will perform. Goals should follow logically from problems that have been identified by assessment and selected by the client in collaboration with others, as being important or meaningful to them. The more specific the description of the problem, the easier it is to write the corresponding goal. Consider the following:

- Mr Cardinal demonstrates low self-esteem.
- Ms Danford demonstrates poor reality testing.

These problem statements are confusing because they do not describe the person's behavior nor provide documented assessment of these client factors. Each could be converted into a statement of a specific behavioral problem by the addition of some observable evidence, qualitative evidence gathered while creating an occupational profile, or documented assessment or performance analysis. Therefore, problem statements that contain observable, describable, or measurable behaviors are preferred. Here are some problem statements that meet this criterion:

- Ms Flint exhibits poor hygiene and self-care as evidenced by disheveled clothing and noticeable body odor.
- Mr Mills reports no regular leisure interests except watching television and drinking.
- Per client report, Ms Woolworth has been fired from many jobs because of arguments with supervisors.

Once the problems have been adequately described, the goals that correspond to them can be written. Goals also must be phrased in terms of how the client will behave or what the client will do once the goal is reached. Examples of goals for the three problem statements are as follows:

- Ms Flint will wash her hair twice a week, bathe daily, and brush her teeth twice every day.
- Mr Mills will attend the activity center two evenings a week and will have dinner with a friend once a week.
- For 1 week, Ms Woolworth will not argue with the occupational therapy professionals and group leaders in her daily activity programs.

These goals have been written in behavioral terms so that all concerned (occupational therapy professional, client, and other staff) will know when the goal has been reached. By contrast, it is impossible to agree on when or whether a goal

such as "Mr Cardinal will have increased self-esteem" has been reached; there is no way to measure the client's success.

RUMBA

Some occupational therapists use the mnemonic RUMBA to evaluate the goal statements they write. RUMBA stands for these points:

Relevant
Understandable
Measurable
Behavioral
Achievable

A goal is **relevant** if it reflects the individual's life situation and future goals. As discussed previously, both client and occupational therapist should agree that the goal is important. Other team members such as the social worker, the psychiatrist, and the nurse, as well as the client's caregiver, significant other, family, and friends will also hopefully support these goals. Nevertheless, even if there is another professional who disagrees with some element of a goal, this may be a situation where the occupational therapy professional needs to utilize skills of advocacy to support occupational goals that are priorities for the client. This is particularly true if the OT and/or OTA have collaboratively agreed with the client that the goal is appropriate, realistic, achievable, and occupation centered. Finally, occupational therapy professionals should keep in mind the client's sociocultural characteristics, expectations, and experiences, as well as their developmental stage in life when considering the relevancy of a client's stated goal priorities. An 18- to 24-year-old may describe their most relevant priority as having a significant other to establish a relationship with. The occupational therapy professional might explain that social skills groups at the day treatment center will help the person learn and develop the skills that they need to meet people and develop relationships with them.

A goal is **understandable** when it is stated in plain language and observable terms. Professional jargon is to be avoided and the goal should be phrased so that the client and others outside of occupational therapy can understand it.

A goal is **measurable** when it contains one or more criteria for success. It is best if each criterion is stated in quantifiable terms (numbers), or if it is stated using qualitative terms, a list of specific observable qualities capable of indicating both client current status and establishing when progress is being made should be completed. For example, "bathing once a day" is more easily measured than "having adequate hygiene." Similarly, it is important to include an estimated date of completion, a time by which the goal should be reached. Thus, the measurable criteria should include any of the *measures* shown in Box 13.3 as well as a *time frame*, or time limit, by which the goal is to be achieved or reassessed.

A goal is **behavioral** when it focuses on what the client must *do* to accomplish the goal. It is **achievable** when it is something that the person is likely to be able to accomplish

---

BOX 13.3 Making Goals Measurable and Time Limited

Measure

- Frequency, or *how often* (eg, twice daily)
- Duration, or *how long* (eg, for 30 min)
- Level of accuracy (eg, with 50% accuracy)
- Number of times (eg, 6 times)
- Level of assistance needed (eg, with standby assistance)

Time Frame

- By specific date (eg, by March 31, 2025)
- By end of specific unit of time (eg, by 30 d)
- After a specified number of sessions (eg, after five sessions)
- By a known milestone (eg, by discharge)

---

within a reasonably short period as defined by the client and the occupational therapist together. For instance, assume the client is a very isolated 24-year-old person who has always lived with their parents and who has never held a job. Getting a job and moving into his own apartment *might* be a future goal but would almost certainly result in client frustration as a more immediate one; an **achievable** goal for that person begins with establishing a plan to try limited travel back and forth to the day treatment center on his own and arriving on time.

The following are some examples of occupational therapy goals developed using the RUMBA criteria:

Performance patterns: occupational roles

- The client will identify the primary functions and tasks of her role as mother of a preschooler by the end of 1 week.
- Within 2 weeks, the client will identify at least two ways in which her disability interferes with her functioning effectively in the role of mother of a preschooler and will identify a minimum of two specific strategies to compensate.
- The client will go with her child to a play date at another parent's home, twice within the next 3 weeks.

Play and leisure: exploration

- The member will identify and discuss at least three interests that are important to him by the end of 2 weeks.
- The client will identify at least three ways to pursue his interest in watercolor painting by the end of the next session.

Instrumental activities of daily living (IADLs): health management

- The client will use the smart phone app or the internet to locate the telephone number and address of a pharmacy near her home, by the end of the next session.
- The client will visit the pharmacy near her home and locate the prescription counter within the next week.
- The client will telephone the pharmacy to make sure that the pharmacy has received the doctor's prescription.

- The client will pick up her prescription medication at the pharmacy, within 2 days.

Communication and interaction performance skills (physicality)

- The member will consistently stand *no closer than 3 feet* from another person when engaged in a work-related conversation by the end of 4 weeks.
- The member will maintain eye contact with the waitress for at least 3 seconds while ordering coffee at the local cafe.

How to Write About Goals That Seem Difficult to Measure

Despite application of the RUMBA criteria, the occupational therapy professional may find that some goals appropriate for persons with psychiatric disabilities are difficult to measure. Abilities such as self-assertion, self-control, and independence (unlike range of motion or muscle strength) cannot be physically measured and quantified. There are at least two ways around this problem. The first is to include behavioral indicators of the desired goal in the criteria. For example, in the case of self-control:

- The client's family will report no violent behaviors during a visit of the client with her family for a meal over the weekend.
- The client will describe at least one constructive way in which she coped with her feelings during the visit with her family over the weekend.

The second way is to develop a rating scale for each goal. Goal attainment scaling (GAS) (31, 45) identifies five levels of achievement for a goal. Two of the levels are higher than what is expected, two are lower than what is expected, and the middle level defines the expected outcome. Table 13.2 gives two examples of how this might be done. GAS provides the client and the team with a clear understanding of what the person is expected to achieve and allows for a form of documentation that is simple and easy to use with goals that can be difficult to measure. Use of GAS has been shown in psychometric evaluations to be effective in distinguishing between clients who have demonstrated progress against those who have not, if the set criteria is objective and measurable (45).

Scott and Haggerty (48) used GAS concepts in a partial hospitalization (outpatient) setting to help clients set their own goals and define their own criteria for success in meeting them. With the use of a paper-and-pencil form, the client was asked to select a goal based on problems identified through evaluation. Next, the client was encouraged to explore and discuss why they chose that particular goal and how it related to the client's immediate and future concerns. Then, the client was asked to state what outcome they would *expect* to achieve. (Scott and Haggerty give the example of a person who is chronically 15 minutes late; the expected outcome is that the person will be 10 minutes late.) Working from this expected outcome, the person then describes

Table 13.2. Goal Attainment Scale for Two Goals: Social Interaction and Health Maintenance

Predicted Attainment	Score	Goals	
		Social Interactions	Increase Exercise to Promote and Support Improvement of A1–C Levels (Type II Diabetes) (Health Maintenance)
Most unfavorable outcome	−2	Speaks to no one except therapist during 3-h session	Does not participate in planned physical exercise
Less than expected outcome	−1	Says hello or other greeting to fellow workers during 3-h training session	Participates in planned physical exercise for <30 min, or 1–2 times per wk
Expected level of outcome	0	Holds sustained, interactive conversation of 200 words or 10 min with one other worker during 3-h session	Participates in planned physical exercise for 30 min, 3 times per wk
Greater than expected outcome	+1	Holds interactive conversation of more than 200 words or 10 min with two or more workers independently or simultaneously during 3-h session	Participates in planned physical exercise for 30 min, 4 times per wk
Most favorable outcome likely	+2	Holds interactive conversation of 500 words or 20 min with three or more workers during 3-h session	Participates in planned physical exercise for 30 min, 4 times per wk

Modified with permission from Ottenbacher, K. J., & Cusick, A. (1990). Goal attainment scaling as a method of clinical service evaluation. *American Journal of Occupational Therapy, 44*(6), 519–525. ©1990 by American Occupational Therapy Association, Inc.

a least favorable outcome and a most favorable one. Finally, outcomes intermediate between the expected one and the extreme ones are described (less favorable, more favorable). Of course, it is not necessary to identify five different points on the rating scale; three points (expected, more than expected, and less than expected) are also sufficient.

Involving Clients in Setting Their Own Goals

Involving clients directly in selecting goals and measuring success is desirable whenever possible. Setting and achieving personal goals contributes to a sense of independence and empowerment. Clients who are not experienced at setting goals will need some assistance in the beginning, especially in choosing achievable and realistic short-term objectives. This is all part of the intervention process. It is worth taking the time to discuss goals with clients and help them identify their own.

Scott and Haggerty (48) point out that not all clients can generate their own goals and attainment scales, and that persons with severe and persistent mental illness, or intellectual disabilities may require various levels of assistance from the occupational therapist. Clients in the acute stages of mental illness have also demonstrated more difficulty monitoring themselves once they have set up the attainment scales, which may be a result of their fluctuating symptoms. The GAS approach seems to be more efficacious for individuals who are more stable medically (17, 45).

To summarize, goals may be written by the OT or the supervised OTA in collaboration with the client and family. A particular client's involvement in selecting and refining goals may be limited to varying degrees by cognitive impairments or psychotic symptoms but the occupational therapy professional must involve the person as much as

possible. Goals must address functional outcomes related to occupational performance. Goals should be relevant to the client's needs and values and stated in terms that the client can understand. Goals should contain some criterion against which success can be measured and they must indicate the behavior the person is to demonstrate. They must include a time frame that is reasonable and that corresponds to the reimbursement guidelines applicable to the situation. Finally, they must be achievable—that is, realistic for this person at this time in life.

SELECTING APPROPRIATE INTERVENTION PRINCIPLES

Once the goals are written, the next task is to figure out how best to reach them; the occupational therapy professional will need to choose an intervention type. The AOTA *OTPF-4* (6) describes six intervention types: occupations and activities, interventions to support occupations, education and training, advocacy, group interventions, and virtual interventions (6). At the beginning of this chapter, we emphasized the importance of identifying the causes of the client's problems as well as the problems themselves. In other words, occupational therapy professionals choose a theoretical perspective, a frame of reference, or a practice model that best explains the client's problems, as a guide in selecting approaches to intervention, types of intervention, and sometimes even specific intervention protocols. To return to the example presented earlier in the chapter, a person may have poor hygiene for any number of reasons . . . .

If the reason for the person's poor hygiene is that they never learned proper grooming and hygiene, the most logical approach and type of intervention would be to teach the client the skills.

If the reason for poor hygiene is that the client forgets the task of grooming, we need to know more about why they are forgetting (organic memory loss, disorganization, depression and lack of focus, experiencing feelings of overwhelm, poor sleep hygiene, or lack of a reinforcing environment are just a few possible reasons); once we perform further assessments, we can figure out a way to help the person remember. Perhaps, visual cues or the assistance of another person is necessary. The occupational therapist might apply the cognitive disabilities model in such a situation.

If the reason for poor hygiene is that the client's skin "feels funny," which prevents them from completing tasks such as brushing their teeth or hair, then we might suspect a sensory processing or sensory modulation problem, which the OT could further evaluate. The point is, the more we know about the cause of the person's problem, the easier it is to select a practice model and intervention approaches and types.

Intangible factors such as self-esteem can, and often should, be considered in this stage of intervention planning. Several of the theories covered in this text are based, at least in part, on ideas about the client's feelings and internal psychodynamics. The client's sense of personal causation (MOHO) or narcissistic needs (object–relations) may provide clues about what principles we might follow. Although these intangibles cannot be directly measured, they are client factors that can help guide our selection of intervention methods. If we believe, for example, that the person in the example is neglecting hygiene because of low self-esteem, and the client's self-esteem has likely been impacted by the fact that the client has been laid off from work for the second time in 18 months, we may plan an intervention that directs our energies toward raising self-esteem, possibly using CBT as an intervention, and help the client procure work opportunities, assuming that the hygiene improvements will follow.

The different theories and practice models discussed in the first section of the text contain principles for organizing our thinking. Allen's Cognitive Disabilities Model (1) is useful for evaluating how well a person with long-term schizophrenia can function in an independent living situation, for example, and for detailing how to modify the environment so that it better supports the person's current level of functioning. However, this theory helps little in designing a work adjustment program for a middle-aged woman suffering from serious depression. The MOHO or the Role Acquisition Model might be a better guide for planning in this case. No one theory is adequate to address every problem, and so it is important to choose the best one for each situation.

THE ROLES OF THE OCCUPATIONAL THERAPIST AND THE OCCUPATIONAL THERAPY ASSISTANT DURING INTERVENTION PLANNING AND DEVELOPMENT

As with all aspects of occupational therapy care and service delivery throughout the occupational therapy process, intervention planning and intervention development is a shared responsibility between the OT and the OTA. Similarly, just as aspects of the client are unique, and contexts inform how the client's therapeutic experience will unfold, contextual influences and other factors will influence the way that the OT and the OTA provide occupational therapy services. Other factors that help determine the practitioners' roles and functions in each circumstance include characteristics such as each occupational therapy professionals' level and type of past experience(s), education (or clinical educational pathways), and specialized training or certifications. Ultimately, state statutes and regulations, as well as individual state-to-state occupational therapy practice acts, with their rules and regulations, help guide the provision of high-quality occupational therapy services. Nevertheless, several essential features remain consistent: (i) as mentioned in Chapter 12, the OTA must be supervised by an OT, and (ii) the OTA may only provide intervention documented and contained in the plan of care constructed by a licensed occupational therapist (4, 8, 40).

SUMMARY

Intervention planning, implementation, and review require the application of clinical reasoning, professional judgment, and collaboration between the occupational therapy professional and the client. The process of intervention planning involves identifying specific problems and functional occupational goals that the client believes are important priorities. Both problems and goals must be stated in terms that are relevant to the client's needs, and the goals must be understandable, measurable, behavioral, and achievable. Above all, goals should be observable and realistic for the client to achieve during their allotted timeframe. These factors are imperative for interventions to be as successful as possible. There are many ways to determine the most appropriate approach and type of intervention that will provide guidance as the client and the occupational therapist collaborate in implementing an intervention during occupational therapy sessions. This chapter introduced the nuts and bolts used to build the initial part of the occupational therapy intervention plan. The reader was introduced to various theories and practice models that contain principles for guiding clinical reasoning and selecting and modifying intervention methods and approaches. In the next chapter, readers will learn more about our profession's unique contribution to supporting clients with mental illness, matching occupational demands to intervention types for improved occupation outcomes.

OT HACKS SUMMARY

O: Occupation as a means and an end

An additional element of the intervention planning phase that occupational therapy professionals must also consider is related to the person's potential future needs and possible future environments. It is in making the transition from one setting to another that consumers are often the most vulnerable and at risk for relapse, or of falling through the cracks in the mental health system. Quality of care necessitates continuity of care. Occupational therapy professionals must anticipate how the individual client will respond to transitions. The occupational therapy professional should obtain permission from the client to speak directly with the occupational therapy professional or other service providers in the next setting about the client's needs. The occupational therapy professional can then establish a brief follow-up after transition to the service provider and/or the client to ensure that the transition has been made and to answer any remaining questions.

T: Theoretical concepts, values, and principles, or historical foundations

As Rogers (44) states: "Simply because a goal appears technically feasible for the patient does not mean that it should be set as a goal." The client has a right to choose. The notion that through human occupation each person becomes what he or she does, and by doing, shapes their own identity has always been at the core of occupational therapy (27). The client should select their own goals, although these may differ from those the occupational therapist might have chosen.

H: How can we Help? OT's role in serving clients with mental illness or mental health needs

According to Cahill and Richardson, "Shared decision making (SDM), or the process by which clients actively work with health care professionals to make informed decisions about health care options, is critical to value-based, client-centered care and representing client preferences as part of the occupational therapy process" (14, para. 1, abstract).

Read more about shared decision-making in this article to consider how to add value to our occupational therapy services: Cahill, S., & Richardson, H. (2022). Shared decision making and reducing the use of low-value occupational therapy interventions. *American Journal of Occupational Therapy, 76*(3), 7603090010.

A: Adaptations

Writing an occupational therapy intervention goal . . .

Goals in an intervention plan should be written so that they describe very clearly **what the person will do**, and **what action the person will perform**. Goals should follow logically from problems that have been identified by assessment and selected by the client in collaboration with others, as being important or meaningful to them. The more specific the description of the problem, the easier it is to write the corresponding goal. Goals should be associated with occupational outcomes! (7, 20)

C: Case study includes

Let us revisit the case example from the beginning of the chapter to learn how occupational therapy services might support Drew, who has been diagnosed with schizophrenia, and his family.

Drew has been stabilized on medication and is in an outpatient day program that includes occupational therapy. The occupational therapy team, including an OTA and an OT, are collaborating with Drew and his family to provide occupational therapy services. The occupational therapy evaluation has been completed, and the occupational therapy team with Drew have determined that the following long-term goals are priorities:

1. To return to college
2. To live in a dorm rather than at home
3. To have friends

On the basis of these goals, the OT and OTA have identified some short-term objectives and discussed them with Drew. These are listed as a, b for the numbered goals to which they correspond:

1a. Sustain attention for 45 minutes in an activity group setting by 2 weeks.
1b. Bathe and complete grooming tasks daily to promote positive social interactions with others in the group by 2 weeks.
2a. Demonstrate ability to make a bed and dust/vacuum a room by 2 weeks.
2b. Clean up after self, cleaning own area, during and after activity group by 2 weeks.
3a. Tolerate the presence of others in the group by 3 days.
3b. Interact with others by sharing and passing materials and tools in activity group by 2 weeks.

Drew will be attending an activity group with four other people. Here, he will work on all objectives except 2a. He will attend a community living group, in a simulated apartment environment, to work on goal 2a.

At the beginning, the occupational therapy team orients Drew to the plan and the planned activities, encouraging him to ask questions. At first, he does not see how attending the activity group has anything to do with returning to college. The OT asks him whether he has to pay attention in college. He then says he continues to have trouble with the voices that distract him, even though the medication has helped "calm them down." With more discussion, Drew agrees that maybe this small group is a good place to practice directing attention to a task and away from the voices. For each of the other objectives, the occupational therapy team spends time with Drew helping him see the connection of the methods to his short- and long-term goals. The OT and the OTA, who cofacilitate the activity group, set aside an additional 20 minutes at the end of each group session for members to express what they did in the group and how it might relate to their goals. The team encourages members to give each other feedback (both positive and constructive), and they model this type of feedback as well.

Over time, Drew improves his personal hygiene but this is an area that Drew continues to need to work on. Sometimes, Drew attended the group and distinctly smelled unwashed and seemed not to have brushed his teeth or combed his hair. Most of the other group members refused to sit near him. This became a focus of private discussion between Drew and the OT team, and smaller more specific objectives were set: to brush teeth daily before coming to group, to bathe daily including underarms and genitals and buttocks, to wash hair once a week, to comb hair daily, and to dress in clean clothing.

The OT team used principles from the Cognitive Disabilities Model and theories of cognitive social learning to guide their clinical reasoning in making decisions. They used the power of the group, especially Mark (the most tolerant and highest functioning group member) to reinforce Drew's improvement in grooming and hygiene.

This case illustration describes only a small portion of the very beginning of an extended intervention program. As Drew continued to improve (quickly in some areas, more slowly in others), the plan was adjusted. Both occupational therapy professionals continued to encourage and validate Drew's progress, to note his achievements, and to facilitate peer feedback. At the end of 3 months, Drew enrolled in one college course and continued to attend the day program on a reduced schedule while still living at home.

Among other things, this case example highlights that providing individual intervention in the context of a group session is "considered the standard in most mental health settings" (50). Another aspect shown in the case study is the effort to encourage Drew to reflect on his own experience and identify issues that interfere with achieving his goals.

K: Knowledge: keeping mental health OT practice grounded in evidence, in occupational science, and in research

As the readers learned in this chapter, sometimes the most challenging part of occupational therapy intervention planning and implementation is knowing where to begin. For our clients, it can be equally challenging to describe and articulate the problems that they are having, especially if they are experiencing difficult side effects of medication, challenging symptoms of mental illness, or difficult emotions. Sometimes it is easier to define or describe a thing by defining or describing what the thing is *not*. However, the client's motivation, and the occupational therapy professional's understanding of the client's readiness for change are critical components to optimal experiences and outcomes in therapy. The level, approach, and type of intervention should match closely to the client's appropriate level of readiness for change, and for optimal therapeutic benefits the motivation to make a change must come from the client. MI can help clients articulate and respond to their own reasons for changing. The occupational therapy professional guides, but the client decides.

Read the article titled, "Ten Things That Motivational Interviewing Is Not," by the authors and creators of the MI method (https://orca.cardiff.ac.uk/id/eprint/30246/1/MILLER 2009.PDF). Choose one of the 10 items and see if you can summarize "Why Motivational Interviewing Is Not."

When used properly, and with training and practice, MI as a communication approach is a useful, evidence-based practice for guiding clients toward strengthening their own motivation to change.

S: Some terms that may be new to you

Not applicable for this chapter.

Reflection Questions

1. One of the recommendations from The AOTA's *Choosing Wisely* List of Ten Things Patients and Providers Should Question is "Don't provide intervention activities that are nonpurposeful (eg, cones, pegs, shoulder arc, arm bike)." How might nonpurposeful intervention activities in a behavioral health or psychiatric setting differ from a physical rehabilitation setting?
2. Describe some of the complexities of OT intervention planning with clients who have psychiatric diagnoses.
3. Which of these factors do you think has the most potential to impact occupational therapy intervention outcomes positively or negatively?
   a. Application of therapeutic reasoning and the amount of experience of the OT professionals
   b. The quality and thoroughness of the OT evaluation
   c. The quality of the therapeutic relationship and collaboration with the client
   Defend your answer.
4. Describe MI. In what ways do you think this evidence-based approach is a good fit for application during the OT process?
5. What is the relationship between MI and the TTM/SCM?
6. Compare and contrast CBT and DBT.
7. Create three OT intervention goals that could be measured using GAS.
8. Explain the factors that influence the role(s) of the occupational therapist and the occupational therapy assistant during intervention planning.
9. Summarize the role(s) that theory and practice models play in OT intervention planning.

REFERENCES

1. Allen, C. (1985). *Occupational therapy for psychiatric diseases: Measurement and management of cognitive disabilities.* Little, Brown, & Company.
2. American Occupational Therapy Association (2023). Evidence-Based Practice. *Choosing Wisely: An update on AOTA's best practice recommendations* (formerly Choosing Wisely®). Retrieved from: https://www.aota.org/practice/practice-essentials/evidencebased-practiceknowledge-translation/aotas-top-10-choosing-wisely-recommendations
3. American Occupational Therapy Association. (2020). AOTA 2020 occupational therapy code of ethics. *American Journal of Occupational Therapy, 74*(Suppl. 3), 7413410005.
4. American Occupational Therapy Association. (2020). Guidelines for supervision, roles, and responsibilities during the delivery of occupational therapy services. *American Journal of Occupational Therapy, 74*(Suppl. 3), 7413410020.
5. American Occupational Therapy Association. (2020). Occupational therapy in the promotion of health and well-being. *American Journal of Occupational Therapy, 74*, 7403420010.
6. American Occupational Therapy Association. (2020). Occupational therapy practice framework: Domain and process—Fourth edition. *American Journal of Occupational Therapy, 74*(Suppl. 2), 7412410010.
7. American Occupational Therapy Association. (2021). Occupational therapy scope of practice. *American Journal of Occupational Therapy, 75*(Suppl. 3), 7513410030.
8. American Occupational Therapy Association. (2021). Standards of practice for occupational therapy. *American Journal of Occupational Therapy, 75*(Suppl. 3), 7513410050.

9. American Psychiatric Association. (2022). *Diagnostic and statistical manual of mental disorders* (5th ed., text rev.). https://doi.org/10.1176/appi.books.9780890425787

10. Beck, A. T. (1964). Thinking and depression II: Theory and therapy. *Archives of General Psychiatry, 10*(6), 561–571.

11. Beck, J. S. (2011). *Cognitive behavior therapy: Basics and beyond* (2nd ed.). Guilford Press.

12. Bonder, B. R. (2022). *Psychopathology and function* (6th ed.). SLACK.

13. Brown, C. (2019). Ecological models in occupational therapy. In B. A. B. Schell & G. Gillen (Eds.), *Willard and Spackman's occupational therapy* (13th ed., pp. 622–632). Lippincott Williams & Wilkins.

14. Cahill, S., & Richardson, H. (2022). Shared decision making and reducing the use of low-value occupational therapy interventions. *American Journal of Occupational Therapy, 76*(3), 7603090010.

15. Christiansen, C., Baum, C., & Bass-Haugen, J. (Eds.). (2005). *Occupational therapy: Performance, participation, and well-being* (3rd ed.). SLACK.

16. Cole, M. B. (2018). *Group dynamics in occupational therapy: The theoretical basis and practice application of group intervention* (5th ed., pp. 285–319). SLACK.

17. Doig, E., Fleming, J., Kuipers, P., & Cornwell, P. L. (2010). Clinical utility of the combined use of the Canadian occupational performance measure and goal attainment scaling. *The American Journal of Occupational Therapy, 64*(6), 904–914.

18. Dunn, W., McClain, L. H., Brown, C., & Youngstrom, M. J. (1998). The ecology of human performance. In M. E. Neistadt & E. B. Crepeau (Eds.), *Willard and Spackman's occupational therapy* (9th ed., pp. 525–535). Lippincott Williams & Wilkins.

19. Ellis, A. (1962). *Reason and emotion in psychotherapy.* Lyle Stuart.

20. Fisher, A. G., & Marterella, A. (2019). *Powerful practice: A model for authentic occupational therapy.* Center for Innovative OT Solutions.

21. Forsyth, K., Taylor, R. R., Kramer, J. M., Prior, S., Ritchie, L., & Melton, J. (2019). The Model of Human Occupation. In B. A. B. Schell & G. Gillen (Eds.), *Willard and Spackman's occupational therapy* (13th ed., pp. 601–621). Lippincott Williams & Wilkins.

22. Gillen, G., Hunter, E. G., Lieberman, D., & Stutzbach, M. (2019). AOTA's top 5 Choosing Wisely© recommendations. *American Journal of Occupational Therapy, 73*(2), 7302420010p1–7302420010p9.

23. Grajo, L. C. (2019). Theory of occupational adaptation. In B. A. B. Schell & G. Gillen (Eds.), *Willard and Spackman's occupational therapy* (13th ed., pp. 633–642). Lippincott Williams & Wilkins.

24. Helfrich, C. A. (2019). Principles of learning and behavior change. In B. A. B. Schell & G. Gillen (Eds.), *Willard and Spackman's occupational therapy* (13th ed., pp. 693–708). Lippincott Williams & Wilkins.

25. Hemphill, B. J., & Urish, C. K. (Eds.). (2020). *Assessments in occupational therapy mental health: An integrative approach* (4th ed.). SLACK.

26. Hill, R., & Dahlitz, M. (2022). *The practitioner's guide to the science of psychotherapy.* W. W. Norton & Company.

27. Hooper, B., & Wood, W. (2019). The philosophy of occupational therapy: A framework for practice. In B. A. B. Schell & G. Gillen (Eds.), *Willard and Spackman's occupational therapy* (13th ed., pp. 43–55). Lippincott Williams & Wilkins.

28. Janiri, D., Moser, D. A., Doucet, G. E., Luber, M. J., Rasgon, A., Lee, W. H., Murrough, J. W., Sani, G., Eickhoff, S. B., & Frangou, S. (2019). Shared neural phenotypes for mood and anxiety disorders: A meta-analysis of 226 task-related functional imaging studies. *JAMA Psychiatry, 77*(2), 172–179.

29. Januszewski, C., & Mahaffey, L. (2020). Assessments used within the Model of Human Occupation. In B. J. Hemphill & C. J. Urish (Eds.), *Assessments in occupational therapy mental health: An integrative approach* (4th ed., pp. 279–305). SLACK.

30. Kielhofner, G. (Ed.). (2002). *A Model of Human Occupation: Theory and application* (3rd ed.). Lippincott Williams & Wilkins.

31. Kiresuk, T. J., & Sherman, R. E. (1968). Goal attainment scaling: A general method for evaluation of comprehensive mental health programs. *Community Mental Health Journal, 4*(6), 443–453.

32. Law, M., Baptiste, S., Carswell, A., McColl, M. A., Polatajko, H., & Pollack, N. (2014). *COPM 5th edition: Canadian occupational performance measure manual* (5th ed.). CAOT Publications: ACE.

33. Lee, J. (2010). Achieving best practice: A review of evidence linked to occupation focused practice models. *Occupational Therapy in Health Care, 24*(3), 206–222.

34. Linehan, M. (1993). *Skills training manual for treating borderline personality disorder.* New Guilford Press.

35. Linehan, M. (1993). *The Cognitive-Behavioral Treatment of borderline personality disorder.* Guilford Press.

36. McKay, M., Wood, J. C., & Brantley, J. (2007). *The dialectical behavior therapy skills workbook: Practical DBT exercises for learning mindfulness, interpersonal effectiveness, emotion regulation & distress tolerance.* New Harbinger Publications.

37. Miller, W. R., & Rollnick, S. (2009). Ten things that motivational interviewing is not. *Behavioural and Cognitive Psychotherapy, 37*(2), 129–140.

38. Miller, W. R., & Rollnick, S. (Eds.). (2013). *Motivational interviewing: Helping people change* (3rd ed.). Guilford Press.

39. Nakamura-Thomas, H., van Antwerp, L. R., Ikiugu, M. N., Scott, P. J., & Bonsaksen, T. (2015). The 4th International MOHO Institute: Summary and reflections. *Ergoterapeuten, 6,* 62–67.

40. Nicholson, J., & Salinas, J. (2022). Occupational therapist/ occupational therapy assistant partnership: Supervision and collaboration. In B. Braveman (Ed.), *Leading and managing occupational therapy services: An evidence-based approach* (3rd ed., pp 252–263). F.A. Davis.

41. Pederson, L. (2015). *Dialectical behavior therapy: A contemporary guide for practitioners.* Wiley-Blackwell.

42. Pederson, L., & Pederson, C. S. (2017). *The expanded dialectical behavior therapy skills training manual: DBT for self-help, and individual & group treatment settings.* PESI Publishing.

43. Reitz, S. M., & Graham, K. (2019). Health promotion theories. In B. A. B. Schell & G. Gillen (Eds.), *Willard and Spackman's occupational therapy* (13th ed., pp. 675–692). Lippincott Williams & Wilkins.

44. Rogers, J. C. (1983). Clinical reasoning: The ethics, science, and art. In R. Padilla & Y. Griffiths (Eds.), *The Eleanor Clarke Slagle Lectures in occupational therapy 1955–2016: A professional legacy, centennial edition* (pp. 265–280). AOTA Press.

45. Ruble, L., McGrew, J. H., & Toland, M. D. (2012). Goal attainment scaling as an outcome measure in randomized controlled trials of psychosocial interventions in autism. *Journal of Autism and Developmental Disorders, 42*(9), 1974–1983.

46. Schkade, J. K., & Schultz, S. (1992). Occupational adaptation: Toward a holistic approach for contemporary practice, part 1. *American Journal of Occupational Therapy, 46*(9), 829–838.

47. Schultz, S., & Schkade, J. K. (1992). Occupational adaptation: Toward a holistic approach for contemporary practice, part 2. *American Journal of Occupational Therapy, 46*(10), 917–926.

48. Scott, A. H., & Haggerty, E. J. (1984). Structuring goals via goal attainment scaling in occupational therapy groups in a partial hospitalization setting. *Occupational Therapy in Mental Health, 4*(2), 39–58.

49. Sokol, L., & Fox, M. G. (2019). *The comprehensive clinician's guide to cognitive behavioral therapy.* PESI Publishing.

50. Sullivan, A., Dowdy, T., Haddad, J., Hussain, S., Patel, A., & Smyth, K. (2013). Occupational therapy interventions in adult mental health across settings: A literature review. *AOTA MHSIS Quarterly, 36*(1), 1–3.

51. Taylor, R. R. (Ed.). (2017). *Kielhofner's Model of Human Occupation: Theory and application.* Wolters Kluwer.

52. Taylor, R. R. (2020). *The intentional relationship: Occupational therapy and use of self.* F.A. Davis.

53. Wong, S. R., & Fisher, G. (2015). Comparing and using occupation-focused models. *Occupational Therapy in Health Care, 29*(3), 297–315.

SUGGESTED RESOURCES

Articles

As the recipient of the *Eleanor Clarke Slagle Lecture* in 1983, Dr Joan Rogers' address, *Clinical Reasoning: The Ethics, Science, and Art,* which was referenced in this chapter, was originally published in the *American Journal of Occupational Therapy.* The lecture in its entirety can be found in the link below. This article is suggested because of the continued relevancy of its core message, particularly regarding applying professional reasoning as we collaborate with clients throughout the occupational therapy process, "the clinician functions as a scientist, ethicist, and artist. The scientific, ethical, and artistic dimensions of clinical reasoning are inextricably intertwined, and each strand is needed to strengthen the line of thought leading to understanding" (REF Rogers, p. 279).

Rogers, J. C. (1983). Clinical reasoning: The ethics, science, and art. *American Journal of Occupational Therapy, 37*(9), 601–616. https://pubmed.ncbi.nlm.nih.gov/6624858/

Videos

This video is about the Spirit of Motivational Interviewing. Spirit is the guide to the ethical practice of using the powerful strategies and techniques of motivational interviewing. This video is 1 of 12 videos that make up an online motivational interviewing course.

The Spirit of Motivational Interviewing Posted by Bill Matulich, https://www.youtube.com/watch?v=APPoKvTPhog

This video features one of the creators of motivational interviewing, Dr Stephan Rollnick, demonstrating one element of the MI method, engaging in a role-play of a brief consultation. The video is produced by BMJ Learning, who are one of the leading providers of medical education for health care professionals with more than 450,000 users worldwide. Readers can find other useful information by subscribing to the BMJ Learning Channel at the link listed under websites.

Motivational interviewing in brief consultations: role-play focusing on engaging, https://www.youtube.com/watch?v=bTRRNWrwRCo&t=1s

Websites

The BMJ learning channel. https://www.youtube.com/user/BMJLearning

The BMJ learning website: Find more clinical and non-clinical peer reviewed content about a variety of health topics. https://new-learning.bmj.com/

Matching Occupational Demands to Intervention Types for Improved Occupational Outcomes

OT HACKS OVERVIEW

O: Occupation as a means and an end

The American Occupational Therapy Association (AOTA's) Philosophical Base of Occupational Therapy (4) states that "Occupational therapy practitioners conceptualize occupations as both a means and an end in therapy. That is, there is therapeutic value in occupational engagement as a change agent, and engagement in occupations is also the ultimate goal of therapy" (para. 3). In this chapter, readers learn more about how the analysis of occupational performance is used in the following:

1. Selecting methods for service delivery
2. Intervention implementation, which is defined by the *Occupational Therapy Practice Framework: Domain and Process, 4th Edition (OTPF-4)* (7) as: "Carry[ing] out occupational therapy intervention to address specific occupations, contexts, and performance patterns and skills affecting performance" (p. 56).

T: Theoretical concepts, values, and principles, or historical foundations

Dr Claudia Allen was the 1987 recipient of the Eleanor Clarke Slagle Lecture. She began her address, *Activity: Occupational Therapy's Treatment Method*, as follows:

Difficulties in explaining the value of using activity as a treatment method have been with us from the beginning (Fields, 1911). During a testimonial dinner in tribute to Eleanor Clarke Slagle, Dr Adolph Meyer (1937) struggled to explain the value of activity. He said, "I should like to voice adequately what so many of my patients have gained through Mrs Slagle and her pupils and what it means for the sufferers, but also for the healthy . . . those with 'time on their hands'" (p. 6). (2, p. 309)

After reading this chapter, how would you describe the value of using activity as an intervention method in modern occupational therapy practice?

H: How can we Help? OT's role in serving clients with mental illness or mental health needs

Activity analysis is the general structure for analyzing and designing an activity to address the specific goals of a particular client. Because activity analysis and occupational performance analysis are such core aspects of occupational therapy, this is a skill set that the occupational therapy professional will frequently use in clinical practice.

A: Adaptations

To use any activity analysis format effectively, the practitioner must understand and know how to apply the principles of adaptation and gradation. **Adaptation** means the modification of the activity to facilitate performance, generally by modifying the task or the environment.

C: Case study includes

Client: Antoine B.

Diagnostic and Statistical Manual of Mental Disorders, Fifth Edition, Text Revision (DSM-5-TR) Diagnosis at Admission: F71, Moderate Intellectual Developmental Disorder

ICD-10-CM: Q90.9, Down syndrome, unspecified

The case study presented at the end of this chapter is about planning intervention activities for a client named Antoine. Antoine is a 40-year-old man with moderate intellectual developmental disorder and Down syndrome. Readers will find a brief occupational profile and an excerpt of one of Antoine's occupational performance analyses, collected and observed by the occupational therapist (OT) to help determine and select appropriate intervention activities to meet Antoine's goals and priorities for occupational therapy services.

K: Knowledge: keeping mental health OT practice grounded in evidence, in occupational science, and in research

Knowledgeable analysis must be the basis of activity selection in intervention if the expectation is to produce the desired therapeutic effect and eventually the occupational outcome.

S: Some terms that may be new to you

Adaptation
Declarative memory

Dynamic performance analysis
Environmental demand
Environmental support
Errorless learning
Gradation
Intervention implementation
Procedural memory
Social conduct/interpersonal skills
Sustained attention
Task-oriented approach/task-specific approach

INTRODUCTION

In Chapter 13, we learned more about the process of developing an intervention plan. We discussed how to integrate the client's priorities into occupation-centered goals. In this chapter, we learn how to connect the unique focus of an intervention by utilizing the most appropriate intervention approach. Furthermore, the reader is introduced to the various types of occupational therapy interventions and strategies that promote matching occupational and activity demands to intervention types to improve client outcomes.

LINKING CLIENT GOALS AND PRIORITIES TO OCCUPATION-FOCUSED INTERVENTION

Look at the goals listed in Table 14.1. These are selected as broad general goals, derived from the *OTPF-4* (7), Mosey's adaptive skills, and other occupation-based practice models (13, 15, 16). Several goals are listed for the areas of occupation and some are further classified by more specific process or performance skills, or other client factors. Each goal may be phrased in a way that indicates an approach focus such as health promotion, remediation or restoration, maintenance, compensation or adaptation, and disability prevention (7). Beginning the goal statement with verbs such as *to develop, to restore,* and *to improve* indicates an emphasis on restoration, remediation, rehabilitation, or habilitation. Maintenance of function is the indicated focus of goals that begin with the words *to maintain ability to,* and prevention is the focus of goals that begin with the words *to prevent deterioration of ability to.*

The list in Table 14.1 is by no means exhaustive. The list is offered to help the reader make connections between what an occupational therapy professional does, how they do it, and how our profession operationalizes the occupational therapy process. The reader should remember three important cautions when referring to this list. First, not every possible goal is listed; do not be discouraged if a goal that you think would be important for a client is missing from this list. Remember, occupational therapy goals are made in collaboration with the client; they are unique to the individual and are based on the unique occupational priorities of each person. The goals listed here are offered as a tool to assist learners in having a starting place for organizing their thoughts. Second, other occupational therapy goals, such as those that relate

to movement functions, may have to be addressed even for clients whose primary diagnosis is psychiatric—for example, the person who has depression and is recovering from a tendon repair following an attempted suicide will need physical restoration as well. Third, many of the listed goals themselves depend on the client first having met smaller or more specific goals or objectives. Writing more specific, individualized, and measurable goals derived from these general goals requires the addition of the other cornerstones of occupational therapy, such as the effective application of therapeutic reasoning and the development of a positive therapeutic relationship with the client (24).

SELECTING INTERVENTION METHODS FOR SERVICE DELIVERY

Once we have chosen the theoretical perspective, model of practice or frame of reference, and the principles that we believe best explain the client's problems, we can choose methods for service delivery based on them. The method specifies the activity or occupation to be used in the intervention, the environment in which it will be performed, and the approach that the therapist will use to present the activity. Each of these—activity, environment, and therapeutic type—is examined separately.

Activity

Activities are chosen depending on the stated principles identified in the intervention plan. Activities are selected primarily for their ability to address the intervention goal(s). We determine this primarily by synthesizing information from the occupational profile with the occupational performance analysis, as well as any other relevant additional assessment information. Knowledgeable analysis must be the basis of activity selection in intervention if the expectation is to produce the desired therapeutic effect. For example, if the practitioner suspects that the person has trouble making decisions because other people have always made decisions on the client's behalf, the occupational therapy professional looks for activities that involve making choices, rather than ones that require absolute adherence to a sequence of rules or directions; cooking and meal prep, gardening, grocery shopping, making home repairs, and many leisure activities could be adapted to fit this principle.

Table 14.1. Examples of General Goals of Occupational Therapy

Focus of Intervention	Goals (to Establish, Restore, Improve, or Maintain Ability to, . . .)
ADL	• Initiate and effectively perform to a socially acceptable level in such activities as personal hygiene and grooming, oral hygiene, bathing or showering, personal device care, dressing, feeding and eating, functional mobility, sexual expression.
IADL: community mobility	• Travel within community on foot and by mechanical transport (bike, car, bus, train).
IADL: financial management	• Use money and other forms of payment. • Budget within one's means. • Plan for financial goals.
IADL: health management	• Develop and maintain physical and psychological health by health and wellness routines, exercise, nutrition, adhering to medication schedule, decreasing health risk behaviors.
IADL: shopping	• Prepare lists. • Locate and select items either in person or over the phone or internet. • Use payment methods such as cash, debit card, credit card, or others. • Apply arithmetic knowledge to money transactions. • Receive, transport, store purchased items.
IADL: meal preparation and cleanup	• Plan and prepare nutritious meals within budget. • Clean up, store leftovers, observe food safety.
IADL: emergency response	• Recognize unsafe situations and respond with effective measures (remedy dangerous condition, call 911, remove self and others from danger).
IADL: home management	• Organize and carry out tasks related to clothing care, cleaning, household maintenance, safety procedures.
IADL: care of others, childrearing	• Provide physical care, nurturance, and appropriate activities for children and others under one's care, including pets.
Rest and sleep	• Meet needs for restorative sleep and rest, eg, by engaging in sleep hygiene.
Education	• Plan and carry out tasks related to schooling, such as homework, study, preparation for tests, extracurricular activities; engage in education on a less formal level to satisfy interests.
Work: employment interests and pursuits	• Identify aptitudes and interests. • Identify and pursue vocational training suited to one's aptitude, interests, and skills.
Work: employment seeking	• Search, identify, and select work opportunities. • Carry out application and interview process. • Evaluate results of application and interview process.
Work: job performance	• Follow directions. • Perform job tasks effectively within the context. • Work neatly and with reasonable attention to detail. • Follow a schedule, maintain attendance, adhere to time standards of the job, and manage time and tasks. • Demonstrate appropriate behaviors in grooming, interpersonal communication, and safety.
Work: retirement planning	• Determine valued goals and interests and pursue them.
Work: volunteer exploration and participation	• Identify volunteer activities of interest. • Perform unpaid activities to benefit others.
Play and leisure: exploration	• Identify interests and skills and find appropriate opportunities to pursue them.
Play and leisure: participation	• Schedule time and follow-through on using leisure to pursue interests.
Social participation	• Interact in ways that are successful within culture and context. • Interact successfully with peers, family members, and community.
Motor performance skills	• Move in environment effectively to accomplish task. • Use objects. • Engage in desired occupations.
Process performance skills	• Manage and modify actions to accomplish desired tasks and occupations. • Use pacing to conserve energy. • Obtain and use knowledge to execute tasks; organize tasks in time by initiating, continuing, sequencing, and completing actions effectively. • Organize space and objects for effective task completion. • Demonstrate flexibility in adapting to changes in tasks and environment. • Adjust self to complete occupational tasks.

(continued)

Table 14.1. Examples of General Goals of Occupational Therapy (*continued*)

Focus of Intervention	Goals (to Establish, Restore, Improve, or Maintain Ability to, . . .)
Social interaction performance skills	• Coordinate behavior so as to effectively convey and receive information in relation to others, eg, turning toward them and engaging in eye contact. • Use gestures, eye contact, physical distance, and personal space in ways that are socially appropriate and effective for communication. • Give and receive information. • Speak, ask, respond, and modulate communication in a manner conducive to task completion. • Interact comfortably with one other person and within a group. • Relate to others with respect. • Collaborate with groups and partners and conform to groups as needed. • Compromise, negotiate, cooperate, and compete with others. • Use facial and bodily gestures, voice tone, and volume to express feelings and ideas. • Assert self.
Performance patterns: habits	• Demonstrate useful habits to support occupational engagement. • Abstain from or diminish involvement in nonproductive or dominating habits.
Performance patterns: routines	• Demonstrate effective routines related to occupational engagement.
Performance patterns: rituals	• Recognize and engage in actions that have a valued symbolic aspect in one's spiritual or cultural tradition.
Performance patterns: roles	• Engage effectively in desired and necessary occupational roles. • Identify, value, and carry out roles within a social context (eg, worker, student, neighbor).
Sensory functions (pertaining to occupational engagement)	• Attend to sensory stimuli. • Correctly interpret sensory stimuli. • Organize information received through senses. • Integrate body parts in reaction to sensory stimuli. • Identify one's own sensory responses and preferences. • Manage one's environment and activities so as to support sensory preferences.
Mental functions (pertaining to occupational engagement)	• Demonstrate alertness and responsiveness to situations in environment. • Locate self with regard to time, place, and person. • Recognize familiar faces. • Concentrate and attend to a task long enough to complete it. • Remember important information and skills. Place information, steps, and concepts in order. Generalize learning to new situations. Make decisions. Solve problems as they arise. Initiate and maintain performance and attention in an activity. Cease an activity when it is appropriate or desirable to do so.
Mental functions: experience of self (pertaining to occupational engagement)	Identify and enact ideas and beliefs important to the self. Perceive, understand, accept, and enact direction of self. Identify and pursue activities that bring pleasure to self.
Mental functions: self-concept and self-awareness (pertaining to occupational engagement)	Accept and embrace self as having value. Identify one's strengths and challenges.
Mental functions: coping (pertaining to occupational engagement)	Identify stress, stress reaction, stressors. Identify, select, and apply stress management strategies.
Mental functions: sense and use of time (pertaining to occupational engagement)	Sequence motor actions in time. Maintain time orientation. Budget and schedule use of time.
Mental functions: self-control (pertaining to occupational engagement)	Recognize one's own behavior and its internal and external causes. Develop awareness of one's emotions as they change. Control feelings and impulses. Take responsibility for one's own behavior. Modify one's behavior as appropriate for situation.

ADL, activities of daily living; IADL, instrumental activities of daily living.

Terminology adapted from: American Occupational Therapy Association. (2020). Occupational therapy practice framework: Domain and process—Fourth edition. *American Journal of Occupational Therapy, 74*(Suppl. 2), 1–87.

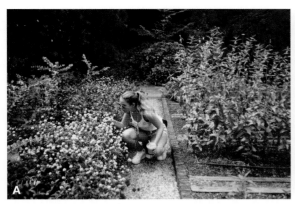
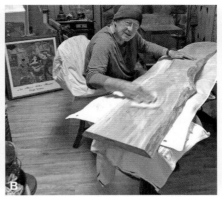
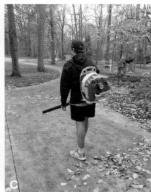

Figure 14.1. Many Typical Activities Such as Gardening (A) or Yard Work (C) Can Be Structured to Address a Client's Occupational Needs. Carpentry Projects and Woodworking (B) Are Examples of Structured Activities That Require Accuracy, Patience, and Skill. Activities With These Parameters Might Help the Client Explore Job-Related Interests and Barriers, While Also Exploring Leisure Interests.

On the other hand, if the person has been fired from many jobs because they did not follow procedures, perhaps an activity with lots of rules and restrictions, consequences for ignoring them, and the inherent rewards that will come with the finished product if the rules and procedures are accurately followed, would be best. An activity with these parameters might help the client explore the job-related barriers to maintaining employment. Many leisure activities could be used in this example. Carpentry projects and woodworking are notoriously unforgiving mediums, or slip casting in ceramics might be appropriate for this. Baking also requires accurate measurement and following directions. Many typical activities such as yard work or gardening can be structured to address a client's occupational needs (Figure 14.1).

Although occupational therapy professionals use many other therapeutic methods (such as cognitive behavioral therapy, use of adaptive equipment, or environmental modifications), activity or engagement in occupation should be included in every intervention plan. Activity and occupation have the power to create change in a way that verbal therapies

simply cannot. When a person actually *does* something, they explore and experience their effect on the world; talking about something is not the same thing as taking action. By participating in activities, people learn about themselves, about their abilities to use tools and materials, about the pleasure of working directly with their hands and bodies and minds, and about the reactions of others to what they have done. They discover, refine, and shape their images of themselves; they discover what they can and cannot do. And they become better at the things they desire to do; see Figure 14.2.

Environment

The conditions under which the intervention activity takes place influence the client's response. "Environmental factors are aspects of the physical, social, and attitudinal surroundings in which people live and conduct their life" (7, p. 36). An individual's home or discharge environment, performance contexts, and the setting for intervention must all be considered. Environments present demands and can also provide

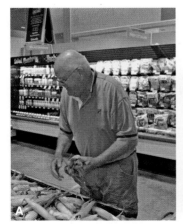
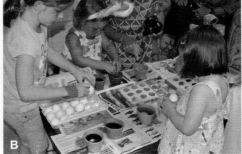
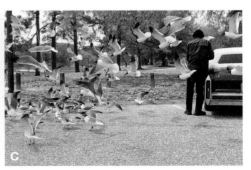

Figure 14.2. When a Person Engages in Occupation Through Doing, They Explore and Experience Their Effect on the World, Even While Performing Everyday Tasks Such as Grocery Shopping (A). Through Occupational Engagement, People Learn About Themselves, About Their Abilities to Use Tools and Materials, About the Pleasure of Working Directly With Their Hands, Bodies, and Minds (B, Children Decorating Eggs). Perhaps Most Importantly, Occupational Participation Provides Feedback About the Reactions of Others to What One Has Done, as the Gentleman in (C) Feeds the Birds at a Local Park as Part of His Daily Routine.

supports for activity performance. An **environmental demand** is an expectation for a certain kind of behavior or action that is evoked by something in the environment. Allen (1, 3) gives the example of the American flag stimulating a person to salute. Another environmental demand might be a family member who expects specific behaviors from the client (eg, the parent who requires their children to place their laundry in a basket). **Environmental support** is a feature of the environment that encourages and assists the individual to perform a particular behavior. A machine that dispenses premeasured packets of detergent and fabric softeners in a laundromat or college dorm laundry room is an example of environmental support.

Environmental supports may also be social or relational in the form of "people or animals that provide practical physical or emotional support, nurturing, protection, assistance, and relationships to other persons in the home, workplace, or school or at play or in other aspects of their daily activities" (7, p. 38). One such example is the case manager who regularly calls on clients to make sure that they have taken their medication. The occupational therapy professional can alter the demands and supports within the environment by adding or removing objects or people, by changing the arrangement of the furniture or the lighting, or in countless other ways. The purpose of this environmental manipulation is to stimulate clients to perform particular activities significant to their important roles, to engage more effectively in occupations, to develop skills, or acquire habits, and to enhance their sense of personal causation by providing opportunities for success. How to modify the environment and choose the proper level of stimulation is discussed within the context of activity analysis and adaptation throughout the remainder of the chapter.

Types of Occupational Therapy Interventions

When selecting which type of occupational therapy intervention to use with a particular client, the occupational therapy professional must consider the client's values, learning style and preferences, motivation, and readiness for change. It is essential that the activities and occupational forms chosen for therapy provide the person with experiences that are pleasurable, and that they reinforce and enhance a sense of competence and mastery (3, 23). To engage the person's interest and drive toward competency, interventions must provide a reasonable challenge. Occupational therapy intervention types include the use of occupations and activities. Targeted interventions related to specific client factors and areas of occupation are further covered in Chapters 17 to 23.

Intervention Implementation: The Roles of the Occupational Therapist and the Occupational Therapy Assistant

Intervention implementation is the enactment of the methods and activities outlined in the intervention plan. Although the OT has the overall responsibility for supervision of intervention implementation, competencies in the educational

programs for occupational therapy assistants (OTAs) ensure that the OTA professional can apply culturally relevant, client-centered, evidence-based, and occupation-centered interventions (6). Not only does this underscore the importance and benefit of the OTA's contribution to the intervention process but it also highlights the critical importance of the collaboration between the OT and the OTA (5).

Whose job is it to select intervention tasks and activities, the OT or the OTA? The answer is both, in collaboration with the client. Although OTs may preserve this responsibility in some practice contexts, more often, the OT calls upon the OTA to propose activities, or to work together in discussing which activities could and should be used for a particular client or group (8).

Regardless of the specific activity or approach employed, intervention should be executed thoughtfully with input from both occupational therapy professionals and with careful attention to the client's interest in and understanding of the intervention. The OTA will often have the responsibility, while carrying out the intervention, to be certain that the person is aware of the purpose of the intervention and should be prepared to continually provide reminders to help the client understand why it is important. Sometimes, clients with cognitive impairments or serious mental illness forget why occupational therapy is important, or they fail to make the connection between the specific intervention activities and how those activities are serving the client's priorities and goals (9, 10). Peloquin (20) provides timeless suggestions for how to help the client link the activities used with their purposes:

1. Explain the purpose of the group or activity.
2. Encourage the client to think about the purpose and ask them to share this view.
3. Discuss the skills used and link them to the activities or tasks performed.
4. Summarize what has transpired.

This four-step process ensures that the occupational therapy professional has verbalized the purposes to the client and has engaged the client in understanding the purpose of the occupational therapy intervention.

TYPES OF OCCUPATIONAL THERAPY INTERVENTIONS

The various types of occupational therapy interventions "facilitate engagement in occupation to enable persons, groups, and populations to achieve health, well-being, and participation in life" (7, p. 4). According to the *OTPF-4*, occupational therapy types include occupations and activities, interventions to support occupations, education and training, advocacy, group interventions, and virtual interventions (7). If we refer to our metaphor of the home as the structure that houses the client's occupational being and day-to-day occupations, in the previous chapter we described the occupational therapy professionals' role in intervention planning as collaborating with our client to do maintenance, or remodeling, repairing, and in some cases rebuilding (similar to deciding an occupational therapy approach), to improve the value and quality of their homes. The types of occupational therapy interventions are the pathways leading to supporting the client's desired changes in occupation. The types of occupational therapy interventions are briefly reviewed next.

Occupations, Activities, and Interventions to Support Occupation

When occupations and activities are chosen and incorporated into intervention for certain clients, the activity itself is constructed around criteria that meet the objectives and goals meant to improve aspects of the clients' underlying priorities and needs. **Occupations** can be either broad or narrow and specific daily life events that are personally relevant to the client's situation and context. **Activities** are described as components of occupations that are ***not specific*** to the client's context and which have aspects that can be objectively described or defined. According to the *OTPF-4*, "Activities as interventions are selected and designed to support the development of performance skills and performance patterns to enhance occupational engagement" (7, p. 59).

Any intervention that supports the client's optimal occupational experience or prepares them for occupational performance may be used as a part of occupational therapy intervention sessions. The *OTPF-4* categorizes these as **Interventions to Support Occupations** (7, p. 59). These interventions that support or enhance occupation can be used either in readying the client for occupation or used simultaneously with the occupation or activity. Lastly, supportive occupational interventions can be introduced or provided in the context of engagement in occupations in the client's home or natural environment to encourage the safety, quality, or efficacy of daily performance in occupation (7). Types of interventions to support occupations include the following:

- Physical agent modalities (PAMs) and mechanical modalities: Any modality, device or technique that prepares the client for occupational performance. For example, the use of thermal agents (heat packs or ice) is sometimes incorporated in therapy to address pain or prepare muscles and joints for movement (with the planned outcome being improved occupational function and engagement in occupation). The occupational therapy professional must only implement interventions that support occupations as preparation for engagement; the use of these modalities in isolation is contrary to the expectations of occupation-focused outcomes (7).
- Orthotics and prosthetics: This category of occupation-supportive intervention includes the creation of devices that the client uses to mobilize, immobilize, or support body structures so that they are more successful in participating in occupations that are most significant to them. An example of this would be a practitioner fabricating a splint that allows a client with carpal tunnel syndrome to more effectively complete tasks at work (7).

- Assistive technology and environmental modifications: An occupational therapy professional can assess, select, and provide training in the use of assistive technology, often applying universal design principles, and making recommendations for changing the environment or the occupation to improve or enhance the client's capacity for occupational engagement (7).
- Wheeled mobility: Advances in technology, engineering, and design have given way to a plethora of seating and positioning products that can be implemented into interventions, allowing clients to maneuver through space more efficiently while also reducing risks for contracture or skin breakdown (7).
- Self-regulation: Self-regulatory interventions are "Actions the client performs to target specific client factors or performance skills. Intervention approaches may address sensory processing to promote emotional stability in preparation for social participation or work or leisure activities or executive functioning to support engagement in occupation" (7, p. 60).

Education and Training and Advocacy

When an occupational therapy professional provides education, or translates knowledge that is useful in helping the client or the client's caregivers develop or acquire behaviors, habits, roles, or routines that promote their well-being and occupational participation, the type of intervention is education. Training is a type of intervention where the occupational therapy professional facilitates the client's acquisition of concrete skills necessary for meeting specific goals in a realistic and ecologically relevant life situation. "Training is differentiated from education by its goal of enhanced performance as opposed to enhanced understanding" (7, p. 60).

The profession of occupational therapy is grounded in the principles of advocacy and so there is a natural progression to have two types of occupational therapy interventions that emerge from advocacy. The *OTPF-4* (7) defines advocacy as efforts that aim to promote occupational justice and enable clients to secure resources that positively impact health and participation. Advocacy efforts can be undertaken by the occupational therapy professional, on behalf of their client, and considered as an intervention type. The second form of advocacy intervention type described by the *OTPF-4* (7) is self-advocacy. In self-advocacy, the client undertakes efforts to advocate for themselves and the occupational therapy professional is in a more supportive role. Self-advocacy is one of the major pillars of the recovery movement, and so practitioners who work in community mental health settings frequently implement this type of occupational therapy intervention (11).

Group Interventions and Virtual Interventions

Group interventions are one of the most widely used intervention types and methods of service delivery in psychosocial settings (13). Group interventions use "distinct knowledge of the dynamics of group and social interaction and leadership techniques to facilitate learning and skill acquisition across the lifespan" (7, p. 62). Chapter 16 is dedicated to further exploring the application of group interventions in occupational therapy practice. Virtual interventions are interventions that allow the delivery of occupational therapy services that are absent of physical contact. The dimensions of these virtual interventions include simulated, real-time, and near real-time technologies to provide telehealth (telecommunication and information technology) and mHealth (ie, mobile app technologies) (7, p. 62).

ANALYZING, ADAPTING, AND GRADING ACTIVITIES

To the casual and uninformed observer, psychosocial aspects of occupational therapy practice may appear deceptively natural and easy. What could be more elementary supporting a client as they are performing everyday activities or arts and crafts projects? Despite appearances, these seemingly natural activities are possible only because the OT or OTA has often spent many hours carefully analyzing and reflecting upon a client's occupational profile, occupational performance analysis, and evaluation data. That clients are willing (motivated) and able to participate in meaningful occupation cannot be taken for granted. Only by selecting activities carefully, analyzing them thoroughly, and adapting and preparing them to match the needs and interests of the clients can occupational therapy professionals create a task environment that motivates clients and enables them to succeed.

This section discusses how to select, analyze, adapt, and grade activities to meet intervention goals for clients with mental health problems. Several methods of activity analysis are described, along with the rationale for choosing one over the others for a particular client or situation. General principles for adapting activities are outlined and examples are given. Finally, the chapter discusses the concept of gradation and considers some traditional methods for grading activities to promote a variety of skills and behaviors.

SELECTION OF ACTIVITIES

Two major factors are considered when selecting an activity. The first is how well it suits its purpose in the occupational therapy intervention process. In some cases, the activity must be modified or structured by the practitioner to suit the situation. Unless the activity is going to help provide assessment data or help the client reach intervention goals, there is no reason to consider it further. The second factor is the match or fit between the activity and the client. Is this client interested in this activity? Is it consistent with the client's values and personal goals? How does the client feel about doing the activity? Is it compatible with the person's age, sex, and sociocultural background? How does it help the client develop or maintain chosen or predicted occupational roles? Can the client do the activity at their current functional level?

Only activities that are well matched to the client should be considered. Although it is often possible to alter the way an activity is performed, or the materials that are used to do

it, these changes cannot be expected to compensate for the client finding the activity irrelevant or uninteresting, and unfortunately some necessary occupations may be considered tedious and boring but they are still are necessary for the client's overall well-being. The skilled practitioner will find ways to explain the purpose of necessary, but not particularly exciting interventions, or they will find other activity substitutions that still target the particular skills needed by the client, to progress their engagement in occupation.

ANALYSIS OF ACTIVITIES

To judge whether an activity will meet goals and be acceptable to the client, one must first analyze the activity. To do this, the occupational therapy professional must take the activity apart, examining each piece against concepts and theories drawn from professional and technical education and clinical experience. Every step of the activity, every tool and material used, and every social interaction it entails, all of these and many other aspects must be examined to determine whether the activity can do what it is meant to do for the client (obviously, an attempt must first be made to capture a holistic and thoughtful understanding of the client and all the client's enmeshed situations and contextual layers). An activity analysis, therefore, is the systematic breakdown of something complex (the activity) into its smaller, simpler parts.

Many formats and procedures have been used by OTs to analyze activities for mental health practice. Some of these are based on particular theories or practice models; these activity analysis formats emphasize specific aspects of the activity that are relevant to a particular theory. When a particular theory or practice model is used to plan intervention, the activity must be analyzed from the same perspective.

If an activity is to be used for assessment rather than intervention, the analysis will determine how well it can measure whatever is to be assessed (19). For instance, if the activity will be used to assess decision-making skills, it must provide choices and decision points. In addition, the occupational therapy professional must anticipate what outcomes and responses are possible, and what these different outcomes suggest about the client's ability to make decisions. The analysis of activities to be used as assessment is always the responsibility of the OT as opposed to the OTA (6). Another type of activity analysis explores all the possibilities and potentials of an activity without reference to a particular intervention goal or client. This may be a useful exercise to help students appreciate the multiple facets of activity and develop a habit of thinking of how activities might be used but it is not sufficiently specific to be useful in a clinical situation (17).

ADAPTATION OF ACTIVITY

Often, the occupational therapy professional will analyze activities so as to adapt them to help a particular client reach an identified intervention goal. **Adaptation** is *a change that facilitates performance.* Adaptation may entail a change in the task or the environment. To analyze the possibilities for adaptation of an activity, the occupational therapy professional must start by identifying and describing the activity as exactly as possible. To illustrate, making a cup of coffee may be adding instant coffee to a cup of boiling water; it may be using a single service coffee pod in an instant coffee maker, or it may be grinding the coffee beans and then using a sophisticated machine to brew an espresso. These are three *different* activities. Thus, the first step in analysis is a complete description of the materials, tools, and procedures used in the activity. Any equipment needed and the kind of environment where the activity will be performed must also be identified.

The second step is to clarify the relationship between the activity and the intervention goals for the client. Why is this a good activity for this client? What purposes does it serve? What functional outcomes does it address? The third step is to analyze further all aspects of the activity that might affect the client's performance and to consider how one could modify or design them to better meet the client's needs. For example, fixing a clogged toilet, sink, or shower drain, or knowing what to do if that situation happens, is a very necessary household maintenance task that people may need to know about when they are learning to live alone. How might this activity be taught, and over how many sessions? Should visual reminders or written procedures be posted somewhere in the bathroom, or is this an activity that the client may need assistance with, and if so, who can help provide support for these types of problems? Is it better for the occupational therapy professional to teach the activity to the client individually or in a small group? These are only a few of the questions to be considered.

Box 14.1 provides a general structure for analyzing and designing an activity to address specific goals of a particular client. Because activity analysis and occupational performance analysis are such core aspects of occupational therapy, this is a skill set that the occupational therapy professional will frequently use in clinical practice. The outline in Box 14.1 can be used as a foundation and other types of analyses can be added when needed (eg, if a specific practice model is used).

BOX 14.1 Activity Analysis Outline

i. General information
  a. Name of activity
  b. Context where this activity will occur (specific setting)
    1. Special features of environment (eg, equipment, safety requirements)
    2. Space per person to do this activity
  c. Breakdown of activity
    1. List of materials and supplies
    2. List of tools and equipment
    3. Cost of materials and supplies for one performance or project
    4. Steps and key points of each step
ii. Fit or match among client, activity, and intervention goals
  a. Relationship of activity to goals
  b. Relationship of activity to client's interests, values, cultural background, age, sex, activity history, occupational roles, current skills and functional level, previous learning, and present and future environment
  c. Motivating reasons for this person to engage in this activity
iii. Time and space factors
  a. Time needed for entire activity (estimate for average person and for this client); if more than one session is needed, estimate number of sessions to complete activity.
  b. Number of steps in the activity and time needed for each step
    1. Minimum sustained attention needed to engage in each step
    2. Opportunity or need to repeat steps
    3. Possibilities for skipping, condensing, or rearranging order of steps
  c. Necessary delays (waiting time)
  d. Demands for rate of performance

  e. Therapist's modifications of environment to facilitate client's performance of activity
    1. Arrangement of furniture to increase or minimize interaction
    2. Provision for task and general lighting
    3. Control of distracting elements (eg, posters, sample projects, noise)
    4. Control of potential dangers in environment
    5. Positioning of client in relation to activity
      a. Placement of activity, tools, and materials
      b. Opportunity or need for client to move about, get up from chair, etc
iv. Materials and tools
  a. Potential hazards and precautions
  b. Sensory stimulation available (visual, auditory, tactile, olfactory, gustatory, kinesthetic)
  c. Physical properties (assess in relation to client's abilities and preferences)
    1. Resistance (strength required)
    2. Pliability and maneuverability of materials
    3. Controllability (ease with which material is controlled)
    4. Messiness
    5. Noisiness
    6. Effects on others present in environment (dust, smells, noise)
v. Processes involved
  a. Degree of difficulty of each step or process
  b. Technical knowledge required
  c. Presence of "magical" transformations or other phenomena that may be difficult for those with cognitive deficits to understand (eg, color change of glaze after firing)
  d. Sensory discrimination required (eg, of colors, textures)

(continued)

BOX 14.1 Activity Analysis Outline (*continued*)

 e. Perceptual demands (eg, for matching, spatial relationships)
 f. Physical factors and demands
  1. Coordination, both fine and gross
   a. Muscular control
   b. Dexterity and manipulative skill
  2. Strength
  3. Endurance
  4. Postural balance and control
  5. Range of motion
 g. Cognitive factors and demands
  1. Attention span and concentration
  2. Orientation to time, place, person, and activity
  3. Memory (need to retain or transfer learning from one situation to another)
  4. New learning required
  5. Prerequisite process skills (eg, literacy, measurement)
  6. Opportunities for reality testing and consensual validation
 h. Social factors and demands
  1. Individual or group activity
  2. Number of people present (staff, clients, family members, others)

 3. Interactions (both possible and necessary)
  a. Level of group interaction skill needed (parallel, project, egocentric–cooperative, cooperative, mature)
  b. Type of interpersonal transactions needed or possible (eg, giving and receiving help, depending on others, sharing tools or materials, cooperating, competing, providing leadership)
  4. Communication needed (how much, whether verbal or nonverbal)
 i. Opportunities and demands for expression
  1. Expression of feeling, in words or symbolically
  2. Exploration and discussion of feelings
vi. Design of instruction
 a. Type of directions (demonstration, oral direction, written direction, or diagrams)
 b. Unit of learning (number of steps taught at one time)
 c. Provisions for particular learning experiences (eg, modeling, feedback, trial-and-error experiences, practice and repetition, reality testing)
 d. External instructional aids provided (eg, stimulation, audiovisual aids, activity sample)
 e. Advance preparation of materials by someone other than client

To use any activity analysis format effectively, the occupational therapy professional must understand and know how to apply the principles of adaptation and gradation. **Adaptation** has many meanings. As discussed previously, for our purposes, it means the modification of the activity to facilitate performance, generally by modifying the task or the environment. Modifications to the task may include changing the tools, materials, directions, procedures, or rules. For instance, cross-stitch is typically done with a needle and thread on cross-stitch material, but other materials, such as yarn or heavier types of string, and different patterns or types of material that are easier to see and easier to manipulate, can be substituted. Projects may also be made smaller or larger. Adaptation of the environment may focus on physical aspects (the room, the lighting, the furniture) or social demands and social support (number of people involved, their demands on the client, the type and degree of assistance they provide). A game that is usually played by two people might be played by two teams instead. Or a person with cognitive disabilities might participate in meal preparation by peeling and cutting carrots as a part of a group rather than cooking independently.

The occupational therapy professional may adapt an activity to enable performance. The client who cannot do the activity in the usual way may be able to do it with modifications. For example, a client with a neurocognitive disorder and poor postural balance might not be able to execute traditional exercises but might be capable of less rigorous exercise while seated in a chair. Or someone with hand tremors, a side effect of some medications, might not be able to paint glaze with a brush on a ceramic project but might instead dip the project in glaze. Another very common example is that some clients with cognitive deficits find it difficult or impossible to start a stitch in leather lacing or knitting or sewing; however, if the therapist or a volunteer starts the stitch for them, they can often be successful in continuing with the stitching.

Another reason the occupational therapy professional might adapt an activity is to change its demands to make it more effective as an intervention. For instance, if the goal is for the client to assert themselves during group activities, the occupational therapy professional might provide fewer supplies and tools so that people have to share. In this task environment, the client must ask for what they need. Of course, activities are not infinitely adaptable. It is hard to change a crossword puzzle into something that can be done by a large group. One might argue that you could project the puzzle onto a screen so that everyone can see it or give each person a copy of the same puzzle or that partners could work in teams, but these adaptations may feel make the activity feel contrived. Adaptations should appear reasonable to the client and should support personal dignity and competence. If a group activity is required, an activity designed to be shared should be selected.

Occupational therapy professionals must possess both flexibility and good judgment to use the principle of adaptation effectively. They must envision the versatility of the activity and imagine how it could be changed. At the same time, however, they need enough common sense to recognize when the adaptation is excessive, impractical, or unacceptable to the client.

GRADATION OF ACTIVITY

Gradation is defined in the *Oxford English Dictionary* as "the process of advancing step by step; the course of gradual progress." In other words, a goal that is out of reach today can be attained by steady, stepwise movement, as shown in Figure 14.3. Gradation has been employed by OTs since the beginning of the profession. The OTA or OT designs a graded activity program so that clients begin where they are capable and make progress as rapidly as possible. Over time, the occupational therapy professional gradually adds new challenges so that clients can develop new abilities by building on what they have already done. Figure 14.3 demonstrates some of the ways that activities might be structured to provide increasing opportunities to make decisions; although 5 steps are shown, as many as 20 or 30 might actually be needed. In addition, choices other than those shown could be used to stimulate decision-making.

It requires imagination and logic to design a graded program of activities for many of the intervention goals common to psychiatric occupational therapy. Improvements in range of motion, increased strength that improves engagement in occupation, or other typical intervention goals of physical rehabilitation are concrete, visible, and easy to measure; they can be graded by performing simple physical procedures such as changing the position of the activity in relation to the client or adding weights, not so with some goals of psychiatric rehabilitation; as discussed several times throughout this text, many important psychiatric goals are intangible and difficult to measure. This imposes a relative uncertainty about how to approach them and how to grade activities to make them easier to reach.

The following sections address some of the ways in which activities can be graded to help clients work toward goals typical of psychiatric occupational therapy programs. These include increased ability and performance in the following areas: attention span; decision-making; problem solving; self-awareness; awareness of others; interaction with others; and independence, self-direction, and self-responsibility.

Attention Span

Attention span may also be called **sustained attention** and may be classified as a mental function or as a performance skill. It is the ability to keep attention focused on a task. A person can be required to work for increasingly long periods. For example, if the client can work for only 15 minutes without being distracted, the program should begin with 15-minute work periods. Gradually, the client would be asked to work for longer times without taking a break: 20, 30, 45 minutes, and so on. The amount by which the period increases and the rate at which the program progresses are based on the client's ability to tolerate increased demands. Generally, the clients should be expected to do as much as they can as quickly as they can, while still being safe and efficient, and to not forget that the quality of the occupational engagement is dependent on how the client experiences the participation (17). Finally, the program should be designed to accommodate day-to-day variations in ability and motivation that may occur because of medication, stress, or other contextual factors.

If a program is designed to help a client increase attention span, other factors that may interfere with this goal should be eliminated. The task should be one that is meaningful, one that the client is capable of doing, and one that really *does* require constant attention over time. If the client feels the task is meaningless, it is not reasonable to expect them to pay much attention to it. If the task is too difficult, the client may be too frustrated or anxious to try to do it for very long. Finally, tasks that take only a short time (eg, making coffee) or that people generally approach casually (picking them up and then stopping them to do something else, as knitting and many other crafts), for example, are not suitable activities for increasing attention span.

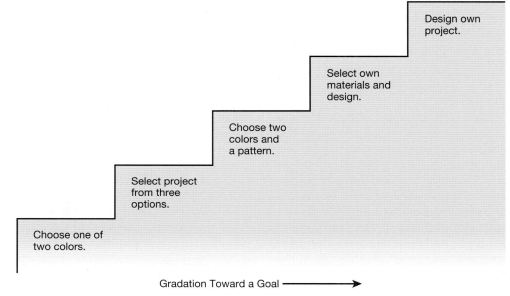

Gradation Toward a Goal ⟶

Figure 14.3. Gradation of Decision-Making. An Example of Gradation Toward a Goal.

Decision-Making

Someone accustomed to having other people take care of life's important details may find making decisions an unfamiliar and difficult process. Two kinds of clients who may find it hard to make even simple decisions are those who have been hospitalized for years and those whose families have controlled their environment and activities. A program to help someone improve their ability to make decisions must logically include many opportunities to face real choices and decide among them. It must also consider family members' resistance to change and must provide strategies to assist the family unit to be more accepting of change.

Some activities are easier than others to structure the number and kinds of choices presented to a client. Most crafts can be approached on a very simple level and then made increasingly complex. Historically, our profession used creative activities as occupational interventions, in part because these activities allow for flexibility in adapting and grading the occupational demands. However, craft activities will not appeal to some clients. Although a craft activity may be a safe place to begin helping a client learn to make decisions, other real-life decisions that are important to the client and functionally relevant must also be prioritized. Furthermore, it is the responsibility of the occupational therapy professional to collaborate with the client to figure out through assessments, development of the therapeutic relationship, collection of information to create an occupational profile, and occupational performance analyses, which activities might forge the route to helping the client develop the necessary skills, or make the appropriate adaptations, to help them move toward accomplishing their goals.

If the problem is that the person is quite inexperienced and does not know how to make decisions, instruction about how to generate alternatives and predict outcomes can be combined with simulations and consistent practice in the client's natural context. In the beginning, the client will not necessarily make sound decisions; but with encouragement to try again, discussion of what happened, and acceptance of the outcome, the client will have the support to refine this skill. Decision-making is an aspect of performance skills, as defined by the *OTPF-4* (7).

Problem Solving

Problem solving is an aspect of process skills and can be graded in a similar manner. One can begin with activities that have minor problems with relatively obvious solutions and little chance of failure. Gradually, more problematic activities and situations can be introduced. As with decision-making, it is important to work with problems that clients face in their everyday lives (eg, what to do when a family member asks for money, or how to get into one's apartment if the keys accidentally get locked inside). Again, specific instruction about how to analyze a problem and generate solutions should be interwoven with opportunities to practice these skills both in simulations and in real life.

Self-Awareness

This skill is associated with mental functions and performance skills (7). Self-awareness is a skill that has many developmental layers. At its most basic, it is the awareness of the body and its effects on the environment. Clients who have severe deficits may need to begin with sensorimotor activities. Usually, however, when we say that someone needs to develop greater self-awareness, we mean that the person is not in touch with their personal interests, talents, attributes, behaviors, and reactions to life events.

A graded program to develop a person's self-awareness and self-concept (ideas about the self) must include both experiences that allow an exploration of one's effect on the world and opportunities to discuss these experiences with other people. The choice of activities should be based on the interests and experience of the client. Almost any activity can be used, although most people agree that you can learn more about yourself through an expressive art activity or a game played with other people than you can from doing an activity in isolation. This suggests that suitable activities must provide either an expressive medium or interaction with others (or, if possible, both). The essential ingredient, however, is the opportunity to verbalize one's ideas and feelings and to receive feedback from others in a safe setting. Thus, it is not the activities that are graded but the way the occupational therapy professional structures the activities to encourage self-reflection and feedback.

Social Conduct and Interpersonal Skills

When we say that someone needs to develop skills in **social conduct** and **interpersonal skills**, we usually mean that the person disregards the needs or rights of other people. For the client to develop in this area, the occupational therapy professional provides activities that require interaction with other people, and that include opportunities to discuss and analyze what happens between them. Thus, as with awareness of self, a program to develop social conduct and interpersonal skills is graded in its demands for reflection, discussion, and analysis. Social conduct and interpersonal skills are associated with emotional regulation (a client factor) and with performance skills.

Clients who are socially isolated or who rely on a few rigid patterns of relating to other people can improve their social skills and comfort through a graded program to increase their level of social interaction. Activities are graded depending on how much involvement with other people is required and on the nature of the involvement. The occupational therapy professional must be careful not to make excessive demands for clients to become involved with other people. Interaction skills take a long time to develop and can improve only when the person is reasonably comfortable. Among the many factors the occupational therapy professional can vary to accommodate the client's needs are the frequency, length, and intensity of involvement with others. Many of these factors are most easily accommodated by implementing group interventions, which are further discussed in Chapter 16.

Independence, Self-Direction, and Self-Responsibility

Programs to help clients develop a greater sense of independence and self-direction require activities that can be graded in terms of how much the client must rely on the occupational therapy professional or other people for help. In other words, the program begins with an activity in which the client requires instruction from the occupational therapy professional. Gradually, as clients acquire more skills and knowledge, they will need the occupational therapy professional less. This does not necessarily mean that the client will ask for less help than at the beginning; often, the occupational therapy professional must initiate a discussion of what the client is able to do without assistance. Clients who are not accustomed to doing things on their own may not recognize that they are able to do so, or that they have done so. In this case, the therapist encourages clients to reflect on what they have done and to think about how little assistance they received. Activities that can be graded to increase independence and self-direction must be ones that require some instruction in the beginning, allow for increased mastery with practice over time, and are complex enough that they include opportunities to develop new skills and to make multiple decisions. Woodworking, leathercraft, and cooking meet these criteria.

MATCHING OCCUPATIONAL AND ACTIVITY DEMANDS TO INTERVENTION TYPES AND APPROACHES: ACTIVITY ANALYSIS BASED ON THEORY

We have discussed in a broad and general way how the principles of adaptation and gradation can be used to tailor an activity to meet the needs of clients of varying skill levels. Within a given practice model, occupational therapy professionals employ theory-based activity analysis. Claudia Allen's Cognitive Disabilities Model (3) is one example. In this model, factors that delineate the difficulty level of a task are matched with factors that are assessed to determine whether an activity is one that the client can perform successfully at a given level of cognitive function, according to the person's assessed cognitive level using the *Allen Cognitive Level Screen 5th Edition* (ACLS-5) (14). Using the same method of analysis, the occupational therapy professional can make an activity less demanding or more demanding.

The occupational therapy professional who is matching activity demands to intervention types, approaches, and client goals should be aware of some important concepts. Directions are instructions given by another person, most often the occupational therapy professional. Verbal directions use words; demonstrated directions instead use physical movements to model or demonstrate what is to be done. The occupational therapy professional may need to use hand-over-hand guidance or otherwise touch the client to teach what is to be done. However, best practices demand that all clients, regardless of their known trauma history,

should be approached applying trauma-informed care principles. One of those important principles of care is to *always* ask permission before placing your hands on a client. For clients who have experienced abuse, violence, or assault, being touched can be a triggering event (13). Physical properties of material objects are the kind of sensory information that the client must respond to in order to perform the activity. The client can act only upon what is known and perceived, so it is important to present the activity in a way that allows the client to understand it and act on it. The occupational therapy professional may need to draw attention to the qualities of objects and tools.

Motor actions are behaviors exhibited by clients. The number of actions, both different actions and repetitions of the same action, are considered. Tool use means whether tools are used and what kind of tools are used to do the activity. Stimulus for motor action refers to the kind of stimulation that will catch the client's attention and interest. The idea is that the stimulus motivates client engagement in the activity. Because the goal is for the client to do something (participate in occupation that they find meaningful), we need to know what kind of stimulation will help the client initiate the task.

Allen (1) explains how to present each of these aspects of the task for each of the six cognitive levels that are part of the Cognitive Disabilities Model. We can use this information to design activities so that clients will be able to find success. A brief description of the cognitive levels and associated interventions follows.

Level 1

The person functioning at level 1 is aware only of what penetrates the threshold of conscious awareness. Therefore, louder than normal, one-to-two-word directions, and physical contact are needed to start the action. It is characteristic that a person at level 1.0 can do only one action at a time and may not repeat it unless prompted. For example, the occupational therapy professional might get the person to bring their spoon to their mouth, by touching their hand and saying "Arm up" in a loud voice. By contrast, the person probably would not mirror the actions of the occupational therapy professional or peers who brought their hand to their mouth, nor would they be likely to follow a verbal request alone (1, 3).

Level 2

Persons at level 2 are aware of their own movements and those of others and can perform simple gross motor actions that have been demonstrated by the therapist. Movement-based and sensorimotor activities can be used. The person will not understand how to use tools but will show interest in simple familiar objects, such as balls and jump ropes. The verbal directions can include names of body parts but the therapist must also demonstrate the desired action. Each demonstration is limited to one action at a time; repetitions or variations on the same action can be introduced (1, 3).

Level 3

The person at level 3 is more aware of surroundings, particularly objects that can be seen and touched. The person enjoys hand movements that are repeated and will participate in activities that have a repetitive manual action. The person enjoys performing the action of the activity but fails to comprehend the end product or goal. For example, the client will string beads but not understand that a necklace or bracelet might be made this way. The directions can include the names of objects used in the action but the action must also be demonstrated. The same action is repeated over and over (1, 3).

Level 4

The person at level 4 is motivated by a desire to do the project rather than by an interest in the motions involved. The person is interested in the color and shape of objects and materials and prefers contrasting colors and clear shapes. The activity can have several steps but each must be demonstrated separately and then performed by the person before the next step is demonstrated. The spoken directions can include adjectives and adverbs that clarify the standards of performance. The person can use simple tools, such as scissors and hammers, but may be confused by tools that hide part of the project, such as when a stapler or hole punch covers the pages (1, 3).

Level 5

Individuals at level 5 can perform most activities that can be demonstrated and the demonstrations can include up to three steps at a time. Because the person at this level is aware of space and depth and the relations between objects, the verbal directions can include prepositions and terms about spatial relationships. Activities that require understanding of a spatial pattern (eg, mosaics) can be introduced. The person can use all hand tools and will spontaneously experiment with different ways to use them to obtain varying results. New learning may be self-initiated (1, 3).

Level 6

At level 6, the individual can understand abstract ideas. Written directions and diagrams can be used and demonstrations may not be required. The possible range of activities is unlimited.

Allen's task analysis methods can be used to select, adapt, and grade activities to make it easier for the person to succeed. For example, arranging and spacing mosaic tiles is a poor choice of activity for someone at level 4 but is perfectly suitable for someone at level 5. A person at level 4 who says they are interested in making a mosaic tile trivet is probably responding to how the project looks rather than the process used to make it. Therefore, the occupational therapy professional can substitute something that gives a similar appearance but requires less complex thought (eg, making a trivet but eliminating spacing and grouting from the process). Allen's work addresses the range of abilities (modes) in each of the six levels and provides details on adapting and grading activities to meet individual task abilities (1, 3).

MATCHING OCCUPATIONAL AND ACTIVITY DEMANDS TO INTERVENTION TYPES AND APPROACHES: DYNAMIC PERFORMANCE ANALYSIS

Analyzing an activity without the client present can introduce errors. The occupational therapy professional may assume that the client possesses skills that they, in fact, do not have. A mismatch between the analysis and the client's actual capacity to perform will result in frustration for the client. Our goal is always to facilitate safe, accurate, and engaged performance; this means we must endeavor to reduce errors and prevent the client from practicing things in ineffective or dangerous ways that risk the development of habits that do not support their optimal occupational engagement.

Dynamic performance analysis (DPA) is a method for analyzing the activity during client performance of the activity (21).

Observation and therapist reflection provide opportunities to reteach and otherwise adapt the activity to enable more effective performance. Figure 14.4 shows the DPA decision-making process of the therapist observing the client perform an activity.

MATCHING OCCUPATIONAL AND ACTIVITY DEMANDS TO INTERVENTION TYPES AND APPROACHES: ANALYSIS FOR A TASK-ORIENTED OR TASK-SPECIFIC APPROACH

The **task-oriented approach** (22) or **task-specific approach** (12) may be used for clients with severe cognitive limitations acquired as a result of a neurocognitive disorder. Because **procedural memory** (remembering how to do things) may be retained even when **declarative memory** (remembering facts) is lost, the person with dementia may be trained to succeed in performing activities and occupations that are familiar and valued. An activity that fits with client and family priorities is chosen. The therapy practitioner analyzes the activity to determine whether it might be possible for the client to perform particular aspects of the occupation.

Analysis includes the client's learning style (eg, visual vs auditory), tolerance for a period of instruction, and possible external contextual memory supports that would be helpful for this person, in this specific activity (such as the presence of others or the use of lists, alarm clocks, or signs). Presentation of the activity is planned to incorporate **errorless learning** so that the client does not experience failure or the confusion of unsuccessful attempts. The client is deterred from the activity (not allowed to proceed) if an error occurs. Instead, the occupational therapy professional intervenes and reinstructs. Thus, every attempt is successful (with the occupational therapy professional's intervention) and is practiced repeatedly until the client can perform the task on their own.

Performer Prerequisites

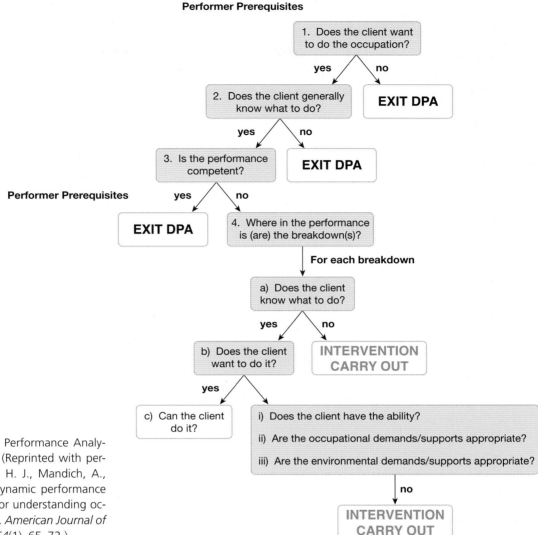

Figure 14.4. Dynamic Performance Analysis (DPA) Decision Tree. (Reprinted with permission from Polatajko, H. J., Mandich, A., & Martini, R. (2000). Dynamic performance analysis: A framework for understanding occupational performance. *American Journal of Occupational Therapy, 54*(1), 65–72.)

FROM EVALUATION TO OUTCOMES: CIRCLING BACK TO OUTCOMES

The *Examples of General Goals of Occupational Therapy* shared in Table 14.1, the format used in the *Activity Analysis Outline* (Box 14.1), and the *Dynamic Performance Analysis Decision Tree* shown in Figure 14.4, might appear highly detailed and complex. However, this is the nature of occupations and of the clients whom we collaborate with. Occupational therapy professionals analyze an activity in detail by considering the individual parts and steps. In occupational therapy practice, we generally begin with the client and the client's goals and then analyze how we can use occupations in interventions in ways that might address their individualized goals. Occupational therapy professionals use techniques of adaptation, changing the task itself, or the environment, to enable or enhance participation in meaningful occupations. To assist clients to reach goals that are more demanding than their current level of abilities, occupational therapy professionals also apply the principle of gradation, or gradual

movement toward a goal by small, successive steps. Adaptation and gradation, based on skillful and thorough activity analysis, task analysis, and occupational performance analysis, permits a range of possibilities for meeting intervention goals. The intervention process culminates with realization of outcomes.

Outcomes are the end result of the occupational therapy process that begins with screening and evaluation. There are essentially two types of outcomes. Some outcomes describe the occupational therapy intervention goals that clients have attained related to engagement in occupation. This type of outcome provides measurable guideposts that can be used in planning interventions and for discharge planning (7). "Other outcomes are experienced by clients when they have realized the effects of engagement in occupation and are able to return to desired habits, routines, roles, and rituals" (7, p. 65). Regardless of the type of outcome, adaptation is a part of all occupational therapy outcomes and analysis helps occupational therapy professionals reflect upon the best way to help the client adapt and thrive.

Case Study – A 40-Year-Old Man With Intellectual Developmental Disorder and Down Syndrome

Client: Antoine B.

DSM-5-TR Diagnosis at Admission

F71   Moderate Intellectual Developmental Disorder

ICD-10-CM

Q90.9 Down syndrome, unspecified

Antoine is a 40-year-old Black male with Down syndrome and moderate intellectual developmental disorder who was referred by his primary medical doctor and his family for evaluation at the community behavioral mental health center near his home. Antoine has lived in a small apartment home for almost 15 years. The apartment home was once used as a rental property and belongs to his parents. It is adjacent to his family's home and has allowed Antoine to live semi-independently while still having family support and supervision. Antoine works 2 days a week at a local hardware store sorting and labeling merchandise and helping in the outdoor gardening area. Antoine has gotten along well with the people he works with and with his vocational rehabilitation specialist; however, he also has a noted history of threatening behavior toward family members, and most recently unintentionally caused a fire in his home apartment kitchen while preparing a meal, forgetting to turn off the burner on his stove. His family reports that he has also forgotten to take his medications several times in the past weeks; they are worried about leaving him unsupervised because his mood becomes negative when he is isolated and has unstructured time. As a part of the initial occupational therapy evaluation, the OT assessed his functional cognitive status to see how that may be impacting his daily activities such as preparing his meals and managing his medications.

Following the evaluation, the team at the community mental health center recommended that Antoine would be the safest if he had some level of support and supervision on the days of the week that he was not working at the hardware store. He and his family decided that Antoine would like to attend an adult day care center 3 days a week. The day center employs an OT and an OTA who collaboratively work with the day clients on a variety of occupations and run various instrumental activities of daily living (IADL) and activities of daily living (ADL) skills groups. Antoine begins to thrive at the center, making new friends and practicing functional independence skills that allow him to perform daily tasks such as meal preparation more safely with appropriate supports. Together with the OT or the OTA, Antoine learned to work in the snack bar and coffee shop at the day center. Part of his responsibility will be counting the money collected each day that he is there and keeping track of the weekly totals for deposit. His OT conducted the following occupational analysis with Antoine to help plan the most effective activities for intervention and to help Antoine develop his skills to perform this new task role. After studying the occupational performance analysis shown in Boxes 14.2 and 14.3, discuss the answers to case study questions given in the OT HACKS Summary.

BOX 14.2 Example A: Activity Analysis

Activity description: performing end of the business day accounting tasks to close out cash register and balance/secure assets in a retail setting

Occupations		
Occupation		**Subcategory**
Activities of daily living		
Instrumental activities of daily living	✓	Financial management; safety and emergency management
Education		
Work	✓	Employment interests and pursuits; job performance and maintenance; volunteer participation
Play		
Leisure		
Social participation	✓	Community participation; peer group participation; friendships
Rest and sleep		
Health management		

1. Objects and their properties required: cash register, money from cash register, pencil, spreadsheet to input numbers (for data entry in computer), key to unlock cash in safe, accounting binder to find numbers and relevant daily tallies
2. Space demands: plenty of space on table to leave room for counting money
3. Social demands: communication with peer or partner to ensure money is being counted accurately

BOX 14.2 Example A: Activity Analysis (*continued*)

4. Sequence and timing:
   (List all steps to complete the entire activity.)

   1. Obtain key to unlock safe.
   2. Grab cash drawer out of safe and place on table.
   3. Go to register and close out for the day.
   4. Obtain number of sales and write down on spreadsheet.
   5. Grab cash drawer out of register and bring to table for counting.
   6. Count all cash in both drawers and write down how much of each kind of money is there (1s, 5s, 10s, 20s, pennies, nickels, dimes, quarters).
   7. Write down amounts.
   8. Place numbers into snack bar database.
   9. Print paper out.
   10. Three-hole punch paper and place in accounting binder under appropriate month tab.
   11. Return both cash drawers to safe and return key.

Body Functions

Function	Essential to Task	Greatly Challenged	Description
Specific Mental Functions			
Higher level cognitive: judgment, concept formation, metacognition, executive functions, praxis, cognitive flexibility, insight	✓		Ability to be cognitively flexible to ensure all money is being accounted for
Attention: sustained attention and concentration; selective, divided, and shifting attention	✓		Ability to maintain attention to task to ensure all money is accounted for
Memory: short-term, working, and long-term memory	✓		Ability to remember how much money is counted
Perception: discrimination of sensations—auditory, tactile, visual, olfactory, gustatory, vestibular, and proprioceptive			
Thought: control and content of thought, awareness of reality, logical and coherent thought	✓		Ability to form thoughts related to counting money accurately and precisely
Sequencing complex movement: regulating speed, response, quality, and time of motor production	✓		Ability to sequence movements to count money and perform tasks in the correct order, completing the task in a reasonable amount of time.
Emotional: regulation and range of emotion, appropriateness of emotions		✓	Ability to control emotions to count money accurately
Experience of self and time: appropriateness and range of emotion, body image, self-concept (instructor role)			
Global Mental Functions			
Consciousness: awareness and alertness, clarity, and continuity of the wakeful state	✓		Ability to be alert and aware to make sure money is counted correctly and steps are being completed in correct order
Orientation: orientation to person and self, place, time, and others	✓		Able to make sure money is protected and aware of surroundings
Temperament and personality: extroversion, introversion, agreeableness, and conscientiousness; emotional stability; openness to experience; self-expression; confidence; motivation; self-control and impulse control; appetite	✓		Able to control impulses to ensure money is corrected and stays where it should
Energy and drive: motivation, impulse control, appetite	✓		Able to control impulse to ensure correct amount of money is being kept safe and counted correctly
Sleep: physiologic process	✓		

(*continued*)

BOX 14.2 Example A: Activity Analysis (*continued*)

Function	Essential to Task	Greatly Challenged	Description
Sensory Functions			
Visual: quality of vision, visual acuity, visual stability, visual field	✓		Able to see money to ensure it is being counted correctly
Hearing: sound detection and discrimination, awareness of location and distance of sounds			
Vestibular: position, balance, secure movement against gravity		✓	Able to move about freely in space to ensure tasks are being completed
Taste: qualities of bitterness, sweetness, sourness, and saltiness			
Smell: sensing odors and smells			
Proprioceptive: awareness of body position and space	✓		Able to be aware of body positioning to move freely around the environment to ensure all tasks are being completed
Touch: feeling of being touched, touching various textures			
Pain: localized and generalized pain			
Temperature and pressure: thermal awareness, sense of force applied to skin			
Neuromusculoskeletal and Movement-Related Functions			
Joint mobility: joint range of motion (ROM)	✓		Able to have wrist ROM to count money and perform fine motor tasks
Joint stability: structural integrity of joint	✓		Able to have wrist stability to count money and perform fine motor tasks
Muscle Functions			
Muscle power: strength	✓		Able to carry cash drawer from safe to table
Muscle tone: degree of muscle tension	✓		Able to carry cash drawer from safe to table
Muscle endurance: sustaining a muscle contraction (repetition)	✓		Able to sustain fine motor movements for, respectively, counting cash and coins
Movement Functions			
Motor reflexes: involuntary reflexes— involuntary contractions of muscles automatically induced by stretching (protective stretch reflex)	✓		Able to use reflexes to contract muscles when performing fine motor tasks
Involuntary movement reactions: postural, body adjustment, and supporting reactions	✓		Able to position self against table and able to utilize fine motor upper extremity (UE) movements
Control of voluntary movement: eye– hand and eye–foot coordination, bilateral integration, crossing midline, fine and gross motor control, oculomotor control	✓		Able to utilize hand–eye coordination to count and visualize money
Gait patterns: movements used to walk			
Voice and Speech; Digestive, Metabolic, and Endocrine Systems; and Genitourinary and Reproductive Systems Functions			
Voice and speech: rhythm and fluency, alternative vocalization functions		✓	Ability to communicate to peer how much money is being counted
Digestive, metabolic, and endocrine systems			
Genitourinary and reproductive systems: urinary, genital, and reproductive functions			

BOX 14.2 Example A: Activity Analysis (*continued*)

Function	Essential to Task	Greatly Challenged	Description
Skin and Related Structures and Functions			
Skin: protection and repair	✓		Protection from pathogens, from money, and paper cuts
Hair and nails	✓		Protection from pathogens

Muscular Analysis of Movement

Muscle	Not Used	Minimally Challenged	Greatly Challenged
Shoulder flexion		✓	
Shoulder extension		✓	
Shoulder abduction		✓	
Shoulder adduction			✓
Shoulder internal rotation			✓
Shoulder external rotation		✓	
Elbow flexion			✓
Elbow extension			✓
Forearm supination			✓
Forearm pronation			✓
Wrist flexion			✓
Wrist extension			✓
Wrist radial deviation			✓
Wrist ulnar deviation			✓
Thumb flexion			✓
Thumb extension			✓
Thumb abduction			✓
Thumb adduction			✓
Thumb opposition			✓
Finger flexion			✓
Finger extension			✓
Finger abduction			✓
Finger adduction			✓
Trunk flexion			✓
Trunk extension			✓
Trunk lateral flexion			✓
Trunk rotation			✓
Lower extremities—describe			

Body Structures

Category	Body Structure	Required for Activity Participation?
Nervous system	Frontal lobe: *Gray Matter Concentration, attention, insight, motivation*	Yes
	Temporal lobe	Yes
	Parietal lobe: *touch, awareness of body position in space*	Yes
	Occipital lobe	Yes
	Midbrain: *execution of learned movements, discrimination of senses, proprioception*	Yes
	Diencephalon: *execution of learned movements, discrimination of senses, proprioception*	Yes

(continued)

BOX 14.2   Example A: Activity Analysis (*continued*)

Body Structures

Category	Body Structure	Required for Activity Participation?
	Basal ganglia: *crossing midline, walking patterns, GMC*	Yes
	Cerebellum: *eye–foot coordination, bilateral integration, crossing midline, muscle tone*	Yes
	Brainstem	Yes
	Cranial nerves	Yes
	Spinal cord: *muscle tone*	Yes
	Spinal nerves	Yes
	Meninges	Yes
	Sympathetic nervous system	Yes
	Parasympathetic nervous system	Yes
Eyes, ears, and related structures	Eyeball: conjunctiva, cornea, iris, retina, lens, vitreous body	Yes
	Structures around the eye: lachrymal glans, eyelid, eyebrow, external ocular muscles	Yes
	Structures of external ear	
	Structures of the middle ear: tympanic membrane, Eustachian canal, ossicles	Yes
	Structures of the inner ear: cochlea, vestibular labyrinth, semicircular canals, internal auditory meatus	Yes
Voice and speech structures	Structures of the mouth: teeth, gums, hard plate, soft palate, tongue, lips	
	Structure of the pharynx: nasal pharynx and oral pharynx	Yes
	Structure of the larynx: vocal folds	
Cardiovascular system	Heart: atria, ventricles	Yes
	Arteries	Yes
	Veins	Yes
	Capillaries	Yes
Immunologic system	Lymphatic system	Yes
	Lymphatic nodes	Yes
	Thymus	Yes
	Spleen	Yes
	Bone marrow	Yes
Respiratory system	Trachea	Yes
	Lungs: bronchial tree, alveoli	Yes
	Thoracic cage	Yes
	Muscles of respiration: intercostal muscles, diaphragm	Yes
Digestive, metabolic, and endocrine systems	Salivary glands	Yes
	Esophagus	Yes
	Stomach	Yes
	Intestines: small and large	Yes
	Pancreas	Yes
	Liver	Yes
	Gallbladder and ducts	Yes
	Endocrine glands: pituitary, thyroid, parathyroid, adrenal	Yes

BOX 14.2 Example A: Activity Analysis (*continued*)

Body Structures

Category	Body Structure	Required for Activity Participation?
Genitourinary and reproductive systems	Urinary system: kidneys, ureters, bladder, urethra	Yes
	Structure of pelvic floor	Yes
	Structure of reproductive system: ovaries, uterus, breast/nipple, vagina and external genitalia, testes, penis, prostate	
Structures related to movement	Bones of cranium	Yes
	Bones of neck region	Yes
	Joints of head and neck	Yes
	Bones of shoulder region	Yes
	Joints of the shoulder region	Yes
	Muscles of the shoulder region	Yes
	Bones of the upper arm	Yes
	Elbow joint	Yes
	Muscles of upper arm	Yes
	Ligaments and fascia of upper arm	Yes
	Bones of the forearm	Yes
	Wrist joint	Yes
	Muscles of the forearm	Yes
	Ligaments and fascia of forearm	Yes
	Bones of the hand	Yes
	Joints of hand and fingers	Yes
	Muscles of hand	Yes
	Ligaments and fascia of hand	Yes
	Bones of the pelvic region	Yes
	Joints of the pelvic region	Yes
	Muscles of the pelvis region	Yes
	Ligaments and fascia of the pelvic region	Yes
	Bones of thigh	
	Hip joint	
	Muscles of thigh	
	Ligaments and fascia of thigh	
	Bones of lower leg	
	Knee joint	
	Muscles of lower leg	
	Ligaments and fascia of lower leg	
	Bones of ankle and foot	
	Ankle, foot, and toe joints	
	Muscles of the ankle and foot	
	Ligaments of fascia of ankle and foot	
	Cervical vertebral column	Yes
	Lumbar vertebral column	Yes
	Sacral vertebral column	Yes
	Muscles of trunk	Yes
	Ligaments and fascia of trunk	Yes

(*continued*)

BOX 14.2 Example A: Activity Analysis (*continued*)

Body Structures

Category	Body Structure	Required for Activity Participation?
Skin and related structures	Areas of skin: head, neck, shoulder, UE, pelvic region, lower extremities, trunk, back	Yes
	Structures of skin glands: sweat and sebaceous	Yes
	Structures of nails: fingernails and toenails	Yes
	Structure of hair	

Performance Skills

Skill Name	Essential to Activity	Required Level to Perform Activity (Low, Moderate, High)	Description
		Motor Skills	
Aligns		Moderate	Aligns to table to ensure posture allows ability to count money effectively
Stabilizes		Moderate	Able to move through the room collecting materials without propping or loss of balance
Positions		Moderate	Positions self appropriately at the table to allow UE movements to be conducive to task
Reaches		Moderate	Extends arm to reach for money and cash drawers
Bends		Low	
Grips		High	Able to grip cash and coins for counting
Manipulates		High	Able to grasp and manipulate cash and coins for counting
Coordinates		High	Uses both hands to count money to allow for no slipping or fumbling
Moves		Moderate	Pushes and pulls cash drawers to make easier for reaching and counting
Lifts		Moderate	Lifts cash drawers
Walks			
Transports		Moderate	Carries cash drawers from place to place
Calibrates		Moderate	Handles paper money appropriately, to not tear bills
Flows		Moderate	Able to demonstrate fluid arm and wrist motions when counting money
Endures			
Paces			
		Process Skills	
Paces		Moderate	Performs task within a reasonable amount of time
Attends		Moderate	Does not get distracted by other clients or environmental stimuli
Heeds		Moderate	Follows protocol in gaining entry to safe
Chooses		Moderate	
Uses		Moderate	Uses cardboard coin holders to hold money while sorting and counting
Handles			
Inquires		Moderate	Asks for assistance when having difficulty
Initiates		High	Puts daily totals into the spreadsheet (database on computer)

BOX 14.2 Example A: Activity Analysis (*continued*)

Performance Skills

Skill Name	Essential to Activity	Required Level to Perform Activity (Low, Moderate, High)	Description
Continues		Moderate	Finishes counting money, continues by adding individual amounts together (using calculator)
Sequences		High	Sorts and counts money from higher bills to lower bills, similar sequence for counting coins
Terminates		Moderate	
Searches/locates			
Gathers			
Organizes		High	Writes down tally for each type of bill or coin, to add all together using a calculator at the end of task
Restores		High	All cash is returned to safe and safe is restored to a locked position.
Navigates			
Notices/responds		High	Notices when there is not enough of a particular bill or coin in daily drawer and responds by making appropriate exchanges with money in the safe to ensure that the next day's drawer is adequate to provide customer change the following day
Adjusts			
Accommodates			
Benefits			

BOX 14.3 Example B: An Excerpt From Antoine's Occupational Performance Analysis (Skills Rating)

Client Name: *Antoine B.*

Date: April 15, 2026

Occupational Therapist or Occupational Therapy Assistant: J. Coffey OTR/L

Client's Goals and Objectives

LTG: Antoine will adjust activities and responsibilities at home and work to the level of his cognitive capacity, asking for help when needed, and cooperating with others who provide assistance or oversight.

Objective 1: In his role as manager of the Adult Day Center Snack Bar & Coffee Shop, Antoine will initiate and complete assigned accounting tasks in 30 min with <3 verbal prompts 75% of the time within 2 mo.

Objective 2: During his time at the Adult Care Center, Antoine will demonstrate use of a systematic approach to problem solving, by linking new recurring activities to existing recurring activities (ie, behavioral chaining) at least 2 times, within 2 wk.

LTG: Antoine will safely and efficiently manage his medications.

Objective 1: Antoine will demonstrate an awareness of times to take medications (2 times daily) and follow through, with a minimum of one verbal prompt, 90% of the time by 1 mo.

Objective 2: In his home setting, Antoine will recognize that his medication is empty and will refill the prescription independently 3/5 times over the next 3 mo.

Task performed/activity description: Client is doing accounting work for the money taken in from the snack bar and coffee shop at the Adult Day Center. Client must count the money in the register by obtaining, tallying, and recording total daily sales; the client must find what the starting cash count was in the register from the prior day, count money in the register, and input the new amount into the computer database, to ensure that the money count is accurate from day to day at the snack bar.

Context where this activity will occur (specific setting): The end of the day closing accounting process takes place in the business office at the Adult Day Center. There is a large worktable in the center of the room where the client can stand or be seated to count the money drawer and tally and record the totals. A basket on the table holds paper, pens, pencils, and calculators. Behind the table, there is a workstation with a computer for Antoine to use to enter the daily totals onto a simplified spreadsheet that has been designed for Antoine to be able to easily enter daily data. The safe is in the closet of the business office. The rooms have adequate lighting and enough space for Antoine to move around while performing his tasks.

(continued)

BOX 14.3 Example B: An Excerpt From Antoine's Occupational Performance Analysis (Skills Rating) (*continued*)

Motor and Process Skill Ratings

Instructions: Circle the rating that best matches the observed quality of performance. Also record the observed performance / rationale for each rating.

Rating (based on level of observed problems):

No = none, **Mi** = mild, **Mo** = moderate, or **Ma** = marked

Performance Skills

Skill Name	Rating				Observed performance/rationale
			Motor Skills		
Aligns	(No)	Mi	Mo	Ma	
Stabilizes	(No)	Mi	Mo	Ma	
Positions	No	(Mi)	Mo	Ma	Sits slightly far from table, some money is beyond his reach, stands to grasp out of reach coins
Reaches	(No)	Mi	Mo	Ma	
Bends	(No)	Mi	Mo	Ma	
Grips	(No)	Mi	Mo	Ma	
Manipulates	No	(Mi)	Mo	Ma	Drops coins 3 times, difficulty with in-hand manipulation
Coordinates	(No)	Mi	Mo	Ma	
Moves	No	(Mi)	Mo	Ma	Does not pull drawer out far enough, has difficulty pulling cash out of drawer
Lifts	(No)	Mi	Mo	Ma	
Walks	(No)	Mi	Mo	Ma	
Transports	No	Mi	Mo	Ma	Almost ran into another client, was looking down at cash tray while walking, instead of watching where he was going
Calibrates	(No)	Mi	Mo	Ma	
Flows	No	(Mi)	Mo	Ma	Some awkward movements when sorting and counting cash (left hand)
Endures	(No)	Mi	Mo	Ma	
Paces	(No)	Mi	Mo	Ma	
			Process Skills		
Paces	No	Mi	(Mo)	Ma	Lost track of the total when counting the $5 dollar bills because he got distracted by a noise in office. Required him to start over (took @ 2 min to get back on track) +2 min
Attends	No	Mi	(Mo)	Ma	Easily distracted, by external noises
Heeds	(No)	Mi	Mo	Ma	
Chooses	(No)	Mi	Mo	Ma	
Uses	No	(Mi)	Mo	Ma	Some difficulty stacking coins in cardboard rolls, pennies would not stack flat
Handles	(No)	Mi	Mo	Ma	
Inquires	No	Mi	(Mo)	Ma	Does not ask for assistance despite having some difficulties during the process
Initiates	(No)	Mi	Mo	Ma	
Continues	No	Mi	(Mo)	Ma	Difficulty entering correct numbers into calculator
Sequences	(No)	Mi	Mo	Ma	
Terminates	(No)	Mi	Mo	Ma	
Searches/locates	No	Mi	Mo	Ma	
Gathers	No	Mi	Mo	Ma	
Organizes	No	(Mi)	Mo	Ma	Transposed numbers when writing down totals
Restores	(No)	Mi	Mo	Ma	

BOX 14.3 Example B: An Excerpt From Antoine's Occupational Performance Analysis (Skills Rating) (*continued*)

Performance Skills

Skill Name	Rating				Observed performance/rationale
Navigates	No	Mi	Mo	Ma	
Notices/ responds	No	(Mi)	Mo	Ma	Notices that there is only one $5 bill, but does not respond by exchanging to prepare for tomorrow's drawer
Adjusts	No	Mi	Mo	Ma	
Accommodates	No	Mi	Mo	Ma	
Benefits	No	Mi	Mo	Ma	

Adapted from: Fisher, A. G., & Marterella, A. (2019). *Powerful practice: A model for authentic occupational therapy* (Appendix D, pp. 371–377). Center for Innovative OT Solutions.

OT HACKS SUMMARY

O: Occupation as a means and an end

In occupational therapy practice, we generally begin with the client and the client's goals and then analyze how we can use occupations in interventions in ways that might address their individualized goals.

T: Theoretical concepts, values, and principles, or historical foundations

In this section of the *OT HACKS* at the beginning of the chapter, the introduction of Dr Claudia Allen's Eleanor Clarke Slagle Lecture address (1987) was shared:

Activity: Occupational Therapy's Treatment Method

"Difficulties in explaining the value of using activity as a treatment method have been with us from the beginning (Fields, 1911). During a testimonial dinner in tribute to Eleanor Clarke Slagle, Dr Adolph Meyer (1937) struggled to explain the value of activity. He said, "I should like to voice adequately what so many of my patients have gained through Mrs Slagle and her pupils and what it means for the sufferers, but also for the healthy . . . those with 'time on their hands' (p. 6)" (2, p. 309).

Now consider this quote from author Annie Dillard:

"How we spend our days is, of course, how we spend our lives. What we do with this hour, and that one, is what we are doing."

After a few moments of reflection, can you describe how these two ideas are related and how they are equally related to occupational therapy practice and occupational performance or activity analysis?

H: How can we Help? OT's role in serving clients with mental illness or mental health needs

Clients with cognitive impairments or serious mental illness sometimes forget why occupational therapy is important, or they fail to make the connection between the specific intervention activities and how those activities are serving the client's priorities and goals. Peloquin (20) provides timeless suggestions for how to help the client link the activities used with their purposes:

1. Explain the purpose of the group or activity.
2. Encourage the client to think about the purpose and ask them to share this view.

3. Discuss the skills used and link them to the activities or tasks performed.
4. Summarize what has transpired.

A: Adaptations

Adaptation is *a change that facilitates performance*. Adaptation may entail a change in the task or the environment. To analyze the possibilities for adaptation of an activity, the occupational therapy professional must start by identifying and describing the activity as exactly as possible.

C: Case study includes

Client: Antoine B.

***DSM-5-TR* Diagnosis at Admission**

F71   Moderate Intellectual Developmental Disorder

ICD-10-CM

Q90.9 Down syndrome, unspecified

Antoine's OT conducted a thorough activity analysis (Example A) and an occupational performance analysis (Example B) with him to help plan the most effective activities for his intervention. After studying the occupational performance analysis, discuss the answers to the case study questions given.

1. Is this a standardized or nonstandardized performance analysis? Provide a rationale for your answer.
2. Describe the relationship between the activity chosen for intervention (performing the accounting tasks for the day center's snack bar and coffee shop), and Antoine's intervention goals.
3. Why is this a good choice of activity specifically for Antoine?
4. What functional outcomes will this intervention serve?
5. Explain how the occupational therapy professional can use occupational performance analysis over time to document changes in the client's occupational participation.

K: Knowledge: keeping mental health OT practice grounded in evidence, in occupational science, and in research

In this study, the researcher's aim was to further explore and describe the occupational performance problems of people with depression or anxiety disorders. How might occupational performance analysis and/or activity analysis be incorporated into this, or other similar future research studies?

Gunnarsson, A. B., Hedberg, A. K., Håkansson, C., Hedin, K., & Wagman, P. (2023). Occupational performance problems in people with depression and anxiety. *Scandinavian Journal of Occupational Therapy, 30*(2), 148–158.

S: Some terms that may be new to you

Adaptation: a change that facilitates performance

Declarative memory: remembering factual information

Dynamic performance analysis: a method for analyzing the activity during client performance of the activity

Environmental demand: an expectation for a certain kind of behavior or action that is evoked by something in the environment

Environmental support: a feature of the environment that encourages and assists the individual to perform a particular behavior

Errorless learning: presentation of an activity where the plan does not allow for the client to experience failure or the confusion of unsuccessful attempts

Gradation: the process of advancing step by step; the course of gradual progress

Intervention implementation: the enactment of the methods and activities outlined in the intervention plan

Procedural memory: remembering how to do something

Social conduct/interpersonal skills: the ways a person regards the needs or rights of other people

Sustained attention: attention span

Task-oriented approach/task-specific approach: an approach where the therapist analyzes the activity to determine whether it is possible for the client with severe cognitive limitations or neurocognitive disorders to perform particular aspects of the occupation, by relying on their procedural memory

Reflection Questions

1. What is the purpose of performing an activity analysis?
2. Describe **activity analysis**.
3. Compare and contrast an activity analysis with an occupational performance analysis.
4. What are the most important factors in selecting an activity for intervention? What is the relationship between choosing an activity for intervention and performing an occupational performance analysis?
5. What is the relationship of activity analysis to theories and practice models?
6. What are some considerations in analyzing an activity to be used in assessment?
7. Why should one describe the activity in detail before beginning to analyze it?
8. List the three main steps in analyzing an activity.
9. Define **adaptation** as the term is used in activity analysis.
10. Discuss reasons why an occupational therapy professional might adapt an activity.
11. Define **gradation** as the term is used in activity analysis.
12. Explain how the occupational therapy professional would grade an activity to help someone increase attention span.

If the person fails to increase their attention span, what aspects of the activity should the therapist consider?
13. Explain how the occupational therapy professional might grade an activity to help someone increase their ability to make decisions.

REFERENCES

1. Allen, C. K. (1985). *Occupational therapy for psychiatric diseases: Measurement and management of cognitive disabilities.* Little, Brown and Company.
2. Allen, C. K. (1987). Activity: Occupational therapy's treatment method. In R. Padilla & Y. Griffiths (Eds.), *The Eleanor Clarke Slagle Lectures in occupational therapy 1955–2016: A professional legacy, centennial edition* (pp. 309–323). AOTA Press.
3. Allen, C. A., Earhart, C. K., & Blue, T. (1992). *Occupational therapy treatment goals for the physically and cognitively disabled.* AOTA Press.
4. American Occupational Therapy Association. (2017). Philosophical base of occupational therapy. *American Journal of Occupational Therapy, 71*(Suppl. 2), 7112410045.
5. American Occupational Therapy Association. (2019). Value of occupational therapy assistant education to the profession. *American Journal of Occupational Therapy, 73*(Suppl. 2), 7312410007p1–7312410007p3.
6. American Occupational Therapy Association. (2020). Guidelines for supervision, roles, and responsibilities during the delivery of occupational therapy services. *American Journal of Occupational Therapy, 74*(Suppl. 3), 7413410020.
7. American Occupational Therapy Association. (2020). Occupational therapy practice framework: Domain and process—Fourth edition. *American Journal of Occupational Therapy, 74*(Suppl. 2), 1–87.
8. American Occupational Therapy Association. (2021). Occupational therapy scope of practice. *American Journal of Occupational Therapy, 75*(Suppl. 3), 7513410030.
9. American Psychiatric Association. (2022). *Diagnostic and statistical manual of mental disorders* (5th ed., text rev.). https://doi.org/10.1176/appi.books.9780890425787
10. Bonder, B. R. (2022). *Psychopathology and function* (6th ed.). SLACK.
11. Brown, C., Stoffel, V. C., & Munoz, J. (2019). *Occupational therapy in mental health: A vision for participation.* F.A. Davis.
12. Ciro, C. (2013). Second nature—Improving occupational performance in people with dementia through role-based, task-specific learning. *OT Practice, 18*(3), 9–12.
13. Cole, M. B. (2018). *Group dynamics in occupational therapy: The theoretical basis and practice application of group intervention* (5th ed.). SLACK.
14. Earhart, C. A. (2014). *Allen diagnostic module: [Revised] manual* (2nd ed.). S & S Worldwide.
15. Fidler, G., & Fidler, J. (1963). *Occupational therapy: A communication process in psychiatry.* Macmillan.
16. Fidler, G., & Velde, B. (1999). *Activities: Reality and symbol.* SLACK.
17. Fisher, A. G., & Marterella, A. (2019). *Powerful practice: A model for authentic occupational therapy.* Center for Innovative OT Solutions.
18. Hansen, B. W., Erlandsson, L. K., & Leufstadius, C. (2021). A concept analysis of creative activities as intervention in occupational therapy. *Scandinavian Journal of Occupational Therapy, 28*(1), 63–77.
19. Hemphill, B. J., & Urish, C. K. (Eds.). (2020). *Assessments in occupational therapy mental health: An integrative approach* (4th ed.). SLACK.
20. Peloquin, S. M. (1988). Linking purpose to procedure during interactions with patients. *American Journal of Occupational Therapy, 42*(12), 775–781.
21. Polatajko, H. J., Mandich, A., & Martini, R. (2000). Dynamic performance analysis: A framework for understanding occupational performance. *American Journal of Occupational Therapy, 54*(1), 65–72.
22. Preissner, K. (2010). Use of the occupational therapy task-oriented approach to optimize the motor performance of a client with cognitive limitations. *American Journal of Occupational Therapy, 64*(5), 727–734.
23. Schell, B. A. B., Gillen, G., Crepeau, E. B., & Scaffa, M. E. (2019). Analyzing occupations and activity. In B. A. B. Schell & G. Gillen (Eds.),

Willard and Spackman's occupational therapy (13th ed., pp. 320–334). Lippincott Williams & Wilkins.

24. Taylor, R. R. (2020). *The intentional relationship: Occupational therapy and use of self.* F.A. Davis.

Suggested Resources

Articles

This scoping review explores the implementation of the video modeling (VM) technique during the intervention process for children and adolescents with special needs. The article provides a snapshot showing how activity and task analysis can be used in modern occupational therapy practice.

Abd Aziz, N., Kadar, M., Harun, D., & Mohd Rasdi, H. F. (2021). Implementation of video modeling in the occupational therapy intervention process for children and adolescents with special needs: A scoping review. *Occupational Therapy in Health Care, 35*(2), 227–244.

The profession of occupational therapy has used creative activities "both as main treatment outcomes (resulting in something tangible) and as a media to achieve certain goals with clients" (18, p. 63) since its earliest days. However, a consistent description or definition of creative activities used in occupational therapy intervention has lacked clarity. This initial study, a concept analysis, sought to investigate and clarify the concept of creative activities used as an intervention (CaI) and to validate the findings in occupational therapy practice.

Hansen, B. W., Erlandsson, L. K., & Leufstadius, C. (2021). A concept analysis of creative activities as intervention in occupational therapy. *Scandinavian Journal of Occupational Therapy, 28*(1), 63–77.

Video

A brief (6:51) YouTube video explanation of the history and use of task analysis, activity analysis, and occupation analysis in occupational therapy. *Analysis—occupation/activity,* posted May 10, 2014 by MMolineuxUni, https://www.youtube.com/watch?v=YOvVNlYspNE

Websites

The Spruce Crafts is a DIY craft and hobby website that offers helpful tips, step-by-step tutorials, and thousands of creative tasks and activities perfect for incorporating into occupational therapy interventions. According to the website, "The Spruce Crafts is part of The Spruce family of sites, including The Spruce, The Spruce Eats, and The Spruce Pets, covering home decor, home repair, recipes, cooking techniques, pets, and crafts." https://www.thesprucecrafts.com/mentally-soothing-diys-4799755

CHAPTER 15

Therapeutic Use of Self

OT HACKS OVERVIEW

O: Occupation as a means and an end

The *Intentional Relationship Model* (IRM) (27) conceptualizes how therapeutic relationship can be applied **as a therapeutic means** to positively impact the client's occupational participation, thus helping them in meeting their occupational goals, hence, **occupation as an end** (27).

T: Theoretical concepts, values, and principles, or historical foundations

Dr Renee Taylor developed the IRM, "a conceptual practice model that provides therapists with a practical set of skills and an interpersonal reasoning approach that requires the use of different modes of communication that a therapist invokes in response to the client's evolving interpersonal characteristics and the inevitably challenging and intense interpersonal events of therapy" (27, p. 11). Taylor formalized the ways that occupational therapy professionals relate to clients through the use of therapeutic modes.

H: How can we Help? OT's role in serving clients with mental illness or mental health needs

The occupational therapy professional who can successfully establish and manage a therapeutic relationship possesses particular skills and characteristics, as does the therapeutic relationship itself, and these traits, skills, and characteristics are referred to as therapeutic qualities. These qualities include empathy, sensitivity, respect, warmth, genuineness, self-disclosure, specificity, and immediacy.

A: Adaptations

To collaboratively develop an intervention with a client, the occupational therapy professional will first need to be able to develop therapeutic rapport. The following are evidence-supported strategies for relating to clients. In this chapter, the reader explores these strategies in greater depth.

- Make initial contacts brief.
- Choose words carefully.
- Be comfortable with silence.
- Encourage by minimal response.
- Listen and observe.
- Summarize and focus.
- Ask for clarification.
- Follow through on promises.

C: Case study includes

Raeann is a 16-year-old female with dual diagnoses: anorexia nervosa, binge-eating/purging type, and generalized anxiety disorder. After reading this chapter and reflecting upon the initial occupational history information of Raeann's case, the reader can consider which approaches, therapeutic modes, or skills may be helpful in developing and maintaining a therapeutic relationship with Raeann, throughout the occupational therapy process, to help her meet her occupational goals most effectively.

K: Knowledge: keeping mental health OT practice grounded in evidence, in occupational science, and in research

Use of therapeutic modes and communication are essential to the development of a therapeutic relationship with clients. Although the therapeutic relationship and the various aspects of therapeutic use of self and therapeutic modes are foundational to occupational therapy practice, a minimum number of studies have been completed to assess the correlation between the use of therapeutic modes of communication (use of self) and the client's participation in rehabilitation. That is the aim of this research. After reading and reflecting upon this research, what conclusions about therapeutic use of self and the therapeutic relationship might one draw from the findings in this study by Fan and Taylor (8)?

S: Some terms that may be new to you

Competence
Countertransference
Immediacy
Intentional Relationship Model (IRM)
Projective identification
Psychosocial assistance
Specificity
Therapeutic modes
Therapeutic use of self
Transference

INTRODUCTION

Wanting to help other people is one reason students choose to enter the helping professions in a field such as occupational therapy. Although occupational therapy professionals help people primarily through use of occupation, they also help them by the way they relate to them and through the development of a therapeutic relationship. By encouraging clients to become more aware of their own abilities and strengths, clients often become more confident and motivated to engage in occupations. Relating to others is a skill used by all health professionals. The ability to listen and communicate are essential. Sometimes, relating to people who have psychiatric disorders requires the occupational therapy professional to heighten their own interpersonal skills and capacity for active listening even further. Unfortunately, people with psychiatric disorders continue to be a marginalized population, and many have had negative or traumatic experiences in their relationships with others. They may be fearful and have trouble expressing themselves. The way that the occupational therapy professional relates to clients, what we say and what we do not say, in words or in actions, affects them (sometimes deeply), whether we are aware of it or not. This interpersonal way of approaching, developing therapeutic rapport and relationship, and the collaboration between the occupational therapy professional and the client is the foundation of one of the cornerstones of our profession, therapeutic use of self (3, 27).

Being aware of oneself and of the client and being able to control what one communicates is called **therapeutic use of self**. It is different from other ways of relating to people because the purpose of the relationship is different (27). Clients expect that the health care providers, in this case the occupational therapy professional, will be able to help them with their problems and facilitate interventions that help remove the barriers they experience when engaging in life's daily occupations. The purpose of the establishment of a therapeutic relationship is to create a safe space, or safe container, where consumers identify their problems, set reasonable goals, and work toward accomplishing those goals. Therapeutic use of self is an occupational therapy professional's planned use of their personality, insights, perceptions, and judgments as part of the therapeutic process (27).

THE THERAPEUTIC RELATIONSHIP

To understand the special nature of the therapeutic relationship, it is helpful to reflect upon some important differences between a therapeutic relationship and a relationship one might have with a friend. The first is that in a friendship, each person expects something from the other. By contrast, in the therapeutic relationship, the client expects to receive help and the therapist expects to give help, but neither expects the help to be returned. Another consideration is that in a friendship, both people are responsible for making sure the relationship is rewarding and mutually satisfying. In a therapeutic relationship, the occupational therapy professional is responsible for using their personality, insights,

perceptions, professional reasoning, and communication skills to develop and maintain a positive and collaborative relationship with the client.

Many sociopolitical and sociocultural events have influenced the way that occupational therapy professionals and clients think about themselves, about the therapeutic relationship, and about their role(s) in the therapeutic relationship (5, 12, 19). A large research study about therapeutic use of self showed that over 82% of 1,000 American Occupational Therapy Association (AOTA) members and practitioners surveyed had agreed that the relationship with the client is the most important factor in the outcome of therapy (28). An even higher percentage agreed that therapeutic use of self is the most important skill for an occupational therapy professional. Those in mental health settings reported more difficulty with dysfunctional interpersonal behaviors from clients (than did practitioners in other settings). However, the study authors cited evidence that suggested that this may have meant that mental health occupational therapy professionals have higher interpersonal skill levels and are therefore more sensitive to client emotions and behaviors (28). Finally, occupational therapy professionals reported feeling that they had not received as much training as they would have liked regarding therapeutic use of self during their occupational therapy education.

Relating to clients effectively, like other skills, comes more easily to some people than to others. Fortunately, it *is* a skill, which, like any other skill, can be developed through effort and practice. Reading about it and understanding the impacts that the therapeutic relationship and use of self can have on a client's success and willingness to participate is only the beginning (8, 27). Developing skills in the art of therapeutic communication and developing therapeutic relationships where therapeutic use of self can be applied to benefit the client is like learning to ride a bicycle; it is mastered only through experience and practicing (25, 26). Still, before attempting to relate to clients, it is helpful to know something about what is expected. This chapter examines the role(s) that occupational therapy staff fulfill and some of the evidence-based approaches and methods they use with people who are experiencing mental illness that interferes with their daily occupations. This chapter also explores some of the therapeutic qualities that clients report as helpful to their success in therapy (8, 20–22) and further explores some techniques that the occupational therapy professional can use to relate to the client effectively (27). Finally, this chapter considers some of the legal and moral aspects of the therapeutic relationship and discusses how to end a therapeutic relationship.

The Intentional Relationship Model and Therapeutic Modes

Dr Renee Taylor developed the Intentional Relationship Model (IRM), "a conceptual practice model that provides therapists with a practical set of skills and an interpersonal reasoning approach that requires the use of different modes of communication that a therapist invokes in response to the client's evolving interpersonal characteristics and the inevitably challenging and intense interpersonal events of therapy" (27, p. 11). Taylor formalized the ways that occupational therapy professionals relate to clients as **therapeutic modes**. The six modes are patterns in which the practitioner applies different styles of interaction in different kinds of situations as appropriate for each client. The six therapeutic modes are advocating, collaborating, empathizing, encouraging, instructing, and problem-solving. Taylor describes why and how the practitioner might choose or use a specific mode. Table 15.1 describes the therapeutic modes and provides additional guidance in their application.

Taylor's IRM (27) conceptualizes how the therapeutic relationship can be applied as a therapeutic means to positively impact the client's occupational participation, thus helping them in meeting their occupational goals, hence, occupation as an end (27). The IRM is guided by four clear assumptions (25, 27):

1. Occupations are the means by which clients effect changes when participating in occupational therapy. "Unlike psychotherapists, who view the process of relating and communicating as the central mechanism of change, occupational therapists view occupational engagement as the central mechanism of change" (15, as cited in 27, p. 9).

2. The client is approached by the occupational therapy professional who has a desire to understand their client's interpersonal characteristics genuinely and more deeply, including their underlying personality and temperament, as well as the dimensional aspects of their current context and life situation.

3. The client's reactions to inevitable interpersonal events within the therapeutic relationship will influence the relationship between client and occupational therapy professional, whether positively or negatively, which is dependent on how the interpersonal events are managed by the occupational therapy professional. The management of interpersonal events and adapting to client interactions consistently within the therapeutic relationship require the occupational therapy professional to effectively apply the most appropriate of the six interpersonal therapeutic modes of communication to specific situations and clients.

4. "These three elements are incorporated into an interpersonal reasoning process that, when effective, will lead to occupational engagement, which represents the fourth and final component of the IRM" (27, p. 11).

Table 15.1. Taylor's Therapeutic Modes Associated With *the Intentional Relationship Model*

Therapeutic Mode	Description	Best Used When
Advocating	Helping the client obtain resources such as housing or education, to improve occupational engagement	The client is no longer symptomatic and has a need to progress beyond the present situation.
Collaborating	Engaging with clients as partners in choosing goals and methods	The client does not see the occupational therapy professional as an authority and is willing to engage in mutual planning. The client can engage as an equal.
Empathizing	Listening to clients, observing body language, observing expressed emotion, validating and reflecting back client perceptions	This mode is used most frequently but should not be an end in itself. Empathizing is helpful with the "difficult" or "unmotivated" client, to learn what contributes to their behavior. It is not helpful when it becomes the main content of therapy.
Encouraging	Emphasizing the positive, reminding clients of success and of their own strengths. Praising efforts and achievements. Engaging with humor and respect. Giving specific constructive feedback. Conveying hope and expectations of client success	Helpful with clients who seem resistant or unmotivated. Be careful not to praise too much but do encourage further effort. Some clients may depend on the therapist or others to evaluate their progress by praising their achievements. Try to facilitate client's own self-evaluation.
Instructing	Coaching, showing, demonstrating, teaching, sharing information, discussing possible outcomes. Setting limits and redirecting behavior are also part of this mode.	Clients do not know how to do something or how to understand something. For clients who need instruction, information, explanations, and professional advice
Problem-solving	Supporting the client in analyzing and thinking through barriers and solutions	Clients need help thinking through possibilities. Helpful when clients can only see one solution. Also when clients engage in either/or, good/bad thinking. This mode may feel very cold and intellectual to the client and should be balanced with other modes such as encouraging and empathizing.

Information selected from:
Dorenberg, M. D., & Taylor, R. R. (2014). The intentional relationship model: A framework for teaching therapeutic use of self. *OT Practice, 19*(17), CE1–CE8.
Taylor, R. R. (2008). *Pain, fear and avoidance: Therapeutic use of self with difficult occupational therapy populations* (Continuing Education on CD). AOTA.
Taylor, R. R. (2020). *The intentional relationship: Occupational therapy and use of self.* F.A. Davis.

THERAPEUTIC QUALITIES

In this section, you learn to recognize some essential qualities of the therapeutic relationship: empathy, sensitivity, respect, warmth, genuineness, self-disclosure, specificity, and immediacy.

Empathy

Empathy is the ability to understand how the other person feels. Taylor (27) defines empathy as being one of the most critical qualities of an occupational therapy professional, providing a broader definition of both empathy as it is captured in psychotherapeutic models and for its everyday application in occupational therapy practice via the *IRM*. "According to the IRM, empathy is defined as the deliberate effort to understand the client's inner experience as a separate and independent ideological, psychological, visceral, cognitive, or emotional perspective as it is reflected in that person's expressed thoughts, feelings, or behaviors" (27, p. 8). The occupational therapy professional not only should try to see the world from the client's point of view by considering their unique interpersonal characteristics but they should also convey what they hear back to the client. Listening to what the client says and encouraging them to say more about it helps the occupational therapy professional understand how the client feels. A client who believes that the occupational therapy professional truly understands their point of view is likely to communicate more and be more motivated in occupational therapy. For empathy to be effective, it must be genuine—that is, the occupational therapy professional must fully enter into the world of the client. Empathy requires a kind of experiential bonding, or "being with" the other person (21).

Sensitivity

In the therapeutic relationship, sensitivity is alertness to the client's needs and awareness of your effect on them. The effective occupational therapy professional is acutely attuned to the client's behaviors, especially facial expressions, and nonverbal behavior. The movements of people's face and body often give a more accurate picture of their true feelings than do the words they use. Behaviors convey mixed feelings, perhaps fear, sadness, or anxiety. By recognizing these, the practitioner can give the person the opportunity to discuss their feelings. When the client is nonverbal or has impairments in cognition, vision, hearing, or movement, it is especially important to be sensitive to body language, facial expression, and eye contact. People diagnosed with autism spectrum disorder, or with intellectual disability or neurocognitive disorders, may need extra time to respond. Facial expression and body language may indicate whether the person has understood or is thinking of something else, for example.

It is also important to recognize that expressing the therapeutic qualities of empathy and sensitivity does not mean that the occupational therapy professional will be able to alleviate a client's expressed emotions or painful problems, and that is not the intent of the professional building these qualities within themselves nor should it be a reason to demonstrate the qualities. Rather, the therapeutic qualities show the client that the occupational therapy professional cares. Dr Thomas Moore (18) states that each of us "can offer care that may improve the situation without necessarily solving the deeper problem" (18, p. 181). He further recommends five simple directives for cultivating therapeutic qualities within oneself:

1. Listen closely.
2. Give advice cautiously.
3. Feedback what you hear at a deeper level.
4. Affirm the person.
5. Help deepen the story (18, p. 181).

Respect

The client requires respect and recognition as a unique individual with personal interests and values that may be quite different from those of the OT professional. Similarly, clients often choose and enjoy with great pleasure the activities that staff may find nonproductive or unhealthful. For example, the occupational therapy professional may identify overspending as a problem for a client who has trouble staying within a budget, although the client does not recognize this as a problem because shopping is an occupation that is meaningful to them. Being "in relationship" with a client requires that the occupational therapy professional willingly look at things from the client's point of view.

Different cultures and generations may have different expectations and boundaries for what the therapeutic relationship between a client and a mental health worker looks like. To engage diverse clients, the practitioner has an ethical responsibility to make every effort to understand and appreciate the values and traditions to which the person is accustomed (1, 5).

Warmth

Warmth is the sense of friendliness, interest, and enthusiasm the therapist conveys. Warmth spreads outward from a person as loving and positive regard. Smiling, eye contact, leaning forward, and other nonverbal behaviors communicate warmth. These behaviors should be genuine but must be used selectively, depending on the situation and the client's ability to tolerate the therapist's warmth. Consistent awareness of client needs in the moment and the therapist's ability to apply the therapeutic modes, as suggested by the IRM, are ways to build and maintain the therapeutic relationship (27). Some people are very uncomfortable about being touched and the therapist must be alert to this. The way the therapist displays warmth must vary with the situation; smiling is often appropriate when praising someone's efforts but perhaps not when listening to a tearful recitation of problems or when confronting a client who has broken the rules of the group. In the latter two situations, the occupational therapy professional's warmth is conveyed through eye contact, body position, and tone of voice.

Genuineness

Genuineness is the ability to be oneself openly. To do this, occupational therapy professionals must first be aware of themselves and be comfortable with who they are. Occupational therapy professionals who have mastered this can say and do what they really mean; their verbal and nonverbal messages say the same thing. They are not afraid of making mistakes, or not knowing the answer to every question and are willing to admit it. They are comfortable saying "I don't know. I can try to find out." They do not need to distance themselves from their clients with an artificially professional authoritative role; they find it easy to be in the role of therapist without being condescending or defensive.

Self-Disclosure

Self-disclosure is the practice of revealing things about oneself. In a therapeutic relationship, the client is often asked to unveil many private facts and feelings. Indeed, clients may be required to reveal so much that, at times, they feel like specimens under a microscope. By letting the client know some facts about themselves, occupational therapy professionals can even the score a little and make the relationship feel more collaborative. It is important, however, to reveal only as much as is needed to make the person more comfortable. Timing is very important; self-disclosure is most helpful when the client has asked for it (verbally or nonverbally) and very detrimental when it interrupts them in the midst of expressing themselves. Also, some clients may see an occupational therapy professional's self-disclosure as unprofessional and offensive.

In addition, it is important to know what *not* to disclose. This includes details about one's personal life, such as one's address and phone number. Unfortunately, some clients want to seek out staff after they are discharged, and this can be difficult (and occasionally dangerous) for the staff member and their family. Finally, whatever is disclosed should be for the client's benefit; the occupational therapy professional must never burden the client with their personal problems.

Specificity

Specificity is the art of stating things simply, directly, and concretely, focusing only on what is relevant. The effective occupational therapy professional points out what is happening without labeling it or turning it into an abstract principle or a value judgment. For example, the occupational therapy professional says, "When you walk away while I am talking to you, I get the feeling that you don't want to hear what I have to say," rather than "You're being hostile." When giving directions, the occupational therapy professional states them in language simple enough to be understood—for instance, telling the client, "Find the center of the block of wood by drawing lines across from corner to corner" rather than

"Find where the right angles meet." Similarly, when helping a client understand what is happening during an activity, the occupational therapy professional should identify relevant details and help the person see them. For example, when the client makes a mistake, becomes upset, and wants to quit the activity, the occupational therapy professional should help them problem-solve so that they see exactly what has to be done to correct the error.

Immediacy

Immediacy is the practice of giving feedback right after the event to which it relates. Clients benefit from learning about their successes and their mistakes while they are happening, rather than later, when they or the occupational therapy professional may have forgotten important details. Immediacy also includes the idea of focusing the person's attention on the here and now. Clients sometimes become preoccupied with things over which they have no control. The more someone ruminates on things that are not happening and that probably will not happen, the more distanced they become from the here and now, and from making real-life decisions and carrying them out. These clients need to become involved in something that is happening presently.

To sum up, the occupational therapy provider should try to cultivate the therapeutic qualities discussed. This is a lifelong project; these qualities cannot be developed overnight. Nor can they be developed by a piecemeal study and practice of their separate parts (eg, listening, leaning forward, trying to maintain eye contact) (22, 27). Rather, these qualities are acquired only by persistent efforts to genuinely understand clients. Once the therapeutic qualities have been developed, they need constant nurturing, evaluation, and refinement. Research studies have documented that regardless of the health professional's training or theoretical orientation, clients get better sooner and with more lasting results when they are treated by health professionals who possess these traits (8, 14).

DEVELOPING THERAPEUTIC QUALITIES

Students and new practitioners may be perplexed by the expectation that they acquire or refine these therapeutic qualities in themselves. From the student's perspective, there may not seem to be a problem. However, we are not always accurate in our assessments of how we seem to others. A gesture or comment that we mean to be warm and understanding may be perceived as pushy, intrusive, and insensitive. How can one resolve this confusion and move toward developing a therapeutic self that is reliable and effective? One key is to improve one's awareness of self. Another is constant examination of one's motives and expectations in relationships with clients.

Many roads lead to increased awareness of self. Some occupational therapy professionals seek mental health therapy or counseling for themselves, to learn about how they are perceived by others and to understand more about their own ways of being in the world. Another way to learn about the self is to ask trusted and honest colleagues to give feedback; these may be fellow students or teachers or supervisors. An acronym for processing feedback is ALOR (ask, listen, observe, reflect), illustrated in Box 15.1. After the fourth step (reflect), one may circle back and begin with the first step (ask) again. Peer supervision is an especially valuable source of feedback; it is easier for many people to hear the message when it comes from a peer (someone of equal status) than from a supervisor. Keeping a journal of reflections on interactions can also be helpful.

Regarding the occupational therapy professional's motivations and expectations, the self-aware therapist is vigilant. Whenever we collaborate with a client to provide a therapy service, we naturally have expectations about the hoped-for client outcomes, but have we paused long enough to reflect upon the process of the therapeutic interactions that lead to positive outcomes? Do we know what we are expecting? And are we fully conscious of what we expect? We may expect clients to benefit from whatever we do with them, or that a person who fits a particular stereotype cannot be reached because they are "unmotivated." We may feel disappointed or angry or otherwise negative when our expectations are not met. If we are not conscious of this, we may act it out in ways that are harmful to clients. Thus, therapists should keep a careful watch over their expectations. In summary, therapeutic qualities are developed by seeking and accepting feedback, by learning about oneself, and by maintaining a conscious awareness of one's motives and expectations.

TECHNIQUES FOR RELATING TO CLIENTS

Although self-knowledge and a genuine willingness to enter the client's world are the foundations of successful therapeutic relationships, it also may help the new practitioner to know some of the specific techniques used by experienced occupational therapy professionals. These are detailed next and rephrased in Box 15.2. Remember that these are suggestions, but the context of some current health care settings will require that the occupational therapy professional adapt some of the strategies, using professional judgment to keep the integrity of the technique securely in place. Also note that these techniques are successful only when applied in the context of a genuinely caring response (20, 22).

1. *When trying to develop a relationship with a new client, try to make the first contacts brief.* Introduce yourself, explain your purpose in getting to know the client, briefly describe what they may gain from occupational therapy, and set a time for your next meeting. If you place yourself for a moment in the client's position, you will understand why they may feel overwhelmed by meeting so many new people at one time, all of them eager to ask questions. Instead, promote trust by orienting the client to occupational therapy and provide a schedule for the first few days.

2. *Use language that conveys what you mean and that will accomplish your purpose.* When attempting to get clients to explore their feelings or give general information about themselves, open-ended questions should be used. Remember that an open-ended question asks for an answer longer than a few words. For example, "What have you been doing today?" is likely to produce a lengthier reply than "Did you go to the exercise group?" On the other hand, a closed question, of which the latter is an example, is more useful when you want to know something specific, such as whether the client has attended the exercise group that you have been encouraging them to try. Similarly, avoid implying that a choice exists if it does not. A client always has a right to deny participation in rehabilitation services; however, in some circumstances, participation in therapy is a condition of a client's safe discharge to home. It is situations such as these that

---

BOX 15.1 Improving Understanding of Self and Others Through ALOR

Ask

Student to supervisor: "I am so upset about my interview with Noelani. I was asking her questions and everything was fine and then she just got up and gave me an angry look and walked off. What did I do wrong?"

Listen

Supervisor: "Well, I wasn't there, so I'm not sure. I have noticed, though, that you sometimes cut people off and finish their sentences for them. You even do this with me. You might try waiting until they finish and then take a breath before you talk again."

Observe

Student watches self during interactions with friends, clients, and colleagues and observes behavior that supervisor described.

Reflect

Student reflects, "Wow, I didn't know I did that. I thought I knew what the person was going to say, but now I see that I didn't."

BOX 15.2 Communication Techniques

- Make initial contacts brief.
- Choose words carefully.
- Be comfortable with silence.
- Encourage by minimal response.
- Listen and observe.
- Summarize and focus.
- Ask for clarification.
- Follow through on promises.

require careful communication from the occupational therapy professional. For example, asking, "Would you like to come to occupational therapy now?" risks angering clients once they learn that it is a necessary condition for safe discharge that they participate. Instead, saying, "It's time for occupational therapy. We will be meeting in the day room," is a better option because it gives clients time to collect their thoughts and get ready for the group. This helps to make it clear to the client there is an expectation from the team that the client attend.

3. *Be comfortable with occasional silences, your own and the client's.* Everyone needs time to collect their thoughts, and clients may need more time because their thinking is slowed by the disease process, or they may be genuinely overwhelmed with an abundance of new information. While you are waiting for the client to answer, observe their nonverbal behavior to determine whether they are confused by the question, have not heard it, or are merely trying to compose an answer. In any case, avoid sending unintentional messages with your body language, implying that you are impatient or in a hurry, such as tapping your feet or looking at your watch, or the door.

4. *Use minimal responses such as "go on" or "uh-huh" to show that you have been listening and to encourage the client to keep talking.* At times, clients find it hard to express themselves or to believe that you are interested, and your encouragement will help them. Remember that minimal responses can also be nonverbal, as with leaning forward or making eye contact.

5. *Actively listen to what the client is communicating.* Words are not everything. Much is conveyed by gesture, eye movement, and a tilt of the head or a tightening or softening or trembling around the mouth. Watch the client carefully (without staring) and feel with the person. Pay attention to nonverbal clues as well as to the words used. What is the message in the nonverbal body language? What else is going on? Be ready to tolerate the client's struggle with uncomfortable feelings. Verbalize what you see. If the client is fidgeting, say, "I notice you're tapping your nails and twirling your hair." This allows the client to say "I always do that when I'm nervous" and thus may help them interpret and understand the behavior. Saying to the client, "You seem nervous" makes the occupational therapy professional seem the authority and the client less likely to wish to communicate or collaborate. It also deprives the person of the opportunity to increase self-awareness by reflecting on these behaviors and the associated feelings.

6. *Try to get the client to focus on one thing at a time.* Clients may have trouble concentrating and may skip from topic to topic or gloss over something painful to avoid dealing with it. By saying "I'd like to go back to what you said about banks making you angry because I think it might have something to do with the problem you said you have sticking to a budget," the occupational therapy professional opens an important topic for a more thorough discussion. Some clients resist this at first, or are too anxious to stay on the topic; if so, the therapist should drop the subject and bring it up at another time.

7. *Ask for clarification when you do not understand something the client has said or done.* Because your purpose is to get the client to explain further, your request should be phrased in a way that does not cause the client to feel defensive. For example, "Would you repeat that? I didn't hear it" is much easier for the client to take (and more polite) than "You really have to talk louder if you expect me to answer you." Likewise, when commenting on something a client has done in an activity, it is better to say "You've glued the pictures so that they face in different directions. I'm not sure I see why. Can you tell me about it?" than "Why did you do that?" It is helpful to give specifics and to state your observations in neutral language.

8. *Promise only what you can deliver.* Clients will take, at their word, any staff member who makes a promise and will be hurt and perhaps angry if the promise is not kept. Occupational therapy professionals, like other staff, are often so busy that they forget or run out of time to do things they sincerely meant to do. The artful occupational therapy professional will leave a way out by saying, for example, "I'll try to bring you some purple yarn this afternoon if I get out of the meeting in time." The occupational therapy professional who cannot keep a promise should go to the client and briefly explain why, indicating whether and when they will be able to do it—for example, "I can't find the purple yarn, but I'll ask my supervisor about it tomorrow morning and let you know." Oftentimes, when the occupational therapy professional follows through with actions, or makes sure to communicate with clients, they are modeling some of the very changes in behavior that the client may be striving toward.

PSYCHOTHERAPEUTIC PRINCIPLES IN THE THERAPEUTIC RELATIONSHIP: TRANSFERENCE AND COUNTERTRANSFERENCE

Transference occurs when one person unconsciously relates to the other as if that person were someone else, usually an important person in their life. For example, a client may begin to act as if the occupational therapy professional is an older brother who always took care of her and helped mediate her conflicts with others. **Countertransference** occurs when the other person unconsciously falls into a role that has been transferred onto them (7). In the example discussed, if the occupational therapy professional began to do special favors for the client and step into her interactions with her peers, this would be an example of countertransference. It would be easy for this occupational therapy professional to fall into the role unconsciously if they had a younger relative or friend for whom they had played this role in the past.

It is crucial to recognize that transference and counter-transference occur on an unconscious level; this makes them very difficult to bring awareness to and even more difficult to actively manage.

If client and occupational therapy professional continue to act out the roles prescribed by the transference, it will be difficult for the client in our example to learn that there are other ways of relating to people who remind them of their brother. The relationship with this occupational therapy professional does not benefit the client's progress in meeting occupational goals. If, on the other hand, the occupational therapy professional can recognize what is going on, they can observe the client's transference to find out more about how the client expects other people to act. Once the occupational therapy professional learns, for example, that one of the client's expectations is that others will defend them when conflicts arise in her relationships, the occupational therapy professional can bring this up for discussion with the client and use the information to inform the client's occupational goals and outcomes. The occupational therapy professional can also, by refraining from entering conflicts between the client and their peers, help them explore other ways of relating to people that will help them learn to solve problems and conflicts by themself. Examples such as this one demonstrate the distinct need for occupational therapy interventions in many psychosocial settings to take place in groups. Any client who has a social interaction skill or aspect of social participation that presents a barrier to their occupational engagement will require the presence of others to facilitate improving their interpersonal skills (7).

There are two ways to identify a transference. The first is to observe your own behavior and study how you relate to the clients, especially noting if you relate differently to (or feel differently about) certain clients. The second is to learn from your supervisor and other staff, who have more objectivity because they are not involved in the immediate situation. Students, beginning occupational therapy professionals, and even experienced staff are sometimes amazed to learn that they have gotten involved in a countertransferential relationship with a client. Certainly, there is no reason to be surprised and even less reason to be ashamed to find out that you have become enmeshed in a client's transference. The patterns and feelings we have developed over many years of dealing with our families and others close to us are so much a part of us that it is natural for them to be set in motion by clients who remind us of important people in our own lives.

Projective Identification: Projection as a Defense Mechanism

The concept of defense mechanisms, and, specifically, **projective identification** originated from the work of Sigmund Freud and his daughter Anna Freud, and their psychoanalytic and psychodynamic theoretical foundations. Later, Melanie Klein's work with object relations theory and Wilfred Bion's work with attachment theory further contributed to psychotherapeutic traditions and principles that are embedded in occupational therapy practice even today (9, 27). Projection is a psychological defense mechanism that people unconsciously use as a means of self-protection. Projective identification occurs when a person attributes their own feelings, desires, or qualities (especially negative ones) to another person, group, animal, or object (9, 31). Many psychologists see the process of projecting things onto another person (object, group) as a means for people to reflect on how they feel about themselves.

Those clients' with low self-esteem, poor agency, or who have been abused, may not feel that they are able to acknowledge or face things about themselves that do not feel good, or are not unacceptable by societal standards. So, people project these unacceptable feelings and desires onto someone else to avoid them (7, 9). Projection is quite similar to transference, except that with projection the client is typically trying to avoid difficult feelings and emotions, whereas transference usually has more to do with the roles of the client and the occupational therapy professional or the person themselves and less about ridding oneself of painful feelings or emotions (11, 16, 17).

OPERATIONALIZING THE THERAPEUTIC RELATIONSHIP IN EVERYDAY OCCUPATIONAL THERAPY PRACTICE

Helping clients return to optimal participation in the meaningful occupations of their lives hinges on being in a therapeutic relationship where awareness is heightened and help toward seeking resources and intervention is present. This is regardless of the client's diagnosis, level, or selected intervention. The therapeutic relationship is a primary factor in combating mental disorders. For this reason, interventions that employ techniques with relational characteristics and structures are becoming popular and successful approaches to address the crisis of increasing numbers of (in particular) aging adults, who are diagnosed (and undiagnosed) with mental health disorders. The World Health Organization (WHO)'s Mental Health Gap Action Programme (mhGAP) is one example of such an intervention. This model helps increase the availability of mental health services for people with neuropsychological, substance abuse, and mild forms of mental health conditions such as depression. Programs such as mhGAP and others similar to it, train lay workers who are not necessarily mental health specialists, to deliver the proper care that occurs within the container of a therapeutic relationship. The client gains psychosocial assistance, assistance with accessing proper mental health care, and medication if deemed necessary (prescribed and administered by a medical doctor), and acts as a sort of peer counselor whose main obligation is to be the other loving person in a safe, attentive, and caring relationship (32). Considering our profession's application of therapeutic use of self, occupational therapy professionals are well suited to receive training and carry out roles and responsibilities such as WHO's mhGAP, thereby advocating for occupational therapy's continued role in mental and behavioral health settings and in emerging areas of occupational therapy practice.

Author Jeff Brown (6) explains one of the potential reasons for the success of programs that bring together someone in need with a safe peer relationship from a loving other person:

> If there is any need that is perpetually unmet on this planet, it is the need to feel seen. To feel seen in our humanity, in our vulnerability, in our beautiful imperfection. When we are held safe in that, a key turns inside of our hearts, freeing us from our isolation, transforming our inner world. If there is anything we can offer each other, it is the gift of sight. "I see you" perhaps the most important words that we can utter to another. (6)

Psychosocial assistance is, at its most simple level, the capacity of the caregiver to "see" the one for whom they are caring at an affective or emotional level.

Many mental health interventions continue to rely upon the traditional medical model paradigm, the trained occupational therapy professional is the "expert," who administers a particular procedure or protocol, or trains the client in its use. Intrapersonal interventions, such as mindfulness, meditation, Yoga, and relaxation techniques, demonstrate unquestionable benefits and are considered evidence-based interventions. Nevertheless, with few exceptions, these interventions do little to tap into the relevance and powerful potential to influence change that so naturally exists in the therapeutic relationship between occupational therapy professional and client, or between the caregiver and the one being cared for (10, 11, 13, 17, 30). Furthermore, "Research on brain development and the maturation of mental processes suggests that patterns of emotional, social, and behavioral functioning involve many brain areas working together rather than in isolation . . .. Numerous researchers have concluded that the nature of the psychotherapeutic relationship, reflecting interconnected aspects of mind, brain, and body operating together in an interpersonal context, predicts outcome more robustly than any specific treatment approach per se" (23, p. 1).

Relational somatic psychotherapy (RSP) (11) is a discipline and model of practice developed by Dr Bob Hilton over the past 50 years in his work as a professional counselor, educator, minister, seminary professor, local trainer, and member of the International Faculty of Bioenergetic Analysis (11). RSP has theoretical roots in Jungian psychotherapy, somatic psychology, classical (Lowenian) bioenergetics, Freudian psychoanalytic approaches, and Gestalt therapy. It continues to be informed by the current influx of research in neuropsychology, neurobiology, and consistent exploration of object relations and attachment theory approaches. Intrinsic and extrinsic changes for the client during the therapeutic process are often experienced somatically, or in and through the body (11).

There are several basic RSP principles that inform this methodology and approach toward healing. First, the human body is understood to be capable of healing itself. "Health" in this paradigm occurs as the result of releasing long-held

tensions and stressors (physical and psychological) that are held within the body (soma). Physical movement facilitates the release of tensions in the body and encourages emotional expression (11, 30). Finally, RSP insists that optimal physical and psychological healing and health happen more effectively in the context of a safe and healthy relationship where both the client and the therapist or caregiver feel that they are safe and, most importantly, where both people in the relationship feel authentically seen and heard (11).

The consideration of using an RSP approach to caring for someone with a mental disorder has the potential to critically impact plans of care in behavioral health care settings and is a wonderful approach for occupational therapy professionals to consider because occupational therapy adds the "doing" element to relational and psychoanalytic aspects of this model through our emphasis on occupation (9). Both the RSP and the occupational therapy models share the insistence that one of the central focuses throughout therapeutic interventions should remain on the intimate attachment and powerful exchanges that occur within the context of authentic and safe interpersonal relationships (9, 11, 27).

THE AMERICAN OCCUPATIONAL THERAPY ASSOCIATION'S CODE OF ETHICS

A code of ethics is a set of principles that guide the practice of a profession. It consists of rules and guidelines about what is considered proper conduct for the professional in their relationship with the general public and with the person receiving their professional services. In occupational therapy, the patient or client is the person to whom the occupational therapy professional has the greatest obligation depending on the trust implied by the client's willingness to be placed under the occupational therapy professional's care (1, 2). The guiding principles of the AOTA's *Occupational Therapy Code of Ethics* (1) are listed in Box 15.3. A less formal and more specific discussion of the obligations of occupational therapy staff toward the clients in their care follows.

Client-Centered Focus

Place the client's interests above your own. The client always comes first. In a fire or other emergency, clients should be helped to leave the building before any staff member sees to their own welfare. Likewise, in less dramatic situations, the occupational therapy professional should attend to the client's needs even if this means they must defer their own. For example, helping a client to the bathroom is more important than talking to a colleague, even if a prearranged meeting had been scheduled.

Goal-Oriented Intervention

Direct your energies toward accomplishing the occupation-centered intervention goals. Every encounter with a client should be related to that client's occupational problems and goals. An evaluation should be carried out in collaboration with the client, and an intervention plan developed and

Principle 1

Occupational therapy personnel shall demonstrate a concern for the safety and well-being and safety of the recipients of their services (beneficence).

Principle 2

Occupational therapy personnel shall refrain from actions that cause harm (nonmaleficence).

Principle 3

Occupational therapy personnel shall respect the right of the individual to self-determination (autonomy, confidentiality, consent).

Principle 4

Occupational therapy personnel shall provide services in a fair and equitable manner (social justice).

Principle 5

Occupational therapy personnel shall provide comprehensive, accurate, and objective information when representing the profession (veracity).

Principle 6

Occupational therapy personnel shall treat colleagues and other professionals with respect, fairness, discretion, and integrity (fidelity).

Based on information from American Occupational Therapy Association. (2020). AOTA 2020 occupational therapy code of ethics. *American Journal of Occupational Therapy, 74*(Suppl. 3), 7413410005 and American Occupational Therapy Association Ethics Commission. (2015). Occupational therapy code of ethics. *American Journal of Occupational Therapy, 69*(Suppl. 3).

documented as soon as possible, so that the client can be made aware of the purpose for and direction of intervention.

Client's Rights

Respect the client's rights, including the right to refuse treatment. The right to refuse intervention is based on the individual's right to determine what is best for their own welfare, as written in the U.S. Constitution. A client can be forced to accept treatment only if they have been involuntarily admitted to the hospital or declared legally incompetent. Treatment in each of these situations requires a special court order that must be renewed periodically. Clients also have a right to receive treatment regardless of their sexual orientation, race, creed, or national origin.

Confidentiality

Respect the confidentiality of the therapeutic relationship. The client has the right, both morally and legally, to expect that information about their condition, personal life, and treatment will be shared only with those directly concerned with

their care. It is *never* appropriate to discuss this information with anyone outside the health care facility or agency.

One should refrain from talking about clients, even to another professional, in public places such as the elevator, the subway, or the cafeteria. Students and beginning occupational therapy professionals often wonder whether they should share with the behavioral health team things that a client has told them. Usually, they should. Some exceptions are obvious—for example, if the client is planning a party or a treat for a staff member. In general, however, there should be no secrets from the treatment team. The occupational therapy professional must actively support the staff in providing the client with the best possible care. Reporting a client's confidential sharing is necessary when the client threatens to harm themselves or someone else; such threats should never be taken lightly.

The client's right to privacy of personal medical information is protected by the Health Insurance Portability and Accountability Act of 1996 (HIPAA) (29). In practical terms, this means that copies of facility's or agency's records may not be shared with teachers or classmates, even if all the apparent identifying information is removed, unless the client has given express written consent for the one-time use. When writing about a client for a class assignment or when discussing the client in a class or seminar, the student must disguise all identifying information so that it is impossible for another person to guess the client's identity. This means changing details such as name, date of birth, place of birth, and perhaps also the national origin, date of immigration, number of children, and so on. When the person is well known (an entertainer or sports figure), the occupation must also be changed.

When working with an adolescent who is 18 years of age or older, HIPAA rules apply because the person is considered an adult. Before the 18th birthday, information about the child or adolescent may be shared with the parent or guardian; however, to maintain a trusting and genuine relationship with the young person, the occupational therapy provider must advise the client that the information can (must) legally be shared (29).

Regarding persons with intellectual disabilities and other cognitive disabilities, HIPAA law permits them to control access to their health information to whatever extent state or local law permits them to act on their own behalf. When in doubt, the occupational therapy professional should consult a supervisor or more senior health care practitioner in the agency with questions related to HIPAA. The HIPAA website provides extensive information as well as answers to frequently asked questions (29). The reader is highly encouraged to view the site and read the questions and answers.

Client Welfare

Safeguard the welfare of clients under your care. Although this principle applies equally to all recipients of occupational therapy services, special precautions are necessary when working with persons with mental disorders because they may harm themselves or others because of confusion, incoordination, impaired thinking, or inability to control their impulses. In inpatient settings, occupational therapy professionals must be consistently alert as to where their clients are and what they are doing. They must take care to account for tools, sharp objects, and other materials that could be used in a suicide attempt or an assault. They must also make sure that confused clients do not get lost or hurt themselves accidentally.

Continuing Education

Maintain your own competence to provide occupational therapy. The client has every right to expect that the occupational therapy professional will provide skillful interventions on the basis of current knowledge, best practices, and evidence in occupational therapy. Consequently, the occupational therapy professional has an obligation to keep up to date on advances in their areas of practice. For continuing certification and renewal of certification by the National Board for Certification in Occupational Therapy (NBCOT), all occupational therapy providers must complete units toward certification of competency (1, 4, 5). In some states, occupational therapy personnel must show evidence of continuing education courses to renew their state licenses or certificates. **Competence** is not synonymous with "years of experience" but is acquired by study and application. Excellent resources for developing and maintaining competency are available at the AOTA and the NBCOT websites.

Standard of Care

Protect the client from negligence, abuse, and substandard care. Most malpractice suits involve situations in which clients were harmed because a health professional failed to attend to their needs or caused them injury, directly or indirectly. For example, the occupational therapy professional could be sued if they were responsible for leading or coleading an activity from which an inpatient client from a locked unit slipped away and later attempted suicide. Similarly, if a client who was confused as a side effect of receiving electroconvulsive therapy was injured while using a power tool in the workshop, the staff member in charge would be held accountable.

A client has the right to a reasonable standard of care. This does not necessarily mean the absolute latest in experimental medical technology but, rather, the kind of care that is usual and considered adequate and customary by most professionals in the field. The client also has a right to receive treatment only from those who are qualified to give it. OTs and occupational therapy assistants (OTAs) should know and follow their job descriptions and AOTA and legal guidelines. Occupational therapy professionals should refuse to perform tasks for which they are not qualified or trained. Most importantly, it is the ethical obligation of occupational therapy professionals to collaborate effectively and efficiently with clients, families, and other health care professionals to provide the highest quality of occupational therapy services possible.

ENDING THE THERAPEUTIC RELATIONSHIP

Saying goodbye is hard, especially when we have grown close to someone or worked with a client for a long time. This is no less true of the therapeutic relationship; new occupational therapy professionals are often surprised not only by the strength of their clients' feelings but by their own feelings as well. Many circumstances can bring an end to the relationship between client and occupational therapy professional: the client's discharge, the client's successful accomplishment of goals, a change of job or living situation for consumer or occupational therapy professional, or a recognition that the client cannot benefit from further interventions. Completion of fieldwork may be the student's first experience of saying goodbye to clients. Ending a relationship can be uncomfortable and difficult, but ending it well can resolve unfinished issues and strengthen the person's confidence to deal with the real demands and opportunities that life brings.

Occupational therapy professionals can help consumers learn and grow even at the end of the relationship. One way is to ask clients to take some time to think about what they have gained from occupational therapy and encourage them to talk about it. Another is to ask the client how they feel about leaving or about the occupational therapy professional leaving. If someone is leaving a group or the group is breaking up, the members should each be given time and encouragement to talk about their feelings, to express what they have gotten out of the group, and to say goodbye to each other.

Sometimes, new practitioners are concerned that saying goodbye takes too much valuable time away from other occupational therapy activities or from the main business of a group. The end of a therapeutic relationship is at least as important as the beginning. The end gives an opportunity for closure and to reinforce whatever gains have been made. In addition, it can help prepare the individual (both consumer and practitioner) to deal with natural losses and terminations in the future.

SUMMARY

The relationship with the occupational therapy professional strongly influences the way clients see themselves and their abilities. At its best, the therapeutic relationship increases clients' confidence and strengthens their will to try new things and become more fully themselves. Such a relationship requires that the occupational therapy professional genuinely and unconditionally experience the world through the client's perspective. Although specific therapeutic qualities can be listed and individual communication techniques can be taught, these by themselves are insufficient. To make a connection with another person that is authentic and powerful requires that occupational therapy professionals be conscious of their feelings and actions and that they take the risk to learn and accept and change themselves. By self-study through counseling and supervision and by thoughtful application of ethical principles, the occupational therapy professional can begin to understand and learn to master this complex and powerful element of occupational therapy practice.

Case Study

Raeann: A 16-Year-Old Female With Anorexia Nervosa, Binge-Eating/Purging Type and Generalized Anxiety Disorder

DSM-5-TR *Diagnoses*

F50.02 Anorexia nervosa, binge-eating/purging type

F41.1 Generalized Anxiety Disorder

Z Codes

Z62.898 Child affected by parental relationship distress

You are an occupational therapy professional working at a specialty pediatric eating disorders outpatient clinic. You work with a team of behavioral specialists, nutritionists, and psychiatric specialists. Raeann was referred by her pediatrician after she revealed some unhealthy eating patterns and behaviors to her counselor at school. These include her hiding and hoarding food, and consuming too much food (binge eating), which leads on occasion to her purging. These patterns began when she was 12 years old, and currently at age 16, Raeann's weight yo-yos between unhealthy highs and unhealthy lows, creating an unhealthy overall pattern and trajectory. Her low self-esteem and difficulty with anxiety and depression, coupled with her family's insecurities with her father's situation (he has, for much of her life, been in prison or rehabilitation for drug addiction), has impacted all her daily occupations. Because of her family history, and the situational contexts associated with her occupational engagement, Raeann is at higher risk for both addiction (currently to food) and at risk for future health problems associated with childhood obesity and disordered eating. You are interested in learning which occupation-based approaches and interventions are the most efficacious for targeting Raeann's insecure attachments with her father, her emotional dysregulation, and her lack of self-esteem—which you believe are the primary contributing factors to her unhealthy eating patterns.

After reflecting on the initial case study details that you have available, answer the following question:

1. Describe which of the therapeutic modes associated with *the IRM* you think you might apply with Raeann throughout the various parts of the OT process? Explain your choices of modes.

OT HACKS SUMMARY

O: Occupation as a means

To make a connection with another person that is authentic and powerful (ie, incorporating the therapeutic use of self, therapeutic relationship) requires that occupational therapy professionals be conscious of their feelings and actions, and that they take the risks to learn, accept, and consistently reflect upon and change aspects of themselves as they grow and learn, before they can authentically encourage clients to do the same.

Occupation as an end

"Only when one is able to truly recognize and understand the individual interpersonal differences and needs of one's clients, as they evolve from session to session and from moment to moment, is one able to characterize oneself as truly client-centered" (27, p. 16).

T: Theoretical concepts, values, and principles, or historical foundations

This continuing professional development article published in the *British Journal of Wellbeing* draws on the literature from the disciplines of occupational therapy, social work, nursing, and psychotherapy to explore the foundation and history of the concept of therapeutic use of self. The authors suggest that before therapeutic use of self can be applied in practice, one must examine and understand its foundational principles. After reading this article, compare and contrast therapeutic use of self in occupational therapy practice versus use of self in other disciplines.

Currid, T., & Pennington, J. (2010). Continuing professional development: Therapeutic use of self. *British Journal of Wellbeing, 1*(3), 35–42.

H: How can we Help? OT's role in serving clients with mental illness or mental health needs

Regardless of the client's diagnosis, level of ability, or type of need, selected occupational interventions are the primary factor in combating mental illness. This helps clients return to optimal participation in the meaningful occupations of their lives. The therapeutic relationship is where awareness is heightened, thus helping the client toward seeking appropriate resources and intervention. For this reason, interventions that employ techniques with relational characteristics and structures are becoming popular and successful approaches to address the crisis of increasing numbers of (in particular) aging adults, who are diagnosed (and undiagnosed) with mental health disorders (32).

A: Adaptations

Many mental health interventions rely on the traditional medical model paradigm that the trained occupational therapy professional is the "expert" who administers a particular procedure or protocol, or trains the client in its use. Intrapersonal interventions, such as mindfulness, meditation, Yoga, and relaxation techniques, demonstrate unquestionable benefits and are considered evidence-based interventions. . . . [but] with few exceptions, these interventions do little to tap into the relevance and powerful potential to influence change that . . . exists in the therapeutic relationship between the occupational therapy professional and the client.

C: Case study includes

Consider the following brief case scenario. (This is based on an actual situation reported to the original author of this text, Dr Mary Beth Early, by a student after the September 11, 2001, terrorist attacks in New York City.)

Imagine that you are an occupational therapy professional working in a community mental health setting. A federal agent approaches you, shows you his identification, and then shows you a picture and asks you if you know the client/person. The agent says that the person, a woman from another country, is wanted for questioning about two of her sons who are suspected of terrorism. The client is well known to you. The agent presses you to say whether you know her and where he might find her. How do you respond? Use the information presented in this chapter regarding HIPAA policies (29) and the AOTA's *Occupational Therapy Code of Ethics* (1) to support your response.

K: Knowledge: keeping mental health OT practice grounded in evidence, in occupational science, and in research

The client has every right to expect that the occupational therapy professional will provide skillful interventions on the basis of the current knowledge, best practices, and evidence in occupational therapy. Consequently, the occupational therapy professional has an obligation to keep up to date on advances in their areas of practice. For continuing certification and renewal of certification by the NBCOT, all occupational therapy providers must complete units toward certification of competency.

S: Some terms that may be new to you

Competence: having the ability to complete a task effectively; competence is acquired through study and application.

Countertransference: occurs when the other person unconsciously falls into a role that has been transferred onto them

Immediacy: practice of giving feedback right after the event to which it relates

Intentional Relationship Model (IRM): "a conceptual practice model that provides therapists with a practical set of skills and an interpersonal reasoning approach that requires the use of different modes of communication that a therapist invokes in response to the client's evolving interpersonal characteristics and the inevitably challenging and intense interpersonal events of therapy" (27, p. 11).

Projective identification: projection is a psychological defense mechanism that people unconsciously use as a means of self-protection. Projective identification occurs when a person attributes their own feelings, desires, or qualities (especially negative ones) to another person, group, animal, or object.

Psychosocial assistance: at its most simple level, the capacity of the caregiver to "see" the one for whom they are caring at an affective or emotional level

Specificity: art of stating things simply, directly, and concretely, focusing only on what is relevant

Therapeutic modes: patterns or methods of communication that the occupational therapy professional applies as a therapeutic means to helping clients reach their occupational goals, incorporating different styles of interactions in different kinds of situations, as appropriate for each client. The six therapeutic modes are advocating, collaborating, empathizing, encouraging, instructing, and problem-solving.

Therapeutic use of self: being aware of oneself, of the client, and being able to control what one communicates

Transference: occurs when one person unconsciously relates to the other as if that person were someone else, usually an important person in their life

Reflection Questions

1. Write your own definition of *therapeutic use of self*.
2. List and describe Taylor's six therapeutic modes. Identify the kind of situation in which each mode may be useful.
3. What are therapeutic qualities? How might they impact occupational therapy practice and the client's experience and performance in occupational therapy?
4. How do you plan to develop your own therapeutic qualities? Be specific.
5. Compare and contrast the methods and approaches for relating to clients discussed in this chapter.
6. Create a scenario that illustrates transference and countertransference.
7. What can one do if one is afraid of a client?
8. Describe helpful ways to end a therapeutic relationship.

REFERENCES

1. American Occupational Therapy Association. (2020). AOTA 2020 occupational therapy code of ethics. *American Journal of Occupational Therapy, 74*(Suppl. 3), 7413410005.
2. American Occupational Therapy Association. (2020). Occupational therapy in the promotion of health and well-being. *American Journal of Occupational Therapy, 74*, 7403420010.
3. American Occupational Therapy Association. (2020). Occupational therapy practice framework: Domain and process—Fourth edition. *American Journal of Occupational Therapy, 74*(Suppl. 2), 7412410010.
4. American Occupational Therapy Association. (2021). Occupational therapy scope of practice. *American Journal of Occupational Therapy, 75*(Suppl. 3), 7513410030.
5. American Occupational Therapy Association. (2021). Standards of practice for occupational therapy. *American Journal of Occupational Therapy, 75*(Suppl. 3), 7513410050.
6. Brown, J. (2009). *Soul shaping: A journey of self-creation.* North Atlantic Books.
7. Cole, M. B. (2018). *Group dynamics in occupational therapy: The theoretical basis and practice application of group intervention* (5th ed.). SLACK.
8. Fan, C. W., & Taylor, R. (2018). Correlation between therapeutic use of self and clients' participation in rehabilitation. *American Journal of Occupational Therapy, 72*(4, Suppl. 1), 7211500036p1.
9. Gibertoni, C. (2013). An occupational therapy perspective on Freud, Klein and Bion. In L. Nicholls, J. C. Piergrossi, C. Gibertoni, & M. Daniel (Eds.), *Psychoanalytic thinking in occupational therapy* (pp. 32–56). Wiley-Blackwell.
10. Hillman, J. (1989). *A blue fire: Selected writings by James Hillman: Introduced and edited by Thomas Moore in collaboration with James Hillman.* HarperCollins.
11. Hilton, R. (2016). *Relational somatic psychotherapy: Collected essays of Robert Hilton, Ph.D.* (Michael Sieck, Ed.). Robert Hilton and Michael Sieck.
12. Hooper, B., & Wood, W. (2019). The philosophy of occupational therapy: A framework for practice. In B. A. B. Schell & G. Gillen (Eds.), *Willard and Spackman's occupational therapy* (13th ed., pp. 43–55). Lippincott Williams & Wilkins.
13. Kearney, M. (2009). *A place of healing: Working with nature and soul at the end of life.* Spring Journal Books.
14. Kerasidou, A., Bærøe, K., Berger, Z., & Caruso Brown, A. E. (2021). The need for empathetic healthcare systems. *Journal of Medical Ethics, 47*(12), 1–5.

15. Kielhofner, G. (2009). Therapeutic reasoning: Using occupational therapy's conceptual foundations in everyday practice. In G. Kielhofner (Ed.), *Conceptual foundations of occupational therapy practice* (4th ed., pp. 281–283). F.A. Davis.

16. LaLa, A. P., & Kinsella, E. A. (2011). Phenomenology and the study of human occupation. *Journal of Occupational Science, 18*(3), 195–209.

17. Moore, T. (2017). *Ageless soul: The lifelong journey toward meaning and joy.* St. Martin's Press.

18. Moore, T. (2021). *Soul therapy.* HarperCollins.

19. Moreno, P. A. R., Delgado, H. P., Leyva, M. J. M., Casanova, G. G., & Montesó, C. P. (2019). Implementing evidence-based practices on the therapeutic relationship in inpatient psychiatric care: A participatory action research. *Journal of Clinical Nursing, 28*(9–10), 1614–1622.

20. Peloquin, S. M. (1989). Sustaining the art of practice in occupational therapy. *American Journal of Occupational Therapy, 43*(4), 219–226.

21. Peloquin, S. M. (1995). The fullness of empathy: Reflections and illustrations. *American Journal of Occupational Therapy, 49*(1), 24–31.

22. Peloquin, S. M. (1995). The issue is: Communication skills: Why not turn to a skills training model? *American Journal of Occupational Therapy, 49*(7), 721–723.

23. *Psychodynamic diagnostic manual.* (2006). A Task Force of the Alliance of Psychoanalytic Organizations.

24. Sabater, V. (2021). *The origin of the famous saying "Know Thyself".* https://exploringyourmind.com/the-origin-of-the-famous-saying-know-thyself/

25. Schwank, K., Carstensen, T., Yazdani, F., & Bonsaksen, T. (2018). The course of self-efficacy for therapeutic use of self in Norwegian occupational therapy students: A 10-month follow-up study. *Occupational Therapy International, 2018,* 2962747.

26. Sheperd, M. M., Cardin, A., Boehne, T. L., Paloncy-Patel, K. A., & Willis, J. K. (2021). Therapeutic use of self and fieldwork experience: An exploration of the art and science of occupational therapy. *Journal of Occupational Therapy Education, 5*(3), 1–18.

27. Taylor, R. R. (2020). *The intentional relationship: Occupational therapy and use of self* (2nd ed.). F.A. Davis.

28. Taylor, R. R., Lee, S. W., Kielhofner, G., & Ketkar, M. (2009). Therapeutic use of self: A nationwide survey of practitioners' attitudes and experiences. *American Journal of Occupational Therapy, 63*(2), 198–207.

29. United States Department of Health and Human Services. (n.d.). *Health information privacy.* https://www.hhs.gov/hipaa/index.html

30. van der Kolk, B. (2014). *The body keeps the score: Brain, mind, and body in the healing of trauma.* Viking Penguin Group.

31. Yalom, I. D., & Leszcz, M. (2020). *The theory and practice of group psychotherapy* (6th ed.). Basic Books.

32. World Health Organization. (2017). *Mental health in older adults.* http://www.who.int/news-room/fact-sheets/detail/mental-health-of-older-adults

SUGGESTED RESOURCES

Article

Sheperd, M. M., Cardin, A., Boehne, T. L., Paloncy-Patel, K. A., & Willis, J. K. (2021). Therapeutic use of self and fieldwork experience: An exploration of the art and science of occupational therapy. *Journal of Occupational Therapy Education, 5*(3). https://doi.org/10.26681/jote.2021.050313

Books

Before an OT professional (or anyone in a helping profession or role) can endeavor to enter a caregiving relationship, develop a therapeutic rapport and relationship with a client, or employ therapeutic use of self, they must make sure that they "Know Thyself." Psychologist Valaria Sabater writes, "As Thomas Hobbes rightly said, 'Whosoever looketh into himself, and considereth what he doth, when he does think, opine, reason, hope, fear, etc, and upon what grounds; he shall thereby read and know, what are the thoughts, and passions of all other men'. In other words, knowing who you are doesn't only help you, it helps you understand others as well" (32, para. 6).

The following books offer a few good places to begin exploring what makes you who you are, so that in turn you can relate to and support others:

Brown, B. (2010). *The gifts of imperfection: Let go of who you think you're supposed to be and embrace who you are.* Hazelden Press.

Brown, B. (2012). *Daring greatly.* Penguin.

Brown, B. (2015). *Rising strong.* Spiegel & Grau; Penguin Random House.

Brown, B. (2017). *Braving the wilderness.* Penguin Random House.

Doyle, G. (2020). *Untamed.* The Dial Press; Penguin Random House LLC.

Video

A very good example of how to establish therapeutic rapport, listen to the client, explore their story! Understanding the Mental Health Needs of Ukrainian Refugees: Olga's Story https://www.who.int/multi-media/details/understanding-the-mental-health-needs-of-ukrainian-refugees--olga-s-story

Website

HIPAA FAQs for professionals. https://www.hhs.gov/hipaa/for-professionals/faq/index.html

Group Concepts and Techniques in OT Practice

OT HACKS OVERVIEW

O: Occupation as a means and an end

There are a variety of different types of groups; in occupational therapy intervention groups, the emphasis is on helping the client improve role performance through promotion, development, or retention of skills. Group interventions as a service delivery mode have the added benefit of offering a format where clients can establish or improve interpersonal skills, communication, and social interaction skills.

T: Theoretical concepts, values, and principles, or historical foundations

Anne Mosey (35, 36), an occupational therapist, was among the first occupational therapy professionals to analyze the development of **group interaction skills**. Mosey defined group interaction skills as the skills that allow a person to consistently be a productive member of a variety of types of primary groups. Through sequential acquisition of the various group interaction subskills, the individuals in the group learn to perform in appropriate group membership roles, thus enhancing their occupational engagement.

H: How can we Help? OT's role in serving clients with mental illness or mental health needs

Occupational therapy professionals frequently utilize group intervention as a service delivery method in psychosocial and behavioral health settings.

As leaders and developers of occupational therapy intervention groups, the occupational therapy professional must have a working knowledge of the typical dynamics that occur at certain stages of group development. This understanding allows the occupational therapy professional to select, design, and apply appropriate intervention activities, to be mindful of individual client concerns, problem behaviors, and member roles. Understanding group dynamics also helps occupational therapy leaders to support the establishment of healthy and productive group culture and norms, making it more possible for the members to reach their individual goals (10).

A: Adaptations

Developing a rich understanding of the therapeutic factors suggested by Yalom and Leszcz (60) offers a method for

intentionally incorporating therapeutic factors of change into the planning and implementation of occupational therapy intervention groups by incorporating psychotherapeutic principles into the group process. Therapeutic factors that are introduced in this chapter include instillation of hope, universality, imparting of information, altruism, the corrective recapitulation of the primary family group, development of socializing techniques, imitative behavior, interpersonal learning, group cohesiveness, catharsis, and existential factors.

C: Case study includes

This chapter includes guidelines and information about how the occupational therapy professional can design and develop therapeutic occupational therapy group interventions. The following is an example of a group protocol developed for clients who are transitioning into the community and are working on independent living skills. In this example, the group members are developing their ability to meal plan, grocery shop, and meal prep.

Sample Group Session Protocol: Grocery Shopping Goals

Members will learn to do the following:

- Use digital coupons and weekly advertising circulars
- Compare prices
- Compose a shopping list based on a menu

Supplies
- Menu from yesterday's group meeting
- Computer or iPads (available from facility)
- Grocery ads
- Paper
- Pencils
- Calculator

Environment
- For this session, meet in the kitchen.
- Have one member write the menu on flip chart using large letters so all members can see.

Introduction
- Reintroduce self and the name of the group.

- As needed, introduce new members to the group.
- Explain why the group is meeting (eg, "You all want to live semi-independently, and this is an important part of community living.").
- Ask a member to describe what was done yesterday (planning a menu for Friday's lunch, which they will be cooking).
- As needed, restate the rules.

Activities

1. "Friday, this group will prepare a lunch for staff and members of the club. There will be 35 people. The budget is $_____. The menu you developed yesterday is posted. Today, we need to plan our shopping. How do you think we should go about this?"

2. Call on members as needed to get discussion going. Focus on member experiences. Give supportive responses and encourage this behavior in members. Then have members list needed ingredients and calculate quantities.

3. "We have only $_____. What shall we do?" Get members to discuss. If members do not come up with ideas, facilitate discussion of prices, coupons, in-store specials, and so on.

4. Explain the concept of comparison shopping (ideally, get a member to do this). Distribute newspapers and circulars, have members work in pairs to search the internet for digital coupons.

5. Help members develop a plan for when to shop (Thursday) and what to buy at each store.

6. When this is done, ask members to clean up the papers in preparation for discussion. Leave sufficient time for sharing of feelings and of process.

Processing and Discussion

- Get the members to talk about what they have learned and about how they feel about what has happened in the group. Allow time for discussion and feedback among members.
- As needed, focus on behaviors of the members (maintain a constructive and positive attitude even when addressing disruptive behaviors).
- Ask members to consider how what they did here might be of use in their own lives.
- Preview the next group meeting.
- Remind members to bring their bus passes for Thursday because the group will be going shopping.

K: Knowledge: keeping mental health OT practice grounded in evidence, in occupational science, and in research

In the *What's the Evidence?* box in this chapter, readers will find one example, among the growing number of studies, that explore the efficacy of therapeutic groups. *Videogame-Based Group Therapy to Improve Self-Awareness and Social Skills After Traumatic Brain Injury* (30) is an intervention study that investigated the efficacy of using different approaches to integrative videogame-based group therapy to improve self-awareness (SA), social skills, and adaptive behaviors among traumatic brain injury (TBI) survivors. The experimental intervention involved weekly 1-hour group sessions conducted over 6 months. To find out more, check out *What's the Evidence?*

S: Some terms that may be new to you

Advisory leadership
Altruism
Catharsis
Cohesiveness
Didactic instruction
Directive leadership
Facilitative leadership
Group
Group dynamics
Group interaction skills
Group process
Group therapy
Group-centered actions
Illumination of process
Individual/egocentric roles
Interpersonal-input
Interpersonal-output
Psychoeducation
Purposeful actions
Self-initiated actions
Social capital
Social network
Social support
Social support groups
Social-emotional roles
Spontaneous actions
Task roles

INTRODUCTION

According to the *American Occupational Therapy Association Practice Framework: Domain and Process*, Fourth Edition (OTPF-4), the term **group** is defined as a "Collection of individuals having shared characteristics or a common or shared purpose (eg, family members, workers, students, others with similar occupational interests or occupational challenges)" (1, p. 77). The OTPF-4 further acknowledges

that a "client" may indicate an individual person, a group, or a population. Occupational therapy professionals frequently utilize group intervention as a service delivery method in psychosocial and behavioral health settings. When occupational therapy professionals facilitate groups, they preserve the focus on client-driven priorities that will support the client being able to engage in the everyday occupations that are meaningful and necessary (5). Although there are a variety of different types of groups, the emphasis in occupational therapy intervention groups is often on helping the client improve role performance through skill development or retention of skills. Group interventions as a service delivery mode have the added benefit of offering a format where clients can improve or establish interpersonal skills, communication, or social interaction skills. The most frequently reported types of groups used in occupational therapy practice are physical activity groups that are aimed at overall wellness, sensory modulation groups, and task-based groups (21).

People live and work in groups. Social interaction skills for relating to others effectively are essential for everyday functioning. Because people with disabilities, regardless of the nature of the disability, may have trouble relating to others, whether individually or in groups, it is important to consider how people generally develop these skills. This chapter explains why and how occupational therapy groups might be used to support the client's optimal occupational engagement across all occupations. A review of group process and group dynamics is included, as is a brief discussion of the necessary components required for developing an occupational therapy intervention group. The chapter concludes with a discussion focused on leading and managing occupational therapy groups. The final sections of the chapter introduce and address some basic adaptations required for specialized types or formats of groups. Specialized groups described include those designed explicitly for clients in acute inpatient settings, and particularly relevant following the COVID-19 pandemic, and the reader is offered a glimpse at the characteristics of group facilitation in virtual contexts and best practices in delivery of services through telehealth initiatives.

The ability to plan, implement, and lead groups effectively is one of the most valuable skill sets that the occupational therapy professional can bring to a psychiatric or behavioral health team. An understanding of how therapeutic groups differ from other kinds of groups, and knowledge about the varied roles and skills needed in a group leader, is essential. These topics, as well as a suggested procedure for designing group sessions as part of a larger organized group protocol, are covered in some detail. As is true for developing other clinical skills, the ability to run a group effectively increases with practice and studious self-reflection. This chapter is designed to prepare the reader to *initiate* this process.

GROUPS IN OCCUPATIONAL THERAPY

Why use groups in occupational therapy practice? How does an occupational therapy professional use groups to most effectively lead to optimal outcomes for the client? And what is **group therapy**? The occupational therapy process is designed to help clients create changes that will enable them to carry out daily life activities as independently, comfortably, and efficiently as possible. If we add this concept to our definition of a group, we may imagine group therapy conceptually as the following: *Group therapy is a planned process for creating changes in individuals by bringing them together for*

this purpose. Group therapy is considered a service delivery mode in occupational therapy practice, and groups can be further categorized by their type or intended purpose. Four commonly recognized types of occupational therapy groups are functional groups, social groups, activity groups, and task groups (1).

Functional Groups

Therapeutic groups are further defined by their intended purpose or outcome. The purpose, and ultimately the goal, of a functional group in occupational therapy is to help individuals to enhance their overall health and wellness through purposeful engagement in occupation (14). In functional groups, experiences are planned to encourage members to adjust the problematic features of their contexts to cope more effectively and, eventually, to adapt a personally satisfying and healthy engagement in everyday life. Functional groups are centered around two primary constructs: adaptation, or the adjustment to one's context, and the occupational behaviors and actions of the group members and the group as a whole. The mechanism of change in functional groups occurs through dynamic action-oriented participation in health-promoting, purposeful occupations that result in the increased likelihood of client adaptation.

Four actions that come together and stimulate adaptation in a functional group are **purposeful actions**, actions that are meaningful to the client; **self-initiated actions**, any actions, verbal or nonverbal, that are initiated by the client; **spontaneous actions**, unplanned or unexpected actions that take place during the group process, the here-and-now experience; and **group-centered action**, occurrences that result from the dynamic and interdependent actions between group members. A functional group model embraces a common group goal but the actions and dynamic interactions among the members produce the learning and, in turn, influence adaptation (27). Essentially, occupational participation becomes the vehicle for learning, change, and growth. In the truest sense, this demonstrates the principle of using occupations as a means, rather than an end. Functional groups can be designed to focus on any occupational area. These groups can be modified to be well suited for the ages and functional levels of group members.

One example of the use of a functional group model in occupational therapy practice is a pilot pretest–posttest intervention study that was designed to evaluate the effects of a functional group–based intervention treatment with preschoolers who have attention deficit hyperactivity disorder (ADHD) (43). The intervention was based on the Cog–Fun treatment approach, which emphasizes the acquisition of executive strategies in the context of occupational performance in common childhood occupations such as play, self-care, and social participation (8, 31). The Cog–Fun approach must be administered by occupational therapists who have achieved the additional Cog–Fun training and certification, and while Cog–Fun is typically implemented with a client and their parent or teacher (dyad), this study expanded the use of the intervention to a group service delivery method (18, 31, 43). The intervention encouraged purposeful actions, self-initiated actions, spontaneous actions, and group-centered actions by teaching six specific executive strategies (I listened, I waited for my turn, I asked for help, I have an idea, I made an effort, and I helped a friend) in a group context.

The findings in this study imply that the use of a group intervention that applies a functional group model, combined with guided parent involvement and training, and focused on executive strategies presented through occupational engagement is effective in meeting occupational goals. Furthermore, this initial study supports the notion that children with executive function difficulties have the potential to improve when their parents are active participants in a dynamic, action-oriented, occupation-centered functional group designed to improve executive function (43).

Social Groups

Human beings are neurologically wired for social connection, and lacking appropriate social connection and support is linked to a myriad of negative health effects. Occupational therapy professionals can assist clients who have mental illness with the management of the symptoms causing occupational disruptions. To do this, practitioners must develop an awareness of how social supports and social support networks are either hindering or contributing to client recovery (45). **Social support** is described as the various sources of help offered to individuals and groups, typically from within their communities. These sources can act as a protective factor against adverse life circumstances, harmful living conditions, and may help the client develop resiliency toward enhancing quality of life. **Social networks** are the relationships and social ties between people that often increase access to social supports or help to mobilize the needed social supports (6).

One of many approaches that occupational therapy professionals can apply as an evidence-based method of service provision for providing opportunities to clients with mental illness is facilitation of **social groups**, also referred to as **social support groups**. Clients who have experienced mental illness need opportunities to form healthy reciprocal relationships in safe contexts (10). Recent research indicates the broad positive impacts of interventions that target the social support needs of these clients by helping them to develop social capital. **Social capital** refers to social support resources, relationships, and support networks that influence a client's overall occupational engagement (46).

There is increasing attention on the valuable contribution of positive social capital on the recovery process for clients with the psychosocial dysfunctions that often characterize conditions such as bipolar disorder, major depressive disorder, schizophrenia, and delusional disorders, among others. It is also well-documented that disability and mental illness that results in occupational disruption negatively impacts both the quality and number of meaningful relationships that a person has. This further contributes to loneliness, social isolation, and stigmatization. Social capital, sometimes understood as social connectedness, promotes recovery through the instillation of therapeutic factors (discussed in later sections of this chapter) so that people with mental illness have increased likelihood of reengaging in meaningful occupational roles and participation. The literature further indicates the potential that these interventions have in helping the client sustain supportive networks that can help with future challenges related to their illness (4, 10, 45).

Nevertheless, the focus of much of the research related to the importance of social support and social networks is aimed at service provision modalities and client adherence to adopting new healthier ways of daily living. There is a paucity of work that examines how people with mental illness who are in recovery can generalize the social supports, reciprocal relationships, and social networks developed through social support groups (and other modes of treatment) into broader forms, and in different forums in the community in more natural and often client-preferred contexts. With that in mind, researchers Brown and Baker (2020) explored aspects of participants' recovery experiences that "went beyond health and social care or those forms of social support which was focused on symptom management and enabled them to venture into other social networks" (4, p. 387).

The purpose of their inquiry was to examine recovery through interviews with 34 participants who had been treated for mental health disorders. The intent of the interviews was to allow the participants to describe their experiences of recovery through the lens of social capital. The researchers focused on the clients' social networks and relationships, and how their social capital changed over the course of their recovery process. The responses of the participants are a powerful example of how development of client social capital that is truly focused on client occupational priorities, and that focuses on occupational outcomes (specifically occupational justice, occupational balance, and quality of life), can be applied in occupational therapy practice to encourage broadening of social engagement and social networks for the client that extend beyond the outcomes of standard clinical interventions (4).

Task Groups

Similar to the social group interventions discussed in the preceding section, the impact of a client's social network and cultural heritage on their behaviors, lifestyle, and occupational engagement cannot be ignored. This has widened the span of traditional treatments and led to the development of, in particular, task-oriented groups. "Such developments are manifested in the gradual melding of sociologic, psychoanalytic, and learning theories and the emerging focus on ego functions and adaptive skills" (15, p. 427). Task-oriented group interventions exist across several disciplines, but task-oriented groups are used as a context for implementing occupational therapy intervention, which is somewhat different from their application in other arenas. When used for occupational therapy, these task groups are uniquely designed and characterized by the production of goods or services resulting from the members of the group working together: planning, developing, or implementing activities or products that will benefit the group as a whole, or sometimes a person or organization outside of the group.

Fidler (15) wrote about how contextually, the occupational therapy small group settings can be planned to mimic a version of life and work situations so that the clients, while performing task roles as a group member, can explore in real time what problems exist in the occupational context of one's work life. "The intent of the task-oriented group is to provide a shared working experience wherein the relationship between feeling, thinking, and behavior; their impact on others and on task accomplishment; and their productivity can be viewed and explored" (15, p. 429). In other words, the primary purpose of the group is not necessarily to complete the task, rather the context of the group becomes the backdrop and the task itself is as follows:

1. A catalyst that elicits work behaviors and work-related communication and interaction with others (15)
2. A strategy for focusing on a client's strengths and limitations regarding work skills and problem-solving (15)
3. A reality-grounded means by which the client's learning gains can be measured (15)

In the past decade, the use of task-oriented groups with clients who have schizophrenia, psychosis, and major depression has expanded and encouraged contribution to the research and literature supporting the intervention strategy for these populations (7, 32, 42). Research indicates that task-oriented groups are helpful to the client with reality testing and the validation of the cause and effect of their function and behaviors on the task process. In task-oriented group work, the responsibility of tasks is shared, and so a member's actions, follow-through, and action or inaction are revealed in terms of the contribution to the group, which reinforces the learning (15).

Activity Groups

Although activity groups are similar to task groups, activity groups differ from other therapy groups in that the *doing*, or participating in a meaningful activity, is the medium through which the group members achieve their goals. Thus, activity groups become laboratories designed so that members can experiment with the occupational roles, skills, interests, and habits that are most meaningful and relevant to their present daily lives. In this model, the most important function of the group leader is to assign members specific tasks and roles that are pragmatic or motivating relative to their everyday life. For example, within the context of a community-based seniors group, in a current events group that uses activities related to the daily newspaper to encourage both social interaction and other client performance skill enhancement (such as improved cognitive function, memory enhancement, or problem-solving), the leader may assign members to a role where each member must act as a daily reporter for their assigned section of the paper. In that way, the role assignment for each member takes into account the job responsibilities of the actual counterpart in that same occupational role (a reporter), while simultaneously taking into account the preferences of the group member (ie, asking the member which section of the newspaper interests them the most—one reads the sports highlights, someone covers international news, and maybe someone even reads or shows a few of the clips from the comics section). Furthermore, social interaction can be encouraged through a structured format; the "activity" at weekly meetings requires members to report on their designated part of the newspaper.

GROUP PROCESS: A REVIEW OF BASIC CONCEPTS

We have all participated in groups that worked well, that reached their goals through the combined efforts of all the members in a way that was relatively satisfying to the members. Likewise, we have all known groups that never seemed to get off the ground, that failed to reach their goals because the members could not work together. Such groups can be psychologically draining for functional people; and for people who are ill, these group experiences pose risks for further exacerbating their condition. What accounts for the difference between these two kinds of group outcomes? Why do some groups succeed while others fail? What ingredients are necessary for a group to be successful, according to the evidence? The answers to these questions are usually found by reflecting more deeply on four core aspects of therapeutic groups: group process, group dynamics, group members and group membership, and group leadership.

When groups are incorporated as a context for treatment in occupational therapy intervention, application of a psychoanalytic approach or method of treatment is common. In the psychoanalytic tradition, personality changes occur when the client explores their interpersonal conflicts and they become gradually willing to reflect more deeply on where their internal conflicts or struggles and how those struggles affect their personality, behavioral responses, and relationships (11, 15, 22). This kind of interpersonal work, of course, begins with the individual; however, it cannot be fully successful without the presence of others. The power of interpersonal learning as a therapeutic factor occurs as the group experience a process together in the "here and now" (15). According to Cole (10), an understanding of the underlying principles of group process will guide the occupational therapy professional in choosing an appropriate intervention approach. However, the difference between a psychotherapeutic group (one that applies the psychoanalytic frame of reference) and other types of groups (support groups, 12-step groups, social skills training groups, or psychoeducational groups) is the emphasis on the "here-and-now" experience (15).

Understanding process provides clues about various group members' emotions and motivations. The occupational therapy professional can, and should, use this information over time to bring the client to an improved level of SA while also strategically helping the group members to use the here-and-now experiences to help one another recognize characteristics within themselves and during interactions. In therapeutic groups this type of self-reflection and exploration occurs because of the interactions between the members (with each other) and between the members and the group leader(s), or occupational therapy professional (10, 60). "[Group] Process is often first understood by what it is not. It is not content. The content of a group is what is done and what is said. . . . [The group process] thrust is what is happening in the group, between and among members, right now. Process concerns the interpersonal relationships among participants" (10, p. 30). **Group process**, then, is defined as the consideration of many aspects; the relationships and interactions between the individual group members and occupational therapy professional, consideration of other contexts (ie, sociocultural, setting of the group, sociopolitical), interpersonal interactions, whole-group elements, and the psyche (or internal psychological world) of the individuals in the group (39, 54, 60).

Experts in the theory and practical application of psychotherapeutic groups, Irvin Yalom and Molyn Leszcz insist that for the "here-and-now" experience to lead to efficacious outcomes for clients, two things must happen. Without both factors occurring, the therapeutic power of group intervention cannot be present. First, the members must be present to experience the things that are happening in the group, in the moment. They begin to develop feelings and relationships with the other group members and with the leader so that "The immediate events of the meeting take precedence over events both in the outside life, and in the distant past of the members" (60, p. 184). The concentration on what is happening in the moment within the group, according to Yalom and Leszcz (60), helps the client transform the group into a social microcosm that can be used as a context for facilitating growth through various therapeutic factors such as catharsis, which are introduced in the next section.

Although the capacity for the clients to experience and remain focused on the in-the-moment transactions is critical, without the second ingredient, which Yalom and Leszcz (60) call "the illumination of process" (60, p. 184), the power of therapeutic change and interpersonal learning within the group will not happen. The **illumination of process** means that the group, over time, does more than experience the "here and now." The group must recognize, examine, and reflect upon process to understand the experience more fully. This self-reflective loop allows members to examine the experiences of the group together (as a microcosm) to study its transactions and make connections. Through this mechanism, the group members rise above merely having very powerful here-and-now experiences. They transcend the experiences by illuminating the process so that they can integrate what they learn into meaningful life situations outside of the group, which leads to improved occupational function and engagement (10, 60).

Therapeutic Factors

An occupational therapy professional applies both therapeutic reasoning and an approach to therapeutic groups that is unique from that of other disciplines. The occupational therapy focus remains on utilizing occupations as the primary route to support improvements in client health. The occupational therapy professional, by creating an occupational profile, and through effective occupational performance analysis and activity analysis, can plan powerful contextually appropriate interventions that help group members improve the qualitative experience and function of engagement in their own daily lives. Developing a rich understanding of the therapeutic factors suggested by Yalom and Leszcz (60) offers a method for intentionally incorporating factors of change into the planning and implementation of occupational therapy intervention groups that incorporate psychotherapeutic principles into the group process. Furthermore, the body of evidence suggests that many of the therapeutic factors have a neurologic foundation, which implies that intentional use of the therapeutic factors has potential to improve neurophysiologic responses, leading to more positive behavioral changes and better functional outcomes for the client (28, 41). The following is a very brief introduction to some of the psychoanalytic therapeutic principles that are at work in an intervention group.

Instillation of Hope

When a client is hopeful that they will receive help from an intervention, treatment, or therapy, evidence indicates that their high expectation is correlated with more positive therapeutic outcomes (60). As an occupational therapy professional is designing and implementing therapeutic groups, maximum effort should be put into increasing the group members' confidence that the group will be helpful to them in reaching their individual occupational goals. The instillation of hope begins even during the planning stages, when the occupational therapy leader is recruiting or selecting members for the group. Throughout the planning stages (pregroup orientation), the therapist can clearly explain what the group is designed to address, which reinforces positive expectations and may help moderate negative preconceived notions of group therapy.

Instillation of hope occurs in more than one way, and one source of hope is distinctive to the group format. Because most therapeutic groups have members who are at different places in their recovery journey and who also often share similar problems, groups provide a firsthand account of how others have improved and are improving because of the occupational therapy. Members who have been present in the group on a longer term basis, or who have benefited from the group, often naturally assume the role of instilling hope by sharing their success stories with skeptical new members (60). Self-help groups emphasize the importance of hopefulness and maintaining the expectation that recovery and a better quality of life is possible. Peer mentors and peer group leaders are powerful reminders to others of hope and potential for wellness that exist when supportive interventions and a support network are in place, *if* the individual commits to doing the work (60).

Universality

At some point in life, most of us will experience the feeling of being alone in a problem we are having, or feeling as if nobody else could possibly understand the kinds of thoughts or emotions that we are having. For clients with mental illness though, extensive social isolation contributes to a heightened sense of being alone, unique in their problems, problematic choices, and typically stigmatized further as a consequence of problematic behavioral responses (60). Universality is the feeling or realization that one is not alone. "For some clients, feeling human among other humans is the beginning of recovery and a central feature of the healing context that group therapists aim to create" (60, p. 16). Universality is significant for the sense of relief a client feels when, despite their complexities, they begin to identify similarities with other members. The occupational therapy professional must consider client factors carefully when developing therapeutic groups. There are instances when members of a more homogeneous group can speak to one another with the authenticity that comes from having firsthand experience with a difficult problem. Evidence indicates that a more homogeneous group with similar experiences can be efficacious for offsetting secrecy and shame in therapeutic groups for sexual abuse survivors and individuals with eating disorders, among others (19, 33, 48).

Imparting Information

Occupational therapy professionals provide information to members of therapeutic groups in a variety of forms and formats, the most common of which is through **didactic instruction**. Didactic instruction is direct instruction about mental health, mental illness, and the psychodynamics of interpersonal relationships (60). Didactic instruction can be used to explain the typical progression or symptoms of an illness or, as in cognitive behavioral therapy (CBT), direct instruction can be given to the client about strategies they can use to change destructive thought patterns. At times, the occupational therapy professional leading the group may provide direct instruction, guidance, or advice. Depending on the type and maturity level of the group, at other times information will be transferred between the group members (10). Literature also supports the notion that participation in an effectively facilitated therapy group has the potential to enhance the client's emotional intelligence skills and capabilities, allowing them to learn about empathy and understand more about the connection between their symptoms, their responses, and their relationships (24, 60). The provision of direct instruction and interpersonal feedback in a more formalized manner is called **psychoeducation**. Many occupational therapy therapeutic group interventions embrace the psychoeducational approach. Yalom and Leszcz (60) advise occupational therapy professionals that when imparting

information, regardless of the type or approach, "The group environment in which learning takes place is important. The atmosphere in all these groups is one of partnership and collaboration rather than prescription and subordination" (60, p. 19).

Altruism

Understanding the therapeutic factors may help occupational therapy professionals maximize the effectiveness of their intervention planning and inform the way that they facilitate groups. **Altruism** is defined as actions taken to promote the welfare of others, despite personal liabilities, risks, or harms to oneself (2, 17). Clients with psychiatric illness are often marginalized. Having lived with the stigma of having a mental illness, this population tends to feel that they do not possess any useful characteristics and they are hesitant that they can be helpful to anyone. Finding a place in a therapeutic group, developing roles and being able to contribute something to the group or to another member promotes a sense of self-worth. "members gain through giving. . . . Being useful to others is refreshing and boosts self-esteem, and it is only group therapy that offers clients such an experience" (60, p. 24).

The Corrective Recapitulation of the Primary Family Group

One of the first and most fundamental group experiences that we encounter is with the primary family. According to the evidence, many clients who enter therapeutic groups have had negative experiences with their primary family (with the exception of clients with posttraumatic stress disorder [PTSD] or other environmental or medical stressors) (60). In structure, the therapy group shares many characteristics of a family unit with its authority figures, peer relationships that may be compared to sibling relationships, and the dynamics, deep intimacy, and strong emotions that may develop over time. The corrective recapitulation of the primary family group allows the client to explore how negative experiences with their primary family have impacted their current state of health. The therapeutic group allows the client to relive negative experiences *correctively* (60). For some clients, working out problems in the safe context of a group that represents their primary family structure provides them with closure of long unfinished business.

Development of Socializing Techniques

Social learning is the development of necessary social skills. Social learning as an approach and as a therapeutic factor is one of the main reasons that occupational therapy professionals implement group interventions. Clients who need support with social skills must have a context in which to learn and practice socialization, hence the occupational therapy literature is full of examples of the use of evidence-based group interventions to enhance social skills so that clients can engage or reengage in meaningful occupations (16, 38, 40).

As mentioned previously, social skills or socializing techniques may be taught using a variety of approaches. Direct instruction may be employed, or in some groups the social learning may be less explicit. Group members can receive feedback about their interpersonal skills or social habits that increase their awareness about how those social habits or patterns have impacted relationships or aspects of their occupational engagement. For some clients, their psychiatric illness has made it difficult for them to establish intimate friendships or relationships; the group may be among the first opportunity that the client has had to receive accurate interpersonal feedback from others (60).

Imitative Behavior

Socialization and a significant amount of social learning happen by watching and imitating the behaviors of instrumental people in our life. Successfully adapting one's behavior and modeling others in ways that are appropriate to the situation and context supports clients' successful occupational participation. Occupational therapy group leaders can incorporate interventions such as role-playing to encourage the development and imitation of useful and appropriate adaptive responses. Imitative behavior as a therapeutic factor is also found in techniques that incorporate assignment of peer mentors, or buddies, to support inclusion and transition back into the community after discharge from psychiatric rehabilitation (60).

Another element of imitative behavior worthwhile to reflect upon is the role that the group leader, facilitator, or therapist plays in shaping the behavior of the group members. The occupational therapy professional who has a successful grasp on facilitating groups, with practice, can incorporate principles of imitative behavior to use in the group. In occupational therapy, this is accomplished through therapeutic use of self and by demonstrating behaviors that provide a good model for clients to imitate. Occupational therapy professional behaviors such as appropriate use of self-disclosure, provision of timely and compassionate feedback, and accepting the group member wherever they are in their illness recovery, all have been shown to positively impact the outcomes of therapy (23, 49, 60).

Interpersonal Learning

Of the therapeutic factors, understanding how to apply interpersonal learning as a therapeutic factor during group work is a high priority. Interpersonal learning can be broken into two subcategories: **interpersonal-input**, when an individual learns how they impact others, and **interpersonal-output**, when an individual learns to change how they interact with others. People need other people to live a life that is healthy and balanced. Human connection and interaction are essential for survival, socialization, and pursuit of a satisfactory life (59, 60). Interpersonal learning directly impacts the development of therapeutic relationships and how the occupational therapy professional demonstrates primary accurate empathy in both individual therapy sessions and

in therapeutic groups. Understanding this complex therapeutic factor is essential in the pursuit of becoming a successful evidence-based leader of therapeutic groups (29, 59). Furthermore, some interpersonal learning processes that encourage client growth are unique to group interventions. This requires the occupational therapy professional to be aware of how to initiate particular aspects of group process through their actions. Interpersonal learning is the primary therapeutic factor in group work that mediates changes in the group members.

The World Health Organization (WHO) developed the Mental Health Gap Action Programme (mhGAP) in 2008. The mhGAP was designed to increase the availability of resources globally to provide more accessible services for people with mental, neurologic, and substance use disorders. In 2010, the *mhGAP Intervention Guide for Mental, Neurological and Substance Use Disorders for Non-specialized Health Settings, Version 1.0* (mhGAP-IG) was established to further amplify the dissemination and implementation of mhGAP objectives (56). The *mhGAP Intervention Guide* provided protocols for use in clinical decision-making and managing prioritized conditions including the following:

- Anxiety
- Depression
- Psychoses and bipolar disorders
- Epilepsy and seizures
- Child and adolescent mental disorders
- Dementia
- Alcohol use disorders
- Drug use disorders
- Self-harm and suicide
- Conditions related to stress and other significant emotional and medical unexplained somatic complaints

Updates to the mhGAP guidelines based on new evidence and research were published in 2015 (57) and followed in 2016 by the publication of the *mhGAP Intervention Guide, Version 2.0*, online application, which reflected the updated guidelines (58). Extensive feedback collected from use of the tool in the field was included to clarify the original version and further increase its usability. According to Shekhar Saxena, Director of the Department of Mental Health and Substance Abuse at the WHO (58), "There is a widely shared but false notion that all mental health interventions are complex and can only be delivered by highly specialized staff. Research in recent years has demonstrated the feasibility of delivery of pharmacologic and psychosocial interventions in non-specialized health-care settings" (58, p. iii).

The therapeutic value of interpersonal learning is that it mediates change through social connections and interpersonal relationships. In group interventions, the relationships and the connections of the group as a social microcosm facilitate the changes in the group members. Interpersonal therapy (IPT) is an evidence-based psychological treatment intervention that focuses on the links between mental health symptoms and interpersonal problems using aspects of interpersonal learning (58). When the WHO developed the mhGAP in 2008 and subsequently published the mhGAP Intervention Guide in 2010, there were recommendations for evidence-based interventions, but few details were given about the interventions themselves or about how to implement them (56, 58). In response, the *Group Interpersonal Therapy for Depression* protocol (IPT adapted for use with groups) was created to provide detailed instructions on how to facilitate group IPT. IPT and CBT are two of the mhGAP's first-line, evidence-based recommendations for intervention (59). Occupational therapy professionals are well prepared to lead IPT groups. The clear directions and suggestions offered in the *Group Interpersonal Therapy for Depression* (59) protocol provide excellent guidance.

Group Cohesiveness

In a variety of therapeutic interventions with individual clients, the literature suggests that a constructive relationship between the therapist and client is essential to positive outcomes. **Group cohesiveness** as a therapeutic factor in groups might be compared to the therapeutic relationship between the client and the occupational therapy professional in individual therapy (60). For all the other therapeutic factors to function, group cohesiveness must be in place. Essentially, group cohesiveness is the broad perspective that includes the interactions and relational bonds that form between the members, that also considers the relationships between the occupational therapy professionals and each of the group members, and finally produces the connections that bond the group to one another as a whole (10, 60). Groups do not typically demonstrate a sense of cohesiveness in the early stages because developing cohesiveness is a process that occurs over time. Cohesiveness is one of the characteristics of the end stage in group development and is frequently seen in mature groups. However, the level of cohesiveness of a group is not fixed. In fact, some degree of early cohesiveness, or the potential for new members or newly formed groups to feel a sense of belongingness in the early stages of group development, is necessary for relationships and bonding to continue to flourish. Lastly, the critical importance of the group leader's attention to the cohesiveness of the group cannot be overstated. "Cohesion requires the therapist's diligent attention to the dynamic interplay of member and group, and *regular* feedback about the state of the group and its members can help focus this attention, alerting the group to threats to group cohesion in the interest of timely therapist responsiveness" (60, p. 85).

Catharsis

From the perspective of the psychoanalytic frame of reference, **catharsis** means that an individual experiences an emotional release. Yalom and Leszcz (60) describe actions characteristic of therapeutic catharsis as the following:

1. The group member being able to get things off their chest
2. The group member being able to express negative and positive feelings toward another group member

3. The group member being able to express negative and positive feelings toward the group leader
4. The group member learning how to express their feelings
5. The group member being able to express what is bothering them rather than internalizing it

In occupational therapy intervention groups, if a client experiences an emotional release and the occupational therapy leader(s) can guide the focus and responses of the group, the possible reasons for the catharsis can be reflected upon, interpreted, and used to mediate positive change for the client (10, 60). If the cathartic expression can be connected to the client learning something about themselves, the therapeutic value of catharsis has been enacted.

Existential Factors

Existential factors are related to all the aspects that a person faces that are a part of existing as a human, a part of the human condition. Many of these factors are conceptual and difficult to capture or describe. Behaviors or learning principles characteristic of existential factors include the recognition that life will sometimes be unfair and that the circumstances of one's life are sometimes unjust. Existential factors can also include things that are difficult for many of us to face, that some painful life events are unavoidable, and that death is an inevitable part of life for all of us. Several existential factors are of relevance to group therapy. Clients must learn that regardless of how much guidance or support that comes from other members of the group, or from the group leader, and no matter how close the group members relationships get, life must be faced alone, and the individual must ultimately take responsibility for the choices that they make and the way that they live their lives (10, 60).

GROUP DYNAMICS AND THE STAGES OF GROUP DEVELOPMENT

Dynamic energies are a function of all groups and they profoundly influence group development. **Group dynamics** consist of all the forces that influence the interactions and interrelationships of the group members. Group dynamics will also eventually impact whether group members experience success within a group intervention setting and the overall outcomes of the group (10, 60). As leaders and developers of occupational therapy intervention groups, the occupational therapy professional must have a working knowledge of the typical dynamics that occur at certain stages of group development. This understanding allows the occupational therapy professional to select, design, and apply appropriate intervention activities, to be mindful of individual client concerns, problem behaviors, and member roles. Understanding group dynamics also helps occupational therapy leaders to support the establishment of healthy and productive group culture and norms (10).

"Familiarity with group development is essential to understanding group process and group dynamics" (60, p. 381). One of the most well-recognized group developmental theories suggests that the stages of group development include the five phases: forming, storming, norming, performing, and adjourning (50, 51). According to Yalom and Leszcz (60), during the initial phase of group development, the forming stage, the members are trying to determine the rationale for therapy and may even ask how this group (and its suggested activities) will help them with their problems. They are simultaneously comparing themselves against others, trying to decide if they will be liked and accepted by others, and thinking about whether there is a role for them in the group. In other words, the decision question at the forming stage is "Am I **in or out** with this group?"

In the storming phase, the members' preoccupation with acceptance and approval, and the need to understand the agenda and rules of the group, passes and are replaced with a conflictual period that is characterized by each member struggling for their desired level of dominance, control, and power. A social order typically emerges. The decision question at the storming stage is "Will I be at the **top or the bottom** of the hierarchy of power and control?" The third stage, or the norming stage of group development, is characterized by the appearance of early stages of group cohesiveness. The decisions and questions of this phase can be thought of as the members being concerned about the relational aspects of the group, "Am I **near or far?**" "The members' primary anxieties have to do with not being liked, not being close enough to others, or being too close to others" (60, p. 391). Finally, in the performing stage, the group moves into a mature level where cohesiveness of the group is apparent, which most effectively allows for therapeutic change to occur for the group members and the group. Table 16.1 summarizes well-evidenced common stages of group development.

Table 16.1. Common Stages of Group Development

Stage of Group Development	Group Member Characteristics and Behaviors	Relationship to the Group Leader and Group Outcomes
Forming "In or out?"	• Orientation to other group members, to the leader, and to the task or goals of the group • Members must decide how to achieve their primary task (ie, the reason they joined the group). • Members attend to social relationships and create a niche for themselves.	• Heavy dependence on the group leader for guidance • The leader should provide direction and structure. • The leader builds safety and trust by offering an agenda of what lies ahead.
Storming "Top or bottom?"	• Characterized by conflict as members challenge: each other, the task, and the rules	• Members often compete for authority and challenge the leader. • Leader manages and contains conflicts with no defensiveness or hostility.
Norming "Near or far?"	• A tentative peacefulness is present in the group; early stages of cohesiveness are noted among members (ie, group against the world). • Members begin to accept and trust one another. • Conflict is mostly avoided, and negativity is suppressed to preserve cohesiveness.[a]	• The leader acts as an encourager, helps keep consistent balance as this stage is characterized by the early stages of the development of cohesiveness.
Performing	• Group members have established stable cohesiveness, are able to experience conflict, discuss the conflict openly, and in most cases problem-solve to reach a resolution (ie, struggles arise not for purposes of gaining power or control but often because of members' internal struggles—true teamwork is demonstrated as members help one another to resolve personal and interpersonal problems).	• A supportive psychosocial and emotional context has been established, encouraging growth and therapeutic change to occur in individual group members and in the group as a whole. • In many cases, the leadership style becomes more facilitative, less restrictive than in other stages.
Adjourning	• Termination of a therapeutic group is an important part of the group development process. • The adjourning of a group can happen for a variety of reasons. • Tuckman and Jensen (51) assert that the task of the members in this stage is to review both positive and negative experiences in the group and evaluate what has been learned. • In this stage, members organize and plan for the future.	• Termination of a group can be difficult for an attuned occupational therapy leader. • Leaders who are open with their feelings and who demonstrate authentic self-disclosure will make the good-byes easier for the members of the group.

[a]Note that for the group to move into a mature group (the performing stage), the group members must be able to openly express both positive and negative feelings and thoughts, to attempt resolution.
Adapted from Cole, M. B. (2018). *Group dynamics in occupational therapy: The theoretical basis and practice application of group intervention* (5th ed.). SLACK; Yalom, I. D., & Leszcz, M. (2020). *The theory and practice of group psychotherapy* (6th ed.). Basic Books.

Group Member Tasks and Roles

In the beginning stages of group formation, members tend to focus on two primary responsibilities:

1. Determining how to achieve the primary task (which is usually the reason that the client has joined the group)
2. Attending to their social relationships in the group, to create a niche for themselves (60)

These two priorities, over time, lead the members to establish roles. If you watch any small group interact for an hour or so, you will see that the individuals in the group behave in very different ways. For example, five students may be studying together for a neuroscience examination. Angie suggests that they ask each other questions; Robert says it would be better to go over the notes. After a few minutes, Tanya asks if they could consider doing both, going over the notes first, and then asking questions. Meanwhile, Marin has gotten coffee for everyone, and Serena is not really paying much attention because she has been copying Angie's notes from a class that she missed. Each student plays a different role in the group. As the study group progresses, they may switch roles or take on new ones. For instance, when the group gets cranky and tired, Angie may suggest taking a break to get something to eat, or Serena may give a motivating pep talk about how important this test is.

Task roles are sometimes thought of as roles that support the broader functioning of the group. Task roles develop in relationship to the group's goals and the problems it must solve to reach them. **Social-emotional roles** are roles that support the emotional and psychosocial needs of both the individual members and the group as a whole (10, 47).

Social-emotional roles can also be considered as **group maintenance roles**. Social-emotional or group maintenance roles are needed to promote and maintain **cohesiveness**, or closeness, among group members. According to the evidence, the cohesive nature of the group is a therapeutic factor that significantly influences the success of both the group and its individual members in reaching their goals (10, 60).

Individual or egocentric roles are oppositional to group process and group progress. These member roles tend to reflect a member using the group as a space to serve their individual needs, to serve their ego (3). Egocentric roles serve the needs of individuals but they also frequently interfere with the group's progress. It is likely that some individuals in every type of group will adopt these destructive roles. It usually signifies a need for increased support and training to develop the individual's more positive group behaviors. However, even people with the skill and ability to take on productive group roles sometimes enact these destructive and negative roles. This may happen if a group is given a task that is not relevant to them, or at the appropriate skill level to match the members' skill sets, or it may indicate a problem with the leader's style or approach, such as the leader who is too dominant or who is too permissive or passive.

Whenever people interact in groups, individual members take on different functional roles. These roles, which help the group work toward its goals and satisfy the needs of the members, are further exemplified in Table 16.2. Examples illustrate how an individual may behave when serving in each role. The examples given in the table are based on interactions within a task-oriented student group that is planning a fundraiser for their student occupational therapy association.

Table 16.2. Group Member Roles

Group Task Roles	Examples
These roles help the group meet its goals.	This student occupational therapy association has planned to do four fundraising events leading up to the national AOTA conference, which is coming to their city this year. A portion of the funds earned will help defray the costs of attending for students who wish to go to the conference.
Initiator-contributor: Suggests new ideas or new ways of looking at a problem	Rob suggests ordering and selling T-shirts as the next fundraising project.
Information seeker: Asks for facts and further explanation of them	Ginny asks Rob to explain what is involved in submitting an order for a shirt customized with their school logo on it.
Opinion seeker: Asks for opinions and feelings about issues under discussion	Nick asks the others whether they think the T-shirts would sell.
Information giver: Provides facts or information from own experience	Maria reports that the DPT Club had really good luck selling T-shirts at the college career fair last month.
Opinion giver: Expresses feelings or beliefs not necessarily based on facts	Nick says he believes that students already have too many T-shirts and that the profit margin probably would not be very good for the number of shirts they would be able to sell. He suggests organizing a golf tournament.
Elaborator: Spells out suggestions by giving examples or developing scenarios of how it might work out	Rob suggests that maybe the group could come up with a few designs and show them to other students. On the basis of their reactions, the group can decide whether the T-shirt idea is a worthy one to pursue.

Table 16.2. Group Member Roles (*continued*)

Group Task Roles	Examples
Coordinator: Pulls ideas together by showing relationship among different ideas expressed	Ginny says it will probably be easier to make decisions based on student interest levels after sharing some potential designs. The proposed golf tournament is a good backup plan.
Orienter: Focuses group on its goals, keeps discussion from wandering off the point, and so on	Michelle reminds the group that they have already completed a car wash, and hosted a silent auction, but that to complete all four fundraisers before the conference, this one needs to take place in the next 8 wk.
Evaluator-critic: Assesses accomplishments of group in relation to some standard	Caleb says all the ideas sound good to him and comments that this group seems far more organized than other student clubs he has been in.
Energizer: Prods or arouses group to act; stimulates and boosts morale	Maria says, "I'm sure that we can get this third fundraiser moving if we all work together, so who wants to start working on a few sample designs to share with other students?"
Procedural technician: Performs routine tasks that help the group accomplish its task	Although Sarah had not been very vocal during the meeting, before the meeting she had reserved the room, arranged for enough chairs, started the coffee, and got the laptop set up to show the meeting agenda and minutes from the last meeting.
Recorder: Tracks and records member suggestions and decisions; acts as the group scribe	Jack keeps minutes of the meeting and e-mails copies to the group members following the meeting.
Social-emotional or group maintenance roles: These roles support the optimal function and maintenance of the group.	**Examples**
Encourager: Praises, accepts, and supports others in group; encourages different points of view	Jack says that Rob's T-shirt idea has good potential and encourages everyone to consider carefully the potential designs and other related details that could really make his idea come to life.
Harmonizer: Settles differences between other members by reconciling disputes or relieves tension by joking	After a heated debate between Nick and Rob about what to charge for the T-shirts, Valerie jokes, "Well, we aren't trying to sell our shirts in an exclusive online boutique, we can't forget that *we* are the target customers, broke graduate students!"
Compromiser: Gives in to a dispute and changes position to preserve group harmony	Nick admits that maybe people cannot afford to pay $25 for a T-shirt; he is willing to compromise at $15, if they can find a company who can help them get to that price point.
Gatekeeper/expediter: Keeps communication going; this may mean asking others to speak or suggesting ways to give everyone a chance to talk	Maria says some people have not spoken yet and she wonders what they think about the T-shirt prices.
Standard-setter: Expresses norms or standards for group	After the heated debate between Nick and Rob, Sarah says, "I think it will be easier to work together if people can try to listen to each other's ideas before we make any decisions."
Group observer/commentator: Records communication of group; offers this record to group for its comment and interpretation; provides interpretations when needed	Maria notes that Nick has snapped at both Rob and Michelle several times today (this is a role the therapist may play).
Follower: Goes along with the general mood and decisions of the group	The student group included 20 people but not all participated in the discussion; the rest listened and voted by a show of hands at the end of the meeting on how to proceed to move the plans forward.
Individual or egocentric roles: These roles are in opposition to the group task roles and could reflect the possibility that an individual member is using the group context to meet personal needs.	**Examples**
Aggressor: Belittles or attacks group members, group, or its purpose; shows disapproval or tries to take credit for actions of others	Tricia says she would be happy to listen to Rob's ideas, but because he never follows through on anything he suggests, she thinks it is a waste of time.

(continued)

Table 16.2. Group Member Roles (*continued*)	
Blocker: Prevents group from progressing, by resisting change, opposing decisions, rehashing dead issues, and so on	Lenore asks why the group always suggests selling "stuff" that nobody needs or wants to buy, and reminds the group that they still have a box of T-shirts that they could not sell from last year.
Recognition-seeker: Calls attention to self by boasting, talking about own talents, insisting on having a powerful position, and so on	Alberto says he only buys T-shirts if they are high quality and have very unique designs. He tells the group that he will bring some of his T-shirts in so that the group will get the right idea of what people will actually buy.
Self-confessor: Expresses personal problems, political ideology, or other concerns to captive audience of group	Ella tells the group that she is so upset by her grade on the anatomy quiz that was just posted that it is all that she really cares about right now. She asks how everyone else did.
Playboy: Is not involved with group; shows dis- interest by clowning around, being cynical, and so on	Amira sits near Alberto, adding comments under her breath that nobody can hear except Alberto. The two whisper comments to one another, and laugh throughout the meeting, ignoring everyone else.
Dominator: Tries to take control by manipulating group or members; tactics may include interrupt- ing, bossiness, flattery, and seduction	Nick interrupts Rob and several other members repeatedly, telling him to "get to the point" and "leave out the boring details."
Help-seeker: Tries to get sympathy of group by acting helpless, victimized, or insecure	Leslie says she is not sure she can really contribute to the discussion or the T-shirt sale, if that is what the group decides to do, exclaiming that, "I had a bad experience selling T-shirts in undergrad, and besides I am terrible at selling things."
Special interest pleader: Pretends to speak on behalf of a particular group but really is using group to express own biases	John says that the group has to make sure all the money is accounted for because, "some people here aren't too responsible."

AOTA, American Occupational Therapy Association. Adapted from Cole, M. B. (2018). *Group dynamics in occupational therapy: The theoretical basis and practice application of group intervention* (5th ed.). SLACK.

GROUP DYNAMICS: THE DEVELOPMENT OF GROUP SKILLS IN DEVELOPMENTAL GROUPS

Everyone knows one or two people who are exquisitely skill- ful in group situations; these rare individuals circulate grace- fully at parties, bring strangers together, and make lonely people feel more comfortable. On the job, or in community groups, these are individuals who can get people organized, give them motivation and direction, take care of uninterest- ing details, and then step back to let others shine. We can all strive to learn something from such people; their personali- ties and skill sets make them unquestionably confident and approachable. They have achieved high levels of interper- sonal communication and group skill. If you survey your col- leagues, classmates, and family, it is very likely that you will find different degrees of group skill among otherwise mature and functional individuals. How do human beings develop this ability to interact effectively with others?

Anne Mosey (35, 36), an occupational therapist, was among the first occupational therapy professionals to ana- lyze the development of **group interaction skills**. Mosey defined group interaction skills as the skills that allow a per- son to consistently be a productive member of a variety of types of primary groups. Through sequential acquisition of the various group interaction subskills, the individuals in the group learn to perform in appropriate group membership roles. This allows the member to engage in decision-making, communicate effectively, recognize and support group

norms, and interact in accordance with these norms. When people develop the ability to effectively maintain their role, the members are more successful in contributing to goal at- tainment, working toward group cohesiveness, and assisting in resolving group conflict. Consequentially, the group as a whole develops maturity; hence, Mosey called these *develop- mental groups* (10, 36, 47).

Nevertheless, these skills are not always developed nat- urally; they are developed through experience and over time. Interpersonal group skills are also influenced by our personalities and individual histories. Furthermore, people with persistent mental illness may need help and support to develop group interaction skills and social skills. Mosey identified five levels of group interaction skill: parallel, proj- ect, egocentric–cooperative, cooperative, and mature. She described the subskills learned at each level and estimated the chronological age at which most typically developing people learn these skills. Her work also described what a group leader, parent, teacher, or an occupational therapy professional may do to help people at each level acquire the subskills needed to progress to the next level. The following sections summarize Mosey's ideas regarding the develop- ment of group interaction skills (34, 36).

Parallel Level

The skill needed at the *parallel level* is the ability to work and play in the presence of others, comfortably, and with an awareness of their presence. This skill is usually learned between the ages of 18 months and 2 years, when the child becomes gradually more comfortable playing around other children. Most of the play is solitary, although the children interact briefly from time to time—for example, to show one another something. For this parallel play to continue for long, however, there must be at least one adult available to give each of the children support, encouragement, and attention when they need it. Problems such as taking toys from the other child or throwing a temper tantrum because one cannot immediately have one's own way are common but must be discouraged if the child is to progress to the next level.

Project Level

The skill learned at the *project level* is the ability to share a short-term task with one or two other people. This skill develops somewhere between ages 2 and 4 years. The child is interested in the task or the game and recognizes that they need other people to do it; therefore, the child is willing to take turns, to share materials, to cooperate, to ask for help, and to give it. Children in this stage are not so much interested in the other people as in the task. The activities shared at this level last for only a short time, usually not more than half an hour, and the child may engage in several activities in succession; each may have different participants. A parent, teacher, or other adult is needed to provide individual attention and to intervene when children have difficulty sharing.

Egocentric–Cooperative Level

The skill at the *egocentric–cooperative level* is awareness of the group's goals and norms and willingness to abide by them. This skill is based on sensitivity to the rules of the group and the rights of self and others in the group. Because children at this stage feel a sense of belonging to and being accepted by the group, they can carry out long-term activities that allow them to experiment with different roles and levels of participation. Differences among group members become apparent as each tries on functional *task* roles needed for the achievement of the various stages of activities (Table 16.2); this provides an opportunity to recognize and reward the achievement of others and to seek recognition for oneself. In theory, these skills are normally acquired somewhere between 5 and 7 years of age. Supervising adults still must provide support and encouragement to meet the esteem needs of group members.

Cooperative Level

The skill at the *cooperative level* is the ability to express feelings within a group and to be aware of and respond to the feelings of others. Thus, individuals at this level can assume group maintenance roles, which support the emotional well-being of the group. This skill usually develops between ages 9 and 12, through participation in groups whose members share some similarities and are approximately the same age. Adults are usually excluded from these groups, which seem to function better on their own. Groups may form spontaneously,

with members selected depending on their similarity to each other. The group's activities or tasks are not viewed as important; instead, the feelings, both positive and negative, of each member on a variety of subjects are the main agenda.

Mature Level

The skill at the *mature level* is the ability to take on a variety of group roles, both task roles and group maintenance roles, as needed in response to changing conditions in a group. This skill is synonymous with the upper end of the continuum of group interaction skill, as defined by Mosey. Mosey stated that this skill is learned between the ages 15 and 18 years, as the adolescent participates in various clubs and groups whose members come from different backgrounds and have different interests and skills. It must be acknowledged, however, that exposure to this experience does not in itself guarantee that the adolescent will develop a mature level of group interaction skill; there are many adults whose behavior in groups is restricted to the few membership roles with which they feel comfortable. The development of group interaction skills may continue into middle and even late adulthood, provided the individual is willing to risk trying out new roles.

Mosey's work recognized that the group member's social interaction skills are developmental in nature and that they develop on a continuum similar to that of other developmental skills, occurring gradually across the lifespan. As the members of a group develop social interaction skills, and these skills become more mature, the group itself goes through a developmental trajectory and begins to be less dependent on the leader. However, for some clients who have experienced a mental health crisis, or for whom there has been persistent mental illness, development of necessary social interaction skills may have been interrupted or diminished, making their skill set less functional than would be expected for their chronological age.

🔍 WHAT'S THE EVIDENCE?

Videogame-Based Group Therapy to Improve Self-Awareness and Social Skills After Traumatic Brain Injury

The experimental intervention study by Llorens et al included 42 traumatic brain injury (TBI) survivors in a longitudinal study with a pre- and posttest assessment. The purpose of the study was to determine the efficacy of using different approaches to integrative videogame-based group therapy to improve SA, social skills, and adaptive behaviors among (TBI) survivors. The experimental intervention involved weekly 1-hour group sessions conducted over 6 months.

Participants were divided into groups of eight people with others who had presented with or had reported similar cognitive conditions. The groups were then further divided into four groups of two. For each group session, pairs of individuals were seated across from one another at conventional tables that had been adapted to include a multitouch screen and converted into a digital game board table. Participants engaged in the videogames by touching elements presented on the tabletop screen. The objective of the video game was to reach the top of a mountain. Each team strove to reach the summit first by correctly answering questions presented on cards as fast as possible, as in a conventional board game.

SA impairment is defined as a reduced ability to evaluate one's strengths and weaknesses, which consequentially creates the ensuing disruptions in a person's occupational engagement. SA impairment is a commonly reported symptom and, by some estimates, is reported in nearly half of all TBI occurrences. Reduced SA heavily impacts emotional regulation, awareness of differences between self and others, creates difficulty in modulating and adapting to, or accepting and responding to other people's perspectives and behaviors. Furthermore, decreased SA hampers the development of social interaction skills, which negatively impacts transition back into the community following a TBI.

Findings in this study showed associated improvements in the development of appropriate social and behavior management skills, which is a common problem for clients who have sustained a TBI. In addition, both participants and their caregivers or families reported that the experimental intervention was motivating and led to loved one's perceptions that the individual demonstrated fewer behavioral disruptions and improved social skills. The authors report the following:

1. Group interventions can offer TBI survivors feedback and support from other individuals with TBI while allowing for the normalization of everyday functioning and social behaviors through engagement with others experiencing similar challenges.
2. Various group programs for SA development have been evaluated in the literature.
3. Game-based formats have also been used to provide feedback and cognitive rehabilitation and results of this study reinforce the effectiveness of game-based programs.
4. Participants reported high levels of engagement and motivation when participating in the program.

Results support the notion that such group-based interventions that target deficits in social cognition and seek to improve client factors that impact interpersonal relationships (such as impairments in SA) may allow participants to learn coping strategies that will further enhance their occupational engagement while also improving their social interaction skills.

Reflection Questions

1. What characteristics of a developmental group are evidenced in this research?
2. Which therapeutic factors do you believe may have been enacted in this group intervention study?
3. Discuss the reasons why it is significant that the participants in the study reported high levels of engagement and motivation. Why is this particularly important for clients with impaired SA?

Llorens, R., Noé, E., Ferri, J., & Alcañiz, M. (2015). Videogame-based group therapy to improve self-awareness and social skills after traumatic brain injury. *Journal of Neuroengineering and Rehabilitation, 12*(37), 1–8.

Dr Mary Donohue's development of the *Social Profile* expanded upon Mosey's work. The *Social Profile* is an assessment tool that can be used to measure social participation, social interaction, and group membership/roles in activity groups across occupational therapy settings (12). Donahue has developed two versions of the *Social Profile*, the children's and the adult/adolescent versions. The tool may be thought of as a profile because it measures the percentage of time that a client (individual or group) spends engaging at (potentially) several levels during a certain individual or group session, or across a longer time period, but within a particular/consistent activity. This is an important construct of this assessment tool considering that groups/group members may simultaneously demonstrate or apply multiple levels while participating in a singular activity, and still be considered functional and appropriate. For example, a group participating in a stress reduction Yoga class may appropriately be interacting at the parallel level, and the members may or may not be able to effectively interact at different levels during other activities. The *Social Profile* is an important measure of cooperation in social and interpersonal situations (12, 20).

The challenge in establishing therapeutic rapport and relationship with a client who presents with weak or poorly developed social interaction skills (ie, developmental group interaction skills) is to remember that the person is likely doing the best that they can and that our responsibility as an occupational therapy professional is to be client-centered enough to creatively find a way to meet them where they are. Carefully planned evidence-based occupational therapy group interventions with strong leadership can utilize therapeutic factors to support the clients' success in restoring or even developing new social interaction skills that will significantly impact the quality of their occupational engagement. The occupational therapy team can structure groups to meet the needs of people at various levels by grading or adapting the tasks, modifying the environmental or contextual features of the group, and by delegating tasks or helping members develop the skills needed to assume various group maintenance (social-emotional) or functional group task roles. In this way, the OT professional can provide a learning environment for all members, regardless of their functional challenges.

OCCUPATIONAL THERAPY GROUP LEADERSHIP

We have just discussed the developmental process by which people learn to interact effectively in group situations. Daily life presents many opportunities for developing and applying group interaction skills across the occupational therapy domain of concern. Social interaction skills, and the necessity for clients to be able to be a functional member of a group, are critical in work situations, in family interactions, in school, and are a significant predictor of the success (or lack of success) of a client's overall social life. To plan, implement, and facilitate a therapeutic intervention group successfully, according to Yalom and Leszcz (2020), one must consider the complexity of the task, "and at every step of the way the group leader should be guided by this question: What must I do to ensure the success of this group?" (60, p. 293). At some level, the effective leader always assumes control over certain aspects of the group. Using therapeutic reasoning, the leader will set group goals, determine the amount of structure and the just-right challenge for each of the members, choose the service delivery methods and modalities, and facilitate the sharing of leadership and group maintenance roles as appropriate (10). In many ways, the style of leadership and the function and roles of the leader depend upon the group interaction skill levels of individual members, and the group as a whole, as well as the purpose for which the group is designed. This is demonstrated in Table 16.3.

The Role of the Leader Throughout Group Development

The leader is responsible for making sure that group members feel safe during the group's activities and that the group and the individual members are supported in meeting their goals. There are three distinct leadership styles that

an occupational therapy professional may use in leading a group: directive, facilitative, or advisory. In **directive leadership**, as the name suggests, the leader takes on a more direct and intentional role by defining the purpose of the group. A directive leader typically completes more of the "front-end" responsibilities and is more hands on in structuring the format of the group. It is especially important for clients who have cognitive deficits and members who may not have the cognitive skills to problem-solve or to make safe decisions, that a more directive leader carefully considers how to pre-match client factors and needs (based on data from the occupational profile, the occupational performance analysis, and other relevant evaluation data) to the activities and tasks that will comprise the group sessions.

Facilitative leadership can be most closely compared to the democratic style, where members often share in the leadership roles and responsibilities and work collaboratively to select the activities. Using this style of leadership, members are encouraged to learn skills through active participation and are encouraged to provide feedback to one another. With leader guidance when needed, groups with a facilitative leader

Table 16.3. Role of the Occupational Therapy Professionals in Developmental Groups

Level of Group Skills	Role of the Occupational Therapy Group Facilitator
Parallel group: Members have limited attention span and may be quite unaware of others; unless encouraged to notice others, they may ignore them and isolate themselves.	1. Explain purpose and activities of group to member. 2. Help person feel accepted, safe, and valued. 3. Support and encourage minimal interaction, such as eye contact and casual conversation. 4. Set limits on disruptive behavior. 5. Help person select simple, short-term activities that are not self-isolating.
Project group: Members express anxiety about working with others, fearing that they will be unable to complete a task or that some other person will take over; issue is whether to trust another person enough to share a task with them.	1. Explain purpose and activities of group to member. 2. Help person feel accepted, safe, and valued. 3. Support and encourage sharing of tasks, cooperation, giving and seeking assistance, and so on. 4. Help members select simple, short-term tasks that can be shared by two or more people. 5. Encourage experimentation with different ways of sharing, members taking different roles.
Egocentric–cooperative group: Members have trouble engaging in long-term tasks with others; problems may include concern with competition, indifference to the rights of others, and inability to ask for and receive recognition.	1. Take on group membership roles only as required by needs of group. 2. Encourage group to function as independently as it can, stepping in only when group cannot proceed without help. 3. Model appropriate expression of needs. 4. Assist development and discussion of norms. 5. Help members feel accepted, safe, and valued.
Cooperative group: Although able to carry out long-term group tasks, people at this level need to expand their ability to express their feelings and be aware of feelings of others.	1. Participate in group or provide advice from sidelines; not an authority figure 2. May help group develop initially 3. May intervene to promote cohesiveness
Mature group: People at this level need to learn to step into roles as needed and to maintain balance between achieving group task and meeting emotional needs of group members.	1. Participate as a member. 2. When necessary, demonstrate group membership roles. 3. Select members to achieve variety and balance in backgrounds, interests, skills, and so on.

Groups are designed to help members acquire the named level of group interaction skill—for example, those in the project-level group do not have project-level skills but are working to develop them.
Adapted with permission from Mosey, A. C. (1973). *Group interaction skills survey. Activities therapy.* Raven Press.

often make their own group decisions. Lastly, in **advisory leadership**, the most hands-off approach, the occupational therapy professional takes on a role similar to that of a consultant, with members asking for input or advice only as needed. Advisory leadership requires a group that is functioning at a mature level because the members serve in many of the leadership roles and assume most of the responsibilities. Advisory leadership is often used to support self-help groups and within community-based practice settings, to support organizations or groups that are motivated to impact social change and seek to affect occupational injustice. In both group situations, the motivation to participate in the group, and to take on roles and responsibilities, comes from the group itself or the individual member's core processes (10).

Core Behaviors, Skills, and Responsibilities of an Occupational Therapy Leader

The success of any group intervention depends very much on what kind of preparation the leader has made. Four areas of planning therapeutic group interventions demand particular attention: knowledge, space, materials, and documentation of protocol, process, and progress (13, 60).

Knowledge refers to how well the leader understands and can analyze the various therapeutic factors and interpersonal interactions in groups to reflect upon how the therapeutic factors and interactions affect the occupational function of the members and the group. Knowledge and awareness of oneself and one's influence on others are critical. Equally important is the leader's knowledge of the task, medium, and intervention type and approach that will be applied or incorporated in the group's primary tasks and activities. It goes without saying that the occupational therapy leader will have difficulty planning for, facilitating, and teaching something that they are unfamiliar or uncomfortable with. Skills that the group leader has not practiced recently may have to be rehearsed before presenting them to the group.

Space refers to the preparation of the area in which the group will meet. In general, the leader should take care of any special arrangements of furniture or equipment before the group arrives. However, having clients participate in or take charge of preparing the space is appropriate for groups at a higher level of functioning.

Materials are any tools, supplies, books, handouts, audiovisual materials, sample projects, and so on that will be needed during the group. These should be prepared in advance by the group leader(s). The specific requirements depend on the type of group and the functional level of the participants. For example, for individuals with intellectual disabilities, or who are functioning at a lower level secondary to symptoms of their mental illness, it may be necessary to prepare separate materials for each person, and to set these up so that each has a separate and defined work area. In higher functioning groups, it may make sense to have the members take out their own projects or materials and obtain and return tools as they need them.

Documentation of protocol, process, and progress are the final items; this consists of the group protocol and session

plan, any necessary attendance record sheets, the group leader's notebook, and any other forms or documents that the leader may need reference to including records of individual client goals and group goals for documenting progress during the group. Except for taking attendance, the leader should avoid writing during the group session but should do so as soon as it is over with. Having a notebook handy in which the behavior of each group member can be briefly noted makes it easier to keep track of each person's progress. If the group is coled, one leader may have primary responsibility for facilitating the group and the other leader can focus on noting the progress and performance of the members, alternating these responsibilities between the two leaders, and between the sessions.

Despite preparation, surprises will occur. Nonetheless, the leader will find it easier to cope with a minor crisis when everything else has been prepared. Writing a session plan for each group meeting helps the leader to be prepared. It is also critical for the occupational therapy group leader to take the time to learn about group process. The trajectory of the developmental level of individuals and of groups should not be thought of rigidly nor as a linear process. Even in higher functioning and more mature groups, threats to the integrity of the group, as well as member conflicts and struggles, or other contextual factors can influence the group, sometimes causing the group to regress from higher levels of function to less mature stages (60). A well-organized group leader has an easier time adapting to challenges and setbacks, and they are far more likely to be attuned to underlying problems of the group members and the group function.

OCCUPATIONAL THERAPY GROUP INTERVENTION DEVELOPMENT

Developing an occupational therapy group–based intervention for clients with mental illness requires particular knowledge, skill, and expertise. Therefore, group protocol development is typically the responsibility of the occupational therapist. Nevertheless, the experienced occupational therapy assistant (OTA) with an interest in psychosocial occupational therapy may also find tremendous satisfaction in collaborating with the OT to develop and deliver occupational therapy intervention groups. The entry-level OTA can collaborate in program development by planning individual activity groups, which can eventually be integrated into the overall program protocol.

Planning an Activity Group

One of the biggest challenges new occupational therapy group leaders encounter in their clinical work is planning and running a new activity group (13). There seem to be so many possibilities that it is hard to focus on just one. Fortunately, there is a logical, step-by-step way of approaching the task:

1. Identify the clients or consumers who need a group.
2. Assess their specific needs and general level of group skills.
3. Identify rules and resources in the setting.

4. Narrow the focus and outline the main goals.
5. Write a group protocol.

Members

The first step in developing a new group is to identify clients who seem to have similar needs or who are experiencing similar barriers to occupational participation. This involves thinking about the clients you are collaborating with and providing occupational therapy services for and then exploring the kinds of group-based therapeutic resources that already exist. You may notice individuals who are not in any occupational therapy groups or who have gaps in their schedules. Or you may perceive that a particular need is not being met by existing groups—for example, clients on a locked unit may not be able to attend sports and exercise, or recreation and leisure groups off the unit, and may benefit from a group that focuses on play and leisure. Or, in an outpatient rehabilitation setting, members with arthritis may find a group on body mechanics and energy conservation helpful, yet one does not exist. A supervisor or coworker may identify a particular need or suggest individuals who would benefit from occupational therapy intervention.

Needs and Skill Level

The second step is to assess the specific needs and general level of group skills of the prospective participants. The occupational therapy professional may have already begun this during the first step. In other words, they may have already noticed a particular need (eg, for social skill development, exercise, or wellness). But what happens if the therapist has identified some individual clients who seem to need the support of others to reach their occupational goals, but are not sure what type of intervention group or approach would be the most beneficial for the clients? In a behavioral mental health or psychosocial setting, it may be helpful to think about the general goals of psychiatric occupational therapy, as introduced in the first section of the text. For example, the occupational therapy professional may have decided that the clients who most need a group are the ones who have a large amount of unstructured time during the day, but whose current level of function excludes them from being able to participate in the currently offered therapeutic groups. The occupational therapy professional may observe that certain clients have poorly established grooming and hygiene habits and show little interest or motivation in leisure activities outside of watching television. From these observations, the therapist may decide that these clients could benefit from a therapeutic group that focuses on self-care or leisure development. Another way to identify the potential need to develop an intervention group is to review the goals for each individual client who is currently receiving occupational therapy services to assess for any similar problems.

Beyond identifying the needs of prospective members, the occupational therapy professional needs to learn how well the potential member can function within a group. Because of other demands, it is not always possible to set up a separate evaluation session for this and the occupational

therapy professional should be prepared instead to observe each person informally or interview other staff who know the person well. Figure 16.1 presents a checklist developed by Mosey (35). It lists behaviors commonly observed in each of the five levels of group interaction skill development. The observer checks off any behaviors that the client demonstrates during the observation. The level of group interaction where the most behaviors are observed is likely to indicate the client's current developmental level of social interaction skill. It is important, however, for the occupational therapy professional to note that it is common for a person to exhibit a few behaviors at the next higher level to their current functional level. Assessing group interaction skills helps inform the occupational therapy professional about the therapeutic potential of the client within a group setting. For example, those at the project level of group interaction skill are not likely to be capable (presently) of engaging in mutual problem-solving through discussion, and those clients will find it easier to learn from short-term, concrete activities individually with the occupational therapy professional, or when partnered with just one other individual who is at a similar skill level.

Other factors that should be considered in addition to group interaction skills include the physical and cognitive capacities of the participants, in particular their attention span, memory, and capacity for new learning. If these skills are limited, you will have to conduct the group and structure the activities in a way that facilitates optimal occupational performance for every member. This may involve integrating compensatory strategies (activity analysis and adaptation are covered in Chapter 14).

Rules and Resources

The third step is to identify the rules and resources of your setting. These may support or limit what is possible. Included are the equipment and materials available, the rooms or other environments that can be used as settings for groups, the role of occupational therapy in the setting, and the rules of the particular facility or agency. If the occupational therapy professional wants to run a group that needs special equipment or materials, they must allow sufficient time to budget, order, and receive what is needed. Space availability can pose a problem; there may be times when the group must meet in a room that does not necessarily suit the purposes. The roles of occupational therapy, other activity therapies, and other professional disciplines in your setting may also constrain what kinds of groups you can run. Finally, it is critical for the occupational therapy professional to observe the rules of the agency or setting; there may be rules about what clients or members can and cannot do, and other rules governing staff. For instance, two staff members may be required to accompany inpatient clients on field trips. If field trips are planned, there will need to be staff available to accompany the group.

Focus and Goals

The fourth step is to narrow the focus of the group and outline its main goals. The clients are likely to have needs in several areas. The occupational therapy professional may have a

Level of Group Interaction Skill	Representative Skill-Level Behaviors
Parallel level	• Engages in some activity but acts as if it is an individual task as opposed to a group activity • Aware of others in the group • Some verbal or nonverbal interaction with others • Appears to be relatively comfortable in this situation
Project level	• Occasionally engages in the group activity, moving in and out according to own whim • Seeks some assistance from others • Gives some assistance when directly asked to do so
Egocentric–cooperative level	• Aware of group's goal relative to the task • Aware of group norms • Acts as if they belong in the group • Willing to participate • Meets esteem needs of others • Able to get others to meet their own esteem needs • Recognizes rights of others • Not overly competitive
Cooperative level	• Makes own wishes, needs, and desires known • Participates in group activity but seems concerned primarily with own needs and needs of others • Able to meet needs other than esteem needs • Tends to be most responsive to group members who are similar to self in some way
Mature level	• Responsive to all group members • Takes on a variety of task roles • Takes on a variety of social and emotional roles • Able to share leadership • Promotes a good balance between task accomplishment and satisfaction of group members' needs

Figure 16.1. Group Interaction Skills Survey. (Adapted with permission from Mosey, A. C. (1973). *Group interaction skills survey. Activities Therapy.* Raven Press.)

number of ideas for potential tasks or activities. Despite the many potential tasks, activities, and needs of the clients, the skilled occupational therapy professional will narrow their focus. This is perhaps the most difficult part of designing a group. The new leader may be tempted to try to meet several different needs in one group, thinking that the group could have 15 minutes of self-care activities, followed by 15 minutes of leisure activities, followed by a 30-minute work activity. Or perhaps the group could do a different activity every time it meets. These examples are obviously a bit unrealistic but they illustrate that trying to meet too many needs at the same time results in a confusing blur of unrelated and, therefore, meaningless activities. It is best to address only one area at a time, although incidental learning in other areas may occur simultaneously. For example, self-care groups may provide opportunities for some socialization and learning of communication skills.

Once you have chosen the focus of the group, you can begin to outline the goals. These goals should be developed from evaluation results and the individual treatment goals of the participants in the group. They should express in general behavioral terms what you hope the members will achieve, goals that these individuals feel are important and that are possible for them to reach.

DEVELOPING AN OCCUPATIONAL THERAPY INTERVENTION PLAN FOR GROUPS

Cole's Seven Step Group Protocol (10) suggests the following steps to be included in most OT group intervention groups: introduction, activity, sharing, processing, generalizing, application, and summary. Box 16.1 provides a more detailed description of what should be included in each of the seven steps of the group process protocol suggested in *Cole's Seven Step Group Protocol*. Group protocols are a method for coordinating the process of planning group interventions. Evaluating each group member's needs is the first step in developing a group intervention. The identification of the client's specific occupational concerns and priorities collected when creating an occupational profile guides the selection of the individual and group goals, activities, structure, and process. Planning a therapeutic group intervention involves the following main elements:

1. Identifying and evaluating the client population
2. Selecting a model of practice, theory, or frame of reference to use in the design of the group intervention
3. Determining a focus area for the intervention based on the client's problem or barrier to occupation
4. Searching for evidence that can be applied to the group intervention
5. Writing a group intervention outline
6. Developing individual group sessions
7. Implementing the group intervention
8. Evaluating the effectiveness of the group intervention

A group protocol is essentially an intervention plan for a specific population, or for individuals who have similar occupational barriers or needs (10).

Most groups consist of weekly sessions that meet 1 to 2 times per week for 4 to 6 weeks, but this is highly dependent on the setting, the type of group, and the needs of the client (60). The group protocol outlines the overall goals of the group and the objectives for each session; typically, for occupational therapy intervention groups, there will be approximately 6 to 10 sessions. It is the occupational therapy leader's responsibility to plan and develop each session in a detailed outline that includes the group membership and size, the session format, areas of occupation or client factors that will be addressed, the intervention type and approach, and a step-by-step description of the therapeutic activity to be used. Details such as the time and place of the meeting, supplies that are needed and their cost, how the environment needs to be prepared, any potential safety issues, and the role of the leader should also be documented.

Finally, the occupational therapy professional has the responsibility to prepare in advance of the group possible strategies for how they may grade and adapt the activities should the need arise, and they must have a plan for evaluating member progress and the progress of the group as a whole (10). The following section provides further discussion about aspects of the group protocol. Readers are also encouraged to refer to Box 16.1 as they begin to develop the session outlines for therapeutic intervention groups.

BOX 16.1 Developing a Group Protocol: Cole's Seven-Step Group Process Protocol

Step 1: Introduction

- Introduce self (name, title, title of the group).
- Have group members introduce themselves.
- Complete a warm-up exercise.
- Communicate expectations of group members.
- Explain purpose of the group clearly.
- Briefly outline the session/structure of the group.

Step 2: Activity

- Timing is not more than one-third of the group session, simple, short activity.
- Consider the physical, social, emotional, and cognitive capabilities of the group members.
- Modify/adapt to suit client needs and goals.
- Clearly present instructions and provide examples or demonstrations as appropriate.
- Get feedback from the group members to be sure they understand the directions.
- Have materials and supplies ready but out of view.
- After activity, collect supplies.

Step 3: Sharing

- Members share their work or experience with the group.
- Role model sharing for group members.
- Make sure that each group member has an opportunity to share.
- Acknowledge each person's contribution verbally or nonverbally.

Step 4: Processing

- Members share their feelings (about each other, about the experience, about their leader) with the group.
- Role model sharing for group members.
- Make sure that each group member has an opportunity to share.
- Acknowledge each person's contribution verbally or nonverbally.

Step 5: Generalizing

- Sum up the group experience in a few general principles.
- Point out like or similar responses.
- Point out contrasts or differences.
- State one or two principles learned from the experience.

Step 6: Application

- Verbalize the meaning or significance of the experience.
- Discuss how principles learned in the group can be applied to everyday life.
- Relate the experience to issues/problems of members.
- Use concrete examples.

Step 7: Summary

- Emphasize the most important aspects of the group.
- Review goals, content, and process of the group.
- Verbally reinforce group's learning (interpersonal, emotional, and cognitive).
- Thank members for their participation.
- End group on time.

Adapted from Cole, M. B. (2018). *Group dynamics in occupational therapy: The theoretical basis and practice application of group intervention* (5th ed.). SLACK.

Writing a Group Protocol

A group protocol is a written plan that describes the goals of a group and the methods by which these goals will be achieved. It is an outline of what will be happening in the group. It is, practically speaking, an intervention plan for the group. Writing a group protocol has several purposes. The first is to communicate with other staff to help them more easily decide whether a particular person is suited for, or may benefit from, the group. The second purpose is to describe the type of individual who may benefit from the group. This helps screen out those whose needs and group skills are not a good match for the group. The third purpose is to clarify the occupational therapy professional's goals, methods, and roles as a leader of the group. Lastly, writing the group protocol helps identify how the therapist will know when a member has achieved the goals they have prioritized. In other words, it helps the occupational therapy professional describe what the clients will be able to do, how their engagement in occupation will be positively impacted, and what the expected occupational outcomes are when the client "graduates" from the group.

The *goals* or *behavioral objectives* of the group should be stated in clear behavioral terms and with as much specificity as possible. They should be relevant to the members' needs and should be set at a level that members can achieve. Some examples of behavioral objectives that meet these requirements are the following:

- To tolerate the presence of others while working on a task as evidenced by staying in the room and refraining from disruptive behavior or disrespectful speech
- To initiate social conversation with others
- To perform simple assembly tasks accurately using written or demonstrated two-step instructions
- To learn basic home maintenance skills that support transition to semi-independent community living

Some groups have goals that involve changes in awareness, attitudes, or values; such goals are very difficult to state in behavioral terms because they focus not on behavior but on internal psychological or cognitive states. Nevertheless, if these are among the main purposes of the group, they should be included. Examples of such goals are the following:

- To increase awareness of one's own safety and that of others, as evidenced by following shop rules and reminding others to do so
- To develop a feeling of personal competence, as evidenced by spontaneous or elicited comments about one's achievements or skills
- To improve awareness of one's effect on others, as evidenced by cooperation in cleanup and sharing of space

Referral criteria describe the characteristics of people who should be referred to the group. The description may include specific skill deficits and prerequisite behaviors. Skill deficits identify the kinds of problems that will be addressed (eg, poor hygiene and grooming). Prerequisite behaviors state minimum skills or behaviors needed to participate successfully in the group (eg, able to tolerate the presence of others or not actively assaultive or suicidal). In some settings and for some groups, each person might be interviewed before entering the group. This may be done by the group leader or by the occupational therapist or assistant who is managing the person's occupational therapy program. These intake procedures can help determine how well the individual meets the referral criteria and at the same time provide an opportunity to introduce the purpose of the group and to engage the person's commitment or interest. The referral criteria should spell out the intake procedure if one is required.

Often, several referral criteria are used to define the population for which a group is designed. Writing clear criteria allows you to define the limits of the group. The following is an example of how such criteria may be written for a low-level task skills group:

- Males and females
- Ages 17 to older than 65 years
- Attention ability of 5 to 15 minutes
- In need of task skill development (eg, concentration, attention to detail, rate of production)
- Not actively assaultive or suicidal

A potential member must meet all the stated criteria to join the group. This ensures that all the group members have similar needs and skill levels, which generally makes the group easier to run.

The *methodology* section is one of the most important sections, giving detail on how the time of the group will be used to achieve the stated objectives. Within this section are commonly included both the media (activities) and method (how the activity or medium is used). *Media* refers to the activities or tasks that will be used to help the members meet their goals within the group. Sometimes only one activity, or medium, is used. For our purposes, *medium* means the same thing as *activity*. Almost any activity can be used in groups (eg, gardening, collating papers, shopping for clothes for work). The theoretical approach or frame of reference will be part of this section, if appropriate (eg, cognitive behavioral).

Method describes how the medium or media will be used to work toward the goals. The method includes the general plan of what will happen in the group.

Defining the role of the leader in the group protocol helps the occupational therapy professional analyze and plan how best to relate to the members of the group. People at different levels of group interaction skill require different levels of involvement from the group leader. Members at the parallel and project levels need much more assistance and supervision than do those at higher levels. Table 16.3 gives more detail on this point.

The *evaluation section* provides for measuring the achievement of the stated purposes of the group. To what extent does it "improve self-esteem" or "increase consistent application of safety procedures"? The choice of evaluation procedure depends on the content of the group, the skills of the members, and the overall quality management plan of the facility or of the occupational therapy department/

behavioral health team. Assessment may be done by surveying the participants' satisfaction with the group or by having a peer occupational therapy professional make independent ratings of members' behavior. Ideally, the assessment used should be an accepted and standardized instrument, and each member should be evaluated before joining the group, and at predetermined specific stages of the group.

Exit criteria describe the demonstrated behaviors or skills of a person who has achieved the goals of the group. These should be quite specific and stated in behavioral terms. In fact, the exit criteria restate the goals of the group in an observable or measurable form. The exit criteria should be so clear that any observer could determine whether a particular person has met them. Possible exit criteria for a low-level task skills group are the following:

- The person works consistently for 40 minutes.
- The person works at an acceptable rate.
- The person maintains given work standards.
- The person shows minimal initiative by asking the therapist questions and spontaneously interacting with peers.

Reasons for discontinuation are the various factors that may cause the leader to discharge a member from the group before they have achieved the goals set in the exit criteria. There are many reasons a particular person may exit the group. Examples include the following:

- The person has been discharged from the treatment setting.
- The person displays uncontrollable assaultive or suicidal behavior.
- The person fails to attend the group on a regular basis.

In summary, writing the group protocol is the final step in designing a group. The protocol describes the goals of the group and the methods by which these goals will be achieved.

Keeping Accurate Records

As mentioned earlier, it is important to keep track of how members are progressing in the group sessions. Some observations that should be noted are any progress toward goals, changes in interactions with others, new problems or behaviors seen, and possible side effects of medication. Even though there may be only a few minutes between the end of the group and the next meeting or group that the leader must attend, it is very important to note observations while they are fresh. Writing one or two words about each group member takes little time, but reviewing several days of such notes can yield valuable insights into the process of the group and the progress of its members (55).

Keeping track of the goals of individual members and reflecting upon their progress in the group provides details that can be incorporated into progress notes. The occupational therapy professional must first be clear about each person's goals and document the goals in a secure format. The Health Insurance Portability and Accountability Act (HIPAA) impacts client privacy regarding personal health information (52). For this reason, the occupational therapy group leader must consider how they can document individual client

progress *and* the care provided to the individual members in the context of a therapeutic group, without compromising the client's protected health information (60). For this reason, best practice supported by the evidence and literature recommends that occupational therapy professionals who apply group intervention should keep a combined, or dual record, where daily notes are written about what happened during the group (a group summary), and a separate file is kept to record the progress of each individual (60).

OTHER MODELS OF PRACTICE FOR OCCUPATIONAL THERAPY GROUP INTERVENTION

Occupational therapy professionals use groups as an intervention method across all practice settings and with clients of any age, who have varying disabilities (9, 37, 53). Groups may follow a specific practice model, approach, or frame of reference (ie, cognitive behavioral, sensory integrative, biomechanical, psychoeducational, or others). When leading a group that is designed for a specific practice model, the protocol should reflect this. The role of the leader, the interventions used, the choice of activities, and other aspects would correspond to the practice model. For example, a group using a cognitive behavioral model would emphasize identifying and disputing unreasonable beliefs that impair the ability to engage in occupations and achieve satisfaction in occupational roles. The leader might, therefore, ask group members to help a member dispute self-defeating ideas. Other members would be encouraged to provide another perspective.

Kaplan (25, 26) advocates the use of *directive groups* with people with severe functional impairments. These individuals cannot generally be scheduled into existing groups as they are disruptive to the other members and obtain little benefit themselves. The purpose of the directive group is to prepare them to function in other groups that are more readily available but that require a higher level of task and social functioning than the person can demonstrate at present. The "directive" aspect of the group refers to the group leaders' active involvement in nurturing, supporting, and facilitating behaviors that lead to understanding the purpose of the group, attending the group for 45 minutes, concentrating enough to participate, and tolerating the presence of others. The protocols and procedures for such directive groups have been well outlined by Kaplan (25, 26). The *five-stage group* is appropriate for people who function at lower cognitive levels. These individuals may be nonverbal, have intellectual disabilities or cognitive deficits, and may be unable to express themselves or to demonstrate appropriate social behavior. Interested readers are referred to the summary of the five-stage group derived from the work of Mildred Ross that appears in the section "OT HACKS" at the end of the chapter (44).

SUMMARY

Regardless of the type of group or the population of the group, occupational therapy interventions should address occupational performance in one way or another. Although some groups may be limited to discussion, this is not the most effective method to address occupational performance because the "doing" aspect of occupational therapy intervention is one of the things that helps distinguish occupational therapy intervention from intervention provided by other disciplines. An occupational component or activity should *always* be included (10). This chapter provides the entry-level occupational therapy professional or student with the basic concepts and methods for developing a new group or leading one that has already been developed. Groups are used in occupational therapy not only because they are cost-effective but also because they provide more varied and extensive learning opportunities than are available in individual interventions. Some barriers to occupation, such as a client's need to develop appropriate social skills, cannot be learned and practiced in isolation. Effective group leadership is a complex task but the underlying skill required is the ability to help clients identify and use the opportunities available in a group context to connect with one another. Occupational therapy group interventions are planned for the overall benefit of the group and the individual, toward promoting their independence and occupational growth.

OT HACKS SUMMARY

O: Occupation as a means and an end

Occupational therapy professionals who wish to plan and implement an occupational therapy therapeutic group can identify a focus for the group using the following four-step guideline:

1. Identify clients who may benefit from a group intervention.
2. Identify the specific needs of the individuals and their general level of group skills.
3. Identify facility or setting parameters including space availability, availability of equipment and materials, the role of occupational therapy in the setting, and rules of the institution.
4. Narrow focus and outline main goals and behavioral objectives.

Modified from Early, M. B. (1981). *T.A.R. Introductory course workbook: Occupational therapy: Psychosocial dysfunction.* LaGuardia Community College.

T: Theoretical concepts, values, and principles, or historical foundations

Dr Mary Donohue's development of the *Social Profile* expanded upon Mosey's work. The *Social Profile* is an assessment tool that can be used to measure social participation, social interaction, and group membership/roles in activity groups across occupational therapy settings (12). The *Social Profile* is an important measure of cooperation in social and interpersonal situations. Using valid and reliable tools such as this allows occupational therapy group leaders to document and further advocate the positive impacts and occupational outcomes of clients' participation in occupational therapy therapeutic groups (12, 20).

H: How can we Help? OT's role in serving clients with mental illness or mental health needs

There are many techniques and strategies the occupational therapy group leader can use to promote interaction in a group. The techniques can be organized by strategies that can be applied using the environment or through modifying leader behaviors, inquiry, or responses. See the following examples.

Environmental or Contextual Applications
- Arrange the group in a circle so that all the participants (including the leader) are at same level and can see each other.
- Position talkative members so that they are next to less talkative members.
- Consider sitting next to members who tend to monopolize or who act out and explain privately to those members that you will help them with this.

Leader Behaviors, Inquiry, or Responses
- Tolerate silence; let time work for you. Some people take a while to think and respond. Give everyone a chance.
- Avoid responding directly to a member question or comment; instead, redirect the question to the entire group or a specific group member.
- When a member has been talking for a while, break eye contact and scan the group; this leads the talker to make eye contact with others and encourages other members to respond.
- Vary your emotional tone depending on what is being said. Use voice dynamics, pacing, and volume to keep the group focused. Let your voice be soft when trying to draw people out.
- Observe the members and be aware of those whose attention may be wandering or whose nonverbal behavior indicates discomfort. Try to draw them in if they appear able to tolerate it.

Specific Questions or Comments the Occupational Therapy Leader Can Use
- "James, what did you think about what Brenda just said?"
- "Iliana, do you agree with what Mira said?"
- "Hmmmn, I wonder if anyone else has something to share on that topic."
- "Josie, you've had a lot to say. Let's see what the others are thinking."

A: Adaptations

The success of any occupational therapy therapeutic group intervention depends on what kind of preparation the leader has made. Four areas of planning therapeutic group interventions demand particular attention: **knowledge**, **space**, **materials**, and **documentation of protocol, process, and progress** (13, 60).

C: Case study includes

This article by Emily Fong and Jenna Yeager, "The Goof Off Group" appeared in *OT Practice* (October, 2022) and is one example of the modern-day use of an occupation-based (play/leisure/social participation), and group (type) therapeutic intervention, complete with a group member profile (ie, mini case review).

https://www.aota.org/publications/ot-practice/ot-practice-issues/2022/the-goof-off-group

K: Knowledge: keeping mental health OT practice grounded in evidence, in occupational science, and in research

A summary of the *Ross's Five-Stage Group—Sensory Integrative Model* (44), an evidence-based technique that can be implemented for people who function at lower cognitive levels.

Stage 1: Opening of session is designed to welcome members and to stimulate as many senses as possible.

Representative Activities
- Say hello by touching feet or elbows.
- Pass bell or other unusual object.
- Show and assist members to handle a manipulative toy.
- Offer scented items.

Stage 2: Movement is used to increase nonverbal communication and expression of feelings; use simple, basic movements; match movements to task abilities of members.

Representative Activities
- Shake hands
- Clapping
- Group in a circle to raise and lower parachute
- Movement with scarves or ropes
- Range of motion (ROM) dance

Stage 3: Visual–motor perceptual activities are presented to increase demands on members to respond more thoughtfully, less automatically; promotes integration between sensory stimulation, movement, and cognition.

Representative Activities
- Games such as Simon Says
- Large floor dominoes
- Relay races
- Pantomime games (eg, pretend to do the laundry or garden)
- Texture matching with eyes occluded

Stage 4: Verbal or symbolic activities are used to enhance cognitive functioning.

Representative Activities
- Making fruit salad (each member contributes)
- Memory games
- Building a tower of cardboard bricks
- Reading a poem together
- Counting and matching games

Stage 5: Closing program provides opportunities to emphasize positive qualities of experience; familiar and relaxing activities are used.

Representative Activities
- Repeat activities from stage 1.
- Shake hands or hold hands.

- Pass out candy or refreshments.
- Say good-bye to each person.

Adapted from Ross, M. (1997). *Integrative group therapy: Mobilizing coping abilities with the five-stage group.* American Occupational Therapy Association.

S: Some terms that may be new to you

Advisory leadership: a more hands-off approach, the occupational therapy professional takes on a role similar to that of a consultant, with members asking for input or advice only as needed

Altruism: actions taken to promote the welfare of others, despite personal liabilities, risks, or harms to oneself

Catharsis: an emotional release

Cohesiveness: closeness among the group members; a sense of solidarity

Didactic instruction: direct instruction about mental health, mental illness, and the psychodynamics of interpersonal relationships (60)

Directive leadership: a style of leadership where the leader takes on a more direct and intentional role in defining the purpose of the group, planning the group, and leading the group; typically a more involved, structured group format

Facilitative leadership: most closely compared to the democratic style, where members often share in the leadership roles and responsibilities and work collaboratively to select the activities

Group: "Collection of individuals having shared characteristics or a common or shared purpose (eg, family members, workers, students, others with similar occupational interests or occupational challenges)" (1, p. 77)

Group dynamics: consists of all the forces that influence the interactions and interrelationships of the group members

Group interaction skills: the skills that allow a person to consistently be a productive member of a variety of types of primary groups

Group process: the consideration of many aspects; the relationships and interactions between the individual group members and therapist, consideration of other contexts (ie, sociocultural, setting of the group, sociopolitical), interpersonal interactions, whole-group elements, and the psyche (or internal psychological world) of the individuals in the group

Group therapy: Group therapy is a planned process for creating changes in individuals by bringing them together for this purpose.

Group-centered actions: occurrences that result from the dynamic and interdependent actions between group members

Illumination of process: the practice that occurs when a group recognizes, examines, and reflects upon its own group process in an effort to understand the experience more fully; this self-reflective loop allows members to examine the experiences of the group together (as a microcosm) to study its transactions and make learning connections.

Individual/egocentric roles: roles that are oppositional to group process and group progress

Interpersonal-input: when the individual learns how they impact others

Interpersonal-output: when an individual learns to change how they interact with others

Psychoeducation: the provision of direct instruction and interpersonal feedback in a more formalized manner

Purposeful actions: actions that are meaningful to the client

Self-initiated actions: any actions, verbal or nonverbal, that are initiated by the client

Social capital: social support resources, relationships, and support networks that influence a client's overall occupational engagement

Social network: the relationships and social ties between people that often increase access to social supports or help to mobilize the needed social supports

Social support: the various sources of help offered to individuals and groups, typically from within their communities

Social support groups: groups that provide the members with opportunities to form healthy reciprocal relationships in safe contexts

Social-emotional roles: roles that support the emotional and psychosocial needs of both the individual members and the group as a whole

Spontaneous actions: unplanned or unexpected actions that take place during the group process

Task roles: roles that support the broader functioning of the group

Reflection Questions

1. How are groups used in occupational therapy intervention? What are some special considerations for planning and implementing a therapeutic group with people who have mental health challenges?
2. Compare and contrast the various types of intervention groups.
3. List ways in which the OT leader of a therapeutic group can improve group cohesiveness. Why is this important?
4. What other therapeutic factors do you believe are the most important in a group intervention context? Please explain your answer.
5. Describe each of the task roles, group maintenance roles, and egocentric roles (Table 16.2). What role(s) do you play in the groups you are a member of?
6. List and describe each of Mosey's five developmental levels of group skills.
7. To develop a higher level of group skill, the person must be placed in a group operating one level above their present level of skill. Please explain why.
8. Outline the responsibilities of the leader in preparing for a therapeutic OT group.
9. What is group protocol and what purposes does it serve? What elements are typically included?
10. What kind of group might be appropriate for cognitively impaired individuals who have very low arousal?
11. In some settings or groups, using a specific practice model or frame of reference is called for and the groups need to be designed to agree with the model. Why do you think this is important?

REFERENCES

1. American Occupational Therapy Association. (2020). Occupational therapy practice framework: Domain and process—Fourth edition. *American Journal of Occupational Therapy, 74*(Suppl. 2), 1–87.
2. Behenck, A., Wesner, A. C., Finkler, D., & Heldt, E. (2017). Contribution of group therapeutic factors to the outcome of cognitive–behavioral therapy for patients with panic disorder. *Archives of Psychiatric Nursing, 31*(2), 142–146.
3. Benne, K. D., & Sheats, P. (1978). Functional roles of group members. In L. P. Bradford (Ed.), *Group development* (2nd ed., pp. 52–61). University Associates.
4. Brown, B., & Baker, S. (2020). The social capitals of recovery in mental health. *Health, 24*(4), 384–402.
5. Burson, K., Fette, C., & Kannenberg, K. (2017). Mental health promotion, prevention, and intervention in occupational therapy practice. *American Journal of Occupational Therapy, 71*(Suppl. 2), 1–19.
6. Bryant, W., Fieldhouse, J., & Bannigan, K. (Eds.). (2014). *Creek's occupational therapy and mental health* (5th ed.). Churchill Livingstone Elsevier.
7. Cechnicki, A., & Bielańska, A. (2009). Understanding and treatment of people suffering from schizophrenia in Kraków. *Archives of Psychiatry and Psychotherapy, 11*(3), 17–25.
8. Cermak, S. A., & Maeir, A. (2011). Cognitive rehabilitation of children and adults with attention deficit hyperactivity disorder. In N. Katz (Ed.), *Cognition, occupation, and participation across the life span: Neuroscience, neurorehabilitation, and models of intervention in occupational therapy* (pp. 223–247). AOTA Press.
9. Champagne, T. (2012). Creating occupational therapy groups for children and youth in community-based mental health practice. *OT Practice, 17*(14), 13–18.
10. Cole, M. B. (2018). *Group dynamics in occupational therapy: The theoretical basis and practice application of group intervention* (5th ed.). SLACK.
11. Cozolino, L. (2006). *The neuroscience of human relationships: Attachment and the developing social brain*. Norton Books.
12. Donohue, M. V. (2013). *Social profile: Assessment of social participation in children, adolescents, and adults*. AOTA Press.
13. Early, M. B. (1981). *T.A.R. Introductory course workbook: Occupational therapy: Psychosocial dysfunction*. LaGuardia Community College.
14. Ezhumalai, S., Muralidhar, D., Dhanasekarapandian, R., & Nikketha, B. S. (2018). Group interventions. *Indian Journal of Psychiatry, 60*(Suppl. 4), S514–S521.
15. Fidler, G. S. (2018). The task-oriented group as a context for treatment. In M. B. Cole (Ed.), *Group dynamics in occupational therapy: The theoretical basis and practice application of group intervention* (5th ed., Appendix A, pp. 427–432) . SLACK.
16. Fox, A., Dishman, S., Valicek, M., Ratcliff, K., & Hilton, C. (2020). Effectiveness of social skills interventions incorporating peer interactions for children with attention deficit hyperactivity disorder: A systematic review. *The American Journal of Occupational Therapy, 74*(2), 7402180070p1–7402180070p19.
17. Greater Good Science Center. (n.d.). *What is altruism?* https://greatergood.berkeley.edu/topic/altruism/definition
18. Hahn-Markowitz, J., Berger, I., Manor, I., & Maeir, A. (2020). Efficacy of cognitive-functional (Cog-Fun) occupational therapy intervention among children with ADHD: An RCT. *Journal of Attention Disorders, 24*(5), 655–666.
19. Heard, E., & Walsh, D. (2023). Group therapy for survivors of adult sexual assault: A scoping review. *Trauma, Violence, & Abuse, 24*(2), 886–898.

20. Hemphill, B. J., & Urish, C. K. (Eds.). (2020). *Assessments in occupational therapy mental health: An integrative approach* (4th ed.). SLACK.

21. Higgins, S., Schwartzberg, S., Bedell, G., & Duncombe, L. (2015). Current practice and perceptions of group work in occupational therapy. *American Journal of Occupational Therapy, 69*(Suppl. 1), 6911510223p1.

22. Hill, R., & Dahlitz, M. (2022). *The practitioner's guide to the science of psychotherapy.* W.W. Norton & Company.

23. Ho, W. W. (2021, September). Therapeutic factors mediating positive mirror effects in group counseling education. *Current Psychology, 42,* 10136–10150.

24. Hussin, U. R., Mahmud, Z., & Karim, D. N. F. M. (2020). Psychoeducation group counselling for emotional intelligence among secondary school female students. *Journal of Counseling, Education and Society, 1*(2), 53–57.

25. Kaplan, K. L. (1986). The directive group: Short-term treatment for psychiatric patients with a minimal level of functioning. *American Journal of Occupational Therapy, 40*(7), 474–481.

26. Kaplan, K. L. (1988). *Directive group therapy.* SLACK.

27. Kielhofner, G. (2009). The functional group model. In G. Kielhofner (Ed.), *Conceptual foundations of occupational therapy practice* (5th ed.). F.A. Davis.

28. Le Doux, J. E., & Brown, R. (2017). A higher-order theory of emotional consciousness. *Proceedings of the National Academy of Sciences of the United States of America, 114*(10), E2016–E2025.

29. Leszcz, M. (2018). The evidence-based group psychotherapist. *Psychoanalytic Inquiry, 38*(4), 285–298.

30. Llorens, R., Noé, E., Ferri, J., & Alcañiz, M. (2015). Videogame-based group therapy to improve self-awareness and social skills after traumatic brain injury. *Journal of Neuroengineering and Rehabilitation, 12*(37), 1–8.

31. Maeir, A., Hahn-Markowitz, J., Fisher, O., & Traub Bar-Ilan, R. (2012). Cognitive-functional (Cog-Fun) intervention in occupational therapy for children aged 5–10 with ADHD: Treatment manual. Faculty of Medicine, School of Occupational Therapy, Hadassah and the Hebrew University.

32. Miklóšová, P., & Stančiak, J. (2020). People with schizophrenia and possibilities of their employment in the work market. *Scientific Journal of Polonia University, 38*(1–1), 166–171.

33. Moreno, J. K. (1994). Group treatment for eating disorders. In A. Fuhriman & G. M. Burlingame (Eds.), *Handbook of group psychotherapy: An empirical and clinical synthesis* (pp. 416–457). Wiley.

34. Mosey, A. C. (1970). The concept and use of developmental groups. *American Journal of Occupational Therapy, 24*(4), 272–275.

35. Mosey, A. C. (1973). *Group interaction skills survey: Activities therapy.* Raven Press.

36. Mosey, A. C. (1986). *Psychosocial components of occupational therapy.* Raven Press.

37. Olson, L. (2006). Activity groups in family-centered treatment: Psychiatric occupational therapy approaches for parents and children. *Occupational Therapy in Mental Health, 22*(3–4), 1–156.

38. Perilli, V., Stasolla, F., Maselli, S., & Morelli, I. (2018). Occupational therapy and social skills training for enhancing constructive engagement of patients with schizophrenia: A review. *Clinical Research in Psychology, 1*(1), 1–7.

39. Postmes, T., Spears, R., & Cihangir, S. (2001). Quality of decision making and group norms. *Journal of Personality and Social Psychology, 80*(6), 918–930.

40. Ranjan, R., Pradhan, K. R., & Wong, J. (2014). Effect of transdisciplinary approach in group therapy to develop social skills for children with Autism spectrum disorder. *Theory and Practice in Language Studies, 4*(8), 1536–1542.

41. Raphael-Greenfield, E., Shteyler, A., Silva, M. R., Caine, P. G., Soo, S., Rotonda, E. C., & Patrone, D. O. (2011, September). Hard-wired for groups: Students and clients in the classroom and clinic. *Mental Health Special Interest Section Quarterly, 34*(3), 1–4.

42. Rashidian, A., Karbalaei-Nouri, A., Haghgoo, H. A., & Hosseinzadeh, S. (2021). Convergent validity and reliability of the Persian version of the Bay Area Functional Performance Evaluation-Task-Oriented Assessment in people with severe psychiatric disorders. *Journal of Rehabilitation Sciences & Research, 8*(1), 36–39.

43. Rosenberg, L., Maeir, A., Yochman, A., Dahan, I., & Hirsch, I. (2015). Effectiveness of a cognitive–functional group intervention among preschoolers with attention deficit hyperactivity disorder: A pilot study. *American Journal of Occupational Therapy, 69*(3), 6903220040.

44. Ross, M. (1997). *Integrative group therapy: Mobilizing coping abilities with the five-stage group.* American Occupational Therapy Association.

45. Salehi, A., Ehrlich, C., Kendall, E., & Sav, A. (2019). Bonding and bridging social capital in the recovery of severe mental illness: A synthesis of qualitative research. *Journal of Mental Health, 28*(3), 331–339.

46. Salehi, A., Harris, N., Coyne, E., & Sebar, B. (2014). Perceived control and self-efficacy, subjective well-being and lifestyle behaviours in young Iranian women. *Journal of Health Psychology, 21*(7), 1415–1425.

47. Scaffa, M. E. (2019). Group process and group intervention. In B. A. B. Schell & G. Gillen (Eds.), *Willard and Spackman's occupational therapy* (13th ed., pp. 539–555). Lippincott Williams & Wilkins.

48. Stice, E., Rohde, P., Butryn, M., Menke, K. S., & Marti, C. N. (2015). Randomized controlled pilot trial of a novel dissonance-based group treatment for eating disorders. *Behaviour Research and Therapy, 65,* 67–75.

49. Taylor, R. R. (2020). *The intentional relationship: Occupational therapy and use of self* (2nd ed.). F.A. Davis.

50. Tuckman, B. (1965). Developmental sequences in small groups. *Psychological Bulletin, 63*(6), 384–399.

51. Tuckman, B., & Jensen, M. (1977). Stages of small-group development revisited. *Group and Organizational Studies, 2*(4), 419–427.

52. United States Department of Health and Human Services. *Health information privacy.* https://www.hhs.gov/hipaa/index.html

53. Wagenfeld, A. (2013). Nature, an environment for health. *OT Practice, 18*(15), 15–18.

54. Wampold, B. (2015). How important are the common factors in psychotherapy? An update. *World Psychiatry, 14*(3), 270–277.

55. Ward, J. D. (2003). The nature of clinical reasoning with groups: A phenomenological study of an occupational therapist in community mental health. *Occupational Therapy in Mental Health, 57*(6), 625–634.

56. World Health Organization. (2010). *mhGAP intervention guide for mental, neurological and substance use disorders in non-specialized health settings—Version 1.0.* Author.

57. World Health Organization. (2015). *Update of the Mental Health Gap Action Programme (mhGAP) guidelines for mental, neurological and substance use disorders.* Author.

58. World Health Organization. (2016). *mhGAP intervention guide for mental, neurological and substance use disorders in non-specialized health settings—Version 2.0.* Author; (WHO/MSD/MER/17.6). License: CC BY-NC-SA 3.0 IGO.

59. World Health Organization and Columbia University. (2016). *Group interpersonal therapy (IPT) for depression* (WHO generic field-trial version 1.0). World Health Organization.

60. Yalom, I. D., & Leszcz, M. (2020). *The theory and practice of group psychotherapy* (6th ed.). Basic Books.

SUGGESTED RESOURCES

Additional Suggested Reading

Brooks, R., Lambert, C., Coulthard, L., Pennington, L., & Kolehmainen, N. (2021). Social participation to support good mental health in neurodisability. *Child: Care, Health and Development, 47*(5), 675–684.

Hassan, S. M., Giebel, C., Morasae, E. K., Rotheram, C., Mathieson, V., Ward, D., Reynolds, V., Price, A., Bristow, K., & Kullu, C. (2020). Social prescribing for people with mental health needs living in disadvantaged communities: The Life Rooms model. *BMC Health Services Research, 20*(19), 1–9.

Miller, J. E. (2020). Feeding group: An interdisciplinary treatment approach for inpatient stroke populations. *OT Practice, 25*(4), 24–25.

Videos

The Work, directed by Jairus McLeary and Gethin Aldous (2017), is a documentary set in Folsom State Prison that tracks inmates during intensive group therapy. The documentary is a powerful example of how group process and group dynamics support human transformation and can elevate functional occupational outcomes for clients using groups as a context for treatment. The documentary can be rented or purchased from a variety of sources, including Amazon Prime Video, https://www.amazon.com/Work-James-McLeary/dp/B077GGWH8P

In this YouTube video, "Support Groups in Action" (14:12), produced by UCSF Memory and Aging Center, caregivers share insights, laughs, and wisdom with each other in a frontotemporal dementia caregiver support group. https://www.youtube.com/watch?v=X_RRbVfM0ck

Websites

Learn more about group therapy by visiting the website of APA's Division 49 (Society of Group Psychology and Group Psychotherapy). https://www.apadivisions.org/division-49/index?_ga=2.174120804.791079307.1666130006-297007853.1653495189

Group Therapy Activities: A list of expressive group therapy ideas for use in mental health settings with groups of various ages, contributed by Gloria Mahin, an expressive arts therapist. Ms Mahin also offers a blog in which she reviews and discusses a variety of expressive arts techniques that can be applied to occupational therapy therapeutic groups. http://www.expressivetherapist.com/group-activities.html

From Domain and Process to Occupational Therapy Practice

In **Section Three** of this text, our focus is on synthesizing what you have learned thus far about the occupational therapy domain and process in mental health as we transition into active and dynamic occupational therapy practices. Section Three *brings us home again* as we discover more about **How to *Do* What We *Do*.** Because occupational participation occurs as an ongoing dynamic transaction that cannot be separated from the situational contexts in which occupations are transacted, reflective consideration throughout the therapeutic process is necessary for all occupational therapy professionals. Nonetheless, within the psychosocial occupational therapy practice arena, participation in occupation for some clients may give rise to intense feelings or significantly impact their behaviors. The client may bring past experiences of trauma, temporal, sociocultural, or other unique client-specific aspects to their occupational engagement.

In psychosocial settings, a client's communication and interaction skills, including their ability to regulate their emotions or to act and react to others appropriately, are considered especially important skill sets. For many clients, these are the factors that will most directly influence and impact successful engagement in occupation and co-occupation, as well as their recovery. So, in Section Three, we emphasize the importance of viewing occupational therapy services from a holistic and transactional perspective. It is critical for the occupational therapy professional to consistently remain aware of how situational elements and client factors are in relationship in such a way that they are perpetually, dynamically, and continuously influencing each other and shaping occupation as a whole (2).

A PARADIGM SHIFT: BRIDGING THE SCIENCE OF OCCUPATION TO THE ART OF OCCUPATIONAL THERAPY PRACTICE

In Chapter 6, readers were introduced to the research and work of occupational therapist and occupational scientist Dr Ann Wilcock, who developed the *Occupational Perspective of Health* (OPH) theoretical model. Although Dr Wilcock's OPH utilized **doing**, **being**, **becoming**, and **belonging** as major constructs of the model, those ideas as concepts significant to occupational therapy have existed in the literature for nearly four decades (1, 3). Yet, despite the ubiquitous nature of the terms, and the scholarly development of Dr Wilcock's *Occupational Perspective of Health* theoretical model, the OPH failed to translate well into everyday occupational therapy practice.

Recognizing the value of Wilcock's work, more recently, researchers Hitch, Pepin, and Stagnitti (3–5) explored the concepts of doing, being, becoming, and belonging as used by Wilcock, to clarify how they are currently understood. Following an in-depth analysis, the researchers developed a renewal of the OPH, calling it the **Pan Occupational Paradigm**, or POP. POP preserves the four dimensions of occupation (doing, being, becoming, and belonging) and

reimagines the current operational definitions of the concepts as follows:

- ***Doing*** is the transaction that occurs as people engage in personally meaningful occupation. People develop the skills required for *doing* over the course of a lifespan. It is implied that *doing* also means that the client is actively engaged in occupations because they are relevant to the client; however, occupations may or may not be healthy or purposeful. *Doing* can be characterized as either overt, meaning it is observable or takes place at the physical level, or implicit as are some mental and spiritual occupations. "Doing follows broadly similar patterns across the population, and humans are able to adapt their doing to greater and lesser degrees according to circumstance" (3, p. 241).
- ***Being*** is the essence of a person. It is who they are occupationally, including their unique psychological, social, spiritual, and physical capabilities. *Being* comprises the values and the significances that clients invest their time in throughout their lives. Occupation may be a central focus of *being*; however, in some ways, *being* also has a spiritual or ethereal quality and can stand alone, independent of occupation as the client learns through self-discovery or is in reflection. "Being is expressed through consciousness, creativity and the roles people assume in life. Ideally, individuals are able to exercise agency and choice in their expression of being, but this is not always possible or even desirable" (3, p. 241).
- ***Becoming*** is aspirational goal-directed growth and development. *Becoming* is a process. *Becoming* means that human beings are ever evolving. This implies that changes occur constantly and, for different reasons, over the course of a lifetime. For example, a couple who have recently adopted a child are constantly *becoming* parents as they experience the joys and challenges inherent in the endeavor of parenting. "Regular modifications and revisions of goals and aspirations help to maintain momentum in becoming, as does the opportunity to experience new or novel situations and challenges" (3, p. 242).
- ***Belonging*** is a feeling of being in relationship, or connected to others. As described previously in Chapter 6, *belonging* is characterized by who (or what) a person is with, and by the interactions and impacts that we have on one another. All this is inextricably embedded in situational context and occupational engagement, which in turn, helps shape a sense of belonging. Hitch et al (3) concluded that "A sense of reciprocity, mutuality, and sharing characterize belonging relationships, whether they are positive or negative" (3, p. 241).

As the researchers continued their analysis and extensive critical review of the OPH, eventually developing the POP, they noticed the emergence of a constantly changing "pattern of prominence . . . where one or more dimensions [of doing, being, becoming, and belonging] were fore grounded at different times and spaces within occupational engagement" (4, p. 259).

This led them to underscore the importance in occupational therapy practice of the occupational therapy professional addressing all dimensions of occupation, while forming therapeutic interventions focused on the dimension that is most foregrounded in a particular phase of a client's life, situation, or context (4).

The researchers state that:

> POP presents the concepts of doing, being, becoming, and belonging, within a conceptual continuum of ill-being and wellbeing as a way to show how occupational therapists promote wellbeing in individuals and communities. As such, it articulates the heritage, culture and expertise of a profession that is wonderfully varied and notoriously difficult to pin down throughout its history. Adoption of POP as a guiding paradigm would not diminish this diversity and flexibility, but rather provide occupational therapy with a robust but unique way of explaining what it does and just how much it can offer. (5, p. 33)

The chapters in Section Three are organized around the *POP* and use ***doing, being, becoming, and belonging*** to articulate how occupational therapy professionals can move intervention plans into action (5, 6).

REFERENCES

1. Fidler, G. S., & Fidler, J. W. (1978). Doing and becoming: Purposeful action and self-actualization. *American Journal of Occupational Therapy, 32*(5), 305–310.
2. Fisher, A. G., & Marterella, A. (2019). *Powerful practice: A model for authentic occupational therapy.* Center for Innovative OT Solutions.
3. Hitch, D., Pepin, G., & Stagnitti, K. (2014). In the footsteps of Wilcock, Part One: The evolution of doing, being, becoming and belonging. *Occupational Therapy in Health Care, 28,* 231–246.
4. Hitch, D., Pepin, G., & Stagnitti, K. (2014). In the footsteps of Wilcock, Part Two: The interdependent nature of doing, being, becoming and belonging. *Occupational Therapy in Health Care, 28*(3), 247–263.
5. Hitch, D., Pepin, G., & Stagnitti, K. (2018). The pan occupational paradigm: Development and key concepts. *Scandinavian Journal of Occupational Therapy, 25*(1), 27–34.
6. Hitch, D., & Pepin, G. (2021). Doing, being, becoming, and belonging at the heart of occupational therapy: An analysis of theoretical ways of knowing. *Scandinavian Journal of Occupational Therapy, 28*(1), 13–25.

Facilitating Recovery Using Biopsychosocial Models to Guide the OT Process

OT HACKS OVERVIEW

O: Occupation as a means and an end

Occupation, as conceptualized here, is defined as "what people do, what they experience in relation to that doing, and their experiencing personal value in that doing" (20, p. 28). In occupational therapy practice, occupations and activities can be used as a way (the means) to develop multiple dimensions of occupation: doing, being, becoming, and belonging. We have an ethical obligation as occupational therapy professionals to ensure that the outcome of occupational therapy services (the end) for the client is safe and an enriching occupational engagement. We also have an ethical and professional obligation to apply occupational reasoning throughout the occupational therapy process. In this chapter, we discuss occupational considerations critical during the intervention phase.

T: Theoretical concepts, values, and principles, or historical foundations

Most people who are suffering with illness (regardless of whether they experience physical or psychosocial problems) simply want to be heard and understood. One of the ways that occupational therapy professionals provide this holistic care is through therapeutic use of self, which is unique to the profession of occupational therapy. Therapeutic use of self is a cornerstone of occupational therapy practice, according to the *Occupational Therapy Practice Framework: Domain and Process, 4th Edition (OTPF-4)* (3).

H: How can we Help? OT's role in collaborating with clients with mental illness or mental health needs

Recall the occupational therapy domain and process metaphor using the home at the beginning of Section Two. The intervention phase can be compared to a time when a client's home (occupational engagement) might require maintenance, remodeling, repairs, and, in some cases, rebuilding. The occupational therapy professional and the client need to work together to identify which part of the home requires intervention and together they must figure out who, what, or how to best help the client to "return home" to meaningful and functional participation in life.

A: Adaptations

From an occupational therapy perspective, our client-centered goal is to support the development of **healthy adaptive responses** so that resulting actions and behaviors are effective at supporting the clients' optimal occupational engagement.

C: Case study includes

A 29-year-old with generalized anxiety disorder

K: Knowledge: keeping mental health OT practice grounded in evidence, in occupational science, and in research

The demand for cost-effective care and documentation of value-added occupational therapy interventions with client-centered outcomes drive the continuing need for occupation-based research that supports knowledge translation. According to the American Occupational Therapy Association (AOTA) (2022), "Scholarly systematic reviews summarize the evidence on a focused question and include information on background research, methodology, and implications for practice" (Retrieved from: https://www.aota.org/practice/practice-essentials/evidencebased-practiceknowledge-translation). The following systematic review is an excellent example of one form of knowledge translation that prompts advocacy for occupational therapy as an accountable member of the multidisciplinary health care team, with unique contributions to promote positive client outcomes.

D'Amico, M. L., Jaffe, L. E., & Gardner, J. A. (2018). Evidence for interventions to improve and maintain occupational performance and participation for people with serious mental illness: A systematic review. *American Journal of Occupational Therapy, 72*(5), 7205190020.

Guided questions for this article appear at the end of the chapter in the section "Knowledge" of the OT HACKS Summary.

S: Some terms that may be new to you

Adverse childhood experiences (ACEs)
Afferent neurons
Akathisia

Assertive behaviors
Assertiveness
Autonomic nervous system
Biopsychosocial model of practice
Biopsychosocial-spiritual model of practice
Central nervous system (CNS)
Cognitive reappraisal
Deficiency needs
Directed mindfulness
Distancing
Efferent neurons
Emotional regulation/emotional dysregulation
Emotions
Expressive suppression
Expressive therapeutic techniques
Exteroceptive awareness
Feelings
Gross's Modal Model of Emotion
Growth needs
Homeostasis
Hypothalamic–pituitary–adrenal (HPA) axis
Information exchange
Interneurons
Interoceptive awareness

Mandala
Maslow's Hierarchy of Needs Theory
Mindfulness-based stress reduction (MBSR)
Mindfulness/mindfulness meditation
Mirror neurons
Parasympathetic nervous system
Peripheral nervous system (PNS)
Physicality
Positive childhood experiences
Redirection
Response modulation
Response variables
Role conflict
Role stress
Self-awareness
Self-concept
Self-esteem
Self-expression
Social prescribing
State mindfulness
Somatic nervous system
Sympathetic nervous system
Trait mindfulness
Values clarification

INTRODUCTION

The **biopsychosocial model** of practice was developed as one way to encourage health care practitioners to consider the multifaceted experiences of the client, as a person instead of as a patient with a diagnosis, while caring for them. From this perspective, the term **person-centered care** and expressions such as **holistic assessment** are derived. Person-centered care is at the heart of the biopsychosocial model and is an approach to practice that views the person in their entirety, each with various levels of needs, priorities, and goals. This model assumes that each person's needs are rooted in their own experiences and are informed by their own personal social determinants of health (58). Some expanded versions of the biopsychosocial model of client care have added spirituality into the model, calling this model the **biopsychosocial-spiritual** model. Spirituality is considered an important part of the human experience and one that health care providers might consider in holistic assessment, and during intervention planning with clients (57). Spirituality, as a part of occupational therapy's scope of practice, although historically difficult for occupational therapy professionals to articulate a common definition, is generally thought of as a person's relationship with the transcendent and it is not limited to organized religion. In occupational therapy practice, well-being is perceived as multidimensional and these dimensions help define our unique human experiences and what gives each of our lives meaning. The *Wellness Model in Community Mental Health*, for example, defines eight dimensions of wellness: the physical, spiritual, social, intellectual, emotional, occupational, environmental, and the financial dimensions (53, 54).

Occupational therapy practice is also influenced by other disciplines as we interact within the modern health care landscape. The research and literature from public health, neuroscience, and positive psychology, among others, can be used to inform occupational therapy. As we collaborate with the client and maintain an occupational focus, we further advocate for our profession. Although the idea that our brain, body, and spirit are intimately connected and able to affect one another is not a new concept, the ongoing development of new research and the flood of evidence surrounding how these connections impact occupational engagement has shifted our perspective significantly, even in the past 10 years.

ANALYZING OCCUPATIONAL PERFORMANCE THROUGH THE BIOPSYCHOSOCIAL LENS

When an occupational therapy team collaborates with the client to gather information for an occupational profile, they must consider many dynamic aspects of the client's life to prioritize the client's desired outcomes. Referring again to our OT domain and process metaphor of the home at the beginning of Section Two, the intervention phase can be compared to a time when a client's home (occupational engagement) might require maintenance, remodeling, repairs, and, in some cases, rebuilding. The occupational therapy professional and the client need to work together to identify which part of the home requires intervention, and together they must figure out who or what can best help them. If the lights are flickering in several of the rooms of the home, and some of the light switches or power outlets are dysfunctional, an electrician might be called in. If the kitchen sink keeps dripping even after the water is turned off, then researching water leaks or consulting with a plumber may help. On the other hand, if a family finds out that they will be welcoming another member of the family, and they want to knock down a few walls and add a new room, they might call a contractor or consider a do-it-yourself project. Imagine if the client needed to consider aspects of the home such as family dynamics, which typically happen within the walls of the home. Sometimes the help that the client needs will include learning new interpersonal or social interaction skills and the relationships that the client has with others will need to be explored.

In many ways, occupational performance, and aspects of the **central nervous system** (CNS), (the brain and spinal cord), and the **peripheral nervous systems** (PNS) can be explored using an analogy similar to the one given. The PNS has two branches, the **somatic system** and the **autonomic system**, which can be further broken down into the **sympathetic nervous system (SNS)** and **parasympathetic nervous system (PSNS)**. It is important for the occupational therapy professional to have a general understanding of key systems and various theories of the overall relationships between the nervous system and other body systems because they will influence client factors and either hinder or support occupational engagement. The nervous system and other body systems have electrical and chemical features that are used to regulate, modulate, and communicate within the body (ie, brain waves, neurons, hormones, neurochemicals, and neurotransmitters). The result of these regulatory functions, communication, and internal relationships, contributes to the complex behaviors demonstrated by clients.

The brain can be mapped and categorized to study how certain structures work (their function/s), or to learn how the areas are connected and dynamically influence each other. Today we also understand more about how they are connected through neural networks to other parts of the body. Just as clients are inextricably linked to occupational engagement in a dynamic relationship within multiple contexts, when assessing a client's occupational needs and planning an intervention, the occupational therapy professional must consider the ways that the nervous system may be influencing the client's thoughts, behaviors, emotions, and relationships with others, in a more comprehensive way. It is imperative that the practitioner includes consideration of the internal exchanges between the nervous system and other body systems and, most importantly, that they examine how the exchanges may be resulting in behaviors that are barriers to the client's occupational participation (14, 26).

To help navigate these complexities, authors and psychotherapists Richard Hill and Matthew Dahlitz, in their cutting-edge text, *The Science of Psychotherapy* (2022), invite practitioners of multiple disciplines to deepen our collective understanding about the interplay and interconnectedness of our biology, physiology, and psychology. In this work, they highlight some of the research that has birthed a new, or perhaps more modern, understanding about the relationships

and the complex, nonlinear connections between the mind and body, as well as the interconnectedness of human beings to each other and to our context.

Several pertinent recent discoveries are highlighted throughout this chapter. They are presented as examples of the ways that a finding from one discipline can influence so many other potential research avenues and theoretical possibilities, both within and across disciplines. The rather accidental discovery of **mirror neurons** is one such example. This has prompted greater understanding of the neurobiological core of empathy and the unspoken, but neurologically powerful connection between people. This is especially true within caring or therapeutic relationships and it is apparent in the context of safe and secure bonding and attachment to others (especially primary caregivers) in early development (14, 25).

> Mirror neurons and the neural networks that they coordinate, work together to allow us to automatically react to, move with, and generate a theory of what is on the mind of others. Thus, mirror neurons not only link networks within us but link us to each other. They appear to be an essential component of the social brain and an important mechanism of communication across the social synapse (14, p. 198).

This research replaces our faulty belief that "every man is an island" and has energized research on social learning, emotional health, trauma informed care, emotional intelligence, and attachment theory, among other topics.

Another strand of research that has expanded our understanding of the mind–body connection is the discovery of specific neurologic pathways where activities of the mind "talk to" the body and can result in biological functional changes or help with regulatory functions. For example, the connection between our digestive system and our brain, via the vagus nerve, it seems, might actually have something to do with what we refer to as "having a gut feeling." Current evidence has helped us develop an awareness about how our immune system can be negatively impacted by stress, anxiety, or depression; and we understand more deeply that the opposite is also possible, feelings of comfort, calm, and contentment, can positively influence our immune system. Lastly, the authors cite the work of Damasio (16), who explained "that the body and how it processes emotion is critical for the mind, and the mind is vitally important for how the body functions" (26, p. 301).

With the principles of holistic, person-centered, multidimensional care in mind, let us revisit occupational therapy's domain of concern. Next, the reader is presented with a review section, *Body Systems and Functions 101*, as a foundation for the remaining intervention chapters. The review highlights some of the body systems and functions that may impact outcomes for clients with mental health diagnoses. We then proceed with a discussion about how emotional context and client and therapist emotions play a significant role in impacting the clients' overall health by introducing key aspects of emotion regulation that the occupational therapy professional should consider during intervention planning. In the final part of the chapter, we revisit the *pan occupational paradigm* (POP) and explain how to incorporate its concepts into everyday occupational therapy practice.

OCCUPATIONAL THERAPY'S DOMAIN OF CONCERN

Throughout this chapter and the remaining chapters, as we consider occupational therapy intervention, the reader will notice that there are areas of occupational therapy practice that overlap with those of other professions. To avoid confusion in presenting our skills and expertise both to clients and to other mental health practitioners, it is useful to review some of the differences between occupational therapy and the other health professions. The following distinctions help clarify the differences while reminding us of our own unique skills and focus (2–5).

- **First**, **occupational therapy professionals are concerned primarily with how people function in their daily life activities and occupations.** Collaborative interventions constructed with our clients that focus on factors related to psychological and psychosocial skills aim to improve clients' ability to function in work, at home, in school, in play or leisure, and in other occupational areas.

- **Second, ours is a "doing" therapy more than a "talking" therapy.** While we do discuss with clients the problems in their lives, and while we do present much information verbally through the delivery of various types of occupational therapy interventions, **the main vehicle for therapeutic intervention in occupational therapy is participation in the occupations or activities themselves. When occupational therapy professionals provide interventions, there should be a clear relationship between meaningful occupation and the client's personal preferences and goals.**

- **Third, because of the nature of some of the skills, habits, roles, and routines that occupational therapy professionals are collaborating with clients to reestablish in pursuit of optimal occupational engagement, we often develop and implement therapeutic group interventions.** Thus, occupational therapy techniques may be presented in a group format singularly or in combination with individualized occupational therapy sessions. Often, to help clients establish specific skills such as time management or stress management, we utilize a psychoeducational or advocacy intervention to determine our approach. These intervention types and approaches may resemble a classroom context, where the occupational therapy team is delivering information through teaching, while actively engaging clients in "the work" that will lead to them applying the information through meaningful participation in occupation. **We generally do not, therefore, use techniques that require long-term, one-on-one verbal interaction.** This is not to say that we do not take the individual into account; **we individualize therapy by fine-tuning our general approach**

to the person's presenting problems and occupational performance issues.

- **Fourth, it is essential to recognize that regarding occupational therapy's domain of concern, certain client factors, mostly categorized as body functions, and even more specifically, as mental functions, will at times overlap with the practice areas of other mental health professionals. What does not change is that our concern is focused on how those client factors are supporting or inhibiting occupational participation** that is meaningful and purposeful to the client. Client factors (specific mental functions) that may overlap with other disciplines, especially in psychiatric or behavioral health settings, include, but are not limited to, perception, thought, expression of emotion and emotion regulation, and the client's experience of self and time. Aspects of global mental functions, another category of client factors, including consciousness, orientation, psychosocial factors that support personal and interpersonal development, temperament and personality, and energy, which includes human drives such as cravings, impulses, motivation, or energy level, may occasionally find shared areas of intervention within interdisciplinary practice.

BODY SYSTEMS AND FUNCTIONS 101

Keeping the human body in **homeostasis**, or balance, is one of the aspects of overall good health and is one of several regulatory functions that results, in large part, from the exchanges between the nervous system and the endocrine system. The exchanges and communication between these two body systems are critical in transporting the electrical and chemical messages back and forth from the body to the brain. These systems also play a fundamental role in regulating metabolism, reproduction, and emotion. When combined with a person's life experiences, culture, and genetics, the interactions between the nervous system and the endocrine system (among other systems) can help give us perspective about complex human behavior.

The Central Nervous System

As previously mentioned, the CNS is made up of three key structures, the brain, the spinal cord, and nerve cells (neurons). The CNS receives sensory information, processes the information, and sends out motor signals. The brain consists of the cerebrum, the cerebellum, and the brainstem. The surface area of the brain is called the cerebral cortex, and the largest part of the brain, primarily responsible for memory, speech, thought, and voluntary behaviors, is called the cerebrum. The cerebrum is further divided into four lobes: the frontal, occipital, parietal, and the temporal. The brain and its structures contribute to overall body functions including thought (planning), movement, memory, sensation, and **awareness** (**interoceptive** and **exteroceptive**).

The cerebrum (cortex) is divided laterally into two asymmetrical parts, or hemispheres: the right hemisphere controls movements on the left side of the body and the left hemisphere controls movements on the right side of the body. Note that the four lobes of the brain run across both hemispheres and work together to manage and carry out the functions of the body. According to the most recent research, the two hemispheres have unique but complementary functions, and while it is possible for humans to lean into a particular way of being in the world, strictly lateralized thinking, what was referred to in the past as "right brained" verses "left brained" thinking, is no longer a concept that is supported. Current evidence suggests that both a horizontal and a lateral perspective are necessary to our understanding of the human brain (26, 39, 41). See Table 17.1 for a brief review of the unique features of the right and left hemispheres.

The brain connects to the spinal cord in the brainstem, and the spinal cord is responsible for sending out messages from the brain to the rest of the body and then transmitting signals back from the body to the brain. Some reflex movements are, however, controlled by spinal pathways and do not require participation from the brain. There are 31 spinal nerves made up of 8 cervical nerves, 12 thoracic nerves, 5 lumbar nerves, 5 sacral nerves, and 1 coccygeal nerve. Lastly, the cells that make up the CNS, called neurons, carry messages and communications throughout the body. The three types of neurons, **efferent neurons**, **afferent neurons**, and **interneurons**, serve a different function. Efferent neurons are motor neurons that carry messages from the brain to the PNS. Afferent neurons are sensory neurons that communicate sensory information to the brain and interneurons are considered association neurons because they connect afferent and efferent neurons to the CNS (1, 12). A discussion about some of the key structures of the brain and their functions follows.

Thalamus and Hypothalamus

The thalamus is a structure with two lobes, one in each hemisphere of the brain. The thalamus rests above the brainstem and is in the middle of your brain. The thalamus contains

specialized nuclei, each responsible for processing different sensory or motor signals received from the body and then sending select information to the cerebral cortex. It is sometimes thought of as a relay station because all information must pass through the thalamus before going to the cortex to be processed and interpreted at a higher level. The thalamus helps regulate sleep, keeps one alert and awake (a part of consciousness), and plays a role in thinking and cognition. The thalamus also serves as a monitor for the flood of sensory information, everything except smell, flowing to the cortex and provides feedback coming from the cortex.

The hypothalamus is below the thalamus and above the brainstem, and it is the portion of the brain primarily responsible for keeping the internal body in homeostasis. The hypothalamus is what links the endocrine system to the nervous system by way of the pituitary gland. The hypothalamus receives a signal from the nervous system and synthesizes and produces neurohormones that either stimulate or inhibit the release pituitary hormones, which in turn calls to action responses from the **hypothalamic–pituitary–adrenal (HPA)** axis toward danger or threats. The hypothalamus and the anterior pituitary gland collaborate to determine a physiologic response in the face of threats. Corticotropin-releasing hormone (CRH) triggers the anterior pituitary gland to release adrenocorticotropic hormone (ACTH) into the bloodstream, which further triggers the release of glucocorticoids such as cortisol from the adrenal cortex above the kidneys to enhance the ability to fight or flee from threats or extreme stress. When the stress lessens, feedback mechanisms in the hypothalamus, the hippocampus, and the pituitary gland can regulate the HPA axis response to stress (7, 21, 26).

The Amygdala

The amygdala is an almond-shaped section of the CNS tissue that contains a large cluster of interconnected nuclei and is in the temporal lobe of the brain. In fact, there are two amygdalae, one in each brain hemisphere. The amygdala is associated with arousal, autonomic responses, fear, processing the emotional significance of encounters, and formulating emotional responses, hormonal secretions, and explicit memory. The major neurotransmitters that modulate the flow of information through the amygdala are norepinephrine, serotonin, dopamine, and acetylcholine. Modern theories of emotion agree about the key role of the amygdala as the primary emotional brain structure responsible for focusing attention on critical stimuli in the environment, appraising sensory information from the context, and assigning the appropriate emotional response (26, 35, 36).

The amygdala also regulates autonomic and endocrine functions, responding with a release of neurohormones to help the hypothalamus activate the body for adequate responses. As a part of the limbic system, together with the regions of the hippocampus, the amygdala clarifies the stimulus and prepares an immediate response, often by processing social cues such as facial recognition and evaluation. This early detection system influences activation of

Table 17.1. Hemispheric Descriptions	
Left Hemisphere	**Right Hemisphere**
Has narrow attention	**Manages broad attention** "…what we attend to comes first through the right hemisphere" (26, p. 16)
Deconstructs " . . . is good at deconstructing things to its parts" (26, p. 16)	**Makes connections** " . . . is good at making connections so that we can appreciate the wholeness of dynamic structures and relationships that change over time" (26, p. 16)
Appreciates • Static • Decontextualized • Inanimate structures and abstractions	**Attuned to emotion** **Empathic** **Intuitive** **Moral**

the fight-or-flight response via efferent projections from its central nucleus to the cortex and subcortical structures. Furthermore, "the largest afferent fibers in the amygdala come from the associative cortical fields of the ventral visual pathway that provides processed information about objects and faces. This information arrives in the lateral nucleus where it is evaluated together with information from other sensory modalities to determine whether it is a known stimulus or a potential threat based on previous experiences" (51, p. 22).

The amygdala is also sometimes associated with the feeling of fear, but the amygdala is more like a first responder to a disaster, it seeks out patterns and evaluates stimuli to prepare the body in case a more immediate response is required. But the amygdala is not the origination point of emotions such as fear; that is a higher order cortical function. "Someone who feels afraid is interpreting the threat detection of the amygdala and other incoming internal and external information in such a way as to have the experience of fear" (26, p. 32). This is particularly important to recognize because the amygdala has a very dense neural network with high synaptic density, hypoactivity of the γ-aminobutyric acid (GABA) neurons, and/or the combination of increased activation of glutamate neurons that hyper-excite the amygdala; both show up behaviorally as anxiety. One of the common features of an anxiety disorder is feeling inappropriately fearful in situations where the threat levels do not pose actual danger (26, 51).

The Hippocampus

The hippocampus is a part of the limbic system. One of its most important jobs is to support the formation of explicit declarative memories that are contextually rooted in a person's experience in time and space. The process of hippocampal transfer of information to the cortex for memory consolidation occurs during long-term, slow wave sleep. As the body transitions through various states, a juxtapose is created between the sharp waves of sleep and bursts of neuronal activity, which creates a metaphoric conversation between the two areas of the brain, the hippocampus and the cortex. This dialogue may be responsible for consolidating memory so that it can be integrated into long-term memory (26). Another major function of the hippocampus is its ability to efficiently retrieve spatial memory (or the qualitative features of memories).

The hippocampus is often implicated with the diagnosis of major depression, bipolar disorder, and borderline personality disorders (BPDs), for which reduced hippocampal volume has been found. Current evidence also suggests that the creation of new neurons, called neurogenesis, which occurs with new learning, happens in the hippocampus. In enriched environments and especially with learning novel, hands-on tasks, the neural circuitry grows with an uptick in the creation of new neurons. The reverse is also true, the hippocampus is sensitive to the impact of stress hormones such as glucocorticoids; and with prolonged exposure to stress, the hippocampus becomes vulnerable to damage, in turn leading to consistently elevated levels of cortisol. The relevance of this to occupational therapy professionals is that we may better understand that a client's inability to manage stress, or their vulnerability to fear responses and weakened ability to regulate their fear response, especially in the face of trauma, may have a neurophysiologic foundation. Furthermore, because, as occupational therapy professionals, the target outcome is occupational engagement, this understanding might help us plan interventions related to areas of occupation, such as sleep hygiene. We have a more clarified understanding about the ways that effective sleep encourages new learning to be consolidated into long-term memory in the hippocampal region of the brain (26).

Divisions of the Neocortex: The Lobes of the Brain

As previously mentioned, the cortex is divided into four lobes: the frontal, occipital, parietal, and the temporal. There are two other important areas to consider, the insula and the cingulate. All areas are represented in both hemispheres of the brain and each one specializes in particular functions. The cortices in the brain do not work in isolation, they work in full collaboration with other areas, and all are in cooperation with neural networks. Beginning with the frontal lobes, whose primary work is to regulate motor behavior, language, executive functioning, abstract reasoning, and directed attention. The occipital lobe is made up of areas responsible for visual processing, whereas the temporal lobe is involved more with auditory processing, receptive language, and memory. The parietal lobe links sensory information and the senses with motor abilities to provide an experience or sensation of one's body in space. Finally, the insula and cingulate cortices support limbic processing, such that information can be integrated and connected to cortical neural networks (14).

The Peripheral Nervous System

The PNS comprises the nerves that are outside the CNS, including nerves that extend to muscles, organs, and other parts of the body. The PNS has four main functions. First, it connects the CNS to the organs, the skin, and the upper and lower extremities. The PNS allows the brain and spinal cord to receive and send information to the other parts of the body. This system carries both sensory and motor information to and from the CNS. Perhaps most importantly, the PNS is responsible for regulating involuntary body functions such as heartbeat and breathing.

The PNS branches off into two parts, the **somatic nervous system** (SoNS) and the autonomic nervous system. The SoNS contains two types of neurons: motor neurons, also referred to as efferent neurons that carry information from the brain and spinal cord to muscle fibers in the body; and sensory neurons, or afferent neurons that carry sensory information to the brain and spinal cord. The autonomic branch of the PNS is responsible for regulating involuntary body functions such as breathing, heart rate, and digestion. The autonomic system takes care of many of the life-sustaining processes without relying on our conscious control.

The autonomic system also further divides itself into two branches or systems, the SNS and the PSNS. The sympathetic branch is responsible for regulating the fight, flight, or freeze response, which signals the body to prepare for response to a threat in the environment. The parasympathetic system is the "rest and digest" system, meaning that once a threat has passed, the parasympathetic system helps the body return to a more normalized state, which both helps conserve energy and supports maintenance of homeostasis when threats are not present (1, 26).

The Endocrine System

The endocrine system is a network of glands and organs that relies on hormones to coordinate and control many significant body functions from metabolism to mood. Some of the organs or glands that comprise the endocrine system were introduced in the previous sections. Fundamental organs and glands of the endocrine system are the hypothalamus, the pineal body, the pituitary gland, the thyroid and parathyroid, the thymus, the adrenal gland, the pancreas, and the ovary and testis. Although it is beyond the scope of this text to go into more detail, it is critical to understand the significant role that the endocrine system plays in emotion regulation through its release and control of hormones. It is also important to recognize that although the endocrine system is not a part of the nervous system, its relationship with the nervous system, particularly through their link in the hypothalamus, plays a significant role in the formulation of emotional and stress responses, and in regulating other functions such as sleep and hunger.

EMOTIONS DEFINED

Because OT performs holistic assessment and places focused attention on how the client factor of emotion impacts occupation (and how occupation impacts emotion), and because emotion is often shared territory with all other disciplines, this is a good starting place for a discussion. Many terms are used to describe emotions and emotional states: feeling, mood, affect, and emotions. Each word has a slightly different meaning. When we speak of **emotions**, we mean not just subjective feelings but also physiologic arousal (activation of neurotransmitters and hormones by the nervous system and the endocrine system) and the expression of this arousal and feelings through behaviors. Emotion arises from each person's internal physiology coupled with an evaluation of a situation and the assessment of that situation in relationship to one's own needs, goals, and prior experiences (24, 49). To be clear, emotional arousal, and further articulating what an emotion feels like, is a complicated and complex process. The current understanding of emotion, emotional regulation, and expression of feelings is constantly evolving but it does not necessarily line up with the classical perspective which is that most people will experience, demonstrate, and translate emotions in a similar way. Nor is there any common set of emotions that produce a particular response. Instead, emotional response is specific to the situational context of the individual; humans spontaneously create emotions in the moment depending on sensory input and predictions made by the brain and nervous system (7, 10, 26).

For example, a person may experience anger (a feeling) and a heightened state of arousal (racing heart, physical agitation) when someone else cuts ahead of them in a line while waiting at the airport to get through baggage check and security. The person wants and needs to be on time for a flight (desired goal). Context is critical to consider in examples such as this because situational contexts are linked to occupational engagement. Some behavioral responses are considered more socially acceptable, and behavioral responses and demonstration of emotion can also be culturally mediated. The relevance of this information throughout intervention from an occupational perspective is that our client-centered goal is to support the development of their healthy adaptive responses so that resulting behaviors are effective at supporting the clients' occupations.

In the example given, the person might respond by speaking harshly to the person who moved in front of them in the line, or the person might even raise their voice. Alternatively, the person might get the attention of airline personnel managing the line, or speak calmly to the person, saying "I don't know if you realize we are in line here, and the back of the line is there." Some individuals might "stuff" the feeling, inwardly being very angry but outwardly showing no reaction, and doing nothing. Others might engage in deep breathing or meditation to reduce the physiologic arousal. Success in meeting one's goals and in social participation is highly dependent on the ability to regulate or control our emotions.

Emotional dysregulation, a difficulty controlling and modulating emotions and related behavior, may be associated with many different mental disorders: BPD, posttraumatic stress disorder (PTSD), substance-related disorders, bipolar disorder, disruptive behavior disorders in children, autism spectrum disorder (ASD), and neurocognitive disorders, to name a few. As we learned in the previous section, the occupational therapy professional must also take into consideration that many diagnoses and the associated symptom of having difficulty modulating and regulating emotions have a neural basis (21, 22, 26). The reader can review the cognitive behavioral theoretical perspective and more about cognitive behavioral therapy (CBT) in Chapters 2 and 13, because this theory is the foundation of Gross's Modal Model of Emotion Regulation (24, 49), which we discuss next.

The **modal model** provides a view of emotion (and emotion regulation) that can be useful for planning intervention in occupational therapy (Figure 17.1). We begin on the left of the figure with the **situation**, which may be external (someone cuts in line and steps in front of you) or internal (the belief that one is always being taken advantage of). The situation gets the person's **attention** because it is in some way related to personal goals and needs. The person begins the process of **appraisal**, in which they assess the meaning of the situation. The appraisal may be very rapid and may not even be conscious, but it gives rise to **emotions**. Emotions lead to

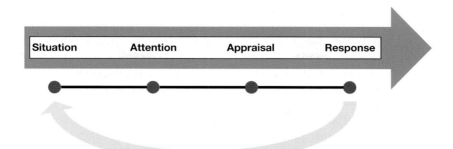

Figure 17.1. The Modal Model of Emotion. (Adapted with permission from Gross, J. J. (2013). Emotion regulation: Conceptual and empirical foundations. In Gross, J. J. (Ed.), *Handbook of emotion regulation* (2nd ed., p. 5, Figure 1.2). Guilford Press.)

behaviors that then affect the situation, and the cycle begins again. This all happens relatively quickly.

Using the given example of someone cutting in line, let us see how this plays out: The situation of someone cutting the line is attended to because it is perceived to interfere with the goals of getting to the gate on time, getting luggage checked, and so on. If the person is already feeling victimized and not respected, the situation may also be attended to because of the underlying feeling that "I can never get this right. People always take advantage of me." The person may then appraise the situation in a variety of ways, ranging from "this is really annoying" to "how dare that person disrespect me?" The emotions aroused may be irritation, frustration, annoyance, anger, or rage (a spectrum of possibilities). The response may be any of those previously described (yelling and verbal abuse, seeking help from airline personnel, expressing oneself assertively, suppressing the feeling, or calming oneself with meditation or breathing).

Accommodating emotionally challenging situations and altering one's behavior to be more effective in meeting one's needs increases the chances for success in occupational performance. In the situation we are using as an example, the occupation is air travel, which might be for leisure or for work. Various strategies can be used to regulate emotions

and behavior. They can be analyzed in relationship to the point or mode in which they are employed. Figure 17.2 illustrates five **emotion regulation processes** that apply to different modes or points in the process:

- Situation selection
- Situation modification
- Attentional deployment
- Cognitive change
- Response modulation

The terms may appear technical and difficult; our aim is to demystify them for the reader. Beginning again on the left, the first point is **situation selection**. Situation selection is used *before* the situation occurs. It is, in a sense, a preventive strategy. For example, knowing that air travel is personally stressful, a person might take the following actions, among others: using the online format to complete precheck- and check-in details the day before travel is to occur; making sure that they allow for possible delays by leaving early for the airport; bringing calming distractions along (eg, a phone app or good book); and if traveling with children, bringing along snacks and toys. Of course, not every eventuality can be predicted or accounted for, but taking actions that make undesirable outcomes less likely is often helpful.

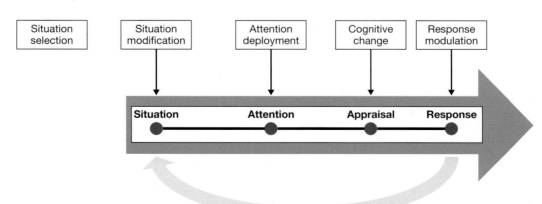

Figure 17.2. The Process Model of Emotion Regulation. (Adapted with permission from Gross, J. J. (2013). Emotion regulation: Conceptual and empirical foundations. In Gross, J. J. (Ed.), *Handbook of emotion regulation* (2nd ed., p. 7, Figure 1.3). Guilford Press.)

Situation modification refers to deliberate changes in the situation as it is occurring. These are changes to the external environment. For example, if the situation is stressful, the person could sit down on the suitcase, or might take out a book, or give the children a snack. Gross (24) alludes to the fact that it is often difficult to differentiate between situation selection and situation modification. What is important for the reader to understand is that different kinds of strategies are available. As stated previously, the person's response alters the situation.

Attentional deployment aims to direct attention away from an emotional situation. We have previously discussed **redirection**, which is a strategy that can be respectfully applied to influence someone else's behavior by directing their attention to something neutral or more pleasant, and away from the distressing situation. This strategy may also be termed **distraction**. Attentional deployment may be applied to the self, as, for example, turning one's attention to something else, playing a game on one's phone, and so on. **Distancing**, or looking at the situation dispassionately as if not personally involved, is another way of deploying attention elsewhere.

Cognitive change (cognitive reappraisal) involves **reappraisal** of the situation to understand it and reduce its emotional power. For example, the person might think about the delay caused by the line cutter as relatively minor or might consider that perhaps that person has an earlier flight and

therefore greater need, or the person might recognize that the internal stressor of "people always take advantage of me" is a cognitive distortion that really does not apply to the current situation. This is sometimes referred to as **reframing**.

Response modulation refers to strategies to control or change the emotional response. Sensory-based modulation techniques may be employed, as can exercise, both of which may be long-term interventions aimed at reducing sensory responsiveness. Nevertheless, in the heat of the moment, the person might use **expressive suppression**, which is an effort to keep their feelings and expression under control by conscious effort, telling oneself to calm down, and so on. Substance use is another method sometimes used to reduce negative emotional states. Suppression and substance use are considered maladaptive and ineffective responses (15, 24). On the other hand, using breathing techniques, meditative and mindfulness practices, and stress management strategies are all considered more adaptive. See also Table 17.2, in which these regulation processes and their uses are summarized. The third column of Table 17.2 shows the skills a person would need to employ in each of the emotion regulation processes. See also the section on key aspects of emotion regulation.

Research regarding health outcomes for those who demonstrate different response strategies, specifically cognitive reappraisal and expressive suppression, toward regulating their emotional response to stress has gotten a boost

Table 17.2. Emotion Regulation Processes and Foundation Skills

Emotion Regulation Process	Used When, Why, and How?	Client Skills Necessary
Situation selection	Before the situation arises; preventive	• Ability to imagine future possibilities • Ability to plan and carry out intentions • When using this strategy for another person such as a child or dependent person, ability to understand how that person is likely to respond
Situation modification	During the emotional situation, to alter the situation, by changing the externals	• Ability to reflect and act quickly and accurately to alter the environment or the task or the objects in the environment
Attentional deployment	During the emotional situation, to direct attention away from the emotional situation so that internal emotional reaction can be shifted or reduced. Strategies include redirection, distraction, refocusing, and distancing.	• Ability to divert attention away from emotions and reactions sufficiently so as to use the strategies • Experience with different strategies • Ability to anticipate which will be effective in a particular situation
Cognitive change	During the situation to change one's thinking about it. Alternatively, after the situation to review what happened and change one's thinking about future similar situations. May apply also to one's beliefs about the self	• Ability to attend to the feelings and the beliefs associated with them • Ability to differentiate feeling states • Ability to imagine other possibilities • Ability to consider other points of view
Response modulation	Late in the situation, after emotions are already aroused, to influence the response behaviors and the internal physiologic arousal. Strategies may include suppression and substance use (both considered maladaptive) and various adaptive strategies such as physical exercise, deep breathing, meditation, self-soothing behaviors, mindfulness activities, sensory strategies, and others.	• Ability to notice, attend to, and identify the feeling and its associated physiologic state • Sufficient experience with adaptive strategies to be able to use them at will • Ability to select which strategies might work best in the particular situation

with the rapid growth and contributions from the body of neurophysiologic and neuropsychological research. Recent literature looks more closely at the efficacy of two emotion regulation response strategies, suppression and reappraisal (24). Suppression negatively impacts health status (eg, increases high blood pressure), seems to reduce positive emotions, and is therefore not considered effective in reducing negative emotions. People who use suppression tend to be more depressed and have more negative feelings about themselves. Suppression is associated with impaired memory, especially regarding emotionally intense situations (24). On the other hand, reappraisal seems to improve memory about emotional or intense situations and to generally increase overall positive emotion, while reducing negative emotion. Reappraisal is also linked to better health outcomes in that it reduces the overfunctioning or does not exacerbate the activity of the SNS. In addition, cognitive reappraisal is an antecedent-focused strategy that can take place before the emotional response. When a client can engage cognitive reappraisal, the trajectory of the emotional response can be positively influenced before the response has begun (ie, preventive or health-promoting approach). Expressive suppression is less adaptive because it is a response-focused strategy, activated once an emotion has been launched, and after the behavioral responses have fully taken place (15).

KEY ASPECTS OF EMOTION REGULATION: A NEUROPHYSIOLOGIC AND COGNITIVE RESPONSE

We have just introduced some emotion regulation processes. Evidence-based programs, strategies, and interventions that can be considered for emotion regulation are introduced shortly. To reason through the occupational therapy process of evaluating and planning interventions with our client, and to avoid confusion about which strategies or programs may be best suited for a particular client, as well as knowing when or how to approach an intervention strategy, the reader is advised to recall the following:

1. Self-awareness is necessary at some level if the person is to develop the skills to regulate their emotions. If the person does not notice that they are experiencing a feeling, and simply acts it out, and afterward cannot explain why they did what they did, then they would not be able to independently learn to apply solution-oriented techniques. In such a case, changes to environment or context, or use of a compensatory approach, may support creating a clear path to positively impact the person's reactions and behavior. Nevertheless, this makes mindfulness-based interventions a logical first step, before moving through other strategies and stages. The importance of mindfulness to emotion regulation is discussed in the next section.
2. Cognitive recognition that one is experiencing feelings is not the same as being able to name the feeling. Having words to attach to feelings states is helpful.

3. However, being able to name the feeling is not sufficient. The person must know regulatory techniques that are personally relevant and useful and they must be able to employ those techniques.
4. Everything takes time. Emotion regulation and emotional intelligence are learned through multiple experiences. Much practice is necessary to develop a habit of being in a mindfulness state and present to one's emotions and feelings.
5. People with cognitive impairments may have more difficulty articulating their feelings and regulating their emotions. A caregiver may offer support by altering the environment or offer cues or distractions so that negative feeling states are reduced and appropriate behavioral responses can be practiced.

THE NECESSITY OF MINDFULNESS

The habit of being mindful is necessary for emotion regulation. What does it mean to be mindful? Jon Kabat-Zinn (32) defines **mindfulness** as "paying attention in a particular way: on purpose, in the present moment, and nonjudgmentally" (p. 4). **Mindfulness meditation** is a disciplined practice in which one develops a dispassionate awareness about what is happening, in their context, which includes being able to reflect upon one's own actions and reactions. With practice, a person learns to withhold judgment and simply notice one's feelings and thoughts without reaction. The **mindfulness-based stress reduction (MBSR)** program is considered the gold standard for meditation practice protocols and was developed by Dr Jon Kabat-Zinn in 1979 (59). Initially, MBSR was developed to target and assist clients with managing their stress but, since its inception, it has evolved into a resource for treating a variety of health problems. The research indicates that MBSR has shown efficacy when used with clients who are experiencing anxiety, depression, pain, immune system dysfunction, and hypertension, to name a few. MBSR incorporates mindfulness meditation to alleviate painful symptoms of physical and psychiatric illnesses. Today, MBSR is offered as an alternative treatment option to clients in many health care settings internationally (40, 59).

It is also important to recognize the difference between **a state of mindfulness**, which is indicated when a person can be mindful in the current moment, and **trait mindfulness**, which is when a person's disposition makes them more likely to have a consistent tendency toward being mindful in everyday life (18). Evidence indicates that both state mindfulness practice and trait mindfulness help reduce the compulsion to change things, improve tolerance of discomfort, and cultivate a sense of contentment, all of which are associated with increasing positive emotions. Mindfulness practices also inform self-acceptance and self-restraint. Commonly recognized mindfulness practices include prayer, meditation, Yoga, Tai Chi, expressive and interpretive dance, or dance movement therapy, Qigong, and reiki, among others (6).

How can the occupational therapy professional utilize mindfulness practices for persons with psychiatric disabilities? The most basic response is to help the client become mindful and to gradually help them remain present in the performance of a task. Being present allows for noticing, observing, reflecting, being contented, and further appreciating that the "doing" of meaningful tasks supports "being." Being engaged in an occupational task in the here and now sometimes helps redirect the client away from negative thoughts and emotional memories of past traumas, and prevents or mediates ruminating about future events, which research indicates keeps many people locked in a negative emotional cycle (22, 23). Helping the client to be present requires that the occupational therapy professional closely attends to the client's experience of the task and listen closely to what the client is saying both verbally and nonverbally through their body language. These are all skills that are aspects of building the therapeutic relationship and the application of therapeutic modes and therapeutic use of self.

Despite the support that mindfulness meditation may offer some clients with psychiatric disorders by providing a strategy to work on emotion regulation, the occupational therapy professional must always analyze the specific client factors and occupational history of the client. This means close collaboration with the client and, many times, also includes working with a multidisciplinary team of professionals. If a client has a history that includes trauma, the occupational therapy provider may choose to engage a method called "directed mindfulness" (22, 44). **Directed mindfulness** is the use of mindfulness in a context where the therapist needs to intentionally direct the client's awareness toward particular elements of the right here, right now experience. The occupational therapy professional will usually choose elements of the situation or task that are considered specifically important to therapeutic goals and occupational outcomes.

The application of directed mindfulness is especially important for clients who have a trauma history. Sometimes, when mindfulness meditation is practiced, clients are instructed to open their minds to receive, nonjudgmentally, whatever comes to mind. Unfortunately, for some clients, the lack of direction for their thoughts places them "at the mercy of the elements of internal experience that appear most vividly in the forefront of consciousness—typically, the dysregulated aspects, such as panic or intrusive images, which cause further dysregulation, or their similar attachment-related patterns" (45, p. 222). Even for clients who do not necessarily have a trauma history, use of directed mindfulness to target emotions, feelings, or body sensations allows opportunities for the client to become aware of their emotions and sensations to begin processing and regulating them. It may also give the occupational therapy professional insight into further activities and interventions that would support the process (22, 45).

Nevertheless, there are some daily occupations such as self-care, for example, that do not at a surface level seem as complex, but which clients need to engage in to maintain good health and where being mindful might help support

efficiency in completing the task. The same is true for tasks where emotion dysregulation is not the primary barrier to completing the task. In these instances, directed mindfulness meditation is very similar to providing verbal cues that encourage the client to focus. The therapist might ask, "What are you thinking about now? Are you paying attention to what you are doing, or are you getting ahead of yourself or thinking about something else?" Therapeutic reasoning may cause the occupational therapy professional to decide to redirect the client, saying something like: "Focus all of your thoughts on what you are doing right here, right now. Just this task." It is worth mentioning that no matter which occupational task the client is participating in, long-term, consistent practice of being in a state of mindfulness can lead to development of the trait of mindfulness (ie, being consistently mindful in everyday life tasks) (18, 56). For example, if a client is preparing a peanut butter sandwich while practicing mindfulness, they will truly see the bread, the jelly, the peanut butter, the knife, the motions involved, and so on. One becomes receptive to the quality of the air, the light, the cool smooth hardness of the knife, the softness of the bread, the fluid spreading of the peanut butter, and all aspects of the things as they really are. Mindfulness opens a path to completely engage in the occupation. Mindfulness is essential for emotion regulation because it allows one to monitor the feelings and behaviors associated with situation, attention, appraisal, and response.

Mindfulness-Based Emotion Regulation Intervention Programs

Mindfulness-based emotion regulation interventions are one type of promising evidence-based strategy for people with psychiatric disorders to learn to utilize. These interventions can also be implemented for helping clients to cope with adjusting to physical and emotional pain, to loss, and to help people cope with grief. Specifically, the effects of mindfulness-based practices show the most consistent evidence of having beneficial effects on depression, pain conditions, smoking cessation, and with addictive disorders (23). Occupational therapy professionals may also work together with a team that employs various identified emotion regulation programs. Here we highlight a few potential programs and strategies to consider applying to support a client when emotion regulation, behavioral change, or increased distress tolerance must be addressed to improve engagement in occupation.

Keep in mind that application of these interventions should clearly, from an occupational therapy perspective, be associated with outcomes of improved engagement in the occupations that the client has prioritized. Although occupational therapy may begin with teaching mindfulness techniques or, for example, implementing a Tai Chi routine with a client, the eventual long-term goal would be that the client is able to use mindfulness techniques such as conscious breathing while at work, when the client feels overwhelmed with too many tasks, or incorporate a Tai Chi routine each evening after work, to help alleviate stress. Ideally, occupational therapy intervention can help the client identify and articulate their feelings, (attention and appraisal), to complete each individual task efficiently, and to the best of their ability, without significantly increasing their blood pressure (response). Therefore, the occupation-based outcome would be considered successful, healthy engagement at work, and perhaps equally important successfully maintaining their employment and health through increased improved occupational balance.

WHAT'S THE EVIDENCE?

The occupation-based intervention *Redesigning Daily Occupations*-10: Long-term impact on work ability for women at risk for or on sick leave

The purpose of this longitudinal cohort study was to investigate whether the occupation-based intervention *Redesigning Daily Occupations* (ReDO)-10 predicts work ability (the ability to successfully and effectively work or return to work) for women with stress-related disorders or complex medical histories who are at risk for, or on sick leave. The study was primarily concerned with exploring the long-term effects of ReDO-10. A brief review of the literature indicates that "Women with families in western societies tend to have double workload with multiple daily occupations to balance" (46). The ReDO-16 program was originally created as an occupation-based group treatment work rehabilitation intervention method. It was designed to improve participants' perceived health, occupational balance, and ability to work efficiently and safely. The program consists of three phases. Phase I focuses on occupational self-analysis. Phase II focuses on setting goals and strategies for change, and phase III is a job placement program that provides opportunities to implement the strategies when work is restarted. Depending on the desired outcome, the program targets people who experience stressor-induced difficulty organizing and carrying out multiple daily occupations.

The primary goal of the original ReDO intervention (known as ReDO-16) was based on the philosophical tenets of self-reflection, psychoeducation, and occupational science. Outcomes for participants included gaining an enhanced understanding of the connection between their "doing" and their health, which would then positively impact their overall well-being. ReDO-16 was later adapted in 2014 to meet the demands of the context of primary care and changed from 20 group sessions to 13 sessions, with removal of the work placement portion of the intervention. This revised or adapted version of the ReDO-16 is called the ReDO-10.

Using the adapted protocol (ReDO-10), the results of the data collected from the current study indicate significant improvement in participants' sense of mastery, perceived well-being, and occupational balance. Nevertheless, at a 12-month follow-up, occupational balance, concrete value, and self-rewarding value were not predictive of work ability but perceived health was found to be predictive of work ability.

1. On the basis of the findings of this intervention study, what is the relationship between self-awareness, occupational patterns, and ability to work or return to work?

2. How do you think that removing the work placement portion from the ReDO-16 intervention to adapt the instrument to be useful in the primary care arena, impacted the results of the intervention, as experienced by the participants?

Olsson, A., Erlandsson, A. K., & Håkansson, C. (2020). The occupation-based intervention REDO™-10: Long-term impact on work ability for women at risk for or on sick leave. *Scandinavian Journal of Occupational Therapy, 27*(1), 47–55.

The RULER Program

RULER is a comprehensive program developed by the Yale Center for Emotional Intelligence for schools and school systems (61). The aim is to cultivate understanding and intelligence in emotional expression and regulation. Teachers, staff, families, and students are involved. RULER stands for:

- R—recognizing emotions in self and others
- U—understanding the causes and consequences of emotions
- L—labeling emotions accurately
- E—expressing emotions appropriately
- R—regulating emotions effectively (61)

The program incorporates a 2-year curriculum used to develop emotion regulation skills and an ongoing program used to ensure that skills are maintained over time. Workshops and a training program in RULER are available, as well as extensive curriculum materials.

The main components of the RULER program are the following:

- Emotion identification and labeling via the **Mood Meter**, in which the degree of emotion is considered and vocabulary to differentiate emotional states is developed.
- Processing a complex emotional situation through **Meta-Moment**, which is a step back to appraise the situation and consider alternatives.
- Conflict management through **Blueprint**, which provides a protocol for considering conflict from all sides of a dispute.

Zones of Regulation

Developed by OT Leah Kuypers, *Zones of Regulation* has its roots in cognitive behavior therapy (34). The zones are based on traffic signs, cuing to rest, go, slow down, or stop:

- Blue zone—REST AREA—a blue rectangle with white lettering—a zone where the client may appear lethargic or lacking in energy but should be considered a place to reenergize and regroup.
- Green zone—GO—a green circle with white lettering—a zone characterized by client alertness and readiness, a zone where learning is possible.
- Yellow zone—SLOW—a yellow diamond with black lettering—a zone in which negative emotions are present

and perhaps increasing, and where it might be appropriate to slow down and appraise.

- Red zone—STOP—a red octagon with white letters—a zone in which feelings are out of control, and where one needs to stop entirely.

Kuypers developed the zones after recognizing that her students with disabilities would connect best with a concrete visual representation of states of feelings and alertness. The program teaches students to self-monitor, begin to recognize what the different states feel like in the body, and to categorize and label their emotional states. In 2011, Kuypers turned the *Zones* framework into a curriculum and published *The Zones of Regulation: A Curriculum Designed to Foster Self-Regulation and Emotional Control*. The original curriculum has now been expanded into two apps, *The Zones of Regulation* and *The Zones of Regulation: Exploring Emotions* (34).

EMOTIONAL REGULATION AND MOTIVATION: THE IMPACT OF PHYSICAL, SOCIAL, PSYCHOLOGICAL, AND SPIRITUAL NEEDS

Another useful perspective during the occupational therapy assessment and intervention planning phase, when thinking about clients whose emotional dysregulation is disrupting their participation in life, is to consider **Maslow's Hierarchy of Needs Theory** (37). Maslow's Hierarchy suggests that people are *motivated* to fulfill basic needs before moving on to other, higher order needs. In essence, Maslow's Hierarchy of Needs is fundamentally a theory of human motivation—which was the title of the paper he first published in 1943 to articulate his theory. Decades later, although some criticisms do exist, the theory continues to be widely recognized and used as a guide in research and practice, especially in the areas of social services and education.

Many people with psychiatric disorders have difficulty identifying and expressing their needs, which can lead to increasing frustration. When a person is unable to identify, express, or gratify their needs, they may also resort to impulsive behaviors as an attempt to manage unrecognized feelings of distress or frustration. Maslow's Hierarchy of Needs has five levels, each built upon the next rising up in the shape of a pyramid. Maslow suggested that lower level needs such as food, water, shelter, and sleep, must be satisfied before people could move on to pursue the needs at the higher levels (although Maslow agreed that the higher level needs may at times take precedence).

The lowest level of the pyramid represents **physiologic needs** and refers to the things that a person needs to survive. **Safety** needs are at the second level; these include psychological safety needs, as well as physical safety needs. At the third level are **love and belongingness** needs; these are the needs to be accepted and loved as a unique human being, unconditionally for what one is. The fourth level is for **esteem** needs, or the need to be recognized by others. **Self-actualization**, or the need to accomplish personal goals, is at the fifth level (37) (Figure 17.3).

Maslow's Hierarchy of Needs theory proposed two types of needs: **deficiency needs** and **growth needs**. Deficiency needs are needs that occur because of deprivation. These deficiency needs are considered the bottom three levels of the pyramid: physiologic needs, safety needs, and love and belongingness needs. Growth needs, according to Maslow, occupy the highest two levels of the pyramid; these are esteem needs and self-actualization needs. The growth needs occur not from being deprived of something but from a person's motivation to grow as a person, and to reach the place where they feel they have achieved their personal goals and potential (42). Maslow's Hierarchy of Needs Theory marks an important paradigm shift in psychological trends. Together with other psychologists such as Carl Rogers, Abraham Maslow's

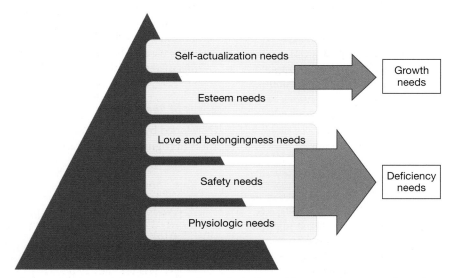

Figure 17.3. Maslow's Hierarchy of Needs. (Adapted from Maslow, A. H. (1943). A theory of human motivation. *Psychological Review, 50*(4), 370–396.)

work ushered in humanistic psychological thought that was person centered and focused on wellness and healthy developmental patterns, very different from the historical emphasis on abnormal behavior and development.

TYING INTERVENTIONS TO ENGAGEMENT IN OCCUPATION

Emotions are intimately connected with needs. Frustration of needs typically leads to negative emotions (anger, depression, fear, boredom, withdrawal, irritability). Need gratification may result in positive emotions (happiness, elation, contentment, pride, relief) but also may generate mixed feelings (guilt, indecision, regret, confusion), especially when there is a conflict between meeting needs at one level while being motivated more toward gratification of higher order needs. Failure to monitor, recognize, and examine one's feelings, current experiences, and needs often contributes to a negative cycle of acting out, or to choosing maladaptive adaptations without understanding the root of the problem or the reasons for one's actions. The next sections of the chapter introduce some of the general targets of intervention that an occupational therapy professional can broadly have in mind during intervention planning. The following client factors and performance skills are not associated with particular mental health diagnoses, nor are they personalized for a unique client, instead they are offered here as common barriers of optimal engagement in occupation and, therefore, are common targets of occupational therapy intervention.

Self-Awareness

Self-awareness is self-knowledge. It is the conscious understanding of internal motivations and feelings and a view of the self as separate from others. Three aspects of self-awareness are discussed (values, interests, and self-concept). Dr Gary Kielhofner (33) defined **values** as "what one finds important and meaningful" (p. 13). Although some people have a clear understanding of their own values, this is not always the case. **Values clarification** is a psychoeducational approach that can be used to help individuals and groups understand their values. Exercises and activities with a written component, such as use of worksheets can be completed individually, but may be more effective in a group format, as members can give and receive feedback. The resources at the end of this chapter provide a link to several ideas for evidence-based activities and interventions that can be implemented for values clarification (see link to Dr Maike Neuhaus's work titled *25 Values Worksheets to Enrich Your Clients' Lives*).

Interests are "what one finds enjoyable or satisfying to do" (33, p. 13). Similar to values, interests are developed through experience. The occupational therapy professional can help clients identify interests using interest checklists or tools such as the *Activity Card Sort* (8) (see Chapter 12), but clients must recognize and have some sense of what the activities are all about for this to be a useful approach. One of the most powerful tools that occupational therapy professionals have at their disposal for clients who cannot identify their interests is to help them explore new hobbies or reinvent hobbies that the client has not participated in for a time because of changes to their life or health status.

The COVID-19 pandemic and the subsequent quarantine changed peoples' lives significantly, negatively impacting mental health across age groups and around the globe. In 2021, the World Health Organization made recommendations underscoring the importance of incorporating strategies for maintaining mental health, which were especially important during the international crisis (60). Beyond the somewhat obvious recommendations for people to keep structure in their day by establishing and maintaining routines and patterns related to eating, sleeping, and exercising, they also recommended finding time to participate in things that bring one joy, to engage in hobbies. Finding time for one's interests during stressful times according to the research, is one way to alleviate or even prevent depression (38). As mentioned in Chapter 16, the significance of social capital to a client's recovery cannot be overstated. **Social prescribing** is a new approach and treatment method being implemented for clients who experience mild to moderate depression, for which antidepressant drugs have proven to be less effective. In social prescribing, medical doctors prescribe unique nonmedical interventions, such as taking up a hobby, as an attempt to help the client improve their mental health state. This creates an excellent opportunity for occupational therapy professionals to enact the social prescription by supporting the client in pursuing hobbies and interests (38).

Self-concept is not only a psychological or biological construct but also a social construct that is influenced by the environment and context. Self-concept can be described as a collection of ideas, feelings, and attitudes that a person has about their own identity, self-worth, capabilities, and limitations (50). This includes ideas, beliefs, feelings, and attitudes about the physical, emotional, and sexual self. Self-concept is acquired through interactions with others and the environment. Childhood experiences and the responses and opinions of family and peers contribute to the development of self-concept, as does the culture. Thus, self-concept is deeply engrained and not easily changed. People may not have a conscious awareness of their ideas and attitudes about themselves. Furthermore, the self-concept may include both positive and negative valuations. Negative valuations tend to undermine effective engagement in occupation because an expectation of failure can become a self-fulfilling prophecy. The person internally believes, "I can't do this; I've never been any good at this," and over time this expectation becomes a belief, and the person fails.

Occupational therapy professionals seek to enable successful engagement in occupation. To do this, we sometimes must help the client recognize that a negative aspect of the self-concept is undermining their ability to function. Once this is recognized, the client may be able to change behavior simply because they recognize how limiting and false the negative valuation has been. However, the client may not appreciate that the negative valuation is incorrect, and then it is necessary to implement strategies to help the client challenge the negativity. As should be clear, interventions related to self-concept must address both **self-awareness** (understanding the self) and **self-esteem** (valuing the self).

PATTERNS: ROLE PERFORMANCE, HABITS, AND ROUTINES IN OCCUPATIONAL ENGAGEMENT

Effective participation in occupations of one's choice is affected by habits and roles, communication skills, and the ability to assert and express oneself. Roles are defined in the *OTPF-4* as "Aspects of identity shaped by culture and context that may be further conceptualized and defined by the client and the activities and occupations one engages in" (3, p. 41). Many ordinary people complain of **role stress** (a feeling that one cannot meet the expectations of one's roles) and **role conflict** (a feeling that expectations for one's roles are in conflict). Again, in planning an intervention that targets either role stress or role conflict, a psychoeducational approach is effective. A group format allows clients to see that others experience the same demands and, at times, others also have feelings of inadequacy. In group situations, the members can help one another recognize that steps can be taken to change or even accept the situation.

Habits and routines may be cultivated to support maintaining emotion regulation during occupational performance. For example, a routine of setting up clothing and meals for the following day before going to bed can engender feeling in control in the morning, while also supporting getting to work on time. A habit of regular meditation or exercise, or writing in a journal enhances well-being and allows for regulation of emotional responses. All the previous examples are potential targeted interventions and all these examples have occupation-based goals and outcomes.

Social Conduct: Communication and Interaction Skills

The concepts of **physicality** (the body language of communication) and **information exchange** (the delivery and receipt of communication) may seem abstract until you collaborate with a client who is having difficulty in this area. Social success requires the use of a complex interrelated skill set that involves things such as gesturing, appropriate use of physical space, the ability to listen and respond, and being able to apply the manners and social customs that match the situation. The number one rule for supporting improvement in the social interaction skills of the client is to provide gentle and specific feedback immediately following a social interaction. It is important to analyze the performance of clients who demonstrate deficient interpersonal or social interaction skills.

Sometimes, the client "knows about" and even understands the desired or acceptable behavior but they misread environmental cues and thus fail to select an effective or appropriate response behavior for achieving the desired result.

The occupational therapy professional can discuss with the client what was happening (the situation) and, through dialogue or even demonstration and role-re-play, determine what the client perceived. Only with repeated experiences and practice, with a trusted loved one or therapist providing friendly observation and feedback, will the client learn to differentiate the expectations of different contexts and environments.

Communication may be verbal and/or nonverbal, clear or confusing, direct or oblique, and effective or ineffective. Clients with mental health problems may need assistance to learn to communicate more effectively, so that others are able to support them and help them meet their needs. Assisting clients with improving their interpersonal communication skills, increases the likelihood of them being more successful in advocating for themselves. Occupational therapy should be concerned with these skill deficits, placing intentional emphasis on how the skill deficit impedes the person's occupational performance and participation. For some clients who have more intense or complex needs, or who have a complicated trauma history, a referral to the psychotherapist or counseling team may be warranted. Although a variety of strategies and approaches have been used to support improved interpersonal communication and social interaction to remove barriers to occupational participation, role play and small group, therapeutic or psychoeducational groups are the most common. Regardless of the medium used, it is most important to help clients analyze their own behavior, to understand what worked and what did not, and to formulate a plan for similar social encounters.

Assertiveness

Assertiveness is the ability to state one's needs, thoughts, and feelings in an appropriate, direct, and honest way. **Assertive behaviors** are actions that reflect a person's priorities and concern for themselves, which include the person having the confidence to stand up for themselves appropriately without experiencing anxiety (ie, using appropriate tone of voice, allowing appropriate response time when making a request, etc) (52). Repeated hospitalization and long involvement with the mental health system may thwart personal assertiveness. Thus, clients may need to acquire or relearn these skills. Assertiveness is similar to other client and personality factors in that it can be considered as a trait or as a state. Assertiveness characteristically runs along a spectrum ranging from excessive agreeableness (submissive) to excessive hostility (aggressive). The intended outcome following an intervention using assertiveness training is that clients become more successful in confidently and appropriately expressing their thoughts, wants, and needs in a variety of contexts (52).

Assertiveness training is a component of social skills training that focuses on teaching the client specific skills of self-advocacy while reducing symptoms of depression, anxiety, and stress. Assertiveness may be approached through a set of structured exercises in assertiveness training using a psychoeducational approach (19, 52). The usual sequence is to begin by defining assertiveness, usually by illustration of assertiveness-based scenarios in a variety of social encounters. The next step is to help clients identify their own assertiveness patterns. This may be done through a questionnaire or a diary or log. Next, obstacles to assertiveness (fear, shyness, self-doubt) are identified and discussed. Homework assignments incorporate the specific assertive behaviors that have been taught and practiced in hypothetical role plays (typically in group sessions over a 6–10-week period). Then, participants are asked to begin applying these new skills in their own lives, and in varying contexts while keeping thought records or diaries. Experiences are reported to the group, which allows the members an opportunity to problem solve and receive feedback (19).

Self-Expression

Self-expression is showing, demonstrating, or revealing one's thoughts, feelings, and needs. Self-expression assumes some awareness of self. For a variety of reasons, many clients need help in this arena. Some have had adverse childhood experiences (ACEs) and experienced extreme emotional deprivation lacking stable or safe attachments and, therefore, habitually suppress or ignore their feelings (9, 43). Others, because of the symptoms of their disease, tend toward extremes of emotion (euphoria and despair) and lack appreciation of the subtle distinctions of emotions in the middle range (eg, contentment, serenity, satisfaction, confusion, mischievousness, shyness, boredom). Occupational therapy has historically included creative activities that facilitate expression of inner thoughts, feelings, beliefs, anxieties, and perceptions. Furthermore, research has indicated over the past several decades the correlation between children who have had ACEs being prone to be at increased risks for adult depression, unstable or poor mental health, and a lack of social and emotional resources into adulthood. We are now learning critical new information about how positive childhood experiences, or (PCEs), especially if they co-occur with ACEs, may lessen the effect of ACEs on adult mental health and interpersonal relationships with family and community. Depending on the needs of the client or family, creative activities may be used to teach basic communication skills, to bolster participation in leisure activities, or to enhance social skills, all of which have the potential to contribute to PCEs (9).

Often, **expressive therapeutic techniques** are used to develop the clients' self-concept and self-identity, their awareness of themselves, and of their own experience of self, feelings, and needs. The degree to which each client expresses themselves and the impact of expressive therapies will be unique to the situation and context. Expressive therapies usually involve some avenue for creativity and can include the use of tools that facilitate self-expression, many times with little need for language (or verbal dialogue). Some common techniques include creating artwork through graphic and fine arts media, such as drawing, painting, and collage, incorporating music, sand-tray playing, drama, dance and movement, and even writing poetry. The key element is using the creative process to help the client achieve their occupational goals by giving them the opportunity to express their internal states in an outward way. "The construction of metaphor through art, music, movement, symbol or some other means becomes a language for activation of the change process—often offering ways to express the inexpressible" (47, p. 56).

A few things to keep in mind when introducing expressive therapies are that these media are unstructured and can feel overwhelming and complex unless the occupational therapy professional imposes some structure. Many clients experience a feeling of overwhelm if presented with too many choices, unfamiliar tools and materials, and a blank canvas or lump of clay. Adult clients may feel insecure or anxious about engaging in art because they feel their work will be seen as childish or unsophisticated, or because they fear it will be analyzed for unconscious content. Many of these potential barriers to implementing expressive therapies can be avoided through careful planning of the activity and by first establishing a safe and trusting therapeutic relationship with the client.

Structured paired or group activities with a specific procedure, purpose, or theme may not only reduce stress but also encourage social participation and enhance self-confidence. For example, one expressive art activity that can be used in a group or with individuals utilizes the symbolism of a **mandala** to encourage self-reflection and awareness. If used in a group, exercises incorporating the mandala establish the importance of unique individual contributions to the whole, or collective. The term mandala is an ancient Sanskrit word, which translates to mean "circle." Historically, the circular form of the mandala had a generative meaning and was associated with a source of life (ie, was symbolic of the womb), but mandalas have been used across cultures and religions to express a variety of aspects of the human experience (11, 17). Dr Carl Jung, arguably one of the fathers of psychotherapy, along with Dr Sigmund Freud, recognized the therapeutic benefits of artistic expression using mandalas. According to Jung, drawing within the circle facilitates a unifying type of meditative space where internal processes of the unconscious could be contained and, with reflection, be brought to consciousness. The mandala, according to Dr Jung was "expression of the self-healing process" (31). Examples of activities that incorporate evidence-based therapeutic use of the mandala can be found in the end of chapter.

Creative writing activities and the study and appreciation of the written word may engage more verbal clients. Clients can perform plays or write and act out plays that they have written, thus learning not only to express ideas but also to identify with the emotions of a particular role. Group work with poetry may include both appreciation and reading of poetry and/or the writing of poetry. Journaling is another widely used intervention strategy. Keeping a daily journal can give clients a structure to record and explore what happens in their lives and how they react to situations and experiences; when clients later review what they have written, they may see patterns that they otherwise might not have recognized. For example, clients may learn that they experience feelings of depression around family holidays or that episodes of tension and outbursts, or changes in their mood at home tend to follow disappointments at work.

AN OCCUPATIONAL THERAPY FRAMEWORK OF CONCEPTS ABOUT SYMPTOMS: INTERVENTION INTO ACTION

Now that the reader has reviewed important concepts related to occupational therapy's domain, this chapter concludes with an introduction of the conceptual framework that is used to guide the reader through each of the remaining chapters. So far in this chapter we have completed a general review of some of the central principles of neurophysiology, provided a brief introduction to emotions and emotional regulation that included the acknowledgment of the importance of mindfulness to nearly all occupational therapy practices. We have discussed the role that motivation, need, client factors and patterns, habits, social interactions, experiences, and relationships have in the dynamics of occupational engagement. Now, let us revisit how we can move the intervention planning and intervention processes into action in everyday occupational therapy practice, using concepts from the *POP*, a theoretical model that was derived from Wilcock's *Occupational Perspective of Health* (OPH) (27–30).

Recall that in the POP model of practice, the occupational therapy professional is urged to address the four dimensions of occupation while forming therapeutic interventions focused on the dimension that is most central to the current phase of a client's life, their needs and priorities and their situation, or context (27). As a reminder, the four dimensions of occupation are as follows:

1. **Doing**: the transaction that occurs as people engage in personally meaningful occupation
2. **Being**: the essence of the person. It is who the person is occupationally, which includes their unique psychological, social, spiritual, and physical characteristics and capabilities.
3. **Becoming**: the aspirational, goal-directed growth and development of a person
4. **Belonging**: a feeling of being in relationship or connected to others; reciprocity, mutuality, and sharing are elements of a sense of belonging, and of belonging relationships.

With these dimensions of occupation in mind, "There is also a need to redefine occupational therapy as a health-care profession that applies meaningful and purposeful activities to help the patient reach functional goals and foster well-being and happiness" (48, p. 11).

When a client has mental health needs or a mental disorder, and they act in uncommon ways or say out of the ordinary things, from the perspective of the medical model, our first reaction may be to label them, or place judgment, while in our mind wondering what their diagnosis is. In doing so,

all that we potentially accomplish is shielding ourselves by seeing the differences between us and them. Unfortunately, often this trajectory leads us toward a line of reasoning that focuses on our own version of what is "normal," rather than toward all the ways that the individual shares similarities with other human beings. The wish of most people who are suffering from illness (regardless of whether they experience physical or psychosocial problems) is simply to be heard and understood. This is a kind of care that is unique to the profession of occupational therapy; it is, in fact, a cornerstone of occupational therapy practice according to the *OTPF-4* (3). Therapeutic use of self, the therapeutic relationship, and an occupational therapy perspective illuminate aspects of the **being dimension** of occupational therapy, allowing us to seek to know the essence of the person, who they are occupationally, just as they are. The reflective and authentic occupational therapy professional learns to step back from initial reactions and examine the reasons behind the client's unusual actions or words.

In most important ways, people with mental health problems are very much like other people. All people have emotional needs, such as the need to belong and to be accepted by other people, the need to be loved and approved of by those around them, and the need to explore and master their environments. These needs are precisely aligned with the characteristics of the **being dimension** and the **belonging dimension** from the POP model. Occupational therapy professionals can initiate a client's sense of belonging by attempting to understand what their priorities and needs are and by developing a therapeutic rapport with the client to figure out how to make them comfortable with us and with themselves. The collaborative nature of occupational therapy practice means that during occupational therapy sessions, the therapist and the client both have a sense of belonging, often a sense of belonging together for the work of therapy.

People with serious or persistent mental illness may not be easy to understand. They still, of course, have basic needs to be loved and accepted but the way that they express these needs may cause other people to be hesitant of them. Consider the following dialogue between an occupational therapy professional and a client in a community day program group that is working on employability skills training:

The occupational therapy professional [observing that the client is getting ready to exit a computer program (document) that they have been working on, and has not saved their work, which would mean that they would lose their progress, and need to begin again.]: "Wait. Don't forget to save your work, so that you can come back to it later, and not have to start all over." [Occupational therapy professional points to the place to save the document on the computer screen.]

The client [irritated and with a raised voice]: "Do you even know what you are doing? I thought you were a therapist not a computer specialist. Are you even a therapy person? You probably don't know anything about computers. It's pathetic. Where's a supervisor? I'm going to tell them that you should not be trying to teach us what to do, when you don't even know how to do it yourself." [Storms off to a corner of the therapy room, stares out the window and begins picking and pulling at their sweater.]

What went wrong here? When the occupational therapy team assesses the here and now events of therapy, we ask questions such as: "What is the client doing?" "What is it that they want to be able to do?" "What should the occupational therapy professional do about it?" These are reflections of the **doing and the being dimensions**, drawn from the perspective of the POP theoretical model. Questions such as "Why is the client reacting this way?" and "What are they feeling?" help us imagine what it must be like to be the client in this circumstance. There are innumerable possible interpretations and the occupational therapy team must be present enough to employ all that they understand about the situational context, the client factors, and what symptoms of their client's mental illness are presenting. This is where professional (or therapeutic) reasoning is critical.

One possible interpretation of this client's behavior is that they felt ashamed about not recognizing that they needed to save their work before leaving the computer, or ashamed at not following the right sequence to complete the task correctly and independently. After all, saving one's work is a more basic word processing skill and one that they had practiced many times. Had they interpreted the occupational therapy professional's comment as a criticism not just of their error but of their entire being? Perhaps they wanted to feel competent; that was why they chose such a basic task to start out with. Maybe the client feels discouraged about how few tasks they have been able to complete independently, making finding employment seem like an impossible goal. Indeed, it could seem to them that they were completely worthless. In this interpretation, it seems that the client displaced their frustration onto the occupational therapy professional. They projected blame because it was too painful for them to face another disappointment. Furthermore, it is so important to recognize the likelihood that everything that happened in the scenario, happened unconsciously; the client's unconscious defense mechanisms protected them from awareness of the (to them) intolerable truth, that they had forgotten an essential step of the task.

With reasoning and reflection, in some ways the client's reaction begins to be understood. Yes, it might be immature, or angry, or rude and unacceptable, but it is a reaction that can lead us to better understand what we might be able to do to support the other dimension of the POP theoretical model, becoming, which is the goal-oriented growth dimension in which the client is motivated toward more successful social interactions that break down the barriers to occupational engagement. The interpretation of the scenario, remember, is just one of many possible ways of understanding what happened, and as the therapist moves through that process, the aspect of belonging with this particular client, in this particular scenario, brings to the forefront the importance of establishing a trusting therapeutic relationship, where therapeutic use of self informs us of our shared humanity.

We all sometimes use defense mechanisms to protect ourselves from facing facts that we find threatening. Perhaps you would have interpreted this client's behavior differently. Many interpretations are possible. The point is that if we take the time and try to know our client through the dimensions of doing, being, becoming, and belonging, it is possible to come to a far deeper understanding of them as unique occupational beings.

Some clients become verbal and combative, as the client in the earlier scenario did, whereas others withdraw, and still others become suspicious. Some may burst into tears and apologize for not getting the steps in the task right. Such reactions, while understandable, may nonetheless seem extreme or inappropriate to the situation. Behaviors such as these are termed *symptoms* because they show that some past experience, problem, disease, or abnormal state is influencing the way that the person acts or responds. Symptoms may be visible behaviors, such as the ones just mentioned, which suggest underlying problems, or they may be subjective feelings reported by the person, such as a feeling of extreme sadness, or experiencing flashbacks of traumatic events in their history that seem very real. Regardless of the nature of the symptoms, it is the symptoms that commonly create barriers to successful occupational participation.

Expressing Unmet Needs or Conflicts

One way to understand the role of symptoms in mental disorders is to recall the concepts of the object relations theory (Chapter 2). According to that theory, the ego mediates the conflicts among the id (needs and primitive drives), the superego (moral principles), and external reality (real-life demands and obstacles). When the ego is not able to solve these conflicts, anxiety results. Anxiety is the most common symptom in psychiatric disorders and it occurs in a wide range of diagnoses. From the perspective of object relations, anxiety is a state of tension and uneasiness caused by conflicts that the ego is unable to resolve. Other common symptoms, such as depression, withdrawal, and hostility, are sometimes just the way the person defends themselves against overwhelming anxiety. It may be helpful to think of these symptoms as maladaptive ego defenses. In other words, the person (consciously perhaps, but most often unconsciously) uses the symptom to reduce anxiety. For example, a person who is angry at their boss and frustrated with their job may develop low back pain; pain allows them to defer unpleasant situations without having to express their anger directly toward their boss.

Although symptoms are sometimes effective for avoiding anxiety, they create other problems and, in many cases, may increase anxiety. A teenage client who feels depressed and insecure about their social skills or appearance may withdraw from their peers, eliminating a potential source of anxiety. As they continue to withdraw, however, peers may consider them less and less socially acceptable, making them seem less approachable, hence increasing the person's anxiety. Whatever symptom the individual displays, though, can usually help us identify what the person needs, what they may be motivated by, and what they are compensating for through their responses.

In another example, a female consumer in a locked psychiatric unit who identifies with a staff member might attempt to copy her clothing and hairstyle, or take on some of the other person's mannerisms. Although one interpretation may be that the client is compensating for a feeling that she herself is inadequate or inferior, this taking on of another person's persona is also a commonly known symptom of several of the personality disorders. Clients who make excuses for (or rationalize) their behavior may be having trouble accepting themselves and meeting responsibilities. And clients who deny feelings or facts that are unpleasant may be protecting themselves from these painful thoughts. This highlights the importance of an occupational therapy professional who works in psychosocial rehabilitation arenas understanding the *Diagnostic and Statistical Manual of Mental Disorder*s (DSM) classifications of diagnoses at some level but, more importantly, knowing what symptoms are commonly associated with a diagnosis, because, again, it is the symptoms that typically interfere with occupational performance.

Symptoms Are Not the Disease

Remember, the symptoms are not the disease. They are only behavioral evidence of the disease. Most of the symptoms discussed in the next chapters occur across diagnostic groups. However, disorders, or diagnoses, can be categorized as being associated with a group of symptoms that commonly occur together. To clarify, this is not unlike the way a diagnosis is made for a physical condition. For example, the client who has a fever, is lethargic, and begins to develop itchy red spots on their skin, who has a history of not having had the chickenpox nor had a vaccine for it, when the doctor finds that the client was recently in contact with a child who had the chickenpox despite having had the vaccine, can reasonably assume the diagnosis is likely the chickenpox. The diagnosis is easier for the doctor to make because the symptoms have occurred together and the doctor has an accurate client medical history. Any one of these symptoms by itself, or in a different combination, with a different history, may lead to a different diagnosis.

A psychiatrist, when evaluating a person and assigning a diagnosis, considers the person's history and presenting symptoms. Although this is similar to the way a doctor might diagnose a case of the chickenpox, there is an important difference; psychiatric disorders are not necessarily explicit or obvious, and many mental health problems do not manifest outward physical signs and symptoms. Although, as you learned in the first sections of this chapter, we have progressed our understanding of mental illness substantially through contributions from neuroscience and advances in the use of psychopharmaceuticals, diagnosing a person with a psychiatric illness is a complex (and sometimes lengthy and shifting) process. A psychiatrist can describe how a client is behaving and can recognize important clues in their history,

but they do not always immediately reach a diagnosis that another psychiatrist would agree with. Indeed, on the next admission, the psychiatrist may reevaluate their own diagnosis and assign a different one. It is not uncommon for someone to have had different diagnoses on different admissions, especially at different hospitals. One wonders whether psychiatric diagnoses are of any use at all? Psychiatrists use diagnoses, a complete medical and personal narrative, and evidence-based research, as a starting place to help them determine what drugs or other treatment protocols would best support the client.

From an occupational therapy perspective, diagnosis may or may not be particularly helpful. Instead, you might find that the individual's behavior and reported symptoms give you more of a handle on the person's situation because they give you clues about what the person needs and desires. Also, because symptoms impair function in predictable ways, they give you clues to where the person may be having difficulty. After all, the purpose of occupational therapy is to help individuals meet their needs, carry on their life activities, and successfully engage in personally meaningful occupation. By identifying the symptom and deciphering the underlying needs and priorities, we collaborate in helping the client take the first step toward getting their needs met, or from the POP theoretical perspective, helping them to become the occupational being that they desire to be, doing the things they wish to do.

Personality and Personal Experiences

Often, particular symptoms that a client demonstrates are more characteristic of the individual's personality than of their diagnosis. To illustrate, someone with a diagnosis of schizophrenia may show obsessive–compulsive behaviors, such as performing bizarre rituals (such as touching doorknobs) or demonstrating obsessive tidiness. Another person, also diagnosed with schizophrenia, may show a different symptom—for example, **akathisia**, a movement disorder frequently associated with schizophrenia that makes it hard for a person to stay still, giving them an urgency to frequently move or walk. Although everyone observing the person can identify the symptom or behavior that is maladaptive, psychiatrists often have difficulty agreeing on why someone has a symptom, and what the underlying process is that is causing it.

Individual Strengths

Throughout the occupational therapy process, it is important to remember that every individual is much more than a bundle of presenting symptoms. Although such behavior may appear to be unreasonable or bizarre, the person likely also has some behaviors or qualities that are supportive and are relative strengths. The person may be able to do crossword puzzles, be a talented artist, or play basketball well. Perhaps you notice that they spontaneously help others who are having difficulty, or that they know extraordinary amounts of sports trivia. An individual's strengths are just as important as their symptoms. In fact, they are more important because they can help the person control and master the symptoms. For example, when a person who is severely depressed and withdrawn finds a way to help another person learn how to make a new recipe or teaches them how to change the oil in their car, or bait a fishing pole, they have done something useful and occupied their time in a productive way. This typically leads to improved mood and to feeling a bit better about themselves. Even if it is for a very short time, the individual may be able to stop thinking about their problems and have a reprieve. When people continue consistently doing something that they feel competent doing, they are likely to feel more in control and, in turn, more able to cope with their problems.

As you continue through the remaining chapters, it is important to remember the concepts we have covered so far:

- Identifying the symptoms and deciphering the underlying need, antecedent event, or environmental stimulus can help in planning interventions that lead to greater levels of independence for the client, particularly in being able to manage their symptoms.
- Symptoms may be seen as an expression of unmet needs (eg, for love and belongingness) or of unresolved conflicts.
- Symptoms are not diagnoses. The same symptom may occur in a variety of diagnoses, and the same symptoms may manifest differently in the people who have the same diagnosis.
- Symptoms are the behavioral or self-reported evidence of underlying psychological or physiologic problems.
- Symptoms may be a response to an event or something in the environment.
- Symptoms are sometimes more related to a person's experiences and underlying personality than to a particular diagnosis.
- Activities selected in response to symptoms should reflect the individual's strengths, interests, goals, occupational roles, and present level of functioning.
- Symptoms are culturally mediated and influenced by situational contexts that are inextricably linked to occupation (20).

APPLYING OCCUPATIONAL THERAPY RESPONSE VARIABLES TO ENABLE DOING, BEING, BECOMING, AND BELONGING

When an occupational therapy professional is collaborating with the client to plan, set goals, and then enact the intervention plan, the therapist can access three distinct tools, or paths. We will call these tools **response variables** because they are intentionally dynamic and changeable to suit the client's unique challenges and needs. The three response variables are therapeutic use of self, deep consideration of contextual influences and environmental perspective on client factors, and how optimal occupational engagement (activity) is defined for each unique client.

Therapeutic Use of Self: Being an Occupational Therapy Professional

Self is defined here in the dimension of being. What it means for us *to be* is associated with the idea that the self is the essence of who we are, "the dimension of being in the POP [model] includes (but is not limited to) identity, personal abilities, roles, creativity and consciousness" (27, p. 14) (29). Not only is the occupational therapy professional interested in the client's ways of being in the world, the occupational therapy professional's ways of being are equally important to consider. Each practitioner's personality; the way they act, react, and interact with others; their unique ways of caring for the people whom they collaborate with; as well as their feelings, thoughts, personalities, and experiences...all this and more defines how they will be in this world, and how they will be as an occupational therapy professional. The essence of their being is what shapes their **therapeutic use of self**, and the therapeutic relationship. The way a person can apply therapeutic modes (55), and adapt their personalities to meet the client as they are, significantly affects clients' self-perception and the occupational therapy process.

As specific symptoms are discussed across the remaining chapters, loose guidelines will be given for how to approach (or shift your interpersonal behavior for) clients who demonstrate particular clusters of symptoms. These guidelines are merely suggestions; they should not be thought of as rules or demands for you to change your way of being. Rather, your relationships with all clients will depend on a warm, interested presence and an open-minded approach that lets them know that they are safe, that you are trustworthy and dedicated to supporting them. Let them know that when they are in occupational therapy, they *belong*. For an occupational therapy professional to develop this type of rapport with clients, they must first be comfortable with themselves and with their own behavior. Any modifications that are made in the occupational therapy professional's actions or behaviors must feel right to them. To feel comfortable in a therapeutic role, it is important not to make unrealistic demands on oneself. Self-care is critical, as is self-compassion. No one is perfect, nor perfectly in control of their responses all the time. The most effective therapists are usually the ones who are in a frame of mind to help their clients by doing the best that they can, while accepting the fact that just like everyone else, they might sometimes make mistakes.

Contextual, Environmental, and Client Factor Considerations

Contextual, environmental, and client factor considerations should be prioritized as the occupational therapist and client collaborate to set client goals and plan interventions. This part of the occupational therapy process is an aspect of the becoming dimension and it includes consideration of the situational contexts in which your interaction with the client will take place for therapy. In addition, this is where the occupational therapy team helps the client to consider what supports or barriers exist in other environments and contexts that impact their participation in the daily activities that are important to them. This is the time to ask the client what they believe that they need to do to become the person who they want to be, doing the things that they want and need to do. This may include the presence or absence of other people, a change in the general noise level, the amount of visual stimulation, the quality of the lighting, the arrangement or modification of the space, the ventilation and temperature, and the presence or absence of animate or inanimate objects. The ones just mentioned are primarily changes in the physical or sensory environment, but they are a good starting place. Contextual and situational elements, client factors, and symptoms that are not explicit, or that the client does not demonstrate in an occupational performance analysis, or is unable to articulate initially, are sometimes discovered over time as the therapeutic relationship grows. This is what makes the dimension of *becoming* a perpetually sustaining aspect of the human experience.

Occupation and Activity: The Doing Dimension

Occupation or activity is the thing that you and the client (and often the group) are *doing*. It is the doing dimension, and it is the dimension that makes occupational therapy unique. Ultimately, the goal of occupational therapy is that people can effectively and safely do what they want and need to do in life. It can range from planting a garden, to writing a résumé, to organizing materials to prepare a meal, or looking at listings for apartments. The possibilities are endless. In selecting activities, it is important that they be based in occupations that are priorities and are valuable (meaningful) to the client. Consider the person's goals, interests, occupational roles, previous skills, and present level of functioning. At times, familiar activities offer security by giving someone an opportunity to demonstrate that they can do something well. At other times, such as when a client is confused and disorganized, familiar activities can make them feel worse because the client either cannot do them at all or cannot do them as well as in the past. The most effective activities are those that the person has chosen, that mean something to them, and that support their goals and occupational roles. Collaboration encourages clients to choose their own activities, activities that are meaningful to them, even if the choice is limited to only two or three options.

RESPONSE STRATEGIES

The remaining chapters present information to help you respond effectively to clients who are experiencing specific symptoms. We hope that this will give both the newly practicing therapist and therapists with many years of experience a fresh perspective and a novel way to guide their occupational therapy practice, ensuring that their emphasis is holistic, occupation centered, and considerate of the multifaceted dimensions of occupation: being, doing, becoming, and belonging. For each cluster of symptoms, the reader will find discussion about application of the four dimensions of occupation suggested by the POP theoretical model (30), coupled with supporting information and evidence-based practices (ie, response strategies) designed to keep occupation as the central focus. The chapters are organized in the following format.

The Doing, Being, and Belonging Dimensions

Focus Questions for the Occupational Therapy Professional to Consider in Developing an Intervention Plan

1. What does it feel like to be a person who is experiencing (*fill in the symptom/s*)?
2. What are some things that a person experiencing (*fill in the symptom/s*) might do, or not do (ie, poor self-care habits)?
3. How can I adjust my way of being (therapeutic use of self) to make the client feel more comfortable about their way of being?
4. What can I do to instill a sense of belonging in occupational therapy that will encourage the client toward setting goals with outcomes that are personally meaningful and relevant to them?

In each of the remaining chapters, this section contains:

- **Definition** of the symptom and a discussion of what it may mean for different individuals (ie, what unmet needs it may be disguising)
- **Diagnosis** or diagnoses in which the symptom commonly occurs
- **Therapeutic use of self** to help the person feel more comfortable and function better by establishing a sense of belonging in the therapeutic relationship

The Doing and Becoming Dimensions

Focus Questions for the OT Professional to Consider in Developing an Intervention Plan

1. What can the client and the occupational therapy team collaboratively do together that will help the client become more functional and effective in the things that are important to them in everyday life?
2. What are the best intervention types and intervention approaches to apply in this therapeutic context (3)?
3. What does the current evidence suggest about the most productive interventions for this diagnosis/set of symptoms?

In each of the remaining chapters, this section contains:

- **Contextual, Environmental, and Client Factor considerations** to meet the person's needs and the OT approach and type of intervention to consider
- **Characteristics of suitable evidence-based activities** and recommended modifications in activities
- **Examples of specific evidence-based activities**

Balanced Health, Wellness, and Recovery: Becoming and Belonging

Focus Questions for the Occupational Therapy Professional to Consider in Developing an Intervention Plan

1. How does the client define success in reaching their goals?
2. How can occupational therapy support the long-term success in the client becoming who they want to be, successfully doing what they want to do?
3. How can occupational therapy support the client's recovery and long-term success in finding community, and feeling a sense of belonging and connectedness?

These ideas are culled from many oral and written sources in occupational therapy; they do not work with every individual, and they should not be applied mechanically. Do not think of these strategies as a cookbook. We cannot approach every person with depression in the same way, no matter what the DSM guidelines may say. Every person must be experienced as unique. Just as when preparing a meal, it is wise to look in the refrigerator before looking in the cookbook; when working with clients, it is important to see what they bring to the situation, before you create their differentiated occupational therapy plan. Remember also that the most powerful intervention is to educate the consumer about symptom management, so that they can monitor symptoms and reduce or eliminate discomfort or barriers to participation. This essential aspect of wellness and health management is introduced in the next section.

Finally, each of the remaining chapters concludes with wellness and health management, or recovery strategies that are related to the symptom clusters relevant to that chapter.

SELF-MONITORING FOR SELF-MASTERY OF SYMPTOMS

Most major psychiatric disorders are lifelong chronic conditions. To enjoy a good quality of life, consumers need to manage their illnesses. Proper diet and nutrition, medication adherence, fitness and exercise, use of social support, and avoidance of triggers and situations that may cause distress are important skills and habits that enhance recovery. Mary Ellen Copeland (13) designed the *Wellness Recovery Action Plan* (WRAP), in which consumers create a "wellness toolbox" to recognize, reduce, and, if possible, eliminate troubling symptoms. The toolbox has the following elements:

- A daily maintenance list (of routines and activities that maintain health)
- A list of personal triggers (events or things that tend to provoke symptoms or relapse) and ways to respond to these
- A list of personal early warning signs and the best ways to respond
- Ways to recognize when symptoms are worsening and ways to respond to this
- A crisis plan or advance directive

Although intended originally for consumers with symptoms of emotional dysregulation, these strategies can be used by anyone for any kind of disruptive illness or situation.

Swarbrick (53, 54), an occupational therapist, has written extensively on wellness and adds to the wellness menu the following additional elements that emphasize the important connection between occupation and health, while also emphasizing the doing, becoming, and belonging dimensions of occupation:

- Productivity
- Participation in meaningful activity

Nevertheless, recovery from mental illness is a process. The consumer does not consider themselves "cured." Instead, they cultivate behaviors and skills to manage the illness and its effects. The role of the health care provider is to help the person in recovery develop and maintain a lifestyle of physical and psychological balance in which symptoms are reduced.

SUMMARY

Symptoms are the behavioral or reported subjective evidence of underlying psychological and physiologic problems. They give us clues about what clients or residents may be experiencing, what they seem to be having trouble with, and what we can do to make them more comfortable. The remaining chapters present some ideas and current best practices about how to respond to those who exhibit specific behaviors or report specific internal experiences that are interfering with their occupational engagement, their daily life activities. Occupational therapy's response and intervention are shaped around three variables: therapeutic use of self; consideration of contextual, environmental, and client factors; and the collaborative process between the occupational therapy professional and the client in selecting and using meaningful activities and occupations to support and enhance occupational participation and well-being.

The information in this chapter and the remaining chapters is intended as a general guide and not as a rigid system of rules. It is also not a substitute to use as a "one-size-fits-all" comprehensive occupational therapy intervention plan because it must be acknowledged that the variety of settings where occupational therapy professionals work, and the individuality of each client, will always influence how the practitioner plans and carries out the intervention. Instead, it is intended to be a useful way to think about the holistic nature of our profession, a way to think about what the occupational therapy professional does, and how we do it. It is also a way of advocating for how occupational therapy contributes to the health and wellness of our clients. Integrating considerations of the dimensions of occupation and occupational engagement: being, doing, becoming, and belonging, as suggested by the POP theoretical model (30) is an ideal way to bridge occupational science and occupational therapy theory into everyday occupational therapy practice by effectively applying response variables.

Case Study

Jennifer Jones: A 33-year-old With Generalized Anxiety Disorder

Jennifer Jones is a 33-year-old Hispanic female who was referred by her primary care doctor to the behavioral health team (BHT) of the outpatient clinic near the community college where she is employed. Jennifer has worked at the community college as an admissions counselor for 5 years and she was promoted 6 months ago to a coordinator position. Jennifer was diagnosed in her early 20s with generalized anxiety disorder (GAD) and reports that her symptoms of anxiety have increased since she began her new job role. Jennifer is married and has two children, a son who is 2-years-old and a daughter who is 4-years-old.

DSM-5-TR Diagnosis at Admission

F41.4   Generalized Anxiety Disorder

Z codes

Z56.1   Change of Job
Z56.6   Other physical and mental strain related to work

Occupational Profile

Mrs Jones was referred to the occupational therapy/BHT by her primary care physician to address her concerns about increased feelings of anxiety, secondary to her diagnosis of GAD.

She reports that her excessive worrying was negatively impacting her performance at work, causing her to miss deadlines, which further increased her anxiety and fear of losing her job. This prompted her to request a leave of absence from her job only a few months after she had been given a promotion. She also reports that her anxiety is interfering with her completion of role-related tasks as a mom and as a wife.

Strengths/Successes

Mrs Jones has a good system of support with friends and family, both of her parents are in good health, and they are able to help with her children when needed. Client reports that for now the family is financially stable. Mrs Jones identified her strengths as being a good mother (when her anxiety is under control), a great cook, loves to make fun meals for her family when she does not feel so fatigued, and she reports that she is good at helping the entering college students decide which coursework to enroll in (good at her job).

Barriers

Currently on a leave of absence from her job, concerned about how long her employer will hold her job. Although she reports having a good network of close friends, she has recently stopped participating socially with her friends because she "doesn't want her anxiety and worrying to ruin everybody else's time." Reports some cognitive changes, difficulty with short term memory, and distractibility. Reports persistent fatigue from worrying that makes her "collapse on the couch with fear." Having trouble with morning routine and parenting tasks (organizing and managing)—getting the kids up, dressed, and to day care—because husband works early shift, and is gone before the children are awake.

Mrs Jones indicates that her priorities are to be able to manage her feelings of anxiety so that she can return to her job and maintain the status of her recent promotion. She also would like to improve the tasks she is responsible for in her role as a mother, particularly preparing dinner for the family, and improve her morning routine to be more efficient and less overwhelmed when getting herself and the children to day care and work.

Goals, objectives, and intervention type and approach are shown in the treatment summary for this case (Table 17.3).

Occupational Therapy Discharge Summary: SOAP Note Format

S: Mrs Jones reports "feeling much more in control of the tasks at work and at home."

O: Client has participated in OP OT 2x/wk/60 min/6 wk. She attended 11/13 group therapy sessions (*ReDO-10* program) and 4/6 individual sessions. Mrs Jones was initially referred to the BHT and OT groups by her primary care physician after having taken a leave of absence from her job because of an exacerbation of her GAD, which was negatively impacting her productivity at work.

A: At the start of care, Mrs Jones's overwhelming worrying and focus on fearful thoughts limited her ability to complete tasks at her job and to complete her instrumental activities of daily living (IADLs), which include caring for her children. Following skilled instruction and consistent participation in the OT *ReDO-10* groups, utilizing assistive technology (mood tracker app) and incorporating mindfulness strategies, Mrs Jones has achieved her goals at this time.

P: Discharge from BHT/OT because of her goals being met (Table 17.4). Mrs Jones will benefit from continued use of scheduling and mood tracker apps and mindfulness practices. Occupational therapist will follow up in 1 month by phone to check on Mrs Jones's functional status. No further services are recommended at this time.

Table 17.3. Occupational Therapy Treatment Summary

Goals	Objectives	Occupational Therapy Intervention Type and Intervention Approach
1. Learn and implement coping skills that result in a reduction of anxiety and worry and improve daily function to return to work and maintain employment.	**1a.** Mrs Jones will develop an awareness of her moods and emotions as they change, by completing the *MindShift CBT* mood tracker and anxiety check-in app on her smart phone, at least twice daily (AM and PM), sharing her results during OT to identify contextual triggers. **1b.** Mrs Jones will identify and describe a minimum of two work-related situations, thoughts, feelings, or actions associated with her anxieties and worries, their impact on her functioning, and document three grounding techniques that she can implement while at work to help resolve them. **1c.** Mrs Jones will participate in at least one mindfulness-based stress reduction group per week to support an overall reduction in her anxiety and to help her manage symptoms.	**1a. Intervention type:** Interventions to support occupations **Intervention approach:** Modify (compensation, adaptation) **1b. Intervention type:** Interventions to support occupations **Intervention approach:** Prevent (disability prevention) **1c. Intervention type:** Education and training **Intervention approach:** Maintain
2. Reestablish effective morning and evening routines to prevent unnecessary stressors that exacerbate symptoms of anxiety	**2a.** Mrs Jones will identify and implement changes to her morning routine, using the strategies she learns through participation in the ReDO OT group sessions. **2b.** Mrs Jones and her husband will complete a weekly meal planner that includes a shopping list of ingredients for 1 wk of meals. They will complete the task each Saturday afternoon, to submit their grocery list online for a pickup of groceries on Sunday afternoon. **2c.** Mrs Jones will meet her need for restorative sleep by creating and enacting a sleep hygiene routine.	**2a. Intervention type:** Education and training **Intervention approach:** Establish, restore (remediation, restoration) **2b. Intervention type:** Interventions to support occupations **Intervention approach:** Modify (compensation, adaptation) **2c. Intervention type:** Occupations and activities **Intervention approach:** Prevent (disability prevention)

Table 17.4. Mrs Jones's Progress Summary

Goal #	SOC Status	Goal	Discharge Status
1. Learn and implement coping skills that result in a reduction of anxiety and worry and improve daily function to return to work and maintain employment.	• Leave of absence from work	• Return to work	• Returned to work 2 wk after SOC. Reports missing work only 1 of the past 20 d (absence was because her child was ill) • Reports daily use of her mood tracker app, and attends meditation group one morning per week at her local YMCA
2. Reestablish effective morning and evening routines to prevent unnecessary stressors that exacerbate symptoms of anxiety.	• Decline in social participation and social activities • Reports feeling frequently fatigued • Decline in completion of IADL tasks	Reestablish effective routines to more successfully complete IADLs and improve the quality of role-related tasks (ie, meal prep, childcare, and self-care).	Goals met

IADL, instrumental activities of daily living; SOC, start of care.

OT HACKS SUMMARY

O: Occupation as a means and an end

Occupations are not just actions. They are actions driven by needs, feelings, and desires, and they generate feelings that act and react with and to physiologic, psychological, and social factors. Being motivated and able to identify, express, and act on one's feelings, needs, and values contributes to a sense of personal identity and improves the quality of one's life. The abilities to assert oneself; manage one's feelings with self-control and dignity; and channel stressors into adaptive responses positively influence successful outcomes and encourage the continual development of useful skills. Although many mental health professionals teach these skills to clients, occupational therapy professionals have a unique perspective, they use occupation (activities) to help the client reach their goals emphasizing functional outcomes in daily life that are personally meaningful and relevant to the individual.

T: Theoretical concepts, values, and principles, or historical foundations

- According to the POP (27), the four dimensions of occupation are as follows:
    1. **Doing:** the transaction that occurs as people engage in personally meaningful occupation
    2. **Being:** the essence of the person. It is who the person is occupationally, which includes their unique psychological, social, spiritual, and physical characteristics and capabilities.
    3. **Becoming:** the aspirational, goal-directed growth and development of a person
    4. **Belonging:** a feeling of being in relationship or connected to others; reciprocity, mutuality, and sharing are elements of a sense of belonging, and of belonging relationships
- Therapeutic use of self, the therapeutic relationship, and an occupational therapy perspective illuminate aspects of the **being dimension** of occupation in occupational therapy practice. This allows us to seek to know the essence of the person, who they are occupationally, just as they are. The reflective and authentic occupational therapy professional learns to step back from initial reactions and assessments and learn as much as possible about what it means to "be" the client whom they are collaborating with in that moment.

H: How can we Help? OT's role in serving clients with mental illness or mental health needs

- We can move the intervention planning and intervention processes into action in everyday occupational therapy practice, using concepts from the *POP*, a theoretical model that was derived from Wilcock's OPH (27, 30).
- Occupational therapy professionals are concerned primarily with how people function in their daily life activities and occupations.
- Occupational therapy is a "doing" therapy more than a "talking" therapy. The main vehicle for therapeutic intervention in occupational therapy is participation in the occupations or activities themselves. When occupational therapy professionals provide interventions, there should be a clear relationship between meaningful occupation and the client's personal preferences and goals.
- Because of the nature of some of the skills, habits, roles, and routines that occupational therapy professionals are collaborating with clients to reestablish in pursuit of optimal occupational engagement, we often develop and implement therapeutic group interventions.
- Occupational therapy's domain of concern is focused on how contextual, environmental, and client factors are supporting or inhibiting their occupational participation.

A: Adaptations

Because one of the primary practices of occupational therapy is to support clients' healthy adaptation to their individualized and contextualized occupational participation, it is critical to recognize that adaptation is inherent in all categories of outcomes (OTPF). Therefore, occupational therapy professionals must also learn to adapt their reasoning to match client priorities to the appropriate outcome.

C: Case study includes

After reading Jennifer Jones's case study and discharge summary, can you think of any evidence-supported caregiver education information or training that the occupational therapy professional could have provided for Mrs Jones's spouse to help facilitate her transition and continued success at work?

K: Knowledge: keeping mental health OT practice grounded in evidence, in occupational science, and in research

D'Amico, M. L., Jaffe, L. E., & Gardner, J. A. (2018). Evidence for interventions to improve and maintain occupational performance and participation for people with serious mental illness: A systematic review. *American Journal of Occupational Therapy, 72*(5), 7205190020.

After reading the *Evidence-Based Practice* (EBP) journal article listed, see if you can answer these questions:

1. Why is it important for an occupational therapy professional to understand the efficacy of specific occupational therapy interventions that benefit individuals with mental illness?
2. According to this systematic review, summarize the evidence for the following types of occupational therapy interventions and approaches:
    a. Occupation based
    b. Psychoeducation
    c. Skills training
    d. Cognition-based interventions
    e. Technology-supported interventions
3. Where do gaps occur in intervention research that informs occupational therapy practice when collaborating with clients with mental illness?
4. According to this systematic review, what is currently the predominant outcome measured in occupational therapy efficacy intervention research studies?
5. What factors make randomized controlled trials of occupational therapy intervention efficacy studies for clients with mental illness difficult to carry out?

S: Some terms that may be new to you

Adverse childhood experiences (ACEs): potentially traumatic events that occur during childhood (0–17 years); examples include (but are not limited to) experiencing abuse, neglect, witnessing violence, or having aspects of the child's environment negatively impact the child's sense of self, sense of safety, trust, or stability—such as having a parent or caregiver who has substance use problems, who has attempted or succeeded at committing suicide, or having family members who are incarcerated

Afferent neurons: Afferent neurons are also called sensory neurons. These nerve fibers bring sensory information from the external environment into the brain. Sensory information may involve the special senses, vision, hearing, smell, or taste, as well as the sense of touch, pain, and temperature.

Akathisia: a neuropsychiatric syndrome associated with psychomotor restlessness, nonproductive movements that are often uncontrollable, and an inability to remain still, sometimes accompanied by agitation or suicidal ideation

Assertive behaviors: actions that reflect a person's priorities and concern for themselves, including having the confidence to stand up for oneself appropriately without experiencing anxiety

Assertiveness: the ability to state one's needs, thoughts, and feelings in an appropriate, direct, and honest way; actions that reflect a person's priorities and concern for themselves, which include the person having the confidence to stand up for themselves appropriately without experiencing anxiety

Autonomic nervous system: The autonomic nervous system is a complex set of neurons that mediate internal homeostasis without conscious intervention or voluntary control. This system innervates most body parts and influences their activity as well as mediating changes to the overall metabolism. It can be divided into the *sympathetic* and *parasympathetic* nervous systems.

Biopsychosocial model of practice: The biopsychosocial model was first introduced by George Engel in 1977; the model suggests that a person's diagnosis does not provide enough information to holistically understand our client. Biological, psychological, and social factors must also be considered.

Biopsychosocial-spiritual model of practice: expanded version of the biopsychosocial model of client care that includes spirituality as an additional dimension

Central nervous system (CNS): The CNS consists of the brain and spinal cord; responsible for integrating and coordinating the activities of the entire body including thought, emotion, sensation, and coordination of movement.

Cognitive reappraisal: a commonly used emotion regulation strategy; an intentional effort to reinterpret (change one's way of thinking about) an emotional situation in a way that alters its meaning and changes its emotional impact

Deficiency needs: needs that occur because of deprivation

Directed mindfulness: use of mindfulness in a context where the occupational therapy professional needs to intentionally direct the client's awareness toward particular elements of the right here, right now experience, or toward reflecting on an idea or solution

Distancing: an attentional deployment strategy. The client attempts to look at a situation dispassionately, as if they are not personally involved.

Efferent neurons: Efferent neurons are also called motor neurons. These nerve fibers carry signals from the brain to the PNS to initiate an action. For example, these motor neurons tell the body to perform an action; for example, they may communicate that you need to remove your hand from a hot pan.

Emotional regulation/emotional dysregulation: controlling and modulating emotions and related behaviors; **emotional dysregulation:** having difficulty controlling and modulating one's emotions and related behaviors

Emotions: Emotions are associated with bodily reactions that are activated through neurotransmitters and hormones released by the brain.

Expressive suppression: a commonly used emotion regulation strategy that involves intentionally changing behavioral responses to emotionally charged situations by hiding, suppressing, or inhibiting emotional responses

Expressive therapeutic techniques: techniques used to develop the clients' self-concept and self-identity, their awareness of themselves, and of their own experience of self, feelings, and needs

Exteroceptive awareness: sometimes called the body schema, awareness about our body in space and movement that comes from the synthesis and integration of exteroceptive signals from the sensory systems—sight, touch, hearing, and from proprioceptive, vestibular, and voluntary motor systems

Feelings: conscious experience of emotional reactions

Gross's Modal Model of Emotion: a process model of emotion that suggests that the generation of emotion occurs in a particular sequence over time

Growth needs: According to Maslow's theory, growth needs occupy the highest two levels of the pyramid, esteem needs and self-actualization needs. These needs arise because an individual is motivated to grow as a person and reach their potential.

Homeostasis: often, though not always, an indication of a system or group of systems being in balance; can also be thought of as "a stable state" (26, pp. 186–187)

Hypothalamic–pituitary–adrenal (HPA) axis: describes the three systems (body structures)—the hypothalamus, the pituitary gland, and the adrenal glands—that interact to try to maintain homeostasis in the body by mediating a response to stressors. The hypothalamus and the anterior pituitary gland collaborate to determine a physiologic response in the face of threats. CRH triggers the anterior pituitary gland to release ACTH into the bloodstream, which further triggers the release of glucocorticoids (cortisol) from the adrenal cortex above the kidneys to enhance the ability to fight or flee from threats or extreme stress. When the stress lessens, feedback mechanisms in the hypothalamus, the hippocampus, and the pituitary gland can regulate the HPA axis response to stress.

Information exchange: the delivery and receipt of communication

Interneurons: neurons that transmit impulses between other neurons, sometimes as part of a reflex arc

Interoceptive awareness: an awareness directed by the communication between body-based sensation and multidimensional cortical oversight. Information about internal physiology is communicated to the brain to strengthen both physical and emotional wellness and to promote effective adaptive responses to stress

Mandala: a Sanskrit word translated to mean "circle." Activities that incorporate the use of mandalas into expressive therapeutic interventions were likely introduced to modern psychiatric practice by Dr Carl Jung, but the use of the circle for ceremonial and other purposes has existed in various forms since ancient times and can be found in nature as well as across cultures and religions.

Maslow's Hierarchy of Needs Theory: Maslow's Hierarchy of Needs Theory suggests that people are motivated to fulfill basic physiologic needs before moving on to other, higher order needs.

Mindfulness-based stress reduction (MBSR): a meditation practice protocol considered to be the gold standard, developed by Dr Jon Kabat-Zinn in 1979 initially to target and assist clients with managing stress, today used to impact a variety of health conditions

Mindfulness/mindfulness meditation: a quality of being conscious or aware of something

Mirror neurons: a specialized type of sensory motor cell located in the brain that is activated when an individual performs an action or observes another individual performing the same action. Thus, the neurons "mirror" others' actions. Mirror neurons may help explain experiences such as empathy and imitation and may provide an explanation for social cognition.

Parasympathetic nervous system (PSNS): The PSNS is part of the nervous system. Responsible for helping a person recover and be at rest, the PSNS is sometimes referred to as the "rest and digest" part of the nervous system and can include digesting food, excreting waste, crying, salivating, or becoming sexually aroused.

Peripheral nervous system (PNS): The PNS consists of all neurons outside the brain and spinal cord. This includes long nerve fibers as well as ganglia made of neural cell bodies. The PNS connects the CNS to various parts of the body.

Physicality: the body language of communication

Positive childhood experiences (PCEs): experiences indicated by the evidence that show promise in supporting the development of resiliency in children despite co-occurring adversities, thereby helping to shape (potentially improve) mental health in adulthood (9)

Redirection: an attentional deployment strategy that can be respectfully applied to influence someone else's behavior by directing their attention to something neutral or more pleasant, and away from a distressing situation; also referred to as distraction

Response modulation: strategies to control or change the emotional response

Response variables: three dynamic and malleable tools or pathways that an OT professional can access during the intervention process to establish a collaborative intervention plan that will meet clients' unique challenges and needs. The three response variables are therapeutic use of self, deep consideration of contextual influences and environmental perspective on client factors, and how optimal occupational engagement (activity) is defined for each unique client.

Role conflict: a feeling that expectations for one's roles are in conflict

Role stress: a feeling that one cannot meet the expectations of one's roles

Self-awareness: understanding the self

Self-concept: a collection of ideas, feelings, and attitudes that a person has about their own identity, self-worth, capabilities, and limitations (Shpig REF)

Self-esteem: valuing the self

Self-expression: showing, demonstrating, or revealing one's thoughts, feelings, and needs. Self-expression assumes some awareness of self.

Social prescribing: Also sometimes referred to as *community referral*, it is a way that health care providers can refer people to a range of local, nonclinical services in an effort to enhance health and quality of life for clients. Social prescribing aims to support people with a wide range of social, emotional, or practical needs to improve mental health and overall wellness. Many occupations could be considered for a social prescription including volunteering, participating in craft or arts activities, task group learning, gardening, cooking, health and fitness or healthy eating advice, and a wide range of leisure activities such as participation in recreational sports.

State mindfulness: a mental state reached through conscious awareness of the right now moment; being aware of and accepting one's feelings, thoughts, and bodily sensations

Somatic nervous system (SoNS): The SoNS, sometimes referred to as the voluntary nervous system, is a part of the PNS. These neurons are associated with skeletal or striated muscle fibers and influence voluntary movements of the body.

Sympathetic nervous system (SNS): The SNS is part of the autonomic nervous system; it regulates the body's involuntary processes. The SNS controls aspects of the body related to the flight-or-fight response, such as mobilizing fat reserves, increasing the heart rate, and releasing adrenaline.

Trait mindfulness: exists when a person's disposition makes them more likely to have a consistent tendency toward being mindful in everyday life

Values clarification: a strategy or an intervention technique that assists clients with increasing their awareness of any values or deeply held beliefs that might influence their lifestyle, decision-making, choices, or behaviors

Reflection Questions

1. Define *symptom* and explain why symptoms are useful guides to understanding client behaviors and feelings.
2. Explain how biopsychosocial or biopsychosocial-spiritual models are similar to occupational models of practice.
3. Using the OT domain and process home metaphor introduced in your text, explain the intervention phase of the OT process.
4. Defend the importance of an occupational therapy professional having a general understanding of the human nervous system.
5. Explain the role of mirror neurons in the communication and social interaction processes between human beings.
6. In your own words, articulate the differences between occupational therapy's domain of concern and the domain of concern in at least one other discipline outside of occupational therapy.
7. Summarize the role of the HPA axis in stress responses.
8. Explain the differences between emotions and feelings and describe emotional dysregulation.
9. Describe how an OT professional might incorporate mindfulness practices into an intervention plan. Why is it important to carefully analyze the incorporation of mindfulness practices into OT interventions?
10. Evaluate and discuss how an OT professional can apply the conceptual model of OT response variables to enable the dimensions of occupation—doing, being, becoming, and belonging—into everyday practice.

REFERENCES

1. Alcamo, E. I., & Krumhardt, B. (2004). *Barron's anatomy and physiology: The easy way* (2nd ed.). Barron's Educational Series.
2. American Occupational Therapy Association. (2020). AOTA 2020 occupational therapy code of ethics. *American Journal of Occupational Therapy, 74*(Suppl. 3), 7413410005.
3. American Occupational Therapy Association. (2020). Occupational therapy practice framework: Domain and process—Fourth edition. *American Journal of Occupational Therapy, 74*(Suppl. 2), 1–87.
4. American Occupational Therapy Association. (2021). Occupational therapy scope of practice. *American Journal of Occupational Therapy, 75*(Suppl. 3), 7513410030.
5. American Occupational Therapy Association. (2021). Standards of practice for occupational therapy. *American Journal of Occupational Therapy, 75*(Suppl. 3), 7513410050.
6. Barnett, J. E. (2020). Complementary, alternative, and integrative interventions in health psychology. In K. Sweeny, M. L. Robbins, & L. M. Cohen (Eds.), *The Wiley encyclopedia of health psychology* (pp. 245–255). John Wiley & Sons.
7. Barrett, L. B. (2017). *How emotions are made: The secret life of the brain.* Houghton Mifflin Harcourt.
8. Baum, C., & Edwards, D. F. (2008). *Activity card sort* (2nd ed.). AOTA Press.
9. Bethell, C., Jones, J., Gombojav, N., Linkenbach, J., & Sege, R. (2019). Positive childhood experiences and adult mental and relational health in a statewide sample: Associations across adverse childhood experiences levels. *JAMA Pediatrics, 173*(11), e193007.
10. Brown, B. (2021). *Atlas of the heart: Mapping meaningful connection and the language of human experience.* Random House.
11. Campenni, C. E., & Hartman, A. (2020). The effects of completing mandalas on mood, anxiety, and state mindfulness. *Art Therapy: Journal of the American Art Therapy Association, 37*(1), 25–33.
12. Carter, R., Aldridge, S., Page, M., & Parker, S. (2009). *The human brain book: An illustrated guide to its structure, function, and disorders.* Dorling Kindersley Limited.
13. Copeland, M. E. (2011). *Wellness recovery action plan for addictions (WRAP).* Peach Press.
14. Cozolino, L. (2006). *The neuroscience of human relationships: Attachment and the developing social brain.* W. W. Norton & Company.
15. Cutuli, D. (2014, September 19). Cognitive reappraisal and expressive suppression strategies role in emotion regulation: An overview on their modulatory effects and neural correlates. *Frontiers in Systems Neuroscience, 8*(Article 175), 1–6.
16. Damasio, A. R. (2005). *Descartes' error: Emotion, reason, and the human brain.* Putnam.
17. Davis, J. (2016). The primordial mandalas of East and West: Jungian and Tibetan Buddhist approaches to healing and transformation. *NeuroQuantology, 14*(2), 242–254.
18. Ding, X., Du, J., Zhou, Y., An, Y., Xu, W., & Zhang, N. (2019). State mindfulness, rumination, and emotions in daily life: An ambulatory assessment study. *Asian Journal of Social Psychology, 22*(4), 369–377.
19. Eslami, A. A., Rabiei, L., Afzali, S. M., Hamidizadeh, S., & Masoudi, R. (2016). The effectiveness of assertiveness training on the levels of stress, anxiety, and depression of high school students. *Iranian Red Crescent Medical Journal, 18*(1), e21096.
20. Fisher, A. G., & Marterella, A. (2019). *Powerful practice: A model for authentic occupational therapy.* Center for Innovative OT Solutions.
21. Fosha, D., Siegel, D. J., & Solomon, M. (Eds.). (2009). *The healing power of emotion: Affective neuroscience, development & clinical practice (Norton series on interpersonal neurobiology)* (A. Schore & D. J. Siegel, Series Eds.). W. W. Norton & Company.
22. Frewen, P., & Lanius, R. (2015). *Healing the traumatized self: Consciousness, neuroscience, treatment (Norton series on interpersonal neurobiology)* (L. Cozolino, A. Schore, & D. J. Siegel, Series Eds.). W. W. Norton & Company.
23. Goldberg, S. B., Tucker, R. P., Greene, P. A., Davidson, R. J., Wampold, B. E., Kearney, D. J., & Simpson, T. L. (2018). Mindfulness-based interventions for psychiatric disorders: A systematic review and meta-analysis. *Clinical Psychology Review, 59*, 52–60.
24. Gross, J. J. (2013). Emotion regulation: Conceptual and empirical foundations. In Gross, J. J (Ed.), *Handbook of emotion regulation* (2nd ed.). Guilford Press.
25. Heller, L., & LaPierre, A. (2012). *Healing developmental trauma: How early trauma affects self-regulation, self-image, and the capacity for relationship.* North Atlantic Books.
26. Hill, R., & Dahlitz, M. (2022). *The practitioner's guide to the science of psychotherapy.* W. W. Norton & Company.
27. Hitch, D., & Pepin, G. (2021). Doing, being, becoming, and belonging at the heart of occupational therapy: An analysis of theoretical ways of knowing. *Scandinavian Journal of Occupational Therapy, 28*(1), 13–25.
28. Hitch, D., Pepin, G., & Stagnitti, K. (2014). In the footsteps of Wilcock, Part one: The evolution of doing, being, becoming and belonging. *Occupational Therapy in Health Care, 28*(3), 231–246.
29. Hitch, D., Pepin, G., & Stagnitti, K. (2014). In the footsteps of Wilcock, Part two: The interdependent nature of doing, being, becoming and belonging. *Occupational Therapy in Health Care, 28*(3), 247–263.
30. Hitch, D., Pepin, G., & Stagnitti, K. (2018). The pan occupational paradigm: Development and key concepts. *Scandinavian Journal of Occupational Therapy, 25*(1), 27–34.
31. Jung, C. G. (1989). *Memories, dreams, reflections.* Random House.
32. Kabat-Zinn, J. (1994). *Wherever you go, there you are.* Hyperion Press.
33. Kielhofner, G. (2008). *A model of human occupation: Theory & application* (4th ed.). Lippincott, Williams, & Wilkins.
34. Kuypers, L. (2011). *The zones of regulation: A curriculum designed to foster self-regulation and emotional control.* https://zonesofregulation.com/resources/
35. LeDoux, J. E. (2020). Thoughtful feelings. *Current Biology, 30*(11), R619–R623.
36. LeDoux, J. E., & Brown, R. (2017). A higher-order theory of emotional consciousness. *Proceedings of the National Academy of Sciences of the United States of America, 114*(10), E2016–E2025.
37. Maslow, A. H. (1943). A theory of human motivation. *Psychological Review, 50*(4), 370–396.
38. McCabe, C. (2011, February 11). The science behind why hobbies can improve our mental health. The Conversation. https://theconversation.com/the-science-behind-why-hobbies-can-improve-our-mental-health-153828
39. McGilchrist, I. (2009). *The master and his emissary: The divided brain and the making of the Western world.* Yale University Press.
40. Niazi, A. K., & Niazi, S. K. (2011). Mindfulness-based stress reduction: A non-pharmacological approach for chronic illnesses. *North American Journal of Medical Sciences, 3*(1), 20–23.
41. Nielsen, J. A., Zielinski, B. A., Ferguson, M. A., Lainhart, J. E., & Anderson, J. S. (2013). An evaluation of the left-brain vs. right-brain hypothesis with resting state functional connectivity magnetic resonance imaging. *PLoS One, 8*(8), e71275.
42. Noltemeyer, A., James, A., Bush, K., Bergen, D., Barrios, V., & Patton, J. (2021). The relationship between deficiency needs and growth needs: The continuing investigation of Maslow's theory. *Children & Youth Services Review, 42*(1), 24–42.
43. Nurius, P. S., Green, S., Logan-Greene, P., & Borja, S. (2015). Life course pathways of adverse childhood experiences toward adult psychological well-being: A stress process analysis. *Child Abuse & Neglect, 45*, 143–153.
44. Ogden, P. (2007). *Beneath the words. A clinical map for using mindfulness of the body and organization of experience in trauma treatment.* Paper presented at Mindfulness and Psychotherapy Conference, Los Angeles, CA.
45. Ogden, P. (2009). Emotion, mindfulness, and movement: Expanding the regulatory boundaries of the window of affect tolerance. In D. Fosha, D. J. Siegel, & M. F. Solomon (Eds.), *The healing power of emotion: Affective neuroscience, development, & clinical practice, Norton series on interpersonal neurobiology* (pp. 204–231). W. W. Norton & Company.
46. Olsson, A., Erlandsson, A. K., & Håkansson, C. (2020). The occupation-based intervention REDO™-10: Long-term impact on work ability for women at risk for or on sick leave. *Scandinavian Journal of Occupational Therapy, (27)*(1), 47–55.
47. Pearson, M., & Wilson, H. (2009). Using expressive arts to work with mind, body and emotions. *Psychotherapy in Australia, 16*(1), 60–69.

48. Royeen, C., Stein, F., Murtha, A., & Stambaugh, J. (2017). Eudemonic care: A future path for occupational therapy? *The Open Journal of Occupational Therapy, 5*(2), Article 13.

49. Scaffa, M. E. (2019). Emotion regulation. In B. A. B. Schell & G. Gillen (Eds.), *Willard and Spackman's occupational therapy* (13th ed., pp. 965–979). Lippincott Williams & Wilkins.

50. Shpigelman, C. N., & HaGani, N. (2019). The impact of disability type and visibility on self-concept and body image: Implications for mental health nursing. *Journal of Psychiatric and Mental Health Nursing, 26*(3–4), 77–86.

51. Šimić, G., Tkalčić, M., Vukić, V., Mulc, D., Španić, E., Šagud, M., Olucha-Bordonau, F. E., Vukšić, M., & R Hof, P. (2021). Understanding emotions: Origins and roles of the amygdala. *Biomolecules, 11*(6), 823.

52. Speed, B. C., Goldstein, B. L., & Goldfried, M. R. (2018). Assertiveness training: A forgotten evidence-based treatment. *Clinical Psychology: Science and Practice, 25*(1), e12216.

53. Swarbrick, M. (2010, January). A wellness model. *Words of Wellness, 3*, 1–3.

54. Swarbrick, M., Tunner, T. P., Miller, D. W., Werner, P., & Tiegreen, W. W. (2016). Promoting health and wellness through peer-delivered services: Three innovative state examples. *Psychiatric Rehabilitation Journal, 39*(3), 204–210.

55. Taylor, R. R. (2020). *The intentional relationship: Occupational therapy and use of self* (2nd ed.). F. A. Davis.

56. Van Gordon, W., & Shonin, E. (2020). Second-generation mindfulness-based interventions: Toward more authentic mindfulness practice and teaching. *Mindfulness, 11*(1), 1–4.

57. Vermette, D., & Doolittle, B. (2022). What educators can learn from the biopsychosocial-spiritual model of patient care: Time for holistic medical education. *Journal of General Internal Medicine, 37*, 2062–2066.

58. Wade, D. T., & Halligan, P. W. (2017). The biopsychosocial model of illness: A model whose time has come. *Clinical Rehabilitation, 31*(8), 995–1004.

59. Wolf, C., & Serpa, J. G. (2015). *A clinician's guide to teaching mindfulness: The comprehensive session-by-session program for mental health professionals and health care providers.* New Harbinger Press.

60. World Health Organization. (2021). *Comprehensive mental health action plan 2013–2030.* Author. License: CC BY-NC-SA 3.0 IGO.

61. Yale University. (2013). *Yale Center for Emotional Intelligence. RULER—Overview.* https://www.rulerapproach.org/how-it-works/overview/

SUGGESTED RESOURCES

Articles

D'Amico, M. L., Jaffe, L. E., & Gardner, J. A. (2018). Evidence for interventions to improve and maintain occupational performance and participation for people with serious mental illness: A systematic review. *American Journal of Occupational Therapy, 72*(5), 7205190020.

Shpigelman, C. N., & HaGani, N. (2019). The impact of disability type and visibility on self-concept and body image: Implications for mental health nursing. *Journal of Psychiatric and Mental Health Nursing, 26*(3–4), 77–86.

- This research study evaluates the impact of disability type, (physical vs psychiatric) and its visibility (outwardly visible to others vs invisible) on the self-concept and body image of people with disabilities.
- Van Gordon, W., & Shonin, E. (2020). Second-generation mindfulness-based interventions: Toward more authentic mindfulness practice and teaching. *Mindfulness, 11*(1), 1–4. In this interesting editorial article, the authors comment on the growing popular use of mindfulness-based interventions (MBIs) in therapy, questioning whether the use of these therapeutic interventions still embody the authenticity and integrity of the traditional contemplative practices from which they arose. They further explore and compare current practices to what they introduce as "Second-Generation Mindfulness-Based Interventions" (p. 1).

Books

Brown, B. (2021). *Atlas of the heart: Mapping meaningful connection and the language of human experience.* Random House. https://www.brenebrown.com

- Dr Brené Brown is a research professor at the University of Houston, where she holds the Huffington Foundation Endowed Chair at the Graduate College of Social Work. She is also a visiting professor in management at the University of Texas at Austin McCombs School of Business. Dr Brown is the author of five #1 New York Times best-selling books about her research findings and work related to courage, vulnerability, shame, and empathy. In her latest book, Atlas of the Heart, Mapping Meaningful Connection and the Language of Human Experience, she translates her research and helps clarify how talking about our experiences helps us connect to one another and gives us courage to understand and find meaning in both our experiences and our emotions.
- Dr Brown is also the host of two excellent podcasts Unlocking Us and Dare to Lead.

Fincher, S. F. (2013). *Coloring mandalas 4: For confidence, energy, and purpose.* Shambhala Press.

- In her therapeutic activity text, *Coloring Mandalas 4: For Confidence, Energy, and Purpose,* the fourth in a series of mandala-inspired meditative coloring books, author, art therapist, and mental health counselor, Susanne Fincher has created a series of mandalas with designs that are associated with being and doing. According to the text description (found on http://www.Amazon.com), "The 'being' mandalas represent a sense of balance, integration, and self-realization. They can be reminiscent of the designs of heraldic shields carried as the emblem of personal power. The 'doing' mandalas represent action, energy, and functioning in the world. These mandalas are associated with creativity, ingenuity, teamwork, and productivity."

Treleaven, D. A. (2018). *Trauma sensitive mindfulness: Practices for safe and transformative healing.* W. W. Norton & Company.

Van der Kolk, B. (2014). *The body keeps the score: Brain, mind, and body in the healing of trauma.* Viking Penguin Group.

- In his work, *The Body Keeps the Score: Brain, Mind, and Body in the Healing of Trauma,* Dr Bessel van der Kolk draws from his vast clinical experience to discuss the impact of trauma on the body, mind, and brain. Van der Kolk explains the complex neurobiology and connection of the human brain–mind–body using plain, easy to understand language and provides useful examples of client case studies with explanations of helpful nonpharmacologic interventions that are evidenced to help victims of PTSD.

Videos

https://www.ted.com/talks/tiffany_watt_smith_the_history_of_human_emotions

- In this Ted Talk, *The history of human emotions,* cultural historian Tiffany Watt Smith describes the language that we use to describe emotion and how that language impacts the way we feel. Watt Smith also places emphasis on the way that our language around emotion is both constantly evolving and culturally mediated (14:20).

https://www.ted.com/talks/lisa_feldman_barrett_you_aren_t_at_the_mercy_of_your_emotions_your_brain_creates_them?language=en

- In this Ted Talk, *You aren't at the mercy of your emotions—your brain creates them,* Dr Lisa Feldman Barrett, distinguished professor of psychology at Northeastern University, with positions in psychiatry and radiology at Massachusetts General Hospital and Harvard Medical School, shares the results of over 25 years of research studying (as the title of her book reads,) how emotions are made (18:20).

https://www.youtube.com/results?search_query=Art+can+heal+ptsd%27s+invisible+wounds

- A powerful Ted Talk, Art can heal PTSD's invisible wounds, featuring Melissa Walker, a creative arts therapist who is helping veterans to engage in creative arts on the journey to healing. Brings to mind one of the most often quoted OT mantras, "Man through the use of his hands as they are energized by mind and will, can influence the state of his own health." Mary Reilly, 1962 (9:48).

Websites

https://www.zonesofregulation.com/free-downloadable-handouts.html

- This is the home website of *Zones of Regulation* created by occupational therapist, Leah Kuypers. In 2011, Kuypers turned the *Zones* framework into a curriculum and published *The Zones of Regulation: A Curriculum Designed to Foster Self-Regulation and Emotional Control.* The original curriculum has now been expanded into two apps, *The Zones of Regulation* and *The Zones of Regulation: Exploring Emotions* (Kuypers, 2013/2015, Selosoft, Inc.www.zonesofregulation.com). Readers will find evidence and research related to the Zones curriculum and can access some free downloadable Zones materials by creating an account.

https://ycei.org/ruler

- This is the link to the Yale Center for Emotional Intelligence (YCEI). The site explains the *RULER program*, (discussed in the chapter), which is a systematic approach to social emotional learning. Other research and resources related to emotion and social learning are also available. In addition, through grant funding, training for several of the programs developed at YCEI, is occasionally offered for free on a first come, first served basis.

https://positivepsychology.com/values-worksheets/

- This link leads to the PositivePsychology.com website and to an article contributed by Dr Maike Neuhaus titled, 25 Values Worksheets to Enrich Your Clients *Lives*. It is rich with ideas, worksheets, and activities to support occupational therapy professionals in implementing interventions focused on values clarification. Several of the values clarification worksheets can be downloaded for free.

https://positivepsychology.com/assertive-communication-worksheets/

- This link leads to the PositivePsychology.com website and to an article contributed by Dr Jeremy Sutton titled, 10 Best Assertive Communication Worksheets and Techniques. It is rich with ideas, worksheets, and activities to support occupational therapy professionals in implementing interventions focused on assertiveness and assertive communication. Several of the worksheets and screening tools can be downloaded for free. Two excellent ones to begin with are the Self-Evaluation Questions for Assertiveness *and the* Rights of Assertiveness Worksheet.

https://www.masterpeacebox.com/post/30-creative-art-therapy-exercises-with-pictures

- This site, MasterPeaceBox.com, offers over 30 great ideas for using expressive art techniques that occupational therapy professionals can incorporate into occupational therapy intervention when helping clients to foster improvements in self-confidence, self-esteem, or self-expression (and many others).

https://intuitivecreativity.typepad.com/expressiveartinspirations/

- This site, Expressive Art Inspirations, is the home website of Shelley Klammer, a depth-oriented psychotherapist and arts educator with the International Expressive Arts Therapy Association. The website offers a wealth of ideas and links to other resources that can be incorporated into occupational therapy interventions. In addition, Ms Klammer offers e-courses for occupational therapy professionals (and others) who may want to learn more about using expressive arts techniques.

https://www.therapistaid.com/therapy-worksheet/mandalas

- This website, Therapist Aid, is an excellent source for a variety of therapist-created worksheets, tips, and ideas. Specifically, this link takes the reader to several free downloadable mandalas.

CHAPTER 18

Targeting Psychological and Social Factors That Influence Occupational Engagement: Being With the Client Who Experiences Anxiety

OT HACKS OVERVIEW

O: Occupation as a means and an end

Before reading this chapter review, the following constructs of the *Pan Occupational Paradigm* (POP) will help occupational therapy professionals (OTPs) bring theory and occupational science into everyday practice (25, 28).

- **Doing:** the transaction that occurs as people engage in personally meaningful occupations
- **Being:** the essence of a person; who the person is occupationally, including their unique psychological, social, spiritual, and physical characteristics and capabilities
- **Belonging:** a feeling of relationship or connection to others, typically involves reciprocity, mutuality, and sharing
- **Becoming:** the aspirational, goal-directed growth and development of a person

T: Theoretical concepts, values, and principles, or historical foundations

Occupational therapy addresses all four interdependent and intricately connected dimensions of occupation (doing, being, belonging, and becoming) throughout the occupational therapy process. However, during occupational therapy intervention planning and implementation, according to the POP, the most authentic therapeutic interventions will be focused on the dimension of occupation that is most foregrounded (central to, or the focal point) in a particular phase of a client's life, situation, or context (26, 27).

H: How can we Help? OT's role in serving clients with mental illness or mental health needs

Cognitive behavior therapy, or CBT, is a widely recognized, evidence-based intervention framework that has been adapted to allow application with a wide variety of diagnostic groups for clients across the lifespan (1, 33, 39). CBT uses a psychotherapy-based approach that draws from the cognitive model. With many diagnoses, use of CBT, especially when combined with other therapies, has become the gold standard intervention to help people with mental health struggles move toward goal-directed growth and

functional recovery. This is also conceptualized by the POP (28) as the dimension of occupation where a person is consistently "becoming" the occupational being who they desire to be (24, 28, 43). OTPs receive education and training in psychosocial and cognitive interventions, allowing for provision of interventions that employ CBT techniques. Among others, a few of these techniques include the management of stress through the development of problem-solving skills, assisting clients with identifying and restructuring automatic thoughts, and helping them acquire coping skills (31).

A: Adaptations

One way for the OTP to "be with" the client who is experiencing anxiety (while also integrating aspects of the being and belonging occupational dimensions into occupational therapy practice) is to enact flexible approaches and responses to the anxious behaviors. The *Intentional Relationship Model* (IRM) (44) is a conceptual practice model and interpersonal reasoning approach that provides therapists with a way to match their use of different therapeutic modes of communication to the client's interpersonal characteristics, needs, and preferences.

C: Case study includes

Our case study is the true story of well-known athlete Kevin Love. Love is a 5-time NBA All-Star, who at the time of the publication of this text plays for the Cleveland Cavaliers. The Cleveland Cavaliers won an NBA championship in 2016. Kevin Love is also an Olympic gold medalist (2012) and was a member of the team that won the International Federation of Basketball (FIBA) World Championship in 2010.

After experiencing a panic attack during an NBA game in 2017, Love decided to share his battle with anxiety and depression in an essay he wrote for *The Players' Tribune* (30). Love's willingness and courage in sharing his story has helped normalize the conversation surrounding mental health. Read Kevin Love's story: https://www.theplayerstribune.com/articles/kevin-love-mental-health

Please find follow-up case reflections and questions in the OT HACKS Summary.

K: Knowledge: keeping mental health OT practice grounded in evidence, in occupational science, and in research

Read this evidence using the following research question as a focus:

How does an OTP-led African drumming group used as an occupational therapy intervention impact the overall feelings of well-being experienced by clients with mood disorders?

After reviewing the article and learning more in this chapter about how the symptoms of mood disorders impact occupational engagement, discuss responses to the *Evidence Application and Translation Questions* found in section "Knowledge" in the *OT HACKS chapter summary*.

S: Some terms that may be new to you

Anxiety
Automatic thoughts
Cognitive distortions
Cognitive restructuring
Emotional resonance
Fear
Intervening (intervention)
Labeling
Mode matching
Mode versatility
Panic attacks
Socratic method
Specifier
Thought record
Witnessing

Plastow, N. A., Joubert, L., Chotoo, Y., Nowers, A., Greeff, M., Strydom, T., Theron, M., & van Niekerk, E. (2018). Brief report—The immediate effect of African drumming on the mental well-being of adults with mood disorders: An uncontrolled pretest–posttest pilot study. *American Journal of Occupational Therapy, 72*(5), 7205345010p1–7205345010p6.

TARGETING SYMPTOMS OF ANXIETY THAT CREATE BARRIERS TO OCCUPATION: THE BEING, DOING, AND BELONGING DIMENSIONS OF OT PRACTICE

BOX 18.1 Intervention Planning Focus Questions: How to Begin

1. What does it feel like to be a person who is experiencing *anxiety*?
2. What are some behaviors that a person experiencing *anxiety* might demonstrate, and how might their behavior, responses, or affect be positively or negatively impacting their occupations?
3. How can I adjust my way of being (therapeutic use of self) to make the client feel more comfortable about their way of being?
4. What can I do to instill a sense of belonging in occupational therapy right now that will encourage the client toward setting goals with outcomes that are personally meaningful and relevant to them?

What Is Anxiety?

Anxiety is a feeling of fear or dread that interrupts typical life functions. It is one of the most common symptoms seen in psychiatric illnesses. According to the *Diagnostic and Statistical Manual of Mental Disorders, Fifth Edition, Text Revision (DSM-5-TR)*, "**Fear** is the emotional response to real or perceived imminent threat, whereas **anxiety** is anticipation of future threat" (6, p. 215). **Panic attacks** are one type of response to fear that is associated with several psychiatric illnesses, including the anxiety disorders (6). It is important to note that anxiety is normal, and, as some argue, even healthy to a certain extent. Most people feel some anxiety, particularly when faced with frightening, challenging, or unpredictable situations. For healthy people, anxiety is an adaptive response to threats. When there is perception of danger, or we feel threatened, our perception triggers the sympathetic nervous system to release stress hormones and adrenaline (43). This nervous system alarm prompts a fight, flight, or freeze physiologic or behavioral response. Our body systems respond in a variety of ways to prepare us to do what we need to do to survive (ie, increased heart rate for greater blood circulation, slowed digestion, and increased metabolic rate to fuel the body for fighting or escaping) (24, 41, 43).

However, anxiety is different from experiencing anxiousness or feeling worried and concerned. Although everyone feels some anxiety, when threats or fears are resolved, or the difficult situation passes, a person who felt worried or anxious is usually able to return to a calm state and experiences decreasing symptoms of anxiety. A person with an anxiety disorder continues to experience symptoms of anxiety, sometimes at continually increasing levels (24). Anxiety becomes pathologic (causing illness) only when it is so extreme and so long lasting that it interferes with effective functioning in daily life.

It is important to reiterate that, to a certain degree, we can think of anxiety as a protective or positive force. If a person awakens to a fire alarm and determines that the closed door to their bedroom has smoke coming in from underneath, the anxiety that the person feels may help them find a safer alternate escape route. Anxiety can also motivate us to attempt new things—for example, your anxiety upon first encountering a new client may prod you to approach and try to talk with them before the more formal occupational therapy evaluation, which could have the benefit of making both people experience less anxiety later.

Anxiety may occur alone, as the primary symptom, or with other symptoms. Sometimes, it causes other symptoms, just as a fever causes malaise, chills, and body aches. For many clients, anxiety masks other emotions such as sadness or fear and anxiety can often be associated with trauma or loss. Because of the complex nature of anxiety, there are innumerable ways that it can manifest. We can recognize when someone is anxious by observing body language and behaviors, and by listening carefully to what the person says (44). Some people worry aloud; they talk incessantly about things that may never happen. Others fidget: they tap their feet, jiggle their legs, bite their nails, pull their hair, tug at their faces, drum the tabletop, and pace the halls. Others express fears about certain places or objects. They may be afraid to go outside or to use the toilet. Some of the most recognizable signs of anxiety are as follows:

- Hesitation when initiating a task or activity
- Sweating, or increased (pressured) breathing
- Changing or higher pitched voice quality
- Self-doubt about an impending performance
- Reports of having a dry mouth when speaking
- Need for frequent approval or reassurance from the OTP or others
- Increases in fatigue, pain, or other physical symptoms (with no other medical explanation)

Regardless of the behaviors through which a person expresses anxiety, the therapeutic objective is generally the same: to control or reduce the experience of anxiety so that the person can participate optimally in valued occupations. OTPs do this by first understanding the general activity demands of the client's preferred occupations through activity analysis and then further tailoring the activity to meet each individual's unique needs (assessing occupational demands). "An important life skill [for the client] is to notice and resolve anxiousness before it becomes anxiety" (24, p. 192).

Referring to our *OT Domain and Process Home* infograph from the introduction to Section II for this example, if Alex (the character who lives in the home) is your client and they need to ascend the set of steps to enter the house, the OTP would first assess the underlying activity demands and think about what is required to get to the top of the steps. Next, the OTP will perform an occupational analysis to observe Alex's occupational performance skills and assess the occupational demands (or what unique requirements exist *for Alex* to be able to ascend the steps) (4, 5, 19). Now imagine that your client Alex has been diagnosed with an anxiety disorder and ascending stairs makes Alex feel anxious. In this situation, Alex's feelings of anxiousness are barriers to participation in occupation and so the anxiousness becomes the target of the intervention. As an approach to intervention (create or promote, establish or restore, maintain, modify, or prevent), the client's desired occupational outcomes will be determined through a collaborative process. However, regardless of approach or outcome, the role of the OTP will involve teaching Alex to recognize or prevent feelings of anxiousness before the anxiousness results in anxiety that would negatively impact further participation in occupations.

Diagnoses in Which Anxiety Is a Common Symptom

The NIH: National Institute of Mental Health (NIMH) reported that in 2017, the prevalence of anxiety disorders (any anxiety disorder) among adults aged 18 or older in the United States was approximately 19.1%. This included the diagnostic groups of panic disorder, generalized anxiety disorder, agoraphobia, specific phobia, social anxiety disorder (social phobia), posttraumatic stress disorder (PTSD), obsessive compulsive disorder, and separation anxiety disorder (34).

As a symptom, anxiety may be found in almost every diagnostic category. Specifically, anxiety may be listed as a **specifier** to further describe the characteristics of a diagnosis. "Specifiers are extensions to a diagnosis that further clarify the course, severity, or special features of a disorder or illness" (38, para. 1). According to the *DSM-5-TR* (6), besides the anxiety disorders, anxiety often accompanies bipolar and related disorders, depressive disorders, trauma and stress-related disorders, substance-related and addictive disorders, schizophrenia spectrum disorders, and illness anxiety disorders.

Strategies for Therapeutic Use of Self

One way for the OTP to "be with" the client who is experiencing anxiety, or demonstrating symptoms of anxiousness, is to enact flexible approaches and responses to the anxious behaviors. In Chapter 15, readers were briefly introduced to Dr Renee Taylor's IRM (44). IRM is a conceptual practice model and interpersonal reasoning approach that provides therapists with a way to match their use of different therapeutic modes of communication to the client's interpersonal characteristics in the moment. Taylor calls this process **mode matching** (44). "*Mode versatility* extends the concept of the mode shift in that it describes the process of trial and error undertaken by an OTP when shifting modes. The aim . . . is ultimately to identify the best-fit mode for the client at that moment in time. To achieve this, you must possess an ability to monitor and read a client's reaction to a particular mode and then utilize the client's reaction as feedback to guide whether to remain in that mode or try a different one" (44, p. 228). Taylor formalized the ways that OTPs relate to clients by applying the appropriate therapeutic mode(s). The six therapeutic modes are patterns in which the practitioner applies different styles of interaction in different kinds of situations, as appropriate for each client, with particular attention paid to situational contexts. The six therapeutic modes are advocating, collaborating, empathizing, encouraging, instructing, and problem-solving (44).

Sometimes clients experience difficult emotions during occupational therapy. Managing the emotional intensity of the therapeutic relationship helps reduce the likelihood that the difficult emotions will interfere with the client's occupational goals or disrupt the therapeutic relationship. Consistent with the principles of the *IRM* (44), the therapist can enact four main approaches to handle emotional intensity and respond to difficult emotions that occur during therapy, such as anxiety. An OTP can approach management of emotional intensity through **witnessing**, **emotional resonance**, **labeling**, or **intervening** (44). Table 18.1 further describes the techniques for managing the emotional dynamics of the therapeutic relationship, specifically for clients who

Table 18.1. Managing the Emotional Dynamics of the Therapeutic Relationship

Intentional Relationship Model (IRM) Suggested Approaches for Responding to Clients' Experience of Difficult Emotions: Anxiety	Definition and How to . . .	Examples of Responses to the Client Experience of Anxiety
Witnessing *Why might I use this response or approach?* • Begin every client interaction by reflecting on the whole client; for OT professionals, this includes surveying the unique situational context and interpersonal circumstances within which the affect or behavior is occurring. • Occupational performance analysis could be thought of as OT's unique form of "witnessing" the client as an occupational being. We witness the doing dimension of occupation in this way.	Observe the client's expression; without use of language, maintain an attitude of nonjudgment and a neutral expression, or one that conveys empathy.	Examples of a witnessing response for a client experiencing anxiety may include: • Demonstrating open body language, including uncrossing arms and opening the palms of the hands, which signifies that the occupational therapy professional is open, willing, and ready to listen to the client • Use of nonverbal cues such as slightly forward-leaning body posture, and nodding the head affirmatively, that help indicate that the professional is present and focused on the client • Maintaining focused attention on the client by using consistent eye contact • Taking a brief walk with the client so that they can move while speaking to the occupational therapy professional can be a particularly helpful way to provide a witnessing response to a client with anxiety who also experiences symptoms of psychomotor agitation
Emotional resonance *Why might I use this response or approach?* • Utilize emotional resonance to clarify the client's emotion. • Resonating with a client's anxiety is effective when the client's worries are realistic and reassurance or other suggestions would be insincere or unrealistic.	Try to feel the same type of emotion as the client and allow your feelings to show through in your expression or in what you say in your response. Emotional resonance is one of the core aspects of therapeutic use of self in occupational therapy.	Examples of showing emotional resonance for anxiety may include the following: • Mirroring a client's affect • Thinking about what might be worrisome for the client and attempting to feel it yourself • Admitting to the client that the situation is worrisome (if indeed you feel that it is)
Labeling *Why might I use this response or approach?* • Utilize labeling to clarify the client's emotion. • Labeling can help clients name and make sense of what they are feeling; some clients experience this as comforting and orienting.	Labeling is to try to describe or name the client's affect or emotional expression using language.	Examples of labeling may include the following: • **Stating what is observed** (eg, "I can see that you are worried about this.") • **Validating what is observed** (eg, "It makes sense you would be feeling worried about this.") • **Giving the client permission to be anxious** (eg, "You look a little uncertain about this—want to review it again?") • **Normalizing the worry** (eg, "A lot of people are reluctant to try this the first time.")
Intervening *Why might I use this response or approach?* • Once anxiety is identified correctly, IRM intervention recommendations may be considered.	Performing some action to intervene, or providing intervention that targets the client's emotional expression. This is often necessary if an emotional expression (of anxiety in this case) has become maladaptive, and is disrupting occupational participation.	IRM intervention recommendations: **Anxiety** 1. Draw more heavily upon **the instructing mode**. Increase the client's comfort level by using increased structure, repetition, guidance, and leadership. 2. Draw upon **the encouraging mode** to offer incentives, provide reassurance, promote self-confidence, and instill hope. 3. Use **the collaborating mode** to make deliberate efforts to increase the client's perceived control (eg, by pointing out the controllable aspects of the situation). 4. Slow the pace of therapy and grade activities more carefully until the client masters and becomes comfortable with less-demanding tasks or activities.

IRM, Intentional Relationship Model: OT, occupational therapy. Adapted from Taylor, R. R. (2020). Establishing intentional relationships. In R. R. Taylor (Ed.), *The intentional relationship: Occupational therapy and use of self* (2nd ed., pp. 225–242). F.A. Davis.

Table 18.2. Flexible Responses to Anxious Behaviors

Behavior	Recommended Response
Ritualistic, compulsive The client carries out unnecessary and what seem to others to be meaningless actions, such as checking for dirt on the threshold of doors before entering/crossing them.	Do not criticize the client's behavior. Instead, recognize that no matter how ridiculous the ritual may seem, it is one that the client uses to cope with anxiety. You can make the person feel more comfortable if you convince them that you are accepting of them no matter what. When considering attachment theories, this is similar to demonstrating an unconditional positive regard for the client.
Phobic, fearful The client is afraid of things that other people do not generally find frightening (eg, being a passenger on a subway, or shopping at a grocery store).	Encourage such clients to talk about their fears; help them focus on exactly what makes them afraid. This is especially important when their fear prevents them from accomplishing tasks needed in their occupational roles.
Intrusive, demanding The client constantly demands attention or interrupts when you are working with others.	Reassure the client that you will be available to help them. Give them a definite time and stick to it. Ignore subsequent interruptions but do not become angry or express irritation.

experience anxiety, according to the principles of the IRM, and provides application examples. Accurate use of the appropriate therapeutic modes and responses is the foundation for application of therapeutic use of self and signifies client-centered practice (44). "Three of the most challenging emotions that clients may exhibit are sadness, anger, and anxiety" (44, p. 229). A discussion about incorporating concepts of the IRM approach when clients experience anxiety follows. Readers can find a similar discussion related to sadness in Chapter 19, and anger in Chapter 22.

According to the IRM, the application of certain therapeutic modes can be especially helpful when responding to clients with anxiety (44). The OTP can draw more heavily upon the **instructing mode** in the initial stages of occupational therapy to increase the client's comfort level. Techniques such as increased structure, repetition, consistent guidance, and sustained leadership may improve the clients' comfort level and reduce feelings of anxiousness. Application of the **encouraging mode** offers the client an incentive to participate in therapy, provides them with reassurance, grows self-confidence, and infuses an attitude of hopefulness. Finally, incorporation of the **collaborating mode** ensures that the OTP is making intentional efforts to raise and improve the client's perceived level of control.

Encourage clients to talk about what is bothering them and to express how they feel. Answer their questions if you can but avoid being drawn into extended discussions of physical symptoms and their possible causes, which could serve to heighten the client's anxiety (44). It helps to focus first on what clients are concerned about, listen to their fears, and then gradually redirect their attention to a neutral topic or something more constructive. Different responses are needed for individuals who express their anxiety through rituals, those who demonstrate specific phobias, or who constantly demand attention. See Table 18.2 for further response recommendations for clients with these special considerations. Finally, it is not unusual for people who are anxious to have trouble focusing (36). The OTP may need to redirect their attention gently and repeatedly to the activity, or grade the intervention activities down until the client experiences

success and feels more comfortable (44, 45). Inattention may also be a signal that the activity is too difficult or not of interest, in which case alternative activities should be explored.

TARGETING SYMPTOMS OF ANXIETY THAT CREATE BARRIERS TO OCCUPATION: THE DOING AND BECOMING DIMENSIONS OF OT PRACTICE

> **BOX 18.2 Intervention Implementation Focus Questions: How to Support Clients' Optimal Engagement in Occupation**
>
> 1. What can the client and the occupational therapy team collaboratively do together that will help the client become more functional and effective in the things that are important to them in everyday life?
> 2. What are the best intervention types and intervention approaches to apply in this therapeutic context?
> 3. What does the current evidence suggest about the most productive interventions for this diagnosis/set of symptoms?

Contextual, Environmental, and Client Factor Considerations for Clients With Symptoms of Anxiety

In general, the therapeutic environment for a person with anxiety should be calm, comfortable, and familiar. People who are inclined to be anxious often become more so when overstimulated by too much noise or too many people. Persons with sensory processing difficulties may first reveal their sensitivities through expression of anxiousness or withdrawal. A context that is different from what the person is used to may also be frightening or quickly become overwhelming. In a new therapeutic environment, one of the most helpful ways to make clients more comfortable is to reduce some of the environmental or contextual "unknowns." Giving clients who are in a new setting a brief tour of the facility and the occupational therapy area, as well as a written or visual schedule for activities, can help them feel more secure and in control and can orient them more effectively to their surroundings.

Characteristics of Interventions That Support Reduced Anxiety

Guide clients to choose their own activity; ask clients what things they find relaxing or what things take their minds off their worries. Help the client select activities that produce a successful result without excessive attention to detail. A project that the person can work on for a while, get up and move about, and come back to later is ideal. Some anxious persons respond well to activities involving a single motor sequence that is repeated (eg, quick point, sanding, bead stringing, crocheting, art activities such as coloring/completing a mandala, and drumming); they seem to use the regular pace of the activity to self-regulate (32, 37). Nevertheless, an activity that is too simple may allow rumination on anxiety-provoking subjects, which means that the OTP must pay careful attention in presenting the just-right challenge and be prepared to quickly grade the activity up for increased difficulty or down for less complexity. Gross motor activities such as aerobic exercise or stretching and relaxation exercises can focus the mind and body and thus reduce the uncomfortable physical symptoms that are exacerbated with anxiety (eg, tense muscles, neck and back aches, racing pulse) (46). Yoga, reiki, Tai Chi, Qigong, and other Eastern practices have been found to be beneficial for reducing stress (9). Meditation, mindfulness, and relaxation exercises, or biofeedback, can also be incorporated into occupational therapy intervention (21, 40, 47). Stress management techniques such as progressive relaxation, incorporating time management systems, and supporting the client in developing leisure skills, may help the person identify stressors and learn self-management strategies that can offset, prevent, or reduce anxiety (9, 15).

Social support such as a conversation with a friend or attendance and participation in a therapeutic activity group can go a long way in easing a client's anxious mind, helping them feel seen and heard, and demonstrating to them that they are not alone in their struggle. Depending on the individual's goals, priorities, and interests, the following activities are a few examples that may be appropriate for clients who are experiencing anxiety.

- *Small, prefabricated woodworking kits*: Those with a small number of pieces (3–5) are best until you are certain the person can handle more.
- *Simple cooking tasks*: For example, making chocolate chip cookies. There are lots of opportunities for the client to move around while cleaning up or waiting for a batch to be done baking.
- *Structured art activities delivered via mobile phone or tablet apps*: Technology apps such as *Zen Color* are free downloadable color by number pages for young adults and adults. Although some of these are solitary tasks, some apps such as *Puzzle Passion—Light* are designed for multiplayer use, offering the client engagement in a structured activity and virtual social connection, simultaneously.

In a scoping review presented by Donnelly and Colleagues (16) published in the *American Journal of Occupational Therapy* in 2021, researchers explored how virtual reality in head-mounted displays (HMD-VR) has been used to treat symptoms of anxiety through virtual reality exposure therapy (VRET). Further, the authors examined how HMD-VR and VRET could be translated for use in psychosocial occupational therapy intervention and practice. Findings from this study suggest that in combination with cognitive behavioral approaches, "HMD-VR can be used by occupational therapy practitioners to simulate ecologically valid environments, evaluate client responses to fearful stimuli, and remediate anxiety though immersion in virtual tasks when participation in natural contexts is unfeasible. Having ecologically valid environments is particularly important for people with anxiety disorders because they need support to cope when they encounter triggers in everyday life environments" (16, p. 1).

Cognitive behavioral approaches to reduce irrational or illogical thoughts help put worries in perspective. Specific evidence-based cognitive behavioral intervention techniques that target symptoms of anxiety are introduced throughout the remainder of the chapter. Activities such as scrapbooking, journal writing, walking meditation, multisensory rooms, and other sensory approaches are additional possibilities (8, 12, 13, 32). Anxiety is a normal response to disaster, occupational disruption, and occupational deprivation. In such situations, the OTP should help clients reestablish normal routines and patterns as much as possible. Occupational therapy may also address needs for sleep hygiene routines, self-care, leisure activities, psychoeducation about stress management, and training in coping skills (18, 22, 23). Occupational therapy interventions that target the symptom of anxiety all share the common characteristic of being designed to help the client establish (or reestablish) occupational balance (3).

Evidence-Based Interventions That Target Symptoms of Anxiety

If we look at the symptoms of anxiety through the lens of the cognitive model, people with anxiety disorders (ie, people with anxiety symptoms that have become pathologic) generally "share this common bias in cognitive processing" (43, p. 114), they have an exaggerated perception of impending threats and they undervalue or underestimate the resources or solutions that they believe they possess to resolve the threatening event or stimuli. "What differentiates the anxiety disorders is the specific content of the fears underlying the anxiety and the ensuing strategies that individuals use to cope" (43, p. 114). The literature suggests that to understand and authentically be present (infusing aspects of the being and belonging dimensions of occupation) with clients who have anxiety disorders, the OTP must make every effort to explore the content of the client's fears. As a part of the occupational therapy process, the OTP helps the client realize that their unproductive behavioral responses, and reactions that they use to cope, have created barriers to their occupational engagement (14, 43).

When a person who is experiencing pathologic anxiety encounters a threatening (or perceived threatening) stimulus, they consider two aspects of the situation: how dangerous is this threat to my situation and do I have the resources or ability to cope with this threat? Invariably, clients with anxiety disorders (although differing in what the fear is that drives the anxiety) will have a vastly overexaggerated sense of fear and will largely dismiss their ability to cope, denying their capacity to draw upon internal or external resources to solve problems that feel like crises. When events or situations of everyday experiences occur, we have thoughts about the occurrence (sometimes called **automatic thoughts**). These automatic thoughts are very important because we experience emotion that is driven by our interpretation of the thoughts. Finally, we respond to our thoughts and feelings through our actions and behaviors. CBT is based on the premise that our thoughts, even irrational or erroneous ones, sometimes referred to as **cognitive distortions**, influence physiologic sensation, how one feels, and how one behaves (10, 43). The central focus of CBT is to help the client become aware of their negative automatic thoughts and then to test the validity of the faulty thoughts to change the behaviors that have led to occupational disruption (7, 20, 31).

CBT includes the therapeutic process of **cognitive restructuring**, which is a variety of psychoeducational and psychotherapeutic techniques used to help identify and challenge irrational, inaccurate, or negative thoughts to positively impact emotions, behaviors, and mood. Cognitive restructuring has been widely applied to the treatment of anxiety disorders and it is an established evidence-based intervention for generalized anxiety disorder, social anxiety disorder, panic disorder, PTSD, and obsessive compulsive disorder (14). Many techniques can be applied to collaborate with the client and help them initiate cognitive restructuring or to work toward development of awareness of their thought patterns. Once the client develops an awareness of their thought patterns, they can progress toward identifying and challenging their cognitive distortions. According to the AOTA *Occupational Therapy Practice Framework, Domain and Process, 4th Edition* (OTPF-4), OTPs who wish to implement CBT into their intervention plan will be applying an education and training type of intervention used for "Imparting of knowledge and information about occupation, health, well-being, and participation to enable the client to acquire helpful behaviors, habits, and routines" (4, 5, p. 61). Cognitive restructuring begins with the OTP using a psychoeducational approach to support the clients' understanding about what cognitive distortions are, and how these false thoughts can negatively impact one's mood, affect, and

behaviors, eventually causing disruption to their engagement in meaningful occupations.

Developing a basic understanding of how our thoughts influence our emotions, sensations, and behaviors is an aspect of both the being and the doing dimensions of occupation. Recall from the POP (25, 28) that the being dimension of occupation is represented in practice when an individual reflects upon who they are as a person, as an occupational being, including their unique psychological, social, spiritual, and physical characteristics and capabilities. Reflection on one's thoughts, emotions, reactions, and behaviors inherently leads them to reflect upon aspects of their way of being in the world. In the early stages of cognitive behavioral therapy, the client is developing an awareness of their thoughts. Once a client has made the connection or begins to understand the relationship between their thoughts, emotions, and behaviors, when the client is ready, they can begin to transition into the doing dimension of occupation. The "doing" part of CBT occurs as the client starts to identify their thoughts so that eventually they can challenge illogical thoughts (cognitive distortions).

Keep in mind that while this is an early step in the cognitive restructuring process, it is likely to be the most difficult phase. It is not easy to be aware of automatic thoughts or of faulty thought patterns. Developing an awareness of thought patterns is a skill that takes practice. It is not logical to think that anyone would be able to stop in the heat of an anxiety-provoking situation to reflect upon the erroneous thoughts that set into motion a moment of extreme anxiousness. Perhaps the most important role for the OTP during this stage is to help the client narrow their focus to the most important cognitive distortions, the ones that are wreaking the most havoc on the client's occupational participation. Often, the most disruptive cognitive distortions are accompanied by negative affect and negative emotions.

From an occupational therapy perspective, an in-depth look at the situational contexts of the client's life, discovered while collecting information to create an occupational profile, will usually yield information about when the symptoms of anxiety are the most prevalent. Asking the client what behaviors are getting in the way of the occupation that they have identified as important, or as a priority to them, is another way to determine when negative emotions are most likely to arise from distorted thought patterns. Once the client and the therapist agree that the client has developed an appropriate level of understanding about the cognitive model and has an awareness of their own thoughts and cognitive distortions, the OTP can introduce a **thought record**. A thought record provides a means for the client to record their experiences or situations and collect data about their thoughts, feelings, and behaviors or responses that surround life situations. OTPs can encourage the client to keep a thought record by building the exercise into their daily habits, roles, and routines. The intent of the thought record is to bring to light cognitive distortions as they occur, so that they can be immediately challenged, and over time the negative emotions and behaviors that result can be extinguished (14, 43).

MANAGING SYMPTOMS OF ANXIETY: THE BECOMING AND BELONGING DIMENSIONS OF OT PRACTICE

> ### BOX 18.3 Focus Questions for Planning Transition, Maintenance, and Long-Term Wellness Plans
>
> 1. How does the client define success in reaching their goals?
> 2. How can occupational therapy support the long-term success in the client becoming who they want to be, successfully doing what they want to do?
> 3. How can occupational therapy support the client's recovery and long-term success in finding community, and feeling a sense of belonging and connectedness?

Social and Emotional Health Promotion and Maintenance for Symptoms of Anxiety

Implementing CBT into an occupational therapy intervention plan is a process. Typically, in the first phase of CBT, cognitive restructuring occurs and clients develop an awareness about the relationship between their thoughts, emotions, physiology, and behavioral responses. The clients learn to identify cognitive distortions, and, with time and practice, they learn to modify the illogical thought processes that feed their anxiety responses and trigger anxiety cycles. When a client develops a level of occupational performance skills that allows them to manage their anxiety using cognitive restructuring techniques, an important part of health promotion and maintenance that occupational therapy can contribute to is providing consistent opportunities for the client to practice applying their skills within the client's natural context during their typical daily occupations, while they are also confronting their underlying fears. This is a critical part of the growth-oriented, ever-evolving, "becoming" dimension of occupation (28).

Many clients with anxiety disorders share an ineffective coping strategy; they avoid any perceived threat that may trigger anxious feelings (43). When a person experiences anxiety that is so overwhelming to them that it negatively impacts their occupational performance, especially if the person has lived for a long time with undiagnosed anxiety, it is common for them to create occupational performance patterns that revolve around avoidance. Performance patterns are "the habits, routines, roles, and rituals . . . associated with different lifestyles and used in the process of engaging in occupations or activities. These patterns are influenced by context and time use and can support or hinder occupational performance" (4, p. 41). Clients with anxiety tend to create performance patterns that allow them to directly avoid what they perceive to be any situation that will provoke anxiety, thereby hindering occupational engagement. When a client with anxiety cannot avoid a situation, they may also engage in a variety of behaviors or rituals that they believe will keep them protected from the anxiety, or somehow help neutralize the feelings of anxiousness. Unfortunately, avoidance is an ineffective coping strategy because it is based on inaccurate thoughts and perceptions. Over time, it holds the person hostage from participating in their valued occupations and prevents new experiences and new learning from occurring, thus reinforcing their inaccurate perceptions because they have had diminished opportunities to face their fears and disprove faulty perception (14, 43).

Because people with pathologic anxiety fail to realize or engage strategies and resources that they may have to cope with potential threats, helping clients clarify and then engage their available resources, regardless of whether those resources are internal or external, is a priority throughout the therapeutic process during occupational therapy. For example, a high school student diagnosed with social anxiety who is in a literature class where the students are asked to find a partner and discuss the scene from a play may need to develop skills in communication or assertiveness. However, a client with a new driving phobia resulting from being a passenger in a car that was involved in a motor vehicle accident may need opportunities to slowly return to driving through brief exposures with an OTP who is a certified driving specialist to become more comfortable before they drive alone, or travel longer routes. Sometimes clients already possess the necessary occupational performance skills to engage in tasks and activities but they need help in recognizing when seeking help from their available resources would prevent increased levels of stress and overwhelm. Some examples of client and contextual factors that could be considered internal resources include mental/cognitive functions, spirituality, coping skills, strengths, personality factors, sense of humor, physical strength, resiliency, self-esteem, and self-confidence.

"Self-confidence is perhaps the most important internal resource to work on within the context of therapy because anxious clients believe they are helpless to do anything about their anxiety, which only exemplifies their self-doubt" (41, p. 117). When clients cultivate self-confidence, their perspective of themselves as capable begins to emerge, literature indicates that their sense of worthiness increases, and their self-questioning doubts about their abilities decrease (42). Self-confidence helps deter unfounded anxiety. Documenting the client's strengths, exploring their internal and external resources, and collaborating with them as they practice accessing support from their resources are all priorities in occupational therapy intervention for clients with anxiety because it reduces the client's self-doubt. "Without self-doubt, anxiety cannot exist" (43, p. 118).

External resources that support maintaining client wellness over time may include any number of structures, people, or social capital in the community, from friends and family to churches or organizations such as the YMCA. However, it is critical as the OTP and client consider longer term mental health and well-being for clients in marginalized populations, or who are socially isolated, that therapeutic goals may need to include building additional resources of support (2).

Importantly, clients' ability to recognize that they have resources available, and knowing how and when to engage the resources, helps lessen their perception that there is a threat (risk of experiencing anxiety) that they do not have the resources (or skills) to survive.

Symptom and Condition Management for Symptoms of Anxiety

People who experience persistent anxiety overestimate the likelihood of something bad happening and they tend to exaggerate how horrific the outcomes to any given scenario will be; a pseudo "worse-case-scenario" way of thinking overcomes their thought processes. For clients with anxiety disorders or obsessive compulsive disorders, automatic thoughts can be so consistently negative and occur with such frequency that the intrusive thoughts make concentrating on tasks very difficult. Pathologic anxiety has the effect of making people catastrophize. "The role of the therapist is to help the client see that those consequences, although unpleasant, may not be as catastrophic as imagined" (43, p. 118). Helping clients examine their catastrophic thinking during therapy by asking exploratory questions like the ones below (43), using cognitive restructuring techniques such as the **Socratic method**, provides a protocol for a healthy process that they can implement later. Furthermore, with practice and habit development, clients can generalize these questions to other aspects of their life to help them prevent stress and deter catastrophic thought patterns.

1. Are these thoughts necessarily true?
2. Are these thoughts consistent with the evidence?
3. What is the worst, best, and most likely outcome?
4. Could you survive the worst outcome, and would it actually be a problem?
5. Are there other ways to think about this situation?
6. Are these thoughts helpful?
7. What might you say to a friend or another person in this situation?
8. What resources do you have within and outside of yourself that are there to help you face this situation?

Coping with anxiety requires us to recognize that there are few certainties in life and that sometimes situations happen that defy our assumptions and our expectations (11, 43). The expression, "no guarantees," comes to mind, and in fact sometimes bad things happen with little or no apparent explanation or reason. Because we cannot guarantee that something bad will not happen, as OTPs working with clients with anxiety, what we can do is help our clients assess the *realistic risks* associated with their fears that provoke anxiety, so that they can manage their symptoms. "When the probability of something bad happening is high, then addressing how to cope with those consequences is warranted. However, it is not helpful to address catastrophic thinking when the probability of the threat is nonexistent or miniscule" (43, p. 117). When clients with anxiety are overwhelmingly preoccupied with catastrophized thinking, they are less available for other

life experiences, which lead to occupational deprivation and imbalance.

Effective Use of Occupation-Centered Outcome Measures

Most clients who experience anxiety disorders have a very difficult time giving up the avoidance behaviors that they have developed over time. For some clients, avoiding situations (or illogical thoughts) that feel threatening starts out as a method to protect them from anxiety (albeit an ineffective method). For other clients, the assumption may be that anxiety is dangerous; therefore, the person attempts to completely terminate and remove all avenues that may lead to anxiety. For the OTP, our primary goal when working with a client who is experiencing pathological anxiety, should not be an outcome that attempts to get rid of anxiety but rather to teach them how to appropriately assess threats, risks, and resources, and reduce stressors to minimize psychological and physiologic "false alarms." Only when clients can begin to face the underlying fears that usually are driving their anxiety can they optimally engage in their chosen occupations (29, 43).

OT HACKS SUMMARY

O: Occupation as a means and an end

When clients with anxiety are overwhelmingly preoccupied with catastrophized thinking, and repeatedly have cognitive distortions that cause them to believe that they do not have the resources or coping skills to survive, their physiologic system (ie, the nervous system) moves into overdrive. These clients become less and less available for other life experiences, which leads to occupational deprivation and imbalance.

Occupational therapy interventions that target the symptom of anxiety all share the common characteristic of being designed to help the client establish (or reestablish) their occupational balance.

The primary goal of occupational therapy with a client who is experiencing pathologic anxiety is to teach them how to appropriately assess threats, risks, and resources, to minimize damage caused by persistent feelings of anxiousness and overworked psychological and physiologic systems. When clients can begin to face the underlying fears, driven by the cognitive distortions that feed anxiety, they generally progress toward optimal engagement in their chosen occupations.

T: Theoretical concepts, values, and principles, or historical foundations

Developing a basic understanding of how our thoughts influence our emotions, sensations, and behaviors is an aspect of both the being and the doing dimensions of occupation. Recall from the POP (28) that the being dimension of occupation is represented in practice when an individual reflects upon who they are as a person, as an occupational being.

Reflection on one's thoughts, emotions, reactions, and behaviors lead the client to reflect upon aspects of their way of being in the world. In the early stages of cognitive behavioral therapy, the client is developing an awareness of their thoughts.

Once a client has made the connection between their thoughts, emotions, and behaviors, they can begin to transition into the doing dimension of occupation. The "doing" part of CBT occurs as the client starts to identify their thoughts, so that eventually they can challenge illogical thoughts (cognitive distortions), working toward more favorable physiologic, affective, and behavioral responses (ie, the becoming aspect of occupation).

H: How can we Help? OT's role in serving clients with mental illness or mental health needs

CBT includes the therapeutic process of **cognitive restructuring**, which is a variety of psychoeducational and psychotherapeutic techniques used to help identify and challenge irrational, inaccurate, or negative thoughts to positively impact emotions, behaviors, and mood. Cognitive restructuring has been widely applied to the treatment of anxiety disorders and it is an established evidence-based intervention for generalized anxiety disorder, social anxiety disorder, panic disorder, PTSD, and obsessive compulsive disorder (14, 17, 18, 35).

A: Adaptations

According to the IRM, the application of certain therapeutic modes can be especially helpful when responding to clients with anxiety (44).

- The OTP can draw more heavily upon the **instructing mode** in the initial stages of occupational therapy to increase the client's comfort level.
- Application of the **encouraging mode** offers the client incentive to participate in therapy, provides them with reassurance, grows self-confidence, and infuses an attitude of hopefulness.
- Incorporation of the **collaborating mode** ensures that the OTP is making intentional efforts to raise and improve the client's perceived level of control, which is typically a high priority for people who suffer from anxiety disorders.

C: Case study includes

Can you answer the following questions related to Kevin Love's story?

1. Describe some of the symptoms of anxiety and depression that Mr Love discusses in his story.
2. How did a lack of early intervention or diagnosis (of Mr Love's anxiety and depression) contribute to occupational performance and participation barriers and problems in various stages of his life?
3. Apply the POP (24) to the information you have regarding Kevin Love's life story. How are the dimensions of doing, being, becoming, and belonging represented in the context of his life?
4. Which dimension of occupation (doing, being, belonging, or becoming) do you believe was foregrounded (central to, or the focal point) in Kevin Love's life when he experienced his first public panic attack in 2017?

5. If you were part of a behavioral mental health team who collaborated with Mr Love during the recovery following his panic attack in 2017, what therapeutic occupation-based interventions might you consider? Please explain your answers.

K: Knowledge: keeping mental health OT practice grounded in evidence, in occupational science, and in research

"Given the experiences of a loss of pleasure and restriction in range of emotions that are typical of depressive disorders, we were particularly pleased to see how much the participants enjoyed the drumming session" (37, p. 4).

"The physical aspect of drumming also contributed to the effectiveness of the intervention" (37, p. 4).

The sample included 13 participants, 3 males and 10 females. Of these, six participants were of mixed ethnicity, and seven participants were described as White. The age range was 33 to 69 years, and the mean age was 45.38. All the participants presented with a mood disorder. Among the findings of the study, the results of the analysis demonstrated a negative correlation between pretest levels of depression (from the Patient Health Questionnaire-9 [PHQ-9]) and anxiety (from the Generalized Anxiety Disorder–7 [GAD-7]), and a mean change in tension, anger, confusion, and depression scores. This essentially signified that participants who were more anxious or depressed showed greater improvement on the subscales of tension, anger, confusion, and depression than did less anxious or depressed participants. The methodology of the study was described as a quasi-experimental, uncontrolled, one-group, pretest–posttest design. Data was collected for six different drumming groups ($N = 13$) using the *Stellenbosch Mood Scale*, the *PHQ–9*, the *GAD–7 Scale*, and the *Enjoyment of Interaction Scale*.

Evidence Application and Translation Questions

1. Describe the contributions of pilot studies such as this to daily occupational therapy practice?
2. Which occupational therapy frame of reference or approach is mentioned as being useful to this type of intervention?
3. Analyze the limitations and implications for future research that the authors of this study report. Choosing only one of the researchers' suggestions, defend why your selection should be the most critical consideration in future studies related to use of drumming as part of a therapeutic intervention?
4. Can you think of ways to make this intervention more explicitly tied to occupation-based goals and outcomes?

S: Some terms that may be new to you

Anxiety: anticipation of future threat

Automatic thoughts: "Thoughts that are instantaneous, habitual, and nonconscious. Automatic thoughts affect a person's mood and actions. Helping individuals to become aware of the presence and impact of negative automatic thoughts, and then to test their validity, is a central task of cognitive [behavioral] therapy" (7, para. 1).

Cognitive distortions: irrational or erroneous (false) thoughts

Cognitive restructuring: the therapeutic process of identifying and challenging irrational, inaccurate, or negative thoughts

Emotional resonance: An approach used by the OTP as a part of the IRM to respond to a client's experience of difficult emotions such as anxiety in the context of a therapeutic relationship; the OTP tries to feel the same type of emotion as the client and allow their feelings to show through in their expression or in what they say in their response. Emotional resonance is a core aspect of therapeutic use of self in occupational therapy practice.

Fear: the emotional response to real or perceived imminent threat

Intervening (intervention): An approach used by the OTP as a part of the IRM to respond to a client's experience of difficult emotions such as anxiety, in the context of a therapeutic relationship; the OTP performs some action to intervene, or provides intervention that targets the client's emotional expression. This is often necessary if an emotional expression (of anxiety in this case) has become maladaptive and is disrupting occupational participation.

Labeling: An approach used by the OTP as a part of the IRM to respond to a client's experience of difficult emotions such as anxiety in the context of a therapeutic relationship; labeling is used to try to describe or help the client name their affective state, their feelings, or emotional expressions, typically using oral or written language.

Mode matching: a way for OTPs to match their use of different therapeutic modes of communication to the client's interpersonal characteristics

Mode versatility: extends the concept of the mode shift (and mode matching), describes the process of trial and error undertaken by a therapist when shifting therapeutic modes; used to identify the best-fit mode for the client at any given moment in time, during therapeutic interactions

Panic attacks: one type of response to fear that is associated with several psychiatric illnesses, including anxiety disorders

Socratic method: A method of instructing a client by asking thoughtful questions; the method can be used as part of the encouraging therapeutic mode and is particularly helpful when a person is challenging their own assumptions or exploring complex ideas.

Specifier: extensions to a diagnosis listed in the *DSM-5-TR* that further clarify the course, severity, or special features of a disorder or illness

Thought record: a tool that the client can use to write down their experiences or situations and record the thoughts, feelings, and behaviors that accompany the situation or experience; frequently used when implementing CBT

Witnessing: An approach used by the OTP as a part of the IRM to respond to a client's experience of difficult emotions such as anxiety in the context of a therapeutic relationship; the OTP will observe the client's expression, without use of language, maintain an attitude of nonjudgment and a neutral expression, or one that conveys empathy.

Reflection Questions

1. Describe the symptom of anxiety and discuss the diagnoses that are commonly associated with symptoms of anxiety.

2. Describe four unique approaches or responses that the OTP can use to support the management of emotional intensity (specifically related to anxiety) within the therapeutic relationship, according to the IRM.

3. Compare and contrast *fear* and *anxiety*. From an occupational perspective, when does anxiety become pathological?

4. Identify and discuss some of the characteristics of appropriate evidence-based interventions that can be considered for a client who is experiencing symptoms of anxiety. Describe one or more intervention activities that would not be appropriate for a client who demonstrates pathological anxiety. Explain the reasons these activities may not be appropriate.

5. The encouraging therapeutic mode is one of the therapeutic modes recommended by the *IRM* as being appropriate to use with clients who experience anxiety. Can you think of situations or moments during occupational therapy sessions that an OTP may need to transition *away* from using the encouraging mode with an anxious client? Defend your answer.

6. Take a moment to consider anxiety-provoking challenges and situations in your own life. What helps you to ease feelings of anxiety? Can you think of any times when anxiety was helpful or even motivating to you?

7. Use images or symbols to describe the relationship between thoughts, behaviors, physiologic response, and emotion. Can you describe how cognitive distortions impact the thought-behavior-response-emotion relationship using only images or symbols?

REFERENCES

1. Åkerblom, S., Perrin, S., Rivano Fischer, M., & McCracken, L. M. (2015). The mediating role of acceptance in multidisciplinary cognitive-behavioral therapy for chronic pain. *Journal of Pain, 16*(7), 606–615.
2. American Occupational Therapy Association. (2020). AOTA 2020 occupational therapy code of ethics. *American Journal of Occupational Therapy, 74*(Suppl. 3), 7413410005p1–7413410005p13.
3. American Occupational Therapy Association. (2020). Occupational therapy in the promotion of health and well-being. *American Journal of Occupational Therapy, 74*(3), 7403420010p1–7403420010p14.
4. American Occupational Therapy Association. (2020). Occupational therapy practice framework: Domain and process—Fourth edition. *American Journal of Occupational Therapy, 74*(Suppl. 2), 1–87.
5. American Occupational Therapy Association. (2021). Occupational therapy scope of practice. *American Journal of Occupational Therapy, 75*(Suppl. 3), 7513410020.
6. American Psychiatric Association. (2022). *Diagnostic and statistical manual of mental disorders* (5th ed., text rev.). https://doi.org/10.1176/appi.books.9780890425787
7. American Psychological Association. *APA Dictionary of Psychology: Automatic thoughts.* https://dictionary.apa.org/automatic-thoughts
8. Bailliard, A. L., & Whigham, S. C. (2017). Linking neuroscience, function, and intervention: A scoping review of sensory processing and mental illness. *American Journal of Occupational Therapy, 71*(5), 7105100040p1–7105100040p18.
9. Barnett, J. E., & Shale, A. J. (2012). The integration of complementary and alternative medicine (CAM) into the practice of psychology: A vision for the future. *Professional Psychology: Research and Practice, 43*(6), 576–585.
10. Beck, J. S. (2011). *Cognitive behavior therapy: Basics and beyond* (2nd ed.). Guilford Press.

11. Brown, B. (2021). *Atlas of the heart: Mapping meaningful connection and the language of human experience.* Random House.

12. Champagne, T., & Sayer, E. (2008). The effects of the use of the sensory room in psychiatry. In T. Champagne (Ed.), *Sensory modulation and environment: Essential elements of occupation* (3rd ed., pp. 252–262). Champagne Conferences.

13. Champagne, T., & Stromberg, N. (2004). Sensory approaches in inpatient psychiatric settings: Innovative alternatives to seclusion and restraint. *Journal of Psychosocial Nursing, 42,* 35–44.

14. Clark, D. A., & Beck, A. T. (2010). *Cognitive therapy of anxiety disorders.* Guilford.

15. D'Amico, M. L., Jaffe, L. E., & Gardner, J. A. (2018). Evidence for interventions to improve and maintain occupational performance and participation for people with serious mental illness: A systematic review. *American Journal of Occupational Therapy, 72*(5), 7205190020p1–7205190020p11.

16. Donnelly, M. R., Reinberg, R., Ito, K. L., Saldana, D., Neureither, M., Schmiesing, A., Jahng, E., & Liew, S.-L. (2021). Virtual reality for the treatment of anxiety disorders: A scoping review. *American Journal of Occupational Therapy, 75*(6), 7506205040.

17. Eakman, A. M., Rolle, N. R., & Henry, K. L. (2017). Occupational therapist delivered cognitive behavioral therapy for insomnia to post-9/11 veterans in college: A wait list control pilot study. *Sleep, 40*(Suppl. 1), A140–A141.

18. Eakman, A. M., Schmid, A. A., Rolle, N. R., Kinney, A. R., & Henry, K. L. (2022). Follow-up analyses from a wait-list controlled trial of occupational therapist–delivered cognitive–behavioral therapy for insomnia among veterans with chronic insomnia. *The American Journal of Occupational Therapy, 76*(2), 7602205110.

19. Fisher, A. G., & Marterella, A. (2019). *Powerful practice: A model for authentic occupational therapy.* Center for Innovative OT Solutions.

20. Franc, I., & Doucet, B. (2020). *Cognitive behavioral therapy interventions to improve or maintain sleep and rest for adults with Parkinson's disease: Systematic review of related literature from 2011–2018* [Critically Appraised Topic]. American Occupational Therapy Association. https://www.aota.org/practice/practice-essentials/evidencebased-practiceknowledge-translation/critically-appraised-topic-alternative-occupational-therapy-interventions-to-improve-sleep-rest-and-adls-for-adults-with-parkinsons-disease

21. Goldberg, S. B., Tucker, R. P., Greene, P. A., Davidson, R. J., Wampold, B. E., Kearney, D. J., & Simpson, T. L. (2018). Mindfulness-based interventions for psychiatric disorders: A systematic review and meta-analysis. *Clinical Psychology Review, 59,* 52–60.

22. Håkansson, C., Gunnarsson, A. B., & Wagman, P. (2021). Occupational balance and satisfaction with daily occupations in persons with depression or anxiety disorders. *Journal of Occupational Science, 30*(1), 1–7.

23. Hemphill, B. J., & Urish, C. K. (Eds.). (2020). *Assessments in occupational therapy mental health: An integrative approach* (4th ed.). SLACK.

24. Hill, R., & Dahlitz, M. (2022). *The practitioner's guide to the science of psychotherapy.* W.W. Norton & Company.

25. Hitch, D., & Pepin, G. (2021). Doing, being, becoming, and belonging at the heart of occupational therapy: An analysis of theoretical ways of knowing. *Scandinavian Journal of Occupational Therapy, 28*(1), 13-25.

26. Hitch, D., Pepin, G., & Stagnitti, K. (2014). In the footsteps of Wilcock, Part one: The evolution of doing, being, becoming, and belonging. *Occupational Therapy in Health Care, 28*(3), 231–246.

27. Hitch, D., Pepin, G., & Stagnitti, K. (2014). In the footsteps of Wilcock, Part two: The interdependent nature of doing, being, becoming and belonging. *Occupational Therapy in Health Care, 28*(3), 247–263.

28. Hitch, D., Pepin, G., & Stagnitti, K. (2018). The pan occupational paradigm: Development and key concepts. *Scandinavian Journal of Occupational Therapy, 25*(1), 27–34.

29. Hooper, B., & Wood, W. (2019). The philosophy of occupational therapy: A framework for practice. In B. A. B. Schell & G. Gillen (Eds.), *Willard and Spackman's occupational therapy* (13th ed., pp. 43–55). Lippincott Williams & Wilkins.

30. Love, K. (2020, September). *To anybody going through it.* The Players' Tribune. https://www.theplayerstribune.com/articles/kevin-love-mental-health

31. McCraith, D. B. (2019). Cognitive beliefs. In C. Brown, V. Stoffel, & J. Munoz (Eds.), *Occupational therapy in mental health: Vision for participation* (pp. 262–279). F.A. Davis.

32. Mouradian, L. E., DeGrace, B. W., & Thompson, D. M. (2013). Art-based occupation group reduces parent anxiety in the neonatal intensive care unit. *American Journal of Occupational Therapy, 67*(6), 692–700.

33. Murphy, S. L., Janevic, M. R., Lee, P., & Williams, D. A. (2018). Occupational therapist–delivered cognitive–behavioral therapy for knee osteoarthritis: A randomized pilot study. *The American Journal of Occupational Therapy, 72*(5), 7205205040p1–7205205040p9.

34. National Institutes of Health, National Institute of Mental Health. (2017, November). *Any anxiety disorder.* https://www.nimh.nih.gov/health/statistics/any-anxiety-disorder

35. National Institutes of Health, National Library of Medicine. (2019, November). Reaching great heights with anxiety and depression. *NIH Medline Plus Magazine.* https://magazine.medlineplus.gov/article/reaching-great-heights-with-anxiety-and-depression

36. Pettersson, R., Söderström, S., Edlund-Söderström, K., & Nilsson, K. W. (2017). Internet-based cognitive behavioral therapy for adults with ADHD in outpatient psychiatric care: A randomized trial. *Journal of Attention Disorders, 21*(6), 508–521.

37. Plastow, N. A., Joubert, L., Chotoo, Y., Nowers, A., Greeff, M., Strydom, T., Theron, M., & van Niekerk, E. (2018). Brief report—The immediate effect of African drumming on the mental well-being of adults with mood disorders: An uncontrolled pretest–posttest pilot study. *American Journal of Occupational Therapy, 72*(5), 7205345010p1–7205345010p6.

38. Purse, M. (2022, July). *Specifiers in bipolar disorder.* verywell mind. https://www.verywellmind.com/what-are-specifiers-379957

39. Radomski, M. V., Giles, G. M., Carroll, G., Anheluk, M., & Yunek, J. (2022). Cognitive interventions to improve a specific cognitive impairment for adults with TBI (June 2013–October 2020). *American Journal of Occupational Therapy, 76*(2), 7613393170.

40. Sabal, R., & Gallagher, R. (2012). Meditation—A mindful approach to promoting occupational performance. *OT Practice, 17*(11), 17–18.

41. Sapolosky, R. M. (2004). *Why zebras don't get ulcers.* Holt Paperbacks.

42. Sokol, L., & Fox, M. G. (2009). *Think confident, be confident: A four-step program to eliminate doubt and achieve lifelong self-esteem.* Penguin.

43. Sokol, L., & Fox, M. G. (2019). *The comprehensive clinician's guide to cognitive behavioral therapy.* PESI Publishing.

44. Taylor, R. R. (2020). *The intentional relationship: Occupational therapy and use of self* (2nd ed.). F.A. Davis.

45. Weinstein, E. C. (2013). Three views of artful practice in psychosocial occupational therapy practice. *Occupational Therapy in Mental Health, 29*(4), 299–360.

46. Wheeler, S., Davis, D., Basch, J., James, G., Lehman, B., & Acord-Vira, A. (2022). Systematic review brief—Physical activity interventions for adults with traumatic brain injury (2013–2020). *American Journal of Occupational Therapy, 76*(Suppl. 2), 7613393140.

47. Wolf, C., & Serpa, J. G. (2015). *A clinician's guide to teaching mindfulness: The comprehensive session-by-session program for mental health professionals and health care providers.* New Harbinger Press.

Suggested Resources

Articles

A fantastic example of how occupational therapy services were brought to life for a specific population who needed mental health support following COVID-19. https://www.aota.org/publications/ot-practice/ot-practice-issues/2022/ot-solution-adolescent-mental-health

A systematic review of the evidence related to occupational therapy interventions/occupational therapy role for supporting clients with anxiety symptoms in inpatient physical rehabilitation settings. Pisegna, J., Anderson, S., & Krok-Schoen, J. L. (2022). Occupational therapy interventions to address depressive and anxiety symptoms in the physical disability inpatient rehabilitation setting: A systematic review. *American Journal of Occupational Therapy, 76*(1), 7601180110.

Books

When Harley *Has Anxiety:* A Fun CBT Skills Activity Book to Help Manage Worries and Fears by Dr Regine Galanti, a licensed clinical psychologist, and illustrated by Vicky Lommatzsch, is a book created for children ages 5 to 9. The story follows Harley the hedgehog who is learning how to manage fears and worries (anxiety) when they interrupt his daily activities. This is an excellent companion that provides the basis for over 45 activities that could be easily incorporated into occupation-centered interventions. Galanti is also the author of the best-selling book, *Anxiety Relief for Teens.*

Videos

Social Anxiety in the Modern World, Dr Fallon Goodman, an Assistant Professor at the University of South Florida and Director of the Emotion and Resilience Laboratory, shares a message based on her research that "Social anxiety is a hefty burden not just on individuals, but society as a whole. Here is the problem—the trend lines are all going in the wrong direction. Each year, more people experience frequent and intense social anxiety. Yet, we know surprisingly little about what social anxiety is and what we can do to address it. In this talk, Dr Fallon Goodman offers three solutions." (~15 minutes) https://www.youtube.com/watch?v=EFhP4wP1TzU

Social Anxiety: ***The Silent Pandemic That Needs a Louder Voice,*** Kyle Mitchell, TEDxTullahoma. "Kyle Mitchell takes us on his own personal journey through teen social anxiety with his 3 simple steps to overcoming it and creating solutions for a happier, healthier life. He is on a mission to help 1 million teens go from socially anxious to socially confident by changing the narrative on mental health." (~16 minutes) https://www.youtube.com/watch?v=g3Cyi3LxdP0

Website

The National Institute of Mental Health (NIMH) offers authoritative information about mental disorders, a range of related topics, and the latest mental health research. https://www.nimh.nih.gov/health

Targeting Psychological and Social Factors That Influence Occupational Engagement: Being With the Client Who Experiences Depression or Mania

OT HACKS OVERVIEW

O: Occupation as a means and an end

Measurable occupation-based outcomes are used to reflect the client's achievement of intervention goals related to enhanced or improved occupational participation.

- Some outcomes use occupation as a means to help clients meet their therapeutic goals as they progress through the occupational therapy process.
- Outcomes that are experienced by clients after they have realized the effects of their engagement in occupation and reflect upon how the participation enabled them to return to their desired habits, roles, routines, and rituals, demonstrate the use of occupation as an end to the therapeutic occupational therapy process (2, 3).

Clients with maladaptive depressive symptoms tend to withdraw from activities and often do not realize the positive impact that engagement in occupation can have on mood until their depressive symptoms have lifted. For these clients in particular, occupation is essential as both a means and an end.

T: Theoretical concepts, values, and principles, or historical foundations

Regardless of the etiology of depression, one common characteristic of depressive symptoms is having negative cognitive biases, or a negative view of the self, one's future, and the world at large (6). Negatively biased thinking is common across depressive and mood disorders and offers a place to begin interventions that incorporate and are guided by the cognitive behavioral frame of reference.

H: How can we Help? OT's role in serving clients with mental illness or mental health needs

According to the Intentional Relationship Model (IRM), there are some occasions during occupational therapy sessions when clients may be more likely to express intense sadness, such as when illness, injury, or trauma has significantly altered one's occupational participation (53). When a client demonstrates sadness during therapy, the occupational therapy professional should *not* discourage or disallow the show of emotions.

However, . . . one complex aspect of responding to a client's demonstration of depressive symptoms is that the occupational therapy professional must apply therapeutic reasoning

and reflect carefully to decide whether there is a need to maintain a more structured emotional boundary with the client. The occupational therapy professional must explore the possibility that the client is experiencing difficulties regulating or controlling emotions that are appropriate to the context and situation, in which case, it is possible that the client needs to become more effective in verbalizing their feelings, rather than consistently expressing displays of intense emotion or becoming too emotionally dependent on others rather than processing the emotions. Collaborating with the client to help them be more aware of their feelings, and to label them, usually prompts more effective emotional regulation (53).

A: Adaptations

Because of low self-confidence and self-esteem, some clients who experience depression tend to blame themselves for whatever goes wrong. This is one reason why **occupational analysis** is such a critical part of the occupational therapy evaluation because the results help clarify how to plan intervention activities that will allow the client to experience success, while still being sufficiently challenged.

C: Case study includes

Myra is a 19-year-old single Latinx woman with a *Diagnostic and Statistical Manual of Mental Disorders, Fifth Edition, Text Revision (DSM-5-TR)* diagnosis of Persistent Depressive Disorder (F34.1) was admitted to the acute admissions crisis ward of a behavioral health hospital after a nearly fatal suicide attempt (pills) following several months of depression, withdrawal, and refusal to leave her mother's house. This is her third hospitalization in 1 year. Myra is medicated with fluvoxamine (Luvox) 100 mg, but her mother reports that Myra is inconsistent with taking her medications.

Read more about the case at the end of the chapter.

K: Knowledge: keeping mental health OT practice grounded in evidence, in occupational science, and in research

Read this evidence by Foster et al (24) using the following research question as a focus:

How does congestive heart failure (CHF) affect participation in daily activity? What is the role of depression and impaired cognitive functioning on daily physical activity?

After reviewing the article and learning more in this chapter about how the symptoms of depression and mania impact occupational engagement, discuss responses to the *Evidence Application and Translation Questions* found in the section "Knowledge" in the *OT HACKS Chapter Summary*.

S: **Some terms that may be new to you**

Affective empathy
Anhedonia
Behavioral activation
Bereavement
Cognitive empathy
Depression
Empathy
Flight of ideas
Grandiosity
Mania
Pressured speech
SIG E CAPSS
Sympathy

TARGETING SYMPTOMS OF DEPRESSION AND MANIA THAT CREATE BARRIERS TO OCCUPATION: THE BEING, DOING, AND BELONGING DIMENSIONS OF OT PRACTICE

BOX 19.1 Intervention Planning Focus Questions: How to Begin

1. What does it feel like to be a person who is experiencing **depression or mania**?
2. What are some behaviors that a person experiencing **depression or mania** might demonstrate, and how might their behavior, responses, or affect be positively or negatively impacting their occupations?
3. How can I adjust my way of being (therapeutic use of self) to make the client feel more comfortable about their way of being?
4. What can I do to instill a sense of belonging in occupational therapy right now that will encourage the client toward setting goals with outcomes that are personally meaningful and relevant to them?

What Is Depression?

Depression *is a feeling of intense sadness, despair, and hopelessness.* Like anxiety, depression, depressive symptoms, or moments of feeling sad occasionally affect most people. Sadness is an appropriate response to painful losses, such as the death of a loved one, being fired from a job, or being rebuffed by a friend. Most people, when they have adequate resources, social connections, and support, recover from these sad feelings and can carry on with their lives (53). Depression becomes pathologic when it lasts longer than most people would consider reasonable and when it interferes with ordinary daily occupations, to the point of disrupting the person's ability to function.

More than 70 changes and updates were made in March 2022 when the DSM-5-TR was published. In fact, many of those modifications were significant to the Depressive Disorders and the Trauma- and Stressor-Related Disorders spectrum of illnesses (5, 12). Some of the changes in the *DSM-5-TR* included the introduction of new symptom codes for suicidal behavior and nonsuicidal self-injury. Because thoughts and attempts of harming oneself are ubiquitous across many diagnostic groups, a section of text appears in the *DSM-5-TR* (5) with each diagnosis titled, "Association of Suicidal Thoughts or Behavior" (5, p. 19). Also, *Unspecified Mood Disorder*, formerly removed in the DSM-IV (4), was brought back in the *DSM-5-TR*. Without having the *Unspecified Mood Disorder* category, when people experienced mood symptoms that did not fit completely in *Bipolar Disorders* or in the *Depressive Disorders,* their mood symptoms were often left undocumented. Finally, a new diagnosis, *Prolonged Grief Disorder,* was added to the chapter on Trauma- and Stressor-Related Disorders of the new text revision (5, 12).

It can be incredibly difficult to distinguish marked symptoms of depression in the context of an individual's grieving process, or **bereavement**. Bereavement is a time of mourning recognized especially following the death of a loved one. Bereavement can be associated with intense emotions and somatic or physical symptoms that share many features similar to the depressive disorders and to trauma stressor disorders (12). This is especially true because what we understand today about grief continues to evolve and we are far more aware that everyone grieves *differently*. Although the literature is full of models that lay out the common stages of grief, people do not often move through the stages of their grief in a linear way. The length of time that a person grieves is a very personal and situationally dependent matter (18, 19, 39). Historically, professionals have been divided on the topic of grief, with some feeling that grieving loss was a "typical period of depression," which should not be diagnosed. However, like other symptoms, when bereavement is extended, and the affective response so intense that routines, habits, roles, and self-care are impacted, grief is considered pathologic and the person is likely to need support to avoid further dysfunction (39). *Prolonged grief disorder* can be diagnosed if the person is experiencing an intense yearning for or preoccupation with the person who has died, more than 1 year past the time of death. Individuals with this diagnosis must also demonstrate three or more of the following symptoms on most days: loneliness, meaninglessness, emotional numbness, identity disruption, denial of loved one's death, avoiding reminders, intense emotional pain, or being unable to resume activities and social connections (5).

The person who is depressed typically demonstrates a cluster of depressive symptoms that are a reflection of their depression. In Chapter 4, the reader was introduced to a helpful way to recall the core symptoms of depression using the acronym, **SIG E CAPSS**, which stands for **Sadness**, a depressed mood or feelings of sadness (daily or most days); **Interest**, anhedonia, loss of enjoyment or interest in occupations or activities that were once pleasurable; **Guilt**, feelings of worthlessness; **Energy loss**, a lack of energy, feelings of fatigue (daily or most days); **Concentration loss**, problems concentrating or difficulty making decisions; **Appetite change**, gain or loss of more than 5% of total body weight within a month, or significant change in appetite; **Psychomotor agitation or slowing**, physical restlessness, agitation, or a change in energy levels that is noticeable to others; **Sleep change**, sleeping too much (hypersomnia), or not sleeping enough (insomnia); and **Suicidality**, persistent thoughts of death, having a plan to commit suicide, or attempting to commit suicide.

The most striking characteristic is usually the depressed mood, which can be accompanied by negatively biased thinking; "clients with depression experience a negative view of the self, the future, and the world" (52, p. 69). They tend to have a self-defeated view of themselves (ie, consider themselves worthless). They have a bleak view of the future, believing that things are unlikely to get better, and their perspective of the world often includes the assumption that they have few resources or people who care about them (6). Because people with depression experience feelings of helplessness, despair, and sometimes guilt, they typically lose interest in people and activities that previously brought joy or pleasure (called **anhedonia**). During occupational therapy, clients may reveal their low opinion of themselves through their words and actions. Comments such as, "I'm stupid," "Leave me alone, I'm not worth helping," or "I can't do anything right," are typically masking feelings associated with depression and anxiety. Many clients with symptoms of depression or depressive disorders will also present with a low frustration tolerance. Because of low self-confidence and self-esteem, some clients who experience depression tend to blame themselves for whatever goes wrong. This is one reason why occupational analysis is such a critical part of the occupational therapy evaluation because the results help clarify how to plan intervention activities that will allow the client to experience success, while still being sufficiently challenged.

There are many theories that address the causes of depression but the truth is that multiple physiologic and psychosocial influences, combined with other causal factors that could contribute to the development of depression, make it an extremely complex problem. Most of the recent evidence suggests that there are at least four factors likely to contribute to depression: neural development, genetics, an individual's immune system (ie, their inflammatory response, histamine reaction, and their gut health, among others), and the vast array of psychosocial factors, including social determinants of health that are inherent to one's context (22, 31). Neurologic evidence suggests that the neurotransmitters, especially serotonin, norepinephrine, and dopamine, change in relationship to one's mood or affective states. Depression is associated with an overall decrease in levels of serotonin in various parts of the brain (37).

Furthermore, in adolescent clients, the natural development of the brain follows a pattern of increase in gray matter beginning around puberty (about 12 years old), followed by a period of selective pruning and increased myelination of the cortical neurons. This creates potential for enormous growth and organization of the brain that is significantly impacted by one's choices, circumstances, attitudes, and experiences. This extreme and quick loss of gray matter volume results in difficulty regulating emotional states and can place the person at a higher risk for suffering from an affective disorder (36, 54). From an occupational therapy perspective, there is tremendous value in supporting the client in the establishment, or reestablishment, of a healthy lifestyle, which is especially important when we plan interventions with teenagers who experience symptoms of depression.

Diagnoses in Which Depression Is a Common Symptom

Depression occurs in a wide range of affective disorders. It is the primary symptom in bipolar disorders and in major depression. Depression is also common in organic mental disorders and frequently is comorbid with schizophrenia. Depressive symptoms and depressive disorders are characteristic of all the personality disorders and often exist with, or are exacerbated by, substance use disorders. As previously discussed, depressive symptoms and episodic depression can be a normal response to personal loss, major changes, or traumatic circumstances, and therefore symptoms of depression are often present during major transitions in people's lives. People with serious or complex physical conditions such as strokes, cardiac conditions, or multiple sclerosis may also experience depression (24, 38, 55). The same may be true of aging individuals who are in the phase of their lives where they are experiencing multiple losses (ie, of spouse, friends, home, physical functions) (14, 26, 42, 43). Regardless of the etiology of depression, the characteristic depressive symptom of having negative cognitive bias, or a negative view of the self, one's future, and the world at large (6), is common across disorders and offers a place to begin interventions that incorporate the cognitive behavioral frame of reference.

Strategies for Therapeutic Use of Self

Depressive symptoms and difficult emotions such as sadness often make people feel particularly alone and isolated. For an occupational therapy professional, therapeutic use of self begins with an understanding of how to engage the appropriate therapeutic response. Two universal ideas are constant when responding to all clients. First, all clients should be met with compassion and empathy. **Empathy** is "the emotional exchange between occupational therapy practitioners and clients that allows more open communication, ensuring that practitioners connect with clients at an emotional level to assist them with their current life situation" (3, p. 20). According to researcher Dr Brené Brown (10), there are at least two components of empathy. One component is focused on the cognitive aspects of empathy such as recognizing and understanding the emotions of the other person; this is called **cognitive empathy**. Cognitive empathy is also known as *perspective taking*, or *mentalizing*. The other component is **affective empathy**. Affective empathy, referred to sometimes as *experience sharing*, is one's own emotional attunement with the other person's experience (10). Brown proposes that meaningful connections with others rely on a combination of compassion and cognitive empathy.

It is important for the occupational therapy professional to be reminded of the difference between *empathy* (an empathic response) and *sympathy* (a sympathetic response). **Sympathy** is defined as expressing genuine **concern or sorrow for someone** who is suffering, **having pity for them**, whereas **empathy** is **connecting with someone's emotions or experiences**. For all clients, the therapist has a goal of creating a collaborative therapeutic relationship and an authentic connection with their client. Empathy is a skill set and a tool that arises from the desire to develop a compassionate understanding about another person's experiences. It is a way to reveal our shared humanity. To properly respond with empathy, the occupational therapy professional must be willing to be present when someone else is suffering, to sit with someone else's pain (10). However, enacting a sympathetic response, particularly with a client who is experiencing maladaptive symptoms of depression, can backfire and unintentionally result in disconnection. As Dr Brown shares, "There is nothing worse than feeling pitied, and we have research to show us why it feels so isolating. Pity involves four elements: a belief that the suffering person is inferior; a passive self-focused reaction that does not include providing help; a desire to maintain emotional distance; and avoidance of sharing in the other person's suffering" (10, p. 120). Several good examples of clients' preferences for being met with compassion and empathy, rather than sympathy, can be drawn from evidence in the medical literature. In multiple studies that have explored clients' reactions to encounters with a sympathetic response versus an empathic response (to either a physical or mental health diagnosis), clients and families responded overwhelmingly that sympathetic responses felt decidedly superficial. Research participants across studies largely found "pity-based" responses unwanted and most preferred empathic responses, seeing those as being more compassionate and helpful (20, 49, 50).

In Chapter 18, the application of the therapeutic modes according to the IRM was introduced (53). Emotions such as grief, sadness, despair, and other strong emotions that

accompany depressive illnesses can feel less isolating and have the potential to be more manageable for the client if they can be shared with a person they trust. This is why the development of therapeutic rapport and the application of therapeutic use of self, through a therapeutic mode that is most appropriate to the circumstances and client's emotional expression, are greatly important. According to the IRM, there are some occasions during occupational therapy sessions when clients may be more likely to express sadness, such as when an illness, injury, or trauma has significantly altered one's occupational participation (53). When a client demonstrates sadness during therapy, the occupational therapy professional should not discourage or disallow the show of emotions. If the occupational therapy professional is able to respond (especially in the beginning phases of a therapeutic relationship) without judgment and with compassionate support, trust is likely to grow within the relationship when authenticity of emotional expression is allowed. The IRM recommends responding to clients' demonstration of sadness with any of the following witnessing actions to promote an empathic response.

- Demonstrate a sense of presence in the occupational therapy space by staying in the room and respectfully listening quietly (53).
- Without making it obvious, checking in with the client by glancing at them briefly, or occasionally looking at the client (not staring) may help the occupational therapy professional determine whether the client wishes to share more, requires time to work through the emotion, or is inviting the therapist to join in the emotion (53).
- Even a simple gesture such as handing a client a tissue demonstrates supportive care without need for a verbal response (53).

Eye contact from the client, especially during their emotional demonstration, can be a sign that the client is giving the occupational therapy professional permission to be more involved in supporting them. According to the recommendation of the IRM, the occupational therapy professional can use labeling what they observe, or show emotional resonance, as appropriate response strategies (53). "When managing sadness, labeling is most appropriate when you wish to preserve an emotional boundary with the client while at the same time showing support and validation for the client's feelings" (53, p. 230).

One complex aspect of responding to a client's demonstration of depressive symptoms that have interfered with occupation is that the occupational therapy professional must use therapeutic reasoning to determine the need to maintain an emotional boundary with the client because they are experiencing difficulties regulating or controlling their emotions. It is also possible that the client needs to become more effective in verbalizing their feelings, rather than becoming too emotionally dependent on others. Collaborating with the client to help them be more aware of their feelings, and to label them, usually prompts more effective emotional regulation (53). Finally, labeling emotions (verbally) can be helpful with clients who seem to have trouble processing or understanding nonverbal, or affective communication. Labeling is a strategy that adds clarity and often aids in avoiding miscommunication.

Although the application of witnessing, labeling, and emotional resonance, recommended by the IRM, are appropriate places to begin, maladaptive depressive symptoms may not be responsive to these approaches. When clients withdraw from the activities in therapy, or if they seek to continue consistent discussion about their worries or problems during an occupational therapy session, with less attention to the goals of occupational therapy, or if their crying is prolonged or chronic, a referral for increased services from other members of the behavioral health team should be considered. However, despite communicating with colleagues in other disciplines, occupational therapy intervention should continue, and so it is critical for occupational therapy professionals to practice reflective thinking and be apprised of strategies for continuing to support clients with depressive symptoms in progressing toward their occupational goals. For these clients, the IRM (53) suggests initiating interventions with the following general characteristics:

- Reassure the client in a way that does not minimize their experience.
- Assume a take-charge attitude so that the client can rely on someone else to take control.
- As part of the dimensions of occupation "being with" and "doing with," if the client is hesitant to initiate their prioritized occupations independently, the therapist can suggest that the client and occupational therapy professional work through the activity together.

Allow clients with depression to talk about what is bothering them; discussion should focus on exactly how they feel and, if they can articulate, why they believe they are feeling this way. The more they understand about their own contributing factors, the more likely they are to be able to do something about it. It is important for the occupational therapy professional to listen and reflect back what they hear clients saying. Not only does this help the client process through their problems by hearing back what they have shared but this type of active listening is also indicative of the occupational therapy professional's empathic response. For clients who are experiencing hopelessness, it is critical that the occupational therapy professional never agree that the situation seems hopeless. Instead, the therapist should provide direction and help with selection of realistic short-term goals and activities that the client can accomplish. Occupational therapy professionals should facilitate the acquisition of habits, routines, and rituals so that clients accomplish certain tasks regularly and can take satisfaction in that. If clients review what they have done each day, either in the evening or the next morning, this can become a ritual that reminds them of success and reinforces habit formation (56).

Clients who are silent and withdrawn present a special challenge. They may try to discourage staff contact by becoming more withdrawn or hostile, and sometimes attempting to flee from the situation. The occupational therapy

professional should not be deterred by these maneuvers into neglecting withdrawn clients. By approaching them many times, each time for only a brief period, the occupational therapy professional demonstrates their acceptance of these clients as they are, including acceptance of their feelings. As clients become more comfortable, most will eventually respond. For example, the occupational therapy professional may visit the client in the client's customary spot and sit quietly, perhaps commenting occasionally about current events or things that have happened in the community or the clinic. After several visits, the client may be willing to attempt a simple activity on a one-on-one basis. Later, group activities can be introduced while simultaneous one-on-one therapy continues concurrently.

In general, occupational therapy professionals should match their tempo to that of the client, regardless of the client's mood. Occupational therapy professionals should be clear when giving any directions to clients and initially avoid giving them too many choices, until more information can be collected to plan the appropriate level of challenge and avoid overwhelming the client. At first, it is often better to present only two activity choices. Occupational therapy professionals should avoid praising what clients accomplish, rather acknowledging their efforts with a simple comment: "It looks like you've finished that. Is there anything more you'd like to do with it?" Clients with depression are usually well aware of the difference between their present level of functioning and their past abilities; excessive praise may make them think they must be in very bad shape. Providing a level of acceptance for whatever their clients can do at the moment, and not pressuring them into doing more than they seem able to tolerate, encourages better engagement in future activities. It is not unusual for people who are depressed not to want to keep projects that they have made. The project may be poorly executed, reminding them of their low energy level and limited attention to detail. The occupational therapy professional should accept the client's decision to reject the project and should refrain from commenting on it further. When the individual who is depressed talks about negative feelings, the occupational therapy professional should not change the subject or try to "cheer up" the client. These approaches deny the importance of the person's feelings and indicate that the therapist does not accept the client as they are.

Clients who are receiving medication may be expected to show a decrease in depressive symptoms (symptom remission) within the first 3 weeks of beginning the pharmacotherapy treatment. It is likely that as the medication begins to titrate, clients may have more energy. However, it is essential to remember that many clients will still experience symptoms of depression, and that despite appropriate medications, there can still be a real risk of suicide; the risk is even greater for those who have previously attempted suicide. Some of the signs that a person may be thinking of suicide include obvious ones such as talking about it or wondering aloud what it would be like to be dead. Others that are less obvious are the appearance of feeling much better for no clear reason and without intervention, or the giving away of personal possessions. The QPR Institute is an organization whose mission is to provide suicide prevention education and training, and ultimately to reduce suicidal behaviors and save lives (46). QPR stands for question, persuade, and refer. The QPR technique is an evidence-based tool that recommends three steps—questioning, persuading, and referring—to prevent suicide before the suicidal person acts. Often compared to being trained in cardiopulmonary resuscitation (CPR), people trained in QPR learn how to recognize the warning signs of a suicide crisis and practice how to question people who may be at risk for suicide so that they can persuade them to get help and refer them to resources (46).

What Is Mania?

Mania *is a disturbance of mood characterized by excessive happiness (euphoria), generosity (expansiveness), irritability, distractibility, impulsivity, and increased activity level.* The manic individual could be compared to someone driving a car at highway speed, while travelling through a 25-mile-per-hour school zone. Everything is speeded up. People who are manic may also appear to be hyperactive and even sometimes seem agitated. They may speak very rapidly (**pressured speech**) and skip from topic to topic (**flight of ideas**). They find it hard to concentrate on any one thing, instead moving from one activity to another; they are often involved in many different activities simultaneously and they may express an unrealistic view of their own abilities, believing that they can accomplish almost anything (**grandiosity**). They may get involved in very risky enterprises and endanger themselves or their families by spending money frivolously, overextending credit, taking expensive trips, extorting money from others, and so on. They seem unaware of or indifferent to the consequences of their actions (16, 28).

People in manic states typically have very poor judgment, which reveals itself in almost everything they attempt. Their style of dress may be eccentric or downright bizarre. One of the most disruptive qualities of people in manic states is their attitude toward and effect on other people. They have a lot of energy and are often overzealous in their flattery of others. Unfortunately, a person who is experiencing mania does not tend to think about the consequences of their behaviors and actions. As with overspending, the manic person may also give extravagant gifts. In the dynamics of their relationships, unsuspecting others can be drawn in by a person with mania because they enjoy the flattery that fuels their own self-esteem, or they may enjoy the expensive gifts that are a result of the client's mania. It has also been noted that people with mania are very sensitive to others' vulnerabilities. For example, they may say that they cannot be helped by a certain new therapist because that person just got out of school and does not have enough experience. If the therapist really feels insecure about this, the person may be able to drive the therapist away and manipulate the self-esteem of other staff members who may feel superior because they have more experience. Using this maneuver (known as splitting) can create staff conflict, which takes the pressure off the client (35).

Another tactic used by individuals in the manic state is upping the ante. The client starts by making what seems like a reasonable, although not necessarily healthy, request (eg, to go outside to the designated smoking area to smoke a cigarette). Once the request is granted, the person asks for something else, and then something else, until they finally make a request that is completely unreasonable (eg, to have everyone stop working and take a break). When the therapist refuses to grant the final request, the person becomes angry and abusive, arguing that the occupational therapy professional is uptight and rigid.

What purposes do these tactics serve? Why is the person who is manic so ready to manipulate others? Some (35) have argued that such individuals are very ambivalent about their need to be taken care of. They need other people, but are frightened of depending on them, and so they arrange to control and manipulate their caregivers. When such a client finally exhausts the patience of the caregivers and the caregivers take control over the client's behavior, the client has the satisfaction of being taken care of without having to ask for it, or seek out help.

Diagnoses in Which Mania Is a Common Symptom

Mania is the primary symptom of a manic episode in the spectrum of bipolar disorders, but it can occur in other disorders as well. In the United States, about 40% of people presenting with depression are later found to have bipolar disorder (32). The bipolar disorders (and thus the symptom of mania) can be comorbid with psychosis, anxiety disorders, attention-deficit hyperactivity disorder (ADHD), and a tendency to misuse drugs and alcohol. During severe episodes of either depression or mania, psychotic symptoms including hallucinations and delusions may be present and will tend to match the client's high (or low) mood (31). Other conditions where mania is often a primary symptom include substance use disorders, schizophrenia, trauma, and certain personality disorders (particularly borderline personality disorder).

Dr Kay Redfield Jamison, a successful psychiatrist and expert on manic-depressive (bipolar) illness, is also a person living with bipolar disorder. In her autobiography, *An Unquiet Mind: A Memoir of Moods and Madness* (34), Jamison shares the power-charged highs and catastrophic lows that threw her into disastrous spending sprees, episodes of violence, resistance to taking her medication, and eventually an attempted suicide. She examines bipolar illness in a highly readable, first-person account of mania.

Strategies for Therapeutic Use of Self

The manic client's ambivalence about relying on other people raises specific issues for the therapeutic relationship. Unfortunately, it can be easy to unintentionally be manipulated by someone who positively impacts one's ego, or who makes them feel special, and the occupational therapy professional should be aware of excessive flattery, keeping ethical and responsible professional duties and boundaries in mind.

Similarly, criticisms of other staff by a client who is experiencing symptoms of mania are often the opening gambit in a game of "You're the only one who can help me."

These clients may demand almost constant attention, praise, and approval from staff members. At the same time, their behavior for which they are seeking approval is often so odd or self-centered that others avoid them. The occupational therapy professional should be cautious when giving any praise or approval to the person who is in a manic state and, instead, firmly and gently focus on how to make the behavior more appropriate through encouragement rather than praise. However, it is also essential to avoid criticizing someone who is manic because the person is very vulnerable and they are likely to have a heightened sensitivity to feeling rejection. Some psychologists argue that mania is the flip side of depression. In other words, the low self-esteem and feelings of despair and hopelessness that characterize depression are often just under the surface of the manic behavior (32).

It is important to be calm, matter of fact, firm, and consistent with the individual who is manic. Setting and enforcing limits on what the person can do shows the client that *someone* is in control, even when the client is not. Such clients may also interpret limit setting as a message that the staff cares enough about them to stop them from hurting themselves. As medication begins to take effect and symptoms diminish, the person who has been manic may become frightened, remembering the bizarre and impulsive behaviors they have engaged in. Reassuring such clients that these behaviors were caused by the illness can make them feel more comfortable. It is important to recognize, though, that people coming out of a manic episode may face legal or financial problems because of their actions during the manic phase and that they may need future support to make reparations. Collaborating or cotreating with a social worker as the client progresses toward improved functional independence can be helpful in reestablishing community or family resources and relationships that may have been negatively impacted during exacerbations of the illness and the manic symptoms.

TARGETING SYMPTOMS OF DEPRESSION AND MANIA THAT CREATE BARRIERS TO OCCUPATION: THE DOING AND BECOMING DIMENSIONS OF OT PRACTICE

> **BOX 19.2 Intervention Implementation Focus Questions: How to Support Clients' Optimal Engagement in Occupation**
>
> 1. What can the client and the occupational therapy team collaboratively do together that will help the client become more functional and effective in the things that are important to them in everyday life?
> 2. What are the best intervention types and intervention approaches to apply in this therapeutic context?
> 3. What does the current evidence suggest about the most productive interventions for this diagnosis/set of symptoms?

Contextual, Environmental, and Client Factor Considerations for Clients' With Symptoms of Depression

The environment should be safe and subdued. In general, the more severe the depression, the less stimulation should be present in the beginning. It may be necessary to reduce the lighting and the noise level and work one-on-one to support the client's focus on the activity. Too much stimulation may cause the client to retreat further. This is particularly true for withdrawn clients, who may not initially be able to tolerate the others in a group situation. As the client becomes more comfortable, the amount of stimulation should be increased gradually; having more materials, supplies, and sample projects visible will increase opportunities for decision-making.

The structure in an inpatient setting may limit opportunities for clients to make even simple choices and decisions. The schedule of daily activities and routines may be limited and is usually predetermined. For example, meals and menus consist of food choices that have been planned with nutritional guidelines and each person's medical profile considered, but the meal schedule and how meals are served may be very different from the client's natural context and, again, offer few opportunities for making choices. Clients with suicidal ideation, or who demonstrate self-injurious behavior, may have very limited choices for the items that they keep in their room, the clothing that they wear, or access to typical utensils and sharp objects that could be used for self-harm. Showering and shaving may be scheduled around a staffing plan that, while ensuring client safety, leaves the clients' routines at the mercy of staff. These factors can further weaken a fragile sense of self-empowerment that is a common characteristic of people who experience the symptoms of depression. Therefore, limited choices (to prevent overwhelming the client) should be presented whenever possible. In a home-based context, merely deciding to rearrange the furniture, or hang up a picture, can increase the client's sense of responsibility, competence, and personal agency.

Characteristics of Interventions That Support Reduced Symptoms of Depression

Start with simple, structured, short-term, familiar activities. Unstructured activities should be avoided because depression tends to deteriorate people's energy and so making decisions feels very taxing. The activities must be short-term ones because the individual who is depressed typically lacks the attention span for a longer activity and works only slowly and intermittently. For the same reason, activities that require rapid responses at particular moments (eg, smart phone applications or games that have a time-limited response rate) should be avoided unless a staff member or volunteer is available to assist the person. Repetitive activities allow the individual to succeed and require minimal new learning because the motions are learned only once and then repeated. Although familiar activities are generally more comfortable, there is a risk that the client will compare present performance with past performance, further damaging self-esteem. Therefore, simple, unfamiliar activities are sometimes preferred, at least initially.

The overarching goal for the first several sessions with planned therapeutic intervention activities (regardless of the client diagnosis) is to find ways to help the person experience success. For the person experiencing depression, even a simple task such as making a phone call to a friend or brushing one's hair can be a first step. Activities are then graded to include more complexity and require more effort as the person becomes more confident and energetic. In the beginning, the activities should be ones that can be done alone, without the need to interact or share tools or materials with others. Thereafter, opportunities for minimal socialization should be presented as soon as the person seems comfortable. Those who are agitated benefit from activities in which they use their hands; this substitutes productive actions for nonproductive ones such as hand wringing and fidgeting. Gross motor activities that permit moving about are also beneficial for clients who are agitated (21, 30).

People who are depressed may avoid crafts, games, and exercise because these activities seem too far away from their current mood orientation. For example, a client who has not had success in finding pleasure in the occupations that they used to enjoy may find the activity that the occupational therapy professional has planned seems too pleasurable. They may perceive that it would be too exhausting to try to bridge the gap between their current low energy, low mood, and a seemingly pleasurable activity. Clients with depressive symptoms may be more willing to accept and participate in an activity that is deemed important and useful to other people, or even to plants or animals. The occupational therapy professional and other staff should try to accept offers of help from clients who experience depressive symptoms to positively reinforce the client's choice toward action. Withdrawal and inactivity are common themes when a person is depressed, and decreased activity usually plays a role in increasing the client's negatively biased thought patterns, dampening overall recovery efforts. **Behavioral activation**, an evidence-based cognitive behavioral intervention strategy, is introduced in the following section and it begins with getting clients activated and socially reconnected (52).

Some clients respond well to activities that others may find tedious, menial, or repetitive (peeling potatoes, mopping the floor, folding laundry, or completing office tasks). However, for some clients, the repetition without high cognitive demands may create a sense of safety and feel very grounding to them. Although clients should be permitted to do these activities according to their preference, other activities should be introduced gradually so that the person does not use the tasks to further isolate. Gross motor activities can help release tension, promote the intake of oxygen, and increase blood flow to the brain. Exercising outdoors in the daytime may increase the levels of certain neurotransmitters (dopamine and serotonin), in part because of the exposure to daylight (sunlight). There is ample evidence that activity can relieve depression (58), but many times the real problem is motivating the individual with depression to attempt it. The person's low energy level is a serious obstacle, but it can sometimes be overcome by simply telling the client that it is time for the activity (eg, "We are going to the gym now." Or "It's time for our walk. Have you got your jacket?").

Precautions against suicide and self-harm should always be observed and during all activities. Although clients who are depressed may feel more in control if they can use sharp tools without harming themselves, the occupational therapy professional must stay alert to this possibility. Even seemingly innocuous objects can be used in a suicide attempt—for example, a client might use a leather belt or the rope pieces from a macramé project in an attempt at hanging. Particularly in inpatient settings, tools and supplies should be accounted for at the beginning and end of every session and before any client leaves the room, even to go to the bathroom. Similarly, when working with clients outdoors or in open or unfamiliar settings, the assistant must stay aware of the whereabouts of all clients. People who experience depressive symptoms may leave the group and are at a higher risk for self-harm.

Experts suggest teaching the consumer to consistently monitor their moods. When clients become proficient in tracking their mood, they benefit by being able to choose to engage in occupations that support the regulation of their mood (ie, participating in activities that are either arousing or calming, depending on need). Clients may feel discouraged when depression recurs, and psychoeducation about the up-and-down patterns of mood disorders gives them the information that they may really need and find helpful. This is especially the case when the information is delivered in a way that the person understands and in the context of a trusting therapeutic relationship (29, 52). Implementing mood monitoring strategies will also assist clients with establishing or reestablishing mindful habits and routines, which can positively impact compliance with medication management.

Activities that teach people with depression to manage stress and advocate for themselves are critically important for recovery. Such activities include exploration of leisure activities, enhancement of leisure skills, assertiveness training, and role-oriented treatment that focuses on the client's prioritized roles. These experiences help clients to unlearn helplessness. Some individuals who are depressed may feel that their lives are monotonous, too dull, too much the same from day to day. They may feel that their lives lack purpose. In these cases, the occupational therapy professional should be alert to any behaviors (verbal or nonverbal) that may indicate interest in something new. The use of interest inventories during the evaluation and intervention planning phases can be helpful for the purposes of exploration.

Evidence-Based Interventions That Target Symptoms of Depression

If the client can identify occupations that they find pleasurable, gratifying, or fulfilling, even if the depressive symptoms have created barriers to those occupations, the occupational therapy professional may wish to "prescribe" gradual reengagement in the identified activities (40, 47, 48). As mentioned earlier, one of the first ways to encourage the client to reengage in occupation is to help them to develop an awareness of their mood patterns. Implementing the use of mood scales can help both client and therapist assess the severity of the depressive symptoms. Realizing the severity and pattern of depressive symptoms provides the occupational therapy professional an entry point for further assessing how the depressive symptoms interfere with occupational performance and participation. There are a variety of formal and informal mood scales. Formal mood assessments such as the Beck Depression Inventory-II (7) or the Burns Brief Mood Survey (11), among others, are objective self-report measurement tools that are considered valid and reliable. Occupational therapy professionals can incorporate these measures into the occupational therapy process using the tool as either a way to screen clients to assess whether a referral should be made to a psychologist or mental health counselor (if one is not already involved) or the tools can be used in combination with occupation-based assessments for intervention treatment planning.

A less formal and equally effective alternative to more formal mood assessments is suggested by authors and psychologists Drs Sokol and Fox (52). They recommend asking clients to provide a subjective rating of their mood using a traditional Likert scale. "Depending on the difficulties that the clients are experiencing, you can ask them to rate their level of irritability, agitation, frustration, anger, anxiety, or hopelessness on a scale from 0 (not at all severe) to 10 (severe)" (52, p. 69). As is true for many mental illnesses, recovery from depression is a lifelong process and relief of symptoms is a necessary precursor to reengaging in occupation. But feeling relief of symptoms from depression can be a slow process and one that occurs over an extended time period. Because it can be a slow or bumpy road to recovery, clients who are experiencing depressive symptoms often cannot distinguish the difference between severe depression (severe depressive symptoms), moderate depression (moderate depressive symptoms), and finally the lifting of the depressive symptoms. Completing daily or weekly mood ratings allows the clients to have a visual log so that they can celebrate even small improvements in mood (52).

In outpatient settings, Sokol and Fox (52) recommend incorporating a brief informal mood assessment or mood check-in at the beginning of an occupational therapy session

each week, and at the end of the session, so that the client can have an opportunity to reflect upon what positively or negatively impacted the mood. Having an intentional mood check at the end of a session with clients who are at an increased or significant risk for self-harm can help remind the practitioner to assess for indicators that a higher level of resources or more immediate intervention is required. If mood assessments are completed consistently throughout the therapeutic process, mood scales can also help the occupational therapy professional analyze the data to determine the efficacy of different intervention approaches, strategies, and intervention types. In inpatient settings, collecting these data across the therapeutic milieu can provide invaluable information to the behavioral health team for planning the client's discharge and transition back into the home or community.

Lastly, when the occupational therapy professional assesses a client's mood through a client-reported self-check at the beginning of a session, the data can be used as an immediate source for adjusting the priorities of individual occupational therapy intervention sessions. For example, if the client reports a low mood, the occupational therapy professional can briefly explore which area of the persons occupations have been most significantly impacted by the low mood since the last occupational therapy session (ie, sleep disruptions, impaired mobility, problematic eating, decreased hygiene or grooming, role disruptions) and then prioritize those occupational goals to target for that session (52). See the examples in Table 19.1 for examples of daily and weekly Likert scales of mood ratings.

Depressive symptoms reduce the client's participation in occupations, which is usually also characterized by withdrawal from social participation. Isolation and negatively biased thinking inhibits recovery. To initiate the evidence-supported method of behavioral activation, the occupational therapy professional needs to begin by learning what a client's daily life looks like at present, so that they can assess and document the client's level of occupational function. "The activity schedule is the tool of choice for getting a behavioral assessment of your client's activity" (52, p. 71). There are a variety of different activity schedule formats that the occupational therapy professional can integrate into occupational therapy intervention; but for the client who is experiencing symptoms of depression (or of mood disorders), it is essential to collect information that gives a clear picture

Table 19.1. Examples of Informal Weekly and Daily Mood Scales

Ask the Client . . .	Use This Likert Scale . . .										
Ask the client to rate their average mood over the past week on whichever specific mood(s) are being tracked and evaluated.	Not at all		Mild			Moderate			Severe		
	0	1	2	3	4	5	6	7	8	9	10
Use this daily log alone or in addition to the weekly mood tracker. Ask the client to keep a daily log of their overall mood.	Poor		Below Average			Average		Good		Excellent	
	0	1	2	3	4	5	6	7	8	9	10

Adapted from Sokol, L., & Fox, M. G. (2019). *The comprehensive clinician's guide to cognitive behavioral therapy.* PESI Publishing.

of both the client's typical daily/weekly activities and their mood during the activities. By collecting this information, the occupational therapist can evaluate the client's level of enjoyment, their sense of self-sufficiency and accomplishment, and the degree of social connection that are associated with the occupations, while also assessing how engagement in the various activities impacts mood (41, 52).

The Model of Human Occupation (MOHO) can be applied to guide intervention planning and implementation for clients who are experiencing the symptoms of depression or mania that are interfering with occupation (23). Several MOHO-based assessment tools that can be used to incorporate an activity schedule with clients exist. These include, among others, the National Institutes of Health (NIH) Activity Record (ACTRE) (25, 27) and the Occupational Questionnaire (OQ) (51). The ACTRE asks the client to record their participation in activities by 30-minute intervals throughout their day. Clients categorize the activities and rate their levels of difficulty in completing the task, recording their pain and fatigue levels, as well as their competence and enjoyment of the activity (25, 27). The OQ (51) is another activity record with a client self-report format that can be used throughout occupational therapy intervention to assess occupational therapy outcomes or to monitor a change in a client's participation (23).

The OQ was designed on the basis of the ACTRE and is essentially a shortened version of it (23, 51). However, the additional requirement of asking the client to identify the type of activity as **work** (paid or unpaid; the occupation of education could also be considered within this category), **daily living tasks** or tasks that are related to one's self-care (ie, activities of daily living [ADLs]; instrumental activities of daily living [IADLs]; or health management), **recreation** including both structured and unstructured tasks and time (play or leisure), or **rest** (rest and sleep) embeds occupational language within the record, offering the occupational therapy professional a way to ensure that occupation consistently remains the focus of the intervention and outcomes (23). The OQ goes on to ask the client to consider how well they feel that they do the activities (occupational competence), how important activities are to them (occupational value and priority), and how much they enjoy them (51). Both the ACTRE (25, 27) and the OQ (51) can be used with adolescents or adults, and either tool can be easily modified to add a simple informal mood rating scale. This would provide the occupational therapy professional and the client an effective tool for collecting data that reflect the relationship between occupational engagement (action), mood, feelings, and behaviors.

Ultimately the goal for the client in completing an activity schedule and the mood scale is for them to be able to use the information that they collected to reflect upon where the barriers to optimal engagement in occupation are the most evident. The evidence reflected by the activity schedule or mood scale typically reveals problems with the clients' performance skills or performance patterns. The activity/mood schedule and scale may uncover behavioral inactivity, an unbalanced schedule, a lack of social interaction, too

much time in bed, or even spending too much time focused on unproductive or destructive behaviors (eg, drug-seeking behaviors for a person with an addiction problem). From the cognitive behavioral theoretical perspective, collaboration with the client to first help them develop an awareness of the problem and understand the purpose and value of setting a schedule can support motivation for action. In some ways, what the client learns by seeing a glimpse of their daily life on paper, in the form of an activity schedule, especially with the guidance of the therapist, becomes a tool that drives the client toward action. Importantly, the schedule "serves as a starting point for intentionally planning activities that clients can gradually begin incorporating into their schedule" (52, p. 75). This also helps the occupational therapy professional when planning interventions because the activities that the client has reported as being associated with elevated mood, per their activity schedule and mood scale, can be prioritized in occupational therapy sessions.

Clients who are experiencing depressive symptoms are usually trapped in a vicious cycle that often begins with the person withdrawing from life. The withdrawal from typical life activities negatively impacts the client's performance patterns across occupational areas (ie, poor self-care, inability to help with typical parenting roles and responsibilities, decreased efficiency at work that may lead to job loss, etc). These barriers to engaging in occupation then perpetuate social isolation that further discourages action or activity. The literature suggests that inactivity and isolation drive a sense of hopelessness that further damages the person's perspective of themselves and of their future (21, 26, 30, 52). According to Sokol and Fox (52), "When clients have no obligation to leave their bed or home, depression continues to prevail" (p. 75). One antidote to this prevailing depression is to implement the principles of *behavioral activation* into the intervention plan. There are seven key concepts for the occupational therapy professional and the client to be aware of for the behavioral activation method to be the most effective. The key concepts of behavioral activation are listed and summarized in Table 19.2. The concepts are also correlated with the possible dimensions of occupation that may be foregrounded during an occupational therapy intervention, according to the Pan Occupational Paradigm (33), when the behavioral activation process is applied (10, 52).

Contextual, Environmental, and Client Factor Considerations for Clients With Symptoms of Mania

Supporting the client to help them control their context and environment to the extent possible is based on a single principle: Clients who experience depressive symptoms and unipolar depression tend to be underresponsive and withdrawn, whereas clients with mania tend to be hyperresponsive to every bit of stimulation presented to them, with a common tendency to fail to recognize their limitations. Therefore, the occupational therapy professional should, first and foremost, eliminate or reduce distractions in the environment or space

Table 19.2. The Key Concepts of Behavioral Activation: An Evidence-Based Intervention for Clients With Depressive Symptoms	
Key Concept 1: Action Precedes Motivation Doing, being, becoming, belonging: Which of these dimension(s) of occupation are represented by this key concept of behavioral activation when applied during occupational therapy intervention?	Decreased motivation and lack of energy are symptoms of depression but they are NOT obstacles to action. Taking action despite experiencing these symptoms is what creates improved energy, increased motivation, and shifts mood to a more positive level.
Key Concept 2: Success Is in the Effort, Not the Outcome Doing, being, becoming, belonging: Which of these dimension(s) of occupation are represented by this key concept of behavioral activation when applied during occupational therapy intervention?	• Outcomes can be impacted by contextual variables that are outside of a person's control. Sometimes effort is not obvious in immediate outcomes. • Depressive symptoms make even small tasks require tremendous effort and make most tasks feel very challenging. • Success is in the doing. • Taking action *is* the SUCCESS, not the outcome.
Key Concept 3: Establish a Goal and Rationale Doing, being, becoming, belonging: Which of these dimension(s) of occupation are represented by this key concept of behavioral activation when applied during occupational therapy intervention?	• When applying a cognitive or cognitive behavioral approach, the specificity of the client's goal is less important than the person "buying-in" or believing that the goal makes sense and is in their best interest. • Collaborate with the client to make a list of the benefits or advantages to working on this goal. When the client helps determine the rationale for the goal, it makes more sense and does not feel like something others are requiring, demanding, or suggesting that they "should do." • A client may remind themselves that "I don't have to do this, but it makes sense to tackle this goal" (52, p. 77).
Key Concept 4: Have a Plan and Put It on the Schedule Doing, being, becoming, belonging: Which of these dimension(s) of occupation are represented by this key concept of behavioral activation when applied during occupational therapy intervention?	• For clients who have experienced significant occupational disruption because of depressive symptoms, the most critical part of any intervention is having a detailed plan of action, and also *scheduling the plan of action*. • To increase the chances that actions will happen, put the activity on the schedule. This creates a visual reminder to the client that they are taking active steps to get better. • Even planned and scheduled events sometimes change or get canceled. Encourage the client to keep rescheduling the activity until it occurs so that they meet their goal.
Key Concept 5: Change Your Self-Talk From "Give-Up" Thoughts, to "Go-To" Thoughts Doing, being, becoming, belonging: Which of these dimension(s) of occupation are represented by this key concept of behavioral activation when applied during occupational therapy intervention?	• Clients with depression often sabotage themselves by avoiding action. "Helping clients mobilize themselves provides the data needed to address the negative biases of depression that get in the way of action" (52, p. 80). • "Give-up" thoughts are automatic thoughts, usually driven by fear or a sense of hopelessness, that sway people from taking action. Examples include thoughts such as "I can't do this," "I'll do it later," or "I don't feel like it" (52). • "Go-to" thoughts are rational, objective, and goal-directed thoughts (52). Clients can learn to change negative thoughts that lead to occupational disruption by practicing replacement of "give-up" thoughts with "go-to thoughts."
Key Concept 6: Take Credit Doing, being, becoming, belonging: Which of these dimension(s) of occupation are represented by this key concept of behavioral activation when applied during occupational therapy intervention?	• Important aspects of people's lives, including their identity, their self-worth, the evaluation of the past, and their choices or decisions for the future, all have the potential to be impacted by comparison. It is human nature to compare ourselves both to our past selves and to other people, but comparison can be the thief of joy, self-confidence, and self-worth (10). • Clients who experience depressive symptoms are especially vulnerable to comparing themselves to other people who are not experiencing obvious external signs of depression, or to their own previously higher levels of function. They tend to negate or minimize any effort or degree of their success. • The occupational therapy professional should encourage the client to celebrate and take credit for every small effort and not wait until the goal is fully met. Explain that celebrating all efforts will silently improve intrinsic motivation and sustain the person until they are able to fully reach their goal.

(continued)

Table 19.2. The Key Concepts of Behavioral Activation: An Evidence-Based Intervention for Clients With Depressive Symptoms (*continued*)

Key Concept 7:
Consider the Reward
Doing, being, becoming, belonging:
Which of these dimension(s) of occupation are represented by this key concept of behavioral activation when applied during occupational therapy intervention?
	• Understanding how systems of rewards affect behavior change is a complex task. Rewards that are tangible, or that are available in a physical sense, called extrinsic or external rewards, are not typically effective for promoting long-lasting, beneficial, behavior change.
	• Intrinsic (or internal) rewards are more efficacious for supporting the client's behavior changes as they battle depressive symptoms. Sokol and Fox (52) suggest the following client self-talk reminders as ways for the client to consider the rewards that maximize long-term recovery:
	  • The reward is the sense of accomplishment that I feel.
	  • The reward is my mood improving.
	  • The reward is the little bit of pleasure that I feel.
	  • The reward is my self-confidence growing.

Adapted from Brown, B. (2021). *Atlas of the heart: Mapping meaningful connection and the language of human experience.* Random House; Hitch, D., Pepin, G., & Stagnitti, K. (2018). The pan occupational paradigm: Development and key concepts. *Scandinavian Journal of Occupational Therapy, 25*(1), 27–34; Sokol, L., & Fox, M. G. (2019). *The comprehensive clinician's guide to cognitive behavioral therapy.* PESI Publishing.

where the occupational therapy session will take place, to the greatest possible extent. For example, in an inpatient unit where the occupational therapy professional leads activities groups, and where the clients may choose a project that they would like to work on, the space should not be cluttered with many examples of finished projects, or have the available choices of interesting materials for completing projects on display. Stimuli such as these are likely to provoke intense interest and it risks encouraging the client to want to try to do everything at once. To avoid this, the occupational therapy professional should strip the environment of everything but what is essential to the activity. Tools and supplies needed for later steps in a project should be kept out of sight until such time as they are needed.

Remember that *anything* can distract the individual who is experiencing mania, which makes their attention to details, directions, and sometimes even to advice from people whom the client trusts, less likely to be heard or followed. Music, other people, cell phones, and even the view from the window can all invite the most intense curiosity and involvement. Distractions should be minimized as much as possible, especially in the acute experience of manic symptoms. If possible, have the person working in their own designated space, preferably one-on-one with the occupational therapy professional, or in a group of no more than 3 to 5 people. Accept that the person is likely to move away from their workstation, allow space for some movement, and use encouragement to draw the client back to the project when possible.

Getting a person who is manic to focus on just one activity is a challenge. Even when the therapeutic relationship has been enacted successfully, the occupational therapy professional may attempt to provide directions or give suggestions or support, and be met with responses from a manic individual that are grandiose, unrealistic, and can seem disrespectful (eg, "I'm very creative. I don't really need to look at the patterns for designs. I already have a design in my mind, and I know how to make beaded jewelry. I'm going to finish at least 10 bracelets so that I can sell them to the nurses

on the unit. I can take orders for more because I am sure everyone will want them when they see my designs."). The occupational therapy professional should not go along with these unrealistic plans and should instead consistently suggest and reinforce a more realistic plan or activity. Set firm limits on the use of supplies and materials initially, so that as the manic behaviors subside, limitations and restrictions can gradually be lessened. This requires constant alertness and patience; the occupational therapy professional is likely to need to calmly remind and redirect the client many times over. As the person's mood becomes more stable, expectations for attention span and decision-making should be increased (8, 57).

The person experiencing mania is likely to resist rules and expectations for performance, implying in effect that "My way is much more creative. Please don't limit my creativity." It is important to avoid getting emotionally involved in discussing why a project should be done a certain way; instead, firmly and briefly explain what has to be done and show the client a sample. If the person insists on doing it differently, there is no point in arguing about it as long as no one is endangered. A sense of humor and the ability for the occupational therapy professional to be adept at perspective taking is very helpful in establishing and maintaining a therapeutic relationship with manic individuals. Because of the common characteristics of mania that include such things as high distractibility, poor judgment, and impulsivity, these clients should be carefully monitored during acute manic episodes to prevent unintentional accidents and injuries.

Characteristics of Interventions That Support Reduced Symptoms of Mania

Because of the high energy level, activities that permit the person to get up and move around are ideal. Short-term activities provide immediate gratification to the person with poor frustration tolerance and inability to wait for results. Allen (1) recommends that activities be portable because the client is likely to want to carry projects around. Activities should be structured and have three or fewer steps. Activities that are unfocused or creative or that require decisions (eg, oil painting) should be avoided during acute episodes. Similarly, activities should not require extensive fine motor coordination or attention to detail. Materials for project work should be easy to manipulate, rather than tedious, loose, or unpredictable (eg, leather, wood, or clay, rather than liquid materials, cloth, or yarn). Because the person who is manic usually needs to develop a longer attention span, provide activities that involve carryover of skills from one day to the next. If the person has expressed an interest in sewing, needlework, or quilting, adapt the activity using different materials. For example, the whipstitch can be done first on leather and later as an embroidery stitch (fabric is floppier and therefore less controllable than leather).

Clients in a manic state may benefit from gross motor exercise because it allows them to move around so that they can channel their excess energy. However, the appropriate staffing plan should be in place before implementing exercise groups with more than three or four members if one is acutely manic; more staff members are needed for larger groups. In later stages, as medication becomes effective, the person coming out of a manic episode can benefit from exploring ways to create and maintain a balanced daily schedule, including ample time for rest and sleep (9). A brief overview of suggested examples of appropriate activities for a client who is experiencing mania is provided in Box 19.3.

Evidence-Based Interventions That Target Symptoms of Mania

The bipolar spectrum of disorders is typically treated with some combination of medication, psychotherapy, and psychoeducation but the research continues to explore the efficacy of various approaches to intervention (31, 32). By and large, the primary treatment for bipolar disorders is medications such as lithium, ketamine, and risperidone; however, the side effects and potential of toxicity with lithium make some medications imperfect for particular clients (8). Group therapy (especially family therapy), behavioral interventions, and educational approaches when combined with medication provide a foundation for continued recovery and improved quality of life (13, 15). However, cognitive behavioral interventions have repeatedly been shown to have higher rates of efficacy than psychoeducational approaches (15, 45). Therefore, the occupational therapy professional can utilize the activities schedule and behavioral activation method as an evidence-based intervention with clients who are manic; however, the goals of the activities schedule are different.

With the manic client, the activities schedule is used in the opposite way than it is implemented with a client who experiences depressive symptoms. The client with mania tends toward overaction, hyperreactivity, usually has an inflated sense of self, an unrealistic or grandiose idea of their abilities, and can be impulsive. An activities schedule can be used to help the client monitor and *decrease* their activities. With the

> ### BOX 19.3 Examples of Intervention Activities Appropriate for Clients Experiencing Mania
>
> As with any other client in an activities or leisure exploration group, it is best to let the client choose the activity. The occupational therapy professional should present only two or, at most, three choices. Ideas about what activities might be appropriate can be obtained from the person's occupational profile, any of the screening or evaluation results, or from the occupational performance analysis.
>
> - **Crafts** that might be considered are copper tooling, stringing beads or making beaded jewelry, and sanding and finishing prefabricated wooden projects. Some clients respond well to small leather projects or weaving with sturdy materials. The occupational therapy professional may need to perform one or more of the steps, especially if they involve fine motor coordination (eg, ending the lacing during a leather or weaving project, or applying a clasp or closure to the beaded jewelry). Projects in which the person's name can be part of the design appeals to some individuals when they are manic.
>
> - **Semistructured activities** can be used with caution. For example, a magazine picture collage will invite chaos unless it is structured; by providing only a few magazines and a pair of scissors at first, then supplying the backing paper after the pictures have been selected and cut out, and the glue only after the pictures have been arranged, the occupational therapy professional will help the client stay in control of what they are doing and increase the likelihood of obtaining a better result.
>
> - **Gross motor activities** such as dance, exercise, and team sports like volleyball can help the client work off energy and allows a productive outlet for the person's symptoms of hyperactivity. Sometimes it is easier to work one-on-one in an exercise activity with the person instead of in a group, and this usually depends upon the setting and the availability of staff.
>
> - **Time management, stress management, and money management activities** may be of use to persons who have recently experienced a manic episode or who have a history of such episodes.

help of the therapist, the activities schedule can also be used to collect data that help the client with mania to develop an awareness of when they are pushing their own boundaries to an unhealthy place (52). When an occupational therapy professional collaborates with a client who is experiencing mania, the following recommendation aligns closely with the goals of occupational therapy intervention because it focuses on improving the client's engagement in daily life through habit training and establishment of healthy patterns and routines. "The best starting point is to normalize sleep, exercise, diet, and thought patterns; take a 20-minute robust walk twice a day, regulate sleep patterns, direct dietary habits toward healthy foods, and encourage positive self-contemplation" (31, p. 197).

MANAGING SYMPTOMS OF DEPRESSION AND MANIA: THE BECOMING AND BELONGING DIMENSIONS OF OT PRACTICE

BOX 19.4 Focus Questions for Planning Transition, Maintenance, and Long-Term Wellness Plans

1. How does the client define success in reaching their goals?
2. How can occupational therapy support the long-term success in the client becoming who they want to be, successfully doing what they want to do?
3. How can occupational therapy support the client's recovery and long-term success in finding community, and feeling a sense of belonging and connectedness?

Social and Emotional Health Promotion and Maintenance for Symptoms of Depression and Mania

Although psychopharmaceutical intervention with medication may help the client to work toward an improved affective state or more consistent mood, clients who have experienced chronic symptoms of depression, anxiety, or mania (bipolar disorders) often require assistance with rebuilding damaged self-esteem and damaged social relationships. According to the Depression and Bipolar Support Alliance (DBSA) (17), wellness can be attained by understanding one's strengths and by finding even small ways to be more active and move forward in one's life. Nevertheless, fighting depressive symptoms and maintaining one's recovery requires commitment because it is a multistep process. Sokol and Fox (52) suggest that the following stages must be present for a client to use action and cognitive behavioral therapy (CBT) strategies to sustain and grow their self-confidence; they must consistently be ready to, **rethink**, **relax**, and **respond**.

In stage 1, the clients learn to practice the techniques of cognitive restructuring and in time can identify their errors in thinking and **rethink** their thoughts, assumptions, and beliefs. Although in the beginning therapy stage 2 seems very difficult, with time the second stage, **relax**, becomes far easier. When a person is more able to identify and modify errors in thought, it becomes easier to replace the unhealthy thoughts with more helpful (and more realistic) thoughts and beliefs. The reduction in negatively biased thinking makes room for more hopeful thoughts, which are commonly followed by experiencing an increase in positive emotions. The occupational therapy professional can help clients promote relaxation (which ushers in positive emotions) by introducing the client to evidence-based techniques for quieting their mind and easing tension in their body. Meditation and mindfulness techniques, diaphragmatic breathing, progressive relaxation, and even time spent with a trusted companion or community, are all well-evidenced techniques for promoting wellness (44). The final stage is that the client must be prepared with a behavioral strategy that they can **respond** to when depressive symptoms try to steal their energy or negative thought patterns rear their ugly head. Similarly, a client who has recovered from a manic episode, and the people in the client's support network, should have a plan for how to recognize and respond to the warning signs that a manic episode may occur (52).

Symptom and Condition Management for Symptoms of Depression or Mania

The DBSA *Wellness Wheel* (17) is an easy-to-use tool that helps give the client a holistic picture of their wellness journey. Furthermore, the tool can be continually used throughout their recovery maintenance. The DBSA *Wellness Wheel* allows the client to inventory their strengths across seven key areas of wellness: spiritual, social, occupational, intellectual, environmental, financial, and physical. The wheel can be created at any point during occupational therapy sessions but is especially helpful for the client to take the resource with them following discharge so that they have a simple tool to continue to remind them to make new goals, and to document and reflect upon their strengths and progress. The DBSA website link is available in the section "Suggested Resources" at the end of the chapter. The website also offers additional resources that clients may find helpful during recovery, including the *DBSA Wellness Wheel COVID-19 Workbook* and a *DBSA Goal Planner* and *Goal Tracker* (17).

Effective Use of Occupation-Centered Outcome Measures

Selection of intervention activities depends on the client's unique treatment goals. For clients with depression, goals may include things such as improving role balance, increasing coping skills, enhancing independent living skills, or improving social skills, among other things, but the occupational therapy professional must always ensure that the outcomes of client goals are infused with occupation. Outcomes that are occupation centered are apparent because they describe the distinct ways that a client's life has been or will be positively impacted through collaboration and participation in occupational therapy intervention (22). Measurable occupation-based outcomes are used to reflect the client's achievement of intervention goals related to enhanced or improved occupational participation. As a reminder, these outcomes use occupation as a means to help clients meet their therapeutic goals as they progress through the occupational therapy process. Outcomes that are experienced by clients after they have realized the effects of their engagement in occupation and reflect upon how the participation enabled them to return to their desired habits, roles, routines, and rituals demonstrate the use of occupation as an end to the therapeutic occupational therapy process (3).

Case

Myra: A 19-Year-Old Female With Depression

DSM-5-TR **Diagnosis at Admission**

F34.1   Persistent Depressive Disorder

Z Codes

Z62.891   Sibling relational problem
Z59.6   Low income
Z63.4   Uncomplicated bereavement

Myra is a 19-year-old single Latinx woman with a *DSM-5-TR* diagnosis of Persistent Depressive Disorder (F34.1). She was admitted to the acute admissions crisis ward of a behavioral health hospital after a nearly fatal suicide attempt (pills) following several months of depression, withdrawal, and refusal to leave her mother's house. This is her third hospitalization in 1 year. Myra is medicated with fluvoxamine (Luvox) 100 mg, but her mother reports that Myra is inconsistent with taking her medications.

Myra is the oldest of three children who are living with their mother. Her father died when she was 13 years old. The client states that she no longer has contact with any friends since her best friend from high school moved from Texas to Florida. She used to socialize with friends and had dated some but was never in a serious relationship.

Myra is a high school graduate and attended college for two semesters, majoring in psychology; she had hoped to enroll eventually in nursing school but quit college to move to Florida with her friend. She stayed there only a few months and returned home, withdrawn and depressed. She subsequently refused to leave her mother's home, leading to this hospitalization.

Myra worked as a nanny and housekeeper in a private residence during her stay in Florida. At present, she has no income of her own and relies on her mother for economic support. She was referred to occupational therapy for a general evaluation of employability skills, leisure interests, and a stress assessment.

The following evaluations or screenings were administered: informal structured activity analysis of self-care routine, to gain insight about her basic occupational performance skills, *Occupational Performance History Interview 2.0* (OPHI-II), Modified Interest Checklist, and Stress Profile.

Occupational Profile Data Collection Interview and Evaluation

The interview revealed little new information. Most of Myra's occupational roles have been as a student. She reported that she enjoyed school and did well there. She expressed no interest, however, in the world of work, stating that she is not interested in going to school or getting a job. She appeared despondent throughout the interview. She was, however, clean, neat, and appropriately groomed.

In a mixed-level general crafts group in which functional skills were assessed, the client worked on a simple mosaic tile task. She completed the task easily, requesting instruction from the therapist only twice. She did not interact with others, isolated herself, and did not respond to casual conversation initiated by the therapist. She expressed indifference about the task, saying she did not care whether she completed it or not. No problems in cognition, memory, or coordination were noted.

Results of the *Modified Interest Checklist* indicated a strong interest in social recreational activities (conversations with friends, gaming, and social media), athletic activities (soccer, working out, swimming), and manual activities (cleaning, crafting, making jewelry).

The *Stress Profile* and follow-up discussion revealed that Myra frequently experiences severe stress that is often exacerbated by frustration over situations in the home environment such as fighting (especially among siblings), rules, financial worries, living conditions, and lack of activity. Myra finds leisure time depressing and feels she has no real accomplishments. She says living at home is too strict and cites her relationship with her mother as particularly stressful. She also reports a strong feeling of loss associated with the death of her father, her own graduation from school, and her separation from her friend who moved to Florida. In addition, Myra discussed her asthma, allergies, and acne. She says she feels ugly. She feels that others do not understand her.

She stated that she would like to have friends and would like to feel better about how she looks. She continued to express that she is not interested in working or going to school.

Please find follow-up case reflections and questions in the section "OT HACKS Summary."

OT HACKS SUMMARY

O: **Occupation as a means and an end**

Selection of intervention activities depends on the client's unique intervention priorities and goals. For clients with depression, goals may include the following:

- Improved role balance
- Increasing coping skills
- Enhancing independent living skills
- Improving or developing social skills
- Learning or improving performance skills
- Increasing active participation in pleasurable and necessary occupations

The occupational therapy professional must always ensure that the outcomes of client goals are infused with occupation. Outcomes that are occupation centered are apparent because they describe the distinct ways that a client's life has been or will be positively impacted through collaboration and participation in occupational therapy intervention (22).

T: **Theoretical concepts, values, and principles, or historical foundations**

The following recommendation aligns closely with the goals of occupational therapy intervention because it focuses on improving the client's engagement in daily life through habit training and establishment of healthy patterns and routines. "The best starting point is to normalize sleep, exercise, diet, and thought patterns; take a 20-minute robust walk twice a day, regulate sleep patterns, direct dietary habits toward healthy foods, and encourage positive self-contemplation" (31, p. 197).

H: How can we Help? OT's role in serving clients with mental illness or mental health needs

Occupational therapy professionals should facilitate the acquisition of habits, routines, and rituals so that clients accomplish certain tasks regularly and can take satisfaction in small achievements. If clients review what they have done each day, either in the evening, or the next morning, this can become a ritual that reminds them of successes and reinforces habit formation (56).

A: Adaptations

- Clients who are experiencing depressive symptoms are usually trapped in a vicious cycle that often begins with the person withdrawing from life.
- Withdrawal from life activities creates occupational imbalance and negatively impacts the clients' performance patterns across occupational areas (ie, poor self-care, inability to help with typical parenting roles and responsibilities, decreased efficiency at work which may lead to job loss, etc).
- These barriers to occupational engagement further perpetuate social isolation and discourage action or activity.
- The literature suggests that inactivity and isolation drive a sense of hopelessness that further damages the person's perspective of themselves and of their future (21, 26, 30, 52).
- Some evidence-based antidotes to combat destructive depressive symptoms (and symptoms of mania) are to implement the principles of *behavioral activation,* use *activities schedules* and *mood tracking,* and eventually apply *cognitive restructuring* techniques into the intervention plan. All these CBT strategies have been shown to be efficacious in treating symptoms of depression and bipolar disorders that interfere with occupation (13, 31, 52).

C: Case study includes

Can you answer the following questions related to Myra's case?

1. After reading and reflecting upon Myra's case, which client factor(s) do you believe that her depressive symptoms are the most reflective of: her emotional status, her cognitive status and motivational level, or her self-concept and self-esteem levels? Defend your answer with evidence of specific problems cited in the case that Myra is experiencing with engagement in occupation.

2. As the occupational therapy professional working with a behavioral health team, what additional information would you like to have to collaborate with her to plan her occupational therapy intervention and set occupation-focused goals with Myra? Please articulate at least three additional questions that you would like to ask Myra, and discuss any further screening or assessment tools that you would like to incorporate during the course of occupational therapy sessions.

3. In an inpatient acute crisis department, it is likely that Myra's length of stay in acute care will extend no more than 3 to 5 days, at which time, depending on her status, she will likely be discharged or transitioned to either an inpatient unit or to a partial hospitalization outpatient program. As her occupational therapy professional during the acute stages of care, explain what you believe are your priorities in this setting while working with Myra? What would you predict as being priorities for future occupational therapy sessions beyond acute care?

4. Discuss why Key Concept 1 of the behavioral activation method, "Action Precedes Motivation" is relevant to planning intervention activities for Myra. Which other key concepts of behavioral activation are significant for intervention planning in Myra's situation? Explain the rationale for your choices.

K: Knowledge: keeping mental health OT practice grounded in evidence, in occupational science, and in research

A few key points are given here:

"The extent of restricted participation in our sample was surprising" (24, p. 310).

" . . . we found that people with CHF experience drastic reductions in participation across all activity domains and that these participation restrictions may, in part, result from executive dysfunction and depressive symptoms" (24, p. 311).

The sample included only 27 participants, 21 males and 6 females. Of these, 15 participants were Caucasian and 12 participants were African American. The age range was 24 to 64 years and the mean age was 49.1. Among the results of the study was an apparent relationship between executive dysfunction and depressive symptoms and reduced participation in a range of life activities including social and family activities, ADL and IADL, and work. Memory and attention did not seem to affect participation. The authors used multiple assessment measures and had access to others, as the study is part of a much larger longitudinal (over time) study of the effects of heart transplantation.

Evidence Application and Translation Questions

1. Is the sample large enough in this study?
2. Where might a study like this be ranked in the levels of evidence?
3. How might you use the information with a client who has CHF?
4. How would you search for other articles addressing similar problems for people with different physical conditions?

S: Some terms that may be new to you

Affective empathy: referred to sometimes as *experience sharing,* is one's own emotional attunement with the other person's experience (10)

Anhedonia: loss of pleasure or inability to feel pleasure

Behavioral activation: an evidence-based cognitive behavioral intervention strategy that promotes action and participation in activity to combat depressive symptoms. Action is the goal, despite a person's lack of motivation or feelings of apathy. Activity is thought to help improve mood and spur further participation (to offset isolation and inactivity).

Bereavement: a time of mourning recognized especially following the death of a loved one

Cognitive empathy: a component of empathy that is focused on the cognitive aspects of empathy such as recognizing and understanding the emotions of the other person (10)

Depression: the experience of having feelings of intense sadness, despair, and hopelessness

Empathy: "the emotional exchange between occupational therapy practitioners and clients that allows more open communication, ensuring that practitioners connect with clients at an emotional level to assist them with their current life situation" (3, p. 20)

Flight of ideas: skipping from topic to topic, with the ideas not being necessarily connected between topics

Grandiosity: an unrealistic view of one's abilities, or a belief that one can accomplish anything (despite realistic limitations and practical barriers)

Mania: a disturbance of mood characterized by excessive happiness (euphoria), generosity (expansiveness), irritability, distractibility, impulsivity, and increased activity level

Pressured speech: very rapid speech

SIG E CAPSS: an acronym for the core symptoms of depression: **Sadness, Interest** (loss of enjoyment or interest in occupations or activities that were once pleasurable), **Guilt, Energy loss, Concentration loss, Appetite change, Psychomotor agitation or slowing, Sleep change,** and **Suicidality**

Sympathy: expressing genuine concern or sorrow for someone who is suffering, having pity for them

Reflection Questions

1. Compare and contrast the symptoms and behaviors associated with depression and mania. How do depressive symptoms most significantly impact occupational engagement?
2. Describe the difference between empathy and sympathy in your own words. Do you think that there are therapeutic contexts where a demonstration of sympathy is more appropriate than a demonstration of empathy? Give an example.
3. Explain why the establishment of healthy habits and routines is such an important part of intervention, particularly when working with adolescents or teenagers who are experiencing depression.
4. Summarize the reasons for using an activity schedule with clients who experience mania or depression.
5. Discuss strategies and interventions that the occupational therapist can apply to screen for and prevent the risk of suicide.
6. Describe the key concepts of behavioral activation. How does behavioral activation relate to the dimensions of occupation: doing, being, becoming, and belonging?
7. How does the application of witnessing, labeling, or emotional resonance, as suggested by the IRM, help guide the occupational therapy professional when responding to a client who is expressing difficult emotions, such as sadness? What is the difference between sadness, bereavement, prolonged grief, and maladaptive sadness?
8. Evaluate and expand upon this statement: "Some psychologists argue that mania is the flip side of depression." In what ways do you agree or disagree with this idea?

REFERENCES

1. Allen, C. K. (1985). *Occupational therapy for psychiatric diseases: Measurement and management of cognitive disabilities.* Little, Brown and Company.
2. American Occupational Therapy Association. (2020). Occupational therapy in the promotion of health and well-being. *American Journal of Occupational Therapy, 74*(3), 7403420010p1–7403420010p14.
3. American Occupational Therapy Association. (2020). Occupational therapy practice framework: Domain and process—Fourth edition. *American Journal of Occupational Therapy, 74*(Suppl. 2), 1–87.
4. American Psychiatric Association. (2000). *Diagnostic and statistical manual of mental disorders* (4th ed., text rev.). American Psychiatric Association.
5. American Psychiatric Association. (2022). *Diagnostic and statistical manual of mental disorders* (5th ed., text rev.). https://doi.org/10.1176/appi.books.9780890425787
6. Beck, A. T., Rush, A., Shaw, B., & Emery, G. (1987). *Cognitive therapy of depression.* Guilford.
7. Beck, A. T., Steer, R. A., & Brown, G. K. (1996). *Manual for the Beck depression inventory-II.* Psychological Corporation.
8. Bonder, B. R. (2022). *Psychopathology and function* (6th ed.). SLACK.
9. Briguglio, M., Vitale, J. A., Galentino, R., Banfi, G., Dina, C. Z., Bona, A., Panzica, G., Porta, M., Dell'Osso, B., & Glick, I. D. (2020). Healthy eating, physical activity, and sleep hygiene (HEPAS) as the winning triad for sustaining physical and mental health in patients at risk for or with neuropsychiatric disorders: Considerations for clinical practice. *Neuropsychiatric Disease and Treatment, 16,* 55–70.
10. Brown, B. (2021). *Atlas of the heart: Mapping meaningful connection and the language of human experience.* Random House Publishers.
11. Burns, D. D. (1995). *Therapist's toolkit: Comprehensive treatment and assessment tools for the mental health professional.* Author.
12. Buser, S., & Cruz, L. (2022). *DSM-5-TR insanely simplified: Unlocking the spectrums within DSM-5-TR and ICD-10.* Chiron Publications.
13. Chen, R., Zhu, X., Capitão, L. P., Zhang, H., Luo, J., Wang, X., Xi, Y., Song, X., Feng, Y., Cao, L., & Malhi, G. S. (2019). Psychoeducation for psychiatric inpatients following remission of a manic episode in bipolar I disorder: A randomized controlled trial. *Bipolar Disorders, 21*(1), 76–85.
14. Chippendale, T., & Bear-Lehman, J. (2012). Effect of life review writing on depressive symptoms in older adults: A randomized controlled trial. *American Journal of Occupational Therapy, 66*(4), 438–444.
15. Costa, R. T., Cheniaux, E., Rangé, B. P., Versiani, M., & Nardi, A. E. (2012). Group cognitive behavior therapy for bipolar disorder can improve the quality of life. *Brazilian Journal of Medical and Biological Research, 45*(9), 862–868.
16. Da Silva, R. D. A., Mograbi, D. C., Bifano, J., Santana, C. M., & Cheniaux, E. (2016). Insight in bipolar mania: Evaluation of its heterogeneity and correlation with clinical symptoms. *Journal of Affective Disorders, 199,* 95–98.
17. Depression and Bipolar Support Alliance. *DBSA Wellness Wheel.* https://www.dbsalliance.org/wellness/wellness-toolbox/dbsa-wellness-wheel/
18. Devine, M. (n.d.). *Everything is not okay* [Audio file]. http://www.refugeingrief.com
19. Devine, M. (2015, July). *Grief: My perspective.* Address at the World Domination Summit; Portland, OR. https://vimeo.com/134620373
20. Eisenberg, N., Eggum, N. D., & Di Giunta, L. (2010). Empathy-related responding: Associations with prosocial behavior, aggression, and intergroup relations. *Social Issues and Policy Review, 4*(1), 143–180.
21. Firth, J., Schuch, F., & Mittal, V. A. (2020). Using exercise to protect physical and mental health in youth at risk for psychosis. *Research in Psychotherapy, 23*(1), 433.
22. Fisher, A. G., & Marterella, A. (2019). *Powerful practice: A model for authentic occupational therapy.* Center for Innovative OT Solutions.

23. Forsyth, K., Taylor, R. R., Kramer, J. M., Prior, S., Ritchie, L., & Melton, J. (2019). The model of human occupation. In B. A. B. Schell & G. Gillen (Eds.), *Willard and Spackman's occupational therapy* (13th ed., pp. 601–621). Lippincott Williams & Wilkins.

24. Foster, E. R., Cunnane, K. B., Edwards, D. F., Moorison, M. T., Ewald, G. A., Geltman, G. M., & Zazulia, A. R. (2011). Executive dysfunction and depressive symptoms associated with reduced participation of people with severe congestive heart failure. *American Journal of Occupational Therapy, 65*(3), 306–313.

25. Frust, G., Gerber, L., Smith, C., Fisher, S., & Shulman, B. (1987). A program for improving energy conservation behaviors in adults with rheumatoid arthritis. *American Journal of Occupational Therapy, 41*(2), 102–111.

26. Garabrant, A. A., & Liu, C.-J. (2021). Loneliness and activity engagement among rural homebound older adults with and without self-reported depression. *American Journal of Occupational Therapy, 75*(5), 7505205100.

27. Gerber, L., & Frust, G. (1992). Scoring methods and application of the activity record (ACTRE) for patients with musculoskeletal disorders. *Arthritis Care and Research, 5*(3), 151–156.

28. Gibbs, M., Winsper, C., Marwaha, S., Gilbert, E., Broome, M., & Singh, S. P. (2015). Cannabis use and mania symptoms: A systematic review and meta-analysis. *Journal of Affective Disorders, 171*, 39–47.

29. Gutman, S. A. (2005). Understanding suicide: What therapists should know. *Occupational Therapy in Mental Health, 21*(2), 55–77.

30. Hearing, C. M., Chang, W. C., Szuhany, K. L., Deckersbach, T., Nierenberg, A. A., & Sylvia, L. G. (2016). Physical exercise for treatment of mood disorders: A critical review. *Current Behavioral Neuroscience Reports, 3*(4), 350–359.

31. Hill, R., & Dahlitz, M. (2022). *The practitioner's guide to the science of psychotherapy.* W.W. Norton & Company.

32. Hirschfeld, R. M., Lewis, L., & Vornik, L. A. (2003). Perceptions and impact of bipolar disorder: How far have we really come? Results of the National Depressive and Manic-Depressive Association 2000 survey of individuals with bipolar disorder. *Journal of Clinical Psychiatry, 64*(2), 61–74.

33. Hitch, D., Pepin, G., & Stagnitti, K. (2018). The pan occupational paradigm: Development and key concepts. *Scandinavian Journal of Occupational Therapy, 25*(1), 27–34.

34. Jamison, K. R. (1995). *An unquiet mind: A memoir of moods and madness.* Vintage Press.

35. Janowsky, D. S., Leff, M., & Epstein, R. S. (1970). Playing the manic game: Interpersonal maneuvers of the acutely manic patient. *Archives of General Psychiatry, 22*(2), 252–261.

36. Joo, Y. Y., Moon, S., Wang, H., Kim, H., Lee, E.-J., Kim, J. H., Posner, J., Ahn, W.-Y., Chol, I., Kim, J.-W., & Cha, J. (2022). Association of genome-wide polygenic scores for multiple psychiatric and common traits in preadolescent youths at risk of suicide. *JAMA Network Open, 5*(2), e2148585.

37. Kaltenboeck, A., & Harmer, C. (2018). The neuroscience of depressive disorders: A brief review of the past and some considerations about the future. *Brain and Neuroscience Advances, 2*, 2398212818799269.

38. Kay, D. B., Tanner, J. J., & Bowers, D. (2018). Sleep disturbances and depression severity in patients with Parkinson's disease. *Brain and Behavior, 8*(6), e00967.

39. Kessler, D. (2020). *Finding meaning: The sixth stage of grief.* Scribner Press.

40. Kielhofner, G. (2017). *A model of human occupation: Theory and application* (5th ed.). Lippincott Williams & Wilkins.

41. Kinney, A. R., Graham, J. E., & Eakman, A. M. (2020). Participation is associated with well-being among community-based veterans: An investigation of coping ability, meaningful activity, and social support as mediating mechanisms. *American Journal of Occupational Therapy, 74*(5), 7405205010p1–7405205010p11.

42. Luke, H. M. (1987). Suffering. In *Old age: Journey into simplicity* (E. V. Rieu, Trans., published by Penguin Classics, pp. 103–112). Parabola Books.

43. Olson, L. M. (2014). BRIGHTEN: An interdisciplinary approach to address depression in older adults. *Mental Health Special Interest Section Quarterly, 37*(2), 1–3.

44. Pandya, S. P. (2019). Meditation for treating adults with bipolar disorder II: A multi-city study. *Clinical Psychology & Psychotherapy, 26*(2), 252–261.

45. Parikh, S. V., Zaretsky, A., Beaulieu, S., Yatham, L. N., Young, L. T., Patelis-Siotis, I., Macqueen, G. M., Levitt, A., Arenovich, T., Cervantes, P., Velyvis, V., Kennedy, S. H., & Streiner, D. L. (2012). A randomized controlled trial of psychoeducation or cognitive-behavioral therapy in bipolar disorder: A Canadian Network for Mood and Anxiety Treatments (CANMAT) study. *The Journal of Clinical Psychiatry, 73*(6), 803–810.

46. Quinnett, P. (2016). *Ask a question, save a life.* QPR Institute: Question. Persuade. Refer. National Registry of Evidence-based Programs and Practices. https://www.qprinstitute.com

47. Seligman, M. E. P. (2002). *Authentic happiness: Using the new positive psychology to realize your potential for lasting fulfillment.* Free Press.

48. Seligman, M. E. P. (2011). *Flourish: A visionary new understanding of happiness and well-being.* Free Press.

49. Shin, W. G., Woo, C. W., Jung, W. H., Kim, H., Lee, T. Y., Decety, J., & Kwon, J. S. (2020). The neurobehavioral mechanisms underlying attitudes toward people with mental or physical illness. *Frontiers in Behavioral Neuroscience, 14*, 571225.

50. Sinclair, S., Beamer, K., Hack, T. F., McClement, S., Raffin Bouchal, S. R., Chochinov, H. M., & Hagen, N. A. (2017). Sympathy, empathy, and compassion: A grounded theory study of palliative care patients' understandings, experiences, and preferences. *Palliative Medicine, 31*(5), 437–447.

51. Smith, N. R., Kielhofner, G., & Watts, J. H. (1986). The relationships between volition, activity pattern, and life satisfaction in the elderly. *American Journal of Occupational Therapy, 40*(4), 278–283.

52. Sokol, L., & Fox, M. G. (2019). *The comprehensive clinician's guide to cognitive behavioral therapy.* PESI Publishing.

53. Taylor, R. R. (2020). *The intentional relationship: Occupational therapy and use of self* (2nd ed.). F.A. Davis.

54. Thompson, P., Vidal, C., Giedd, J. N., Gochman, P., Blumenthal, J., & Nicholson, R., Toga, A. W., & Rapoport, J. L. (2001). Mapping adolescent brain change reveals dynamic wave of accelerated gray matter loss in very early-onset schizophrenia. *Proceedings of the National Academy of Sciences of the United States of America, 98*(20), 11650–11655.

55. Weaver, L. L., Page, S. J., Sheffler, L., & Chae, J. (2013). Minimal depression: How does it relate to upper-extremity impairment and function in stroke? *American Journal of Occupational Therapy, 67*(5), 550–555.

56. Weinstein, E. C. (2013). Three views of artful practice in psychosocial occupational therapy. *Occupational Therapy in Mental Health, 29*(4), 299–360.

57. Wootton, T. (2009). *Bipolar in order: Looking at depression, mania, hallucination, and delusion from the other side.* Bipolar Advantage.

58. Working off depression. (2005). *Harvard Mental Health Letters, 22*(6), 6–7.

SUGGESTED RESOURCES

Articles

An excellent advocacy resource, a single-page brochure from the National Institute of Mental Health, Teen Depression: *More than just moodiness.* The brochure provides a simplified, plain language Q & A format, asking "Do I have depression?" and "How do I get help for depression?" This brochure could serve as a conversation guide for occupational therapy professionals and other caregivers to screen for symptoms of depression. https://www.nimh.nih.gov/sites/default/files/documents/health/publications/teen-depression/Teen_Depression_More_Than_Just_Moodiness_2022.pdf

Steede, K., & Gough, R. (2022). Service user experiences of occupational therapy in acute mental health settings: A qualitative evidence synthesis. *Occupational Therapy in Mental Health, 38*(4), 364–382.

Books

The Science of Unbreakable Things (2018) by Tae Keller is a book written for young readers but with a poignant grown-up message about living with a family member who is experiencing depression. The main character, Natalie, enters a science contest convinced that winning the contest will help her solve her most important problem and answer her bigger question—how to help her mother, and "cure" her mom's severe depression.

Charlie and the Dog Who Came to Stay (2021) by Dr Ruth Spence and Kimiya Pahlevan. Spence, a psychologist, tells the story in this children's book imagining depression as a dog that follows the main character Charlie around. The story also includes tips to help manage depression.

Comics and graphic novels are excellent resources to build into occupational therapy group or individual interventions and are appreciated by clients of all ages. This one is especially good because the author reveals, in her graphic novel, her own experiences with anxiety and depression, and how she got on the road to recovery making her daily mental health a mindful priority: *Everything is Okay* (2022) by Debbie Tung.

Videos

The U.S. Department of Health and Human Services, Substance Abuse and Mental Health Services Administration (SAMHSA) website offers a plethora of resources including brief video profiles (1–3 minutes each) of people discussing what it is like living with mental illness and what recovery looks like for them.

Profile: Mike V., *Living with Major Depression.* https://www.youtube.com/watch?v=LaPwuaw_Rz0

Profile: Phil Y., *Living with Bipolar Disorder.* https://www.youtube.com/watch?v=zj4s532wTxE

John Green is the successful author of *Looking for Alaska* (2005); *The Fault in Our Stars* (2012); *Papertowns* (2008); *Turtles All the Way Down* (2017); *An Abundance of Katherines* (2006); *The Anthropocene Reviewed: Essays on a Human-Centered Planet* (2021), and a list of coauthored books, including *Will Grayson Will Grayson* (2010), coauthored with David Levithan, which debuted at #3 on the *New York Times* bestseller list for children's chapter books, and was the first book starring gay characters ever to appear on the list. Green is also a screenwriter, cohost with his brother Hank, of the Vlogbrothers YouTube channel, a philanthropist, and a champion for mental health advocacy. John Green is also

diagnosed with obsessive compulsive disorder and experiences anxiety. His works give voice to the real experiences of mental illness. These two brief videos glimpse how Green has found ways to not only make his own recovery a way of life but also to advocate for others by sharing ways that he has found to, as he says, "remember to be awesome."

The 60 Minutes (Season 52, Episode 18) interview with Author John Green: *Reaching Young Adults with Mental Illness* (13 minutes). https://www.cbs.com/shows/video/Kq3fZJqcWCbR4yyx7U5txxWLzjestHqv/

My Truly Mortifying Self-Talk (3:14): In this brief video, Green uses storytelling and humor to describe one of the go-to strategies he uses to successfully move through stressful daily situations–self talk (drawn from his years of participating in Cognitive Behavioral Therapy). https://www.youtube.com/watch?v=XDcpy8_AL3w

Websites

SAMHSA website offers a plethora of resources, including links to pages specifically focused on mental health prevention, recovery, and health promotion to support clients with mental illness and their loved ones in living qualitatively improved lives. There is also a link (see later) to a fact sheet that is associated with each disorder presented in the "*Living Well with . . .* " series, which is an excellent resource for clients and their loved ones.

Living Well with *Bipolar Disorder* web page—https://www.samhsa.gov/serious-mental-illness/bi-polar

Understanding Bipolar Disorder Fact Sheet—https://www.samhsa.gov/sites/default/files/understanding-bipolar-disorder.pdf

Living Well with *Major Depressive Disorder* web page—https://www.samhsa.gov/serious-mental-illness/major-depression

Understanding Major Depressive Disorder Fact Sheet—https://www.samhsa.gov/sites/default/files/understanding-major-depressive-disorder.pdf

The DBSA is a leading national organization that focuses on mood disorders, including depression and bipolar disorder. DBSA's mission is to provide hope, help, support, and education to improve the lives of people who have mood disorders. The DBSA website is full of evidence-driven resources and information for the health care provider, client, caregiver, and community, including a national directory (by zip code) of more than 400 support groups for people experiencing affective mood disorders. https://www.dbsalliance.org/

CHAPTER 20

Targeting Psychological and Social Factors That Influence Occupational Engagement: Being With the Client Who Experiences Hallucinations, Delusions, and Paranoia

OT HACKS OVERVIEW

O: Occupation as a means and an end

Ultimately, the goal of intervention for treatment of symptoms of psychosis is for the client to have increased opportunities to successfully participate in their preferred (and necessary) occupations (2, 3). This increases their chances of achieving their goals and aspirations. Increasing opportunities for clients to successfully participate in their occupations is the equivalent of using occupational therapy as a means; achieving the client's goals through participation in occupation is the use of occupation toward an end.

T: Theoretical concepts, values, principles, or historical foundations

In terms of the social and emotional impacts of living with psychotic disorders, the occupational therapy professional (OTP) has a responsibility to include the client and the caregivers, support network, or family of the consumer, throughout the stages of the occupational therapy process (1, 2).

This is particularly critical for clients with schizophrenia spectrum disorders and those who experience the symptoms of psychosis.

There is strong evidence that having a supportive network and support system is fundamental to positive and enduring recovery.

H: How can we Help? OT's role in collaborating with clients with mental illness or mental health needs

Responding with empathy is critical in all occupational therapy interventions. But understanding or even imagining what it feels like to experience psychotic symptoms such as auditory hallucinations is one of the most difficult things for OTPs to do. Most of us have not experienced sensations like these. As you read more about responding to clients with these experiences, reflect upon the role of occupational therapy in supporting more optimal occupational engagement for this group of clients.

A: Adaptations

OTPs can incorporate the principles of Cognitive Behavioral Therapy for Psychosis (CBTp) and Recovery-Oriented Cognitive Therapy (CT-R) into their practice as part of a holistic occupational therapy plan for clients who experience psychotic disorders or symptoms. Learn more about these two evidence-based interventions in this chapter.

C: Case study includes

This 54-year-old unmarried Caucasian woman, Laura, was admitted to the acute admissions ward on court certification following action by her neighbors. Commitment papers state that the client has been complaining of people doing things against her; she is suspicious of her neighbors and has been breaking windows. Client has had two previous psychiatric hospitalizations, in 2017 for 3 months and in 2021 for 6 months. Diagnosis is schizophrenia (F20.9). Client also has chronic phlebitis in both legs. Prescribed medication includes olanzapine (Zyprexa) 10 mg, doxepin (Sinequan) 100 mg tid, and docusate (Colace) 100 mg.

Read more about the case at the end of this chapter.

K: Knowledge: keeping mental health OT practice grounded in evidence, in occupational science, and in research

Read this evidence by Magliano et al (27) using the following research question as a focus:

Do nonpsychiatric medical specialists (NPMS) use different approaches or have different perceptions of dangerousness and social distance requirements for clients with schizophrenia and depression?

After reviewing the article and learning more in this chapter about how the symptoms of hallucinations, delusions, or paranoia impact occupational engagement, discuss responses to the *Evidence Application and Translation Questions* found in the section "Knowledge" in the OT HACKS Chapter Summary.

S: Some terms that may be new to you

Delusion

Delusions of persecution

Erotomania

Hallucination

Idea of reference

Megalomania/delusions of grandeur

Mood congruent
Paranoia
Paranoid delusions
Paranoid ideation

Somatic delusions
Thought insertion
Thought withdrawal

TARGETING SYMPTOMS OF HALLUCINATIONS, DELUSIONS, AND PARANOIA THAT CREATE BARRIERS TO OCCUPATION: THE BEING, DOING, AND BELONGING DIMENSIONS OF OT PRACTICE

BOX 20.1 Intervention Planning Focus Questions: How to Begin

1. What does it feel like to be a person who is experiencing *hallucinations, delusions, or paranoia*?
2. What are some behaviors that a person experiencing *hallucinations, delusions, or paranoia* might demonstrate, and how might their behavior, responses, or affect be positively or negatively impacting their occupations?
3. How can I adjust my way of being (therapeutic use of self) to make the client feel more comfortable about their way of being?
4. What can I do to instill a sense of belonging in occupational therapy right now that will encourage the client toward setting goals with outcomes that are personally meaningful and relevant to them?

Introduction

In Chapter 4, readers were introduced to some of the common diagnoses that clients present with during occupational therapy practice. The schizophrenia spectrum and other psychotic disorders, as conceptualized in the *Diagnostic and Statistical Manual of Mental Disorders, Fifth Edition, Text Revision (DSM-5-TR)*, are characterized by the presence of at least one positive symptom (4, 12). Recall that the symptoms of psychotic disorders can be categorized into three groups: positive, negative, and disorganized. Positive symptoms include any behaviors or characteristics that are abnormally present for the person, such as hallucinations, delusions, or paranoia. Negative symptoms include any behaviors or characteristics that are lacking or missing, such as the client's lack of ability to initiate plans, express emotion, or find pleasure, and behaviors such as withdrawing from others (social isolation). The disorganized symptoms include confused and disordered thinking and speech, difficulty with thinking logically, and, occasionally, the demonstration of bizarre movements or behaviors (24).

Diagnoses in Which Hallucinations, Delusions, and Paranoia Are Common Symptoms

The schizophrenia and psychotic disorders spectrum is a class of mental disorders that are marked by symptoms of abnormal thinking and perceptions that often seriously disrupt occupational participation, not only for the person with the disorder but also for the caregivers and families who love and support the individual (20, 33). Unfortunately, the lack of understanding surrounding these diagnoses, as well as the misused or misguided language and terminology expressed when discussing the diagnoses and symptoms, only serves to further confuse the situation and exacerbate the stigma for people living with the diseases. It is especially important for the OTP to become familiar with the nuances that distinguish the differences in the terms and to apply the appropriate language and terminology in documentation and interpersonal communication (24).

A **psychotic disorder** is a diagnosable psychological condition. The psychotic disorders include schizophrenia, which is the most common; schizoaffective disorder, which includes both psychotic and mood symptoms; schizophreniform disorder; delusional disorder; brief psychotic disorder; substance-induced psychotic disorder; bipolar psychosis or bipolar disorder with psychotic features; postpartum psychosis; psychotic depression; and age-related psychosis.

Psychosis is a symptom (or a family of symptoms), demonstrable or describable effects that can accompany *both* psychotic disorders *and* other conditions. Confusion is furthered when there is no clear understanding that the symptoms of psychosis can be present with several other illnesses or conditions, even though those disorders are not necessarily classified as psychotic disorders. Some conditions where symptoms of psychosis could emerge include the use of or withdrawal from psychedelic drugs, alcohol, or other illicit drugs, exposure to extreme stress, trauma, or grief, and illnesses where a person has experienced a high fever or stroke (24, 35). Additional diseases or conditions that may produce psychotic symptomology include, but are certainly not limited to, bipolar disorders, brain tumors (especially tumors of the pituitary gland), viral encephalitis, temporal lobe epilepsy, cerebral syphilis, multiple sclerosis, Huntington disease, AIDS, and narcolepsy (20).

When a person experiences an episode of psychosis, the way their brain processes information interferes with the person's perception of reality. These departures from reality are sometimes called "psychotic breaks." Psychotic breaks vary in length. They can be brief and temporary or they may recur at other times throughout one's life (13). Of importance, psychotic symptoms that happen secondary to substance use or withdrawal or psychosis that is associated with an organic medical condition are very different from psychotic episodes from the primary psychotic disorders such as schizophrenia. These psychotic episodes have different etiologies, characteristics, courses, and onset. If the underlying medical condition(s) are treated, or the offending substance is ceased, the symptoms of psychosis will typically diminish over time (35).

What Are Hallucinations?

Clients who experience psychosis might see, hear, or believe things that are not real. *A* **hallucination** *is a sensory experience that does not correspond to external reality.* A person who is hallucinating sees, hears, feels, smells, or tastes things that are not there. It is important to realize, however, that most hallucinations and delusions are an extension of hyper-acute senses and the brain's challenges in both interpretation and appropriate response to the stimuli. Most delusions and hallucinations are understandable reflections of what the hallucinating person's brain is experiencing. They appear unreal or even bizarre to others, but to the person experiencing them, the hallucinations are not only real to them but are also part of a logical and coherent pattern (20). Some common hallucinations are hearing voices (auditory hallucinations), seeing animals, people, or lights and shadows, or experiencing burning or crawling sensations on the skin. Auditory or sound hallucinations occur the most frequently. People who are hallucinating may hear voices telling them to do things (called command hallucinations) or criticizing them, or they may hear music or strange sounds, or someone calling their name. They may perceive a sound as much louder or softer than it really is. Visual hallucinations are also common and may involve seeing walls move, having one's face look strange in the mirror, or thinking that people look transparent or flat. Gustatory (taste) and olfactory (smell) hallucinations, which are less common, often affect clients with temporal lobe epilepsy; usually, the hallucinated taste or smell is very unpleasant. Tactile (touch) hallucinations may be of itching or burning or a feeling that insects are crawling on or biting one's skin, or at times feel as though someone is touching the client, when no one is present.

Clients usually find hallucinations troubling, frightening, and uncomfortable, and many times they develop beliefs related to the hallucinations. Without intervention, they can form elaborate ways to reinforce their false beliefs. The strong beliefs and the compensatory patterns, habits, rituals, and routines that they implement to support (or allay the fears associated with) their hallucinations are what disrupt their participation in occupation far more than the hallucinations themselves.

What Are Delusions?

A **delusion** *is a belief that is contrary to reality as experienced by others in one's cultural group.* Delusions may or may not be based on reality, but regardless of the extent of connection to reality, the person's delusion cannot easily be corrected by reasoning with the individual. According to Beck et al (6), delusions of thought are the result of information processing biases that are applied in response to a person's threatening beliefs about themselves or the world. When a person with delusions is faced with (oftentimes irrelevant) contextual situations or information, they ascribe personal meaning to the information. This is called **self-referential bias**. Then, the person attempts to make up an explanation of the situation where the actions or thoughts of others are intentionally and maliciously directed at them; this is called **intentionalizing bias**. Lastly, the person will attribute the whole situation to an external cause, and this is called an **externalizing bias** (5, 35).

From the perspective of the cognitive model, these three biases, when combined, skew information and distort reality, causing development of the delusion (5, 35). Take, for example, the person who experiences delusional symptoms and who happens to walk past a table at a restaurant where a family is having lunch. When one of the children shares a funny story, the person with delusions hears the other members of the family laugh and attributes a meaning to their laughter (self-referential bias). The person then assumes that everyone in the restaurant is laughing at him and judging him because of the amount of food that he is carrying on his tray (intentionalizing bias) and that all this is because of his recent weight gain (externalizing bias).

People who experience delusions may believe, for example, that television shows and newspaper stories have special messages for them, or that automobile license plates contain a secret code that they must decipher to save the world. These beliefs are called **ideas of reference**. Or a woman may believe that the FBI (Federal Bureau of Investigation) is taking thoughts out of her brain (**thought withdrawal**) or putting strange ones in (**thought insertion**). She may feel as if she were being followed (**delusions of persecution**) or that she has special powers (**megalomania** or **delusions of grandeur**). Other common delusions include **erotomania** (the delusion that someone is in love with you) and **somatic delusions** (belief that something horrible is wrong with one's body). Some delusions may appear to have some basis in reality. As an example, consider a woman (with a family history of cancer) who believes she has cancer despite multiple physical examinations and tests and reassurance from her doctors.

A delusion is a false belief that is peculiar to the individual. It thus differs from a cultural belief, which, although odd, may be embraced by an entire nation or ethnic group. For example, people in some Caribbean countries believe that pulling on babies' limbs when they are bathed will make them taller, stronger, and better coordinated when they grow up. As another example, Australian Aboriginal people believe that the physical world that we experience while awake is less powerful, and in a sense less real, than the dream world of sleep. Students sometimes find it hard to remember the difference between a delusion and a hallucination. A delusion is an inaccurate thought or idea. (*Hint: **d**elusion is a wrong i**d**ea.*) By contrast, a hallucination is a false perception, sensory experience, or feeling. A person does not have to hear or see something that is not there to have a delusional idea; a delusion may be based on real-life events; it is the *interpretation* of these events that is odd. For example, the person may think that the newscaster on television who seems to look them right in the eye while summarizing a story knows all about the person and is sending a special message. What the person actually sees and hears is no different from what any viewer would see; it is the interpretation that is different.

The content and quality of delusions can sometimes reveal information about a client's needs, their occupational identity, or their occupational history, which makes the OTP's presence, attunement, and responses to the client exceptionally important (36). For example, delusions in which one is highly sought after, or regarded as highly admired and special, could be indicative of the client's feelings of inferiority, inadequacy, or hopelessness. From an attachment theory perspective that focuses on the emotional, psychological, and physiologic bonds that develop between an infant and their primary caregiver, secure attachment establishes feelings of safety and security (9). Some evidence has recently appeared in the literature that suggests that delusions of persecution and the symptom of paranoia may be related to insecure attachments and convey a defensive strategy that, to some extent, masks poor self-esteem and pathologic self-doubt (9, 38).

What Is Paranoia?

Paranoia *is a type of thinking in which persecutory and grandiose ideas predominate.* General suspiciousness is usually called **paranoid ideation**, whereas very extreme and unbelievable ideas (such as that the attorney general and the police are out to get one) are termed **paranoid delusions**. Individuals who are paranoid feel suspicious of those around them; they are constantly alert and concerned about whether others are harassing them, persecuting them, taking advantage of them, or treating them unfairly. They keep themselves aloof and distant from others, often subjecting family and would-be friends to repeated "tests" of loyalty. One way to think about paranoia is as a defense against rejection. By believing that others are out to get them, these clients protect themselves from rejection. This keeps them from developing relationships in which they fear they may get hurt. Similarly, they avoid experiencing their low self-esteem by instead thinking that they are special in some way. Individuals who are paranoid seem to need to believe that they are better, more moral, and more self-sufficient than other ordinary people. Ironically, it is these actions, thoughts, and behaviors that reinforce their delusions and contribute to the vicious cycle of further withdrawing and disconnecting them from social supports and connections who could help them reality test their ideas. They are often afraid of losing their independence and they cannot imagine having to rely on others for help.

The type, level of intensity, and frequency of psychotic symptoms are highly individualized, and each person's experience with psychosis is unique. The type of hallucination, delusion, or paranoia may also differ by condition or circumstance, "it has been argued that different symptoms of psychosis, such as paranoia and hallucinations, may reflect different cognitive and emotional mechanisms in response to different kinds of adverse life experiences" (38, p. 1495). For example, auditory hallucinations are common in schizophrenia; voices may comment on the client's behavior or their character, sometimes in insulting or demeaning ways. In schizophrenia, the hallucinations seem unrelated to the person's mood; however, in bipolar disorders, auditory hallucinations may also be present and tend to be **mood congruent**. This means that the voices say things that are consistent with the person's mood (eg, telling the depressed person that they are bad, worthless, or suggesting self-harm). Delusions may be present in any of the psychotic disorders: schizophrenia, bipolar disorder (both manic and depressive phases), and neurocognitive disorders. They may occur in certain personality disorders (schizotypal personality, paranoid personality), in eating disorders or somatic disorders, and even in people who have no other known psychopathology.

Strategies for Therapeutic Use of Self

Responding with empathy is critical in all occupational therapy interventions. But understanding or even imagining what it feels like to experience psychotic symptoms, such as auditory hallucinations, is one of the most difficult things for the OTP to do. Most of us have not experienced such sensations. However, an important principle of empathy according to Dr Brené Brown (11) is that we are not required to have shared the same or similar experience as someone else for us to be able to demonstrate compassion and empathy. We do not have to "walk a mile in their shoes," as Brown puts it. Instead, we need to learn how to listen to the story they tell about what it is like in their shoes and believe them even when it does not match or is not the same as one's own experiences (11).

When a client experiences psychosis, their perception of reality is in disarray. The OTP should recognize that a person experiencing psychosis may find it difficult to tell what is real from what is not real, and this requires an understanding that the delusions and hallucinations are *very real* to the person experiencing them (7). Because of that, it is important to not dismiss, minimize, or argue with the person about their delusions and hallucinations. The varying symptoms can be unrelenting and stressful, causing disorganization of thoughts that make concentration difficult or impossible. The combined impacts of the symptoms usually lead to frustration, a great deal of fear and distrust, and a generally heightened suspicion of the person's environment and context (including sometimes even suspicion of people whom the client has previously known and trusted—their friends, significant other, and family) (24).

Feelings of fear and distrust can lead to the client isolating themselves or withdrawing from their typical occupations (24, 37). This is often the situation upon which the OTP must find a way to build a therapeutic relationship. Regardless of whether the OTP is working with the client in the acute stages of psychosis, or in later stages when psychotic symptoms are actively controlled with medication or other therapies, when a person has experienced psychosis, it is essential to meet them where they are because "the individual might maintain worries or compensatory strategies established during the psychotic episode" (35, p. 229). Creating a context where a client feels safe is the first step in developing a sense of trust. The therapist might say, for example, "I believe that what you are experiencing is very frightening and you are safe here" (8). The key is to try to empathize with how the person *feels* about their beliefs and experiences, withholding any judgments about the content of their beliefs and experiences. Emphasis is on acknowledging to the person that what they are experiencing is real to them, without confirming or denying their hallucinations or delusions. Another example of this type of response is stating "I accept that you hear voices or see things in that way, but it's not like that for me."

Although it is not necessary to have experienced symptoms of psychosis for the OTP to respond in an empathic way, there are increasing opportunities for OTPs to become better prepared to treat clients in the mental health population, through fieldwork opportunities and simulated experiences. One simulation program called the *Hearing Voices That Are Distressing* (HVTAD) *simulation* (15) is being incorporated into some occupational therapy educational experiences to help increase empathy for clients with mental illnesses, and, in this case, clients with auditory hallucinations. Results of a qualitative analysis in one program that incorporated the simulated experience of auditory hallucinations into their occupational therapy curriculum showed that the students who participated found the simulation to be an effective means of broadening their perspective and preparing them to work with clients in this group (30).

In the acute phases of psychosis, having the client who is hallucinating repeat a word or phrase that is comforting and positive may help reduce the length, frequency, and intrusiveness of hallucinations (26). For example, the person might say, "I am safe here," or "I have done the best I can. It's good enough." Other strategies include either increasing or decreasing external stimulation, depending on what works, or has historically worked for each client (in circumstances where an accurate history is available). Beyond the acute stages of psychosis, and once a therapeutic relationship of trust is built with a therapist, identifying simple and successful crisis intervention techniques, learning to recognize the warning signs, practicing coping mechanisms, and making plans to help remember and apply them during a crisis or episode, can become a primary and ongoing goal of intervention and management of the disease (26).

Whenever possible, try to redirect the person's attention to an activity or something else that is reality based. In responding to clients who are experiencing any of the symptoms of psychosis, OTPs can practice perspective taking by listening with interest while keeping the focus on what is happening and what people are doing in the present moment. It is pointless to try to convince people with delusional thinking that their delusions are not true; doing so usually serves to further alienate the person. The perspective of a person experiencing paranoia has been described by consumers as feeling like everything around them is dangerous, that anyone or anything can feel like a threat to their safety and uncertain sense of self (20). The OTP should avoid approaching them suddenly, from behind, or in a manner that might be perceived as threatening. Finally, avoid confronting, criticizing, blaming, joking, laughing at, or using sarcasm with the person experiencing psychosis.

Body language and verbal and nonverbal messages are also important considerations in the therapeutic context. It is recommended that the OTP avoid facing the person directly and instead sit to the side or at an angle. Similarly, sustained eye contact may be frightening to the person and should be avoided in the acute stages of psychosis (8). Some of the same aspects of applying a trauma-informed approach to delivery of care are useful when working with clients who experience psychosis. Do not touch the person without asking their permission. The therapist and other health care professionals, especially those who are unfamiliar to the person, should try to minimize body language that shows distress and control their nervous behaviors (eg, jiggling legs, fidgeting, or speaking too quickly) as much as possible. If the person is sitting down, do not stand over them or hover near them. Any directions or statements made by the OTP should be clear, consistent, and unambiguous.

In certain stages of therapeutic intervention, or in certain settings, group therapy is common, which will introduce another set of contextual and therapeutic relationship considerations. Frequently, a person in an activity group who is feeling paranoid will separate from others or try to strike up a special relationship with a staff member, to feel a bit more in control. Some OTPs believe that allowing and encouraging this special relationship helps the person adjust faster to the group. The person can be given a special role (passing out supplies, taking attendance) that makes them feel important. The individual who is paranoid is commonly threatened by competition, so competitive games and situations in which one person is compared with another should be avoided until the group has arrived at a more mature level (39). A person who is experiencing paranoia or other psychotic symptoms may require extra time before engaging in activities. Maintaining a good relationship with the person and repeatedly inviting them to join while tolerating them not doing so may eventually result in success (28). The client may, over time, change their mind and their behaviors as they develop relationships and trust in other members of the group, and in the OTP (39).

The question of who is in control of a situation is a real concern for the person who is feeling paranoid; experiences of hallucinations or delusions degrade trust. When a client experiences paranoia, the OTP can reassure them that they do not see any threats and that the OTP will stay with them if it helps them to feel safe. If it is safely possible, the OTP can encourage the client to move away from whatever is causing their fear. It is imperative to tell the person what you are going to do **before** doing it, for example, that you are going to get out your cell phone. If it is necessary for the client's safety to give them directives, give the person simple directions and ample time to respond; for example: "Sit down, and let's talk about it." If it is within the scope of one's role, it is helpful to stay with the person in the initial stage of an episode of paranoia, but remaining at a distance that is comfortable for the OTP and the client is essential. Many times, just slowing down the pace can help the OTP think more reflectively about moving through a situation and imagine how their actions may be perceived by a client who is paranoid. For example, head off the encouragement of the person's paranoia by not whispering to or about them, and certainly not to another professional. Likewise, be mindful of one's own actions and behaviors and do not use body language that could exacerbate paranoia, such as approaching the person with your hands in your pockets or behind your back or standing over or too close to them.

TARGETING SYMPTOMS OF HALLUCINATIONS, DELUSIONS, AND MANIA THAT CREATE BARRIERS TO OCCUPATION: THE DOING AND BECOMING DIMENSIONS OF OT PRACTICE

BOX 20.2 Intervention Implementation Focus Questions: How to Support Clients' Optimal Engagement in Occupation

1. What can the client and the occupational therapy team collaboratively do together that will help the client become more functional and effective in the things that are important to them in everyday life?
2. What are the best intervention types and intervention approaches to apply in this therapeutic context?
3. What does the current evidence suggest about the most productive interventions for this diagnosis/set of symptoms?

Contextual, Environmental, and Client Factor Considerations for Clients' With Symptoms of Hallucinations, Delusions, or Paranoia

Many of those who hallucinate do so when they are under stress, especially in environments that are too stimulating for them. Sometimes, just moving the person to a quieter, less overwhelming area will make the hallucinations diminish or ease their intensity. Therefore, in general, the environment should be calm, quiet, and nondistracting. On the other hand, clients should not be permitted to isolate themselves from other people entirely because hallucinations may increase in the absence of any other stimulation. In fact, associating with other people, especially conversing with them, tends to block auditory hallucinations and increase focus on reality. MacRae (26) reported that a client successfully limited his hallucinations by going on a planned walk as soon

as the voices began. For delusions, the environment can be relatively stimulating and should provide opportunities for the person to gradually get involved in activities. Finally, the person who is paranoid is easily threatened by changes in the environment; therefore, the environment and the schedule should be kept as stable and consistent as possible. When changes are anticipated (eg, a new paint job, a rearrangement of furniture for a special event), the client should be prepared well in advance, and, if possible, be a part of making changes and decisions.

It is common for individuals who are paranoid to deliberately isolate themselves from other people. This is a self-protective measure that the OTP should tolerate and support until the person feels more comfortable. Social contact should never be forced on any client and can be particularly harmful for a client who is experiencing symptoms of paranoia. After an initial period of isolation, they should be encouraged to join others in a group; usually, they will first take on the role of a watchful observer or "special assistant" described earlier. Gradually, after repeated exposure to the same people, the client who is paranoid may begin to relate more spontaneously. Because the person experiencing paranoia commonly feels vulnerable, easily threatened, and frightened, there is some potential for the person to demonstrate an adverse response to others. Staff should follow the safety guidelines appropriate to their setting and develop an understanding of the recommendations for deescalating a hostile situation or aggressive client, which are covered in Chapter 22.

Characteristics of Interventions That Support Reduced Symptoms of Hallucinations, Delusions, or Paranoia

Simple, highly structured activities that encourage involvement and interaction with a few other trusted people are recommended. The structure prevents clients from drifting away into a private world and the presence of other people tends to focus them on reality. If possible, the activity should require some minimal interaction with others, if only to ask for a tool. The person who is hallucinating should not be permitted to work alone, apart from the group. Activities should not demand attention to detail or fine motor coordination initially because the person may still be distracted occasionally by the hallucinations and they are often focused on the goal of learning how to minimize their symptoms.

Some therapists advocate activities that strongly stimulate the senses. They argue that flooding the person's auditory channels with music or rhythmic songs may help block auditory hallucinations (34). However, it is also acknowledged that hallucinations in some people seem to get worse when other stimulation is increased, as if the hallucination is trying to compete for the person's attention. The most useful information about how a given activity affects a particular individual is obtained from that person. By watching how someone reacts and listening to what they say, the OTP can usually learn enough about the effects of the activity to determine whether it is working or how it needs to be changed.

All activities should be suited to the person's intellectual and developmental level. Of course, the activities should be appropriate to the person's occupational roles and reflect their interests and the person should be supported in selecting their own activity. For a client who is experiencing paranoia, activities must be ones the person can control. Structured activities involving controllable materials (eg, leather work) are recommended. Before presenting any activity, the OTP should make sure that it is appropriate for the person's cognitive level and sufficiently complex to engage and maintain their interest. In the beginning, activities should be individual and done independently without need for help or instructions. People with neurocognitive disorders who demonstrate paranoia will have cognitive impairments; great care should be taken in selecting activities of interest that the person can perform successfully. Other than those with neurocognitive disorders, most people who are paranoid can follow diagrams and written directions. Unless there is reason to suspect that a person is suicidal or hostile, it is best to hand over the tools at the beginning of the session rather than requiring them to come and ask for each one individually. Further examples of activities that may be appropriate for individuals who are experiencing the symptoms of psychosis can be found in Box 20.3.

Evidence-Based Interventions That Target Symptoms of Hallucinations, Delusions, or Paranoia

According to the Department of Psychiatry's Best Practices in Schizophrenia Treatment Center, (BeST), at Northeast Ohio Medical University (7), there are six evidence-supported best practices that are helpful in providing support and services to people with schizophrenia and other psychotic disorders. These include (a) the provision of coordinated specialty care for first-episode psychosis (FEP), (b) family education and support, (c) CBTp, (d) integrated primary and mental health care, (e) cognitive enhancement therapy (CET), and (f) pharmacotherapy for schizophrenia. A brief description and discussion of each of these best practice approaches and interventions follows. It should be noted that OTPs have the essential knowledge and skills required to incorporate these techniques and approaches into occupational therapy interventions.

Coordinated Specialty Care for First-Episode Psychosis

The provision of coordinated specialty care means using a team approach to address and treat early psychosis. Coordinated specialty care is multidimensional and embraces shared decision-making between specialists, families, and the client. Although coordinated specialty care programs may differ, coordinated care should always contain the following essential components: individual or group

> **BOX 20.3 Examples of Appropriate Activities for Clients Who Are Experiencing Hallucinations, Delusions, or Paranoia**
>
> **For Clients Who Are Experiencing Hallucinations**
>
> - *Simple, structured, short-term activities* might include coloring "stained-glass" (nonreligious) pictures, discussing specific current events, preparing lunch, or assembling wood kits. Familiar, necessary life tasks, such as doing laundry or housework, can also be used when relevant to the individual's interests and occupational roles.
>
> - *Activities with appropriate sensory stimulation* include those involving music, dance, or drumming, watching films, or cooking and eating.
>
> **For Clients Who Are Experiencing Delusions**
>
> - Some intellectually challenging verbal activities include board games, current events discussion, crossword puzzles, and word games. Chess and computer games might also be used. Aspects of the person's usual occupations should be incorporated wherever possible—for example, a real estate agent can take photographs of buildings and interiors, or help develop presentation materials in a supported employment situation; or an office assistant could perform office-related tasks, or teach peers to use a word-processing program. Expressive activities such as dancing, writing poetry, and journaling are often recommended as helpful by people who have experienced the symptoms (consumers). Care should be used with regard to internet-based activities because of the possibility of the person searching for material that supports the delusions.
>
> **For Clients Who Are Experiencing Paranoia**
>
> - *Wood, leather, or metal projects* constructed according to written instructions are sufficiently complex to challenge the individual. The project shown is a good example. Other possibilities include high-level clerical tasks (organizing files, using computerized databases), design tasks, jewelry making, photography, and puzzles. As with delusions, care should be used with regard to internet-based activities because of the possibility of the person searching for material that supports or increases the paranoid ideation.

psychotherapy; family support and education programs; medication management; supported employment and education services; and case management. Within the specialty coordinated care concept, there is potential for many emerging roles for OTPs. See further descriptions of the components of coordinated specialty care for clients with psychosis or psychotic disorders in Table 20.1.

In a systematic review that described the evidence for efficacy of early intervention services to improve and maintain the occupational participation in youths at risk for serious mental illness, early detection, targeted interventions, and improved access to care were shown to be effective in reducing the negative impacts of illnesses such as schizophrenia, bipolar disorders, and major depression (32). In the same study, a critical analysis of the evidence identified four

Table 20.1. Components of Coordinated Specialty Care for Clients With Psychosis or Psychotic Disorders

Component of Coordinated Specialty Care With Potential Roles for Occupational Therapy	Description
Individual or group psychotherapy	Individual therapy is tailored to a person's recovery goals. Cognitive and behavioral therapy focuses on developing the knowledge and skills necessary to build resilience and cope with aspects of psychosis while maintaining and achieving personal goals.
Family support and education programs	Programs that teach family members about psychosis as well as coping, communication, and problem-solving skills
Medication management	Medication management involves health care providers tailoring medication to a person's specific needs by selecting the appropriate type and dose to help reduce psychosis symptoms.
Supported employment and education services	Supported employment and education services aim to help individuals return to work or school using the support of a coach to help people achieve their goals.
Case management	Case management allows people with psychosis to work with a case manager to address practical problems and improve access to needed support services.

Adapted from National Institute of Mental Health. (2022, October). *Recovery after an initial schizophrenia episode (RAISE)*. NIMH Information Resource Center. https://www.nimh.nih.gov/research/research-funded-by-nimh/research-initiatives/recovery-after-an-initial-schizophrenia-episode-raise

primary categories of intervention typically used with clients who experience psychosis, or psychotic symptoms, each with moderate levels of evidence to support their effectiveness: cognitive remediation (CR), CBT, supported education and supported employment (SE/E), and family psychoeducation (FPE). This emerging evidence can be used to guide occupational therapy intervention planning for adolescents and young adults experiencing FEP (32).

Family Support and Education

Current literature suggests that the more information that families and caregivers have regarding psychosis and psychotic disorders, the better they can understand the disease and advocate for help and resources for themselves and their loved one (20). This makes family support and education a key ingredient of coordinated specialty care. The monthly meetings of community support groups such as the ones offered by local chapters of the National Alliance on Mental Illness (NAMI) are a rich source of support for clients and their families. More formalized educational programs such as "Family-to-Family," a free 8-week course developed by Joyce Burland and the Vermont Chapter of NAMI, are also offered (29). The courses are taught by NAMI-trained family members who, in many cases, have been through experiences with their own loved one. "Family-to-Family" has experienced tremendous success, is considered an evidence-based intervention, and to date has been taught in 49 states to more than 300,000 people. The resource is updated yearly and has been translated into Spanish, Italian, Mandarin, Vietnamese, and Arabic. Evaluations of the course indicate its usefulness in reducing stress and improving problem-solving by family members (20, 29).

Cognitive Behavioral Therapy for Psychosis

The use of CBT in the treatment of psychosis and schizophrenia spectrum diagnoses, referred to as CBTp, has been studied for nearly 25 years (35). CBT draws from the theoretical perspective of the cognitive model, which subscribes to the belief that a person's thoughts influence their emotions and behavior. The same principle applies for clients experiencing psychosis or psychotic symptoms (35). The person with a schizophrenia spectrum diagnosis or who is experiencing enduring symptoms of psychosis typically is operating from a core set of beliefs that cause them to see the world as rejecting and dangerous, and themselves as broken and defeated. Because symptoms of psychosis make the person feel that they are constantly in danger, they tend to be hypervigilant, which eventually negatively impacts their cognitive performance skills (ie, memory, planning, and attention). CBTp is the main cognitive behavioral intervention that has been tested for targeting delusions and other positive symptoms of schizophrenia, such as hallucinations, that create barriers to occupations (19).

In the past decade, research on the use of CBTp has expanded to include its use with clients who experience negative symptoms of psychosis (10). This new branch of CBTp is called CT-R (5, 10). Researchers Paul Grant and Aaron Beck (22), in a collaborative effort to further understand the negative symptoms of schizophrenia, proposed that rather than the negative symptoms of schizophrenia happening because of cognitive deficits, what possibly linked the person's occupational deficits and the negative symptoms together are their false, dysfunctional, and catastrophizing beliefs about themselves and the world. In several studies, the researchers targeted these defeatist beliefs to have the client try to modify them and found that modifying these negative beliefs significantly impacted occupational function, avolition (or apathy), and positive symptoms (10, 22). Further research indicated that the positive impacts of this approach and intervention were maintained in a 6-month follow-up study (23). This initial discovery laid the foundation for changing the focus of intervention to what would evolve into the three main parts of the CT-R.

These parts are engagement and activation of the adaptive mode, identification of aspirations for the future, and action through activity scheduling (10). In part 1 of CT-R, the collaborative therapeutic relationship provides the backdrop for activating a network of beliefs that inhibit or neutralize the client's symptom-related dysfunctional beliefs. This is thought to help them increase their access to their cognitive resources that then activates what this model calls an adaptive mode. Interestingly, the activation of an adaptive mode takes place through *engagement in activities*. In other words, from an occupational therapy perspective, occupation is being used as a means to activate an adaptive mode. However, the developers of CT-R caution that activation of an adaptive mode is only one part of the initial step; the role of the therapy professional is to help the person energize their adaptive mode. "Energizing the adaptive mode requires repeated activity, based on the person's interests, that increases energy over time and lead to easier access of the adaptive mode. Ultimately, the individual can begin to project a future" (5, p. 28). Again, from an occupational therapy perspective, this is comparable with the use of occupation as an end, helping the individual move toward satisfying occupational engagement and quality of life.

When the client has improved access and use of their cognitive performance skills, they are often better able to identify their aspirations for their future. Talking about their dreams and hopes for their future will drive the person's energy and increased activation. When this happens, the client can start the process of changing long-term goals and dreams into smaller stepstone objectives that they can accomplish right away with the support of the OTP or the behavioral health team (10). In the last stage of the CT-R process, the clients' level of motivation driven by their engagement in activities, and the reflection on their aspirations, helps individuals start planning to repeat and evaluate the activities that they have attempted (ie, the occupations that they have engaged in). The OTP can help the person evaluate any new potential activities that the person wants to try so that they can add them to their daily schedule. "Over the course of treatment, the activity is formalized into an activity schedule and the therapist helps the individual identify the benefits of the activity on motivation, distress, mood, and success" (10, para. 10). The CT-R model treats the symptoms of psychosis (such as hallucinations, delusions, communication problems, trauma reactions, self-injurious behaviors, or substance abuse) as obstacles to engagement, aspiration, or taking action—the three parts of the CT-R process. When these obstacles happen, the team works together with the client to neutralize

the challenge for the client to be able to keep moving toward their aspirational goals (5).

One study incorporating many of the principles of CT-R (5) developed a parallel, single-blind, randomized controlled trial to test a program called the *Feeling Safe Programme* against a care protocol modeled to mirror the nonspecific effects of seeing a mental health counselor, which the study termed the "befriending programme" (19). If participants received the befriending programme, therapists were trained to respond to the client in the ways that a friend may respond to their needs. To control for differences in the characteristics of the professionals, the same group of therapists delivered either the Feeling Safe protocol or the befriending protocol. All other aspects of typical care continued throughout the duration of the trial. The purpose of the research study was to determine whether targeted cognitive therapy would lead to clinical changes in clients' experiences of disruptive persecutory delusions more so than with the nonspecific relationship benefits of befriending (or the nonspecific effects of seeing a mental health therapist). The participants were people with persistent persecutory delusions in the context of nonaffective psychosis diagnoses (19).

Clients were randomly assigned to either the Feeling Safe Programme protocol or the befriending programme protocol. Each intervention was delivered to individual clients over a 6-month time frame. After an initial clinical interview used to assess a recent episode of delusional thinking, the clients in the Feeling Safe Programme protocol could choose and help formulate a plan of the learning modules that they wanted to participate in to help them move toward their life aspirations. All the modules in the Feeling Safe Programme address factors that help maintain regular life functions, which for these participants had been disrupted because of delusions. The modules offered in the Feeling Safe Programme were improving sleep, reducing worry, increasing self-confidence, reducing the impact of voices, improving reasoning processes, and feeling safe enough. Typically, three to four modules were completed, on the basis of each client's preference and personalized plan. However, "all patients were encouraged to complete the feeling safe enough module (this module related to the dropping of safety-seeking behaviours in behavioural tests to reduce threat beliefs and build safety beliefs) before the end of treatment" (19, p. 684).

The Feeling Safe Programme included a focus on evaluating safety, addressing sleep dysfunction, worry, and positive self-beliefs, or the "maintenance factors" that are necessary for successful recovery and occupational engagement. Findings indicated that although clinical improvements were associated with both the Feeling Safe Programme and the befriending protocol, targeted cognitive therapy (the Feeling Safe Programme) led to large clinical changes in persecutory delusions that were greater than the nonspecific relationship benefits of the befriending programme. The authors noted, "We believe these results show that if a proven theoretical model is translated into focused intervention techniques that are implemented intensively—within an intervention framework that explicitly addresses the multifactorial complexity of causation in psychosis and patient preference—then major improvements in treatment outcomes are possible" (19, p. 702).

The CT-R model aligns well with an occupational therapy perspective. OTPs can incorporate the principles of CBTp and CT-R into their practice as part of a holistic occupational therapy plan for clients who experience psychotic disorders or symptoms (32). OTPs who are interested in learning more, or who wish to receive further training with CBTp or CT-R, can find ways to do so, including the link to the Beck Institute of Cognitive Behavioral Therapy, listed in the section "Suggested Resources" at the end of this chapter.

Cognitive Enhancement Therapy

Another evidence-based intervention is CET. CET was developed by Gerard Hogarty, a researcher and an expert in the treatment of schizophrenia. CET is a performance-based, developmental approach to the rehabilitation of neurocognitive and social cognition deficits (14). For clients with a diagnosis of schizophrenia or schizoaffective disorders, CET can be implemented as an intervention that supports their recovery phase. Many clients, even when their symptoms are stabilized with the use of medication, find their recovery a struggle and are unsuccessful at achieving the level of independence that they desire. Their illness continues to make social connections and social participation very problematic. Finding and maintaining employment or vocational training also tends to consistently be a challenge throughout recovery (20, 25). CET incorporates structured groups and technology-based exercises to assist clients with increasing their mental stamina, improving information processing skills, and supporting negotiation of spontaneous unrehearsed social challenges (25). The components of social cognition, including a focus on perspective taking and helping the person appraise the situational context and social environment, are synthesized with neurocognitive training and small social groups to achieve improvements in performance-based skills (14, 25).

MANAGING SYMPTOMS OF HALLUCINATIONS, DELUSIONS, AND PARANOIA: THE BECOMING AND BELONGING DIMENSIONS OF OT PRACTICE

> **BOX 20.4 Focus Questions for Planning Transition, Maintenance, and Long-Term Wellness Plans**
>
> 1. How does the client define success in reaching their goals?
> 2. How can occupational therapy support the long-term success in the client becoming who they want to be, successfully doing what they want to do?
> 3. How can occupational therapy support the client's recovery and long-term success in finding community, and feeling a sense of belonging and connectedness?

Social and Emotional Health Promotion and Maintenance for Symptoms of Hallucinations, Delusions, and Paranoia

Individuals with mental illness are consistently marginalized in society today. Although consumers, mental health advocates, and researchers are working tirelessly to explore ways to support this group more effectively, the task is often daunting. For individuals who experience schizophrenia or schizophrenia spectrum disorders and the symptoms of psychosis, a more thorough understanding of how the dynamics of social participation and emotion regulation impact occupational engagement is needed to continue to develop interventions that target social integration and participation. In a recent ethnographic research study, the social participation of young adults following their FEP was explored (17). The purpose of the research was to further understand perceived opportunities for social participation for adolescents following FEP and to identify the sociocultural mechanisms that facilitate or hinder the experience of social participation for these clients. This initial exploratory study suggested five factors that impacted social participation for the participants: social norms and expectations, the person's sense of obligation or responsibility to others, participants' occupational histories and relationships before their illness/diagnosis, changes in the environment or context, and the type of participation available. After experiencing an episode of psychosis, the participants' personal factors and the social factors impacted their sense of belonging and their life course in complex ways. The researchers suggest, as many other mental health advocates agree, that the complex relationship between the client's unique personal factors and the sociocultural context must be the point of intervention. "Occupation is the medium through which this relationship can be examined and addressed to promote social participation and belonging" (13, 17, p. 69).

In terms of the social and emotional impacts of living with psychotic disorders, the OTP has a responsibility to include the client and the caregivers, support network, or the family of the consumer throughout the stages of the occupational therapy process. This is particularly critical for these clients given the evidence that having a strong support network is fundamental to positive recovery (20, 32). The effects of caring for relatives diagnosed with schizophrenia can produce a significant burden on the caregiver. The burden of care is reported to be characterized by experiences of anxiety, fear, sadness, sleeplessness, loss of appetite, loss of libido, and episodic depression (4, 33).

OTPs can provide evidence-supported interventions to help caregivers cope with their stressors, incorporating relaxation and mindfulness techniques that both the client experiencing psychotic symptoms and the caregiver or family members can participate in (21). Family support groups provide caregivers with a forum for sharing feelings of isolation and frustration and discussing common caregiving problems while facilitating empathic social connections. A systematic review of 53 randomized controlled trials concluded that family interventions decreased the frequency of client relapse and reduced hospital admissions. The positive outcomes were attributed to psychosocial family interventions that improved problem-solving skills and emotional regulation skills that further reduced levels of expressed emotion, stress, and family burden (31). Essentially, "the degree and quality of social support that caregivers received was very important in helping them to manage their stressful caregiving activities, and ultimately prevent or reduce the threat of negative psychological symptoms [for the caregiver]" (33, p. 100).

Symptom and Condition Management for Symptoms of Hallucinations, Delusions, and Paranoia

Managing health requires extensive time and effort, especially in the context of illnesses with complex manifestation of symptoms, such as psychosis. Health management is an important occupation that is critical to recovery from the burden of experiencing psychotic symptoms such as hallucinations and delusions. However, health management in long-term recovery can also threaten to disrupt occupational gains by disrupting participation in other important or preferred daily life activities. This further builds upon the already heavy burden of illness. In some cases, the literature suggests that having a diagnosis of schizophrenia, or any of the diseases of the schizophrenia spectrum, and engaging in health management occupations further embeds the illness (and its complex symptoms) into one's identity (18, 20). Researchers Fox and Bailliard (18) found this to be characteristic of young adults following FEP. Specifically, they found that for the participants in their study, the occupation of managing a new diagnosis in the immediate stages after FEP hindered the person's social participation and created a kind of transitional space in the trajectory of their lives. Some study participants reported being or feeling trapped in the transitional space, and so they put their life goals aside to focus on managing the illness. Other study participants reported using the transition time to learn more about their condition, grow, and move toward transformation (18).

OTPs certainly have a responsibility to help clients who experience psychotic symptoms that disrupt occupations to incorporate important health management occupations into their daily lives. People with psychosis are less physically active than are other members of the general population, on average spending as much as 11 hours per day being sedentary (16). Sedentary behaviors and lack of physical activity are linked to increased mortality, cardiovascular disease, cancer, and type 2 diabetes. Inactivity has a significant impact on psychosocial functioning, short-term memory, sleep, depression, and the negative symptoms of psychosis (16). Occupational therapy providers can incorporate the principles of behavioral activation (35), discussed in Chapter 19, to encourage sedentary clients to establish and participate in even brief periods of physical activity that will sustain management of their health and recovery efforts.

Providing education, and practicing with the client to support the establishment of healthy habits and routines, and collaborating with the client so that they can be as independent as possible with tasks such as medication management, or scheduling and attending medical appointments, are invaluable. However, OTPs should be reflective and mindful of encouraging occupational balance because the literature suggests that overemphasizing health management can hinder social participation and negatively impact a client's quality of life (18).

Effective Treatment Goals and Use of Occupation-Centered Outcome Measures

Ultimately, the goal of intervention for treatment of symptoms of psychosis is for the client to have increased opportunities to successfully participate in their preferred (and necessary) occupations. This increases their chances of achieving their goals and aspirations (32, 35, 36). Increased participation leads to increased motivation and improved functioning. For clients who experience symptoms such as hallucinations, delusions, or disordered thinking, increased occupational participation reduces distress. There are three general categories of beliefs that clients attribute their psychotic symptoms (hallucinations) to: control, credibility, and power (35). The client who believes that their hallucinations "get to decide," or are in control of when they happen or appear, will tend to isolate themselves as a compensatory behavior. They believe that isolation protects them from the symptoms happening while they are in social situations or out in public. This compensatory behavior, isolating oneself, creates a vicious cycle because evidence indicates that isolation increases anxiety and increases the likelihood of hallucinating. Control beliefs are most often associated with dysfunction (35).

When a person hallucinates, they firmly believe that their hallucinations are credible sources of the truth. Giving the voices credibility makes the person having this experience somewhat vulnerable to also experiencing paranoid behaviors. Because clients lend credibility to the voices, they tend to be vigilant in listening and monitoring for incoming messages out of fear that missing them would be catastrophic. If the messages are believed to be reliable, there is no reason to check the accuracy of their thoughts and beliefs. The content of hallucinations can be overwhelmingly frightening, and often threatening or demanding (as is the case with command hallucinations). If clients believe that the voices or hallucinations have the power to follow through on their threatening messages, the person will often seek ways to defuse the threat to prevent it from happening, sometimes engaging in a ritual such as praying. Alternatively, the person may seek to stop the hallucination by complying with the demands of the voice (35). Current evidence suggests that one of the most effective treatment interventions is to target the person's beliefs around the control, credibility, and power of their hallucinations (6, 35). For OTPs, engagement in occupations provides an intervention context to be able to perform "behavioral experiments," as a way to collect evidence that tests their false beliefs about control, credibility, and power. Once clients begin to have more successful occupational participation, their maladaptive beliefs can be better understood and they can further challenge themselves to engaging in activities that reduce their symptoms (2, 35).

Case Study

Laura: A 54-Year-Old Female With Schizophrenia

DSM-5-TR Diagnosis at Admission

F20.9   Schizophrenia

Z Codes

Z62.891   Sibling relational problem
Z59.2   Discord with neighbor, lodger, or landlord
I80.01   Phlebitis and thrombophlebitis of superficial vessels of lower extremities

This 54-year-old unmarried Caucasian woman, Laura, was admitted to the acute admissions ward on court certification following action by her neighbors. Commitment papers state that the client has been complaining of people doing things against her; she is suspicious of her neighbors and has been breaking windows. Client has had two previous psychiatric hospitalizations, in 2017 for 3 months and in 2021 for 6 months. Diagnosis is schizophrenia (F20.9). Client also has chronic phlebitis in both legs. Prescribed medication includes olanzapine (Zyprexa) 10 mg, doxepin (Sinequan) 100 mg tid, and docusate (Colace) 100 mg.

At admission, Laura was groomed poorly and dressed in dirty clothing. She appeared anxious, tense, and somewhat confused. Her speech was coherent but at times irrelevant. She denied hearing voices and denied having said that her food was poisoned. She said she had no idea why she was hospitalized other than the ill will of her neighbors.

Occupational Profile Data Collection Interview and Evaluation

Laura is the third child in a family of eight and was raised in a rural section of northern New York State near the Canadian border. She has never married. She lives alone in an apartment with two cats. She has a 10th-grade education and has held numerous jobs, mostly in the food service industry. She says she is now retired and living on Supplemental Security Income (SSI).

Client was referred to occupational therapy 2 weeks after admission for evaluation of functional living skills and assessment of needs in relation to discharge planning. Evaluation instruments included a structured interview, the *Comprehensive Occupational Therapy Evaluation (COTE)* scale, and a functional living skills evaluation.

Laura arrived on time for the interview and each of the subsequent evaluation sessions. Although her hair was often slightly disheveled, she was otherwise clean and neat. She was cooperative in the interview and spoke at length about her apartment, the "things" (she refused to further define what she meant), and her two cats. She expressed sorrow over the death of her mother 5 years ago and seemed to have some unresolved feelings. She mentioned that she does not see her family; she feels positively about one of her brothers who lives in California but expressed hostility toward another brother who lives nearby. She spoke angrily of her neighbors, stating that she feels persecuted and that they pick on her, are stealing from her, and say bad things

about her. She also mentioned that the neighborhood children harass her.

She said she neither has friends nor wants them. She said she is not interested in learning anything new to fill leisure hours, although she does enjoy solitary activities. The only group activity she expressed interest in was bingo. She was unaware of local resources and activity programs for retired people and said she was not interested in them.

Comprehensive Occupational Therapy Evaluation

The *COTE* scale was used to rate the client's performance of a simple craft activity (magazine picture collage). The client worked at moderate speed and an acceptable level of activity. She appeared oriented to place, person, and time. She expressed concern about why certain other persons were not present or were late for the evaluation, which was administered in a group.

Client was responsive and appropriate in her conversation, but many interactions were either dependent or impulsive. For example, she repeatedly asked for help, extra directions, and materials that she could obtain herself. Other clients appeared to view this as an attention-getting device and several made negative remarks to the effect that she took needed attention from them. Laura also made comments that were unrelated to the conversation.

Client needed no encouragement to engage in the activity; and after receiving repeated directions, which she requested, she was able to follow through and complete the task. She worked neatly, in an organized manner; coordination and concentration were more than adequate for the task. She was able to make decisions and solve minor problems encountered in the activity despite her requests for assistance in other less difficult areas. She appeared highly motivated by the activity and expressed interest in other crafts displayed in the occupational therapy room.

Functional Living Skills Evaluation

Laura demonstrated an ability to function independently in the following areas: use of medication, use of her savings account, organization and cleaning of her home, selection of clothing and laundry and clothing maintenance, and single-serving cooking. She was unable to identify the correct response to several household emergencies, including what to do if the lights went out or if she smelled gas. She was able to use her cell phone to find emergency phone numbers but reports that she frequently forgets to charge her phone or turn it on, and so it is not available when she needs it sometimes. Laura demonstrates decreased literacy levels, which prevents her from writing simple messages or reading a bus schedule. She apparently relies on others to tell her when and where to take the bus, but she has a good knowledge of the public transportation system. She states that she does have a budget and could demonstrate how to break down her monthly income into weekly budgets. However, she was unable to demonstrate or explain how to make correct change from $20 and she could not figure the sales tax.

Please find follow-up case reflections and questions in the section "OT HACKS Summary."

Commonly Used Acronyms

With the growing need for more CMHCs and CSC, OTPs can find opportunities in a variety of these settings. As a member of a multidisciplinary care team, it will become increasingly important for the OTP to be proficient in recognizing commonly used acronyms such as the ones found here.

ACE: Adverse childhood experience
BARS: Behaviorally Anchored Rating Scale
BPRS: Brief Psychiatric Rating Scale
CAB: Core Assessment Battery
CBT: Cognitive behavioral therapy
CBTp: Cognitive Behavioral Therapy for Psychosis
CT-R: Recovery-Oriented Cognitive Therapy
CHR: Clinical high risk (for psychosis)
CMHC: Community mental health center
CSC: Coordinated specialty care
CSI: Colorado Symptom Index

DUP: Duration of untreated psychosis
EASA: Early Assessment and Support Alliance
EPINET: Early Psychosis Intervention Network
ESMI: Early serious mental illness
FEP: First-episode psychosis
MHBG: Community Mental Health Block Grant
PCL-5: PTSD Checklist for *DSM-5*
QPR: Questionnaire about the process of recovery
SAMHSA: Substance Abuse Mental Health Services Administration
SMHA: State Mental Health Authority

Reprinted with permission from Kazandjian, M., Neylon, K., Ghose, S., George, P., Masiakowski, N. P., Lutterman, T., & Rosenblatt, A. (2022, November). *State snapshot 2021–2022: Early psychosis programming across the United States* (p. 5). https://nationalepinet.org/wp-content/uploads/2022/12/EPINET_State_Snapshot_FINAL_508_COMPLIANT.pdf

OT HACKS SUMMARY

O: Occupation as a means and an end

Although the benefits of using antipsychotic medications in the treatment of schizophrenia and psychotic disorders cannot be denied, medication alone is not sufficient for achieving optimal recovery outcomes. A comprehensive treatment program includes rehabilitation as well. Clients with psychotic symptomology vary widely in their priorities and needs; this is largely dependent on the severity of their symptoms and how those symptoms have altered their occupational engagement. Nevertheless, these clients share a common need to address the following fundamental and basic priorities (20):

- Money
- Food
- Housing
- Employment
- Friendship (social connection)
- Medical care

Each of these fundamental needs can inform the way an OTP uses occupation as either a means or an end (1, 3).

T: Theoretical concepts, values, and principles, or historical foundations

FIRST: Demonstrate Empathy!

"Before addressing these specific problems, it should be noted that one concept underlies all rehabilitation efforts—hope. If the individual with schizophrenia has hope, then rehabilitation efforts are likely to succeed. If the person has no hope, these efforts are likely to fail" (20, p. 206).

ALWAYS . . . Be Hopeful and Instill HOPE!

H: How can we Help? OT's role in serving clients with mental illness or mental health needs

With the growing need for more community mental health centers (CMHCs) and coordinated specialty care (CSC), OTPs can find opportunities in a variety of these settings. As a member of a multidisciplinary care team, it will become increasingly important for the OTP to be proficient in recognizing commonly used acronyms such as the ones found in the box given earlier. What other skills or traits can you think of that might be helpful to an OTP who is a member of a multidisciplinary behavioral health team?

A: Adaptations

What is CBTp? **CBTp** is a structured intervention similar to CBT that has been adapted to address the symptoms of psychosis such as delusions, depression, hallucinations, mania, negative symptoms, sleep difficulties, and hopelessness. Targeted CBTp interventions can address client factors such as interpersonal problems, isolation, motivation/volition, social skills, self-esteem, and medication adherence. CBTp involves establishing a collaborative therapeutic relationship, developing a shared understanding of the problem, setting goals, and teaching the person techniques or strategies to reduce or manage the symptoms that create barriers to occupational engagement. Clients learn specific strategies to reduce distress and improve occupational balance and function. Specific CBTp approaches include cognitive restructuring, behavioral experiments/reality testing, and self-monitoring and coping skills training.

What is CT-R? **CT-R** is an extension of CBTp. CBTp was originally developed to address positive symptoms of psychosis (hallucinations and delusions) to help people regain their lives. CT-R is a related treatment approach designed to promote empowerment, recovery, and resiliency in individuals with serious mental health conditions. It focuses on activating adaptive modes of living, developing meaningful aspirations, and engaging in personally meaningful activities to bring about one's desired life (5).

C: Case study includes

Can you answer the following questions related to Laura's case?

1. How do you interpret the client's interest in bingo? In what ways is this helpful in developing social and interpersonal skills? Explain. What other activities are similar

to bingo but offer greater opportunities for social inter-action? In what ways could the OTP alter the environ-ment or the activity to increase opportunity for social interaction?

2. The physician wants to know whether Laura can function well enough on her own to return to her own apartment or should be placed in a supervised living situation. For-mulate a recommendation and justify it with evidence from the case history. Indicate any further evaluations or information that you think are needed or believe will help in making this determination. Document your recommen-dations in the form of a note suitable for the client's chart.

3. The client seems not to have worked in a while and says she is retired, at age 54. What are the arguments for and against exploring whether she wants to begin some sort of part-time employment?

K: Knowledge: keeping mental health OT practice grounded in evidence, in occupational science, and in research

A few key points are given here:

"People with mental disorders have greater morbidity and mortality due to physical health problems compared to the general population" (as cited in 27, p. 1078).

"People diagnosed with schizophrenia have higher rates of metabolic diseases, cardiovascular problems, obesity, and osteoporosis" (as cited in 27, p. 1078).

"In depression, higher prevalence of type 2 diabetes melli-tus, stroke and myocardial infarction are observed" (as cited in 27, p. 1078).

". . . even in medical services, there is prejudice and dis-crimination against people with mental disorders, which may negatively influence medical-patient relationships, and the accessibility and quality of treatment" (as cited in 27, p. 1078).

The sample included 211 NPMS. Participants "were asked to complete a revised version of the *Opinions on mental disorders Questionnaire* (OQ) after reading, at random, a clinical description of either schizophrenia (Appendix A) or depression (Appendix B). . . . 114 NPMS completed the OQ after reading a clinical description of schizophrenia and 97 completed the same questionnaire after reading a clinical description of depression" (as cited in 27, p. 1080).

The findings indicated: "NPMS have both similarities and dif-ferences in their views of people diagnosed with schizophre-nia and depression. Specialists seem to have similar level of skepticism regarding the capacities of these clients to report their health problems to doctors" (as cited in 27, p. 1082).

"Specialists considered people with schizophrenia to be less capable than those with depression of taking care of their own physical health problems, mainly in their capacity to adhere to treatments" (as cited in 27, p. 1083).

Evidence Application and Translation Questions

1. On the basis of this piece of evidence, describe how stigma and prejudice against people with psychosis or psychotic symptoms can negatively impact the clients' overall health?

2. What level of evidence is this study?

3. What are some of the strengths and limitations of this study?

4. In the introduction of this study, the authors cite an ear-lier 2015 study by Welch and colleagues that found that, "physicians often alerted colleagues about clients' mental disorders, influencing colleagues' expectations" (as cited in 27, p. 1078). Which of the American Occupational Therapy Association (AOTA) Ethical Codes (1) would this behavior violate if an OTP demonstrated a similar behav-ioral response?

S: Some terms that may be new to you

Delusion: a belief that may or may not be based on reality

Delusions of persecution: persistent, troubling, false be-liefs that one is about to be harmed or mistreated by others in some way

Erotomania: false belief (delusion) that someone is in love with you

Hallucination: a sensory experience that does not corre-spond to external reality; hallucinations can include seeing, hearing, feeling, smelling, or tasting things that are not there

Idea of reference: false belief that irrelevant occurrences or details in the world relate directly to oneself

Megalomania/delusions of grandeur: false belief that one has special powers or when one believes that they have more power, wealth, smarts, or other grandiose traits than are actually true

Mood congruent: auditory hallucinations that are consis-tent with the person's mood

Paranoia: thoughts and feelings of being threatened in some way, even if there is little or no evidence to support the thoughts, feelings, and suspiciousness

Paranoid delusions: extreme and unbelievable ideas or be-liefs, typically focused on suspiciousness

Paranoid ideation: heightened general suspiciousness

Somatic delusions: a false belief that one's internal or ex-ternal bodily functions are abnormal or that something is physically, biologically, or medically wrong with them

Thought insertion: false belief that someone or something in inserting thoughts into one's brain (a type of delusion)

Thought withdrawal: false belief that someone or some-thing is taking thoughts out of one's brain (a type of delusion)

Reflection Questions

1. Differentiate the term psychotic disorder from psychosis. Why does the careful use of language matter when we describe or discuss symptoms and diseases?

2. Compare and contrast the positive, negative, and the disordered symptoms of psychosis. Which category of client symptoms do you feel would be the most difficult for you, as an OTP, to plan targeted interventions for? Explain your reasoning.

3. Describe the relationship between CBTp and CT-R.

4. Explain how the components of CT-R correspond with similar occupational therapy principles of using occupation as a means and as an end during the therapeutic process.

5. Which dimension of occupation—doing, being, becoming, or belonging—do you think is the most troublesome for clients who experience symptoms of psychosis? Provide a rationale for your response.

6. What are three general categories of beliefs that clients attribute their psychotic symptoms (ie, hallucinations) to, and what compensatory behaviors are associated with those beliefs?

7. Why or how might the occupation of health management lead to occupational disruption?

Rᴇꜰᴇʀᴇɴᴄᴇꜱ

1. American Occupational Therapy Association. (2020). AOTA occupational therapy code of ethics. *American Journal of Occupational Therapy, 74*(Suppl. 3), 7413410005.
2. American Occupational Therapy Association. (2020). Occupational therapy in the promotion of health and well-being. *American Journal of Occupational Therapy, 74*, 7403420010.
3. American Occupational Therapy Association. (2020). Occupational therapy practice framework: Domain and process—Fourth edition. *American Journal of Occupational Therapy, 74*(Suppl. 2), 1–87.
4. American Psychiatric Association. (2022). *Diagnostic and statistical manual of mental disorders* (5th ed., text rev.). https://doi.org/10.1176/appi.books.9780890425787
5. Beck, A. T., Grant, P., Inverso, E., Brinen, A. P., & Perivoliotis, D. (2021). *Recovery-oriented cognitive therapy for serious mental health conditions* (Kindle ed.). The Guilford Press.
6. Beck, A. T., Rector, N. A., Stolar, N., & Grant, P. (2009). *Schizophrenia: Cognitive theory, research, and therapy.* Guilford Press.
7. Best Practices in Schizophrenia Treatment (BeST) Center. (n.d.). *Tips for engaging individuals with psychotic illness in treatment.* Department of Psychiatry, Northeast Ohio Medical University. https://www.neomed.edu/wp-content/uploads/BST_first-engaging-tips.pdf
8. Boland, R., & Verduin, M. (2021). *Kaplan & Sadock's concise textbook of clinical psychiatry.* Lippincott Williams & Wilkins.
9. Branjerdporn, G., Hussain, B., Roberts, S., & Creedy, D. (2022). Uncovering the model and philosophy of care of a psychiatric inpatient mother-baby unit in a qualitative study with staff. *International Journal of Environmental Research and Public Health, 19*(15), 9717.
10. Brinen, A. P., & Beck, A. T. (2016). *Cognitive behavioral therapy for psychosis (CBTp) and recovery-oriented therapy (CT-R): What is the difference?* Beck Institute for Cognitive Therapy. https://beckinstitute.org/blog/cbtp-and-ct-r-what-is-the-difference/
11. Brown, B. (2021). *Atlas of the heart: Mapping meaningful connection and the language of human experience.* Random House Publishers.
12. Buser, S., & Cruz, L. (2022). *DSM-5-TR insanely simplified: Unlocking the spectrums within DSM-5-TR and ICD-10.* Chiron Publications.
13. Carey, E. (2018, September 28). *Psychosis.* Healthline. Https://www.healthline.com/health/psychosis
14. Cognitive Enhancement Therapy. (n.d.). *The official site for research, training, and implementation.* Retrieved June 06, 2023, from https://www.cognitiveenhancementtherapy.com/
15. Deegan, P. (2006). *Hearing voices that are distressing curriculum: Complete training and curriculum package.* National Empowerment Center.
16. Diamond, R., Bird, J. C., Waite, F., Bold, E., Chadwick, E., Collett, N., & Freeman, D. (2022). The physical activity profiles of patients with persecutory delusions. *Mental Health and Physical Activity, 23*, 100462.
17. Fox, V. (2019). An exploration of social participation of young adults following a first psychotic episode. *Journal of Occupational Science, 27*(3), 69–81.
18. Fox, V., & Bailliard, A. L. (2021). Liminal space of first-episode psychosis: Health management and its effect on social participation. *American Journal of Occupational Therapy, 75*(6), 7506205090.
19. Freeman, D., Emsley, R., Diamond, R., Collett, N., Bold, E., Chadwick, E., Isham, L., Bird, J. C., Edwards, D. Kingdon, D., Fitzpatrick, R., Kabir, T., & Waite, F. (2021). Comparison of a theoretically driven cognitive therapy (the Feeling Safe Programme) with befriending for the treatment of persistent persecutory delusions: A parallel, single-blind, randomised controlled trial. *The Lancet Psychiatry, 8*(8), 696–707.
20. Fuller Torrey, E. (2019). *Surviving schizophrenia: A family manual* (7th ed.). HarperCollins.
21. Goldberg, S. B., Tucker, R. P., Greene, P. A., Davidson, R. J., Wampold, B. E., Kearney, D. J., & Simpson, T. L. (2018). Mindfulness-based interventions for psychiatric disorders: A systematic review and meta-analysis. *Clinical Psychology Review, 59*, 52–60.
22. Grant, P. M., & Beck, A. T. (2009, July 1). Defeatist beliefs as a mediator of cognitive impairment, negative symptoms, and functioning in schizophrenia. *Schizophrenia Bulletin, 35*(4), 798–806.
23. Grant, P. M., Bredemeier, K., & Beck, A. T. (2017). Six-month follow-up of recovery-oriented cognitive therapy for low-functioning individuals with schizophrenia. *Psychiatric Services, 68*(10), 997–1002.
24. Hill, R., & Dahlitz, M. (2022). *The practitioner's guide to the science of psychotherapy.* W.W. Norton & Company.
25. Hogarty, G. E., Flesher, S., Ulrich, R., Carter, M., Greenwald, D., Pogue-Geile, M., Kechavan, M., Cooley, S., DiBarry, A., Garrett, A., Parepally, H., & Zoretich, R. (2004). Cognitive enhancement therapy for schizophrenia: Effects of a 2-year randomized trial on cognition and behavior. *Archives of General Psychiatry, 61*(9), 866–876.
26. MacRae, A (1997). The model of functional deficits associated with hallucinations. *American Journal of Occupational Therapy, 51*(1), 57–63.
27. Magliano, L., Ruggiero, G., Read, J., Mancuso, A., Schiavone, A., & Sepe, A. (2020). The views of non-psychiatric medical specialists about people with schizophrenia and depression. *Community Mental Health Journal, 56*(6), 1077–1084.
28. Maloney, S. M., & Griffith, K. (2013). Occupational therapy students' development of therapeutic communication skills during a service-learning experience. *Occupational Therapy in Mental Health, 29*(1), 10–26.
29. National Alliance on Mental Illness Florida. (2023). *NAMI: Family-to-family program.* Retrieved June 17, 2023, from https://namiflorida.org/support-and-education/mental-health-education/nami-family-to-family/
30. Ozelie, R., Panfil, P., Swiderski, N., & Walz, E. (2018). Hearing voices simulation: Impact on occupational therapy students. *The Open Journal of Occupational Therapy, 6*(4), Article 10.
31. Pharoah, F., Mari, J., Rathbone, J., & Wong, W. (2010). Family intervention for schizophrenia. *Cochrane Database of Systematic Reviews, 12*, 1–166.
32. Read, H., Roush, S., & Downing, D. (2018). Early intervention in mental health for adolescents and young adults: A systematic review. *American Journal of Occupational Therapy, 72*(5), 7205190040.
33. Riley-McHugh, D., Brown, C. H., & Lindo, J. (2016). Schizophrenia: Its psychological effects on family caregivers. *International Journal of Advanced Nursing Studies, 5*(1), 96–101.
34. Seraphine, P. L. (2019, September). Self-regulation through drumming: A brain-body model for optimizing mental health. *The Science of Psychotherapy Magazine*, 4–17.
35. Sokol, L., & Fox, M. G. (2019). *The comprehensive clinician's guide to cognitive behavioral therapy.* PESI Publishing.
36. Tan, B. L., Zhen Lim, M. W., Xie, H., Li, Z., & Lee, J. (2020). Defining occupational competence and occupational identity in the context of recovery in schizophrenia. *American Journal of Occupational Therapy, 74*(4), 7404205120.
37. Taylor, R. R. (2020). *The intentional relationship: Occupational therapy and use of self* (2nd ed.). F.A. Davis.
38. Wickham, S., Sitko, K., & Bentall, R. P. (2015). Insecure attachment is associated with paranoia but not hallucinations in psychotic patients: The mediating role of negative self-esteem. *Psychological Medicine, 45*(7), 1495–1507.
39. Yalom, I. D., & Leszcz, M. (2020). *The theory and practice of group psychotherapy* (6th ed.). Basic Books.

Suggested Resources

Articles

Tan, B. L., Zhen Lim, M. W., Xie, H., Li, Z., & Lee, J. (2020). Defining occupational competence and occupational identity in the context of recovery in schizophrenia. *American Journal of Occupational Therapy, 74*(4), 7404205120.

McCarthy, K., Gottheil, K., Villavicencio, E., & Jeong, H. (2021). Exploring voice hearers' occupational experience of romantic and sexual relationships. *The Open Journal of Occupational Therapy, 9*(1), 1–17.

Books

Beck, A. T., Grant, P., Inverso, E., Brinen, A. P., & Perivoliotis, D. (2021). *Recovery-oriented cognitive therapy for serious mental health conditions.* The Guilford Press.

This book describes CT-R, an evidence-based approach that empowers people who are experiencing symptoms of psychosis, or who have diagnoses such as schizophrenia, to build a life of increased independence and freedom from their symptoms. CT-R provides innovative strategies to help individuals shift from a "patient" mode to a more adaptive mode of living where their strengths, talents, and abilities are recognized. This is an excellent resource for the OTP who works in a behavioral or psychosocial setting. It contains resources that can be incorporated into occupational therapy sessions, as well as case examples, reproducible worksheets, and several tip sheets relevant to COVID-19 and telehealth.

Fuller Torrey, E. (2019). *Surviving schizophrenia: A family manual* (7th ed.). HarperCollins.

This book, originally published in 1983, is in its 7th edition. It describes the nature, causes, symptoms, treatment, and course of schizophrenia. The author presents both the lived experience of the client and the perspective of the family. This is an excellent resource that includes the latest research findings related to schizophrenia, as well as information about positive courses and options for treatment.

My Brother Adam: A Journey With Schizophrenia by Linda Onyilofor and Nneka Onyilofor, a mother and daughter team whose biographies and more information about their story, and their journey loving and caring for someone with schizophrenia, can be found on their website: https://mybrotheradam.com/

Videos

Interacting With Someone in Psychosis: Advice Series. A conversation with the cofounder and host of the Living Well With Schizophrenia YouTube Channel (The home page for Living Well With Schizophrenia is linked in the Websites resources) (approximately 6 minutes). https://www.youtube.com/watch?v=kOyiLKMEnMk

Cognitive Behavioral Therapy for Schizophrenia—Video Series with leading researcher Dr David Kingdon. http://schizophrenia.com/?p=632

Websites

Schizophrenia.com is an internet community that was founded in 1995 and is dedicated to provide high-quality information, support, and education to the family members, caregivers, and individuals whose lives have been impacted by schizophrenia. According to their home page, the web community was founded in memory of John Chiko, who suffered from schizophrenia. The staff of Schizophrenia.com is dedicated to improving the lives of all individuals and families suffering from schizophrenia and in speeding the research progress toward a cure.

The Early Assessment and Support Alliance (EASA) provides information, support, and resources to young people experiencing symptoms of psychosis for the first time, and offers a wide range of resources for people who love and care for a person who is experiencing the symptoms of psychosis. https://easacommunity.org/index.php

Early Psychosis Intervention Network (EPINET) is a national learning health care system for early psychosis. EPINET links early psychosis clinics through standard clinical measures, uniform data collection methods, data sharing agreements, and integration of client-level data across service users and clinics. Clients and their families, clinicians, health care administrators, and scientific experts partner within EPINET to improve early psychosis care and conduct large-scale, practice-based research. https://nationalepinet.org/

Initiated in 2019 and sponsored by the National Institute of Mental Health (NIMH), the EPINET initiative includes 8 Regional Hubs, over 100 early psychosis clinics across 17 states, and the EPINET National Data Coordinating Center (ENDCC).

Living Well With Schizophrenia https://www.livingwellwithschizophrenia.org/

The Beck Institute for Cognitive Behavioral Therapy https://beckinstitute .or

Targeting Psychological and Social Factors That Influence Occupational Engagement: Being With the Client Who Experiences Cognitive Deficits, Confusion, or Impaired Memory

OT HACKS OVERVIEW

O: Occupation as a means and an end

In some ways, cognition can be seen as a means to an end. Cognition describes the mental processes (such as attention, memory, and executive function) that a person employs to perceive and make sense of information so that they can use the information for specific tasks and purposes. This chapter focuses on application of the occupational therapy process targeting the symptoms of cognitive impairment and cognitive decline that create problems with occupational performance and present obstacles to participation.

T: Theoretical concepts, values, and principles, or historical foundations

In her 1961 Eleanor Clarke Slagle Lecture, Mary Reilly stated that "Man, through the use of his hands, as they are energized by mind and will, can influence the state of his own health." Today, that is among the top 10 most frequently cited quotes in occupational therapy literature (17).

For clients with cognitive impairment activities that are somewhat familiar and interesting to the client, and that also occupy the person's hands with a purposeful task (ie, the *doing* dimension of occupation) serve to alleviate boredom *and* distract attention away from disruptive or unsafe behavioral responses, which, particularly in moderate to late stages of major neurocognitive disorders (NCDs), become increasingly common.

H: How can we Help? OT's role in serving clients with mental illness or mental health needs

Because of occupational therapy's holistic perspective and focus on overall occupational participation (rather than isolated performance skills or client factors), especially considering occupational therapy's incorporation of analysis of the person's performance patterns, habits, roles, and routines, the occupational therapy professional (OTP) has an increased likelihood of detecting and documenting the subtle changes that occur when clients experience cognitive impairment or decline.

A: Adaptations

Research suggests a high correlation between cognitive function and a person's performance of activities of daily living (ADLs). This highlights the critical need for OTPs to make the assessment of a client's functional status while completing ADLs and instrumental activities of daily living (IADLs) a critical priority when working with clients experiencing cognitive impairments.

In planning interventions, the OTP must differentiate permanent or progressive cognitive deficits from those that are temporary or fluctuating, particularly with regard to choosing the intervention type and approach that will be most appropriate for the needs of the client (ie, remedial and restorative approaches vs compensatory techniques and maintenance approaches).

The OTP's ability to be highly organized and prepared, as well as possessing the ability to shift between several relevant activities that all have been planned as purposeful in helping the client progress toward their occupational goals, are some of the characteristics of occupational therapy intervention that lead to positive outcomes.

C: Case study includes

Mrs Anderson is a 72-year-old Caucasian female admitted to Green Manor, a skilled nursing facility. Mrs Anderson has a *Diagnostic and Statistical Manual of Mental Disorders, Fifth Edition, Text Revision (DSM-5–TR)* diagnosis of Alzheimer disease (AD; G30.9), and major NCD due to AD with behavioral disturbance (F02.81). Depressed mood was also noted. Mrs Anderson, who has cerebral atherosclerosis (I67.2) and congestive heart failure (I50.4), was first diagnosed with AD 3 years ago. Until admission, she was cared for at home by her husband of 45 years. However, Mrs Anderson has become weaker and incontinent, and Mr Anderson, who is 74 years old, is not strong enough to help his wife transfer from bed to commode, so it was necessary to place her in a specialized memory care unit of the skilled nursing facility.

Read more about the case at the end of the chapter.

Read this evidence, a systematic review brief by Hildebrand and Mack, using the following research question as a focus:

What is the evidence for the effectiveness of interventions within the scope of occupational therapy practice for caregivers of people who have had a stroke that facilitate maintaining participation in the caregiver role?

After reviewing this systematic review and learning more in this chapter about how the symptoms of cognitive deficit, memory impairment, or confusion impact occupational engagement, discuss responses to the *Evidence Application and Translation Questions* found in the *"OT HACKS Chapter Summary, Knowledge"* section.

S: **Some terms that may be new to you**

Alertness
Attention
Attention deficits
Attention span
Backward chaining
Clouding of consciousness
Cognition
Cognitive deficit
Comprehension
Concentration
Confabulation
Cuing devices
Disorganization
Disorientation/confusion
Distractibility
Dressing apraxia
Emotional prosody
Etiology
Executive function
External memory aids
Impaired judgment
Inattention
Judgment
Labile
Long-term memory
Low arousal
Memory
Memory impairment
Orientation
Problem-solving
Short-term memory
Sundowning syndrome
Wayfinding (wandering)
Working memory

TARGETING SYMPTOMS OF COGNITIVE DEFICITS THAT CREATE BARRIERS TO OCCUPATION: THE BEING, DOING, AND BELONGING DIMENSIONS OF OT PRACTICE

BOX 21.1 Intervention Planning Focus Questions: How to Begin

1. What does it feel like to be a person experiencing the symptoms of deficits in cognition, including *confusion, impaired memory, attention deficits, or disorganization*?
2. What are some behaviors that a person experiencing *confusion, impaired memory, attention deficits, or disorganization* might demonstrate, and how might their behavior, responses, or affect be positively or negatively impacting their occupations?
3. How can I adjust my way of being (therapeutic use of self) to make the client feel more comfortable about their way of being?
4. What can I do to instill a sense of belonging in occupational therapy, right now, that will encourage the client toward setting goals with outcomes that are personally meaningful and relevant to them?

Cognition describes the mental processes that a person employs to perceive and make sense of information so that they can use the information for specific tasks and purposes. The main mental processes that comprise cognition are **attention**, **memory**, and **executive function** (13). This chapter focuses on application of the occupational therapy process targeting the symptoms of cognitive impairment and cognitive decline that are typical with major and mild NCDs. The chapter also details barriers to occupation presented by cognitive deficits that create problems with attention and disorganization (or disorganized thinking) and which can be core features of both NCDs and other psychiatric diagnoses (eg, attention deficit hyperactivity disorder [ADHD] and intellectual disabilities [IDs]). Cognitive deficits and impairments that interfere with occupational performance and participation affect many diagnostic groups. Even clients with conditions whose main symptoms are more closely associated with symptoms of psychosis (ie, schizophrenia) or mood (eg, depressive and bipolar disorders) can experience occupational disruption because of cognitive impairment. Therefore, the reader will also be introduced to restorative, remedial, compensatory, and adaptive strategies and approaches that can help OTPs collaborate with clients and their care partners in assessing and addressing cognitive concerns.

Beginning in the *DSM-5* series, the term *Dementia* was replaced by the term *Neurocognitive Disorder (NCD)*. There are two spectrums of illness associated with NCDs, according to the *DSM-5-TR* (9), the *Mild Neurocognitive Disorders* and the *Major Neurocognitive Disorders*. These two spectrums represent a wide range of functional levels and are further organized according to subtypes based on the **etiology** (cause) of the NCD. The subtypes of the NCDs include traumatic brain injury (TBI), HIV infection, Parkinson disease (PD), prion disease, vascular disorders (eg, stroke), Huntington disease, substance-induced dementia, Lewy bodies, and AD (9, 14). Each of the illnesses and their constellation of symptoms will be unique to the individual client; however, these disorders share some commonalities in both symptoms and in course. First, most of the NCDs are degenerative, meaning that functional decline should be expected (although the nature and timeline of the decline can vary widely). Next, cognitive impairment, and especially deterioration of executive function over time, is a common characteristic shared by people who are diagnosed with NCDs. "Neural tissue is damaged by neurodegenerative diseases and by injury, and some treatments have side effects that exacerbate and even initiate other problems" (32, pp. 228–229).

Confusion and Impaired Memory as Symptoms of Cognitive Impairment

As stated earlier, cognition is comprised of three major components—attention, memory, and executive function—all of which contribute to "thinking." Perhaps most important to OTPs, thinking is an integral part of "doing," or necessary for engaging in occupation. A **cognitive deficit** is an impairment or anomaly in one or more of the mental processes needed for thinking. Some of these processes are orientation, alertness, concentration, attention span, memory, comprehension, judgment, and problem-solving. **Orientation** is knowledge of where one is, what time it is (hour, day, date, season), and who one is. This is sometimes called orientation to time, place, and person and abbreviated as orientation ×3 (meaning orientation in three spheres of information). Problems in this area are described as **disorientation** or **confusion**. Generally, disorientation to time alone is the least severe form; disorientation to place and time is more severe; and disorientation to person, place, and time indicates the most significant impairment.

Alertness is awareness of the immediate context and environment. Problems with alertness may be described generally as **low arousal** (seemingly unaware of stimulation), **clouding of consciousness** (meaning literally that the person seems to be in a fog), or impairment of a specific aspect of alertness. Concentration and attention span, for example, are aspects of alertness. **Concentration** is the ability to focus one's mental energies on the task at hand. The intensity of focus is the primary concern. **Attention span** is the length of time that concentration can

be maintained. Impairment in attention span may be described as **distractibility** (meaning a tendency to lose focus because other stimuli catch one's interest) or **inattention** (usually meaning the inability to pay attention even though little or no competing external stimulus is present). Strategies for responding to these symptoms and addressing specific cognitive deficits that interfere with occupational participation are introduced and discussed throughout the chapter.

Memory is the ability to recall past information, knowledge, and events. Problems in remembering important information are called, in general, **memory impairment**. Health professionals commonly distinguish between short-term memory and long-term memory to indicate the difference between memory of events from months or years ago (**long-term memory**) and memory of more recent events (**short-term memory**). Thus, the ability to remember one's date of birth or the names of one's children reflects long-term memory and the ability to remember whether one had lunch or where one's eyeglasses are reflects short-term memory. **Working memory** refers to short-term memory that is stored for a brief period for a specific purpose; it is memory for information that needs to be worked with temporarily, usually only for a short period of time, such as remembering a phone number until one can enter the information into the cell phone, or listening to directions to arrive at a location a short time later. As a member of an interdisciplinary behavioral health team, it is imperative for the OTP to be familiar with the various types of memory and to also have clarity about which type of memory is being discussed with regard to each client.

Higher order cognitive skills such as comprehension (understanding), concept formation, categorization, judgment, problem-solving, or decision-making are sometimes called **executive function** (13, 18, 46, 59). **Comprehension** is the ability to understand. Comprehension is composed of many skills including the ability to recognize words; to identify objects; to place things in order by time, size, or some other quality; to extract essential information from a spoken or written passage; and to classify, sort, or group objects in a logical manner (18). Comprehension depends on the development of concepts, or **concept formation**. We can think of concepts as containers for experiences—for example, our concept of *dog* includes many varieties and sizes of dog; when we see a four-legged animal, we compare it to other items in the concept *dog* to see whether it belongs in this container. A person's ability to comprehend depends on the number of concepts available and the way that concepts can be organized and categorized. To illustrate, an unsophisticated concept of *muscle* might refer just to physical strength (ie, "they are strong, they have got muscles"). A student of physical medicine or anatomy has a far more sophisticated conceptualization—in fact, a highly organized group of concepts—including a more complex understanding of what "muscle" could mean in a variety of contextualized situations.

Because of the complexity of the comprehension process, the cause of a client's problems with comprehension may not be apparent and could be multifactorial. Language skills and communication abilities, prior education, exposure to trauma, adverse childhood experiences, occupational deprivation, and life experiences all have the potential to impact a person's level of understanding and comprehension. Physiologic changes to the neurologic system caused by brain injury, insult, illness, infection, or exposure to harmful substances or chemicals in the body can also impair a person's level of comprehension. Problems with comprehension are usually described as an **inability to comprehend**.

Judgment is the ability to recognize and comply with established social norms and standard procedures, and to use what most people refer to as "common sense." Like comprehension, a client's judgment may reflect their occupational history and is often influenced by social determinants of health. Using inappropriate language in a workplace setting, for example, indicates poor judgment. Problems in judgment are usually referred to as **impaired judgment**; some examples are driving while intoxicated, or making sexual innuendoes to coworkers, and even more simple behavioral responses, choices such as exiting a fire escape door that is clearly marked with a sign that says "NO EXIT," especially when the written sign is accompanied by a graphic to further deter people. **Problem-solving** is the ability to recognize, analyze, and ultimately figure out solutions to problems that arise during everyday activity. Some examples of problems that most people must solve are budgeting money and getting from place to place. Most adults living independently need to figure out how to pay for things such as repair of the water heater or the purchase of weekly groceries. When the car breaks down or the train is delayed, an alternative way of transporting oneself must be found. Living on one's own in the community depends on the ability to solve problems such as these. Because cognitive impairments have such a profound effect on a person's ability to function independently, they are discussed several times throughout this text.

The loss of personal autonomy and independence in everyday life that often occurs when one experiences cognitive decline or cognitive deficits is profoundly disturbing. People who realize that their thinking is not as clear as it once was, or that they have forgotten and left a pot burning on the stove (more than once), may become very frightened and anxious. They may begin to check things many times over or engage in ritualistic actions. Or they may become anxious, agitated, and even belligerent or aggressive. Commonly, long-term memory and recall of events from many years ago are intact, but when occupational performance begins to suffer as an individual participates in their typical ADLs or IADLs, it can be indicative of future problems with short-term memory or working memory deficits (25, 46). "The loss of independence begins with a decline in the IADL (ie, shopping, using the media, managing money, among others), which require interaction with the environment, cognitive skills, and social interaction" (46, pp. 1–2). These initial experiences of

occupational disruption and the corresponding negative emotions may even cause the person to make up stories to hide their problems. This is called **confabulation**.

Cognitively impaired individuals also experience symptoms of depression; it is not always clear whether the depression is the cause of the cognitive problems, or the result. Many aspects of cognition are impacted, for example, by symptoms of major depressive disorder (MDD), including attention, decision-making, problem-solving, language, and memory (59). The symptoms of depression and the cognitive deficits interact with each other in a negative way; the more severe the problems in thinking and remembering, the more intense the levels of depressive symptoms become. Likewise, the more depressed the person is, the more likely they are to forget things and have trouble concentrating. Thus, symptoms of depression and cognitive problems are in a relationship, fueling each other, and often locking the person who is suffering in a vicious cycle that leads to diminished quality of life. Unfortunately, without intervention, the individual may become more depressed and, thus, more cognitively impaired as time goes by (35, 59).

Poor quality or insufficient amounts of sleep also contribute to cognitive deficits because of sleep's powerful influence on overall health. Clients with neurologic illnesses or NCDs such as PD are often especially affected by frustrating patterns of sleep, which tend to directly impact their mood, behavior, and thinking processes (32, 52). The literature indicates that approximately 25% to 30% of people who are diagnosed with PD develop dementia related to executive dysfunction that causes varied levels of confusion, disorganization, and language disruption (32). "Limitations might be more apparent in complex daily activities like eating, dressing, shopping and gardening because the attention load and mental flexibility required for these activities can further constrain motor performance" (44, p. 932). Sleep disruption and fatigue during the day in clients with neurocognitive impairments restrict participation in work, leisure, and social participation. The persistent fatigue experienced by people with PD is one of the main factors attributed to these clients disengaging from employment at an early age (44).

According to the Alzheimer's Association (4), mild cognitive impairment (MCI), which impacts over 20% of community-dwelling older adults, is also characterized by changes in memory and cognition. Language deficits, emotional dysregulation, disorientation, difficulty in making decisions, and apraxia can all be symptoms of MCI (12, 18, 32). Unfortunately, in the preliminary or initial stages of neurodegenerative disease, these mild symptoms can be very subtle (32). Because of occupational therapy's holistic perspective and focus on occupational engagement (and not on isolated performance skills or client factors), especially considering occupational therapy's analysis of the person's performance patterns, habits, roles, and routines, the OTP may have an increased likelihood of detecting these subtle changes. Disruption of sleep, for example, in individuals with MCI is associated with an increased timeline in the progression toward

AD and increased levels and intensity of their symptoms of dementia (including cognitive impairments) (53).

Furthermore, some individuals with cognitive problems have very **labile** emotions. This means that they rapidly shift from being calm and appearing comfortable to crying or laughing, sometimes uncontrollably (12). For example, an elderly nursing home resident who remembers the death of a childhood pet may suddenly burst into tears, or a client with a TBI might demonstrate characteristics of passivity in one moment and aggression or grief in the next (32). Emotional dysregulation can be a contributing factor in exacerbating or amplifying disorientation. People who are disoriented frequently get lost, especially in strange new environments such as hospitals and nursing homes. They are likely to consistently need help finding their rooms and their way to the bathroom, therapy gym, dining room, or other places. The OTP should be highly cognizant of the needs of these individuals given the vulnerability of their condition.

Problems in carrying out motor actions during daily tasks are often associated with cognitive deficits as well (32, 40). These may be more or less severe and can be analyzed according to Allen's Cognitive Levels (1, 2), among other tools, such as the Routine Task Inventory–Expanded (RTI-E) (37) or the Performance Assessment of Self-Care Skills (PASS) (33). **Dressing apraxia** is one example of a problematic barrier to occupational function caused by the inability to carry out a motor action. Dressing apraxia is characterized by difficulty with the instinctive ability to don and doff clothing. An example of dressing apraxia would be the client putting on a t-shirt backward or dressing only one side of their body. Clients who have experienced a cerebrovascular accident (CVA; often associated with right parietal lobe lesions) may demonstrate problems with visual perception, spatial abilities, categorizing, matching, and have difficulty with cancellation tasks, indicative of visual inattention. In fact, research suggests a high correlation between cognitive functioning and the performance of ADLs, which makes the assessment of a client's functional status in completing ADLs and IADLs a critical priority when working with clients experiencing cognitive impairments (12, 46).

Clients with poor judgment usually do not recognize (or have insight) that their judgment is impaired. Similarly, they do not usually recognize when their behaviors, actions, or decisions are inappropriate (sometimes attributed to disinhibition). A client trying to wash their hair in the water fountain or leaving their room without being fully dressed is displaying behaviors that demonstrate poor judgment likely to be rooted in a lack of awareness. Depending on the level of impairment and the stage of progression of the disease, clients may engage in behaviors considered to be defense mechanisms against the anxiety, distress, or frustration that they are feeling, or the consequences that they feel would happen if they recognized what they had done (ie, feelings of embarrassment, guilt, or shame). Some clients who experience moments of clarity may try to laugh off their peculiar or disruptive responses or behaviors and others may try to prevent further criticism and become argumentative.

Diagnoses With the Common Symptoms of Confusion or Impaired Memory

Because cognition is a multifaceted concept with a wide variety of contributing factors, and because science is consistently advancing our understanding of how certain conditions impact our overall health, it is not advantageous to determine which diagnostic groups may experience some level of cognitive deficit. Cognitive deficits occur to varying degrees in many psychiatric disorders. That being said, there are certain diagnostic groups who are more likely to experience cognitive impairment, for example, they are always found in NCDs. In these disorders, which include AD, the impairment is usually severe and progressive, meaning that it gets worse over time. A few exceptions to the progressive nature of NCDs are vascular disorders, which may or may not be progressive, TBIs that do not tend to be progressive, and substance-induced NCDs that will be progressive if the substance use continues, and which may have caused permanent cognitive changes, but again will not necessarily progress if the substance use is discontinued. Cognitive deficits can be associated with some neurodevelopmental disorders, including ID, ADHD, autism spectrum disorder, and specific learning disorders. Cognitive impairment is also more likely to be comorbid with depressive disorders, anxiety disorders, bipolar disorders, trauma and stress disorders, and sleep–wake disorders (9, 14, 32).

In addition, cognitive impairments can arise from physical disease. Any disease that impairs circulation affects the brain because less blood (and, therefore, less oxygen) is available to the central nervous system. Brain infections and trauma to the head can result in cognitive problems that may be permanent or transient. Drugs and alcohol affect brain chemistry and therefore can cause cognitive deficits. Prolonged or extensive alcohol use is associated with an organic mental disorder characterized by permanent impairment of intellectual abilities. Some prescription medications, including several used for treatment of psychiatric disorders, can cause temporary cognitive deficits that disappear when the medication is discontinued. Finally, clients receiving electroconvulsive therapy (ECT) as a treatment for depression usually are disoriented and have short-term memory loss for several days after receiving treatments. With time, these cognitive functions usually recover, although the person may never be able to remember events that occurred around the time of the treatments (8). In planning interventions, it is essential to differentiate permanent or progressive disabilities from those that are temporary, particularly regarding choosing the intervention type and approach that is most appropriate for the needs of the client (7, 30, 51).

Strategies for Therapeutic Use of Self for Clients With Confusion or Impaired Memory

General rules for approaching the person with cognitive deficits are difficult to prescribe. Different individuals function at different levels; some forget only an occasional fact or today's date, whereas others are so disoriented that they think Nixon is president or that they are in a factory rather than in a nursing home. It is important to approach each person as an individual and to make every effort to keep your comments and directions matched to the person's present level of function. The OTP can accomplish this by using communication that is full of simple explanations, reminders, cues, gestures, and frequent reassurances (49).

Because being disoriented can be very frightening, be sure to remind these clients frequently of where they are and who you are. For someone with severe memory impairment (this includes those receiving ECT), it may be necessary to repeat information each time you see the person. Wearing a nametag with your name and title in large print can sometimes help. Keep in mind that disoriented clients may have trouble finding the bathroom; orient them to this and any other important aspects of the environment to minimize risks to their safety. Other information that clients may need to know includes the time of day, what is happening now, and what will be happening next. Do not express impatience or irritation if the person still does not seem to become oriented. Do not argue with the client or get preoccupied with who is right and what the facts are. It is equally important for the person with significant memory loss not to attempt to rationally explain the disappearances of the person's possessions; instead, offer to look for the item and then distract the client toward switching to another activity or less distressing topic (49). It is important to avoid startling the person because this may further disorient the person and provoke negative behaviors (39). If the person has trouble following or responding to verbal direction, use demonstration and gesture instead. Presenting a person with an object, for example, a hairbrush, may be a more effective cue than requesting them to brush their hair.

Although people with cognitive impairment may demonstrate inappropriate behaviors because of poor judgment, poor impulse control, limited control of bodily functions, or a lack of insight, the OTP should consistently display a warm and accepting attitude, keeping their own mood as consistent as possible. Try to speak by keeping the pitch of your voice low (in a deeper range) because auditory processing for the client is more accurate in the lower ranges of pitch (39). Develop and maintain an awareness of your tone of voice, body language, and any unintended emotion that they might convey. Avoid being patronizing or condescending. Clients who cannot understand your words are likely to read your body language more accurately (39).

Punitive or threatening responses are never appropriate regardless of how inconvenient, offensive, or unpleasant a person's behavior has been. Instead, the OTP should kindly, but firmly, explain what is expected and then guide clients toward more acceptable and appropriate behaviors. Timeliness is essential; intervene immediately when clients do something wrong or inappropriate, help them correct or resolve the problematic event in the moment, then and there.

If corrective actions take place too long after the behavioral incident, the OTP risks having the client not know what they are referring to, ultimately heightening the client's confusion, anxiety, and level of fear.

Literature indicates that the capabilities of the person with NCD may vary by time of day (sometimes worse in the evening) and may change from day to day (32, 39). In some disorders, such as PD, there are setbacks on one day and better, improved behavioral responses and functioning the next day. It can be unpredictable. Whenever clients are given directions, whether on how to do an activity or how to get from one place to another, the directions should reflect the five *C*s: *calm, clear, concise, concrete,* and *consistent.* Speak in a calm tone of voice, articulating the words clearly. You may have to speak more slowly than you do usually but your tone of voice should be respectful, not patronizing, or impatient. Whatever you have to say, make it brief; the person's attention span is likely to be short. Use common everyday language, not abstract or difficult words that are hard to understand. Finally, use the same words every time you give the directions. Repeat the directions as needed at the same speed and in the same respectful tone.

Incorporating the person's own words can be helpful. To illustrate, if a man asks where you put his "specs," use this word rather than *glasses* or *eyeglasses* when you tell him where to find them. If you expect the person to remember the directions and use them later, have them repeat the directions to you. Better yet, write them down or make sure that the client writes them down (assuming the client has adequate vision and sufficient cognitive level and literacy). Be sure to match your tempo to what the person seems able to handle. The person who is cognitively impaired may take a while to respond; it just takes them longer to process ideas and information.

If a client is already upset, the OTP needs to be especially careful. Impulsive, aggressive acting out that results in harm to the client or to a staff member is possible when the person is in extreme distress. Empathy, simplicity, and a positive physical approach provide a good strategy and one likely to succeed in calming the person and reducing the negative behavior (39). Approach the person within their own field of vision. Approach slowly. Speak slowly and use simple language. Do not say too much. Do not give too much information. Try to figure out what the person might be experiencing. Use reflection of feeling, a client-centered technique, to identify or restate the feeling you are sensing from the person ("You seem very upset," or "You seem worried," or "Something seems to be making you angry. What is it?"); make sure that your body language is consistent with a helpful, listening attitude. Give the person ample time to respond and express themselves. Do not rush. When the person seems ready, attempt to redirect attention to another activity or topic of interest to the person. Be prepared to step away and give the person more time if this approach does not work the first time (39, 49).

Challenging Behaviors Associated With Neurocognitive Disorders

People with NCDs may demonstrate some challenging behaviors that are frustrating for families, care partners, and staff. Some of these challenging behaviors include wayfinding (or wandering); sleeplessness (or sundowning syndrome); argumentative, aggressive, or angry behaviors; incontinence; hoarding or rummaging behaviors; repetitive questioning; and general mistrust or suspiciousness (49). The behaviors are all thought to have a relationship to the person's feelings of distress or anxiety (29). It is believed that the various forms of dementia cause changes in the brain that kill nerve cells (called neurotoxicity) and negatively impact the person's ability to function. Damage to specific neurotransmitters results in these challenging behaviors (29).

Wayfinding or wandering behavior includes aimless movement that does not appear to have purpose but it has been suggested, and most experts agree, that wandering does serve as a way of communicating something (3, 49). It may be a response to an unmet physiologic need that is making the person uncomfortable (eg, needing to go to the bathroom) or the person may be bothered by an environmental or contextual discomfort such as the noise level, temperature, or even particular smells (10, 27). It can be extremely frustrating for care partners to try to assess the reasons for their loved one's wandering because the communication abilities of people with cognitive deficits are typically impaired. Nevertheless, "The person with dementia is unsettled in some way and begins to wander as an expression of something that they can perform" (29, p. 560). To minimize the likelihood that the person gets lost or hurt, it is important to create a safe area for them to be able to walk, when possible.

Sundowning (sundowning syndrome) refers to a cluster of symptoms (drowsiness, disorientation, confusion, aggression) that result in behaviors such as restlessness, pacing, attempts by the person to "go home," increased tearfulness, and at times increased symptoms of psychosis that may include hallucinations or delusions. The symptoms and behaviors of sundowning syndrome occur in the late afternoon or after sundown when it becomes dark. The literature indicates that there may be some physiologic causes for the characteristic behaviors (such as exhaustion from disrupted sleep patterns, reduced sunlight and ability to see, hunger or thirst with an inability to communicate those needs, or a reduction in the efficacy of pain medications) (24, 29). For many families, the evenings are full of busy routines such as making an evening meal or preparing for the following day. For individuals who experience sundowning symptoms, some experts have suggested that the person's loss of role identity during what has historically been a productive time may be one reason why behaviors escalate at the end of the day (24). ADLs such as bathing, toileting, or grooming may also become increasingly difficult in the late afternoons or evenings (24).

Argumentative, agitated, or aggressive behaviors may be a response in the mild to moderate stages of dementia to anything that is perceived as a threat, or to the perception that one is not being permitted to do what one wants. However, as the disease progresses, the client's ability to process internal cues and external stimuli to express their needs decreases, which in turn drives higher levels of frustration, anxiety, and agitation (3, 25, 29). Unfortunately, these behaviors are common in moderate to severe stages of dementia with 40% to 60% of individuals experiencing some level of agitation (29). **Rummaging** or **hoarding behaviors** are often a result of the context around the person becoming less familiar to them, or objects that were once familiar no longer being recognized as familiar. Thus, as aspects of their memory decline, it causes the person to consistently look for something that they have misplaced or cannot find (49). Hoarding behaviors associated with dementia are often referred to as "agitation behaviors" because the accompanying disinhibition causes people to collect and hide random items that do not belong to them (29).

In the middle and late stages of AD, **incontinence** of the bowel and bladder is not uncommon. Incontinence is typically caused by one of three things, comorbid medical conditions or deteriorating physiologic systems, medications or diuretics, and environmental or clothing management obstacles (3). Medical conditions such as a stroke, diabetes, PD, or a urinary tract infection can all be causes of, or exacerbate, incontinence. Sometimes the person is unable to get to the bathroom in time because of a physical disability or they may lack urinary sensation and fail to recognize the urge to go to the bathroom. Medications used to alleviate anxiety or aid with sleep can relax the muscles of the bladder, leading to incontinence. Finally, some people with dementia are unable to find the location of the bathroom or have difficulty with clothing management. One of the most important first tasks in addressing incontinence is to determine the cause; performing an occupational analysis can assist with making this determination (3, 29, 49).

Attention Deficits and Disorganization as Symptoms of Cognitive Impairment

Attention deficits are problems in directing attention to a task or in sustaining attention for a reasonable length of time. **Disorganization** is a lack of planning and order or an apparent inability to follow a plan. Disorganization interferes with successful completion of activities. Attention deficits and disorganization are often associated with other cognitive impairments, as previously described. However, because the general management of these symptoms is different, they are discussed here separately.

Clients may have trouble concentrating on a task or paying attention to it over time for several reasons. They may be distracted by hallucinations, memories, physical pain, or other internally generated stimuli, or by things around them in the external environment. There are five types of attention. **Sustained attention** allows a person to persist with their attention for a relatively long, continuous, or uninterrupted length of time. **Selective attention** permits the individual to be selectively attentive to a particular stimulus while also ignoring other distractions. **Alternating attention** allows focus to switch between tasks based on which task is a priority. **Focused attention** is necessary when complete focus to task is suddenly required in a short span of time. Finally, **divided or limited attention** is similar to selective attention except that the individual's cognitive resources are divided among different tasks (41). Individuals with cognitive deficits characterized by inattention may process information more slowly than do other people; by the time they figure out what is happening, something else is going on, and they have trouble keeping up with the pace of the information in their context. Clients who have trouble paying attention are also more likely to have trouble with organization.

However, another possible cause of disorganization is overstimulation. Often, if the environment is overstimulating, the client has difficulty focusing on one thing at a time because there is so much that catches their attention (ie, deficits in selective attention, which is a common characteristic of other symptoms and conditions such as mania). Still another cause of disorganization is poor judgment, as evidenced by the client trying to do too many things at one time. In addition, someone may appear disorganized if they lack the skills or knowledge to perform the activity. To illustrate, someone who has done little cooking will have trouble assembling the necessary ingredients and implements and carrying out the steps of a recipe efficiently, and they are likely to perform the activity more slowly than someone who is accustomed to doing it.

Diagnoses in Which Attention Deficits and Disorganization Are Common Symptoms

Both attention deficits and disorganization are indicative of cognitive deficits that occur across the subtypes of NCDs. Attention deficits and disorganization are also symptoms in some neurodevelopmental disorders, psychotic disorders, substance abuse disorders, bipolar disorders, acquired brain disorders (such as TBI, stroke, transient ischemic attacks [TIAs]), and depressive disorders, among others (42, 59). Even otherwise healthy individuals are likely to have impaired attention and to be disorganized when they are under significantly high or extensive stress or have experienced trauma (32).

Strategies for Therapeutic Use of Self: Attention Deficits and Disorganization

It can be exceedingly difficult to get the attention of someone with severe cognitive impairment. Be alert to nonverbal behavior. Gestures and grunts may indicate pain or, in some cases, the opposite may be true, and the person may use gestures to indicate their curiosity or interest in an activity. Body positioning, restlessness, and facial expression may give clues as to the person's psychological and physiologic state. Clients who are disorganized or are having trouble paying attention to a task may simply not be capable of participating in a particular task at the designated time. The OTP must draw upon their pragmatic reasoning to determine when and whether

the client should be directed to another simpler activity. If, during an activity, it becomes necessary to grade the activity down, or to switch activities altogether, the new activity should be introduced in a matter-of-fact manner with a seamless transition to avoid having a negative impact on the client's level of personal competence and agency. The OTP might, for example, say, "I think that we should save this for another day; I still have a few details that I need to work out for this project. Can you try this one instead?" The goal is to help the client feel comfortable and competent within the limits of their present abilities.

Glantz and Richman (28) point out that many behaviors that look like a problem or deficit can be seen as strengths if rephrased and looked at from a more positive perspective using a strengths-based approach. For example, the person who has a limited attention span may still be able to attend to a task that interests them, or one that they are familiar with, for a more substantial amount of time. Similarly, the person who works in an unsafe manner in an unstructured context may be able to achieve work safety if a structured environment is provided and set-up assist is available. It is essential to confirm and reaffirm to clients their strengths and the capacity to initiate, participate, and successfully complete occupations; this enhances independence.

TARGETING SYMPTOMS OF COGNITIVE DEFICITS THAT CREATE BARRIERS TO OCCUPATION: THE DOING AND BECOMING DIMENSIONS OF OT PRACTICE

> **BOX 21.2 Intervention Implementation Focus Questions: How to Support Clients' Optimal Engagement in Occupation**
>
> 1. What can the client and the occupational therapy team collaboratively do together that will help the client become more functional and effective in the things that are important to them in everyday life?
> 2. What are the best intervention types and intervention approaches to apply in this therapeutic context?
> 3. What does the current evidence suggest about the most productive interventions for this diagnosis/set of symptoms?

Contextual, Environmental, and Client Factor Considerations for Clients With Confusion, Memory, or Attentional Deficits

A large amount of research evidence and specific suggestions exist on environmental management for cognitive impairments related to dementia, TBI, schizophrenia, and other psychiatric disorders (2, 25, 28, 36). Three main principles are used to modify the environment. First, control the environment to maximize safety. Second, use the environment to cue desired behavior. Third, avoid environmental cues that may trigger undesirable behavior (28). If the environment is unsafe in any way, correct this immediately (but using calm movements to avoid startling the person). Remove anything in the environment that might be cuing the undesired behavior. When the person seems relaxed and comfortable, introduce items that might cue redirection of attention to a neutral or positive activity, preferably something of interest to the person (28).

Cognitively impaired individuals, perhaps more than any other group of clients, need a consistent and well-designed environment. Good lighting will help keep the person oriented and prevent falls. Even at night, lighting should be kept bright enough that the person can see their surroundings and find familiar items (using night-lights, when necessary). Colored lines (whether tiled, taped, or painted) on the floor leading to the bathroom and other frequently used areas are also good orientation aids. Because people with cognitive impairments rely so much on structure and routine in the external environment to help them stay organized, they are very sensitive to any changes. Therefore, the environment should be kept the same from day to day; this is true of the occupational therapy practice setting, as well as the person's living area. The OTP can further support the establishment of trust with the client and help them develop a sense of control by asking the client's permission if something in the immediate environment must be moved or changed (49).

Locations should be clearly marked with signs. Large print should be used. Pictographs or pictorial symbols may be more easily recognized than words; an example is a picture of a knife, fork, and plate on the door of the dining room. Signs or symbols on residents' doors may help them find their rooms; making the sign can be a good project for the client to participate in. Clients with cognitive impairment may need a staff member to label, mark, or color-code objects in their rooms to help them find them. In general, the environment should be simplified and all needed objects and locations should be clearly marked. Items that are often needed should be made visible, whereas items that are rarely used, or that may distract, should be out of the sight of the client.

External memory aids such as a large clock, large calendar, and a radio, television, or smart device can be extremely useful because they help orient the client to time, place, and often to current events. External memory aids are especially useful when they are embedded in the clients' naturalistic environment and incorporated consistently into their routine. When clients must remember to do things at a certain time, the OTP can help the client and the caregiver to implement and learn to use **cuing devices** such as programmable alarm watches, smart phones, or iPads. Even low-tech and inexpensive kitchen timers can be used by caregivers as an auditory cuing device. Many electronic devices store specific kinds of information; however, when such devices are difficult for the client to learn to use, and the client cannot retrieve necessary or desired information, they are of little value. Devices that require new learning will require training and this may be frustrating and unsuccessful for the person with significant cognitive impairment, or one who is in the later stages of cognitive decline (15).

The question of how much sensory stimulation should be available in the environment is fascinating and much debated. Research has shown that people with mental illness experience atypical sensory processing and that they have difficulty with sensory modulation (11). Current evidence further suggests that "the sensory qualities of the physical environment can be adapted to promote the occupational engagement of adults with mental illness" (11, p. 11). This has contributed to the increase in strong levels of evidence about the efficacy of using sensory rooms in inpatient psychiatric settings to reduce the incidence of seclusion and the use of restraints, as well as its capacity to reduce agitation and symptoms of anxiety in clients with AD and other major NCDs (11, 34). Clinicians agree that any stimulation presented should be clear and unambiguous. For example, when music is used, it should be played on a good quality sound system rather than through speakers with poor sound quality.

Another factor to be considered in designing an environment for someone with cognitive impairments is its similarity or dissimilarity to the person's home environment. Ideally, the person should remain at home as long as possible, using compensatory devices and the support of other people. When entering the hospital or other facility, not only are such clients often seriously ill and in psychological distress but their distress is also further exacerbated by the strangeness of the environment. Residents' discomfort can sometimes be lessened if they are allowed to keep mementos of home in the room. They should also be encouraged to set up their belongings in whatever way makes sense for them, as this will encourage carryover of dressing, hygiene, grooming, and other self-care or ADL routines (34). Creating a special personal space that is filled with the client's familiar things where they can retreat if they are overwhelmed, or are experiencing confusion, will not only encourage them to rest but is also likely to encourage feelings of safety and security (49). Finally, when someone is planning to return home or is to transfer to another facility, the future environment must also be considered. Teaching of new skills or reinforcement of old skills should take place in an ecologically relevant context or in an environment as similar as possible to the future one (23).

For the person who experiences deficits of attention, distractions can be reduced by having the person work alone in the initial stages of a task and by considering a reduction in the environmental stimuli. The OTP should limit the tools and supplies to those needed for the immediate step or task. If the person is distracted by internally generated stimuli (eg, hallucinations), more intensive extraneous stimulation may be necessary and preferable for the client to be successful in maintaining their attention. In a systematic review of the efficacy of environmental intervention for people with AD and other major NCDs, Jensen and Padilla (34) reported that classical and favorite music played in the background may reduce stereotypical and disruptive behaviors in persons with dementia, "strong evidence supports the use of ambient music other than at mealtimes" (34, p. 6). In using music, careful observation of the effects on clients' functional performance is essential because it is also possible for music to be distracting, confusing, and overstimulating.

Characteristics of Intervention Activities and Recommended Modifications for Clients With Confusion, Memory, or Attentional Deficits

In many situations, the OTP will need to distract or divert the attention of clients with cognitive deficits. For this reason, it is essential for the OTP to be consistently prepared with a range of high-interest activities that are positive or functional, within the person's range of abilities, or, alternatively, something that is—if not preferable—at minimum, familiar. Preparation and the practitioner's ability to shift between relevant activities that have been planned as purposeful in helping the client progress toward their goals is the main priority for intervention. For example, if a client had worked in a retail job in a department store as a past occupation, the OTP might have on hand a basket of colorful scarves near the person, and if distraction or a diversion of their attention became necessary, may ask the client if they would help fold them. This activity is likely to be somewhat familiar and interesting to this client and the occupying of the person's hands with a purposeful task (ie, the doing dimension of occupation) will both alleviate boredom and distract attention away from disruptive or unsafe behavioral responses. Another example is asking the person to take a walk with you back to the day room, or to the person's room, or asking them to help with a safe kitchen task such as watering a kitchen windowsill herb garden.

An activity that is a co-occupation is preferable to a solitary activity in almost all circumstances with clients who experience cognitive impairments, as it introduces social interaction, makes the person feel useful, and invites conversation. A few careful and brief observations of the client at other times of the day or in other contexts (outside of therapy), may help the OTP see whether the person is attracted to particular people, places, activities, or objects that may indicate a valued former occupation or activity. Ridge and Robnett (45) give the example of a client who kept trying to enter the nursing station to take a pen. An occupational therapy fieldwork student observed this. While working with the client later, she gave him a pen, which he used skillfully. He had once been an animation artist.

In a scoping review of sensory processing and mental illness by Bailliard and Whigham (11), the researchers found that adults with mental illness experience atypical neurophysiologic responses to auditory and visual sensory stimuli. These atypical responses are associated with deficits in **emotional prosody** or being able to recognize emotion through tone. Impaired sensory processing was also found to negatively impact cognitive performance skills including self-regulation and attention to task (11). Particularly in adults with schizophrenia, basic visual deficits such as in detecting visual contrast, maintaining a steady gaze on a fixed target, and demonstrating abnormal scanning patterns, resulted in deficits in the person's ability to read (11). Finally, the literature has also suggested that remedial interventions targeting sensory processing skills may positively influence cognitive performance and result in cognitive gains that would enhance overall occupational performance.

Yet, despite the ever-evolving understanding and awareness about the problems that adults with mental illness experience because of their sensory deficits, very little translational research that examines and makes the connection between the person's sensory deficits and their functional occupational performance exists (11). "Studies in psychiatry, neuroscience, and occupational therapy have only begun to explore the implications of sensory deficits for function, albeit not on occupational performance" (11, p. 9). Although the need to expand this type of research is ongoing, for occupational therapy interventions to continue to maintain their focus on occupational outcomes (rather than on isolated client factors or performance skills), evidence continues to support the implementation of interventions that incorporate compensatory strategies for individuals with cognitive deficits. This includes interventions that target sensory deficits, for example, "a systematic review study on nonpharmacologic interventions to reduce neuropsychiatric and behavioral symptoms [in clients with Alzheimer's Disease] has shown modest scientific evidence on its effects with aromatherapy, phototherapy, ambient music and multisensory stimulation interventions" (12, p. 939).

The person's prognosis is another primary consideration when the OTP is assessing and planning activities that target cognitive impairments that disrupt occupation. Some cognitive impairments are transitory, fluctuating, or responsive to treatments that allow reestablishment of new gains (or new learning) and the person is expected to be able to improve or sometimes even regain full function (eg, post-ECT memory impairment). These clients should be given simple, structured, short-term activities that are relevant to their interests to help them maintain their abilities and self-confidence until they recover and reestablish or rehabilitate function. Activities that can be finished within 1 day are preferable in the acute stages; the person may refuse to work on a project 2 days in a row if they do not remember it. Once cognitive functions begin to return to normal (or typical for that particular client), the person should be quickly reintroduced to familiar activities and skills that they need in their occupational roles. This is a remedial or restorative approach to intervention (6, 7).

Other conditions and symptoms of cognitive deficit are somewhat more permanent, although not necessarily progressive, for example, major NCD that is substance induced (ie, dementia associated with alcoholism), or the executive dysfunction associated with ADHD. For these individuals, the specific cognitive deficits must be identified and analyzed in relation to previous or expected developmental occupational roles. Then the person can be taught ways to adapt to the disability within these roles or to find new occupational roles and tasks more appropriate to the present condition. These are also considered to be remedial and restorative approaches to intervention (7). The general idea in these adaptive remedial or restorative approaches is to simplify and reintroduce (establish or reestablish) known activities by teaching processing and self-monitoring strategies, rather than introduce novel occupations or occupational roles. A third group of (primarily) neurocognitive conditions, unfortunately, are permanent and progressive; the person will become less and less able to function over time. These clients need help to maintain, for as long as possible, whatever skills remain. This represents a maintenance approach to intervention (7). The client should be encouraged to be as independent as they can, while they can. Activities can be adjusted and readjusted over time using adaptive or compensatory approaches and modeled to include characteristics of occupations that are familiar, relevant, or necessary (7). Participation in self-care is important in helping clients with NCDs to retain a sense of dignity and self-esteem. Gitlin and Corcoran (26) provide specific suggestions to modify objects and tasks to improve occupational performance. Ciro (16) explains how to analyze the person's occupational performance and teach tasks that are specific to familiar and valued roles. In general, the idea is to reduce complexity and make the task clear and obtainable.

Some general guidelines apply to interventions of all clients who experience cognitive impairments. First, unfamiliar and complex activities should be avoided because of their tendency to add to confusion, which leads to decreased frustration tolerance. Activities that require independent decision-making may overwhelm someone with impaired judgment; on the contrary, activities that involve simple choices (eg, between two colors or two food items) can build confidence. The OTP should help these clients carry out the activities that they prioritize and value. Even for severely disoriented clients, encouraging safe physical activities with the necessary levels of assistance, such as touring around the halls and practicing safe travel within the treatment facility, are appropriate for building confidence (49). Some clients who have mild confusion or impaired memory find it helpful to write things down. They can be encouraged to always carry a notebook or planner with them; designing and organizing the notebook can be an ongoing activity and it offers a low-tech option for use as a compensatory tool.

For persons who have been evaluated with the Allen Cognitive Level Screen-5 (ACLS-5) (20) or the Allen Diagnostic Module (21, 22), intervention activities should be matched to the appropriate level of challenge that is correlated with the person's functional cognitive level. Observation of performance will help guide the OTP in determining whether to increase or decrease the level of difficulty. Allen (1, 2) recommends that tasks be within the person's current ability; the OTP should intervene rapidly to provide a less demanding activity if the person shows signs of confusion, frustration, or discomfort.

Interventions that support improved attention to task and organization should include simple, well-delineated activities that have a definite sequence and initially consist of

BOX 21.3 Examples of Appropriate Activities for Confusion or Memory Deficits

- *Current events discussions* are designed to help the person stay oriented and involved in community events to the extent that they are able.
- *Life tasks* should emphasize self-care and whatever other tasks are the most necessary for each client to remain as independent as possible, also while retaining their best QoL (eg, cooking, housework, laundry, shopping).
- *Familiar crafts and hobbies* can help bolster self-confidence when the ability to do more complex tasks has been lost.
- *Short walks or shopping excursions* provide variety, exercise, and a sense of added purpose.

very few steps. The OTP may need to do the more difficult steps for the person, using a **backward-chaining strategy**, or working backward in the steps to reach a goal. Activities that are creative or that have flexible standards or goals should be avoided; they increase the potential and likelihood for breaks in attention that can lead to disorganization (and increased frustration). For clients with fluctuating levels of attention, meditation, or other somatic activities that invoke the connection between the mind and body (eg, Yoga, Tai Chi, or breathing techniques) can help develop the ability to sustain attention over time (47, 58). Meditation can be used as an intervention that supports occupation, for example, before beginning an activity that requires focused attention (7). Boxes 21.3 to 21.5 provide further examples of appropriate activities or adaptive technology that can be considered to support clients who experience cognitive impairments that limit their occupational participation.

BOX 21.4 Knowledge Translation and Evidence-Informed Occupational Therapy Intervention Summary: Assistive Technology for Clients With Neurocognitive Disorders

Approach to Intervention (19)

- OTPs can use a future-oriented approach to help clients find effective technology supports.
- Helping clients develop habits and skills to use the technology in earlier stages of dementia improves the ease of use in later stages of dementia.

Strategies Applied (19)

1. Storing redundant information
2. Retrieving information more immediate to the time when it is needed
3. "Outsourcing" tasks
   A. Setting up memory cues or reminders (eg, birthday reminders)
   B. Establishing automatic processes such as Autopay for bills
4. Use of technology to minimize the appearance of cognitive deficits in social situations

Bottom Line for Occupational Therapy Intervention in Action

"Occupational therapy practitioners should work with people with mild and moderate dementia to develop habits and routines that incorporate technology, and ease continued participation in daily occupations and everyday activities" (15, p. 36)

Types of Assistive Technology That Care Partners Used With People With Neurocognitive Disorders (Dementia) (50)

1. **Safety and security devices** (tracking devices and bed alarms were the most frequently used in this category.)
2. **Devices that helped with the following:**
   A. **Memory:** Medication reminders, timed alarms
   B. **Orientation:** Reminiscence tools, calendars
   C. **Social participation:** Photo button phone
   D. **Leisure:** Simplified remote control

Bottom Line for Occupational Therapy Intervention in Action

"Care partners of people with dementia should be provided with education about AT that is commercially available and addresses safety and security, memory, orientation, social participation, and leisure" (15, p. 36).

Facilitators of Incorporating Assistive Technology (38)

1. Care partners' desire to use assistive technology (AT)
2. Technology with simple interfaces
3. Increased safety, independence, well-being, and communication

Barriers to Assistive Technology Use (38)

1. Cost
2. Client not wishing to use AT
3. Complex interfaces
4. Timing of when the technology is introduced in the context of the stage or level of neurocognitive decline that the client is experiencing

Medical Outcomes of Assistive Technology Use (38)

1. Improved cognitive abilities
2. Improved memory
3. Improved mood and behavior
4. Improved overall health

Bottom Line for Occupational Therapy Intervention in Action

"Occupational therapy practitioners should use low-cost AT with simple interfaces with people with dementia and their care partners, based on goals and contextual factors, to improve these medical outcomes" (15, p. 37).

Evidence-Based Interventions That Target Cognitive Deficits or Impairment

Evidence-based interventions that target cognitive deficits or impairments should never be assumed to also be automatically occupation centered. In fact, most interventions that target aspects of cognition are not explicitly occupation focused. This serves as an important reminder that one of the best ways to advocate for the benefits of occupational

---

BOX 21.5 Examples of Appropriate Activities for Attention Deficits and Disorganization

- *Simple craft projects*
- *Self-care* and *life tasks needed in the person's occupational roles* are typically prioritized highly. For example, helping a person who does the most cooking in the household to organize their kitchen will probably be more important to them than learning a new craft of activity (unless it is for the purpose of leisure exploration).
- *Provision of compensatory skills training in safety and emergency procedures* may make the difference in allowing the person to remain in their home or community and able to age in place more effectively.
- *Coping skills and stress management techniques* can be modified to suit the level of the person's understanding (their cognitive abilities). These intervention types help the client control anxiety and emotional arousal that further interferes with cognition.
- *Computer games* that reinforce specific cognitive skills may also be used.
- *Mindfulness meditation* and focused activities that have a meditative quality, such as Yoga or Tai Chi, can help the person develop an attitude of attention, as well as remain calm (58).

---

therapy intervention is to consistently use occupational performance analysis and engagement in occupation as a means to helping clients reach their goals. The first priority then for OTPs to consider when targeting cognitive impairments as a focus for intervention is how barriers to occupational participation or problems with occupational performance are directly linked to the cognitive deficit, skill, or impairment. Next, the evidence-informed practitioner should maintain knowledge of current recommendations, evidence, and research related to the impacts that cognitive impairments (as symptoms of psychiatric disability) have on occupational performance and participation (5).

There are two main techniques evidenced to support occupational therapy interventions that target cognitive impairments, remediation, and compensation. Remedial interventions target the cognitive impairment and the focus of the intervention is on improving a specific cognitive skill or set of skills; thus, the focus is on an aspect of the client (7, 13). However, in compensatory strategies and approaches, OTPs focus on adaptation of the context, environment, task, or method of client training and education, to compensate for the cognitive impairment; thus, the emphasis is on changing an aspect of something outside of the client with the goal of improving the clients' ability and experience of engaging in valued occupations (7, 13). OTPs can apply a variety of evidence-based models of practice when there is sufficient information to show that the clients' occupational dysfunction results from the negative impacts of cognitive deficits. The key to determining both approach and intervention technique often lies in appropriate assessment of where the breakdown in performance skills exists during occupational performance. "To best describe and document functional cognitive changes, clients must complete standardized performance-based measures, . . . or therapist-constructed tasks to assess breakdowns in performance skills during cognitively complex IADLs such as cooking, medication, and money management" (56, p. 3). Table 21.1 summarizes samples from the literature of a few of the currently available evidence-based techniques being incorporated into occupational therapy assessment and interventions targeting cognitive impairments that impact occupation.

Table 21.1. From the Literature: Evidence to Support Intervention Strategies That Target Cognitive Impairment

Technique or Strategy	Sample of Evidence From the Literature
Cognitive Remediation Cognitive remediation techniques are focused on improving specific cognitive performance skills such as memory, attention, or problem-solving so that clients can more successfully engage in their prioritized daily occupations. Repetition and rehearsal are embedded in interventions to provide the client with experiential opportunities to engage in practicing the use of cognitive skills, which over time are thought to promote neurologic changes (changes in the brain).	Trapp, W., Landgrebe, M., Hoesl, K., Lautenbacher, S., Gallhofer, B., Günther, W., & Hajak, G. (2013). Cognitive remediation improves cognition and good cognitive performance increases time to relapse—Results of a 5-year catamnestic study in schizophrenia patients. *BMC Psychiatry, 13*(1), 1–9.
Appropriate Population Cognitive remediation has been found to be effective in improving basic cognitive skills that are maintained over time with populations that include people with diagnoses of schizophrenia, affective mood disorders, and eating disorders (13).	
Cognitive–Functional Therapy for Adults (Cog-Fun A) Cog-Fun A is a metacognitive–functional intervention for adults with ADHD that targets self-awareness and executive function in occupational contexts. The Cog-Fun A intervention was developed on the basis of the widely successful and highly efficacious Cognitive–Functional (Cog-Fun) intervention for young children with ADHD, and adapted to explore its use with adults with ADHD.	Kastner, L., Velder-Shukrun, Y., Bonne, O., Bar-Ilan, R. T., & Maeir, A. (2022). Pilot study of the Cognitive–Functional Intervention for Adults (Cog-Fun A): A metacognitive–functional tool for adults with attention deficit hyperactivity disorder. *American Journal of Occupational Therapy, 76*(2), 7602205070.
Appropriate Population Adults with attentional deficits, or executive dysfunction, or who have been diagnosed with ADHD or TBI	
Valid, Reliable, Accurate, and Ecologically Relevant Assessment of Cognitive Impairment That Is Linked to Occupation-Based Interventions *Relevant Guideposts Include* • Use of performance-based assessments that include real-world objects or tasks allow OTPs to link observed performance to the underlying performance skills (and impairments). Particularly with the assessment of executive function, OTPs need to be able to reflect upon how deficits of executive function impact daily occupational function. • Consider use of cognitive adaptation strategies. Cognitive adaptation strategies can be incorporated when a person's cognitive impairments are progressive and cognitive remediation is no longer helpful. In cognitive adaptation, the environment or task is adapted to compensate for the cognitive impairment (13).	Nadler Tzadok, Y., Eliav, R., Portnoy, S., & Rand, D. (2022). Establishing the validity of the internet-based Bill-Paying Task to assess executive function deficits among adults with traumatic brain injury. *American Journal of Occupational Therapy, 76*(4), 7604205110. Watters, K., Marks, T. S., Edwards, D. F., Skidmore, E. R., & Giles, G. M. (2021). A framework for addressing clients' functional cognitive deficits after COVID-19. *American Journal of Occupational Therapy, 75* (Suppl. 1), 7511347010. Wesson, J., Clemson, L., Crawford, J. D., Kochan, N. A., Brodaty, H., & Reppermund, S. (2017). Measurement of functional cognition and complex everyday activities in older adults with mild cognitive impairment and mild dementia: Validity of the Large Allen's Cognitive Level Screen. *American Journal of Geriatric Psychiatry, 25*(5), 471–482.
Appropriate Population Adults with executive function deficits	
Cognitive Orientation to Daily Occupational Performance (CO-OP) Approach Originally developed for children with developmental coordination disorder, CO-OP (43) applies a four-step problem-solving strategy to assist with the acquisition of motor-based performance skills. The four steps can then be applied to an occupation-based goal that is specific to the client (13). The four steps are as follows: 1. Goal: What do you want to do? 2. Plan: How will you go about doing it? 3. Do: Carry out the plan. 4. Check: Did the plan work out? Does the plan need to be modified?	Skidmore, E. R., Butters, M., Whyte, E., Grattan, E., Shen, J., & Terhorst, L. (2017). Guided training relative to direct skill training for individuals with cognitive impairments after stroke: A pilot randomized trial. *Archives of Physical Medicine and Rehabilitation, 98*(4), 673–680. Skidmore, E. R. (2017). Functional cognition: Implications for practice, policy, and research. *The American Journal of Geriatric Psychiatry, 25*(5), 483–484.
Appropriate Population Children with neurodevelopmental disabilities (developmental coordination disorder, ADHD), or adults with neurocognitive disorders or cognitive impairments	

ADHD, attention deficit hyperactivity disorder; OTP, occupational therapy professional; TBI, traumatic brain injury.

MANAGING SYMPTOMS OF COGNITIVE DEFICITS

> **BOX 21.6 Focus Questions for Planning Transition, Maintenance, and Long-Term Wellness Plans**
>
> 1. How does the client define success in reaching their goals?
> 2. How can occupational therapy support the long-term success in the client becoming who they want to be, successfully doing what they want to do?
> 3. How can occupational therapy support the client's recovery and long-term success in finding community, and feeling a sense of belonging and connectedness?

Social and Emotional Health Promotion and Maintenance for Symptoms of Cognitive Deficits

When a client is diagnosed with an NCD, or experiences the symptoms of cognitive deficit, one of the first questions that the therapist can reflect upon is, "Who needs help, assistance, or support?" Care and concern for the client's priorities and their safety is central to the occupational therapy process, "but there is also the human system surrounding the client, including family, spouse, friends at work or school, and a social community" (32, p. 228). Consideration of this network is essential to promoting and maintaining the wellness and health of clients with neurocognitive conditions or cognitive impairment related to other conditions.

Functional cognition has been described as the integration of "everyday task performance and underlying cognitive skills" (57, p. 471). From an occupational therapy perspective, the best way to measure functional cognition is through performance observation when the client is engaging in ADLs, especially if the client is engaging in complex activities with high cognitive demands. Observing the client performing IADLs such as medication management, bill paying, or grocery shopping in their natural environment allows the OTP to collaborate with the client to manage their symptoms to promote ongoing wellness and independence throughout their course of intervention (23, 48).

SUMMARY

Evidence from extensive research indicates that there are moderate correlations between occupational dysfunction resulting from cognitive deficits and clients' functional outcomes (46, 54, 55). According to Trapp and Colleagues (55), who studied the use of cognitive remediation to improve the cognitive performance of clients with schizophrenia, cognitive performance appears to be linked to social skills, social problem-solving, and a myriad of other social behaviors. It is likely that successfully functioning within one's community is also related to cognitive performance. Furthermore, research consistently confirms that cognitive performance impacts the probability that a client

with cognitive impairment will be able to return to work, school, and other valued or necessary occupations or social roles (42, 55, 59).

To summarize, the outcomes, outcome measures, and goals for each client who experiences cognitive impairment will largely depend on the extent of cognitive impairment, the status or prognosis for the client's condition, the type of cognitive deficit, and the priorities of the client. Although the variability in the level and type of cognitive deficit associated with particular diagnostic groups are significant, cognitive impairment is a symptom of many psychiatric conditions. One of the benefits of establishing a strong therapeutic relationship with the client is that the OTP can, over time, develop a rich understanding of the unique nature of each client that will further guide and enhance their professional reasoning and judgment (6, 7).

Attempting to understand and accept the unique nature of each client while projecting a sense that they belong, and that they can be exactly as they are in each moment, represents aspects of the "being" and "belonging" dimensions of occupation that highlights a unique contribution of the profession of occupational therapy to the care of these individuals. Cognitive deficits can seriously impair a person's ability to function. The person with cognitive deficits may have a wide range of behavioral and emotional reactions in response to the change or decline in function. When working with these clients, it is important to consider all aspects of their health and occupational engagement, and to use valid and reliable means to evaluate cognitive skills that are still intact, so that a strengths-based approach can be engaged in supporting the reestablishment, remediation, restoration, or maintenance of function, thereby supporting their pursuit of optimal engagement in everyday life.

> **Case Study**
>
> **Mrs Anderson: A 72-Year-Old Female With Alzheimer Disease**
>
> *DSM-5-TR Diagnosis at Admission*
>
> G30.9 Alzheimer disease
>
> F02.81 Major neurocognitive disorder due to possible Alzheimer disease with behavioral disturbance
>
> *ICD-10-CM*
>
> I67.2 Cerebral atherosclerosis
>
> I50.4 Congestive heart failure
>
> **Z code**
>
> Z59.3 Problem related to living in a residential institution
>
> Mrs Anderson is a 72-year-old, Caucasian female admitted to Green Manor, a skilled nursing facility, with a *DSM-5 TR* diagnosis of AD (G30.9), and major NCD due to possible AD with behavioral disturbance (F02.81). Depressed mood was also noted. Mrs Anderson, who has cerebral atherosclerosis (I67.2) and congestive heart failure (I50.4), was first diagnosed with AD 3 years ago. Until admission, she was

cared for at home by her husband of 45 years. However, Mrs Anderson has become weaker and incontinent, and Mr Anderson, who is 74 years old, is not strong enough to help his wife transfer from bed to commode, so it was necessary to place her in a specialized memory care unit of the skilled nursing facility.

Occupational Profile Data Collection Interview and Evaluation

Mrs Anderson is of Norwegian ancestry; her religion is Lutheran, and her faith is very important to her. She was the fifth of nine children and is the only one still living. She has a high school diploma and was employed for 29 years as the office manager in a local manufacturing business. The Andersons have one son, aged 51, who lives in another state. According to Mr Anderson, his wife used to enjoy needlework, bridge, and gardening, activities that she slowly abandoned as her illness became more severe. During the final 6 months that Mrs Anderson remained at home, her husband took care of all the cooking, cleaning, and household management. According to him, she complained constantly that he was not doing a good enough job, that she did not like his cooking, and so on. The following evaluations were attempted: structured interview and mental status examination, functional range of motion (ROM) examination, and functional daily living skills evaluation.

At interview, Mrs Anderson was found seated in a wheelchair in her room. The wheelchair was the wrong size and the footrests too high. Her shoulders were elevated and protracted because of poor positioning. Mrs Anderson was well groomed and neatly dressed. Conference with the nursing staff revealed that her husband comes in early every morning to help with dressing and grooming. Mrs Anderson was able to state her name and knew she was in some sort of institution. She did not know the correct date, gave a month in a different season, and said the year was 2012 (10 years ago). When asked how she came to be in the home, she replied that she had come here for a job interview. ("They need someone to do the scheduling and payroll.") She then said that she decided not to take the job. ("Who'd want to work in a place like this?")

Mrs Anderson incorrectly answered 7 of 10 questions on the mental status examination; recent memory and fund of general information seemed particularly impaired. She could follow a one-step command but not two steps. Her speech was clear and her hearing apparently unimpaired. Mrs Anderson wears glasses.

Functional ROM examination confirmed that Mrs Anderson could not walk, even with a walker, because of poor endurance and poor balance. She had full range in most motions of the upper extremities but was unable to raise her arms above the level of her shoulders; range was more impaired on the right than on the left. Grasp was very weak.

Functional Daily Living Skills Evaluation

Functional daily living skills evaluation showed that Mrs Anderson had sufficient pinch and coordination to button and unbutton garments with front closures. She needed assistance to don and doff clothing because of ROM impairments. She was unable to bathe or care for her teeth and

hair without assistance but seemed aware of the need for help, and asked for it. She complained that she could not see, which the staff understood to mean that her glasses needed cleaning. She could feed herself if the tray was prepared (eg, meat cut up). Sitting balance was poor and Mrs Anderson could not perform transfers unassisted.

Please find follow-up case reflections and activities in the "OT HACKS Summary" section.

OT HACKS SUMMARY

O: **Occupation as a means and an end**

Outcomes, outcome measures, and goals for each client who experiences cognitive impairment will largely depend on items such as the following:

- The extent of cognitive impairment
- The status or prognosis for the client's condition
- The type of cognitive deficit and its impact on occupational performance or participation
- The client's occupational history and situational context
- The priorities of the client

One of the best ways to advocate for the benefits of occupational therapy intervention is to consistently use occupational performance analysis and engagement in occupation as a means to helping clients reach their goals.

T: **Theoretical concepts, values, and principles, or historical foundations**

Attempting to understand and accept the unique nature of each client while projecting a sense that they belong, and that they can be exactly as they are in each moment, represents aspects of the "being" and "belonging" dimensions of occupation that highlight a unique contribution of the profession of occupational therapy to the care of individuals with cognitive deficits.

H: **How can we Help? OT's role in serving clients with mental illness or mental health needs**

There are two main techniques evidenced to support occupational therapy interventions that target cognitive impairments, *remediation*, and *compensation*. Remedial interventions target the cognitive impairment and the focus of the intervention is on improving a specific cognitive skill or set of skills; thus, the focus is on an aspect of the client (7, 13). However, in compensatory strategies and approaches, OTPs focus on adaptation of the context, environment, task, or method of client training and education, to compensate for the cognitive impairment; thus, the emphasis is on changing an aspect of something outside of the client with the goal of improving the clients' ability and experience of engaging in valued occupations (7, 13).

A: **Adaptations**

For clients experiencing cognitive impairment:

- When the OTP gives directions, whether on how to do an activity or how to get from one place to another, the directions should reflect the five *Cs: calm, clear, concise, concrete,* and *consistent.*

- When it becomes necessary to grade an activity down, or to switch activities altogether, the new activity should be introduced in a matter-of-fact manner with a seamless transition. This ensures that the change will not discourage the client and have a negative impact on the client's level of personal competence and agency.

- The goal is to help the client feel comfortable and competent, achieving their potential within the limits of their present abilities.

C: Case study includes

Try these activities related to Mrs Anderson's case!

1. Write an occupational therapy intervention plan, including goals and activities. *Hint:* The plan should focus on maintaining rather than improving function and should allow for deterioration in the resident's condition. State which activities are to be individual and which in a group. In your plan, consider the following areas: ADLs, leisure, and social participation. Also consider possible gross motor or sensory activities. Be specific and detailed in your plan.

2. Assuming the resident's functional level declines, at what point would you recommend that occupational therapy be discontinued? Identify specific behavioral and functional impairments that would indicate that the resident cannot benefit from further intervention. Write a discharge plan (discontinuance from occupational therapy), including recommendations and directions for the nursing staff.

K: Knowledge: Keeping mental health OT practice grounded in evidence, in occupational science, and in research

A few key points are given here:

- "To facilitate positive experiences, health professionals can use CBT techniques to assist caregivers in adopting problem-solving and coping strategies." (31, p. 1)

- "Problem-solving training paired with other CBT techniques, such as cognitive restructuring, reframing, or relaxation, can help alleviate symptoms of depression and physical complaints in caregivers. Occupational therapy professionals are well suited to deliver interventions using problem-solving training and other CBT techniques . . . ." (31, p. 4)

Evidence Application and Translation Questions

1. Describe the purpose of a systematic review brief. How is a systematic review brief different from a full systematic review?

2. Where is a full systematic review typically ranked in the levels of evidence?

3. According to this systematic review brief, why are OTPs well suited to deliver cognitive behavioral therapy (CBT) techniques to caregivers of people who have had a stroke?

4. Summarize the strength of the evidence for using CBT techniques with caregivers of people who have experienced a stroke.

S: Some terms that may be new to you

Alertness: awareness of the immediate environment

Attention: proficiently expending cognitive resources to take in the information necessary to accomplish a task, purpose, or goal

Attention deficits: problems in directing attention to a task or in sustaining attention for a reasonable length of time

Attention span: the length of time that a person can maintain their concentration

Backward chaining: a technique that involves the OTP (or parent or other care partner) completing the more difficult steps of a task for a person who is attempting to master or practice a new skill or process; backward chaining is working backward in the steps toward reaching a goal, provision of assistance is thought to promote success and enhance self-confidence and personal agency within the client.

Clouding of consciousness: meaning literally that the person seems to be in a fog

Cognition: the mental processes (attention, memory, executive function and their subsets of skills) that a person employs to perceive and make sense of information, so that they can use the information for specific tasks or purposes

Cognitive deficit: an impairment or a defect in one or more of the mental functions needed for thinking

Comprehension: the ability to understand

Concentration: the ability to focus one's mental energies on the task at hand

Confabulation: "stories," often made up to cover or hide problems with short-term memory

Cuing devices: devices that help clients to remember to do something at a certain time, such as an alarm on a smart phone

Disorganization: a lack of planning and order or an apparent inability to follow a plan; disorganization interferes with successful completion of activities.

Disorientation/confusion: problems with orientation

Distractibility: a tendency to lose focus because another stimulus catches one's interest

Dressing apraxia: problems in carrying out motor actions, often associated with cognitive deficits; in *dressing apraxia*, the person has trouble carrying out the proper sequence of actions to get dressed.

Emotional prosody: recognition of emotion through tone

Etiology: cause, or origin

Executive function: higher order cognitive skills such as comprehension (an understanding), concept formation, categorization, judgment, problem-solving, or decision-making

External memory aids: items such as large clocks or wall calendars that help orient a client to time and current events

Impaired judgment: problems with judgment

Inattention: the inability to pay attention even though no competing external stimulus is present

Judgment: the ability to recognize and comply with established social norms and standard procedures and to use what most people refer to as "common sense"

Labile: rapidly shift from being calm and appearing comfortable to crying or laughing uncontrollably

Long-term memory: memory of events from months or years ago

Low arousal: problems with alertness; seemingly unaware of stimulation

Memory: ability to recall past events and knowledge

Memory impairment: problems remembering past information

Orientation: knowledge of where one is, what time it is (hour, day, date, season), and who one is with

Problem-solving: the ability to recognize, analyze, and ultimately figure out solutions to problems that arise during everyday activity

Short-term memory: memory of more recent events

Sundowning syndrome: refers to a cluster of behaviors (drowsiness, disorientation, confusion, aggression) that occur in the late afternoon that may have physiologic causes (such as exhaustion, reduced ability to see because of reduced illumination, or hunger or thirst)

Wayfinding (wandering): a challenging behavior associated with NCDs; moving away from one's home or current surroundings (ie, away from the skilled nursing or assisted living facility)

Working memory: short-term memory that is stored for a brief period

Reflection Questions

1. Describe the symptoms of NCDs.
2. List and describe the subtypes of NCDs. How are the subtypes of the NCDs categorized in the *DSM-5-TR*?
3. How do the symptoms of NCDs impact a person's daily occupations?
4. List and describe the three major components of cognition.
5. What is the relationship between cognition (or the associated mental processes and cognitive performance skills) and occupational engagement?
   - Please formulate your answer avoiding the use of occupational therapy jargon, as if you were providing the response to members of a behavioral health team comprising colleagues from other disciplines.
6. Evaluate possible ways that clients' inability to comprehend information or difficulty with judgment may in some ways be a reflection of their occupational history.
7. Explain backward chaining. Recommend appropriate situations when this technique may be helpful.
8. Choose one evidence-supported intervention strategy that targets cognitive impairment from Table 21.1. In your words summarize the key principles of the strategy or technique.

REFERENCES

1. Allen, C. K. (1992). Professional judgment. In C. K. Allen, C. A. Earhardt, & T. Blue (Eds.), *Treatment goals for the physically and cognitively disabled*. AOTA Press.
2. Allen, C. K., Blue, T., & Earhardt, C. A. (1997). *Understanding cognitive performance modes*. Allen Conferences.
3. Alzheimer's Association. (2020). https://www.alz.org
4. Alzheimer's Association. (2020). *Mild cognitive impairment (MCI)*. https://www.alz.org/alzheimers-dementia/what-is-dementia/related_conditions/mild-cognitive-impairment
5. American Occupational Therapy Association. (2020). AOTA 2020 occupational therapy code of ethics. *American Journal of Occupational Therapy, 74*(Suppl. 3), 7413410005p1–7413410005p13.
6. American Occupational Therapy Association. (2020). Occupational therapy in the promotion of health and well-being. *American Journal of Occupational Therapy, 74*(3), 7403420010.
7. American Occupational Therapy Association. (2020). Occupational therapy practice framework: Domain and process—Fourth edition. *American Journal of Occupational Therapy, 74*(Suppl. 2), 1–87.
8. American Psychiatric Association. (2019, July). *What is electroconvulsive therapy (ECT)?* https://www.psychiatry.org/patients-families/ect
9. American Psychiatric Association. (2022). *Diagnostic and statistical manual of mental disorders* (5th ed., text rev.). https://doi.org/10.1176/appi.books.9780890425787
10. Andrews, J. (2017). "Wandering" and dementia. *British Journal of Community Nursing, 22*(7), 322–323.
11. Bailliard, A. L., & Whigham, S. C. (2017). Linking neuroscience, function, and intervention: A scoping review of sensory processing and mental illness. *American Journal of Occupational Therapy, 71*(5), 7105100040.
12. Bernardo, L. D. (2018). Older adults with Alzheimer's disease: A systematic review about the occupational therapy intervention in changes of performance skills. *Cadernos Brasileiros de Terapia Ocupacional, 26*(4), 926–942.
13. Brown, C. (2019). Cognition. In C. Brown, V. C. Stoffel, & J. P. Munoz (Eds.), *Occupational therapy in mental health: A vision for participation* (2nd ed., pp. 281–300). F.A. Davis.
14. Buser, S., & Cruz, L. (2022). *DSM-5-TR insanely simplified: Unlocking the spectrums within DSM-5-TR and ICD-10*. Chiron Publications.
15. Cahill, S. (2022). Assistive technology interventions for people with dementia and their care partners, research update. *OT Practice, 27*(9), 36–37.
16. Ciro, C. (2013). Second nature: Improving occupational performance in people with dementia through role-based, task-specific learning. *OT Practice, 18*(3), 9–12.
17. Clark, F. (2012, Spring). Mary Reilly 1916–2012. *USC Chan Magazine*. University of Southern California (USC). https://chan.usc.edu/news/magazine/spring2012/mary-reilly-1916-2012
18. da Cruz Morello, A. N., Lima, T. M., & Brandão, L. (2017). Language and communication non-pharmacological interventions in patients with Alzheimer's disease: A systematic review of communication intervention in Alzheimer. *Dementia & Neuropsychologia, 11*(3), 227–241.
19. Dixon, E., Piper, A. M., & Lazar, A. (2021, May 8–13). *Taking care of myself as long as I can: How people with dementia configure self-management systems* [Research article]. CHI Conference on Human Factors in Computing Systems, Yokohama, Japan.
20. Earhart, C. A. (2014). *Allen diagnostic module: [Revised] Manual* (2nd ed.). S&S Worldwide.
21. Earhart, C. A. (2015). *Using Allen diagnostic module—2nd edition assessments*. S&S Worldwide. https://cdn.s48888.com/share/S52_How_to_use_the_Allen_Diagnostic_Module.pdf
22. Earhart, C. A., & McCraith, D. B. (2020). Cognitive disabilities model: Allen cognitive level screen-5 and Allen diagnostic module (2nd edition) assessments. In B. J. Hemphill & C. J. Urish (Eds.), *Assessments in occupational therapy mental health: An integrative approach* (4th ed., pp. 179–210). SLACK.
23. Fisher, A. G., & Marterella, A. (2019). *Powerful practice: A model for authentic occupational therapy*. Center for Innovative OT Solutions.
24. Forbes, R. (2011). Easing agitation in residents with 'Sundowning syndrome' behaviour. *Nursing and Residential Care, 13*(7), 345–347.
25. Gitlin, L. N., Arthur, P., Piersol, C., Hessels, V., Wu, S. S., Dai, Y., & Mann, W. C. (2018). Targeting behavioral symptoms and functional decline in dementia: A randomized clinical trial. *Journal of the American Geriatrics Society, 66*(2), 339–345.
26. Gitlin, L. N., & Corcoran, M. A. (2005). Appendix B: Examples of environmental strategies for targeted management areas. In L. N. Gitlin & M. A. Corcoran (Eds.), *Occupational therapy and dementia care: The home environmental skill-building program for individuals and families*. AOTA Press.

27. Gitlin, L. N., Kales, H. C., Lyketsos, C., & Plank, E. (2012). Managing behavioral symptoms in dementia using nonpharmacological approaches: An overview. *Journal of the American Medical Directors Association, 308*(19), 2020–2029.

28. Glantz, C., & Richman, N. (2007). Occupation-based, ability-centered care for people with dementia. *OT Practice, 12*(2), 10–16.

29. Grillo, D. M., & Anderson, R. (2020). Overview of behaviors in dementia. In C. R. Martin & V. R. Preedy (Eds.), *Genetics, neurology, behavior, and diet in dementia* (pp. 555–567). Academic Press.

30. Hemphill, B. J., & Urish, C. K. (Eds.). (2020). *Assessments in occupational therapy mental health: An integrative approach* (4th ed.). SLACK.

31. Hildebrand, M., & Mack, A. (2022). Interventions using cognitive–behavioral therapy techniques for caregivers of people with stroke (January 1, 1999–December 31, 2019). *American Journal of Occupational Therapy, 76*(3), 7603393040.

32. Hill, R., & Dahlitz, M. (2022). *The practitioner's guide to the science of psychotherapy.* W. W. Norton & Company.

33. Holm, M. B., & Rogers, J. C. (2020). The performance assessment of self-care skills. In B. J. Hemphill & C. J. Urish (Eds.), *Assessments in occupational therapy mental health: An integrative approach* (4th ed., pp. 359–370). SLACK.

34. Jensen, L., & Padilla, R. (2017). Effectiveness of environment-based interventions that address behavior, perception, and falls in people with Alzheimer's disease and related major neurocognitive disorders: A systematic review. *American Journal of Occupational Therapy, 71*(5), 7105180030p1–7105180030p10.

35. Judd, L. L., Akiskal, H. S., Zeller, P. J., Paulus, M., Leon, A. C., Maser, J. D., Endicott, J., Coryell, W., Kunovac, J. L., Mueller, T. I., Rice, J. P., & Keller, M. B. (2000). Psychosocial disability during the long-term course of unipolar major depressive disorder. *Archives of General Psychiatry, 57*(4), 375–380.

36. Katz, N. (2005). *Cognition and occupation across the life span* (2nd ed.). AOTA Press.

37. Katz, N. (2020). Routine task inventory-expanded. In B. J. Hemphill & C. J. Urish (Eds.), *Assessments in occupational therapy mental health: An integrative approach* (4th ed., pp. 211–221). SLACK.

38. Kruse, C. S., Fohn, J., Umunnakwe, G., Patel, K., & Patel, S. (2020). Evaluating the facilitators, barriers, and medical outcomes commensurate with the use of assistive technology to support people with dementia: A systematic review literature. *Healthcare, 8*(3), 278.

39. McKay, H., & Hanzaker, M. M. (2013). Dementia care communication: A toolbox for professionals and families. *OT Practice, 18*(3), CE1–CE8.

40. Michels, K., Dubaz, O., Hornthal, E., & Berga, D. (2018). "Dance therapy" as a psychotherapeutic movement intervention in Parkinson's disease. *Complementary Therapies in Medicine, 40*, 248–252.

41. Mind Help. (n.d.). *Attention.* https://mind.help/topic/attention/

42. Nadler Tzadok, Y., Eliav, R., Portnoy, S., & Rand, D. (2022). Establishing the validity of the internet-based Bill-Paying Task to assess executive function deficits among adults with traumatic brain injury. *American Journal of Occupational Therapy, 76*(4), 7604205110.

43. Polatajko, H. J., Mandich, A., & McEwen, S. E. (2011). Cognitive orientation to daily occupation (CO-OP): A cognitive-based intervention for children and adults. In N. Katz (Ed.), *Cognition, occupation, and participation across the life span: Neuroscience, neurorehabilitation, and models of intervention in occupational therapy* (3rd ed., pp. 299–322). AOTA Press.

44. Radder, D. L., Sturkenboom, I. H., van Nimwegen, M., Keus, S. H., Bloem, B. R., & de Vries, N. M. (2017). Physical therapy and occupational therapy in Parkinson's disease. *International Journal of Neuroscience, 127*(10), 930–943.

45. Ridge, E., & Robnett, R. (2009). In their own words: The emotional experience of individuals with Alzheimer's disease. *OT Practice, 14*(8), 16–21.

46. Romero-Ayuso, D., Cuerda, C., Morales, C., Tesoriero, R., Triviño-Juárez, J. M., Segura-Fragoso, A., & Gallud, J. A. (2021). Activities of daily living and categorization skills of elderly with cognitive deficit: A preliminary study. *Brain Sciences, 11*(2), 213.

47. Sabel, R., & Gallagher, R. (2012). Meditation: A mindful approach to promoting occupational performance. *OT Practice, 17*(11), 17–18.

48. Skidmore, E. R. (2017). Functional cognition: Implications for practice, policy, and research. *The American Journal of Geriatric Psychiatry, 25*(5), 483–484.

49. Smith, J., & MacRae, A. (2019). Mental health of older adults. In A. MacRae (Ed.), *Cara and MacRae's psychosocial occupational therapy: An evolving practice* (4th ed., pp. 225–241). SLACK.

50. Sriram, V., Jenkinson, C., & Peters, M. (2019). Informal carers' experience of assistive technology use in dementia care at home: A systematic review. *BMC Geriatrics, 19*(1), 1–25.

51. Taylor, R. R. (2020). *The intentional relationship: Occupational therapy and use of self* (2nd ed.). F.A. Davis.

52. Tester, N. J., & Foss, J. J. (2018). Sleep as an occupational need. *American Journal of Occupational Therapy, 72*(1), 7201347010p1–7201347010p4.

53. Torossian, M., Fiske, S. M., & Jacelon, C. S. (2021). Sleep, mild cognitive impairment, and interventions for sleep improvement: An integrative review. *Western Journal of Nursing Research, 43*(11), 1051–1060.

54. Trace, S., & Howell, T. (1991). Occupational therapy in geriatric mental health. *American Journal of Occupational Therapy, 45*(9), 833–838.

55. Trapp, W., Landgrebe, M., Hoesl, K., Lautenbacher, S., Gallhofer, B., Günther, W., & Hajak, G. (2013). Cognitive remediation improves cognition and good cognitive performance increases time to relapse—Results of a 5 year catamnestic study in schizophrenia patients. *BMC Psychiatry, 13*(1), 1–9.

56. Watters, K., Marks, T. S., Edwards, D. F., Skidmore, E. R., & Giles, G. M. (2021). A framework for addressing clients' functional cognitive deficits after COVID-19. *American Journal of Occupational Therapy, 75*(Suppl. 1), 7511347010p1–7511347010p7.

57. Wesson, J., Clemson, L., Crawford, J. D., Kochan, N. A., Brodaty, H., & Reppermund, S. (2017). Measurement of functional cognition and complex everyday activities in older adults with mild cognitive impairment and mild dementia: Validity of the large Allen's Cognitive Level Screen. *American Journal of Geriatric Psychiatry, 25*(5), 471–482.

58. Wolf, C., & Serpa, J. G. (2015). *A clinician's guide to teaching mindfulness: The comprehensive session-by-session program for mental health professionals and health care providers.* New Harbinger Press.

59. Woo, Y. S., Rosenblat, J. D., Kakar, R., Bahk, W.-M., & McIntyre, R. S. (2016). Cognitive deficits as a mediator of poor occupational function in remitted major depressive disorder patients. *Clinical Psychopharmacology and Neuroscience, 14*(1), 1–16.

SUGGESTED RESOURCES

Articles

Baptista, C., Afonso, R. M., & Silva, A. R. (2022). Practitioners' knowledge, acceptability and use of external memory aids with individuals with cognitive deficits: An exploratory study. *Neuropsychological Rehabilitation, 33*(5), 1–19.

Objective of Study: External memory aids (EMAs) are within the most effective cognitive rehabilitation techniques, having demonstrated a positive impact in terms of memory functioning in individuals with multiple cognitive deficits. Despite its proven efficacy, there is yet poor dissemination of these techniques in clinical settings. The current study aims to evaluate the level of knowledge, degree of use, and usage expectations of EMAs by health practitioners who are responsible for implementing these techniques.

Tofani, M., Ranieri, A., Fabbrini, G., Berardi, A., Pelosin, E., Valente, D., Fabbrini, A., Costanzo, M., & Galeoto, G. (2020). Efficacy of occupational therapy interventions on quality of life in patients with Parkinson's disease: A systematic review and meta-analysis. *Movement Disorders Clinical Practice, 7*(8), 891–901.

Objective of Study: To review studies assessing the efficacy of occupational therapy interventions on quality of life in clients with Parkinson disease.

Kastner, L., Velder-Shukrun, Y., Bonne, O., Bar-Ilan, R. T., & Maeir, A. (2022). Pilot study of the Cognitive–Functional Intervention for Adults (Cog-Fun A): A metacognitive–Functional tool for adults with attention deficit hyperactivity disorder. *American Journal of Occupational Therapy, 76*(2), 7602205070.

Objective of Study: To determine the preliminary effectiveness of the Cognitive–Functional Intervention for Adults (Cog-Fun A), a meta-cognitive–functional occupational therapy tool for the improvement of occupational performance (OP) and quality of life (QoL) in adults with attention deficit hyperactivity disorder (ADHD).

Books

My Stroke of Insight by Jill Bolte Taylor: On December 10, 1996, Jill Bolte Taylor, a 37-year-old Harvard-trained brain scientist experienced a massive stroke in the left hemisphere of her brain. As she observed her mind deteriorate to the point that she could not walk, talk, read, write, or recall any of her life—all within 4 hours—Taylor alternated between the euphoria of the intuitive and kinesthetic right brain, in which she felt a sense of complete well-being and peace, and the logical, sequential left brain, which recognized she was having a stroke and enabled her to seek help before she was completely lost. It would take her 8 years to fully recover. This is her story. A link to her TED Talk: https://www.ted.com/talks/jill_bolte_taylor_my_stroke_of_insight

Still Alice by Lisa Genova: In Genova's *New York Times* bestselling novel, an accomplished woman slowly loses her thoughts and memories to Alzheimer disease—only to discover that each day brings a new way of living and loving. *Still Alice* became a major motion picture in 2015 and is available online to rent or purchase.

LEFT Neglected by Lisa Genova: From neuroscientist and bestselling author Lisa Genova comes a story of resilience in the face of a devastating diagnosis. After a motor vehicle accident (MVA) leaves a vibrant mother in her thirties with a traumatic brain disorder called "left neglect," she learns what truly matters most in life.

Videos

Alive Inside: Social worker Dan Cohen, through his nonprofit organization Music and Memory, advocates for the use of music therapy with individuals with dementia. https://tubitv.com/movies/533167/vivos-adentro-sub-esp?start=true&utm_source=google-feed&tracking=google-feed

My Father, My Brother, and Me: In 2004, journalist Dave Iverson received the same news that had been delivered to his father and older brother years earlier: He had Parkinson disease, a degenerative neurologic disorder that affects about 1 million Americans. In a FRONTLINE and ITVS joint production, Iverson sets off on a personal journey to explore the scientific, ethical, and political debates that surround Parkinson disease, which was at the center of the ongoing controversy over embryonic stem cell research. Iverson talks to scientists on the cutting edge of new cures and therapies for Parkinson disease as well as a number of other major neurologic conditions. And he has intimate conversations with fellow Parkinson sufferers such as actor Michael J. Fox and writer Michael Kinsley. https://www.pbs.org/wgbh/frontline/documentary/parkinsons/

Websites

American Parkinson Disease Association: https://www.apdaparkinson.org/
Alzheimer's Association: https://www.alz.org/
National Council on Aging: https://www.ncoa.org/
National Institutes of Health, National Institute on Aging: https://www.nia.nih.gov/

Targeting Psychological and Social Factors That Influence Occupational Engagement: Being With the Client Who Experiences Anger, Hostility, or Aggression

OT HACKS OVERVIEW

O: **Occupation as a means and an end**

Novaco's Affective Stress Reaction Anger Intervention Model (25) is introduced as a frame of reference that can provide guidance to occupational therapy professionals (OTPs) in targeting problematic anger in interventions while using occupation as a means and as an end to improve occupational participation. One element of the model is given here:

The occupational therapy professional develops assignments that are embedded in the client's typical daily occupations that the client can complete between occupational therapy sessions to practice newly acquired coping strategies (away from the clinic or other relevant setting) (occupation as a means). The client can keep a time diary to record their responses to difficult or anger provoking situations that occur throughout the week, so that a performance-based self-report can be shared with the occupational therapy professional. This step further invests the client in taking responsibility to make successful changes (occupation as an end).

T: **Theoretical concepts, values, and principles, or historical foundations**

Referring to the *Pan Occupational Paradigm* (POP), a client's anger can be reflected upon as it applies to the dimensions of occupation—*doing, being, becoming*, and *belonging* (16). In other words, an OTP may ask the client the following:

1. "How does your anger affect what you do?"—*Doing dimension*
2. "What role does anger play in your day-to-day life, especially when it comes to making decisions and completing the things that you want and need to do?"—*Being dimension*
3. "How does your anger cause problems for you in reaching your goals?"—*Becoming dimension*
4. "What do you think other people who know you very well might say about your anger? Do you think that your anger impacts other people, how?"—*Belonging dimension*

H: **How can we Help? OT's role in serving clients with mental illness or mental health needs**

All OTPs will, at some point, have the experience of collaborating with a client who is angry (whether or not their anger is disruptive of occupation or necessarily problematic). This chapter highlights some of the goals and outcomes associated with assessing, targeting, and addressing problematic anger when it interferes with the pursuit of the clients' prioritized occupations.

A: **Adaptations**

The dual capacity of anger to impact occupation either positively or negatively demonstrates its adaptive function. Furthermore, anger is ubiquitous in psychiatric illnesses, and is, according to the evidence, highly predictive of important functional outcomes.

C: **Case study includes**

Jada is a 17-year-old Alaskan Native female who was diagnosed with oppositional defiant disorder (ODD), adolescent-onset type (F91.2) when she was 14 years old following repeated school truancies and suspensions from school for fighting and physical aggression toward others. More recently, 8 months ago, Jada was the victim of an attack and sexual assault by two men who have not yet been identified. Jada was subsequently diagnosed with posttraumatic stress disorder (PTSD).

Read more about the case at the end of the chapter.

K: **Knowledge: keeping mental health OT practice grounded in evidence, in occupational science, and in research**

Read this evidence by Nurenberg et al using the following research question as a focus:

How do the equine-assisted psychotherapy (EAP) and canine-assisted psychotherapy (CAP) forms of animal-assisted therapy (AAT) compare with standard treatments for hospitalized clients with psychiatric problems in affecting violent or regressed behaviors?

After reviewing the article and learning more in this chapter about how the symptoms of anger, aggression, or hostility impact occupational engagement, discuss responses to the *Evidence Application and Translation Questions* found in the "OT HACKS Chapter Summary, Knowledge" section.

S: Some terms that may be new to you

Aggression
Anger
Assertiveness
Hostility
Violence

TARGETING SYMPTOMS OF EMOTIONAL DYSREGULATION: ANGER, HOSTILITY, OR AGGRESSION THAT CREATE BARRIERS TO OCCUPATION: THE BEING, DOING, AND BELONGING DIMENSIONS OF OT PRACTICE

BOX 22.1 Intervention Planning Focus Questions: How to Begin

1. What does it feel like to be a person who is experiencing *anger, hostility, or aggression?*
2. What are some behaviors that a person experiencing *anger, hostility, or aggression* might demonstrate, and how might their behavior, responses, or affect be positively or negatively impacting their occupations?
3. How can I adjust my way of being (therapeutic use of self) to make the client feel more comfortable about their way of being?
4. What can I do to instill a sense of belonging in occupational therapy right now that will encourage the client toward setting goals with outcomes that are personally meaningful and relevant to them?

The complex nature and various conceptualizations of anger make it very difficult to compose a unified or singular definition. This has led to long-standing debates about the multifaceted emotion, especially about whether anger is a primary emotion or a secondary emotion that could be hiding other, more difficult to express emotions (5). To date, there are no commonly shared criteria for differentiating between pathologic anger and physiologic anger. "In-fact, there are several elements that constitute anger, as well as that support and modulate its expression: arousal, cognition, anger regulation, physiological and behavioral display. Moreover, when anger is induced, various networks are activated" (21, p. 189). This further adds to the complexities of the subject and causes many experts to question when typical anger becomes more intense anger, and what the bar is for that intensity to become pathologic anger or rage (5, 15, 21). What characteristics of the person, their history, and their situational context impact the ways that people express their anger? For OTPs, the domain of concern extends those questions one step further to explore how pathologic or problematic anger is disrupting participation in everyday occupations and in

everyday life. This chapter introduces aspects of anger that are important considerations for planning and implementing occupational therapy interventions with clients who experience angry emotions. Some of the primary aspects of anger that are introduced within the chapter include physiologic arousal, cognitive reprocessing, environmental/contextual stimuli, and behavioral reactions, or modes of response (8, 25, 32, 35).

What Are Symptoms of Anger, Hostility, or Aggression?

It is important to begin with a brief, but thorough look at the complex emotion of anger and to differentiate anger from hostility and aggression. **Anger** *is a strong feeling of displeasure.* There are a variety of models where each conceptualizes anger differently. From the cognitive behavioral and motivational models of emotion come two perspectives of anger:

1. Anger arises from a person's evaluation that a wrongdoing has occurred and the individual's subsequent desire to counteract, or "right," the wrongdoing.
2. From the motivational model comes the notion that anger can be considered an approach emotion because it is often the response triggered when a person approaches completion of a task or goal, but then experiences failed attempts to reach the goal, or complete the task (8).

Anger can also be distinguished by levels of intensity (from mildly annoyed to raging). Furthermore, anger can exist in several forms including *emotion, mood,* or *temperament.* Anger in the form of emotion is largely an experience that occurs briefly and temporarily (episodic). When anger can be maintained at a mostly mild level of intensity, but has a longer duration, it can be thought of as an aspect of a person's mood. If a person is prone to continuous or consistent feelings of anger, it is often considered to be a part of the person's temperament (8).

From a purely psychological view of anger, a core concept is the distinction between an *experience of anger,* which is an individual's subjective feelings of anger, and *expression of anger,* or the way that anger is demonstrated or communicated (32). **Hostility** *is an unfriendly and threatening attitude directed toward other people.* Literature indicates that an expression of hostility is usually a "pattern of frequent occurrence that suggests dispositional rather than situational anger" (8, p. 125). In other words, an expression of hostility as an angry response is not necessarily purely a response to an unjust situation but is likely to be, at least in part, a characteristic of the person's disposition (or temperament) (8). **Aggression** *is an attack on a person or object with an intention to cause hurt; aggression can be verbal, physical, or both.* One consequence of aggression is **violence**; violence is behavior that intentionally ends with physical injuries or damage to people (the victims), places, or things (destruction of property).

Hostility, aggression, and violence can all be indicators that the typical emotion of anger has become pathologic (8), and, for the OTP, these are also likely to indicate the kind of pathologic anger that will interfere with optimal occupational performance and participation. That being said, however, remember that each person's combination of physiologic processes, experiences, and expressions of anger are as unique as the client themselves; "anger, whether functional or dysfunctional, can certainly occur in the absence of aggressive or violent [and hostile] behavior and vice-versa" (8, p. 125). OTPs, when assessing a client's pathologic anger relevant to occupational disruption, occupational deprivation, occupational injustice, or, conversely, when assessing any benefits of appropriate anger (ie, enhanced motivation, increased problem-solving, or adaptive function), will require the application of substantial professional judgment to determine the most appropriate type and approach for intervention.

Before discussing some of the reasons that clients become angry, hostile, or aggressive, one final distinction needs to be clarified. It is essential to distinguish aggression from assertiveness, which are frequently confused concepts. **Assertiveness** is the direct expression of one's feelings, needs, and desires. Assertiveness has come to be synonymous with "sticking up for oneself." There are situations in which a person must be both assertive and aggressive. For example, in New York City, parking spaces are at such a premium that it is quite common for two drivers to want the same space. What should the driver who arrived first do? To secure the space, it may be necessary to get out of the car and argue about it. Many New York City car owners consider this assertiveness appropriate and typical of the "driving culture" of the city.

When the OTP is working with individuals who are verbally or physically aggressive, it is important to distinguish between ordinary (culturally endorsed) self-assertiveness and inappropriate aggression. Although almost everyone feels angry at times, and sometimes with good reason, most people can control their feelings and avoid acting them out. Those who are unable to express their feelings in words may resort to violence. The literature consistently confirms that this is especially true for people with a history of abuse or other adverse childhood experiences (15, 27, 37). Clients who become verbally abusive or physically violent may be expressing any of a variety of unmet needs. They may feel threatened or hemmed in, physically or psychologically.

Aggression and violence in psychiatric treatment settings is concerning for both the client and for the health professionals and care team. Not only do incidents of aggression harm the victim but they are also often unavoidable witnesses to acts of aggression in locked units or facilities with limited space. All this leads to emotional, financial, and legal consequences that further impact the quality of life for everyone involved (19). Psychiatric treatment settings are often crowded and clients may find the physical press of other people and the lack of privacy overwhelming. Similarly, they may feel confined and frustrated by the rules and restrictions that often realistically include locked doors and limited time or access to being outdoors (4, 19). From an attachment theory or object relations perspective, hostility and aggression could be seen as a self-protective defense mechanism; by keeping others at a distance, the person's unconscious belief is that they make rejection less likely, if not impossible (14).

In one study, Lamanna and colleagues (19) explored and compared inpatient and clinician perspectives on the factors affecting verbal and physical aggression by inpatients with psychiatric issues. This study and its revelations are unique in several ways that are helpful to understanding and applying an occupational therapy perspective of anger and aggression. Referring to the POP, a client's anger can be reflected upon as it applies to the dimensions of occupation, *doing, being, becoming,* and *belonging* (16). In other words, an OTP may ask the client, "How does your anger affect what you do?"; "What role does anger play in your day-to-day life, especially when it comes to making decisions and completing the things that you want and need to do?"; "How does your anger cause problems for you in reaching your goals?"; and, "What do you think other people who know you very well might say about your anger? Do you think that your anger impacts other people?"

Returning our attention to the study by Lamanna et al, previous works had mostly explored health care providers' perspectives on acts of aggression, or captured administrative data from psychiatric units, but had failed to explore or incorporate the inpatient clients' perspectives and insights (19). Studies such as this one help us grow more accustomed to asking questions with depth and they show the importance of presence and engaged active listening as part of an intentional therapeutic relationship that leads to development of authentic client-centered interventions (9, 36). In this qualitative exploration, the researchers used an interpretive theoretical framework and qualitative interviewing methods to seek and examine the study of participants' perspectives (of both the clients and the clinicians). "The interpretive approach focuses on understanding participants' interpretation of events and processes in their settings and the meanings that they hold" (19, p. 2). Six themes emerged from the participant data, each categorized as either personal or organizational factors that can impact an aggressive response. Three of the themes were central to the clients' personal experiences and their interpersonal relationships, including major life stressors, experience of illness, and interpersonal connections with clinicians. Three of the themes were related to organizational processes, including physical confinement and behavioral restrictions, engagement with clinicians, and treatment decisions (19). Table 22.1 highlights the responses of some of the participants in this study. A link to the full research article can be found in the Suggested Resources section.

The findings of the research introduced in the previous section highlight several important aspects of anger and

aggression as a symptom to consider when planning intervention. First, some individuals use physical or verbal aggression (which can escalate into violence) as a way of venting frustration, of letting off steam; often, such people find it difficult to identify their feelings or to express themselves in words. OTPs can incorporate techniques such as cognitive restructuring, thought blocking, and cognitive reframing, all associated with cognitive behavioral therapy (CBT)

Table 22.1. Patient and Provider Perspectives of Aggression in Psychiatric Settings: Taking a Closer Look at Client-Centered Care

Category and Theme	What Participants Shared . . .
Personal factors	
• **Major life stressors**	"The whole day was just devoted to being upset because of my kids: I didn't know where they were." (Client 05) "You don't know what [clients have] been through outside the hospital . . . they check your medical history. Other than that, what do they know?" (Client 10) "They thought I was aggravated. No kidding, my mom just had a heart attack, and I am stuck in the hospital . . . I can't get anybody to get me out of here." (Client 07)
• **Experience of illness**	Interviewer question: What are the common reasons that clients show aggression to other clients? "Paranoia is a big one . . . people become paranoid of other people staring at them or if they are talking to themselves." (Clinician 01) "I was upset, because it's telling me to follow, but I don't want to follow . . . the voice [said] to do this, do that, but I do not want to follow, so I just throw things." (Client 03) "A client who is manic might not have control of their emotions. Even the personality disorders, they have difficulty with controlling their emotions." (Clinician 06)
• **Interpersonal connections with clinicians**	"It was just a bad moment . . . They were really sweet to me . . . I really appreciated their concern for me." (Client 13) "If someone just kind of brings it down, simplifies it, and empathizes with them . . . [clients] are much more receptive to that . . . a staff member might respond to agitated behavior or anger with inappropriate tone, body language, those kinds of things, and that makes things worse." (Clinician 02) "I seriously think I'm having a stroke . . . don't automatically write off the patient as not knowing what they are talking about because they're in the nut ward." (Client 06)
Organizational factors	
• **Physical confinement** • **Behavioral restrictions**	Interviewer question: What are some common reasons clients show aggression? "Feeling trapped in hospital when they are in fact trapped in hospital, because they're on an involuntary certificate." (Clinician 08) Regarding behavioral restrictions, a clinician participant (unidentified) commented: "I think they feel like their . . . concerns are not being heard or understood. I think that stimulates frustration or inability and it builds . . . " Interviewer question: What can cause that? "Wanting things that can't really be granted – for example, belongings, clothes." (Clinician 09) "It's about freaking out over an item that I can't have, because they took away my freedom." (Client 09) "It drives you nuts, it's so boring . . . you have to have some kind of distraction. Then if you don't, then you just start getting aggressive. I think that's what happens with a lot of people." (Client 06) "Lack of activity is what I have heard from patients. Like they said 'I am just so bored' after an [aggressive] incident." (Clinician 01)
• **Lack of engagement with clinicians** • **Treatment decisions**	"When they disagree with treatment and they have to take it as a result of . . . the legal issues. I think they feel quite let down, and like we're plotting against them." (Clinician 09) "She didn't tell me what kind of pills or nothing, she just said 'take the pills, you have to take these pills'. I said 'I'm not taking any pills', so she called the security guard . . . I'm not going to take something I don't know." (Client 08) Interviewer question: Have staff ever done anything to make you feel more upset? "Telling me to calm down when I have nothing to help me to calm down."(Client 09)

Adapted from Lamanna, D., Ninkovic, D., Vijayaratnam, V., Balderson, K., Spivak, H., Brook, S., & Robertson, D. (2016). Aggression in psychiatric hospitalizations: A qualitative study of patient and provider perspectives. *Journal of Mental Health, 25*(6), 536–542.

into occupation-based intervention plans. CBT is the most widely researched intervention used to target affective states and traits and help clients become more aware of their anger triggers and their angry thought patterns, so that they can eventually develop new, more healthy thought patterns (21). This process is undertaken not to eliminate the anger emotion but to help them recognize when their thoughts are resulting in faulty conclusions, or are encouraging angry, destructive, hostile, or aggressive behavioral responses that impede occupation. Reframing angry thoughts allows the client to channel their anger more appropriately (31).

Clients who experience anger and demonstrate aggressive behaviors may not have developed any constructive channels for expressing their feelings (eg, sports, hobbies, exercise, meditation, prayer), or they may not have access to constructive outlets for their anger, similar to what the participants in the research study expressed. But both groups of participants in the aforementioned study, the clinicians and the clients, also suggested that some demonstrations of aggression were "connected to mental illness itself . . . Elements of mental illness cited to be important included type and acuity of symptoms, reduced emotional resilience, frustration with specific symptoms and perceived effects or side-effects of medications. Symptoms including paranoia or psychosis were universally identified by clinicians as a factor contributing to aggression" (19, p. 3).

Diagnoses in Which Anger, Hostility, or Aggression Are Common Symptoms

Anger is a central diagnostic feature in six *DSM-5-TR* disorders (3). These are intermittent explosive disorder (IED), borderline personality disorder (BPD), bipolar disorder (BD), disruptive mood dysregulation disorder (DMDD), PTSD, and ODD (3, 8). Anger has also been associated, as a symptom, with other psychiatric disorders including psychotic disorders (such as schizophrenia or schizoaffective disorders), major depressive disorder (MDD), attention deficit hyperactivity disorder (ADHD), and some major neurocognitive disorders. Substance users and persons with antisocial personality disorder may also show hostility.

There are a few other factors that OTPs should keep in mind regarding anger, aggression, and hostility. Some neurocognitive disorders are disinhibiting, meaning that the person no longer feels bound by customary social taboos or expectations. Particularly in clients with memory impairments or those who experience disinhibition caused by other neurocognitive dysfunctions such as traumatic brain injury (TBI), aggressive or angry responses are often outside the individual's conscious awareness and therefore may not be responsive to restorative or remedial occupational therapy intervention approaches (39). The occupation of sleep, more specifically sleep deprivation or disruption, significantly influences the intensity, form, expression, and experience of irritability and frustration that can lead to anger or aggression. Sleep disruption is consistently linked with anger, aggression, and violence (18). By amplifying negative affect, angry

feelings, perceptions of threat, and hostile thoughts, sleep disruption increases the likelihood that an individual will demonstrate aggressive behaviors. As previously mentioned, impaired inhibition, poor impulse control, and reduced capacity of executive function that affect problem-solving and decision-making are all possible consequences of sleep deprivation that could contribute to a client's aggressive or hostile response (18). Finally, any person may become angry, hostile, and even violent if sufficiently provoked; and anger can be a normal or culturally mediated (whether or not appropriate to the current situation) response to illness and disability (20, 33, 34).

Strategies for Therapeutic Use of Self to Help Symptoms of Anger, Hostility, and Aggression

OTPs should be sensitive to the emotions of all clients and they should be generally alert to external signs that a client is feeling tense, threatened, or suspicious. Body language and nonverbal behavior can often reveal clues to their affective state. For example, stiffness or rigidity in the set of the mouth or the shoulders may signify heightened anger or anxiety. Threatening gestures and the destruction of property or objects, no matter how small or insignificant, are also considered external signs of frustration or anger. The sooner the possibility of aggression is detected, the more likely that the impending behavior can be deterred through appropriate response and use of de-escalation or diversion approaches and techniques.

The general approach and overarching goal is to get clients who experience disruptive anger or demonstrate aggression to talk about what is bothering them, to identify their feelings, and to help them use words or other appropriate channels to express their feelings, rather than channeling anger into hostility, aggression, or violence that will further disrupt occupational engagement (31, 38). It is critical not to respond in kind, no matter how insulting or provocative the person's behavior might be (36). If the person is in a heightened state of anxiety, or demonstrates high levels of energy such as the ones expressed in a manic client, it can help to integrate calming, grounding activities that will help slow the individual and soothe anxiety. Strategies such as the broken record technique, where the OTP repeats the same calming words several times, can be especially effective for this purpose (33).

It is equally important when a client demonstrates angry or aggressive responses to try to speak to the person privately, avoiding a public display that may make them feel more threatened or embarrassed. Encourage the client to discuss their feelings. Tell them exactly what must be corrected about any inappropriate behaviors or responses, making sure that the instruction is directed only at the current situation. An explanation of why they are being redirected that focuses on how their behavior is affecting you and the other people present is essential to supporting a client's progress toward demonstrating appropriate responses and behaviors that are assertive without being overly aggressive. Finally, giving the client some alternatives for appropriately handling their angry feelings, after they have learned to be more aware of them, is the key to supporting new practices (22, 30). Importantly, be thoughtful in your interactions with clients, doing your best to avoid any statements or behaviors that may be perceived as punitive or critical; these approaches are humiliating and tend to escalate aggressiveness (19).

TARGETING SYMPTOMS OF ANGER, HOSTILITY, OR AGGRESSION THAT CREATE BARRIERS TO OCCUPATION: THE DOING AND BECOMING DIMENSIONS OF OT PRACTICE

> **BOX 22.2 Intervention Implementation Focus Questions: How to Support Clients' Optimal Engagement in Occupation**
>
> 1. What can the client and the occupational therapy team collaboratively do that will help the client become more functional and effective in the things that are important to them in everyday life?
> 2. What are the best intervention types and intervention approaches to apply in this therapeutic context?
> 3. What does the current evidence suggest about the most productive interventions for this diagnosis/set of symptoms?

Contextual, Environmental, and Client Factor Considerations for the Symptoms of Anger, Hostility, and Aggression

Because of the potential for violence, hostile or aggressive individuals may have to be isolated from others who irritate them; this is especially the case for forensic units such as prisons. While speaking to hostile or potentially violent clients, the OTP should stand 4 or 5 feet away and to the side, not facing the person directly. This position gives the person adequate personal space and is considered a nonconfrontational approach. It is not safe or advisable to be alone with someone who has a history of violence or is likely to become violent. Similarly, regardless of the layout or arrangement of a room, be sure that the door is left open and position yourself so that you are closer to the door than is the client. Do not touch the client without permission and always explain your actions if the client seems uncomfortable or demonstrates signs of paranoia. Even what you intend as a comforting touch can be misperceived, misinterpreted, or misunderstood as threatening. Give thoughtful consideration to the therapeutic space, removing all sharp objects and other potential weapons from the area.

Characteristics of Intervention Activities and Recommended Modifications for Symptoms of Anger, Hostility, or Aggression

Unfortunately, there is no handy formula for choosing activities for the person who is experiencing anger or hostility.

Often, activities such as art, dance, drumming, or physical exercise permit the person to express feelings in a socially acceptable way; these mediums seem especially useful for clients with poor verbal skills because they do not rely on verbal expression and communication performance skills. Avoid activities that require moderate or high levels of frustration tolerance and attention to detail. For obvious reasons, eliminate activities that involve sharp tools or small, heavy, or throwable objects. Activities that use repetitive motions may help some people organize and self-regulate so that they have better control of their feelings. Addressing the stress that is fueling the hostile, angry, or aggressive state by introducing stress management techniques is another option.

When angry, a person experiences a high level of physiologic arousal (eg, increased heart rate, respiration, energy) that interferes with rational thinking and problem-solving. Aggressive clients may not be consciously aware that this is happening, or may not know that they can learn to recognize, monitor, and control this arousal by implementing relaxation and stress management techniques. Furthermore,

> **BOX 22.3 Examples of Appropriate Activities for Anger, Hostility, and Aggression**
>
> - *Active sports* and other gross motor activities such as dance are useful for releasing tension.
> - *Sanding a large wood project* involves repetitive gross motor movements; it is an example of an activity that might help reduce tension. Preparing and painting a wall or a large surface is another activity with similar qualities.
> - *Meal prep activities such as peeling potatoes, kneading dough, shucking corn, or cleaning tasks such as vacuuming, folding laundry, or scrubbing* also involve repetitive movements that can be therapeutic in alleviating stress. The tools used should be chosen with careful consideration of the clients' safety; for example, a potato peeler with a rounded point should be selected (rather than a knife). Activities that involve sharp or potentially dangerous tools (eg, woodworking, metal hammering) should be used only when both therapist and client feel comfortable that the client has demonstrated active self-control over their angry or aggressive responses.
> - *Anger management* (12, 13, 35) and *conflict resolution training* (11) may benefit those who have problems managing, controlling, and expressing anger. Such training gives the person the skills of preplanning a response to angry feelings, identifying anger when it occurs, problem-solving to handle anger, and empathizing with and forgiving the other party (13).
> - *Assertiveness training* provides skills that use reason and verbal expression to meet needs.
> - *Use of social media* in occupational therapy interventions that target symptoms of anger, aggressiveness, or hostility should be closely monitored to reduce the chances that the person may express anger, hostility, and so on to someone online.

they may benefit from specific stress management strategies, such as learning to monitor and reduce activity demands and to increase resources to deal with stressful situations. Training in assertiveness skills (learning to use words and reason) can replace the habit of expressing rage while also preventing escalation to violence. A helpful outline with steps for the OTP to consider when designing an occupational therapy intervention plan that targets problematic anger is provided in Box 22.4. The guidelines are based on the work of anger researcher Dr Raymond Novaco and his *Affective Stress Reaction Anger Model* (23–25, 35). Novaco's work provides an excellent frame of reference for reflecting upon and considering the many complex aspects of anger that have the potential to negatively impact occupational engagement.

BOX 22.4 Novaco's Affective Stress Reaction Anger Intervention Model: A Frame of Reference Outline for Targeting Problematic Anger in Occupational Therapy Intervention

i. *Assess whether a client's anger is adaptive or maladaptive* by asking questions about the frequency, intensity, duration and consequences of the anger episodes. What occupations (activities) does the anger episode negatively impact?

ii. *Assess the client's motivation and readiness for change.*

iii. *Assess the client's awareness of their actual arousal levels* (physiologic state, eg, heart rate, breathing, experience of pain, and other somatic symptoms).

iv. *Assess their understanding of the dynamics of arousal during a state of anger.*

v. *Overarching goals of treatment*
   a. Increase the clients' resources for coping with stress.
   b. If possible, decrease the demands made on the client.

vi. *Two-step treatment procedure*
   a. Increase the clients' awareness of the relationship between anger and stress
   b. Increase, thereby, the client's effective use of stress management techniques for coping with anger-producing situations.

vii. *Six-stage treatment process*
   a. Explain the treatment approach to the client. This includes the following:
      1. The clients' responsibility for their own changes
      2. Stress and its relationship to anger
      3. The anger factors: *physiologic arousal, cognitive processing, environmental stimuli*, and *behavioral reactions* (or modes of response)
      4. The use of anger to cue task-oriented stress management behaviors
   b. The therapist plans activities that will increase the clients' awareness of their own arousal, cognitions, environment, and behaviors during episodes of anger.
   c. The therapist may be required to model adaptive coping strategies for handling stress and anger, especially when changes in behavior are necessary.
   d. The therapist employs rehearsal techniques to support the clients' rehearsal of these procedures.
   e. The therapist supplies the client with feedback on their performance after the rehearsal of the procedures.
   f. The therapist develops assignments that are embedded in the client's typical daily occupations that the client can complete between occupational therapy sessions to practice newly acquired coping strategies (away from the clinic or other relevant setting). The client can keep a time diary to record their responses to difficult or anger-provoking situations that occur throughout the week, so that a performance-based self-report can be shared with the therapist. This step further invests the client in taking responsibility to make successful changes.

viii. *Treatment objectives for physiologic arousal*
   a. To increase the client's awareness of their actual level of arousal during episodes of anger
   b. To increase the client's use of arousal control methods for lowering arousal during episodes of anger
      1. For enhancing general awareness of various arousal levels, clients can participate in occupations that provide opportunities for them to experience and label sensations associated with high and low states of arousal.
      2. The client is then provided with opportunities to practice arousal control by having them intentionally apply arousal reduction techniques or activities following arousal-producing activities or occupations.

ix. *Treatment objectives for cognitive processing and behavioral reactions*
   a. Teach clients to increase their recognition of the signs of anger-producing stress and then work up to help them control their thoughts during episodes of stress that occur during daily occupations.
   b. The primary objective of working with the client's behavioral reactions and responses is to teach them stress management skills that allow them to cope with anger-related stressors in a more healthy and appropriate way.

Adapted from Grogan, G. (1991). Anger management: Part 1. A perspective for occupational therapy. *Occupational Therapy in Mental Health, 11*(2–3), 135–148; Grogan, G. (1991). Anger management: Part 2. Clinical applications for occupational therapy. *Occupational Therapy in Mental Health, 11*(2–3), 149–171; Novaco, R. (1979). The cognitive regulation of anger and stress. In P. Kendall & S. Hollen (Eds.), *Cognitive-behavioral interventions: Theory, research, and procedures* (pp. 241–285). Academic Press; Novaco, R. (1985). Anger and its therapeutic regulation. In M. Chesney & R. Rosenman (Eds.), *Anger and hostility in cardiovascular disorders* (pp. 203–226). Hemisphere Publishing; Novaco, R. (1986). Anger as a clinical and social problem. In R. Blanchard & C. Blanchard (Eds.), *Advances in the study of aggression* (Vol. 2, pp. 1–67). Academic Press; Taylor, E. (1988). Anger intervention. *American Journal of Occupational Therapy, 42*(3), 147–155.

Evidence-Based Intervention Activities: Symptoms of Anger, Frustration, and Hostility

As readers learned in Chapter 16, there are a variety of different types of groups that OTPs use during occupational therapy intervention. When applied as an intervention type, the emphasis in occupational therapy groups is on helping the client improve role performance through promotion, development, or retention of skills. Group interventions as a service delivery mode have the added benefit of offering a format where clients can establish or improve interpersonal skills, communication, and social interaction skills, which are all likely to be affected when a client experiences pathologic anger.

In 2019, the Substance Abuse and Mental Health Services Administration (SAMHSA) updated and released its publication (originally published in 2002), *Anger Management for Substance Use Disorder and Mental Health Clients: A Cognitive-Behavioral Therapy Training Manual* (28). An abundance of research findings has confirmed the reliability and efficacy of CBT in the treatment of addiction, anxiety, depression, and trauma disorders, besides even having been adapted to be applicable and effective for some psychotic disorders such as schizophrenia (28, 31, 38). There are four types of CBT that are commonly used in evidence-based interventions that target anger. These include relaxation training, cognitive interventions (interventions that target cognitive processes), communication skills interventions (such as assertiveness training or conflict resolution training), and combined intervention (which is the integration of two or more CBT intervention techniques that target multiple response variables) (28).

The treatment model presented in SAMHSA's protocol and guidelines is designed to be delivered in a group format and is described as "a combined CBT approach that employs relaxation, cognitive, and communication skills interventions. This combined approach presents group members with options that draw upon these different interventions and then encourages them to develop an individualized anger control plan using as many techniques as possible" (28, p. 1). The protocol includes a facilitation guide and curriculum that is designed to be delivered across 12 sessions. This resource is available to download for free from SAMHSA (find link included in the Suggested Resources section) and is especially valuable for new OTPs who are orienting themselves to working in behavioral or psychiatric settings.

Another evidence-supported intervention that has been shown to reduce problematic anger and aggressive behaviors that exist with conditions such as conduct disorder and PTSD is therapeutic drumming, especially when used as part of a therapeutic drumming circle (or group intervention) (17, 29). As one example, a study by a group of occupational therapists (OTs) in South Africa that incorporated therapeutic drumming with a small group of adolescent girls who had been diagnosed with conduct disorder for the purposes of determining the short-term effects of a group drumming intervention on aggression found that group drumming demonstrated promising results that support the short-term reduction of aggression symptoms (behaviors) in adolescents with conduct disorder (17). According to Dr Pamela Seraphine, the developer of neurorhythmic trauma therapy (NRTT), a specialized neurobiologically informed somatic approach for recovery from PTSD and complex trauma, "Drumming offers a comprehensive, adaptive and widely accessible method of physical and mental training that assists with self-development and. . . . improves self-regulation of an individual's cognition, emotions, and behaviors through top-down and bottom-up mechanisms" (29, pp. 5–6).

HEALTH MANAGEMENT AS AN OCCUPATION: THE BECOMING AND BELONGING DIMENSIONS

> **BOX 22.5 Focus Questions for Planning Transition, Maintenance, and Long-Term Wellness Plans**
>
> 1. How does the client define success in reaching their goals?
> 2. How can occupational therapy support the long-term success in the client becoming who they want to be, successfully doing what they want to do?
> 3. How can occupational therapy support the client's recovery and long-term success in finding community and feeling a sense of belonging and connectedness?

Health Promotion and Maintenance: Managing the Symptoms of Anger, Hostility, or Aggression

OTPs can play an important role in supporting clients in reducing occupational disruption that occurs because of frequent or intense anger, aggression, or hostility. When experiences of problematic anger are reduced and occupational participation is enhanced, the overall health of the individual is improved, including their quality of life (28). There are several recommended strategies for helping clients with problematic anger or aggressive tendencies to manage their anger following treatment, as a way to encourage their continued optimal health. Expert clinicians, researchers, and other health care professionals unanimously agree that the provision of ongoing anger management support is essential for the maintenance of appropriate anger management skills and practices, as well as for further reducing the intensity and frequency of problematic anger (1, 28). With burgeoning research related to violence prevention, another way that OTPs can advocate for the overall well-being of their clients is by promoting early intervention strategies that target aggressive behaviors and dysfunctional social skills (particularly as related to patterns of family or domestic violence, bullying, or other adverse childhood experiences) (6, 7, 15). In fact, Hisar et al found that "more anger control difficulties among anger dimensions and poor problem-solving skills in the family were identified as predictors of bullying behavior" (15, p. 62).

The impact of treating the "whole" client, in all the dimensions of occupation, and with consideration of all of their situational contexts, cannot be overstated (9, 16).

Effective Use of Occupation-Centered Outcome Measures With Symptoms of Anger, Hostility, or Aggression

The Occupational Therapy Practice Framework Domain and Process, 4th Edition (OTPF-4) (2) categorizes emotional regulation and range of emotions, as well as the appropriateness of emotions, including anger, as client factors. The OTPF-4 (2) even further classifies emotional regulation as a specific mental function. As a client factor, anger and the behavioral expressions of anger can manifest in positive ways such as encouraging problem-solving, or being a motivating factor that becomes the impetus for creating change. However, the opposite side of anger, problematic anger, and its offshoots— aggressive behaviors, hostility, and, certainly, violence—can present OTPs with some of the most challenging problems in the intervention of a person's disrupted occupations. The dual capacity of anger to impact occupation either positively or negatively demonstrates its adaptive function. Furthermore, anger is ubiquitous in psychiatric illnesses and is, according to the evidence, highly predictive of important functional outcomes (8).

Regardless of an OTP's chosen practice setting or area of specialization, all OTPs will at some point have the experience of collaborating with a client who is angry (whether or not their anger is disruptive of occupation or necessarily problematic). This chapter has highlighted some of the goals and outcomes associated with assessing, targeting, and addressing problematic anger when it interferes with the pursuit of the clients' prioritized occupations. Perhaps Dr Brené Brown (5) summarizes most eloquently the ways that anger has potential to impact (positively or negatively) occupation used as a means, or occupation used as an end (ie, occupation involved as a person is working toward a goal and the outcomes related to the achievement or lack of achievement toward goals). "Anger is a catalyst. Holding on to it will make us exhausted and sick. Internalizing anger will take away our joy and spirit; externalizing anger will make us less effective in our attempts to create change and forge connection. It's an emotion that we need to transform into something life giving: courage, love, change, compassion, justice" (5, p. 224). This seems to land right in the heart of occupational therapy's scope of practice!

Case Study

Jada: A 17-Year-Old Female With Oppositional Defiant Disorder and Posttraumatic Stress Disorder

DSM-5-TR Diagnoses at Admission

F43.10 Posttraumatic stress disorder, with delayed expression

F91.2 Oppositional defiant disorder, adolescent-onset type

Z Codes

Z55.3 Underachievement in school

Z55.4 Educational maladjustment and discord with teachers and classmates

Z65.4 Victim of crime

Z72.0 Tobacco use disorder—mild

Jada is a 17-year-old Alaskan Native female who was diagnosed with ODD, adolescent-onset type (F91.2) when she was 14 years old following repeated school truancies and suspensions from school for fighting and physical aggression toward others. More recently, 8 months ago, Jada was the victim of an attack and sexual assault by two men who have not yet been identified. Jada was attacked as she left her job at a nearby mall. In the months following the assault, Jada's problems with anger and her reactive externalizing symptoms became significantly worse, resulting in increasing problems at school and at home. Jada was subsequently diagnosed with PTSD.

A recent incident that included accusations of Jada participating in cyberbullying triggered her involvement with the juvenile mental health court system, a diversion court for juvenile offenders with mental health diagnoses, in her community. Jada's family, her school counselor, her psychiatrist, and her court-appointed mental health advocate all believe that it would be best for her to participate in an intensive inpatient stay at the local behavioral health hospital so that she could eventually reengage in school and graduate on time. Jada is argumentative and continues to resist being admitted to the inpatient rehabilitation hospital, insisting that "it would be better if I could just be home-schooled or go to virtual school to finish the rest of high school." However, her mother, who works full-time, would not be able to be available to monitor Jada and is unwilling to consider that option.

Finally, the mental health court judge explained to Jada that because of the seriousness of the cyberbullying accusation against her, a successful completion of a minimum of 6 weeks of participation in an inpatient behavioral health program was a requirement for her to be able to safely return to home or to school. Reluctantly, Jada agreed to enter the program.

The community-based behavioral health hospital where Jada will participate in her rehabilitation has a behavioral health team that includes two OTPs, an OT and an occupational therapy assistant (OTA), a licensed clinical social worker, a psychiatric nurse, a licensed mental health counselor (LMHC), a psychiatrist, and several psychologists. Upon admission, each relevant team member contributes to the initial intake information by completing screening and assessment forms containing client data pertinent to specific therapeutic findings and goals. According to Gately and Borcherding (10), "Functional problem statements in a mental health practice setting are traditionally divided into two parts. The problem itself is stated in one or two words, such as *chemical dependence, noncompliant behavior,* or *suicide risk.* The behavioral manifestations that follow define the areas of occupation and the contributing factors involved" (10, p. 284)

Listed here are excerpts of the OTP's findings from Jada's initial occupational therapy screening, evaluation, intervention planning, and goal-setting, beginning with the problems ("What is disrupting Jada's occupational participation?")

and behavioral manifestations ("What behaviors contribute to the problem that is causing occupational disruption?").

Formulating Goals by Identifying the Barriers to Occupational Participation

Problem: Anger

Behavioral Manifestations: demonstrates aggressive behaviors at school, shows little remorse for hurtful verbal and physical attacks on others, places unfounded blame on others, participated in cyberbullying of a peer (reference, juvenile mental health court documents in client file)

Problem: ineffective communication and faulty core beliefs/schema (Jada stated, "People are mean, and the world is mean.")

Behavioral Manifestations: decreased ability to complete tasks with others or in small groups; not completing assignments at school, inattention to social cues and inappropriate and disrespectful responses particularly to authority figures and her peers; demonstrates online-bullying behaviors as a defense for displaced anger and emotions

Problem: Noncompliant behaviors

Behavioral Manifestations: interference with typical age-appropriate occupational tasks (eg, without addressing these problems, Jada cannot get her driver's license, and is less likely to graduate on time from high school); dismisses or intentionally ignores or denies rules, laws, related to smoking/vaping in public places, suspended twice for vaping at school, places her at higher risk for problems with criminal justice system

Problem: increased suicide risk (secondary to being a victim of sexual assault)

Behavioral Manifestations: has reported suicidal ideation (without a plan) to both her mother and her school counselor since she was attacked. Jada stated that she "get[s] so angry all of the time about everything, because I can't do anything to change what those men did to me, and now I don't even want to be here anymore."

Jada's Long-Term Goals and Short-Term Behavioral Objectives for Occupational Therapy

LTG 1: Jada will demonstrate improved anger management skills to enhance successful participation in school-related activities within 6 weeks, or by discharge.

- *STBO 1*: Jada will identify her anger triggers through completion of an anger diary.
- *STBO 2*: Using her identified "Anger Triggers," Jada will identify five or more strategies to help her manage her anger.
- *STBO 3*: Jada will demonstrate application of a minimum of two of the anger management strategies in her activity and life skills group by discharge.
  LTG 2: To enhance her social participation, by discharge Jada will demonstrate improved coping strategies that help her regulate her emotions and improve interpersonal relationships at home, work, and at school.
- *STBO 1*: Jada will demonstrate the use of at least one grounding exercise or technique that she can safely and effectively implement to cope with her intense emotional responses, to both expected and unexpected frustrations.

- *STBO 2*: Jada will participate in at least two planned team-based community outings and activities with her peers in the life skills group, to practice identifying and implementing effective communication, using appropriate levels of assertiveness, to express her emotions and opinions, and to get her needs met.
- *STBO 3*: Jada will respond appropriately a minimum of 3 times to a peer's suggestion, comment, or constructive feedback, during group meal planning, ADL/IADL intervention group, or life skills groups.
- *STBO 4*: Following a role-play activity that focuses on assertive versus aggressive responses, Jada will reflect upon and describe what she learned from the activity during her weekly individual counseling session with the LMHC.

Please find follow-up case reflections and questions in the "OT HACKS Summary" section.

OT HACKS SUMMARY

O: **Occupation as a means and an end**

Perhaps Dr Brené Brown (5) summarizes most eloquently the ways that anger has potential to impact (positively or negatively) occupation used as a means, or occupation used as an end (ie, occupation involved as a person is working toward a goal and the outcomes related to the achievement or lack of achievement toward goals).

"Anger is a catalyst. Holding on to it will make us exhausted and sick. Internalizing anger will take away our joy and spirit; externalizing anger will make us less effective in our attempts to create change and forge connection. It's an emotion that we need to transform into something life giving: courage, love, change, compassion, justice" (5, p. 224).

T: **Theoretical concepts, values, and principles, or historical foundations**

There are a variety of models where each conceptualizes anger differently. From the cognitive behavioral and motivational models of emotion come two perspectives of anger:

1. Anger arises from a person's evaluation that a wrongdoing has occurred and the individual's subsequent desire to counteract, or "right," the wrongdoing.
2. From the motivational model comes the notion that anger can be considered an approach emotion because it is often the response triggered when a person approaches completion of a task or goal but then experiences failed attempts to reach the goal, or complete the task (8).

H: **How can we Help? OT's role in serving clients with mental illness or mental health needs**

The general approach and overarching goal is to get clients who experience disruptive anger or demonstrate aggression to talk about what is bothering them, to identify their feelings, and to help them use words or other appropriate channels to express their feelings, rather than channeling anger into hostility, aggression, or violence that will further disrupt occupational engagement.

A: Adaptations

OTPs can incorporate techniques such as cognitive restructuring, thought blocking, and cognitive reframing, all associated with CBT, into occupation-based intervention plans. CBT is the most widely researched intervention used to target affective states and traits and help clients become more aware of their anger triggers and their angry thought patterns, so that they can eventually develop new, more healthy thought patterns.

C: Case study includes

Can you answer the following questions related to Jada's case?

1. What strategies or contextual factors can you think of that would support or promote Jada's participation in more healthy occupations?
2. What strategies can the OTP use to assess Jada's strengths?
3. How can the OTP collaborate with Jada's mother?
4. Suggest ideas for incorporating occupational engagement (ie, specific activities) in Jada's life skills group. What community-based outings or projects might be appropriate for clients with similarities to Jada?
5. Discuss what factors (outside of standardized or objective measurement results) might suggest that Jada is progressing with her goals and is becoming more adequately prepared for her transition back to home and school.

What role or roles might occupational therapy potentially have in Jada's follow-up or transitional care post her discharge?

K: Knowledge: Keeping mental health OT practice grounded in evidence, in occupational science, and in research

A few key points are given here:

"Animal-assisted therapy (AAT), most frequently used with dogs, is being used increasingly as an adjunctive alternative treatment for psychiatric patients. AAT with larger animals, such as horses, may have unique benefits" (26, p. 80).

"Participants were randomly selected to receive 10 weekly group therapy sessions of standardized equine-assisted psychotherapy (EAP), canine-assisted psychotherapy (CAP), enhanced social skills psychotherapy, or regular hospital care" (26, p. 80).

"Our findings suggest that EAP may be beneficial for a broad range of psychiatric patients with extended hospitalizations" (26, p. 85).

The sample included 90 participants who were clients in a 500-bed state psychiatric hospital, all of whom had been hospitalized for a minimum of 2 months. The mean age of the participants was 44 years. The participants all had recent in-hospital violent or highly regressed behavior. Seventy-six percent had diagnoses of schizophrenia or schizoaffective disorder, and 56% had been committed involuntarily for civil or forensic reasons.

Evidence Application and Translation Questions
1. What type of study is this?
2. What level of evidence would this study be considered?
3. How do the researchers define aggressive or regressed behavior for the purposes of this study?

4. Why do the authors of this study believe that the psychiatric status of the participants (ie, high levels of psychiatric disability requiring long-term hospitalization) make this particularly important evidence to consider?
5. What do the findings suggest about the possible differences between EAP and CAP?

S: Some terms that may be new to you

Aggression: an attack on a person or object; aggression can be verbal, physical, or both.

Anger: a strong feeling of displeasure; a complex and multidimensional emotion

Assertiveness: the direct expression of feelings and desires, could be synonymous for "sticking up for oneself"

Hostility: an unfriendly and threatening attitude directed toward other people

Violence: Violence is behavior that intentionally ends with physical injuries or damage to people (the victims), places, or things (destruction of property).

Reflection Questions

1. Discuss the concepts (symptoms) of anger, hostility, aggression, and violence.
2. How does your personal context or culture mediate how you handle stress-induced anger?
3. Can you remember a time in the past, based on what you now understand about anger, when you believe that you may have demonstrated any of these responses or reactions (anger, hostility, or aggressiveness) as symptoms of anger? If you choose, discuss what you felt angry about.
4. Describe the difference between aggressive behavior and assertive behavior.
5. Create an "image only" collage using cutouts from old magazines to provide a visual representation of your personal anger triggers. This is an excellent intervention that can be applied with clients who are working on awareness of their anger triggers in everyday life. To make the collage even more "OT specific" (ie, on the basis of habits, roles, routines, and time use), divide the collage into three sections, placing visuals for "Morning Anger Triggers" "Daytime Anger Triggers" and "Nighttime Anger Triggers" in three different sections.
6. Review the findings from the Lamanna et al study in Table 22.1. Categorize the six major themes from the study: major life stressors, experience of illness, interpersonal connections with clinicians, physical confinement and behavioral restrictions, lack of engagement with clinicians, and treatment decisions into the dimension of occupation (doing, being, becoming, and belonging) that you feel the theme best represents. Be prepared to explain the rationale for your categorization.
7. What is the relationship between the occupation of sleep and anger or aggression?
8. Briefly describe and summarize the main principles of *Novaco's Affective Stress Reaction Anger Intervention Model.*

REFERENCES

1. American Occupational Therapy Association. (2020). Occupational therapy in the promotion of health and well-being. *American Journal of Occupational Therapy, 74*(3), 7403420010p1–7403420010p14.
2. American Occupational Therapy Association. (2020). Occupational therapy practice framework: Domain and process—Fourth edition. *American Journal of Occupational Therapy, 74*(Suppl. 2), 1–87.
3. American Psychiatric Association. (2022). *Diagnostic and statistical manual of mental disorders* (5th ed., text rev.). https://doi.org/10.1176/appi.books.9780890425787
4. Antonysamy, A. (2013). How can we reduce violence and aggression in psychiatric inpatient units? *BMJ Open Quality, 2*(1), 1–3.
5. Brown, B. (2021). *Atlas of the heart: Mapping meaningful connection and the language of human experience.* Random House.
6. Durham, T. A., Byllesby, B. M., Lv, X., Elhai, J. D., & Wang, L. (2018). Anger as an underlying dimension of posttraumatic stress disorder. *Psychiatry Research, 267*, 535–540.
7. Ebrahimi, T., Aslipoor, A., & Khosrojavid, M. (2019). The effect of group play therapy on aggressive behaviors and social skills in preschool children. *Quarterly Journal of Child Mental Health, 6*(2), 40–52.
8. Fernandez, E., & Johnson, S. L. (2016). Anger in Psychological disorders: Prevalence, presentation, etiology and prognostic implications. *Clinical Psychology Review, 46*, 124–135.
9. Fisher, A. G., & Marterella, A. (2019). *Powerful practice: A model for authentic occupational therapy.* Center for Innovative OT Solutions.
10. Gateley, C. A., & Borcherding, S. (2017). *Documentation manual for occupational therapy: Writing SOAP notes* (4th ed., pp. 183–196). SLACK.
11. Gibson, D. (1986). Theory and strategies for resolving conflict. *Occupational Therapy in Mental Health, 5*(4), 47–62.
12. Grogan, G. (1991). Anger management: Part 1. A perspective for occupational therapy. *Occupational Therapy in Mental Health, 11*(2–3), 135–148.
13. Grogan, G. (1991). Anger management: Part 2. Clinical applications for occupational therapy. *Occupational Therapy in Mental Health, 11*(2–3), 149–171.
14. Heller, L., & LaPierre, A. (2012). *Healing developmental trauma: How early trauma affects self-regulation, self-image, and the capacity for relationship.* North Atlantic Books.
15. Hisar, T., Kızılkurt, Ö. K., & Dilbaz, N. (2021). The effect of anger and family functions on bullying behavior in individuals with substance use disorder between the ages of 15 and 25. *Alpha Psychiatry, 22*(1), 61–66.
16. Hitch, D., Pepin, G., & Stagnitti, K. (2018). The pan occupational paradigm: Development and key concepts. *Scandinavian Journal of Occupational Therapy, 25*(1), 27–34.
17. Janse van Rensburg, E., Hatting, R., van Rooyen, C. M., Chelin, M. B., van der Merwe, C., Putter, L., Herholdt, J., van Druten, J., Taylor, M., & Buitendag, T. (2016). The short-term effect of a group drumming intervention on aggressive behaviour among adolescent girls diagnosed with conduct disorder. *South African Journal of Occupational Therapy, 46*(2), 16–22.
18. Krizan, Z., & Herlache, A. D. (2016). Sleep disruption and aggression: Implications for violence and its prevention. *Psychology of Violence, 6*(4), 542–552.
19. Lamanna, D., Ninkovic, D., Vijayaratnam, V., Balderson, K., Spivak, H., Brook, S., & Robertson, D. (2016). Aggression in psychiatric hospitalizations: A qualitative study of patient and provider perspectives. *Journal of Mental Health, 25*(6), 536–542.
20. Managing and averting anger. (2002). *Harvard Mental Health Letter, 18*(12), 6–7.
21. Manfredi, P., & Taglietti, C. (2022). A psychodynamic contribution to the understanding of anger—The importance of diagnosis before treatment. *Research in Psychotherapy (Milano), 25*(2), 587.
22. Marshall, C. A., McIntosh, E., Sohrabi, A., & Amir, A. (2020). Boredom in inpatient mental healthcare settings: A scoping review. *British Journal of Occupational Therapy, 83*(1), 41–51.
23. Novaco, R. (1979). The cognitive regulation of anger and stress. In P. Kendall & S. Hollen (Eds.), *Cognitive-behavioral interventions: Theory, research, and procedures* (pp. 241–285). Academic Press.
24. Novaco, R. (1985). Anger and its therapeutic regulation. In M. Chesney & R. Rosenman (Eds.), *Anger and hostility in cardiovascular disorders* (pp. 203–226). Hemisphere Publishing.
25. Novaco, R. (1986). Anger as a clinical and social problem. In R. Blanchard & C. Blanchard (Eds.), *Advances in the study of aggression* (Vol. 2, pp. 1–67). Academic Press.
26. Nurenberg, J. R., Schleifer, S. J., Shaffer, T. M., Yellin, M., Desai, P. J., Amin, R., Bouchard, A., & Montalvo, C. (2015). Animal-assisted therapy with chronic psychiatric inpatients: Equine-assisted psychotherapy and aggressive behavior. *Psychiatric Services, 66*(1). 80–86.
27. Pournaghash-Tehrani, S. S., Zamanian, H., & Amini-Tehrani, M. (2021). The impact of relational adverse childhood experiences on suicide outcomes during early and young adulthood. *Journal of Interpersonal Violence, 36*(17–18), 8627–8651.
28. Reilly, P. M., & Shopshire, M. S. (2019, October). *Anger management for substance use disorder and mental health clients: A cognitive–behavioral therapy manual.* SAMHSA Publication No. PEP19-02-01-001. Substance Abuse and Mental Health Services Administration.
29. Seraphine, P. L. (2019, September). Self-regulation through drumming: A brain-body model for optimizing mental health. *The Science of Psychotherapy Magazine*, 4–17.
30. Singh, N. N., Lancioni, G. E., Karazsia, B. T., Winton, A. S., Singh, J., & Wahler, R. G. (2014). Shenpa and compassionate abiding: Mindfulness-based practices for anger and aggression by individuals with schizophrenia. *International Journal of Mental Health and Addiction, 12*(2), 138–152.
31. Sokol, L., & Fox, M. G. (2019). *The comprehensive clinician's guide to cognitive behavioral therapy.* PESI Publishing.
32. Spielberger, C. D., Reheiser, E. C., & Sydeman, S. J. (1995). Measuring the experience, expression, and control of anger. *Issues in Comprehensive Pediatric Nursing, 18*(3), 207–232.
33. Stancliff, B. L. (1996). Anger: How this emotion affects your patient, you, and the rehab process. *OT Practice, 1*(8), 36–45.
34. Suh, H. W., Lee, K. B., Chung, S. Y., Park, M., Jang, B. H., & Kim, J. W. (2021). How suppressed anger can become an illness: A qualitative systematic review of the experiences and perspectives of Hwabyung patients in Korea. *Frontiers in Psychiatry, 12*, 637029.
35. Taylor, E. (1988). Anger intervention. *American Journal of Occupational Therapy, 42*(3), 147–155.
36. Taylor, R. R. (2020). *The intentional relationship: Occupational therapy and use of self* (2nd ed.). F.A. Davis.
37. Thulin, E. J., Heinze, J. E., & Zimmerman, M. A. (2021). Adolescent adverse childhood experiences and risk of adult intimate partner violence. *American Journal of Preventive Medicine, 60*(1), 80–86.
38. Wheeler, S., Davis, D., Basch, J., James, G., Lehman, B., & Acord-Vira, A. (2022). Cognitive behavioral therapy interventions for adults with traumatic brain injury (2013–2020). *American Journal of Occupational Therapy, 76*(Suppl. 2), 7613393160.
39. Wheeler, S., Davis, D., Basch, J., James, G., Lehman, B., & Acord-Vira, A. (2022). Education and skills training interventions for adults with traumatic brain injury (TBI) (Dates of review: 2013–2020). *American Journal of Occupational Therapy, 76*(Suppl. 2), 7613393120.

SUGGESTED RESOURCES

A link to the Substance Abuse and Mental Health Services Administration (SAMHSA) publication and resource guide for *Anger Management for Substance Use Disorder and Mental Health Clients: A Cognitive-Behavioral Therapy Training Manual.* https://store.samhsa.gov/sites/default/files/d7/priv/anger_management_manual_508_compliant.pdf

Articles

Lamanna, D., Ninkovic, D., Vijayaratnam, V., Balderson, K., Spivak, H., Brook, S., & Robertson, D. (2016). Aggression in psychiatric hospitalizations: A qualitative study of patient and provider perspectives. *Journal of Mental Health, 25*(6), 536–542.

The Use of Anger Scale in Clinical Practice and a Test of Its Reliability and Validity

Pan, A. W., & Chen, T. J. (2019, August). The use of anger scale in clinical practice and a test of its reliability and validity. *American Journal of Occupational Therapy, 73* (4_Suppl. 1), 7311500048p1.

Impact of Service Dogs on Family Members' Psychosocial Functioning

Bibbo, J., Rodriguez, K. E., & O'Haire, M. E. (2019). Impact of service dogs on family members' psychosocial functioning. *The American Journal of Occupational Therapy, 73*(3), 7303205120p1–7303205120p11.

Books

The Dialectical Behavior Therapy Skills Workbook by Matthew McKay, PhD, Jeffrey C. Wood, PSY.D, and Jeffrey Brantley, MD

Managing Negative Emotions: How to Deal With Anger, Anxiety, and Irritation Anywhere and Anytime, 2nd edition. By Byron Neal

Coping Skills for Teens Workbook: 60 Helpful Ways to Deal With Stress, Anxiety, and Anger by Janine Halloran, MA., LMHC & Amy Maranville (Editor)

101 Trauma-Informed Interventions: Activities, Exercises and Assignments to Move the Client and Therapy Forward By Linda Curran, BCPC, LPC, CACD, CCDP-D

Videos

Dr Pamela Seraphine is the developer of neurorhythmic trauma therapy (NRTT), a specialized neurobiologically informed somatic approach for recovery from posttraumatic stress disorder (PTSD) and complex trauma. In this interview, Dr Seraphine discusses her philosophy of drumming for trauma therapy. https://www.youtube.com/watch?v=GWvzuC-1imE&t=17s

The reader can find out more about Dr Seraphine at https://www.drpamelaseraphine.com/

Robert Whittaker is the creator of *Polar Warriors*, a YouTube channel dedicated to helping individuals, families, and friends who struggle with, or know someone living with, bipolar disorder. Whittaker is diagnosed with bipolar disorder, and his channel offers a unique consumer perspective of what the symptoms (one of which is anger associated with mania) of his illness feel like and how they can disrupt his everyday life. He also provides tools, tips, and discussions to help others better understand the experience of bipolar disorder. In this video, Whittaker shares *10 Powerful Anger Management Techniques: Help Dealing With Anger and Rage,* https://www.youtube.com/watch?v=QrJeW9381ms (~30 minutes).

Polar Warriors. (2018, May 7). *10 Powerful Anger Management Techniques: Help Dealing With Anger and Rage.* [Video]. YouTube. https://www.youtube.com/watch?v=QrJeW9381ms

When Roger Rodriguez, a flight medical technician and later a flight nurse for the U.S. Navy and the U.S. Air Force, came home from duty with posttraumatic stress disorder (PTSD), his family's dreams were shattered. In this video-based case study, titled *Pot of Gold*, Roger, his family, and his therapist explain how PTSD treatment got him back on track and made him and his family stronger. https://www.youtube.com/watch?v=rY9g_E7V8ho&t=24s

AboutFace Veterans. (2021, August 27). *Pot of Gold.* [Video]. YouTube. https://www.youtube.com/watch?v=rY9g_E7V8ho&t=24s

Websites

The International Bipolar Foundation: https://ibpf.org/

AboutFace Veterans: https://www.ptsd.va.gov/apps/AboutFace/

Learn more about PTSD from veterans who have been there. This website features excellent 1- to 3-minute video clips of veterans of all ages and their loved ones discussing what the experience of PTSD was like for them.

StopBullying.gov A federal government website managed by the U.S. Department of Health and Human Services. https://www.stopbullying.gov/

CHAPTER 23

Targeting Psychological and Social Factors That Influence Occupational Engagement: Being With the Client Who Experiences Symptoms From Substance-Related or Addictive Disorders

OT HACKS OVERVIEW

O: Occupation as a means and an end

Occupation should be used as the target (or aim) of the intervention and as the means for reaching the target.

T: Theoretical concepts, values, and principles, or historical foundations

" . . . the scientific basis for occupational therapy must come from theoretical proposals, the definition of professional roles, and scientific research" (42, p. 6).

H: How can we Help? OT's role in serving clients with mental illness or mental health needs

A person is *not* their condition, and perhaps in no other disease or disorder is that statement more pertinent to reflect upon than with substance-related and addictive disorders.

A: Adaptations

The best ways for occupational therapy to reenter and remain an indispensable part of the network of people who support clients with substance-related problems or addiction to be able to return to optimal occupational engagement in life is by . . .

Learn more in this chapter!

C: Case study includes

Ms Little is a 21-year-old African American who identifies as female. Ms Little sought treatment after the Department of Child Protective Services threatened to place her two children, a boy aged 6 and a girl aged 2, into a crisis foster home. She stated that her neighbor reported her for leaving her children alone. Ms Little and her partner recently separated and she is unemployed. She reports that she cannot make enough money working to afford her bills

and childcare. Client has consumed various substances (primarily alcohol and marijuana) since age 14. She has tried speed and diazepam (Valium) and has also, more recently used cocaine.

Read more about the case at the end of the chapter.

K: Knowledge: keeping mental health OT practice grounded in evidence, in occupational science, and in research

Read this evidence by Brown and Knowles using the following research question as a focus:

What are the sensory processing preferences of individuals recovering from addictions as measured by the *Adolescent/ Adult Sensory Profile* (17, 18)?

After reviewing the article and learning more in this chapter about how the symptoms of substance-related and addictive disorders impact occupational engagement, discuss responses to the *Evidence Application and Translation Questions* found in the "OT HACKS Chapter Summary, Knowledge" section.

S: Some terms that may be new to you

Abstinence

Addiction

Addiction medications

Opiate

Opioid

Substance use

Substance use disorder (SUD)

Withdrawal

Withdrawal management

TARGETING SYMPTOMS OF SUBSTANCE-RELATED AND ADDICTIVE DISORDERS THAT CREATE BARRIERS TO OCCUPATION: THE BEING, DOING, AND BELONGING DIMENSIONS OF OCCUPATIONAL THERAPY PRACTICE

BOX 23.1 Intervention Planning Focus Questions: How to Begin

1. What does it feel like to be a person who is experiencing **withdrawal from substance use or addiction?**
2. What are some behaviors that a person experiencing **withdrawal from substance use or addiction** might demonstrate and how might their behavior, responses, or affect be positively or negatively impacting their occupations?
3. How can I adjust my way of being (therapeutic use of self) to make the client feel more comfortable about their way of being?
4. What can I do to instill a sense of belonging in occupational therapy right now that will encourage the client toward setting goals with outcomes that are personally meaningful and relevant to them?

The general paradigm shifts toward client-centered, collaborative, and more engaged practice that has occurred across the health care landscape has also reached the treatment and care of many people whose lives have been impacted by *substance-related* and *addictive disorders*. Unfortunately, addiction continues to be a global problem and the treatment and recovery from problematic substance use is, as the reader will learn more about in this chapter, an extremely complex and challenging process. Although the challenges for people in recovery are many, the likelihood that relapses will happen are well-documented; but for people with substance-related and addictive disorders (and especially if they also have co-occurring serious mental illness [SMI]), the reward for facing that challenge (every single day . . .) is that they have a chance to regain their lives. Throughout this text, occupational therapy professionals have been encouraged to use the American Psychiatric Association's *Diagnostic and Statistical Manual of Mental Disorders, 5th Edition Text Revision (DSM-5-TR)* (7) as one among many reference tools that can be used to learn more about some of the conditions that affect people's overall health, and thus their engagement in occupation. But a person is *not* their condition, and perhaps in no other disease or disorder is that statement more pertinent to reflect upon than the category of substance-related and addictive disorders.

In a systematic review of aspects linking theoretical models, occupational therapy practice, and research findings, to the understanding of addiction and treatment provided by occupational therapy, Rojo-Mota and colleagues (42) sought to explore and answer three essential questions: Does occupational therapy have its own theoretical and conceptual framework to explain the phenomena of addiction? Does it have its own protocols focused on achievement of strictly occupational objectives? Does it provide data on the implementation of its techniques in treating people with addiction? (42). Occupational therapy has historical connections working within psychiatric settings and we have tremendous potential to provide interventions grounded in occupational science and evidence as part of a multipronged approach to the treatment of psychiatric conditions through the use of occupation and occupational outcomes. However, experts in the field highlight the need for increased evidence that focuses on *how* occupational therapy professionals are engaging with people with SUDs (and the associated behaviors). They further acknowledge the demand for expansion of empirical research that focuses on the efficacy of occupational therapy interventions with these clients, as well as the need to translate and disseminate our work (11, 42, 43, 54).

There is an urgent need for our profession to remember our historical connections and to reenter our places on health care teams that support clients who experience substance-related or addictive disorders. In 2020, there were more than 92,000 drug overdose deaths in America; this equates to a practically 30% increase over the prior year, with the fastest increases in occurring in Black and Latino populations (1, 24, 32). Of these nearly 92,000 drug overdose deaths, 75% involved an **opioid** (20). The best ways for occupational therapy to reenter and remain an indispensable part of the network of people who support a person with substance-related problems or addiction in being able to return to optimal occupational engagement in life is by "using occupation as the means and aim of the intervention according to scientific principles. . . . the scientific basis for occupational therapy must come from theoretical proposals, the definition of professional roles, and scientific research" (42, p. 2).

What Are Substance-Related and Addictive Disorders?

Substance use is a way of describing the use of psychotropic substances, including medications, alcohol, or other illegal drugs (with the exception of nicotine). *Substance use* is the preferred terminology, rather than "drug use" or "drug and alcohol use" (10). **Substance use disorder (SUD)** is characterized by a cluster of cognitive, behavioral, and physiologic symptoms indicating that the individual continues to use alcohol, nicotine, and other drugs despite significant related problems; the diagnostic criteria for SUD are designated by the *DSM-5-TR* (7, 10). As a reminder, substance use disorder appeared in the *DSM-5* series replacing substance dependence and substance abuse from the DSM-IV (10, 19).

According to the American Society of Addiction Medicine (ASAM) (8), **addiction** is "a treatable, chronic medical disease involving complex interactions among brain circuits, genetics, the environment, and an individual's life experiences. People with addiction use substances or engage in behaviors that become compulsive and often continue despite harmful consequences. Prevention efforts and treatment approaches for addiction are generally as successful as those for other chronic diseases" (9, p. 2). **Withdrawal management** is new terminology for what was once referred to as *detoxification*. Withdrawal management is the medical, psychological, and psychosocial care of individuals who are experiencing withdrawal symptoms resulting from stopping or otherwise reducing their use of substance(s). Withdrawal management is a process that includes mitigating the physiologic and psychological features of withdrawal and also interrupting the momentum of habitual and compulsive use in persons with SUD (10, 35, 60).

The ASAM's mission is to "be the physician-led professional community for those who prevent, treat, and promote remission and recovery from the disease of addiction, and to provide resources for continuing innovation, advancement, and implementation of addiction science and care" (8, "About ASAM, Our Mission"). In their role as such a leader, the ASAM has created a vast array of tools, resources, and evidence-based criteria, guidelines, and recommendations that aim to foster consistency and evidence-driven person-centered addiction care in the United States (8, 19). Both the *DSM-5-TR*, published in 2022 (7), and the ASAM (24) acknowledge the biopsychosocial nature of substance use and addiction in terms of etiology of the disease and for

determining and achieving successful assessment, intervention, and care options for these individuals.

Taking a closer look, as recommended by the ASAM's *Criteria* (35) during the holistic evaluation of an individual who is at risk for or who is experiencing problems related to substance use, six dimensions should be evaluated. This multidimensional assessment (Figure 23.1) also guides service planning and treatment across settings and levels of care (ie, the *ASAM Continuum of Care*, Figure 23.2). Referring to the ASAM *Criteria* (35) and *Six Dimensions of Multidimensional Assessment* (Figure 23.1), each dimension lays out specific aspects of what occupational therapy professionals might think of as the person's "occupational life" that should be considered in planning an effective path that leads to successful recovery. *Dimension One* assesses the client's acute intoxication and withdrawal potential by exploring their past and current experiences of substance use and withdrawal. *Dimension Two* assesses the client's biomedical conditions and complications to explore their health history and current physical health needs. *Dimension Three* assesses the person's emotional, behavioral, and cognitive conditions and complications for the purpose of exploring their mental health history and current cognitive and mental health needs. *Dimension Four* assesses the client's readiness to change and explores their preparedness for and interest in changing

AT A GLANCE: THE SIX DIMENSIONS OF MULTIDIMENSIONAL ASSESSMENT

ASAM's Criteria uses six dimensions to create a holistic, biopsychosocial assessment of an individual to be used for service planning and treatment across all services and levels of care. The six dimensions are:

DIMENSION 1
Acute Intoxication and/or Withdrawal Potential
Exploring an individual's past and current experiences of substance use and withdrawal

DIMENSION 2
Biomedical Conditions and Complications
Exploring an individual's health history and current physical health needs

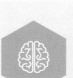

DIMENSION 3
Emotional, Behavioral, or Cognitive Conditions and Complications
Exploring an individual's mental health history and current cognitive and mental health needs

DIMENSION 4
Readiness and Change
Exploring an individual's readiness for and interest in changing

DIMENSION 5
Relapse, Continued Use or Continued Problem Potential
Exploring an individual's unique needs that influence their risk for relapse or continued use

DIMENSION 6
Recovering/Living Environment
Exploring an individual's recovery or living situation, and the people and places that can support or hinder their recovery

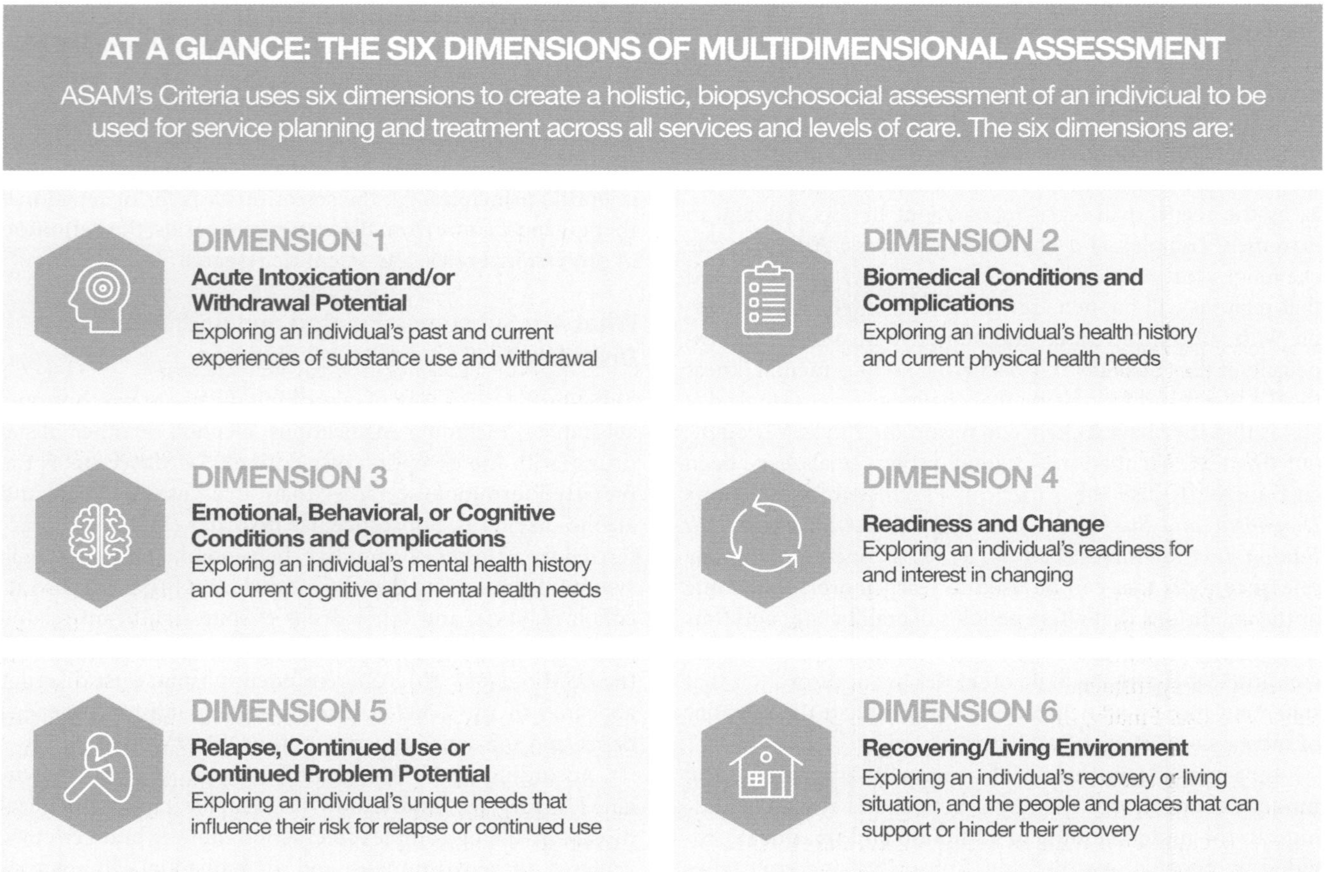

Figure 23.1. American Society of Addiction Medicine: The Six Dimensions of Multidimensional Assessment. (From https://www.asam.org/docs/default-source/quality-science/final---asam-toolkit-speaking-same-language.pdf?sfvrsn=728c5fc2_2 - page=13)

ASAM CONTINUUM OF CARE

▶ **ADULT**

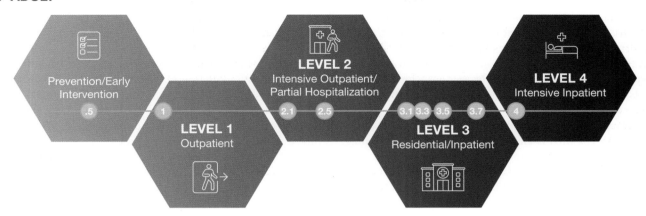

.5	Early Intervention
1	Outpatient Services
2.1	Intensive Outpatient Services
2.5	Partial Hospitalization Services
3.1	Clinically Managed Low-Intesity Residential Services

3.3	Clinically Managed Population-Specific High-Intensity Residential Services
3.5	Clinically Managed Medium-Intensity Residential Services
3.7	Medically Monitored High-Intensity Inpatient Services
4	Medically Managed Intensive Inpatient Services

▶ **ADOLESCENT**

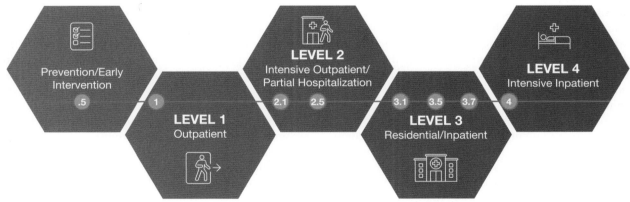

.5	Early Intervention
1	Outpatient Services
2.1	Intensive Outpatient Services
2.5	Partial Hospitalization Services

3.1	Clinically Managed Low-Intesity Residential Services
3.5	Clinically Managed Medium-Intensity Residential Services
3.7	Medically Monitored High-Intensity Inpatient Services
4	Medically Managed Intensive Inpatient Services

Figure 23.2. The American Society of Addiction Medicine (ASAM): Continuum of Care. (From https://www.asam.org/docs/default-source/quality-science/final---asam-toolkit-speaking-same-language.pdf?sfvrsn=728c5fc2_2 - page=13)

(ie, motivation level). *Dimension Five* assesses the individual's risk for relapse, continued use, or their potential for continued problems, to investigate the individual's unique needs that may influence their risk for relapse or continued substance use. Finally, in *Dimension Six*, the person's recovery/living environment should be evaluated to explore their recovery living situation and the people and places that can support or hinder their recovery (24).

For occupational therapy practitioners, the *ASAM's Six Dimensions of Assessment* (Figure 23.1) are essential to understand because the ASAM *Criteria* (35) is the most widely used set of evidence-based criteria in the United States for

the placement and assessment of individuals with problematic substance use or SUD (24). If occupational therapy professionals are to have an effective and active role in collaborating with and helping this group of clients, and we are interested in having a metaphorical seat at the table, it is imperative that we not only recognize the "items on the menu" but that we also are generally informed about why the menu items were placed on the menu and how the food is to be prepared.

Evidence is plentiful indicating the positive impact that an interdisciplinary approach can have in the treatment of SUDs and this often begins with opportunities for interprofessional education, which are increasingly frequent (53, 57). However, beyond participating in experiences of interprofessional education, it is also helpful to acquire a working knowledge of the guiding principles of the various conceptual models used to frame interventions for clients with SUD. Getting to know the targets of intervention and having a general idea of differing practices helps control for duplicated services and further encourages development of the most effective plan and course of intervention for each individual's unique needs. According to Wasmuth et al (53), there are three broad primary conceptual models of addiction, each with its own relative understanding about the etiology of addiction, which in turn dictates what is targeted during treatment planning. **Psychological models** understand addictions to primarily be a consequence of maladaptive cognitive processes and behaviors. **Neurobiologically based models**' interpretation of addiction puts forth ideas that addiction is essentially a pathologic alteration in neurochemistry and neurobiology, an outcome of chronic drug use. **Sociologic models** share some commonalities with psychological models and place focused emphasis on the individual's risk factors such as poverty, comorbid conditions, and other personal factors or social determinants of health, which then tend to interfere with sociocultural participation (53).

As the ASAM's *Six Dimensions of Multidimensional Assessment* (24) suggest and advocate, the right combination of these biopsychosocial models and approaches, when matched appropriately to the unique needs of the individual, are evidenced to support successful outcomes in the care and treatment of SUDs and substance misuse (35, 53). Nevertheless, as with many complex or chronic diseases, intervention and care for problematic substance use (addiction) is not typically a "cure." Rather, the intended outcome is for the addiction to be able to be effectively managed. Effective management of this chronic disease enables people to lessen the negative neurobiological, psychological, and sociologic impacts of the SUD so that they can regain control of their lives. Even with promising treatments and rapidly developing new understanding of the "science of addiction," relapse rates for this chronic illness are similar to the relapse rates for other chronic illnesses such as hypertension and asthma. The relapse rates for individuals with SUD can be as high as 40% to 60% of those who have been diagnosed (37).

The high relapse rates and barriers to addiction recovery services for clients with problematic substance use has prompted a significant amount of research in occupational science and occupational therapy about how to best support improved recovery from addiction, remove barriers to treatment and rehabilitation, and improve the efficacy of occupational therapy interventions with this group of clients (23, 33, 56). From an occupational therapy perspective, people are thought to be "deeply embedded in the context of their occupational life, which shape not only their surroundings but also their personal identities, values, and personal roles" (53, p. 607). This dynamic and transactional relationship between a person, their situational contexts, and occupation

(occupational engagement) means that occupation both informs, and is informed by, what the person considers as meaningful, how they respond, communicate, and relate to others and to themselves, and how their everyday life is organized and carried out (4, 21, 53).

A study by Wasmuth et al (53), for example, explored the concept of addiction-as-occupation to analyze how this concept might align with the experiences of a small group of people with addiction(s). The ongoing development of the concept (addiction-as-occupation) and the addition of several related or similar studies have provided occupational therapy professionals with some important insights regarding the potential role or roles(s) of occupational therapy with the intervention of SUDs (52–55). When addiction is viewed by the client as a primary occupation, despite the application and success of other evidence-based interventions such as the use of medication to reduce cravings (called **medication-assisted treatment**, or **MAT**) or cognitive behavioral therapy (CBT) interventions, the person may still feel the stressful void that is left when the occupation of addiction is halted or abandoned. This is known as an occupational deficit, "some of the challenges of addiction recovery align with the challenges that all individuals face when prevented from participating in primary occupations" (53, p. 607). By understanding addiction as an occupation, practitioners can support the client as they face the challenges inherent to recovery. This can be initiated by exploring from an occupational perspective how problematic substance use leads to occupational disruption, often, although not always, in recognizable stages with predictable characteristics and patterns (52).

This pattern of behavior that occurs when addiction becomes a primary occupation, continues to be verified in the literature, "The occupations to which individuals were addicted became necessary to maintain their personal identities and existence, but also contributed to much conflict and distress, leading participants into frustrating life situations where they ultimately felt little agency or freedom" (52, p. 20). But how does this happen? Of course, experience with any illness is personal and unique to the individual and their context, but when occupational disruption associated with problematic substance use occurs, a distinct pattern is typically apparent (although perhaps not necessarily until the negative impacts of the addiction become explicit). Substance use and its associated behaviors gradually begin to occupy increasing amounts of the person's time, leading to their time use and the accompanying thoughts, emotions, and behaviors being organized around the substance use. Substance use is then sustained by establishing habits, roles, and routines where substance use is the central focus.

Over time, substance use becomes a primary occupation that creates in the person a sense of self and identity associated with the substance use. Like other primary occupations, it soon becomes enmeshed and tightly woven into the fabric of the person's life, negatively impacting other dimensions of occupation. The challenges of recovery from substance use and addiction are many, but imagining addiction-as-occupation illuminates the fact that recovery requires "an entire restructuring of the individual's occupational life; it calls for opportunities to engage in new occupations geared specifically toward reshaping social lives, identities, habits, roles and routines" (52, p. 21). Table 23.1 summarizes the potential impacts and risk indicators of addiction-as-occupation on the various dimensions of occupation.

Table 23.1. The Impacts of Addiction-as-Occupation on Dimensions of Occupation

When meaningful and necessary occupations or activities are given up, or gradually replaced with activities that are important for maintaining the problematic substance use or addiction, it is important to consider these actions and behaviors as occupational risk indicators. The person is at risk for experiencing occupational disruption, occupational alienation and deprivation, and, eventually, dangerous and unhealthy occupational imbalance. Occupational risk indicators may be warnings that substance misuse is developing, has developed, or is reemerging (such as with relapse). Occupational risk indicators that are symptoms of substance-related and addictive disorders can be expressed across the occupational dimensions as aspects of doing, being, belonging, and becoming. However, it is only through collaboration with the client and evaluation of the indicators in all four dimensions that the impacts of these symptoms on a person's overall occupational function may be assessed. They can then be used to set occupation-based goals and plan and implement occupational interventions. Examples of a few occupational risk indicators in each dimension are given here.

Description of Occupational Dimension	Occupational Risk Indicators for Substance-Related and Addictive Disorders
Doing is the transaction that occurs as people engage in personally meaningful occupation. People develop the skills required for *doing* over the course of a lifespan. It is implied that *doing* also means that the client is actively engaged in occupations because they are relevant to the client; however, occupations may or may not be healthy or purposeful. *Doing* can be characterized as either overt, meaning it is observable or takes place at the physical level, or implicit as are some mental and spiritual occupations.	The risk indicators associated with the *doing* dimension are most often observable actions or behaviors that answer the following general inquiry: What kinds of things are you (the client) **doing differently** now than you have in the past (at home, at work, at school, in your free time, for fun etc)? Examples of symptoms (indicators) of substance misuse in the *doing* dimension of occupational engagement: • Raising money or making deals to obtain drugs • Demonstrations of impaired cognitive function demonstrated as poor decision-making, or lack of judgment during the performance of occupations (eg, driving while under the influence of drugs, or completing tasks at work while under the influence, placing self and others at risk) • Hiding the drugs or related paraphernalia • Stealing from others to purchase drugs • Sleeping too much or too little • Decreased or halted completion of self-care, grooming, or hygiene tasks • Decreased quality and completion of occupational tasks, particularly IADLs such as home maintenance, grocery shopping, or maintenance of finances
Being is the essence of a person. It is who they are occupationally including their unique psychological, social, spiritual, and physical capabilities. *Being* comprises the values and the significances that clients invest their time in throughout their lives. Occupation may be a central focus of *being*; however, in some ways, *being* also has a spiritual or ethereal quality, and can stand alone, independent of occupation as the client learns through self-discovery or is in reflection. "Being is expressed through consciousness, creativity and the roles people assume in life. Ideally, individuals are able to exercise agency and choice in their expression of being, but this is not always possible or even desirable." (29, p. 241)	The risk indicators associated with the *being* dimension are most often qualities and characteristics that express what is important to the client. They are unlikely to be directly observable and are equally difficult to bring into dialogue—but can often be detected by the way the person chooses to spend their time and by the roles that they fulfill and describe as being important to them. **Aspects of being help define who the person most authentically is and how they move through life.** Rather than a general inquiry question, look for expressions of creativity (or lack of opportunities to creatively express themselves), and assess the person's sense of agency (capacity to "try again" to be successful, to persevere, to be resilient, to problem-solve, to maintain self-confidence, and to push forward). Examples of symptoms (indicators) of substance misuse in the *being* dimension of occupational engagement: • Pervasive amounts of time are spent pursuing, obtaining, and using the substance • Removing barriers to their planned substance use regardless of the negative impact on valued roles (eg, canceling or being absent from typical family activities or routines) • Missing school or work obligations secondary to recovering from the effects of substance use • Expressing a sense of worthlessness or lack of purpose • Expressing a loss of the sense of self or personal agency, eg, "I don't know who I am any more . . . "; "I can't go on like this"; "I don't know what I want"; "I can't do this anymore"; "I have let everyone down"; "I always mess things up." All these statements express both a struggle with the person's way of being in the world as a person who is addicted and are *clear* indications of **suicidal ideation**. Hearing the depth of a client's expressions is a professional responsibility of all health care professionals (2). **If a client's revelations remotely indicate the threat of self-harm, ask them more questions, stay with them if possible, and connect them to suicide prevention resources.**

(continued)

Table 23.1. The Impacts of Addiction-as-Occupation on Dimensions of Occupation (*continued*)

Description of Occupational Dimension	Occupational Risk Indicators for Substance-Related and Addictive Disorders
Belonging is a feeling of being in relationship, or connected to others and is characterized by who (or what) a person is with, and by the interactions and impacts that we have on one another. All of these connections are inextricably embedded in situational context and occupational engagement, which in turn, helps shape a sense of belonging. Hitch et al (29) concluded that "A sense of reciprocity, mutuality, and sharing characterize belonging relationships, whether they are positive or negative." (p. 241)	The risk indicators associated with the *belonging* dimension are associated with the human need to feel connected to others and to experience feelings of acceptance and inclusion. They answer the following general inquiry: Where and with whom do I (the client) feel **safe** or **at peace** and **experience a sense of fitting in**? Examples of symptoms (indicators) of substance misuse in the *belonging* dimension: • Seeking persons with whom to participate in drug-related activities, often while rejecting time with loved ones • Ignoring or disengaging from healthy relationships with people who object to drug use and its associated behaviors • Identifying with a person or group of people whose primary commonality is substance use
Becoming is aspirational goal-directed growth and development. *Becoming* is a process. *Becoming* means that human beings are ever evolving. This implies that changes occur constantly, and for different reasons, over the course of a lifetime. For example, a couple who have recently adopted a child are constantly *becoming* parents as they experience the joys and challenges inherent in the endeavor of parenting. "Regular modifications and revisions of goals and aspirations help to maintain momentum in becoming, as does the opportunity to experience new or novel situations and challenges." (29, p. 242)	The risk indicators associated with the *becoming* dimension are associated with goal-directed movement and adaptive functioning that allows for positive change and flexibility, even in the face of challenges. The *becoming* dimension supports growth and encourages occupational balance and optimal engagement in one's prioritized occupations. It answers the following general inquiries: What does it mean for you to "get better"? How does "getting better" look and feel? What do you want to put in your past that will help you move forward? Examples of symptoms (indicators) of substance misuse in the *becoming* dimension: • Organizing one's daily occupations around drug seeking and drug use • Creating contexts and situations that will enable or support drug use

IADLs, instrumental activities of daily living. Adapted from Blank, A., Finlay, L., & Prior, S. (2016). The lived experience of people with mental health and substance misuse problems: Dimensions of belonging. *British Journal of Occupational Therapy, 79*(7), 434–441; Fisher, A. G., & Marterella, A. (2019). *Powerful practice: A model for authentic occupational therapy.* Center for Innovative OT Solutions; Hitch, D., Pepin, G., & Stagnitti, K. (2014). In the footsteps of Wilcock, Part One: The evolution of doing, being, becoming and belonging. *Occupational Therapy in Health Care, 28*(3), 231–246.

Diagnoses Often Comorbid With Substance Use Disorders

The *2021 National Survey on Drug Use and Health* (45, 48) from the Substance Abuse and Mental Health Services Administration (SAMHSA) estimates that approximately 9.2 million adults in the United States have a **co-occurring disorder**. The term *co-occurring disorder* is used almost exclusively to mean that a person experiences coexistence of both a mental disorder and an SUD, including any combination of two or more SUDs and mental disorders as identified in the *DSM-5-TR* (7, 36, 49). Still, because language matters, it is important to be able to identify and distinguish between three terms that are frequently used interchangeably, but that have subtle differences: **co-occurring disorder** (described earlier) is synonymous with the term **dual diagnosis**. Both dual diagnosis and co-occurring disorder(s) (which is the preferred and currently recommended terminology according to SAMHSA) refer to a person experiencing two or more conditions at the same time, that coexist as distinct, independent, and separate diagnoses, rather than one of the diagnoses causing a cluster of symptoms. The terms **comorbid condition** or **comorbid disorder** differ slightly in meaning because they describe conditions (or diagnoses) that can

exist either simultaneously or describe that the onset of one of the conditions precedes or follows the other(s) (41).

People with psychiatric illness are more likely to have a co-occurring SUD, but the opposite is also true, people with substance-related or addictive disorders have increased likelihood of experiencing psychiatric illnesses (36, 49). Considering that substance-related and addictive disorders have few boundaries in terms of who they impact, occurring across the lines of socioeconomic status, culture, and age, occupational therapy professionals are increasingly likely to collaborate with clients whose occupations and occupational identity have been disrupted by substance-related or addictive disorders. This is true whether or not they co-occur with other psychiatric illnesses and regardless of the practice area or setting.

Although all people are susceptible to developing or experiencing a substance-related or addictive disorder, people with SMI are particularly vulnerable to co-occurring SUDs. SMI is defined (in the United States) as a person experiencing, at any time during the preceding year, a diagnosable mental, behavioral, or emotional disorder that causes serious functional impairment that significantly interferes with or limits one or more major life activities (36). The SAMHSA identifies some of the psychiatric disorders that commonly co-occur with SUDs as the following: anxiety disorders; schizophrenia spectrum and other psychotic disorders; bipolar and related disorders; depressive disorders (specifically, major depressive disorder); disruptive, impulse control, and conduct disorders; trauma- and stressor-related disorders (specifically posttraumatic stress disorder [PTSD]); and attention deficit hyperactivity disorder (46, 49). Other research, including contributions from occupational therapy and occupational science, confirm the high prevalence of co-occurring SUD with many of these conditions, thus reinforcing the demand to ensure holistic, person-centered, and evidence-informed occupational therapy evaluations and interventions. In one recent literature review exploring occupational interventions, for example, the authors noted, "The frequency with which the BDI [Beck Depression Inventory] appeared as an outcome measure may be a reflection of high rates of comorbidity between addictive disorders and depression. For instance, studies suggest that nearly one third of persons with major depressive disorder also have a substance use disorder" (54, p. 7).

Strategies for Therapeutic Use of Self

As much of researcher Dr Brené Brown's work confirms, human beings seem to be hardwired for connection with others (15, 16). One aspect of the occupational dimension of belonging, as described in occupational science and occupational therapy literature, is the human need for connection to others, which most agree is intimately associated with people's desire for acceptance and belonging. From an occupational perspective, belonging is understood as the interpersonal connections between people as they engage in occupations (14, 28, 30, 51, 58). Hitch et al (29) concluded that "A sense of reciprocity, mutuality, and sharing characterize belonging relationships, whether they are positive or negative" (29, p. 241).

Much of the evidence available in the literature points to the critical importance of social connections and participation for successful recovery from SUDs and for prevention of relapse (54). For example, Wasmuth and colleagues found in a systematic review of occupation-based intervention for addictive disorders that although the *Beck Depression Inventory II* (BDI-II) (13) and the *Addiction Severity Index* (ASI) (34) detected effect sizes of social participation interventions to be poor, "all social participation interventions found significant between group differences favoring social participation over the control or comparison group" (54, p. 7). This suggests that one of the most valuable contributions of occupational therapy interventions when collaborating with these clients may be helping the client to identify and build performance skills that support more positive and satisfying social connections. Moreover, the distinguishing characteristic of successful occupational therapy social participation interventions is ensuring that those skills are built and practiced in ecologically relevant real-life situations and contexts (ie, occupational performance in authentic occupations, with clear occupation-based goals and outcomes) (21, 52, 54).

DOING AND BECOMING DIMENSIONS: SUBSTANCE-RELATED AND ADDICTIVE DISORDERS, AND WITHDRAWAL MANAGEMENT

> **BOX 23.2 Intervention Implementation Focus Questions: How to Support Clients' Optimal Engagement in Occupation**
>
> 1. What can the client and the occupational therapy team collaboratively do together that will help the client become more functional and effective in the things that are important to them in everyday life?
> 2. What are the best intervention types and intervention approaches to apply in this therapeutic context?
> 3. What does the current evidence suggest about the most productive interventions for this diagnosis/set of symptoms?

Evidence-Based Practice: Characteristics of Intervention for Substance-Related and Addictive Disorders

With at least 25% of people who live with SMI experiencing a co-occurring SUD, the question of when or where (ie, which area of occupational therapy practice, or which setting) the occupational therapy professional will collaborate with these clients, becomes a mute-point . . . it is only a matter of time. The far more important questions become, "How does the occupational therapy professional best approach collaboration with **this** client, with **this** set of occupational circumstances?" More importantly, "What are the most efficacious ways to support this person's return to their occupational priorities?" On the basis of an overarching review of recent evidence, comprehensive support is noted for acknowledgment that for individuals in recovery, and for those who are facing withdrawal from addiction and moving toward recovery, "Didactic interventions—interventions that involve skills training or some other element of [psychoeducational approach or direct] instruction—may be helpful for learning new strategies to use in addiction recovery, but evidence suggests that putting newly learned skills into practice [in realistic life contexts] is a challenge for this population" (54, p. 3).

On the other hand, occupation-based interventions encourage real-time application of the newly acquired skills while the client is challenged to respond to contextually relevant life situations. Meeting and progressing through challenges as they actually occur in the clients' natural environments (when possible) gives the person an opportunity to put into action newly learned skills (the doing dimension of occupation and the becoming dimension of occupation), which then provides the client with experiences of mastery. This occupationally relevant practice challenges and bolsters a sense of self-efficacy, self-confidence, and self-esteem, as well as a sense of agency within the client (all of these associated with the being dimension of occupation).

Intervention-focused research continues to inform the way that substance-related and addictive disorders are most effectively approached, and providing these clients with a pathway toward reengaging in their occupational life remains the overall goal of occupational therapy intervention. Occupational therapy professionals must rise to the challenge of advocating for the incorporation of occupation-based approaches. Overwhelming amounts of diverse interdisciplinary research and evidence suggest that the most efficacious treatment plans for successful long-term outcomes for people who experience substance-related and addictive disorders involve a well-planned and well-articulated care plan that should include both valid and reliable occupational therapy assessments and interventions tailored to the individual's specific needs. A brief introduction and discussion of several evidence-based strategies and approaches that have been shown to be effective for clients with substance use and addiction problems follows. Bear in mind that these approaches and strategies are not inherently occupationally focused. The occupational therapy professional must consistently be mindful of integrating evidence-based strategies and approaches into occupational therapy interventions by embedding them in occupation. The vehicle for doing that is to utilize occupation as a means, or occupation as an end.

Interventions from the cognitive behavioral theoretical continuum are well researched and show positive and reliable results with this population, particularly as part of a comprehensive plan that may include MAT (generally prescribed by the psychiatrist). Furthermore, intervention plans that integrate behavioral components have demonstrated success in treating specific conditions that often co-occur with SUDs (27, 44, 49). CBT is intended to help the individual adjust harmful or untrue beliefs and self-talk, often referred to as automatic thoughts, which result in maladaptive behaviors. CBT is widely used by occupational therapy professionals who work in mental health settings. Further, the literature shows strong efficacy for applying CBT with individuals with SUDs. In addition, CBT is considered the most effective approach when working with children and adolescents who experience anxiety and mood disorders (38, 44).

Dialectical behavior therapy or DBT was originally designed specifically for reducing self-harm behaviors such as suicidal ideation, suicide attempts or urges, cutting, and drug use that were common in borderline personality disorder. DBT teaches the individual distress tolerance, a way to notice distressing feelings and thoughts, but not to act on them. Although DBT is still one of the few treatments that is effective for individuals who meet the criteria for borderline personality disorder, it has now been researched and found to be effective with several other psychiatric diagnoses (38–40). Assertive Community Treatment (ACT) programs apply principles of behavioral treatment to SMIs such as schizophrenia and bipolar disorder, as well as using it with co-occurring substance use. ACT was briefly introduced and discussed in earlier chapters of the text and is characterized by things that separate this intervention from other approaches to case management. First, ACT is highly individualized. The clients' overall health and daily life is managed using a team-based approach (typically comprising a multidisciplinary team), with teams who have smaller caseloads, making contact with each client more robust (38).

CBT, DBT, and ACT are all primarily individualized approaches (focused on one client), whereas the following approaches and strategies incorporate small groups as a primary element of the intervention. Therapeutic communities (TCs) are a common form of long-term residential treatment for people who are diagnosed with, or struggle with, SUDs. They focus on the "resocialization" of the individual, often using broad-based community programs as active components of treatment. TCs are appropriate for populations with a high prevalence of co-occurring disorders and for individuals who are involved with the criminal justice system, individuals who are homeless, and other vulnerable populations such as adolescents who are runaways (47, 50).

Integrated group therapy (IGT) is a treatment developed specifically for people with co-occurring bipolar disorder and SUD. IGT is aimed at addressing problems that are common to both these specific disorders. IGT is most indicated in combination with MAT. Lastly, contingency management (CM) or motivational incentives (MI) are intervention strategies that can be combined with or added to other treatment modalities. What is sometimes referred to as a token economy, or voucher system, is put into place to reward patients who practice healthy behaviors and reduce unhealthy behaviors, including refraining from smoking and drug use. Incentive-based treatments have been found to be effective for improving treatment compliance and reducing the use of tobacco and other unhealthy drugs (37, 38).

HEALTH MANAGEMENT AS AN OCCUPATION: THE BECOMING AND BELONGING DIMENSIONS AND RECOVERY

> **BOX 23.3 Focus Questions for Planning Transition, Maintenance, and Long-Term Wellness Plans**
>
> 1. How does the client define success in reaching their goals?
> 2. How can occupational therapy support the long-term success in the client becoming who they want to be, successfully doing what they want to do?
> 3. How can occupational therapy support the client's recovery and long-term success in finding community, and feeling a sense of belonging and connectedness?

Health Promotion and Symptom Management: From Prevention to Recovery

Health promotion always begins with prevention (3). According to the World Health Organization (WHO), every 10 seconds a person dies from alcohol-related causes (59). This alarming statistic was one of the factors that prompted the SAFER Initiative. SAFER is an acronym for the top five most cost-effective interventions to reduce alcohol-related harm (59).

1. **S**trengthen restrictions on alcohol availability.
2. **A**dvance and enforce drinking and driving counter measures.
3. **F**acilitate access to screening, brief interventions, rehabilitation, and treatment.
4. **E**nforce bans or comprehensive restrictions on alcohol advertising, sponsorship, and promotion.
5. **R**aise prices on alcohol through excise taxes and pricing policies.

Global public health campaigns such as the SAFER Initiative often drive change on a larger scale. Sometimes global crises or public health emergencies also propel action. Such was the case when the COVID-19 pandemic occurred. Although we will not know the long-term effects on people's mental and physical health for many years, the pandemic was the primary impetus for the now widely used availability of telehealth services, including telehealth services for the treatment of psychiatric disorders (12, 25, 31).

One way for occupational therapy professionals to facilitate our clients' ongoing health and recovery from SUDs so that we can impact changes and advocate for health promoting occupations on a smaller scale is to have a working knowledge of best practices in addiction to screening, brief interventions, rehabilitation, and treatment resources (5). The availability of resources to help prevent relapses and support maintaining and managing recovery are gradually improving and increasing. For example, a mobile medical application was approved by the U.S. Food and Drug Administration (FDA) in 2017 and was introduced as the first mobile medical application to help treat SUDs (22). The intention is for the client to use it with outpatient therapy to treat alcohol, cocaine, marijuana, and stimulant use disorders (although it is not effective in the treatment of opioid addiction). The mobile medication application device delivers CBT to patients to teach and encourage building skills that benefit the treatment of SUDs. The secondary objective of the mobile medical application was targeting adherence to outpatient therapy, or therapeutic groups, to improve attendance and retention in rehabilitation and recovery programs.

Researchers Ryan and Boland, in a scoping review of occupational therapy interventions applied with people with SUDs, found that "Occupational therapy appears to be a good fit within most addiction treatment settings . . . occupational therapy interventions are most supportive when intervention goes beyond the teaching of skills, to prioritise occupational engagement" (43, p. 110). This again reinforces the importance of using occupational therapy interventions that focus on the dimensions of occupation, rather than on specific client factors. This is the unique contribution of occupational therapy (21, 28, 30, 58).

Summary

Now we return to where we began this final chapter of the text. It is a fitting place to conclude both the chapter and the text because the questions that Rojo-Mota and colleagues

(42) pondered in their systematic review of the literature surrounding the role of occupational therapy and occupational science in the treatment of addiction are perhaps the quintessential questions that should be the focus of occupational therapy's role across *all* illnesses (42). Rojo-Mota et al sought to find answers to the following three questions:

1. Does occupational therapy have its own theoretical and conceptual framework to explain the phenomena of addiction?
2. Does it have its own protocols focused on achievement of strictly occupational objectives?
3. Does it provide data on the implementation of its techniques in treating people with any problem, diagnosis, or disability? (42)

The relevance of continuing to explore answers to these questions may be even more significant for occupational therapy professionals who aspire to work in psychiatric or behavioral health settings. In the face of a national and international crisis related to substance-related disorders, ranging from the opioid addiction crisis to the current alarming misuse of fentanyl that has caused tragic death and loss for too many (26), occupational therapy professionals have a professional and ethical responsibility to clarify and advocate for the distinct benefits and unique roles that occupational therapy can play in supporting clients through these and other illnesses (2, 6).

Case Study

Ms Little: A 21-Year-Old Female With Multiple Substance Use Disorders, Bulimia, and Borderline Personality Disorder

DSM-5-TR Diagnosis at Admission

F14.20	Cocaine use disorder (severe)
F50.2	Bulimia nervosa
F60.3	Borderline personality disorder
F12.11	Cannabis use disorder (in early remission)
F15.10	Amphetamine-type substance use disorder (mild)
F10.11	Alcohol use disorder (in early remission)

Z Codes

Z56.0	Unemployment
Z59.6	Low income
Z69.011	Encounter for mental health services for perpetrator of parental child neglect
Z72.9	Problem related to lifestyle

Ms Little is a 21-year-old African American who identifies as female. Ms Little sought treatment after the Department of Child Protective Services threatened to place her two children, a boy aged 6 and a girl aged 2, into a crisis foster home. She stated that her neighbor reported her for leaving her children alone. Ms Little and her partner recently separated and she is unemployed. She reports that she cannot make enough money working to afford her bills and childcare. Client has consumed various substances (primarily alcohol and marijuana) since age 14. She has tried speed and diazepam (Valium), and has also, more recently, used cocaine.

Occupational Profile Data Collection Interview and Evaluation

Client reports that she has used crack for the past 9 months and denies the use of any other substances except an "occasional drink." Client admitted to selling her food stamps to obtain money. She was never married and does not receive financial support from the fathers of her children. Ms Little was observed purging food in the bathroom of the care unit and has admitted to episodic purging "to control weight."

Ms Little described herself as a good student in high school until her drug use became more important than studying. She has a high school diploma but did not attempt any postsecondary education, as she felt she could not afford it. Client's parents both drank and were physically abusive to one another. Ms Little denies physical or sexual abuse of self or siblings by parents. Client reported she cooks, cleans, and takes care of all household management independently. She stated she has been "out of control" since she began using crack 9 months ago, smoking "hundreds of dollars-worth 1 to 2 days per week at friends' homes or crack houses." She admitted to leaving the children alone twice over the past month and expressed great distress that she would do such a thing. She also admitted to having slept with crack dealers to obtain drugs. Client stated that she knows she has to get clean or she will lose her children. She has never obtained a driver's license but does have a car of her mother's that she drives. She has no friends except other users, and other than drug use, her only leisure activity is watching movies with her kids. Ms Little stated that she feels depressed much of the time and has no energy.

Goals, objectives, and interventions are shown in the treatment summary for this case (Table 23.2).

Occupational Therapy Discharge Summary (3 Weeks After Admission)

Ms Little has been inconsistent with treatment recommendations throughout the 3 weeks. She argued that she didn't need a driver's license but became willing to apply for one after this issue was addressed repeatedly by occupational therapy

professional and other members of the treatment team. Client and occupational therapist collaborated to create a schedule for specific study times, and she obtained her license 18 days after admission. She expressed pride at this accomplishment.

Client initially refused to identify leisure activities for herself but after several community out-trips, began to identify enjoyable leisure interests such as putt-putt golf, swimming, movies, hiking, and eating out. Client selected as family interests board games, making cookies, and going to parks and *Chick-Fil-A*. She met with the vocational rehabilitation counselor and completed the application. Occupational therapy assistant (OTA) sent all records to the counselor, who has confirmed that client is eligible for assistance and employability skills training. One of her sisters has committed to keeping her children for her so that she can attend school when the time comes. Client appeared enthusiastic and stated that an opportunity for education and job preparation gives her hope. She identified a list of job interests and strengths, which was communicated to the counselor.

A goal to increase assertive behavior was added to the intervention plan after client described how much difficulty she has saying "no" to peers. She role-played situations, was initially too aggressive, but, after practice, was able to express herself calmly but firmly. She introduced herself to other women at 12-step meetings and spent time with two women volunteer alumnae who shared their recovery experiences with her.

Client participated in the exercise program only after much encouragement from staff. Treatment team and occupational therapy professional met with her several times to emphasize the importance of her following directions and increasing exercise participation. This client will continue to meet with the occupational therapy team twice a week to work on incorporating leisure into her routine to improve occupational balance, to continue to improve assertiveness, as well as to ensure exercise adherence for wellness management and stress relief.

Please find follow-up case reflections and questions in the "OT HACKS Summary" section.

Table 23.2. Occupational Therapy Intervention Summary

Goals	Objectives	Occupational Therapy Intervention Given
1. To obtain a driver's license	1. Client will spend 1 h a day studying driver's manual and take her driver's test before discharge.	1. Individual occupational therapy as needed
2. Reestablish healthy lifestyle choices, habits, patterns (reduction of destructive habits)	2a. Client will identify for pursuit after discharge five leisure activities appropriate for a sober lifestyle (by 2 wk) 2b. Client will introduce herself to at least two women per night at 12-step meetings. 2c. Client will identify at least five healthy activities to pursue with children at home or in the community (by 2 wk).	2a. Leisure education 1 × wk; community out-trip 1 × week 2b. Nightly 12-step meeting; leisure education assignment 2c. Leisure education 1 × wk; community out-trip 1 × wk
3. To obtain job, educational training	3a. Client will meet with vocational rehabilitation counselor (by 1 wk) 3b. Client will identify job and educational training interests (by 1 wk)	3a. Occupational therapy referral to vocational rehabilitation 3b. Individual occupational therapy sessions
4. To improve energy level and overall health, and decrease cravings for substance(s)	4a. Client will complete exercise assessment (by 3 d). 4b. Client will participate in daily exercise program for 20 min initially (by 4 d, increasing to 45 min by 2 wk).	4a. Individual occupational therapy assessment 4b. Daily structured exercise program

OT HACKS SUMMARY

O: Occupation as a means and an end

The approaches and strategies that are commonly applied in psychiatric or behavioral health settings are not inherently occupationally focused. The occupational therapy professional must consistently be mindful of integrating evidence-based strategies and approaches into occupational therapy interventions by embedding them in occupation.

The vehicle for doing that is to utilize occupation as a means or occupation as an end.

T: Theoretical concepts, values, and principles, or historical foundations

There are three broad primary conceptual models of addiction, each with differing assumptions of the origin of the addiction:

Psychological models understand addictions to primarily be a consequence of maladaptive cognitive processes and behaviors.

Neurobiologically based models' interpretation of addiction puts forth ideas that addiction is essentially a pathologic alteration in neurochemistry and neurobiology, an outcome of chronic drug use.

Sociologic models share some commonalities with psychological models and place focused emphasis on the individual's risk factors (eg, poverty, comorbid conditions, and other personal factors or social determinants of health), which then tend to interfere with sociocultural participation (53).

H: How can we Help? OT's role in serving clients with mental illness or mental health needs

By understanding addiction as an occupation, practitioners can support the client as they face the challenges inherent to recovery. This can be initiated by exploring from an occupational perspective how problematic substance use leads to occupational disruption, often, although not always, in recognizable stages, with predictable characteristics and patterns (52).

A: Adaptations

- Recovery from substance-related and addictive disorders requires an entire restructuring of the individual's occupational life.
- Opportunities to engage in new occupations in ecologically relevant contexts that are geared specifically toward reshaping social lives, identities, habits, and roles and routines, will be required. Planning, designing, providing, and supporting these opportunities is the unique contribution of the occupational therapy professional.

C: Case study includes

Can you answer the following questions related to Ms Little's case?

1. What are this client's occupational roles now? What occupational roles might this client acquire for the future? What are her occupational performance strengths? In what areas does she have difficulty?

2. In Table 23.2, the occupational therapy intervention is stated in general terms. Describe in detail the methods and approaches that you believe will be most helpful to the client.

3. What additional community supports or aftercare strategies would be helpful for this client?

K: Knowledge: keeping mental health OT practice grounded in evidence, in occupational science, and in research

A few key points are given here:

"People with psychiatric conditions often experience sensations differently. . . ." (18, para. 1).

"The findings indicate that people in recovery for addiction tend towards a sensation avoiding preference" (18, para. 5).

The study included only 31 participants; 30 males and 1 female. Of these, 82% were Caucasian, 6% were African American, 9% were Latino, and one participant did not report race. The mean age of the participants was 31.7. The large majority (28 of the participants) reported using multiple substances, with only 3 participants reporting use of a single substance.

Evidence Application and Translation Questions

1. This study is reported as a descriptive study. How do descriptive studies such as this inform occupational therapy practice?

2. Where might a study like this be ranked in the levels of evidence?

3. Besides characterizing the drug use of the participants in the sample, what else could be learned by including the Drug History Questionnaire along with the Adolescent/Adult Sensory Profile (17)?

4. The authors of the study discuss the need for sensory-informed interventions. How might the conclusion in this descriptive study inform intervention planning?

S: Some terms that may be new to you

Abstinence: Intentional and consistent restraint from the pathologic pursuit of reward and/or relief that involves the use of substances and other behaviors. These behaviors may involve, but are not necessarily limited to, substance use, gambling, video gaming, or compulsive sexual behaviors. Use of FDA-approved medications for the treatment of SUD is consistent with abstinence (10).

Addiction: Addiction is a treatable, chronic medical disease involving complex interactions among brain circuits, genetics, the environment, and an individual's life experiences. People with addiction use substances or engage in behaviors that become compulsive and often continue despite harmful consequences (9).

Addiction medications: Medications specifically indicated for and prescribed to treat SUDs (eg, buprenorphine for opioid use disorder, varenicline for tobacco use disorder), both as an initial lifesaving and motivational engagement strategy (ie, withdrawal management) as well as part of a long-term treatment plan similar to other chronic diseases such as bipolar disorder or diabetes (9).

Opiate: Opiate refers to opioids derived from the naturally occurring alkaloid compounds produced in the opium poppy, *Papaver somniferum*, and includes morphine, codeine, and thebaine (9).

Opioid: Opioid is a term that designates all compounds, natural and synthetic, exogenous and endogenous, that bind to and activate any of the opioid receptors (9).

Substance use: Used instead of "drug use" or "drug and alcohol use," this term refers to the use of psychotropic substances, which may include illegal drugs, medications, or alcohol (with the exception of nicotine). This does not refer to nicotine (10).

Substance use disorder (SUD): It is marked by a cluster of cognitive, behavioral, and physiologic symptoms indicating that the individual continues to use alcohol, nicotine, and other drugs despite significant related problems. Diagnostic criteria are given in the *DSM-5-TR* (7, 10).

Withdrawal: symptoms resulting from stopping or otherwise reducing use of substance(s) such as caffeine, nicotine, alcohol, medications, or other psychotropic drugs (10)

Withdrawal management: This is the medical, psychological, and psychosocial care of individuals who are experiencing withdrawal symptoms resulting from stopping or otherwise reducing their use of substance(s). The process includes mitigating the physiologic and psychological features of withdrawal and also interrupting the momentum of habitual and compulsive use in persons with SUD; withdrawal management was once referred to as *detoxification* (10, 35, 60).

Reflection Questions

1. Write a definition for SUD using only occupational science or occupational therapy terminology.
2. Describe *withdrawal management*. What are some of its essential features?
3. Explain the significance of the ASAM's *Six Dimensions of Multidimensional Assessment*.
4. Evaluate this metaphor:
   "If occupational therapists are to have an effective and active role in collaborating with and helping this group of clients, and we are interested in having a metaphorical seat at the table, it is imperative that we not only recognize the 'items on the menu,' but that we also are generally informed about why the menu items were placed on the menu, and how the food is to be prepared."
   What is your interpretation of its meaning?
5. Compare and contrast the ASAM's *Continuum of Care* (see Figure 23.2) for an adult who experiences substance-related or addictive disorders, with the continuum of care for adolescents.
   a. How do you think the role(s) of an occupational therapy professional would be similar, and/or different, with regard to collaborating with an interdisciplinary team and client within the adolescent, versus the adult, continuum?
   b. Do you think that occupational therapy professionals have more potential roles in one or the other continuums of care?

6. Evaluate and articulate the relationship between occupational risk indicators for substance-related and addictive disorders and the aspects of the dimensions of occupation: doing, being, belonging, and becoming.
7. Does reflecting upon addiction-as-occupation shape how you understand or perceive problematic substance use? Why or why not?

REFERENCES

1. Ahmad, F. B., Cisewski, J. A., Rossen, L. M., & Sutton, P. (2023). *Provisional drug overdose death counts*. National Center for Health Statistics. Designed by L. M. Rossen, A. Lipphardt, F. B. Ahmad, J. M. Keralis, & Y. Chong. https://www.cdc.gov/nchs/nvss/vsrr/drug-overdose-data.htm
2. American Occupational Therapy Association. (2020). AOTA 2020 occupational therapy code of ethics. *American Journal of Occupational Therapy, 74*(Suppl. 3), 7413410005.
3. American Occupational Therapy Association. (2020). Occupational therapy in the promotion of health and well-being. *American Journal of Occupational Therapy, 74*(3), 7403420010.
4. American Occupational Therapy Association. (2020). Occupational therapy practice framework: Domain and process—Fourth edition. *American Journal of Occupational Therapy, 74*(Suppl. 2), 1–87.
5. American Occupational Therapy Association. (2021). Occupational therapy scope of practice. *American Journal of Occupational Therapy, 75*(Suppl. 3), 7513410030.
6. American Occupational Therapy Association. (2021). Standards of practice for occupational therapy. *American Journal of Occupational Therapy, 75*(Suppl. 3), 7513410050.
7. American Psychiatric Association. (2022). *Diagnostic and statistical manual of mental disorders* (5th ed., text rev.). https://doi.org/10.1176/appi.books.9780890425787
8. American Society of Addiction Medicine. (n.d.). *About ASAM 2022–2025 strategic plan*. https://www.asam.org/about-us/about-asam/strategic-plan
9. American Society of Addiction Medicine. (2019). *Definition of addiction*. https://www.asam.org/docs/default-source/quality-science/asam's-2019-definition-of-addiction-(1).pdf?sfvrsn=b8b64fc2_2
10. American Society of Addiction Medicine. (2020). *The ASAM clinical practice guidelines on alcohol withdrawal management*. https://sitefinitystorage.blob.core.windows.net/sitefinity-production-blobs/docs/default-source/quality-science/the_asam_clinical_practice_guideline_on_alcohol-1.pdf?sfvrsn=ba255c2_0
11. Amorelli, C. (2016). Psychosocial occupational therapy interventions for substance-use disorders: A narrative review. *Occupational Therapy in Mental Health, 32*(2), 167–184.
12. Arafat, M. Y., Zaman, S., & Hawlader, M. D. H. (2021). Telemedicine improves mental health in COVID-19 pandemic. *Journal of Global Health, 11*, 03004.
13. Beck, A. T., Steer, R. A., & Brown, G. K. (1996). BDI-II, *Beck Depression Inventory: Manual* (2nd ed.). Boston: Harcourt Brace.
14. Blank, A., Finlay, L., & Prior, S. (2016). The lived experience of people with mental health and substance misuse problems: Dimensions of belonging. *British Journal of Occupational Therapy, 79*(7), 434–441.
15. Brown, B. (2012). *Daring greatly*. Penguin.
16. Brown, B. (2021). *Atlas of the heart: Mapping meaningful connection and the language of human experience*. Random House.
17. Brown, C., & Dunn, W. (2002). *Adolescent-adult sensory profile: User's manual: Therapy skill builders*. Pearson.
18. Brown, C., & Knowles, R. L. S. (2021). Sensory processing preferences for people recovering from addictions. *American Journal of Occupational Therapy, 75*(Suppl. 2), 7512500001p1.
19. Buser, S., & Cruz, L. (2022). *DSM-5-TR insanely simplified: Unlocking the spectrums within DSM-5-TR and ICD-10*. Chiron Publications.
20. Centers for Disease Control and Prevention. (n.d.). *Opioids basics*. Retrieved August 8, 2023, from https://www.cdc.gov/opioids/basics/index.html

21. Fisher, A. G., & Marterella, A. (2019). *Powerful practice: A model for authentic occupational therapy.* Center for Innovative OT Solutions.

22. Food and Drug Administration. (2017, September 14). *FDA permits marketing of mobile medical application for substance use disorder.* https://www.fda.gov/NewsEvents/Newsroom/PressAnnouncements/ucm576087.htm

23. Godoy-Vieira, A., Soares, C. B., Cordeiro, L., & Campos, C. M. S. (2018). Inclusive and emancipatory approaches to occupational therapy practice in substance-use contexts. *Canadian Journal of Occupational Therapy, 85*(4), 307–317.

24. Guyer, J., Traube, A., & Deshchenko, O., of Manatt Health Strategies; in collaboration with ASAM and Well Being Trust. (2021, November 9). *Speaking the same language: a toolkit for strengthening patient-centered addiction care in the United States.* American Society of Addiction Medicine. https://www.asam.org/asam-criteria/toolkit. Published November 9, 2021.

25. Haque, S. N. (2021). Telehealth beyond COVID-19. *Psychiatric Services, 72*(1), 100–103.

26. Hicks, T. (2022, November 18). *Why Fentanyl vaccine could be a game changer for opioid epidemic.* https://www.healthline.com/health-news/why-fentanyl-vaccine-could-be-a-game-changer-for-opioid-epidemic

27. Hill, R., & Dahlitz, M. (2022). *The practitioner's guide to the science of psychotherapy.* W. W. Norton & Company.

28. Hitch, D., & Pepin, G. (2021). Doing, being, becoming, and belonging at the heart of occupational therapy: An analysis of theoretical ways of knowing. *Scandinavian Journal of Occupational Therapy, 28*(1), 13–25.

29. Hitch, D., Pepin, G., & Stagnitti, K. (2014). In the footsteps of Wilcock, Part one: The evolution of doing, being, becoming and belonging. *Occupational Therapy in Health Care, 28*(3), 231–246.

30. Hitch, D., Pepin, G., & Stagnitti, K. (2018). The pan occupational paradigm: Development and key concepts. *Scandinavian Journal of Occupational Therapy, 25*(1), 27–34.

31. Hoel, V., von Zweck, C., Ledgerd, R., & World Federation of Occupational Therapists. (2021). Was a global pandemic needed to adopt the use of telehealth in occupational therapy? *Work, 68*(1), 13–20.

32. Katz, J., & Sanger-Katz, M. (2021, July 14). It's huge, it's historic, it's unheard-of: Drug overdose deaths spike. *The New York Times.* https://www.nytimes.com/interactive/2021/07/14/upshot/drug-overdose-deaths.html

33. Mattila, A. M., Santacecilia, G., & LaCroix, R. (2022). Perceptions and knowledge around substance use disorders and the role of occupational therapy: A survey of clinicians. *Substance Abuse: Research and Treatment, 16*, 11782218221130921.

34. McLellan, A. T., Kushner, H., Metzger, D., Peters, R., Smith, I., Grissom, G., Pettinati, H., & Argeriou, M. (1992). The fifth edition of the addiction severity index. *Journal of Substance Abuse Treatment, 9*(3), 199–213.

35. Mee-Lee, D., Shulman, G. D., Fishman, M., Gastfriend, D. R., Miller, M. M., & Provence, S. M. (Eds.). (2013). *The ASAM criteria: Treatment for addictive, substance-related, and co-occurring conditions.* Lippincott Williams & Wilkins.

36. National Institute of Drug Abuse. (2022, September 27). *Part 1: The connection between substance use disorders and mental illness.* https://nida.nih.gov/publications/research-reports/common-comorbidities-substance-use-disorders/part-1-connection-between-substance-use-disorders-mental-illness

37. National Institute of Drug Abuse. (2022, March 22). *Treatment and recovery.* https://nida.nih.gov/publications/drugs-brains-behavior-science-addiction/treatment-recovery

38. National Institute of Drug Abuse. (2023, January 26). *Advancing addiction science and practical solutions.* https://nida.nih.gov/publications/drugs-brains-behavior-science-addiction/advancing-addiction-science-practical-solutions

39. Pederson, L. (2015). *Dialectical behavior therapy: A contemporary guide for practitioners.* Wiley-Blackwell.

40. Pederson, L., & Pederson, C. S. (2017). *The expanded dialectical behavior therapy skills training manual: DBT for self-help, and individual & group treatment settings.* PESI Publishing.

41. Poston, L. (2022, August 15). *Dual diagnosis, co-occurring disorders, & comorbidity: What's the difference?* Ria Health [Blog]. https://riahealth.com/blog/dual-diagnosis-co-occurring-disorders-comorbidity-whats-the-difference/

42. Rojo-Mota, G., Pedrero-Pérez, E. J., & Huertas-Hoyas, E. (2017). Systematic review of occupational therapy in the treatment of addiction: Models, practice, and qualitative and quantitative research. *American Journal of Occupational Therapy, 71*(5), 7105100030.

43. Ryan, D. A., & Boland, P. (2021). A scoping review of occupational therapy interventions in the treatment of people with substance use disorders. *Irish Journal of Occupational Therapy, 49*(2), 104–114.

44. Sokol, L., & Fox, M. G. (2019). *The comprehensive clinician's guide to cognitive behavioral therapy.* PESI Publishing.

45. Substance Abuse and Mental Health Services Administration. (2021). *Highlights for the 2021 National Survey on Drug Use and Health.* https://www.samhsa.gov/data/sites/default/files/2022-12/2021NSDUHF FRHighlights092722.pdf

46. Substance Abuse and Mental Health Services Administration. (2021). *Treating concurrent substance use among adults.* SAMHSA Publication No. PEP21-06-02-002. National Mental Health and Substance Use Policy Laboratory. Substance Abuse and Mental Health Services Administration. https://store.samhsa.gov/sites/default/files/pep21-06-02-002.pdf

47. Substance Abuse and Mental Health Services Administration. (2022). *Community engagement: An essential component of an effective and equitable substance use prevention system.* SAMHSA Publication No. PEP22-06-01-005. National Mental Health and Substance Use Policy Laboratory. Substance Abuse and Mental Health Services Administration. https://store.samhsa.gov/sites/default/files/pep22-06-01-005.pdf

48. Substance Abuse and Mental Health Services Administration. (2022). *Key substance use and mental health indicators in the United States: Results from the 2021 National Survey on Drug Use and Health.* HHS Publication No. PEP22-07-01-005, NSDUH Series H-57. Center for Behavioral Health Statistics and Quality, Substance Abuse and Mental Health Services Administration. https://www.samhsa.gov/data/sites/default/files/reports/rpt39443/2021NSDUHNNR122322/2021NSDUHNNR122322.htm

49. Substance Abuse and Mental Health Services Administration. (2023). *Co-Occurring disorders and other health conditions.* Updated January 25, 2023, from https://www.samhsa.gov/medications-substance-use-disorders/medications-counseling-related-conditions/co-occurring-disorders

50. Substance Abuse and Mental Health Services Administration. (2023). *Expanding access to and use of behavioral health services for people experiencing homelessness.* SAMHSA Publication No. PEP22-06-02-003. National Mental Health and Substance Use Policy Laboratory. Substance Abuse and Mental Health Services Administration. https://store.samhsa.gov/sites/default/files/pep22-06-02-003.pdf

51. Taylor, R. R. (2020). *The intentional relationship: Occupational therapy and use of self* (2nd ed.). F.A. Davis.

52. Wasmuth, S., Brandon-Friedman, R. A., & Olesek, K. (2016). A grounded theory of veterans' experiences of addiction-as-occupation. *Journal of Occupational Science, 23*(1), 128–141.

53. Wasmuth, S., Crabtree, J. L., & Scott, P. J. (2014). Exploring addiction-as-occupation. *British Journal of Occupational Therapy, 77*(12), 605–613.

54. Wasmuth, S., Pritchard, K., & Kaneshiro, K. (2016). Occupation-based intervention for addictive disorders: A systematic review. *Journal of Substance Abuse Treatment, 62*, 1–9.

55. Wasmuth, S., Outcalt, J., Buck, K., Leonhardt, B., Vohs, J., & Lysaker, P. (2015). Metacognition in persons with substance abuse: Findings and implications for occupational therapists. *Canadian Journal of Occupational Therapy, 82*(3), 150–159.

56. Wilburn, V. G., Hoss, A., Pudeler, M., Beukema, E., Rothenbuhler, C., & Stoll, H. B. (2021). Receiving recognition: A case for occupational therapy practitioners as mental and behavioral health providers. *The American Journal of Occupational Therapy, 75*(5), 7505090010.

57. Wilburn, V. G., Stoll, H. B., Fodstad, J. C., Chase, A., & Douglas, C. M. (2020). Utilizing student consultation to promote incorporation of occupational therapy in a pediatric behavioral health unit. *Journal of Occupational Therapy Education, 4*(2), 1–16.

58. Wilcock, A. A., & Hocking, C. (2015). *An occupational perspective of health* (3rd ed.). SLACK.
59. World Health Organization. (n.d.). *SAFER: A safer world free from alcohol related harms. An alcohol-control initiative of the WHO and its partners.* https://www.who.int/initiatives/SAFER/about
60. World Health Organization. (2009). *Clinical guidelines for withdrawal management and treatment of drug dependence in closed setting.* https://apps.who.int/iris/handle/10665/207032

SUGGESTED RESOURCES

Articles

Kotera, Y., Green, P., & Sheffield, D. (2021). Positive psychology for mental wellbeing of UK therapeutic students: Relationships with engagement, motivation, resilience and self-compassion. *International Journal of Mental Health and Addiction, 20,* 1611–1626.

Rawat, H., Petzer, S. L., & Gurayah, T. (2021). Effects of substance use disorder on women's roles and occupational participation. *South African Journal of Occupational Therapy, 51*(1), 54–62.

Ribeiro, J., Mira, E., Lourenço, I., Santos, M., & Braúna, M. (2019). The intervention of occupational therapy in drug addiction: A case study in the comunidade terapêutica clínica do Outeiro–Portugal. *Ciência & Saúde Coletiva, 24*(5), 1585–1596.

Zhang, X. (2022). A study of occupational therapy strategies and psychological regulation of students' internet addiction in the mobile social media environment. *Occupational Therapy International, 2022,* 7598471.

The Substance Abuse and Mental Health Services Administration (SAMHSA) and its Policy Lab, The National Mental Health and Substance Use Policy Laboratory, present *The Evidence-Based Resource Guide Series* as tools for any entity (ie, health care providers and practitioners, health profession educators, policy makers, administrators, or leaders) that is considering an intervention for their community. The guides were designed to address different topics, be applicable to specialized populations or areas of behavioral mental health and substance abuse, and were created by panels of experts. Each guide contains modules and resources, "to improve health outcomes for people at risk for, experiencing, or recovering from mental health and/or substance use disorders" (51, p. IV). The references (with links) listed here are just a few examples highlighting some of the available topics. The resources are free to download. The complete library of guides can be found here: https://www.samhsa.gov/resource-search/ebp

Expanding Access to and Use of Behavioral Health Services for People Experiencing Homelessness https://store.samhsa.gov/sites/default/files/pep22-06-02-003.pdf

Substance Abuse and Mental Health Services Administration. (2023). *Expanding access to and use of behavioral health services for people experiencing homelessness.* SAMHSA Publication No. PEP22-06-02-003. National Mental Health and Substance Use Policy Laboratory. Substance Abuse and Mental Health Services Administration.

Community Engagement: An Essential Component of an Effective and Equitable Substance Use Prevention System. https://store.samhsa.gov/sites/default/files/pep22-06-01-005.pdf

Substance Abuse and Mental Health Services Administration. (2022). *Community engagement: An essential component of an effective and equitable substance use prevention system.* SAMHSA Publication No. PEP22-06-01-005. National Mental Health and Substance Use Policy Laboratory. Substance Abuse and Mental Health Services Administration.

Treating Concurrent Substance Use Among Adults. https://store.samhsa.gov/sites/default/files/pep21-06-02-002.pdf

Substance Abuse and Mental Health Services Administration. (2021). *Treating concurrent substance use among adults.* SAMHSA Publication No. PEP21-06-02-002. National Mental Health and Substance Use Policy Laboratory. Substance Abuse and Mental Health Services Administration.

Preventing Marijuana Use Among Youth. https://store.samhsa.gov/sites/default/files/pep21-06-01-001.pdf

Substance Abuse and Mental Health Services Administration. (2021). *Preventing marijuana use among youth.* SAMHSA Publication No. PEP21-06-01-001. National Mental Health and Substance Use Policy Laboratory. Substance Abuse and Mental Health Services Administration.

Books

Alcoholics Anonymous Big Book, 4th Edition by Bill Walton, first published in 1939, outlines the 12 steps synonymous with Alcoholics Anonymous's plan for healing from addiction. The 12 steps have become a cornerstone in many other programs that help individuals break free from the many types of addiction (ie, food, harmful drugs, sex, gambling, gaming).

Soulbriety by Dr Elisa Hallerman. Dr Elisa Hallerman is the founder of Recovery Management Agency—an agency devoted to helping addicts heal their addictions by reawakening their souls. Hallerman uses her knowledge of depth psychology and her personal experience as a recovering addict to help others reconnect with soul, find meaning, and live their purpose.

Mindfulness for Alcohol Recovery: Making Peace With Drinking by Lewis David and Antonia Ryan. Lewis David is a therapist who specializes in addiction and alcohol abuse. In his text, David provides a step-by-step guide to helping individuals who may have already started to address their drinking habits and problems but who need supportive tools to help them maintain and continue to be successful.

Recommended Books for Use in Bibliotherapy:

Terry: My Daughter's Life-and-Death Struggle With Alcoholism by George Mc Govern

Betty Ford: First Lady, Women's Advocate, Survivor, Trailblazer by Lisa McCubbin with Forward by Susan Ford Bales

Leave Out the Tragic Parts by Dave Kindred

The Big Fix: Hope After Heroine by Tracey Helton Mitchell

Videos

Lily Fang's animation, *Susan's Brain,* is part of a free online course produced by HarvardX and Harvard Health Publications. The course, The Opioid Crisis in America, challenges preconceptions about addiction and about who can become addicted to opioids, and this animation illustrates changes in the brain that lead to addiction (4:37). *This Is What Happens to Your Brain on Opioids: Short Film Showcase.* https://www.youtube.com/watch?v=NDVV_M__CSI

This short animation won a Special Prize in the Rehabilitation Category of the World Health Organization's 3rd Annual Health for All Film Festival in 2022. It chronicles recovery and rehabilitation from brain injury caused by addiction (2:55). https://www.youtube.com/watch?v=GA6M4vMA5mI&list=PL9S6xGsoqIBWgGc1i29H8_MqiWAltgeZL&index=1

In this short film, Nikhil, a drug addict, struggles to overcome addiction while at the same time his mother discovers a damaged plant in the garden and tries to bring it back to health. The film is a beautiful (and accurate) portrayal and metaphor that shows the growth and healing, as well as the struggles that accompany addiction (6:41). https://www.youtube.com/watch?v=kGLT9THy-UI&list=PL9S6xGsoqIBWgGc1i29H8_MqiWAltgeZL&index=8

Websites

U.S. Department of Health and Human Services, Substance Abuse and Mental Health Services Administration (SAMHSA). https://www.samhsa.gov/

Alcoholics Anonymous. https://www.aa.org/

Al-Anon Family Groups (Support Group for friends, families, and relatives of alcoholics). https://al-anon.org/

Narcotics Anonymous World Services. https://na.org/

American Society of Addiction Medicine. https://www.asam.org/

Index

Note: Page numbers followed by *f*, *t*, or *b* indicate figures, tables, or boxed text, respectively

Human trafficking, 199
Hyperactivity, 124, 145, 149
Hypersomnolence disorder, 140
Hypervigilance (tense alertness), 139, 149
Hypocretin deficiency, 140
Hypomania, 131, 149
Hypopnea, 141, 149
Hypothalamic–pituitary–adrenal (HPA),
    432, 453
Hypothalamus, 432

I

IADLs. *See* instrumental activities of daily
    living
ICD-10-CM. *See* International Classification
    of Diseases, Tenth Edition, Clinical
    Modification
ICF. *See* International Classification of
    Functioning, Disability and Health
id, 26, 31
Idea of reference, 462, 503
Idiosyncratic symbols, 28
IEP. *See* Individualized Education Plan
Illumination of process, 403, 421
ILS. *See* Independent Living Scales
Imitation, 71
Imitative behavior, 405
Immediacy, 388, 396
Immigration experience, 181–182
Impaired judgment, 509, 521
Impaired memory, 506–519
    diagnoses with the common symptoms
        of, 510
    evidence-based interventions that target,
        517–518
    intervention activities and recommended
        modifications for, 515–517
    targeting symptoms of, 507–513
    therapeutic use of self for clients with,
        510–511, 513
Imparting information, 404
Implementation science, 287
Impulsivity, 124, 149
Inability to comprehend, 509
Inattention, 124, 508, 521
Inclusion, 183, 216
Incoherence, 126
Incontinence, 512
Independence, 369
Independent Living Scales (ILS), 325
Individual/egocentric roles, 408, 421
Individualized Education Plan (IEP), 160, 238
Individual needs, 217
Individual strengths, 446–447
Inductive-based professional reasoning, 287,
    290
Infancy and childhood, mental health during,
    157–161
    development, 157–158
    "liking" pleasure, 157
    mental health factors in, 158–159
    occupational therapy, 159–161
    "wanting" desire, 157
Infant-Toddler Sensory Profile, 94
Infection control
    in common areas, 266
    and safety for specific situations, 266–269
Information exchange, 442, 453

Initiative or guilt, 33
Initiative versus guilt, 32
Inmate, 226
Inpatient commitment, 269
Inpatient settings, 233–236
    acute care inpatient units, 233
    behavioral units, 234
    forensic settings, 234–235
    long-term care inpatient units, 233–234
    transitional services, 235–236
Insomnia disorder, 140
Instructing mode, 462
Instrumental activities of daily life with a
    cognitive emphasis (CIADLs), 327
Instrumental activities of daily living (IADLs),
    130, 350
Integration scholarship, 281, 290
Intellectual disability (ID), 122
Intensive Psychiatric Rehabilitation Services
    Units, 237
Intensive psychiatric rehabilitation treatment
    (IPRT), 11
Intentional Relationship Model (IRM),
    385–386, 396
Intentionalizing bias, 492
Interaction and intervention, methods and
    models of, 180–216. *See also* caregivers;
    community-based intervention; Kawa
    model; occupational adaptation (OA)
    model; recovery; societal issues
    biopsychosocial model, 189–190
    community mental health centers
        (CMHCs), 192–193
    cultural differences in diagnosis, 182
    culture, 181
    digital literacy, 202
    diversity, 182
    equity, 182–183
    financial literacy, 202
    functional literacy, 202
    gender diversity and identity, 182
    health literacy, 201
    immigration experience, 181–182
    inclusion, 183
    Kawa model, 183, 185–187
    literacy, 201–202
    mental health literacy, 202
    model of human occupation, 183–185
    occupational adaptation (OA) model, 183
    occupational justice, 183
    personal factors, 181–183
    practice models in occupational therapy,
        183–190
    stigma, 183
Interaction levels, 81
Interactive reasoning, 287, 290, 299–300
Interests, 88, 441, 473, 487
Intermittent schedules, 35, 38
Internalized roles, 80, 88
*International Classification of Diseases, Tenth
    Edition, Clinical Modification* (ICD-10-CM),
    115, 117
    mental health F code subcategories, 117,
        117b
*International Classification of Functioning,
    Disability and Health* (ICF), 119
Internet, concerns related to, 258
Interneurons, 432, 453

Interoception, 96, 106
Interoceptive awareness, 431, 453
Interpersonal-input, 405, 421
Interpersonal learning, 405–406
Interpersonal-output, 405, 422
Interpersonal skills, 368
Interpersonal therapy (IPT), 405
Interrater reliability, 320, 331
Intervening (intervention), 460, 468
Intervention goal, writing, 349
Intervention type and approach, determining,
    336–352
    approaches to intervention, 341–342
    appropriate intervention principles,
        selecting, 351–352
    asking the right questions, 339–340
    clients in setting their own goals, 351
    clinical inquiry, 339, 339b
    cognitive behavioral continuum, 346–348
    dialectical behavior therapy (DBT),
        347–348
    intervention goal, writing, 349
    motivational theories and motivational
        interviewing, 343–346
    motivational theories, 343
    occupational therapist role, 352
    occupational therapy assistant role, 352
    Person–Environment–Occupational
        Performance (PEOP), 348
    planning follows from evaluation results,
        340–341
    planning, 338–339
    psychiatric occupational therapy, general
        goals of, 348–349
    RUMBA, 349–351
    social learning, social cognitive theories
        and behaviorism, 346–348
    theory, practice models, and the
        occupational therapy process, 342–343
    therapeutic reasoning, 339–340
Intervention types, matching occupational
    demands to, 357–381, 382
    activities selection, 364
    activity analysis based on theory, 369–370
    adaptation, 364–366
    analyzing, 364
    client goals/priorities and occupation-
        focused intervention, linking, 358
    dynamic performance analysis (DPA), 370
    from evaluation to outcomes, 371–381
    gradation, 364, 367–369
    for improved occupational outcomes,
        357–381
    intervention methods selection for service
        delivery, 358–362. *See also* service
        delivery, Intervention methods selection
        for
    task-oriented approach, 370
    task-specific approach, 370
Intervention, 231
    and engagement in occupation, 441–442
Interview, 320–324
Intimate partner violence, 196, 218
In vivo, 207, 218
IPRT. *See* intensive psychiatric rehabilitation
    treatment
IPT. *See* Interpersonal therapy
IRM. *See* Intentional Relationship Model